The GALE
ENCYCLOPEDIA
of MEDICINE

The GALE ENCYCLOPEDIA of MEDICINE

VOLUME

3

G-M

DONNA OLENDORF, CHRISTINE JERYAN, KAREN BOYDEN, EDITORS
MARY K. FYKE, ASSOCIATE EDITOR

GALE

DETROIT · LONDON

The GALE ENCYCLOPEDIA of MEDICINE

STAFF

Donna Olendorf, Christine Jeryan, Karen Boyden, *Editors*
Mary K. Fyke, *Coordinating Editor (Electronic Manuscript)*
Robyn V. Young, *Coordinating Editor (Images)*
Regie A. Carlton, *Coordinating Editor (Advisors, Contributors)*
Alesia Lawson, *Editorial Assistant*

Bridget Travers, Jacqueline Longe, Kristine M. Krapp, Pamela Proffitt, *Contributing Editors*
Zoran Minderovic, *Associate Editor*

Susan Trosky, *Permissions Manager*
Shalice Shah-Caldwell, *Permissions Associate*
Keasha Jack-Lyles, *Permissions Assistant*
Mary Grimes, *Image Cataloger*

Victoria B. Cariappa, *Research Manager*
Maureen Richards, *Research Specialist*

Mary Beth Trimper, *Production Director*
Evi Seoud, *Assistant Production Manager*
Deborah Milliken, *Production Assistant*

Cynthia Baldwin, *Product Design Manager*
Michelle DiMercurio, *Art Director*
Barbara Yarrow, *Graphic Services Manager*
Randy Bassett, *Image Database Supervisor*
Robert Duncan, Mike Logusz, *Imaging Specialists*
Pamela A. Reed, *Imaging Coordinator*

James Edwards, *Editorial Technical Specialist*
Jeffery Muhr, *Programmer Analyst*
Jeffery Chapman, *Programmer Analyst*

Indexing provided by Synapse, the Knowledge Link Corporation
Illustrations by Electronic Illustrators Group, Fountain Hills, Arizona
Tables by Mark Berger, Standley Publishing, Ferndale, Michigan

Gale encyclopedia of medicine / Donna Olendorf, Christine Jeryan, and Karen Boyden, editors.
    v. < >. cm.
    Includes bibliographical references and index.
    ISBN 0-7876-1868-3 (set). — ISBN 0-7876-1869-1 (vol. 1). —
ISBN 0-7876-1870-5 (vol. 2). — ISBN 0-7876-1871-3 (vol. 3). —
ISBN 0-7876-1872-1 (vol. 4). — ISBN 0-7876-1873-X (vol. 5)
    1. Internal medicine—Encyclopedias. I. Olendorf, Donna.
II. Jeryan, Christine, 1951- . III. Boyden, Karen. IV. Gale Research Company.
RC41.G35 1999
616'.003—dc21
98-37918
CIP

CONTENTS

PLEASE READ - IMPORTANT INFORMATION

INTRODUCTION

The *Gale Encyclopedia of Medicine (GEM)* is a one-stop source for medical information on nearly 1,500 common medical disorders, conditions, tests, and treatments, including high-profile diseases such as AIDS, Alzheimer's disease, cancer, and heart attack. It uses language that laypersons can understand, so users are not confused by medical jargon. The *Gale Encyclopedia of Medicine* fills a gap between basic consumer health resources, such as single-volume family medical guides, and highly technical professional materials.

SCOPE

Almost 1,500 full-length articles are included in the *Gale Encyclopedia of Medicine*, including 905 disorders/conditions, 235 tests/procedures, and 352 treatments/therapies. Many common drugs are also covered, with generic drug names appearing first and brand names following in parentheses, eg. acetaminophen (Tylenol). Articles follow a standardized format that provides information at a glance. Rubrics include:

Disorders/Conditions	Tests/Treatments
Definition	Definition
Description	Purpose
Causes & symptoms	Precautions
Diagnosis	Description
Treatment	Preparation
Alternative treatment	Aftercare
Prognosis	Risks
Prevention	Normal/Abnormal results
Resources	Resources
Key terms	Key terms

In recent years there has been a resurgence of interest in holistic medicine that emphasizes the connection between mind and body. Aimed at achieving and maintaining good health rather than just eliminating disease, this approach has come to be known as alternative medicine. The *Gale Encyclopedia of Medicine* includes a number of general essays on alternative therapies, ranging from Chinese tra-

ditional medicine to homeopathy and from meditation to aromatherapy. In addition to full essays on alternative therapies, the encyclopedia features specific **Alternative treatment** sections for diseases and conditions that may be helped by complementary therapies.

INCLUSION CRITERIA

A preliminary list of diseases, disorders, tests, and treatments was compiled from a wide variety of sources, including professional medical guides and textbooks, as well as consumer guides and encyclopedias. The general advisory board, made up of public librarians, medical librarians, and consumer health experts, evaluated the topics and made suggestions for inclusion. The list was sorted by category and sent to *GEM* medical advisors, certified physicians with various medical specialities, for review. Final selection of topics to include was made by the medical advisors in conjunction with Gale editors.

ABOUT THE CONTRIBUTORS

The essays were compiled by experienced medical writers, including physicians, pharmacists, nurses, and other health care professionals. *GEM* medical advisors reviewed the completed essays to insure that they are appropriate, up-to-date, and medically accurate.

HOW TO USE THIS BOOK

The *Gale Encyclopedia of Medicine* has been designed with ready reference in mind:

- Straight **alphabetical arrangement** allows users to locate information quickly.

- Bold faced terms function as **print hyperlinks** that point the reader to related entries in the encyclopedia.

- A list of **key terms** is provided where appropriate to define unfamiliar words or concepts used within the context of the essay.

- **Cross-references** placed throughout the encyclopedia direct readers to where information on subjects without their own entries can be found. Synonyms are also cross-referenced.

- Valuable **contact information** for organizations and support groups is included.

- **Resources section** directs users to sources of further medical information.

- A comprehensive three-level **general index** allows users to easily target detailed aspects of any topic, including Latin names.

GRAPHICS

The *Gale Encyclopedia of Medicine* is enhanced with 620 illustrations, including photos, charts, and customized line drawings.

ACKNOWLEDGEMENTS

The editors would like to thank the following individuals for their assistance with manuscript review for the *Gale Encyclopedia of Medicine*: Stephen S. Arnon, MD, who reviewed the "Botulism" essay on behalf of Infant Botulism Treatment and Prevention Program, Department of Health Services, State of California; Sandra C. Belmont, MD, who reviewed the "Corneal transplant" essay on behalf of the American Academy of Opthalmology; Carolyn M. Das who reviewed the "Cerebral palsy" essay for accuracy, tone, and currency; and Denise Jackson and Margaret Mazurkiewicz who reviewed the "Autism" essay for accuracy, tone, and currency.

ADVISORY BOARD

A number of experts in the library and medical communities provided invaluable assistance in the formulation of this encyclopedia. Our advisory board performed a myriad of duties, from defining the scope of coverage to reviewing individual entries for accuracy and accessibility. We would therefore like to express our appreciation to them:

MEDICAL ADVISORS

A. Richard Adrouny, MD, FACP
Medical Oncology-Hemtology
Chairman, Cancer Care, Community
Hospital of Los Gatos-Saratoga
Los Gatos, CA

Laurie Barclay, MD
Neurological Consulting Services
Tampa, FL

Rosalyn Carson-DeWitt, MD
Durham, NC

Robin Dipasquale, ND
Clinical Faculty
Bastyr University
Seattle, WA

Faye Fishman, OD
Randolph, NJ

J. Gary Grant, MD
Pacific Grove, CA

L. Anne Hirschel, DDS
Medical/dental Writer
Southfield, MI

Larry I. Lutwick MD, FACP
Director, Infectious Diseases
VA Medical Center, Brooklyn, NY
Professor of Medicine
SUNY-Health Science Center at Brooklyn

Ralph M. Myerson, MD, FACP
Clinical Professor of Medicine
Allegheny University Health Sciences Center
Philadelphia, PA

Ronald Pies, MD
Clinical Professor of Psychiatry, Tufts University
    School of Medicine, Boston, MA
Lecturer on Psychiatry, Harvard Medical School,
    Cambridge, MA

Lee A. Shratter, MD
Staff Radiologist
The Permanente Medical Group
Richmond, CA

Amy B. Tuteur, MD
Sharon, MA

LIBRARIAN ADVISORS

Maureen O. Carleton, MLIS
Medical Reference Specialist
King County Library System
Bellevue, WA

Elizabeth Clewis Crim, MLS
Collection Specialist
Prince William Public Library, VA

Valerie J. Lawrence, MLS
Assistant Librarian
Western States Chiropractic College
Portland, OR

Barbara J. O'Hara, MLS
Adult Services Librarian
Free Library of Philadelphia
Philadelphia, PA

Alan M. Rees, MSLS
Professor Emeritus
Case Western Reserve University
Cleveland, OH

CONTRIBUTORS

Janet Byron Anderson
Linguist/Language Consultant
Rocky River, OH

Howard Baker
Medical Writer
North York, Ontario

Laurie Barclay, MD
Neurological Consulting Services
Tampa, FL

Jeanine Barone
Nutritionist, Exercise Physiologist
New York, NY

Julia R. Barrett
Science Writer
Madison, WI

Donald G. Barstow, RN
Clincal Nurse Specialist
Oklahoma City, OK

Barbara Boughton
Health and Medical Writer
El Cerrito, CA

Maury M. Breecher, PhD
Health Communicator/Journalist
Northport, AL

Ruthan Brodsky
Medical Writer
Bloomfield Hills, MI

Tom Brody, PhD
Science Writer
Berkeley, CA

Leonard C. Bruno, PhD
Medical Writer
Chevy Chase, MD

Richard H. Camer
Editor

International Medical News Group
Silver Spring, MD

Rosalyn Carson-DeWitt, MD
Durham, NC

Lata Cherath, PhD
Science Writing Intern
Cancer Research Institute
New York, NY

Lisa Christenson, PhD
Science Writer
Hamden, CT

Geoffrey N. Clark, DVM
Editor
Canine Sports Medicine Update
Newmarket, NH

David A. Cramer, MD
Medical Writer
Chicago, IL

Tish Davidson
Medical Writer
Fremont, CA

Dominic De Bellis, PhD
Medical Writer/Editor
Mahopac, NY

Lori De Milto
Medical Writer
Sicklerville, NJ

Laura M. Deming, RN
Director, Pediatric and Perinatal Services
Olsten Health Services
Houston, TX

Robert S. Dinsmoor
Medical Writer
South Hamilton, MA

Martin W. Dodge, PhD
Technical Writer/Editor
Centinela Hospital and Medical Center
Inglewood, CA

David Doermann
Medical Writer
Salt Lake City, UT

Altha Edgren
Medical Writer
Medical Ink
St. Paul, MN

Karen Ericson, RN
Medical Writer
Estes Park, CO

Janis Flores
Medical Writer
Lexikon Communications
Sebastopol, CA

Risa Flynn
Medical Writer
Culver City, CA

Paula Ford-Martin
Medical Writer
Chaplin, MN

Rebecca J. Frey
Editor, Writer
Appleton & Lange
New Haven, CT

Cynthia L. Frozena, RN
Nurse, Medical Writer
Manitowoc, WI

Ron Gasbarro, PharmD
Medical Writer
New Milford, PA

Julie A. Gelderloos
Biomedical Writer
Playa del Rey, CA

Harry W. Golden
Medical Writer
Shoreline Medical Writers
Old Lyme, CT

Alison Grant
Medical Writer
Averill Park, NY

Kapil Gupta, MD
Medical Writer
Winston-Salem, NC

Maureen Haggerty
Medical Writer
Ambler, PA

Carol Halsted, PhD
Professor of Dance
Oakland University
Rochester, MI

Ann M. Haren
Science Writer
Madison, CT

Caroline Helwick
Medical Writer
New Orleans, LA

Sally J. Jacobs, EdD
Medical Writer
Los Angeles, CA

Cindy L. A. Jones, PhD
Medical Writer
Palisade, CO

David Kaminstein, MD
Medical Writer
West Chester, PA

Beth Kapes
Medical Writer
Bay Village, OH

Christine Kuehn Kelly
Medical Writer
Havertown, PA

Joseph Knight, PA
Medical Writer
Winton, CA

Mary Jeanne Krob, MD, FACS
Physician Advisor
Blue Cross of Western Pennsylvania
Pittsburgh, PA

Jennifer Lamb
Medical Writer
Spokane, WA

Richard H. Lampert
Senior Medical Editor
W.B. Saunders Co.
Philadelphia, PA

Jeffrey P. Larson, RPT
Physical Therapist
Sabin, MN

Jill Lasker
Medical Writer
Midlothian, VA

Kristy Layman
Music Therapist
East Lansing, MI

Victor Leipzig, PhD
Biological Consultant
Huntington Beach, CA

Lorraine Lica, PhD
Medical Writer
San Diego, CA

John T. Lohr, PhD
Assistant Director, Biotechnology Center
Utah State University
Logan, UT

Larry Lutwick, MD, FACP
Director, Infectious Diseases
VA Medical Center
Brooklyn, NY

Adrienne Massel, RN
Medical Writer
Beloit, WI

Ruth E. Mawyer, RN
Medical Writer
Charlottesville, VA

Mercedes McLaughlin
Medical Writer
Phoenixville, CA

Betty Mishkin
Medical Writer
Skokie, IL

Susan Montgomery
Medical Writer
Milwaukee, WI

Louann W. Murray, PhD
Medical Writer
Huntington Beach, CA

Laura Ninger
Medical Writer
Weehawken, NJ

Nancy J. Nordenson
Medical Writer
Minneapolis, MN

Teresa Norris, RN
Medical Writer
Ute Park, NM

Lisa Papp, RN
Medical Writer
Cherry Hill, NJ

Collette Placek
Medical Writer
Wheaton, IL

J. Ricker Polsdorfer, MD
Medical Writer
Phoenix, AZ

Toni Rizzo
Medical Writer
Salt Lake City, UT

Martha Robbins
Medical Writer
Evanston, IL

Richard Robinson
Medical Writer
Tucson, AZ

Nancy Ross-Flanigan
Science Writer
Belleville, MI

Belinda Rowland, PhD
Medical Writer
Voorheesville, NY

Karen Sandrick
Medical Writer
Chicago, IL

Joyce S. Siok, RN
Medical Writer
South Windsor, CT

Genevieve Slomski, PhD
Medical Writer
New Britain, CT

Stephanie Slon
Medical Writer
Portland, OR

Linda Wasmer Smith
Medical Writer
Albuquerque, NM

Elaine Souder, PhD
Medical Writer
Little Rock, AR

Lorraine Steefel, RN
Medical Writer
Morganville, NJ

Kurt Sternlof
Science Writer
New Rochelle, NY

Dorothy Stonely
Medical Writer
Los Gatos, CA

Bethany Thivierge
Biotechnical Writer/Editor
Technicality Resources
Rockland, ME

Carol Turkington
Medical Writer
Lancaster, PA

Amy B. Tuteur, MD
Medical Advisor
Sharon, MA

Ellen S. Weber, MSN
Medical Writer
Fort Wayne, IN

Karen Wells
Medical Writer
Ponte Vedra Beach, FL

Kathleen D. Wright, RN
Medical Writer
Delmar, DE

Mary Zoll, PhD
Science Writer
Newton Center, MA

Jon Zonderman
Medical Writer
Orange, CA

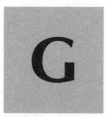

G

G6PD deficiency *see* **Glucose-6—phosphate dehydrogenase deficiency**

Galactorrhea

Definition

Galactorrhea is the secretion of breast milk in men, or in women who are not breastfeeding an infant.

Description

Lactation, or the production of breast milk, is a normal condition occurring in women after delivery of a baby. Many women who have had children may even be able to express a small amount of breast milk from the nipple up to two years after **childbirth.** Galactorrhea, or hyperlactation, however, is a rare condition that can occur in both men and women, where a white or grayish fluid is secreted by the nipples of both breasts. While this condition is not serious in itself, galactorrhea can indicate more serious conditions, including hormone imbalances or the presence of tumors.

Causes & symptoms

Causes

Galactorrhea is associated with a number of conditions. The normal production of breast milk is controlled by a hormone called prolactin, which is secreted by the pituitary gland in the brain. Any condition that upsets the balance of hormones in the blood or the production of hormones by the pituitary gland or sexual organs can stimulate the production of prolactin.

Often, a patient with galactorrhea will have a high level of prolactin in the blood. A tumor in the pituitary gland can cause this overproduction of prolactin. At least 30% of women with galactorrhea, menstrual abnormalities, and high prolactin levels have a pituitary gland

tumor. Other types of **brain tumors,** head injuries, or **encephalitis** (an infection of the brain) can also cause galactorrhea.

Tumors or growths in the ovaries or other reproductive organs in women, or in the testicles or related sexual organs of men, can also stimulate the production of prolactin. Any discharge of fluid from the breast after a woman has passed **menopause** may indicate **breast cancer.** However, most often the discharge associated with breast cancer will be from one breast only. In galactorrhea both breasts are usually involved. The presence of blood in the fluid discharged from the breast could indicate a benign growth in the breast tissue itself. In approximately 10–15% of patients with blood in the fluid, carcinoma of the breast tissue is present.

A number of medications and drugs can also cause galactorrhea as a side-effect. Hormonal therapies (like **oral contraceptives),** drugs for treatment of depression or other psychiatric conditions, tranquilizers, morphine, heroin, and some medications for high blood pressure can cause galactorrhea.

Several normal physiologic situations can cause production of breast milk. Nipple stimulation in men or women during sexual intercourse may induce lactation, for women particularly during or just after **pregnancy.**

Even after extensive testing, no specific cause can be determined for some patients with galactorrhea.

Symptoms

The primary symptom of galactorrhea is the discharge of milky fluid from both breasts. In women, galactorrhea may be associated with **infertility,** menstrual cycle irregularities, hot flushes, or **amenorrhea**—a condition where menstruation stops completely. Men may experience loss of sexual interest and **impotence. Headaches** and visual disturbances have also been associated with some cases of galactorrhea.

Diagnosis

Galactorrhea is generally considered a symptom which may indicate a more serious problem. Collection of a thorough medical history, including pregnancies, surgeries, and consumption of drugs and medications is a first step in diagnosing the cause of galactorrhea. A **physical examination,** along with a breast examination, will usually be conducted. Blood and urine samples may be taken to determine levels of various hormones in the body, including prolactin and compounds related to thyroid function.

A mammogram (an x ray of the breast) or an ultrasound scan (using high frequency sound waves) might be used to determine if there are any tumors or cysts present in the breasts themselves. If a tumor of the pituitary gland is suspected, a series of computer assisted x rays called a **computed tomography scan** (CT scan) may be done. Another procedure which may be useful is a **magnetic resonance imaging** (MRI) scan to locate tumors or abnormalities in tissues.

Treatment

Treatment for galactorrhea will depend on the cause of the condition and the symptoms. The drug bromocriptine is often prescribed first to reduce the secretion of prolactin and to decrease the size of **pituitary tumors.** This drug will control galactorrhea symptoms and in many cases may be the only therapy necessary. Oral estrogen and progestins (hormone pills, like birth control pills) may control symptoms of galactorrhea for some women. Surgery to remove a tumor may be required for patients who have more serious symptoms of headache and vision loss, or if the tumor shows signs of enlargement despite drug treatment. **Radiation therapy** has also been used to reduce tumor size when surgery is not possible or not totally successful. A combination of drug, surgery, and radiation treatment can also be used.

Galactorrhea is more of a nuisance than a real threat to health. While it is important to find the cause of the condition, even if a tumor is discovered in the pituitary gland, it may not require treatment. With very small, slow-growing tumors, some physicians may suggest a ''wait and see'' approach.

Prognosis

Treatment with bromocriptine is usually effective in stopping milk secretion, however, symptoms may recur if drug therapy is discontinued. Surgical removal or radiation treatment may correct the problem permanently if it is related to a tumor. Frequent monitoring of hormone status and tumor size may be recommended.

Prevention

There is no way to prevent galactorrhea. If the condition is caused by the use of a particular drug, a patient may be able to switch to a different drug that does not have the side-effect of galactorrhea.

Resources

BOOKS

''Galactorrhea.'' In *Cecil Textbook of Medicine.* 20th ed. Philadelphia, PA: W.B. Saunders Company, 1996, pp. 1318-1319.

''Galactorrhea.'' In *Current Medical Diagnosis & Treatment 1998,* 37th ed. Stamford, CT: Appleton & Lange, 1998, p. 1033.

''Galactorrhea (Hyperprolactinemia).'' In *Professional Guide to Diseases,* 5th ed. Springhouse, PA: Springhouse Corporation, 1995, pp. 974-975.

''Galactorrhea.'' In *The Merck Manual of Diagnosis and Therapy.* Edited by Robert Berkow, et al. Rahway, NJ: Merck Research Laboratories, 1992, pp. 1065-1067.

Altha Roberts Edgren

Galactosemia

Definition

Galactosemia is an inherited disease where the transformation of galactose to glucose is blocked, allowing galactose to increase to toxic levels in the body. If galactosemia is untreated, high levels of galactose cause vomiting, **diarrhea,** lethargy, low blood sugar, brain damage, **jaundice,** liver enlargement, **cataracts,** susceptibility to infection, and **death.**

Description

Galactosemia is a rare but potentially tragic disease that kills very young babies. However, thanks to an understanding of the root of the problem, infant death from galactosemia can be prevented by giving simple tests to newborns.

KEY TERMS

Casein hydrolysate—A preparation made from the milk protein casein, which is hydrolyzed to break it down into its constituent amino acids. Amino acids are the building blocks of proteins.

Catalyst—A substance that changes the rate of a chemical reaction, but doesn't itself get changed by the reaction.

Enzyme—A protein catalyst; one of the two kinds of biological catalysts, which are exceedingly specific. Each different enzyme only catalyzes one or two specific reactions.

Galactose—A sugar that contains six carbons in its chemical structure. It is similar to glucose and is toxic in high levels.

Glucose—A sugar with six carbon molecules. It is of central importance in energy metabolism and is a part of many other biological molecules, for example lactose, sucrose (table sugar), cellulose, starch, and dextran.

Lactose—A sugar made up of of glucose and galactose. It is the primary sugar in milk.

Metabolic pathway—A sequence of chemical reactions that lead from some precursor to a product, where the product of each step in the series is the starting material for the next step.

Metabolism—The sum of all the chemical reactions that take place in living organisms (whether they use energy or not; whether they build large molecules from small ones or break large molecules into smaller ones).

Recessive trait—An inherited trait or characteristic that is outwardly obvious only when two copies of the gene for that trait are present, as opposed to a dominant trait where one copy of the gene for the dominant trait is necessary to display the trait.

Galactosemia is an inborn error of metabolism. "Metabolism" refers to all the chemical reactions that take place in living organisms. A metabolic pathway is a series of reactions where the product of each step in the series is the starting material for the next step. Because of energy barriers, essentially none of the reactions in organisms occur at any measurable rate unless a catalyst (a compound that affects the rate of a chemical reaction) is present. Most catalysts in organisms, including those required for the transformation of galactose to glucose in humans, are enzymes (large protein molecules). Their ability to function depends on their structure, and their structure is determined by the deoxyribonucleic acid (DNA) sequence of the genes that encode them. Inborn errors of metabolism are caused by defective genes.

Sugars are sometimes called "the energy molecules," and galactose and glucose are both sugars. For galactose to be utilized for energy, it must be transformed into something that can enter the metabolic pathway that converts glucose into energy (plus water and carbon dioxide). This is important for infants because they typically get most of their nutrient energy from milk, which contains a high level of galactose. Each molecule of lactose, the major sugar constituent of milk, is made up of a molecule of galactose and a molecule of glucose, and so galactose makes up 20% of the energy source of a typical infant's diet.

Three enzymes are required to convert galactose into glucose-1-phosphate (a phosphorylated glucose that can enter the metabolic pathway that turns glucose into energy). Each of these three enzymes is encoded by a separate gene. If any of these enzymes fail to function, galactose build-up and galactosemia result. Thus, there are three types of galactosemia with a different gene responsible for each.

Each of the forms of galactosemia is inherited as a recessive trait, which means that galactosemia is only present in individuals with two defective copies of one of the three genes. This also means that carriers, with one copy of a defective recessive gene, will not be aware that they are carrying a defective gene (unless they have had a genetic test), as it is masked by the normal gene they also carry and they have no symptoms of the disease. If two carriers of the same defective gene have children, the chance of any of their children getting galactosemia (the chance of a child getting two copies of the defective gene) is 25% for each **pregnancy.**

Every cell nucleus in a person's body has two copies of each gene (with some exceptions that are not relevant to galactosemia). For each step in the conversion of galactose to glucose, if only one of the two copies of the gene controlling that step is normal, enough functional enzyme is made so that the pathway is not blocked at that step. Thus, if a person has galactosemia, both copies of the gene coding for one of the enzymes required to convert glucose to galactose are defective.

Causes & symptoms

Galactosemia I

Galactosemia I (also called classic galactosemia), the first form to be discovered, is caused by defects in both copies of the gene that codes for an enzyme called galactose-1-phosphate uridyl transferase (GALT). The frequency of occurrence of this form of galactosemia in the United States is about one in every 50,000–70,000 births. There are 30 known different mutations in this gene that cause GALT to malfunction.

Newborns with galactosemia I appear normal when first born, but after they are given milk for the first time, symptoms appear. They include vomiting, diarrhea, lethargy (sluggishness or fatigue), low blood glucose, jaundice (a yellowing of the skin and eyes), enlarged liver, protein and amino acids in the urine, and susceptibility to infection, especially from gram negative bacteria. Cataracts (a grayish white film on the eye lens) can appear within a few days after birth. People with galactosemia frequently have symptoms as they grow older even though they have been given a galactose-free diet. These symptoms include speech disorders, cataracts, ovarian atrophy and **infertility** in females, learning disabilities, and behavioral problems.

Galactosemia II

Galactosemia II is caused by defects in both copies of the gene that codes for an enzyme called galactokinase (GALK). The frequency of occurrence of galactosemia II is about one in 100,000–155,000 births.

Galactosemia II is less harmful than galactosemia I. Babies born with galactosemia II will develop cataracts at an early age unless they are given a galactose-free diet. They do not generally suffer from liver damage or neurologic disturbances.

Galactosemia III

Galactosemia III is caused by defects in the gene that codes for an enzyme called uridyl diphosphogalactose-4-epimerase (GALE). This form of galactosemia is very rare.

There are two forms of galactosemia III, a severe form, which is exceedingly rare, and a benign form. The benign form has no symptoms and requires no special diet. However, newborns with galactosemia III, including the benign form, have high levels of galactose-1-phosphate that show up on the initial screenings for elevated galactose and galactose-1-phosphate. This situation illustrates one aspect of the importance of follow-up enzyme function tests. Tests showing normal levels of GALT and GALK allow people affected by the benign form of galactosemia III to enjoy a normal diet.

The severe form has symptoms similar to those of galactosemia I, but with more severe neurological problems, including seizures. Only two cases of this rare form had been reported as of 1997.

Diagnosis

The diagnostic test for galactosemia is quick and straightforward; almost all states require that all newborns be tested. Blood from a baby who is two to three days old is usually first screened for high levels of galactose and galactose-1-phosphate. If either of these compounds is elevated, further tests are performed to find out which enzymes (GALT, GALK, or GALE) are present or missing.

Naturally, if there is a strong suspicion that a baby will have galactosemia, galactose is removed from their diet right away. In this case, an initial screen for galactose or galactose-1-phosphate will be meaningless. In the absence of galactose in the diet, this test will be negative whether the baby has galactosemia or not. In this case, tests to measure enzyme levels must be given to find out if the suspected baby is indeed galactosemic.

In addition, galactosemic babies who are refusing milk or vomiting will not have elevated levels of galactose or galactose phosphate, and their condition will not be detected by the initial screen. Any baby with symptoms of galactosemia (for example, vomiting) should be given enzyme tests.

Treatment

Galactosemia I and II are treated by removing galactose from the diet. Since galactose is a break-down product of lactose, the primary sugar constituent of milk, this means all milk and foods containing milk products must be totally eliminated. Other foods like legumes, organ meats, and processed meats also contain considerable galactose and must be avoided. Pills that use lactose as a filler must also be avoided. Soy-based and casein hydrolysate-based formulas are recommended for infants with galactosemia.

Treatment of the severe form of galactosemia III with a galactose-restricted diet has been tried, but this disorder is so rare that the long-term effects of this treatment are uncertain.

Prognosis

It is critically important that all newborn babies be tested for galactosemia because the prognosis for any baby with galactosemia I who doesn't start a galactose-free diet within the first five days of life is tragic. About 75% of the untreated babies die within their first two weeks. On the other hand, with treatment, a significant proportion of people with galactosemia I can lead nearly normal lives, although speech defects, learning disabilities, and behavioral problems are common. In addition, cataracts due to galactosemia II can be completely prevented by a galactose-free diet.

Prevention

Since galactosemia is a genetic disease, it cannot be prevented. Prospective parents can undergo **genetic testing** to determine if they are carriers of the defective genes causing the disease and use that information to conduct family planning. Children born with galactocemia should be put on a special diet right away, to reduce the symptoms and complications of the disease.

Resources

BOOKS

Ng, Won G., Thomas F. Roe, and George N. Donnell. "Carbohydrate Metabolism." In *Emery and Rimoin's Principles and Practice of Medical Genetics*, 3rd. ed., edited by David L. Rimoin, J. Michael Connor, and Reed E. Pyeritz. New York: Churchill Livingstone, 1998.

ORGANIZATIONS

Association for Neuro-Metabolic Disorders. 5223 Brookfield Lane, Sylvania, OH 43560. (419) 885-1497.

Metabolic Information Network. P.O. Box 670847, Dallas, TX 75367-0847. (214) 696-2188 or (800) 945-2188.

Parents of Galactosemic Children, Inc. 2148 Bryton Dr., Powell OH 43065. http://www.galactosemia.org/index.htm.

OTHER

"GeneCards: Human Genes, Proteins and Diseases." http://bioinfo.weizmann.ac.il/cards/.

"Vermont Newborn Screening Program: Galactosemia." http://www.vtmednet.org/~m145037/vhgi_mem/nbsman/galacto.htm.

Lorraine Lica

Gallbladder cancer *see* **Biliary tract cancer**

Gallbladder disease *see* **Cholecystitis**

Gallbladder nuclear medicine scan

Definition

A nuclear medicine scan of the gallbladder is used to produce a set of images that look like x rays. The procedure uses a small amount of radioactive dye which is injected into the body. The dye accumulates in the organ, in this case, the gallbladder. A special camera called a scintillation or gamma camera produces images based on how the dye travels through the system and how the radiation is absorbed by the tissues. The procedure is also called cholescintigraphy or a hepatobiliary scan.

Purpose

A nuclear medicine scan can be used to diagnose disease and to find abnormalities in a body organ. A gallbladder scan can detect **gallstones,** tumors, or defects of the gallbladder. It can also be used to diagnose blockages of the bile duct that leads from the gallbladder to the small intestine. Unlike ultrasound, a gallbladder nuclear medicine scan can assess gallbladder function.

Precautions

Women who are pregnant or breastfeeding should tell their doctors before a scan is performed. Some medications or even eating a high fat meal before the procedure can interfere with the results of the scan.

Description

The gallbladder is a small pear-shaped sac located under the liver. The liver produces bile, a yellowish-green mixture of salts, acids, and other chemicals, that are stored in the gallbladder. Bile is secreted into the small intestine to help the body digest fats from foods.

Gallbladder disease, **gallstones, cancer,** or other abnormalities can cause **pain** and other symptoms. A gallbladder condition might be suspected if a patient has chronic or occasional pain in the upper right side of the abdomen. The pain may be stabbing and intense with sudden onset or it may be more of a dull, occasional ache. Loss of appetite, **nausea and vomiting** can also occur. **Fever** may indicate the presence of infection. **Jaundice,** a yellowing of the skin and whites of the eyes, may also indicate that the gallbladder is involved.

A gallbladder nuclear medicine scan may be used to diagnose gallstones, blockage of the bile duct or other abnormalities, and to assess gallbladder functioning and inflammation (**cholecystitis**). The scan is usually performed in a hospital or clinical radiology department. The patient lies on an examination table while a small amount of radioactive dye is injected into a vein in the arm. This dye circulates through the blood and collects in the gallbladder. As the dye moves through the gallbladder, a series of pictures is taken using a special camera called a *scintillation* or *gamma camera*. This procedure produces images that look like x rays. The test usually takes one to two hours to complete, but can last up to four hours.

The results of the scan are read by a radiologist, a doctor specializing in x rays and other types of scanning techniques. A report is sent, usually within 24 hours, to the doctor who will discuss the results with the patient.

Preparation

The patient may be required to withhold food and liquids for up to eight hours before the scan.

Aftercare

No special care is required after the procedure. Once the scan is complete, the patient can return to normal activities.

Risks

Nuclear medicine scans use a very small amount of radioactive material, and the risk of radiation is minimal. Very rarely, a patient may have a reaction to the dye material used.

Normal results

A normal scan shows a gallbladder without gallstones. There will be no evidence of growths or tumors, and no signs of infection or swelling. The normal gallbladder fills with bile and secretes it through the bile duct without blockages.

Abnormal results

An abnormal scan may show abnormal gallbladder emptying (suggesting gallbladder dysfunction or inflammation), or gallstones in the gallbladder or in the bile duct. The presence of tumors, growths or other types of blockages of the duct or the gallbladder itself could also appear on an abnormal scan.

Resources

BOOKS

"Common nuclear scan and why they are performed." in *The Consumer's Medical Desk Reference.* New York, NY: Hyperion, 1995.

"Hepatic scans." in *Infectious Diseases,* Second edition, Philadelphia, PA: W.B. Saunders Company, 1998.

OTHER

Gallbladder function study. Website: http://www.largnet.uwo.ca/nucmed/proto/file27.htm.

Gallbladder scan, radioisotope. Website: http://infonet.med.cornell.edu/Lab/radiology/NMED_Gallbladder_scan_Radioisotope.htm.

Nuclear medicine. Website: http://www.wrapc.com/nuclexam.htm.

Altha Roberts Edgren

Gallbladder surgery *see* **Cholecystectomy**

Gallbladder ultrasound *see* **Abdominal ultrasound**

Gallbladder x rays

Definition

This is an x-ray exam of the gallbladder (GB), a saclike organ that stores bile which is located under the liver. The study involves taking tablets containing dye (contrast) which outline any abnormalities when x rays are taken the following day. The test was once the standard for diagnosing diseases of the GB such as **gallstones;** however in recent years it is not used as often due to advances in diagnostic ultrasound.

Purpose

This test, also known as an oral cholecystogram or OCG, is usually ordered to help physicians diagnose disorders of the gallbladder, such as gallstones and tumors, which show up as solid dark structures. It is performed to help in the investigation of patients with upper abdominal **pain.** The test also measures gallbladder function, as the failure of the organ to visualize can signify a non-functioning or diseased gallbladder. The gallbladder may also not visualize if the bilirubin level is over 4 and the study should not be performed under these circumstances.

Precautions

Your physician must be notified if you are pregnant or allergic to iodine. Patients with a history of severe kidney damage, have an increased risk of injury or side effects from the procedure. In those cases, ultrasound is commonly used instead of the x-ray examination. Some people experience side effects from the contrast material (dye tablets), especially **diarrhea.** During preparation for the test, patients should not use any **laxatives.** Diabetics should discuss the need for any adjustment in medication with their physician.

KEY TERMS

Bile—A yellow-green liquid produced by the liver, which is released through the bile ducts into the small intestines to help digest fat.

Bilirubin—A reddish-yellow pigment formed from the destruction of red blood cells, and metabolized by the liver. Levels of bilirubin in the blood increase in patients with liver disease or blockage of the bile ducts.

Ultrasound—A non-invasive procedure based on changes in sound waves of a frequency that cannot be heard, but respond to changes in tissue composition. It requires no preparation and no radiation occurs; it has become the "gold standard" for diagnosis of stones in the gallbladder, but is less accurate in diagnosing stones in the bile ducts. Gallstones as small as 2 mm can be identified.

Description

The exam is performed in the radiology department. The night before the test, patients swallow six tablets (one at a time) that contain the contrast (x-ray dye). The following day at the hospital, the radiologist examines the gallbladder with a fluoroscope (a special x ray that projects the image onto a video monitor). Sometimes, patients are then asked to drink a highfat formula that will cause the gallbladder to contract and release bile. X rays will then be taken at various intervals. There is no discomfort from the test. If the gallbladder is not seen, the patient may be asked to return the following day for x rays.

Preparation

The day before the test patients are instructed to eat a highfat lunch (eggs, butter, milk, salad oils, or fatty meats), and a fat-free meal (fruits, vegetables, bread, tea or coffee, and only lean meat) in the evening. Two hours after the evening meal, six tablets containing the contrast medium, are taken, one a time. After that, no food or fluid is permitted until after the test.

Aftercare

No special care is required after the study.

Risks

There is a small chance of an allergic reaction to the contrast material. In addition, there is low radiation exposure. X rays are monitored and regulated to provide the minimum amount of radiation exposure needed to produce the image. Most experts feel that the risk is low compared with the benefits. Pregnant women and children are more sensitive to the risks of x rays, and the risk versus benefits should be discussed with the treating physician.

Normal results

The x ray will show normal structures for the age of the patient. The gallbladder should visualize, and be free of any solid structures, such as stones, polyps, etc.

Abnormal results

Abnormal results may show gallstones, tumors, or cholesterol polyps (a tumor growing from the lining that is usually noncancerous). Typically stones will "float" or move around as the patient changes position, whereas tumors will stay in the same place.

Resources

BOOKS

Levenson, Deborah E. and Fromm, Hans. "Oral Cholecystogram." In *Hepatology: A Textbook of Liver Disease,* edited by David Zakim and Thomas D. Boyer et al. Philadelphia: W.B. Saunders Company. 1996, p.1883.

Zeaman, Robert K. "Oral Cholecystography." In *Bockus Gastroenterology*, edited by William S. Haubrich et al. Philadelphia: W.B. Saunders Company. 1995, pp. 208-211.

OTHER

Gall Bladder Exam from Harvard Medical School. http://www.bih.harvard.edu/radiology/Modalities/Xray/xraysSubdivsf/gallbl.html.

Gallstones from NIDDK. http://www.niddk.nih.gov/health/digest/pubs/gallstns/ gallstns.htm.

Information on Gallstone Disease from the University of Connecticut Health Center. http://www6.uchc.edu/zakko/info-gsd.htm.

Oral cholecystogram from healthanswers.com. http://www.healthanswers.com/database/ami/converted/003821.html.

David S Kaminstein

Gallium scan of the body

Definition

A gallium scan of the body is a nuclear medicine test that is conducted using a camera that detects gallium, a form of radionuclide, or radioactive chemical substance.

KEY TERMS

Benign—Not cancerous. Benign tumors are not considered immediate threats, but may still require some form of treatment.

Gallium—A form of radionculide that is used to help locate tumors and inflammation (specifically referred to as GA67 citrate).

Malignant—This term, which is usually used to describe a tumor, means cancerous, becoming worse and possibly growing.

Nuclear medicine—A subspecialty of radiology used to show the function and anatomy of body organs. Very small amounts of radioactive substances, or tracers, are detected with a special camera as they collect in certain organs and tissues.

Radionuclide—A chemical substance, called an isotope, that exhibits radioactivity. A gamma camera, used in nuclear medicine procedures, will pick up the radioactive signals as the substance gathers in an organ or tissue. They are sometimes referred to as tracers.

Purpose

Most gallium scans are ordered to detect tumors in the body or to study the liver. Gallium is known to settle in certain organs and tissues, and also to accumulate in inflamed tissues and abnormal organs. Gallium scans are sometimes used to evaluate **cancer** following **chemotherapy** or **radiation therapy.**

Precautions

Children and women who are pregnant or breast-feeding are only given gallium scans if the potential diagnostic benefits will outweigh the risks.

Description

The patient will usually be asked to come to the testing facility 24–48 hours before the procedure to receive the injection of gallium. Sometimes, the injection will be given within only four to six hours of the study or as many as 72 hours before the procedure. The timeframe is based on the area or organs of the body being studied.

For the study itself the patient lies very still for approximately 30–60 minutes. A camera is moved across the patient's body to detect and capture images of concentrations of the gallium. The camera does not give off radiation, but picks up signals from any accumulated

areas of the radionuclide. In most cases, the patient will be lying down throughout the procedure. Back (posterior) and front (anterior) views will usually be taken, and sometimes a side (lateral) view is used. The camera may occasionally touch the patient's skin, but will not cause any discomfort. A clicking noise may also be heard throughout the procedure, but this sound is only the scanner's registering of radiation.

Preparation

The intravenous injection of gallium is done in a separate appointment prior to the procedure. Generally, no special dietary requirements are necessary. However, sometimes the physician will ask that the patient have light or clear meals within a day or less of the procedure. Many patients will be given **laxatives** or an **enema** prior to the scan to eliminate any residual gallium from the bowels.

Aftercare

There is generally no aftercare required following a gallium scan. However, women who are breastfeeding who have a scan will be cautioned against breastfeeding for four weeks following the exam.

Risks

There is a minimal risk of exposure to radiation from the gallium injection, but the exposure from one gallium scan is generally less than exposure from x rays.

Normal results

A radiologist trained in nuclear medicine or a nuclear medicine specialist will interpret the exam results and compare them to other diagnostic tests. It is normal for gallium to accumulate in the liver, spleen, bones, and large bowel.

Abnormal results

An abnormal concentration of gallium in areas other than those where it normally concentrates may indicate the presence of disease. Concentrations may be due to inflammation or the presence of tumor tissue. Often, additional tests are required to determine if the tumors are malignant or benign.

Even though gallium normally concentrates in organs such as the liver or spleen, abnormally high concentrations will suggest certain diseases and conditions. For example, Hodgkin's or non-Hodgkin's lymphoma may be diagnosed or staged if there is abnormal gallium activity in the lymph nodes. After a patient receives cancer treatment, such as radiation therapy or chemotherapy, a gallium scan may help to find new or recurring tumors or to record regression of a treated tumor. Physicians can narrow causes of liver problems by noting abnormal gallium activity in the liver. Gallium scans also can diagnose lung diseases or a disease called **sarcoidosis,** in the chest.

Resources

BOOKS

Fischbach, Frances T. *A Manual of Laboratory and Diagnostic Tests.* Philadelphia, PA: Lippincott-Raven Publishers, 1996.

Illustrated Guide to Diagnostic Tests. Springhouse, PA: Springhouse Corporation, 1998.

ORGANIZATIONS

American Cancer Society. 1599 Clifton Road NE, Atlanta, GA 30329. (404) 320-3333. http://www.cancer.org.

American College of Nuclear Medicine. P.O. Box 175, Landisville, PA 31906. (717) 898-6006.

American Liver Foundation. 1425 Pompton Avenue, Cedar Grove NJ 07009. 1-800-GO LIVER (465-4837). http://gi.ucsf.edu/ALF/serv.html.

Society of Nuclear Medicine. 1850 Samuel Morse Drive, Reston, VA 10016. (703) 708-9000. http://www.snm.org.

OTHER

A Patient's Guide to Nuclear Medicine. University of Iowa Virtual Hospital. http://www.vh.org/Patients/IHB/Rad/NucMed/PatGuideNucMed/PatGuideNucMed.html.

Teresa G. Norris

Gallstone removal

Definition

Also known as cholelithotomy, gallstone removal is the medical procedure that rids the gallbladder of calculus buildup.

Purpose

The gallbladder is not a vital organ. Its function is to store bile, concentrate it, and release it during digestion. Bile is supposed to retain all of its chemicals in solution, but commonly one of them crystallizes and forms sand, gravel, and finally stones.

The chemistry of gallstones is complex and interesting. Like too much sugar in solution, chemicals in bile will form crystals as the gallbladder draws water out of the bile. The solubility of these chemicals is based on the concentration of three chemicals, not just one—bile

> ### KEY TERMS
>
> **Cholecystectomy**—Surgical removal of the gallbladder.
>
> **Cholelithotomy**—Surgical incision into the gallbladder to remove stones.
>
> **Contrast agent**—A substance that causes shadows on x rays (or other images of the body).
>
> **Endoscope**—One of several instruments designed to enter body cavities. They combine viewing and operating capabilities.
>
> **Jaundice**—A yellow color of the skin and eyes due to excess bile that is not removed by the liver.
>
> **Laparoscopy**—Surgery through pencil-sized viewing instruments and tools so that incisions need be less than half an inch long.

acids, phospholipids, and cholesterol. If the chemicals are out of balance, one or the other will not remain in solution. Certain people, in particular the Pima tribe of Native Americans in Arizona, have a genetic predisposition to forming **gallstones.** Scandinavians also have a higher than average incidence of this disease. Dietary fat and cholesterol are also implicated in their formation. Overweight women in their middle years constitute the vast majority of patients with gallstones in every group.

As the bile crystals aggregate to form stones, they move about, eventually occluding the outlet and preventing the gallbladder from emptying. This creates symptoms. It also results in irritation, inflammation, and sometimes infection of the gallbladder. The pattern is usually one of intermittent obstruction due to stones moving in and out of the way. All the while the gallbladder is becoming more scarred. Sometimes infection fills it with pus—a serious complication.

On occasion a stone will travel down the cystic duct into the common bile duct and get stuck there. This will back bile up into the liver as well as the gallbladder. If the stone sticks at the Ampulla of Vater, the pancreas will also be plugged and will develop **pancreatitis.** These stones can cause a lot of trouble.

Bile is composed of several waste products of metabolism, all of which are supposed to remain in liquid form. The complex chemistry of the liver depends on many chemical processes, which depend in turn upon the chemicals in the diet and the genes that direct those processes. There are greater variations in the output of chemical waste products than there is allowance for their cohabitation in the bile. Incompatible mixes result in the formation of solids.

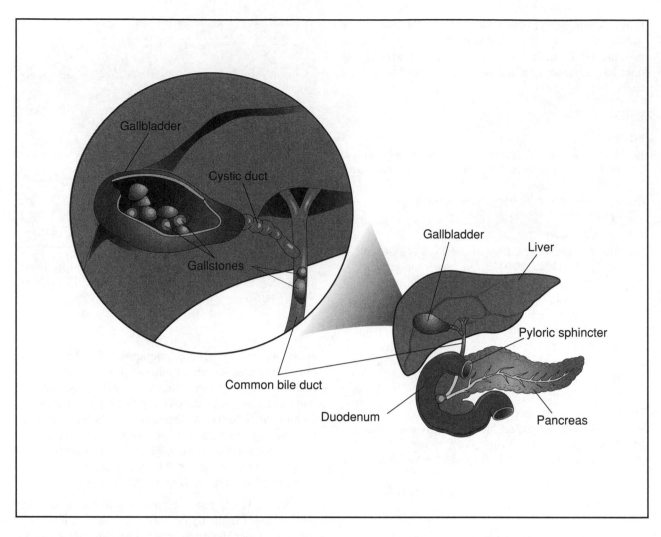

Gallbladder

Cystic duct

Gallstones

Gallbladder   Liver

Pyloric sphincter

Common bile duct

Duodenum   Pancreas

Gallstone removal, also known as cholelithotomy, usually involves the surgical removal of the entire gallbladder, but in recent years the procedure done by laparoscopy has resulted in smaller surgical incisions and faster recovery time. (*Illustration by Electronic Illustrators Group.*)

Gallstones will cause the sudden onset of **pain** in the upper abdomen. Pain will last for 30 minutes to several hours. Pain may move to the right shoulder blade. Nausea with or without vomiting may accompany the pain.

Precautions

Individuals suffering from **sickle cell anemia,** children, and patients with large stones may seek other treatments.

Description

Laparoscopic cholecystectomy

Surgery to remove the entire gallbladder with all its stones is usually the best treatment, provided the patient is able to tolerate the procedure. Over the past decade, a new technique of removing the gallbladder using a laparoscope has resulted in quicker recovery and much smaller surgical incisions than the six-inch gash under the right ribs that used to be standard. Not everyone is a candidate for this approach.

If a stone is lodged in the bile ducts, additional surgery must be done to remove it. After surgery, the surgeon will ordinarily leave in a drain to collect bile until the system is healed. The drain can also be used to inject contrast material and take x rays during or after surgery.

Endoscopic retrograde cholangiopancreatoscopy (ERCP)

A procedure called endoscopic retrograde cholangiopancreatoscopy (ERCP) allows the removal of some bile duct stones through the mouth, throat, esophagus, stomach, duodenum, and biliary system without the need for surgical incisions. ERCP can also be used to inject contrast agents into the biliary system, providing superbly detailed pictures.

Cholelithotomy

Rare circumstances require different techniques. Patients too ill for a complete **cholecystectomy** (removal of the gallbladder), sometimes only the stones are removed, a procedure called cholelithotomy. But that does not cure the problem. The liver will go on making faulty bile, and stones will reform, unless the composition of the bile is altered.

Ursodeoxycholic acid

For patients who cannot receive the laparoscopic procedure, there is also a nonsurgical treatment in which ursodeoxycholic acid is used to dissolve the gallstones. Extracorporeal shock-wave **lithotripsy** has also been successfully used to break up gallstones. During the procedure, high-amplitude sound waves target the stones, slowly breaking them up.

Preparation

There are a number of imaging studies that identify gallbladder disease, but most gallstones will not show up on conventional x rays. That requires contrast agents given by mouth that are excreted into the bile. Ultrasound is very useful and can be enhanced by doing it through an endoscope in the stomach. CT (**computed tomography scans**) and MRI (**magnetic resonance imaging**) scanning are not used routinely but are helpful in detecting common duct stones and complications.

Aftercare

Without a gallbladder, stones rarely reform. Patients who have continued symptoms after their gallbladder is removed may need an ERCP to detect residual stones or damage to the bile ducts caused by the stones before they were removed. Once in a while the Ampulla of Vater is too tight for bile to flow through and causes symptoms until it is opened up.

Resources

BOOKS
Bennett, J. Claude and Fred Plum, ed. *Cecil Textbook of Medicine.* Philadelphia: W. B. Saunders, 1996, pp. 812-816.

Bilhartz, Lyman E. and Jay D. Horton. "Gallstone disease and its complications." In *Sleisenger & Fordtran's Gastrointestinal and Liver Disease.* Edited by Mark Feldman, et al. Philadelphia: W. B. Saunders, 1998, pp. 948-972.

Friedman, Lawrence J. "Liver, biliary tract and pancreas." In *Current Medical Diagnosis and Treatment.* Edited by Lawrence M. Tierney Jr., et al. Stamford, CT: Appleton & Lange, 1996, pp. 652-7.

Hoffmann, Alan F. "Bile secretion and the enterohepatic circulation of bile acids." In *Sleisenger & Fordtran's Gastrointestinal and Liver Disease.* Edited by Mark Feldman, et al. Philadelphia: W. B. Saunders, 1998. pp. 937-948.

Isselbacher, Kurt J. and Norton Greenberger. "Disorders of the gallbladder and bile ducts." In *Harrison's Principles of Internal Medicine.* Edited by Kurt Isselbacher, et al. New York: McGraw-Hill, August 1997, pp. 1505-9.

Mulvihill, Sean J. "Surgical management of gallstone disease and postoperative complications." In *Sleisenger & Fordtran's Gastrointestinal and Liver Disease.* Edited by Mark Feldman, et al. Philadelphia: W. B. Saunders, 1998. pp. 973-984.

Paumgartner, Gustav. "Non-surgical management of gallstone disease" In *Sleisenger & Fordtran's Gastrointestinal and Liver Disease.* Edited by Mark Feldman, et al. Philadelphia: W. B. Saunders, 1998. pp. 984-993.

J. Ricker Polsdorfer

Gallstones

Definition

A gallstone is a solid crystal deposit that forms in the gallbladder, which is a pear-shaped organ that stores bile salts until they are needed to help digest fatty foods. Gallstones can migrate to other parts of the digestive tract and cause severe **pain** with life-threatening complications.

Description

Gallstones vary in size and chemical structure. A gallstone may be as tiny as a grain of sand or as large as a golf ball. Eighty percent of gallstones are composed of cholesterol. They are formed when the liver produces more cholesterol than digestive juices can liquefy. The remaining 20% of gallstones are composed of calcium and an orange-yellow waste product called bilirubin. Bilirubin gives urine its characteristic color and sometimes causes **jaundice**.

KEY TERMS

Acalculous cholecystitis—Inflammation of the gallbladder that occurs without the presence of gallstones.

Bilirubin—A reddish-yellow waste product produced by the liver that colors urine and is involved in the formation of some gallstones.

Celiac disease—Inability to digest wheat protein (gluten), which causes weight loss, lack of energy, and pale, foul-smelling stools.

Cholecystectomy—Surgical removal of the gallbladder.

Cholecystitis—Inflammation of the gallbladder.

Choledocholithiasis—The presence of gallstones within the common bile duct.

Cholelithiasis—The presence of gallstones within the gallbladder.

Cholesterolosis—Cholesterol crystals or deposits in the lining of the gallbladder.

Common bile duct—The passage through which bile travels from the cystic duct to the small intestine.

Gallstone ileus—Obstruction of the large intestine caused by a gallstone that has blocked the intestinal opening.

Lithotripsy—A nonsurgical technique for removing gallstones by breaking them apart with high-frequency sound waves.

Gallstones are the most common of all gallbladder problems. They are responsible for 90% of gallbladder

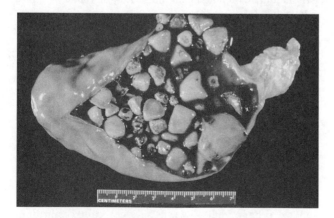

A specimen of a gallbladder with stones. *(Custom Medical Stock Photo. Reproduced by permission.)*

and bile duct disease, and are the fifth most common reason for hospitalization of adults in the United States. Gallstones usually develop in adults between the ages of 20 and 50; about 20% of patients with gallstones are over 40. The risk of developing gallstones increases with age—at least 20% of people over 60 have a single large stone or as many as several thousand smaller ones. The gender ratio of gallstone patients changes with age. Young women are between two and six times more likely to develop gallstones than men in the same age group. In patients over 50, the condition affects men and women with equal frequency. Native Americans develop gallstones more often than any other segment of the population; Mexican-Americans have the second-highest incidence of this disease.

Definitions

Gallstones can cause several different disorders. Cholelithiasis is defined as the presence of gallstones within the gallbladder itself. Choledocholithiasis is the presence of gallstones within the common bile duct that leads into the first portion of the small intestine (the duodenum). The stones in the duct may have been formed inside it or carried there from the gallbladder. These gallstones prevent bile from flowing into the duodenum. Ten percent of patients with gallstones have choledocholithiasis, which is sometimes called common-duct stones. Patients who don't develop infection usually recover completely from this disorder.

Cholecystitis is a disorder marked by inflammation of the gallbladder. It is usually caused by the passage of a stone from the gallbladder into the cystic duct, which is a tube that connects the gallbladder to the common bile duct. In 5–10% of cases, however, cholecystitis develops in the absence of gallstones. This form of the disorder is called acalculous cholecystitis. Cholecystitis causes painful enlargement of the gallbladder and is responsible for 10–25% of all gallbladder surgery. Chronic cholecystitis is most common in the elderly. The acute form is most likely to occur in middle-aged adults.

Cholesterolosis or cholesterol polyps is characterized by deposits of cholesterol crystals in the lining of the gallbladder. This condition may be caused by high levels of cholesterol or inadequate quantities of bile salts, and is usually treated by surgery.

Gallstone **ileus,** which results from a gallstone's blocking the entrance to the large intestine, is most common in elderly people. Surgery usually cures this condition.

Narrowing (stricture) of the common bile duct develops in as many as 5% of patients whose gallbladders have been surgically removed. This condition is characterized by inability to digest fatty foods and by abdominal pain, which sometimes occurs in spasms. Patients with stricture of the common bile duct are likely to recover after appropriate surgical treatment.

Causes & symptoms

Gallstones are caused by an alteration in the chemical composition of bile. Bile is a digestive fluid that helps the body absorb fat. Gallstones tend to run in families. In addition, high levels of estrogen, insulin, or cholesterol can increase a person's risk of developing them.

Pregnancy or the use of birth control pills can slow down gallbladder activity and increase the risk of gallstones. So can diabetes, **pancreatitis,** and **celiac disease.** Other factors influencing gallstone formation are:

- Infection
- **Obesity**
- Intestinal disorders
- **Coronary artery disease** or other recent illness
- Multiple pregnancies
- A high-fat, low-fiber diet
- Smoking
- Heavy drinking
- Rapid weight loss.

Gallbladder attacks usually follow a meal of rich, high-fat foods. The attacks often occur in the middle of the night, sometimes waking the patient with intense pain that ends in a visit to the emergency room. The pain of a gallbladder attack begins in the abdomen and may radiate to the chest, back, or the area between the shoulders. Other symptoms of gallstones include:

- Inability to digest fatty foods
- Low-grade **fever**
- Chills and sweating
- **Nausea and vomiting**
- **Indigestion**
- Gas
- Belching.
- Clay-colored bowel movements.

Diagnosis

Gallstones may be diagnosed by a family doctor, a specialist in digestive problems (a gastroenterologist), or a specialist in internal medicine. The doctor will first examine the patient's skin for signs of jaundice and feel (palpate) the abdomen for soreness or swelling. After the basic **physical examination,** the doctor will order **blood counts** or blood chemistry tests to detect evidence of bile duct obstruction and to rule out other illnesses that cause

fever and pain, including stomach **ulcers, appendicitis,** and **heart attacks.**

More sophisticated procedures used to diagnose gallstones include:

- Ultrasound imaging. Ultrasound has an accuracy rate of 96%.
- Cholecystography (cholecystogram, gallbladder series, gallbladder x ray). This type of study shows how the gallbladder contracts after the patient has eaten a high-fat meal.
- Fluoroscopy. This imaging technique allows the doctor to distinguish between jaundice caused by **pancreatic cancer** and jaundice caused by gallbladder or bile duct disorders.
- Endoscopy (ERCP). ERCP uses a special dye to outline the pancreatic and common bile ducts and locate the position of the gallstones.
- Radioisotopic scan. This technique reveals blockage of the cystic duct.

Treatment

Watchful waiting

One-third of all patients with gallstones never experience a second attack. For this reason many doctors advise watchful waiting after the first episode. Reducing the amount of fat in the diet or following a sensible plan of gradual weight loss may be the only treatments required for occasional mild attacks. A patient diagnosed with gallstones may be able to manage more troublesome episodes by:

- Applying heat to the affected area.
- Resting and taking occasional sips of water.
- Using non-prescription forms of **acetaminophen** (Tylenol or Anacin-3).

A doctor should be notified if pain intensifies or lasts for more than three hours; if the patient's fever rises above 101°F (38.3°C); or if the skin or whites of the eyes turn yellow.

Surgery

Surgical removal of the gallbladder (**cholecystectomy**) is the most common conventional treatment for recurrent attacks. Laparoscopic surgery, the technique most widely used, is a safe, effective procedure that involves less pain and a shorter recovery period than traditional open surgery. In this technique, the doctor makes a small cut (incision) in the patient's abdomen and removes the gallbladder through a long tube called a laparoscope.

Nonsurgical approaches

LITHOTRIPSY

Shock wave therapy (**lithotripsy**) uses high-frequency sound waves to break up the gallstones. The patient can then take bile salts to dissolve the fragments. Bile salt tablets are sometimes prescribed without lithotripsy to dissolve stones composed of cholesterol by raising the level of bile acids in the gallbladder. This approach requires long-term treatment, since it may take months or years for this method to dissolve a sizeable stone.

CONTACT DISSOLUTION

Contact dissolution can destroy gallstones in a matter of hours. This minimally invasive procedure involves using a tube (catheter) inserted into the abdomen to inject medication directly into the gallbladder.

Alternative treatment

Alternative therapies, like non-surgical treatments, may provide temporary relief of gallstone symptoms. Alternative approaches to the symptoms of gallbladder disorders include homeopathy, **Chinese traditional herbal medicine,** and **acupuncture.** Dietary changes may also help relieve the symptoms of gallstones. Since gallstones seem to develop more often in people who are obese, eating a balanced diet, exercising, and losing weight may help keep gallstones from forming.

Prognosis

Forty percent of all patients with gallstones have "silent gallstones" that produce no symptoms. Silent stones, discovered only when their presence is indicated by tests performed to diagnose other symptoms, do not require treatment.

Gallstone problems that require treatment can be surgically corrected. Although most patients recover, some develop infections that must be treated with **antibiotics.**

In rare instances, severe inflammation can cause the gallbladder to burst. The resulting infection can be fatal.

Prevention

The best way to prevent gallstones is to minimize risk factors. In addition, a 1998 study suggests that vigorous **exercise** may lower a man's risk of developing gallstones by as much as 28%. The researchers have not yet determined whether physical activity benefits women to the same extent.

Resources

BOOKS

The Editors of Time-Life Books. *The Medical Advisor: The Complete Guide to Alternative and Conventional Treatments.* Alexandria, VA: Time Life, Inc., 1996.

Gottlieb, Bill, editor. *New Choices in Natural Healing.* Emmaus, PA: Rodale Press, Inc., 1995.

Shaw, Michael, senior editor. *Everything You Need to Know About Diseases.* Springhouse, PA: Springhouse Corporation, 1996.

PERIODICALS

"Exercise Prevents Gallstone Disease." *Journal Watch* (April 15, 1998): 63-64.

ORGANIZATIONS

National Digestive Diseases Clearinghouse (NDDIC). 2 Information Way, Bethesda, MD 20892-3570. http://www.niddk.nih.gov/health/digest/nddic.htm.

National Institute of Diabetes and Digestive and Kidney Disorders of the National Institutes of Health. Bethesda, MD 20892. http://www.niddk.nih/gov/.

OTHER

Gallbladder Problems. http://www.sleh.com/fact-d04-gall.html (3 March 1998).

Gallstones. http://www.geisinger.edu/ghs/pubtips/G/Gallstones.htm (17 April 1998).

Gallstones. http://www.thriveonline.com/health/Library/illsymp/illness 229.html (6 April 1998).

Oral cholecystogram, Gallbladder Series. http://www.healthgate.com/HealthGate/free/dph/static/dph.0178.sht ml (17 April 1998).

Maureen Haggerty

Gamete intrafallopian transfer *see*
Infertility therapies

Gamma globulin electrophoresis *see*
Immunoelectrophoresis

Gammaglobulin

Definition

Gammaglobulin is a type of protein found in the blood. When gammaglobulins are extracted from the blood of many people and combined, they can be used to prevent or treat infections.

Purpose

This medicine is used to treat or prevent diseases that occur when the body's own immune system is not effective against the disease. When disease-causing agents enter the body, they normally trigger the production of antibodies, proteins that circulate in the blood and help fight the disease. Gammaglobulin contains some of these antibodies. When gammaglobulins are taken from the blood of people who have recovered from diseases such as **chickenpox** or hepatitis, they can be given to other people to make them temporarily immune to those diseases. With hepatitis, for example, this is done when someone who has not been vaccinated against hepatitis is exposed to the disease.

Description

Gammaglobulin, also known as immunoglobulin, immune serum globulin or serum therapy, is injected either into a vein or into a muscle. When injected into a vein, it produces results more quickly than when injected into a muscle.

Recommended dosage

Doses are different for different people and depend on the person's body weight and the condition for which he or she is being treated.

Precautions

Anyone who has had unusual reactions to gammaglobulin in the past should let his or her physician know before taking the drugs again. The physician should also be told about any **allergies** to foods, dyes, preservatives, or other substances.

People who have certain medical conditions may have problems if they take gammaglobulins. For example:

• Gammaglobulins may worsen heart problems or deficiencies of immunoglobin A (IgA, a type of antibody)

• Certain patients with low levels of gammaglobulins in the blood (conditions called agammaglobulinemia and hypogammaglobulinemia) may be more likely to have side effects when they take gammaglobulin.

Side effects

Minor side effects such as **headache,** backache, joint or muscle **pain,** and a general feeling of illness usually go away as the body adjusts to this medicine. These problems do not need medical attention unless they continue.

Other side effects, such as breathing problems or a fast or pounding heartbeat, should be brought to a physician's attention as soon as possible.

Anyone who shows the following signs of overdose should check with a physician immediately:

• Unusual tiredness or weakness

• **Dizziness**

• Nausea

• Vomiting

• **Fever**

• Chills

• Tightness in the chest

• Red face

• Sweating.

Interactions

Anyone who takes gammaglobulin should let the physician know all other medicines he or she is taking and should ask whether interactions with gammaglobulin could interfere with treatment.

Nancy Ross-Flanigan

Gamma-glutamyl transferase test *see* **Liver function tests**

Ganglion

Definition

A ganglion is a small, usually hard bump above a tendon or in the capsule that encloses a joint. A ganglion is also called a synovial **hernia** or synovial cyst.

Description

A ganglion is a non-cancerous cyst filled with a thick, jelly-like fluid. Ganglions can develop on or beneath the surface of the skin and usually occur between the ages of 20 and 40.

Most ganglions develop on the hand or wrist. This condition is common in people who bowl or who play handball, raquetball, squash, or tennis. Runners and athletes who jump, ski, or play contact sports often develop foot ganglions.

Causes & symptoms

Mild sprains or other repeated injuries can irritate and tear the thin membrane covering a tendon, causing fluid to leak into a sac that swells and forms a ganglion.

Ganglions are usually painless, but range of motion may be impaired. Flexing or bending the affected area can cause discomfort, as can continuing to perform the activity that caused the condition.

Cysts on the surface of the skin usually develop slowly but may result from injury or severe strain. An internal ganglion can cause soreness or a dull, aching sensation, but the mass cannot always be felt. Symptoms sometimes become evident only when the cyst causes pressure on a nerve or outgrows the membrane surrounding it.

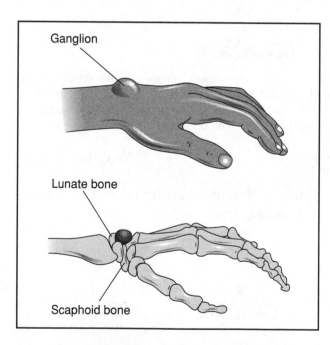

Ganglion

Lunate bone

Scaphoid bone

A ganglion is a non-cancerous cyst filled with a thick, jelly-like fluid. Ganglions can develop on or beneath the surface of the skin, most likely on the hand or wrist, although runners and skiers often develop them on the foot. (Illustration by Electronic Illustrators Group.)

Diagnosis

Diagnosis is usually made through physical examination as well as such imaging studies as x ray, ultrasound, and **magnetic resonance imaging** (MRI). Fluid may be withdrawn from the cyst and evaluated.

Treatment

Some ganglions disappear without treatment, and some reappear despite treatment.

Acetaminophen (Tylenol) or other over-the-counter **analgesics** can be used to control mild pain. Steroids or local anesthetics may be injected into cysts that cause severe pain or other troublesome symptoms. Surgery performed in a hospital operating room or an outpatient facility, is the only treatment guaranteed to remove a ganglion. The condition can recur if the entire cyst is not removed.

A doctor should be notified if the surgical site drains, bleeds, or becomes

• Inflamed

• Painful

• Swollen or if the patient feels ill or develops:

• Head or muscle aches

• **Dizziness**

• **Fever** following surgery.

The patient may bathe or shower as usual, but should keep the surgical site dry and covered with a bandage for two or three days after the operation. Patients may resume normal activities as soon as they feel comfortable doing so.

Prognosis

Possible complications include excessive post-operative bleeding and infection of the surgical site. Calcification, or hardening, of the ganglion is rare.

Prevention

Exercises that increase muscle strength and flexibility can prevent ganglions. Warming and cooling down before and after workouts may also decrease the rate of developing ganglions.

Resources

BOOKS

Taylor, Robert B., editor. *Family Medicine Principles and Practice.* New York, NY: Springer Verlag, 1994.

OTHER

Foot ganglion. http://www.thriveonline.com/health/Library/ sports/sport141.html (25 May 1998).

Hand or wrist ganglion. http://www.thriveonline.com/health/ Library/pedillsymp/pedillsymp184.html (25 May 1998).

Maureen Haggerty

Gangrene

Definition

Gangrene is the term used to describe the decay or death of an organ or tissue caused by a lack of blood supply. It is a complication resulting from infectious or inflammatory processes, injury, or degenerative changes associated with chronic diseases, such as **diabetes mellitus.**

Description

Gangrene may be caused by a variety of chronic diseases and post-traumatic, post-surgical, and spontaneous causes. There are three major types of gangrene: dry, moist, and gas (a type of moist gangrene).

Dry gangrene is a condition that results when one or more arteries become obstructed. In this type of gangrene, the tissue slowly dies, due to receiving little or no blood supply, but does not become infected. The affected area becomes cold and black, begins to dry out and wither, and eventually drops off over a period of weeks or months. Dry gangrene is most common in persons with advanced blockages of the arteries (arteriosclerosis) resulting from diabetes.

Moist gangrene may occur in the toes, feet, or legs after a crushing injury or as a result of some other factor that causes blood flow to the area to suddenly stop. When blood flow ceases, bacteria begin to invade the muscle and thrive, multiplying quickly without interference from the body's immune system.

Gas gangrene, also called myonecrosis, is a type of moist gangrene that is commonly caused by bacterial infection with *Clostridium welchii, Cl. perfringes, Cl. septicum, Cl. novyi, Cl. histolyticum, Cl. sporogenes*, or other species that are capable of thriving under conditions where there is little oxygen (anaerobic). Once present in tissue, these bacteria produce gasses and poisonous toxins as they grow. Normally inhabiting the gastrointestinal, respiratory, and female genital tract, they often infect thigh amputation **wounds,** especially in those individuals who have lost control of their bowel functions (incontinence). Gangrene, incontinence, and debility often are combined in patients with diabetes, and it is in the

amputation stump of diabetic patients that gas gangrene is often found to occur.

Other causative organisms for moist gangrene include various bacterial strains, including *Streptococcus* and *Staphylococcus*. A serious, but rare form of infection with Group A *Streptococcus* can impede blood flow and, if untreated, can progress to synergistic gangrene, more commonly called necrotizing fasciitis, or infection of the skin and tissues directly beneath the skin.

Chronic diseases, such as diabetes mellitus, arteriosclerosis, or diseases affecting the blood vessels, such as **Buerger's disease** or **Raynaud's disease,** can cause gangrene. Post-traumatic causes of gangrene include compound **fractures, burns,** and injections given under the skin or in a muscle. Gangrene may occur following surgery, particularly in individuals with diabetes mellitus or other long-term (chronic) disease. In addition, gas gangrene can be also be a complication of dry gangrene or occur spontaneously in association with an underlying **cancer.**

In the United States, approximately 50% of moist gangrene cases are the result of a severe traumatic injury, and 40% occur following surgery. Car and industrial accidents, crush injuries, and gunshot wounds are the most common traumatic causes. Because of prompt surgical management of wounds with the removal of dead tissue, the incidence of gangrene from trauma has significantly diminished. Surgeries involving the bile ducts or intestine are the most frequent procedures causing gangrene. Approximately two-thirds of cases affect the extremities, and the remaining one-third involve the abdominal wall.

Symptoms

Areas of either dry or moist gangrene are initially characterized by a red line on the skin that marks the border of the affected tissues. As tissues begin to die, dry gangrene may cause some **pain** in the early stages or may go unnoticed, especially in the elderly or in those individuals with diminished sensation to the affected area. Initially, the area becomes cold, numb, and pale before later changing in color to brown, then black. This dead tissue will gradually separate from the healthy tissue and fall off.

Moist gangrene and gas gangrene are distinctly different. Gas gangrene does not involve the skin as much, but usually only the muscle. In moist or gas gangrene, there is a sensation of heaviness in the affected region that is followed by severe pain. The pain is caused by swelling resulting from fluid or gas accumulation in the tissues. This pain peaks, on average, between one to four days following the injury, with a range of eight hours to several weeks. The swollen skin may initially be blis-

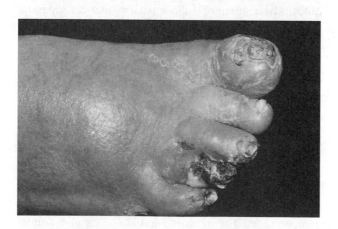

A close-up of gangrene in the toes of a diabetic patient.
(Photo Researchers, Inc. Reproduced by permission.)

tered, red, and warm to the touch before progressing to a bronze, brown, or black color. In approximately 80% of cases, the affected and surrounding tissues may produce crackling sounds (crepitus), as a result of gas bubbles accumulating under the skin. The gas may be felt beneath the skin (palpable). In wet gangrene, the pus is foul-smelling, while in gas gangrene, there is no true pus, just an almost "sweet" smelling watery discharge.

Fever, rapid heart rate, rapid breathing, altered mental state, loss of appetite, **diarrhea,** vomiting, and vascular collapse may also occur if the bacterial toxins are allowed to spread in the bloodstream. Gas gangrene can be a life-threatening condition and should receive prompt medical attention

Diagnosis

A diagnosis of gangrene will be based on a combination of the patient history, a **physical examination,** and the results of blood and other laboratory tests. A physician will look for a history of recent trauma, surgery, cancer, or chronic disease. Blood tests will be used to determine whether infection is present and determine the extent to which an infection has spread.

A sample of drainage from a wound, or obtained through surgical exploration, may be cultured with oxygen (aerobic) and without oxygen (anaerobic) to identify the microorganism causing the infection and to aid in determining which antibiotic will be most effective. The sample obtained from a person with gangrene will contain few, if any, white blood cells and, when stained (with Gram stain) and examined under the microscope, will show the presence of purple (Gram positive), rod-shaped bacteria.

X ray studies and more sophisticated imaging techniques, such as **computed tomography scans** (CT) or **magnetic resonance imaging** (MRI), may be helpful in making a diagnosis since gas accumulation and muscle death (myonecrosis) may be visible. These techniques, however, are not sufficient alone to provide an accurate diagnosis of gangrene.

Precise diagnosis of gas gangrene often requires surgical exploration of the wound. During such a procedure, the exposed muscle may appear pale, beefy-red, or in the most advanced stages, black. If infected, the muscle will fail to contract with stimulation, and the cut surface will not bleed.

Treatment

Gas gangrene is a medical emergency because of the threat of the infection rapidly spreading via the bloodstream and infecting vital organs. It requires immediate surgery and administration of **antibiotics.**

Areas of dry gangrene that remain free from infection (aseptic) in the extremities are most often left to wither and fall off. Treatments applied to the wound externally (topically) are generally not effective without adequate blood supply to support wound healing. Assessment by a vascular surgeon, along with x rays to determine blood supply and circulation to the affected area, can help determine whether surgical intervention would be beneficial.

Once the causative organism has been identified, moist gangrene requires the prompt initiation of intravenous, intramuscular, and/or topical broad-spectrum antibiotic therapy. In addition, the infected tissue must be removed surgically (**debridement**), and amputation of the affected extremity may be necessary. Pain medications (**analgesics**) are prescribed to control discomfort. Intravenous fluids and, occasionally, blood **transfusions** are indicated to counteract **shock** and replenish red blood cells and electrolytes. Adequate hydration and nutrition are vital to wound healing.

Although still controversial, some cases of gangrene are treated by administering oxygen under pressure greater than that of the atmosphere (hyperbaric) to the patient in a specially designed chamber. The theory behind using hyperbaric oxygen is that more oxygen will become dissolved in the patient's bloodstream, and therefore, more oxygen will be delivered to the gangrenous areas. By providing optimal oxygenation, the body's ability to fight off the bacterial infection are believed to be improved, and there is a direct toxic effect on the bacteria that thrive in an oxygen-free environment. Some studies have shown that the use of hyperbaric oxygen produces marked pain relief, reduces the number of amputations required, and reduces the extent of surgical debridement required. Patients receiving hyperbaric oxygen treatments must be monitored closely for evidence of oxygen toxicity. Symptoms of this toxicity include slow heart rate, profuse sweating, ringing in the ears, **shortness of breath, nausea and vomiting,** twitching of the lips/cheeks/eyelids/nose, and convulsions.

The emotional needs of the patient must also be met. The individual with gangrene should be offered moral support, along with an opportunity to share questions and concerns about changes in body image. In addition, particularly in cases where amputation was required, physical, vocational, and **rehabilitation** therapy will also be required.

Prognosis

Except in cases where the infection has been allowed to spread through the blood stream, prognosis is generally favorable. Anaerobic wound infection can progress quickly from initial injury to gas gangrene within one to two days, and the spread of the infection in the blood stream is associated with a 20–25% mortality rate. If recognized and treated early, however, approximately 80% of those with gas gangrene survive, and only 15–20% require any form of amputation. Unfortunately, the individual with dry gangrene most often has multiple other health problems that complicate recovery, and it is usually those other system failures that can prove fatal.

Prevention

Patients with diabetes or severe arteriosclerosis should take particular care of their hands and feet because of the risk of infection associated with even a minor injury. Education about proper **foot care** is vital. Diminished blood flow as a result of narrowed vessels will not lessen the body's defenses against invading bacteria. Measures taken towards the reestablishment of circulation are recommended whenever possible. Any abrasion, break in the skin, or infection tissue should be cared for immediately. Any dying or infected skin must be removed promptly to prevent the spread of bacteria.

Penetrating abdominal wounds should be surgically explored and drained, any tears in the intestinal walls closed, and antibiotic treatment begun early. Patients undergoing elective intestinal surgery should receive preventive antibiotic therapy. Use of antibiotics prior to and directly following surgery has been shown to significantly reduce the rate of infection from 20–30% to 4–8%.

Resources

BOOKS

Berkow, Robert and Andrew Fletcher. *The Merck Manual of Diagnosis and Therapy.* Merck Research Laboratories, 1992.

Brunner, Lillian and Doris Suddarth. *The Lippincott Manual of Nursing Practice.* J.B. Lippincott Company, 1991.

Wyngaarden, James B., Lloyd H. Smith, and J. Claude Bennett. *Cecil Textbook of Medicine.* W.B. Saunders Company, 1992.

PERIODICALS

Basoglu, M., et al. "Fournier's Gangrene: Review of Fifteen Cases." *American Surgeon* (November 1997):1019-1021.

Garcia-Olmo, D., et al. "Postoperative Gangrenous Peritonitis After Laparoscopic Cholecystectomy: A New Complication for a New Technique." *Laparoscopic and Endoscopic Surgery* (June 1997): 179-180.

Howse, Elizabeth A. "Meleney's Synergistic Gangrene: A Case Study." *Critical Care Nurse* (December 1995): 59-64.

Laor, E., et al. "Outcome Prediction in Patients with Fournier's Gangrene." *Journal of Urology* (July 1995): 89-92.

Pizzorno, R., et al. "Hyperbaric Oxygen Therapy in the Treatment of Fournier's Disease in Eleven Male Patients." *Journal of Urology* (September 1997): 837-840.

Kathleen Dredge Wright

Gas embolism

Definition

Gas embolism, also called air **embolism,** is the presence of gas bubbles in the bloodstream that obstruct circulation.

Description

Gas embolism may occur with decompression from increased pressure; it typically occurs in ascending divers who have been breathing compressed air. If a diver does not fully exhale upon ascent, the air in the lungs expands as the pressure decreases, overinflating the lungs and forcing bubbles of gas (emboli) into the bloodstream. When gas emboli reach the arteries to the brain, the blood blockage causes unconsciousness. Gas embolism is second only to drowning as a cause of **death** among divers.

Gas embolism may also result from trauma or medical procedures such as catheterization and open heart surgery that allow air into the circulatory system.

Causes & symptoms

Gas embolism occurs independent of diving depth; it may occur in as little as 6 ft of water. It is frequently caused by a diver holding his breath during ascent. It may also result from an airway obstruction or other condition that prevents a diver from fully exhaling.

The primary sign of gas embolism is immediate loss of consciousness; it may or may not be accompanied by convulsions.

Diagnosis

Any unconscious diver should be assumed to be the victim of gas embolism, regardless of whether consciousness was lost during or promptly after ascent. A doctor may also find pockets of air in the chest around the lungs and sometimes a collapsed lung from overinflation and rupture. Coughing up blood or a bloody froth around the mouth are visible signs of lung injury.

KEY TERMS

Compressed air—Air that is held under pressure in a tank to be breathed underwater by divers. A tank of compressed air is part of a diver's scuba (self-contained underwater breathing apparatus) gear.

Compression—An increase in pressure from the surrounding water that occurs with increasing diving depth.

Decompression—A decrease in pressure from the surrounding water that occurs with decreasing diving depth.

Emboli—Plural of embolus. An embolus is something that blocks the blood flow in a blood vessel. It may be a gas bubble, a blood clot, a fat globule, a mass of bacteria, or other foreign body. It usually forms somewhere else and travels through the circulatory system until it gets stuck.

Hyperbaric chamber—A sealed compartment in which patients are exposed to controlled pressures up to three times normal atmospheric pressure. Hyperbaric treatment may be used to regulate blood gases, reduce gas emboli, and provide higher levels of oxygen more quickly in cases of severe gas poisoning.

Recompression—Restoring the elevated pressure of the diving environment to treat gas embolism by decreasing bubble size.

Treatment

Prompt **recompression treatment** in a hyperbaric (high-pressure) chamber is necessary to deflate the gas bubbles in the bloodstream, dissolve the gases into the blood, and restore adequate oxygenated blood flow to the brain and other organs. Recompression by returning the diver to deeper water will not work, and should not be attempted. The patient should be kept lying down and given oxygen while being transported for recompression treatment.

Before the diver receives recompression treatment, other lifesaving efforts may be necessary. If the diver isn't breathing, artificial respiration (also called mouth-to-mouth resuscitation or rescue breathing) should be administered. In the absence of a pulse, **cardiopulmonary resuscitation (CPR)** must be performed.

Prognosis

The prognosis is dependent upon the promptness of recompression treatment and the extent of the damage caused by oxygen deprivation.

Prevention

All divers should receive adequate training in the use of compressed air and a complete evaluation of fitness for diving. People with a medical history of lung cysts or spontaneous collapsed lung (**pneumothorax**), and those with active **asthma** or other lung disease must not dive, for they would be at extreme risk for gas embolism. Patients with conditions such as **alcoholism** and drug abuse are also discouraged from diving. Individuals with certain other medical conditions such as diabetes may be able to dive safely with careful training and supervision.

Resources

BOOKS

Martin, Lawrence. *Scuba Diving Explained: Questions and Answers on Physiology and Medical Aspects of Scuba Diving.* Flagstaff, AZ: Best Publishing, 1997.

ORGANIZATIONS

American College of Hyperbaric Medicine. P.O. Box 25914-130, Houston, TX 77265. (713) 528-5931. http://www.hyperbaricmedicine.org.

Divers Alert Network. The Peter B. Bennett Center, 6 West Colony Place, Durham, NC 27705. (919) 684-8111. (919) 684-4326 (diving emergencies). (919) 684-2948 (general information). http://www.dan.ycg.org.

Undersea and Hyperbaric Medical Society. 10531 Metropolitan Avenue, Kensington, MD 20895. (301) 942-2980. http://www.uhms.org.

Bethany Thivierge

Gas gangrene *see* **Gangrene**

Gastrectomy

Definition

Gastrectomy is the surgical removal of all or part of the stomach.

Purpose

Gastrectomy is performed for several reasons, most commonly to remove a malignant tumor or to cure a perforated or bleeding stomach ulcer.

Description

Gastrectomy for cancer

Removal of the tumor, often with removal of surrounding lymph nodes, is the only curative treatment for various forms of gastric (stomach) **cancer.** For many patients, this entails removing not just the tumor but part of the stomach as well. The extent to which lymph nodes should also be removed is a subject of some debate, but some studies show additional survival benefit associated with removal of a greater number of lymph nodes.

Gastrectomy, either total or subtotal (also called partial), is the treatment of choice for gastric adenocarcinomas, primary gastric lymphomas (originating in the stomach), and the rare leiomyosarcomas (also called gastric **sarcomas).** Adenocarcinomas are by far the most common form of **stomach cancer** and are less curable than the relatively uncommon lymphomas, for which gastrectomy offers good odds for survival.

After gastrectomy, the surgeon may ''reconstruct'' the altered portions of the digestive tract so that it continues to function. Several different surgical techniques are used, but, generally speaking, the surgeon attaches any remaining portion of the stomach to the small intestine.

Gastrectomy for gastric cancer is almost always done by the traditional ''open'' surgery technique, which requires a wide incision to open the abdomen. However, some surgeons use a laparoscopic technique that requires only a small incision. The laparoscope is connected to a tiny video camera that projects a picture of the abdominal contents onto a monitor for the surgeon's viewing. The stomach is operated on through this incision.

The potential benefits of laparoscopic surgery include less postoperative **pain,** decreased hospitalization, and earlier return to normal activities. The use of laparoscopic gastrectomy is limited, however. Only patients with early stage gastric cancers or those whose surgery is only intended for palliation—pain and symptomatic relief rather than cure—should be considered for this minimally invasive technique. It can only be performed by surgeons experienced in this type of surgery.

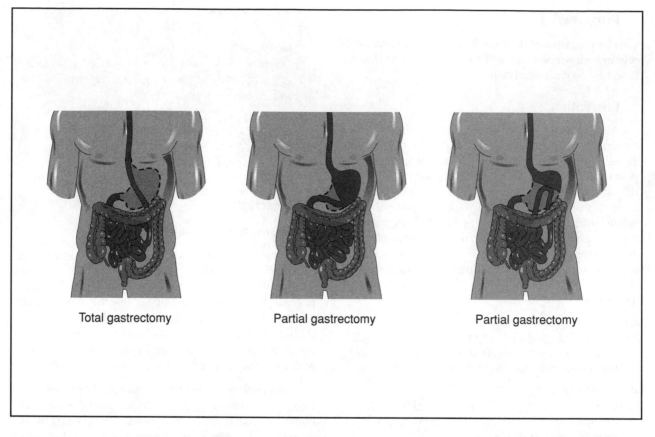

Total gastrectomy   Partial gastrectomy   Partial gastrectomy

Gastrectomy, the surgical removal of all or part of the stomach, is performed primarily to remove a malignant tumor or to cure a bleeding stomach ulcer. Following the gastrectomy, the surgeon may reconstruct the altered portions of the digestive tract so that it continues to function. *(Illustration by Electronic Illustrators Group.)*

Gastrectomy for ulcers

Gastrectomy is also occasionally used in the treatment of severe peptic ulcer disease or its complications. While the vast majority of peptic **ulcers** (gastric ulcers in the stomach or duodenal ulcers in the duodenum) are managed with medication, partial gastrectomy is sometimes required for peptic ulcer patients who have complications. These include patients who do not respond satisfactorily to medical therapy, those who develop a bleeding or perforated ulcer, and those who develop pyloric obstruction, a blockage to the exit from the stomach.

The surgical procedure for severe ulcer disease is also called an antrectomy, a limited form of gastrectomy in which the antrum, a portion of the stomach, is removed. For duodenal ulcers, antrectomy may be combined with other surgical procedures that are aimed at reducing the secretion of gastric acid, which is associated with ulcer formation. This additional surgery is commonly a **vagotomy,** surgery on the vagus nerve that disables the acid-producing portion of the stomach.

Preparation

Before undergoing gastrectomy, patients may need a variety of tests, such as x rays, **computed tomography scans** (CT scans), ultrasonography, or endoscopic biopsies (microscopic examination of tissue), to assure the diagnosis and localize the tumor or ulcer. **Laparoscopy** may be done to diagnose a malignancy or to determine the extent of a tumor that is already diagnosed. When a tumor is strongly suspected, laparoscopy is often performed immediately before the surgery to remove the tumor; this avoids the need to anesthetize the patient twice and sometimes avoids the need for surgery altogether if the tumor found on laparoscopy is deemed inoperable.

Aftercare

It is important to follow any instructions that have been given for postoperative care. Major surgery usually requires a recuperation time of several weeks.

Risks

Surgery for peptic ulcer is effective, but it may result in a variety of postoperative complications. After gastrectomy, as many as 30% of patients have significant symptoms. An operation called highly selective vagotomy is now preferred for ulcer management, and is safer than gastrectomy.

After a gastrectomy, several abnormalities may develop that produce symptoms related to food intake. This happens largely because the stomach, which serves as a food reservoir, has been reduced in its capacity by the surgery. Other surgical procedures that often accompany gastrectomy for ulcer disease can also contribute to later symptoms: vagotomy, which lessens acid production and slows stomach emptying, and **pyloroplasty,** which enlarges the opening between the stomach and small intestine to facilitate emptying of the stomach.

Some patients experience light-headedness, heart **palpitations** or racing heart, sweating, and **nausea and vomiting** after a meal. These may be symptoms of "dumping syndrome," as food is rapidly "dumped" into the small intestine from the stomach. This is treated by adjusting the diet and pattern of eating, for example, eating smaller, more frequent meals, and limiting liquids.

Patients who have abdominal bloating and pain after eating, frequently followed by nausea and vomiting, may have what is called the afferent loop syndrome. This is treated by surgical correction. Patients who have early satiety (feeling of fullness after eating), abdominal discomfort, and vomiting may have bile reflux **gastritis** (also called bilious vomiting), which is also surgically correctable. Many patients also experience weight loss.

Reactive **hypoglycemia** is a condition that results when blood sugar becomes too high after a meal, stimulating the release of insulin, about two hours after eating. A high-protein diet and smaller meals are advised.

Ulcers recur in a small percentage of patients after surgery for peptic ulcer, usually in the first few years. Further surgery is usually necessary.

Vitamin and mineral supplementation is necessary after gastrectomy to correct certain deficiencies, especially vitamin B_{12}, iron, and folate. Vitamin D and calcium are also needed to prevent and treat the bone problems that often occur. These include softening and bending of the bones, which can produce pain, and **osteoporosis,** a loss of bone mass. According to one study, the risk for spinal **fractures** may be as high as 50% after gastrectomy.

Depending on the extent of surgery, the risk for postoperative **death** after gastrectomy for gastric cancer has been reported as 1–3% and the risk of non-fatal complications as 9–18%.

Normal results

Overall survival after gastrectomy for gastric cancer varies greatly by the stage of disease at the time of surgery. For early gastric cancer, the five-year survival rate is up to 80–90%; for late-stage disease, the prognosis is bad. For gastric adenocarcinomas that are amenable to gastrectomy, the five-year survival rate is 10–30%, depending on the location of the tumor. The prognosis for patients with gastric lymphoma is better, with five-year survival rates reported at 40–60%.

Most studies have shown that patients can have an acceptable quality of life after gastrectomy for a potentially curable gastric cancer. Many patients will maintain a healthy appetite and eat a normal diet. Others may lose weight and not enjoy meals as much. Some studies show that patients who have total gastrectomies have more disease-related or treatment-related symptoms after surgery and poorer physical function than patients who have subtotal gastrectomies. There does not appear to be much difference, however, in emotional status or social activity level between patients who have undergone total versus subtotal gastrectomies.

Resources

BOOKS

"Disorders of the Stomach and Duodenum." In *The Merck Manual*. Whitehouse Station, NJ: Merck & Co., Inc., 1992.

"Stomach and Duodenum: Complications of Surgery for Peptic Ulcer Disease." In *Steisenger & Fordtran's Gastrointestinal and Liver Disease*, edited by Mark Feldman et al. Philadelphia: W.B. Saunders Co., 1998.

OTHER

Mayo Health Oasis. http://www.mayohealth.org/mayo/askdiet/htm/new/qd971203.htm.

Caroline A. Helwick

Gastric acid determination

Definition

Gastric acid determination, also known as stomach acid determination, gastric analysis, or basal gastric secretion, is a procedure to evaluate gastric (stomach) function. The test specifically determines the presence of gastric acid, as well as the amount of gastric acid secreted. It is often done in conjunction with the gastric acid stimulation test, a procedure that measures gastric acid output after injection of a drug to stimulate gastric acid secretion.

KEY TERMS

Achlorhydria—An abnormal condition in which hydrochloric acid is absent from the secretions of the gastric glands in the stomach.

Pernicious anemia—One of the main types of anemia, caused by inadequate absorption of vitamin B_{12}. Symptoms include tingling in the hands, legs, and feet, spastic movements, weight loss, confusion, depression, and decreased intellectual function.

Zollinger-Ellison syndrome—A rare condition characterized by severe and recurrent peptic ulcers in the stomach, duodenum, and upper small intestine, caused by a tumor, or tumors, usually found in the pancreas. The tumor secretes the hormone gastrin, which stimulates the stomach and duodenum to produce large quantities of acid, leading to ulceration. Most often cancerous, the tumor must be removed surgically; otherwise total surgical removal of the stomach is necessary.

Purpose

The purpose of the gastric acid determination is to evaluate gastric function by measuring the amount of acid as suctioned directly from the stomach. The complete gastric acid determination includes the basal gastric secretion test, which measures acid secretion while the patient is in a **fasting** state (nothing to eat or drink), followed by the gastric acid stimulation test, which measures the secretion of gastric acid for one hour after injection of pentagastrin or a similar drug that stimulates gastric acid output. The Gastric acid stimulation test is done when the basal secretion test suggests abnormalities in gastric secretion. It is normally performed immediately afterward.

The basal gastric secretion test is indicated for patients with obscure gastric **pain,** loss of appetite, and weight loss. It is also utilized for suspected peptic (related to the stomach) ulcer, severe stomach inflammation (**gastritis**), and Zollinger-Ellison (Z-E) syndrome (a condition in which a pancreatic tumor, called a gastrinoma, stimulates the stomach to secrete excessive amounts of acid, resulting in peptic ulcers). Because external factors like the sight or odor of food, as well as psychological **stress,** can stimulate gastric secretion, accurate testing requires that the patient be relaxed and isolated from all sources of sensory stimulation. Abnormal basal secretion can suggest various gastric and duodenal disorders, so further evaluation requires the gastric acid stimulation test.

The gastric acid stimulation test is indicated when abnormalities are found during the basal secretion test. These abnormalities can be caused by a number of disorders, including duodenal ulcer, **pernicious anemia,** and gastric **cancer.** The test will detect abnormalities, but x rays and other studies are necessary for a definitive diagnosis.

Precautions

Because both the basal gastric secretion test and the gastric acid stimulation test require insertion of a gastric tube (intubation) through the mouth or nasal passage, neither test is recommended for patients with esophageal problems, **aortic aneurysm,** severe gastric hemorrhage, or congestive **heart failure.** The gastric acid stimulation test is also not recommended in patients who are sensitive to pentagastrin (the drug used to stimulate gastric acid output).

Description

This test, whether performed for basal gastric acid secretion, gastric acid stimulation, or both, requires the passage of a lubricated rubber tube, either by mouth or through the nasal passage, while the patient is in a sitting or reclining position on the left side. The tube is situated in the stomach, with proper positioning confirmed by fluoroscopy or x ray.

Basal gastric acid secretion

After a wait of approximately 10–15 minutes for the patient to adjust to the presence of the tube, and with the patient in a sitting position, specimens are obtained every 15 minutes for a period of 90 minutes. The first two specimens are discarded to eliminate gastric contents that might be affected by the stress of the intubation process. The patient is allowed no liquids during the test, and saliva must be ejected to avoid diluting the stomach contents.

The four specimens collected during the test constitute the *basal acid output.* If analysis suggests abnormally low gastric secretion, the gastric acid stimulation test is performed immediately afterward.

Gastric acid stimulation test

After the basal samples have been collected, the tube remains in place for the gastric acid stimulation test. Pentagastrin, or a similar drug that stimulates gastric acid output, is injected under the skin (subcutaneously). After 15 minutes, a specimen is collected every 15 minutes for one hour. These specimens are called the *poststimulation specimens.* As is the case with the basal gastric secretion test, the patient can have no liquids during this test, and must eject saliva to avoid diluting the stomach contents.

Preparation

The patient should be fasting (nothing to eat or drink after the evening meal) on the day prior to the test, but may have water up to one hour before the test. **Antacids,** anticholinergics, cholinergics, alcohol, H_2-receptor antagonists (Tagamet, Pepcid, Axid, Zantac), reserpine, adrenergic blockers, and adrenocorticosteroids should be withheld for one to three days before the test, as the physician requests. If pentagastrin is to be administered for the gastric acid secretion test, medical supervision should be maintained, as possible side effects may occur.

Aftercare

Complications such as nausea, vomiting, and abdominal distention or pain are possible following removal of the gastric tube. If the patient has a **sore throat,** soothing lozenges may be given. The patient may also resume the usual diet and any medications that were withheld for the test(s).

Risks

There is a slight risk that the gastric tube may be inserted improperly, entering the windpipe (trachea) and not the esophagus. If this happens, the patient may have a difficult time breathing or may experience a coughing spell until the tube is removed and reinserted properly. Also, because the tube can be difficult to swallow, if a patient has an overactive gag reflex, there may be a transient rise in blood pressure due to **anxiety.**

Normal results

Reference values for the *basal gastric secretion test* vary by laboratory, but are usually within the following ranges:

- Men: 1–5 mEq/h
- Women: 0.2–3.8 mEq/h.

Reference values for the *gastric acid stimulation test* vary by laboratory, but are usually within the following ranges:

- Men: 18–28 mEq/h
- Women: 11–21 mEq/h.

Abnormal results

Abnormal findings in the *basal gastric secretion test* are considered nonspecific and must be evaluated in conjunction with the results of a gastric acid stimulation test. Elevated secretion may suggest different types of **ulcers;** when markedly elevated, Zollinger-Ellison syndrome is suspected. Depressed secretion can indicate gastric cancer, while complete absence of secretion (achlorhydria) may suggest pernicious anemia.

Elevated gastric secretion levels in the *gastric acid stimulation test* may be indicative of duodenal ulcer; high levels of secretion again suggest Zollinger-Ellison syndrome.

Resources

BOOKS

Cahill, Mathew. *Handbook of Diagnostic Tests.* Springhouse, PA: Springhouse Corporation, 1995.

Jacobs, David S. *Laboratory Test Handbook,* 4th ed. Hudson, OH: Lexi-Comp Inc., 1996.

Pagana, Kathleen Deska. *Mosby's Manual of Diagnostic and Laboratory Tests.* St. Louis: Mosby, Inc., 1998.

Janis O. Flores

Gastric acid stimulation test *see* **Gastric acid determination**

Gastric carcinoma *see* **Stomach cancer**

. . . .

Gastric emptying scan

Definition

A gastric emptying scan (GES) is an x-ray exam using special radioactive material that allows physicians to identify abnormalities related to emptying of the stomach. Diseases that involve changes in the way the stomach contracts (motility disorders) are best diagnosed by this test.

Purpose

The study is used most frequently to evaluate patients who have symptoms suggestive of decreased, delayed, or rapid gastric emptying, and no visible abnormality to explain their symptoms.

Symptoms pointing to a delay in gastric emptying are non-specific, and may be due to a number of causes, such as **ulcers,** diabetes, tumors, and others. These symptoms include nausea, upper abdominal bloating, and at times vomiting. Another significant symptom is called "early satiety," which means feeling full after eating only a small amount of food. In some patients, weight loss is also present. In addition to symptoms, the finding of a large amount of material in the stomach after an overnight fast suggests abnormal emptying, but does not distinguish between an actual blockage or an irregularity in gastric contractions. It is therefore essential to find out what is causing material to remain in the stomach.

KEY TERMS

Endoscopy—The examination of the inside of an organ with an instrument that has a light at the end of it and an optical system for examination of the organ.

Motility—Motility is spontaneous movement. One example is the automatic stomach contractions that move the food content along from the stomach into the intestines. A motility disease is one that involves changes in the way the stomach contracts.

Since many diseases can produce the above symptoms, structural lesions (such as tumors or regions of narrowing or scar tissue) need to be ruled out first. This is usually done by upper gastrointestinal series test or by endoscopy (examination of the inside of an organ, in this instance the stomach, with an instrument that has a light at the end of it and an optical system for examination of the organ). Once it is clear that a mechanical or physical lesion is not the cause of symptoms, attempts to document an abnormality in the nervous or muscular function of the stomach is then begun. GES is usually the first step in that evaluation.

Precautions

The exam should not be performed on pregnant women, but is otherwise quite safe. Since eggs are usually used to hold the radioactive material, patients should notify their physician if they are allergic to eggs. However, other materials can be used in place of an egg.

Description

Gastric emptying scans have undergone several changes since the initial studies in the late 1970s. During the study, patients are asked to ingest an egg sandwich containing a radioactive substance (for example, technetium) that can be followed by a special camera. The emptying of the material from the stomach is then followed and displayed both in the form of an image, as well as the percentage emptied over several hours (generally two and four hours). Studies are in progress using substances that are not radioactive, but this procedure is not available to the patient as of yet.

Preparation

The only preparation involved is for the patient to fast overnight before the test.

Risks

The radiation exposure during the study is quite small and safe, unless the patient is pregnant.

Normal results

There are several different measurements considered normal, depending on the radioactive material and solid meal used. The value is expressed as a percentage of emptying over a period of time. For a technetium-filled egg sandwich, normal emptying is 78 minutes for half the material to leave the stomach, with a variation of 11 minutes either way.

Abnormal results

GES scan studies that show emptying of the stomach in a longer than accepted period is abnormal. Severity of test results and symptoms do not always match; therefore, the physician must carefully interpret these findings. Diabetic injury to the nerves that supply the stomach (called diabetic gastroparesis) is one of the most common causes of abnormal gastric motility. However, up to 30% of patients have no obvious cause to explain the abnormal results and symptoms. These cases are called idiopathic (of unknown cause). GES is often used to follow the effect of medications used for treatment of motility disorders.

Resources

BOOKS

Camilleri, Michael and Charlene M.Prather. ''Gastric Motor Physiology and Motor Disorders.'' In *Sleisenger & Fordtran's Gastrointestinal and Liver Disease,* edited by Mark Feldman, et al. Philadelphia: W.B. Saunders Company, 1997, pp. 572-586.

Maurer, Alan H., Leon S. Malumd, and Robert S.Fisher. ''Radionuclide Scintigraphy of the Gastrointestinal Tract.'' In *Bockus Gastroenterology,* edited by William S. Haubrich, et al. Philadelphia: W.B. Saunders Company, 1995, pp. 221-238.

PERIODICALS

Quigley, Eamonn M.M. ''Gastric and Small Intestinal Motility in Health and Disease.'' *Gastroenterology Clinics of North America* (March 1996): 113-145.

ORGANIZATIONS

American Pseudo-obstruction and Hirschprung's Disease Society. http://www.tiac.net/users/aphs/.

David S. Kaminstein

Gastric lavage *see* **Stomach flushing**

Gastric stapling *see* **Obesity surgery**

Gastric ulcers *see* **Ulcers**

Gastrinoma

Definition

Gastrinomas are tumors associated with a rare gastroenterological disorder known as Zollinger-Ellison syndrome (ZES). They occur primarily in the pancreas and duodenum (beginning of the small intestine) and secrete large quantities of the hormone gastrin, triggering gastric acid production that produces **ulcers.** They may be malignant (cancerous) or benign.

Description

Gastrinomas are an integral part of the Zollinger-Ellison syndrome (ZES). In fact, ZES is also known as gastrinoma. This syndrome consists of ulcer disease in the upper gastrointestinal tract, marked increases in the secretion of gastric acid in the stomach, and tumors of the islet cells in the pancreas. The tumors produce large amounts of gastrin that are responsible for the characteristics of Zollinger-Ellison syndrome, namely severe ulcer disease. Although usually located within the pancreas, they may occur in other organs.

Gastrinomas may occur randomly and sporadically, or they may be inherited as part of a genetic condition called multiple endocrine neoplasia type 1 (MEN-1) syndrome. About half of persons with MEN-1 have gastrinomas, which tend to be more numerous and smaller than tumors in sporadic cases.

About half of ZES patients have multiple gastrinomas, which can vary in size from 1–20 mm. Gastrinomas found in the pancreas are usually much larger than duodenal gastrinomas. About two thirds of gastrinomas are malignant (cancerous). These usually grow slowly, but some may invade surrounding sites rapidly and metastasize (spread) widely. Sometimes, gastrinomas are found only in the lymph nodes, and it is uncertain whether these malignancies have originated in the lymph nodes or have metastasized from a tumor not visible in the pancreas or duodenum.

There is some evidence that the more malignant form of gastrinomas is more frequent in larger pancreatic tumors, especially in females and in persons with a shorter disease symptom duration and higher serum gastrin levels.

Causes & symptoms

Most persons with gastrinomas secrete profound amounts of gastric acid, and almost all develop ulcers, mostly in the duodenum or stomach. Early in the course of the disease, symptoms are typical of peptic ulcers, however once the disease is established, the ulcers become more persistent and symptomatic, and may respond poorly to standard anti-ulcer therapy. Abdominal **pain** is the predominant symptom of ulcer disease. About 40% of patients have **diarrhea** as well. In some patients, diarrhea is the primary symptom of gastrinoma.

Diagnosis

Persons with gastrinomas have many of the same symptoms as persons with ulcers. Their levels of gastric acid, however, are usually far greater than those in common ulcer disease. Gastrinomas are usually diagnosed by a blood test that measures the level of gastrin in the blood. Patients with gastrinomas often have gastrin levels more than 200 pg/mL, which is 4–10 times higher than normal. Serum gastrin levels as high as 450,000 pg/mL have occurred.

When the serum gastrin test does not show these extremely high levels of gastrin, patients may be given certain foods or injections in an attempt to provoke a response that will help diagnose the condition. The most useful of these provocative tests is the secretin injection test (or secretin stimulation or provocative test), which will almost always produce a positive response in persons with gastrinomas but seldom in persons without them.

Surgically, gastrinomas are often difficult to locate, even with careful inspection. They may be missed in at least 10–20% of patients with ZES. Gastrinomas are sometimes found only because they have metastasized and produced symptoms related to the spread of malignancy. Such metastasis may be the most reliable indication of whether the gastrinoma is malignant or benign.

Diagnostic imaging techniques help locate the gastrinomas. The most sophisticated is an x-ray test called radionuclide octreotide scanning (also known as somatostatin receptor scintigraphy or 111In pentetreotide SPECT). A study by the National Institutes of Health (NIH) found this test to be superior to other imaging methods, such as **computed tomography scan** (CT) or **magnetic resonance imaging** (MRI), in pinpointing the location of tumors and guiding physicians in treatment.

Approximately half of all gastrinomas do not show up on imaging studies. Therefore, exploratory surgery is often recommended to try to locate and remove the tumors.

Treatment

Therapy for gastrinomas should be individualized, since patients tend to have varying degrees of disease and symptoms. Treatment is aimed at eliminating the overproduction of gastric acid and removing the gastrin-producing tumors.

Drugs

Gastrinomas may not be easily treated by the standard anti-ulcer approaches. The medical treatment of choice is with drugs called proton pump inhibitors, such as omeprazole or lansoprazole, daily. These drugs are potent inhibitors of gastric acid. High doses of H-2 receptor antagonists may also reduce gastric acid secretion, improve symptoms, and induce ulcer healing. These drugs must be continued indefinitely, since even a brief discontinuation will cause ulcer recurrence. **Antacids** may provide some relief, but it is usually not longlasting or healing.

Surgery

Because of the likelihood that gastrinomas may be malignant, in both sporadic tumors and those associated with the inherited MEN-1 syndrome, surgery to locate and remove gastrinomas is frequently advised. It is now known that complete surgical removal of gastrinomas can cure the overproduction of gastrin, even in patients who have metastases to the lymph nodes. Surgery in patients with MEN-1 and ZES, however, remains controversial since the benefit is less clear.

Freedom from disease after surgery is judged by improved symptoms, reduced gastric acid production, reduced need for drug therapy, normalization of serum gastrin levels, and normalization of results from the secretin stimulation test and imaging studies.

Prognosis

Medical therapy often controls symptoms, and surgery may or may not cure gastrinoma. About 50% of ZES patients in whom gastrinomas are not removed will die from malignant spread of the tumor. In patients with gastrinomas as part of MEN-1 syndrome, the cure rate is extremely low.

A NIH study of patients who had surgical removal of gastrinomas found that 42% were disease-free one year after surgery and 35% were disease-free at five years. Disease recurrences can often be detected with a serum gastrin test or secretin stimulation test.

When gastrinomas are malignant, they often grow slowly. The principal sites of metastasis are the regional lymph nodes and liver, but they may also spread to other structures. About one quarter of patients with gastrinomas have liver metastases at the time of diagnosis. This appears to be more frequent with pancreatic gastrinomas than duodenal gastrinomas.

Metastases of malignant gastrinomas to the liver is very serious. Survival five years after diagnosis is 20–30%, however patients with gastrinomas found only in the lymph nodes have been known to live as long as 25 years after diagnosis, without evidence of further tumor spread. In fact, the life expectancy of patients with gastrinomas that have spread to the lymph nodes is no different from that of patients with gastrinomas that cannot even be found at surgery for about 90%, five years after diagnosis.

Resources

BOOKS

Friedman, Lawrence S., and Walter L. Peterson. "Peptic Ulcer and Related Diseases." In *Harrison's Principles of Internal Medicine*. Edited by Anthony S. Fauci, et al. New York: McGraw-Hill, 1998.

PERIODICALS

Delcore R., and S.R. Friesen. "The Place for Curative Surgical Procedures in the Treatment of Sporadic and Familial Zollinger-Ellison Syndrome." *Current Opinion in General Surgery* (1994): 69-76.

Meko, J.B., and J.A. Norton. "Management of Patients with Zollinger-Ellison Syndrome." *Annual Review of Medicine* 46 (1995): 395-411.

ORGANIZATIONS

National Digestive Diseases Information Clearinghouse. 2 Information Way, Bethesda, MD 20892-3570. (301) 654-3810. http://www.niddk.nih.gov/health/digest/nddic.htm.

Caroline A. Helwick

Gastritis

Definition

Gastritis commonly refers to inflammation of the lining of the stomach, but the term is often used to cover a variety of symptoms resulting from stomach lining inflammation and symptoms of burning or discomfort. True gastritis comes in several forms and is diagnosed using a combination of tests. In the 1990s, scientists discovered that the main cause of true gastritis is infection from a bacterium called *Helicobacter pylori* (*H. pylori*).

Description

Gastritis should not be confused with common symptoms of upper abdominal discomfort. It has been associated with resulting **ulcers,** particularly peptic ulcers. And in some cases, chronic gastritis can lead to more serious complications.

Nonerosive H. pylori gastritis

The main cause of true gastritis is *H. pylori* infection. *H. pylori* is indicated in an average of 90% of patients with chronic gastritis. This form of nonerosive gastritis is the result of infection with *Helicobacter pylori* bacterium, a microorganism whose outer layer is resistant to the normal effects of stomach acid in breaking down bacteria.

The resistance of *H. pylori* means that the bacterium may rest in the stomach for long periods of times, even years, and eventually cause symptoms of gastritis or ulcers when other factors are introduced, such as the presence of specific genes or ingestion of **nonsteroidal anti-inflammatory drugs** (NSAIDS). Study of the role of *H. pylori* in development of gastritis and peptic ulcers has disproved the former belief that **stress** lead to most stomach and duodenal ulcers and has resulted in improved treatment and reduction of stomach ulcers. *H. pylori* is most likely transmitted between humans, although the specific routes of transmission were still under study in early 1998. Studies were also underway to determine the role of *H. pylori* and resulting chronic gastritis in development of gastric **cancer.**

KEY TERMS

Duodenal—Refers to the duodenum, or the first part of the small intestine.

Gastric—Relating to the stomach.

Mucosa—The mucous membrane, or the thin layer which lines body cavities and passages.

Ulcer—A break in the skin or mucous membrane. It can fester and pus like a sore.

Erosive and hemorrhagic gastritis

After *H. pylori*, the second most common cause of chronic gastritis is use of nonsteroidal anti-inflammatory drugs. These commonly used pain killers, including **aspirin,** fenoprofen, ibuprofen and naproxen, among others, can lead to gastritis and peptic ulcers. Other forms of erosive gastritis are those due to alcohol and corrosive agents or due to trauma such as ingestion of foreign bodies.

Other forms of gastritis

Clinicians differ on the classification of the less common and specific forms of gastritis, particularly since there is so much overlap with *H. pylori* in development of chronic gastritis and complications of gastritis. Other types of gastritis that may be diagnosed include:

- Acute stress gastritis—the most serious form of gastritis which usually occurs in critically ill patients, such as those in intensive care. Stress erosions may develop suddenly as a result of severe trauma or stress to the stomach lining.

- Atrophic gastritis is the result of chronic gastritis which is leading to atrophy, or decrease in size and wasting away, of the gastric lining. Gastric atrophy is the final stage of chronic gastritis and may be a precursor to gastric cancer.

- Superficial gastritis is a term often used to describe the initial stages of chronic gastritis.

- Uncommon specific forms of gastritis include granulomatous, eosiniphilic and lymphocytic gastritis.

Causes & symptoms

Nonerosive H. pylori gastritis

H. pylori gastritis is caused by infection from the *H. pylori* bacterium. It is believed that most infection occurs in childhood. The route of its transmission was still under study in 1998 and clinicians guessed that there may be more than one route for the bacterium. Its prevalence and distribution differs in nations around the world. The presence of *H. pylori* has been detected in 86–99% of patients with chronic superficial gastritis. However, physicians are still learning about the link of *H. pylori* to chronic gastritis and peptic ulcers, since many patients with *H. pylori* infection do not develop symptoms or peptic ulcers. *H. pylori* is also seen in 90–100% of patients with duodenal ulcers.

Symptoms of *H. pylori* gastritis include abdominal **pain** and reduced acid secretion in the stomach. However, the majority of patients with *H. pylori* infection suffer no symptoms, even though the infection may lead to ulcers and resulting symptoms. Ulcer symptoms include dull, gnawing pain, often two to three hours after meals and pain in the middle of the night when the stomach is empty.

Erosive and hemorrhagic gastritis

The most common cause of this form of gastritis is use of NSAIDS. Other causes may be **alcoholism** or stress from surgery or critical illness. The role of NSAIDS in development of gastritis and peptic ulcers depends on the dose level. Although even low doses of aspirin or other nonsteroidal anti-inflammatory drugs may cause some gastric upset, low doses generally will not lead to gastritis. However, as many as 10–30% of patients on higher and more frequent doses of NSAIDS, such as those with chronic arthritis, may develop gastric ulcers. In 1998, studies were underway to understand the role of *H. pylori* in gastritis and ulcers among patients using NSAIDS.

Patients with erosive gastritis may also show no symptoms. When symptoms do occur, they may include **anorexia nervosa,** gastric pain, **nausea and vomiting.**

Other Forms of Gastritis

Less common forms of gastritis may result from a number of generalized diseases or from complications of chronic gastritis. Any number of mechanisms may cause various less common forms of gastritis and they may differ slightly in their symptoms and clinical signs. However, they all have in common inflammation of the gastric mucosa.

Diagnosis

Nonerosive H. pylori gastritis

H. pylori gastritis is easily diagnosed through the use of the urea breath test. This test detects active presence of *H. pylori* infection. Other serological tests, which may be readily available in a physician's office, may be used to detect *H. pylori* infection. Newly developed versions offer rapid diagnosis. The choice of test will depend on cost, availability and the physician's experience, since nearly all of the available tests have an accuracy rate of 90% or better. Endoscopy, or the examination of the stomach area using a hollow tube inserted through the mouth, may be ordered to confirm diagnosis. A biopsy of the gastric lining may also be ordered.

Erosive or hemorrhagic gastritis

Clinical history of the patient may be particularly important in the diagnosis of this type of gastritis, since its cause is most often the result of chronic use of NSAIDS, alcoholism, or other substances.

Other forms of gastritis

Gastritis that has developed to the stage of duodenal or gastric ulcers usually requires endoscopy for diagnosis. It allows the physician to perform a biopsy for possible malignancy and for *H. pylori*. Sometimes, an upper gastrointestinal x-ray study with barium is ordered. Some diseases such as Zollinger-Ellison syndrome, an ulcer disease of the upper gastrointestinal tract, may show large mucosal folds in the stomach and duodenum on radiographs or in endoscopy. Other tests check for changes in gastric function.

Treatment

H. pylori gastritis

The discovery of *H. pylori's* role in development of gastritis and ulcers has led to improved treatment of chronic gastritis. In particular, relapse rates for duodenal and gastric ulcers has been reduced with successful treatment of *H. pylori* infection. Since the infection can be treated with **antibiotics,** the bacterium can be completely eliminated up to 90% of the time.

Although *H. pylori* can be successfully treated, the treatment may be uncomfortable for patients and relies heavily on patient compliance. In 1998, studies were underway to identify the best treatment method based on simplicity, patient cooperation and results. No single antibiotic had been found which would eliminate *H. pylori* on its own, so a combination of antibiotics has been prescribed to treat the infection.

DUAL THERAPY

Dual therapy involves the use of an antibiotic and a proton pump inhibitor. Proton pump inhibitors help reduce stomach acid by halting the mechanism that pumps acid into the stomach. This also helps promote healing of ulcers or inflammation. Dual therapy has not been proven to be as effective as triple therapy, but may be ordered for some patients who can more comfortably handle the use of less drugs and will therefore more likely follow the two-week course of therapy.

TRIPLE THERAPY

As of early 1998, triple therapy was the preferred treatment for patients with *H. pylori* gastritis. It is estimated that triple therapy successfully eliminates 80–95% of *H. pylori* cases. This treatment regimen usually involves a two-week course of three drugs. An antibiotic such as amoxicillin or tetracycline, and another antibiotic such as clarithomycin or metronidazole are used in combination with bismuth subsalicylate, a substance found in the over-the-counter medication, Pepto-Bismol, which helps protect the lining of the stomach from acid. Physicians were experimenting with various combinations of drugs and time of treatment to balance side effects with effectiveness. Side effects of triple therapy are not serious, but may cause enough discomfort that patients are not inclined to follow the treatment.

OTHER TREATMENT THERAPIES

Scientists have experimented with quadruple therapy, which adds an antisecretory drug, or one which suppresses gastric secretion, to the standard triple therapy. One study showed this therapy to be effective with only a week's course of treatment in more than 90% of patients. Short course therapy was attempted with triple therapy involving antibiotics and a proton pump inhibitor and seemed effective in eliminating *H. pylori* in one week for more than 90% of patients. The goal is to develop the most effective therapy combination that can work in one week of treatment or less.

MEASURING H. PYLORI TREATMENT EFFECTIVENESS

In order to ensure that *H. pylori* has been eradicated, physicians will test patients following treatment. The breath test is the preferred method to check for remaining signs of *H. pylori*.

Treatment of erosive gastritis

Since few patients with this form of gastritis show symptoms, treatment may depend on severity of symptoms. When symptoms do occur, patients may be treated with therapy similar to that for *H. pylori*, especially since some studies have demonstrated a link between *H. pylori* and NSAIDS in causing ulcers. Avoidance of NSAIDS will most likely be prescribed.

Other forms of gastritis

Specific treatment will depend on the cause and type of gastritis. These may include prednisone or antibiotics. Critically ill patients at high risk for bleeding may be treated with preventive drugs to reduce risk of acute stress gastritis. If stress gastritis does occur, the patient is treated with constant infusion of a drug to stop bleeding. Sometimes surgery is recommended, but is weighed with the possibility of surgical complications or **death.** Once torrential bleeding occurs in acute stress gastritis, mortality is as high as greater than 60%.

Alternative treatment

Alternative forms of treatment for gastritis and ulcers should be used cautiously and in conjunction with conventional medical care, particularly now that scientists have confirmed the role of *H. pylori* in gastritis and ulcers. Alternative treatments can help address gastritis symptoms with diet and nutritional supplements, herbal medicine and **ayurvedic medicine.** It is believed that zinc, vitamin A and beta-carotene aid in the stomach lining's ability to repair and regenerate itself. Herbs thought to stimulate the immune system and reduce inflammation include echinacea (*Echinacea* spp.) and goldenseal (*Hydrastis canadensis*). Ayurvedic medicine involves **meditation.** There are also certain herbs and nutritional supplements aimed at helping to treat ulcers.

Prognosis

The discovery of *H. pylori* has improved the prognosis for patients with gastritis and ulcers. Since treatment exists to eradicate the infection, recurrence is much less common. As of 1998, the only patients requiring treatment for *H. pylori* were those at high risk because of factors such as NSAIDS use or for those with ulcers and other complicating factors or symptoms. Research will continue into the most effective treatment of *H. pylori*, especially in light of the bacterium's resistance to certain antibiotics. Regular treatment of patients with gastric and duodenal ulcers has been recommended, since H. pylori plays such a consistently high role in development of ulcers. It is believed that *H. pylori* also plays a role in the eventual development of serious gastritis complications and cancer. Detection and treatment of *H. pylori* infection may help reduce occurrence of these diseases. The prognosis for patients with acute stress gastritis is much poorer, with a 60 percent or higher mortality rate among those bleeding heavily.

Prevention

The widespread detection and treatment of *H. pylori* as a preventive measure in gastritis has been discussed but not resolved. Until more is known about the routes through which *H. pylori* is spread, specific prevention recommendations are not available. Erosive gastritis from NSAIDS can be prevented with cessation of use of these drugs. An education campaign was launched in 1998 to educate patients, particularly an aging population of arthritis sufferers, about risk for ulcers from NSAIDS and alternative drugs.

Resources

BOOKS

Burton Goldberg Group. *Alternative Medicine: The Definitive Guide.* Puyallup, WA: Future Medicine Publishing, Inc., 1994.

LaMont, J. Thomas. *Gastrointestinal Infections, Diagnosis and Management.* Marcel Dekker, Inc. 1997.

PERIODICALS

Podolski, J. L. "Recent advances in peptic ulcer disease: H. pylori infection and its treatement." *Gastroenterology Nursing* 19 (4): 128-136.

ORGANIZATIONS

National Digestive Diseases Information Clearinghouse (NDDIC). 2 Information Way, Bethesda, MD 20892-3570. http://www.niddk.nih.gov

OTHER

American College of Gastroenterology. http://www.acg.org.
Health Answers. http://www.healthanswers.com.

Teresa G. Norris

Gastroduodenostomy (Billroth I) *see* **Ulcer surgery**

Gastroenteritis

Definition

Gastroenteritis is a catchall term for infection or irritation of the digestive tract, particularly the stomach and intestine. It is frequently referred to as the stomach or intestinal flu, although the **influenza** virus is not associated with this illness. Major symptoms include **nausea and vomiting, diarrhea,** and abdominal cramps. These symptoms are sometimes also accompanied by **fever** and overall weakness. Gastroenteritis typically lasts about three days. Adults usually recover without problem, but children, the elderly, and anyone with an underlying disease are more vulnerable to complications such as **dehydration.**

Description

Gastroenteritis is an uncomfortable and inconvenient ailment, but it is rarely life-threatening in the United States and other developed nations. However, an estimated 220,000 children younger than age five are hospitalized with gastroenteritis symptoms in the United States annually. Of these children, 300 die as a result of severe diarrhea and dehydration. In developing nations, diarrheal illnesses are a major source of mortality. In 1990,

---

---

approximately three million **deaths** occurred worldwide as a result of diarrheal illness.

The most common cause of gastroenteritis is viral infection. Viruses such as rotavirus, adenovirus, astrovirus, and calicivirus and small round-structured viruses (SRSVs) are found all over the world. Exposure typically occurs through the fecal-oral route, such as by consuming foods contaminated by fecal material related to poor sanitation. However, the infective dose can be very low (approximately 100 virus particles), so other routes of transmission are quite probable.

Typically, children are more vulnerable to rotaviruses, the most significant cause of acute watery diarrhea. Annually, worldwide, rotaviruses are estimated to cause 800,000 deaths in children below age five. For this reason, much research has gone into developing a vaccine to protect children from this virus. Adults can be infected with rotaviruses, but these infections typically have minimal or no symptoms.

Children are also susceptible to adenoviruses and astroviruses, which are minor causes of childhood gastroenteritis. Adults experience illness from astroviruses as well, but the major causes of adult viral gastroenteritis are the caliciviruses and SRSVs. These viruses also cause illness in children. The SRSVs are a type of calicivirus and include the Norwalk, Southhampton, and Lonsdale viruses. These viruses are the most likely to produce vomiting as a major symptom.

Bacterial gastroenteritis is frequently a result of poor sanitation, the lack of safe drinking water, or contaminated food—conditions common in developing nations. Natural or man-made disasters can make underlying problems in sanitation and food safety worse. In developed nations, the modern food production system potentially exposes millions of people to disease-causing bacteria through its intensive production and distribution methods. Common types of bacterial gastroenteritis can be linked to *Salmonella* and *Campylobacter* bacteria; however, *Escherichia coli* 0157 and *Listeria monocytogenes* are creating increased concern in developed nations. **Cholera** and Shigella remain two diseases of great concern in developing countries, and research to develop long-term vaccines against them is underway.

Causes & symptoms

Gastroenteritis arises from ingestion of viruses, certain bacteria, or parasites. Food that has spoiled may also cause illness. Certain medications and excessive alcohol can irritate the digestive tract to the point of inducing gastroenteritis. Regardless of the cause, the symptoms of gastroenteritis include diarrhea, nausea and vomiting, and abdominal **pain** and cramps. Sufferers may also experience bloating, low fever, and overall tiredness. Typically, the symptoms last only two to three days, but some viruses may last up to a week.

A usual bout of gastroenteritis shouldn't require a visit to the doctor. However, medical treatment is essential if symptoms worsen or if there are complications. Infants, young children, the elderly, and persons with underlying disease require special attention in this regard.

The greatest danger presented by gastroenteritis is dehydration. The loss of fluids through diarrhea and vomiting can upset the body's electrolyte balance, leading to potentially life-threatening problems such as heart beat abnormalities (arrhythmia). The risk of dehydration increases as symptoms are prolonged. Dehydration should be suspected if a **dry mouth,** increased or excessive thirst, or scanty urination is experienced.

If symptoms do not resolve within a week, an infection or disorder more serious than gastroenteritis may be involved. Symptoms of great concern include a high fever (102° F [38.9°C] or above), blood or mucus in the diarrhea, blood in the vomit, and severe abdominal pain or swelling. These symptoms require prompt medical attention.

Diagnosis

The symptoms of gastroenteritis are usually enough to identify the illness. Unless there is an outbreak affecting several people or complications are encountered in a particular case, identifying the specific cause of the illness is not a priority. However, if identification of the infectious agent is required, a stool sample will be collected and analyzed for the presence of viruses, disease-causing (pathogenic) bacteria, or parasites.

Treatment

Gastroenteritis is a self-limiting illness which will resolve by itself. However, for comfort and convenience, a person may use over-the-counter medications such as Pepto Bismol to relieve the symptoms. These medications work by altering the ability of the intestine to move or secrete spontaneously, absorbing toxins and water, or altering intestinal microflora. Some over-the-counter medicines use more than one element to treat symptoms.

If over-the-counter medications are ineffective and medical treatment is sought, a doctor may prescribe a more powerful anti-diarrheal drug, such as motofen or lomotil. Should pathogenic bacteria or parasites be identified in the patient's stool sample, medications such as **antibiotics** will be prescribed.

It is important to stay hydrated and nourished during a bout of gastroenteritis. If dehydration is absent, the drinking of generous amounts of nonalcoholic fluids, such as water or juice, is adequate. **Caffeine,** since it increases urine output, should be avoided. The traditional BRAT diet—bananas, rice, applesauce, and toast—is tolerated by the tender gastrointestinal system, but it is not particularly nutritious. Many, but not all, medical researchers recommend a diet that includes complex carbohydrates (e.g., rice, wheat, potatoes, bread, and cereal), lean meats, yogurt, fruit, and vegetables. Milk and other dairy products shouldn't create problems if they are part of the normal diet. Fatty foods or foods with a lot of sugar should be avoided. These recommendations are based on clinical experience and controlled trials, but are not universally accepted.

Minimal to moderate dehydration is treated with oral rehydrating solutions that contain glucose and electrolytes. These solutions are commercially available under names such as Naturalyte, Pedialyte, Infalyte, and Rehydralyte. Oral rehydrating solutions are formulated based on physiological properties. Fluids that are not based on these properties—such as cola, apple juice, broth, and sports beverages—are not recommended to treat dehydration. If vomiting interferes with oral rehydration, small frequent fluid intake may be better tolerated. Should oral rehydration fail or severe dehydration occur, medical treatment in the form of intravenous (IV) therapy is required. IV therapy can be followed with oral rehydration as the patient's condition improves. Once normal hydration is achieved, the patient can return to a regular diet.

Alternative treatment

Symptoms of uncomplicated gastroenteritis can be relieved with adjustments in diet, herbal remedies, and homeopathy. An infusion of meadowsweet (*Filipendula ulmaria*) may be effective in reducing nausea and stomach acidity. Once the worst symptoms are relieved, slippery elm (*Ulmus fulva*) can help calm the digestive tract. Of the homeopathic remedies available, *Arsenicum album*, ipecac, or *Nux vomica* are three said to relieve the symptoms of gastroenteritis.

Probiotics, bacteria that are beneficial to a person's health, are recommended during the recovery phase of gastroenteritis. Specifically, live cultures of *Lactobacillus acidophilus* are said to be effective in soothing the digestive tract and returning the intestinal flora to normal. *L. acidophilus* is found in live-culture yogurt, as well as in capsule or powder form at health food stores. The use of probiotics is found in folk remedies and has some support in the medical literature. Castor oil packs to the abdomen can reduce inflammation and also reduce spasms or discomfort.

Prognosis

Gastroenteritis is usually resolved within two to three days and there are no long-term effects. If dehydration occurs, recovery is extended by a few days.

Prevention

There are few steps that can be taken to avoid gastroenteritis. Ensuring that food is well-cooked and unspoiled can prevent bacterial gastroenteritis, but may not be effective against viral gastroenteritis.

Resources

BOOKS

Midthun, Karen, and Albert Z. Kapikian. "Viral Gastroenteritis." In *Gastrointestinal and Hepatic Infections,* edited by Christina Surawicz and Robert L. Owen. Philadelphia: W.B. Saunders Company, 1995.

PERIODICALS

Farthing, M., et al. "The Management of Infective Gastroenteritis in Adults." *Journal of Infection* 33 (1996): 143.

Gorbach, Sherwood L. "Efficacy of *Lactobacillus* in Treatment of Acute Diarrhea." *Nutrition Today* 31 (6) (December 1996): 195.

Hart, C. Anthony, and Nigel A. Cunliffe. "Viral Gastroenteritis." *Current Opinion in Infectious Diseases* 10 (1997): 408.

Moss, Peter J., and Michael W. McKendrick. "Bacterial Gastroenteritis." *Current Opinion in Infectious Diseases* 10 (1997): 402.

Subcommittee on Acute Gastroenteritis. "Practice Parameter: The Management of Acute Gastroenteritis in Young Children." *Pediatrics* 97 (March 1996): 424.

Julia Barrett

Gastroenterostomy *see* **Ulcer surgery**

Gastroesophageal reflux *see* **Heartburn**

Gastrointestinal bleeding studies *see* **GI bleeding studies**

Gastrointestinal study *see* **Liver nuclear medicine scan**

Gastrojejunostomy (Billroth II) *see* **Ulcer surgery**

Gastrostomy

Definition

Gastrostomy is a surgical procedure for inserting a tube through the abdomen wall and into the stomach. The tube is used for feeding or drainage.

Purpose

Gastrostomy is performed because a patient temporarily or permanently needs to be fed directly through a tube in the stomach. Reasons for feeding by gastrostomy include **birth defects** of the mouth, esophagus, or stomach, and problems sucking or swallowing.

Gastrostomy is also performed to provide drainage for the stomach when it is necessary to bypass a long-standing obstruction of the stomach outlet into the small

---

KEY TERMS

Endoscopy—A procedure in which an instrument containing a camera is inserted into the gastrointestinal tract so that the doctor can visually inspect the gastrointestinal system.

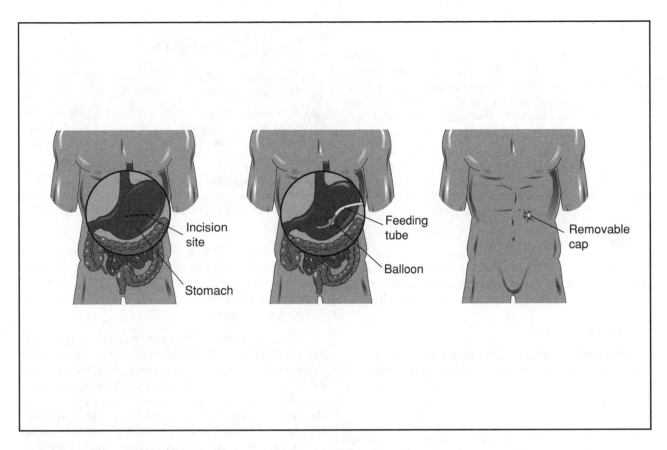

Gastrostomy is a procedure in which the surgeon makes an opening into the stomach and inserts a feeding tube for feeding or for drainage. *(Illustration by Electronic Illustrators Group.)*

intestine. Obstructions may be caused by peptic ulcer scarring or a tumor.

Precautions

Gastrostomy is a relatively simple procedure. As with any surgery, patients are more likely to experience complications if they are smokers, obese, use alcohol heavily, or use illicit drugs. In addition, some prescription medications may increase risks associated with anesthesia.

Description

Gastrostomy, also called gastrostomy tube insertion, is surgery performed by a general surgeon to give an external opening into the stomach. Surgery is performed either when the patient is under general anesthesia—where the patient feels as if he is in a deep sleep and has no awareness of what is happening—or under local anesthesia. With local anesthesia, the patient is awake, but the part of the body cut during the operation is numbed.

A small incision is made on the left side of the abdomen; then, an incision is made through the stomach. A small, flexible, hollow tube, usually made of polyvi-nylchloride or rubber, is inserted into the stomach. The stomach is stitched closed around the tube, and the incision is closed. The procedure is performed at a hospital or free-standing surgery center.

The length of time the patient needs to remain in the hospital depends on the age of the patient and the patient's general health. In some cases, the hospital stay can be as short as one day, but often is longer. Normally, the stomach and abdomen heal in 5–7 days.

The cost of the surgery varies, depending on the age and health of the patient. Younger, sicker patients require more intensive, thus more expensive, care.

Preparation

Prior to the operation, the doctor will perform endoscopy and take x rays of the gastrointestinal tract. Blood and urine tests will also be performed, and the patient may meet with the anesthesiologist to evaluate any special conditions that might affect the administration of anesthesia.

Aftercare

Immediately after the operation, the patient is fed intravenously for at least 24 hours. Once bowel sounds are heard, indicating that the gastrointestinal system is working, the patient can begin clear liquid feedings through the tube. Gradually feedings are increased.

Patient education concerning use and care of the gastrostomy tube is very important. Patients and their families are taught how to recognize and prevent infection around the tube, how to feed through the tube, how to handle tube blockage, what to do if the tube pulls out, and what normal activities can be continued.

Risks

There are few risks associated with this surgery. The main complications are infection, bleeding, dislodgment of the tube, stomach bloating, nausea, and **diarrhea**.

Normal results

The patient is able to eat through the gastrostomy tube, or the stomach can be drained through the tube.

Resources

BOOKS

Griffith, H. Winter. *Complete Guide to Symptoms, Illness, & Surgery.* 3rd edition. New York: The Body Press/Perigee, 1995.

OTHER

Healthanswers. ''Stomach Tube Insertion.'' www.healthanswers.com/database/ami/converted/ 002937.html.

Tish Davidson

. . . .
Gaucher disease

Definition

Gaucher disease is a rare genetic disorder that results in accumulation of fatty molecules called cerebrosides. It can have serious effects on numerous body organs including the liver, spleen, bones, and central nervous system. Treatments based on molecular biology are becoming available, but are very expensive.

Description

Gaucher disease was first described by the French physician Philippe Gaucher in 1882. Gaucher disease is the most common of a class of diseases called lysosomal

---

---

storage diseases, each of which is characterized by the accumulation of a different chemical substance. Gaucher disease is characterized by a wide array of different symptoms and the severity of the disease ranges from undetectable to lethal.

Three forms of the disease are recognized: types I, II, and III. Type I is by far the most common and shows the mildest symptoms. It is non-neuronopathic, meaning that the nervous system is not attacked. The onset of type I can occur at any age in childhood or adult life. Type II, the infantile form, is neuronopathic; nervous system effects are severe, and victims often die within the first year of life. Type III most often has its onset during childhood and has some of the features of both the adult and infantile forms.

The three forms also differ in that type I is most common in persons of eastern European Jewish descent. Among this population, the disease occurs ar a rate of 1 in 450 live births, making it the most common genetic disease affecting Jewish people. The other two types are about equally frequent in all ethnic groups. Type II occurs at a rate of 1 in 100,000 live births, while Type III is estimated to occur in 1 in 50,000 live births.

Causes & symptoms

Gaucher disease is caused by the absence, or near absence, of activity of an enzyme called glucocerebrosidase (GC), also known as acid β-glucosidase. The normal action of GC is to break down a common molecule called glucocerebroside. If not broken down, glucocerebroside accumulates in certain cells to levels that can cause damage, especially in the spleen, liver, and bone. The common link among these organs is that they house a cell type called the macrophage (any large cell that surrounds and consumes a foreign substance, such as bacteria, in the body). The cellular structures in which glucocerebroside accumulates are called lysosomes.

Lack of the enzyme is caused by a mutation in the glucocerebrosidase gene. The gene is autosomal, that is, it is located on a non-sex chromosome. It is recessive, meaning that two defective gene copies must be inherited, one from each parent, for the disease to manifest itself.

The results are widespread in the body and include excessive growth of the liver and spleen (hepatosplenomegaly), weakening of bones, and, in acute cases, severe nervous system damage. Many patients experience "bone crises," which are episodes of extreme **pain** in their bones.

There is a wide array of other problems that occur with Gaucher disease, such as anemia (fewer than normal red blood cells). Just how these other symptoms are caused is not known. Nor is it known why some patients have very mild disease and others have much more significant problems. Even identical twins with the disease can have differing symptoms.

Diagnosis

Diagnosis of Gaucher disease, based initially on the symptoms described above, can be confirmed by microscopic, enzymatic, and molecular tests. When biopsy tissue (tissue removed surgically from a problem area) is examined under the microscope, cells will appear swollen and will show characteristic features of the cytoplasm (part of the cell body along with the nucleus) and nucleus. Enzyme assays will show deficiency of the enzyme, GC. Molecular analysis of DNA samples will show structural defects in the gene for GC. Diagnosis can be performed prenatally (before birth) using **amniocentesis** or **chorionic villus sampling.**

Diagnosis as to which of the three types of Gaucher disease an individual has is based on the symptoms, rather than on test results.

Treatment

Until recently, only supportive therapy could be offered. **Analgesics** are used to control pain. Orthopedic treatment is used for bone **fractures.** In some cases, surgical removal of the spleen may be necessary.

Several treatments for anemia have been used, including vitamin and iron supplements, blood **transfusions,** and bone marrow transplants.

The newest form of treatment for Gaucher disease is enzyme replacement therapy, in which GC can be administered intravenously. The enzyme can be prepared either by purification from placentas (alglucerase) or by recombinant DNA manufacturing techniques (imiglucerase). Either way, the cost of treatment is enormous.

Early results indicate that enzyme replacement is effective at reducing most Gaucher symptoms. The notable exception is neurologic damage in type II disease, which remains unimproved by this treatment.

Many questions remain about enzyme replacement therapy in regard to dosage, method, and frequency of administration. The treatment program may need to be crafted individually for each patient.

Prognosis

A patient's expected lifespan varies greatly with the type of Gaucher disease. Infants with type II disease have a lifespan of about two years. Patients with types I and III disease have highly variable outcomes with some patients dying in childhood and others living full lives. Little is known about the reasons for this variability.

Prevention

No prevention is possible for a genetic condition like Gaucher disease. **Genetic counseling** is advised for individuals with the disease and for those related to a Gaucher patient.

Resources

PERIODICALS

Baranger, John A. et.al. "Enzymatic and molecular diagnosis of Gaucher disease." *Clinics in Laboratory Medicine,* 15 (4)(December 1995): 899-913.

Grabowski, Gregory A. "Current issues in enzyme therapy for Gaucher disease." *Drugs* 52 (2)(August 1996): 159-167.

NIH Technology Assessment Conference. "Gaucher disease: current issues in diagnosis and treatment." *JAMA* 275 (7)(February 12, 1996): 548-553.

ORGANIZATIONS

Alliance of Genetic Support Groups. 4301 Connecticut Ave. NW, Suite 404, Washington, D.C. 20008. (202) 966-5557, (800) 336-4363.

National Gaucher Foundation. 11140 Rockville Pike, Suite 350, Rockville, MD 20852-3106. (800) 925-8885. www.gaucherdisease.org.

National Organization for Rare Disorders. P.O. Box 8923, New Fairfield, CT 06812-1783..

G. Victor Leipzig

Gemfibrozil *see* **Cholesterol-reducing drugs**

Gender identity disorder

Definition

The psychological diagnosis gender identity disorder (GID) is used to describe a male or female that feels a strong identification with the opposite sex and experiences considerable distress because of their actual sex.

Description

Gender identity disorder can affect children, adolescents, and adults. Individuals with gender identity disorder have strong cross-gender identification. They believe that they are, or should be, the opposite sex. They are uncomfortable with their sexual role and organs and may express a desire to alter their bodies. While not all persons with GID are labeled as transsexuals, there are those who are determined to undergo sex change procedures or have done so, and, therefore, are classified as transsexual. They often attempt to pass socially as the opposite sex. Transsexuals alter their physical appearance cosmetically and hormonally, and may eventually undergo a sex-change operation.

Children with gender identity disorder refuse to dress and act in sex-stereotypical ways. It is important to remember that many emotionally healthy children experience fantasies about being a member of the opposite sex. The distinction between these children and gender identity disordered children is that the latter experience significant interference in functioning because of their cross-gender identification. They may become severely depressed, anxious, or socially withdrawn.

Causes & symptoms

The cause of gender identity disorder is not known. It has been theorized that a prenatal hormonal imbalance may predispose individuals to the disorder. Problems in the individual's family interactions or family dynamics have also been postulated as having some causal impact.

The *Diagnostic and Statistical Manual of Mental Disorders*, Fourth Edition (*DSM-IV*), the diagnostic reference standard for United States mental health professionals, describes the criteria for gender identity disorder as an individual's strong and lasting cross-gender identification and their persistent discomfort with their biological gender role. This discomfort must cause a significant amount of distress or impairment in the functioning of the individual.

DSM-IV specifies that children must display at least four of the following symptoms of cross-gender identification for a diagnosis of gender identity disorder:

- A repeatedly stated desire to be, or insistence that he or she is, the opposite sex.
- A preference for cross-dressing.
- A strong and lasting preference to play make-believe and role-playing games as a member of the opposite sex or persistent fantasies that he or she is the opposite sex.
- A strong desire to participate in the stereotypical games of the opposite sex.
- A strong preference for friends and playmates of the opposite sex.

Diagnosis

Gender identity disorder is typically diagnosed by a psychiatrist or psychologist, who conducts an interview with the patient and takes a detailed social history. Family members may also be interviewed during the assessment process. This evaluation usually takes place in an outpatient setting.

Treatment

Treatment for children with gender identity disorder focuses on treating secondary problems such as depression and **anxiety,** and improving self-esteem. Treatment may also work on instilling positive identifications with the child's biological gender. Children typically undergo psychosocial therapy sessions; their parents may also be referred for family or individual therapy.

Transsexual adults often request hormone and surgical treatments to suppress their biological sex characteristics and acquire those of the opposite sex. A team of health professionals, including the treating psychologist or psychiatrist, medical doctors, and several surgical specialists, oversee this transitioning process. Because of the irreversible nature of the surgery, candidates for sex-change surgery are evaluated extensively and are often required to spend a period of time integrating themselves into the cross-gender role before the procedure begins. Counseling and peer support are also invaluable to transsexual individuals.

Prognosis

Long-term follow up studies have shown positive results for many transsexuals who have undergone sex-change surgery. However, significant social, personal, and occupational issues may result from surgical sex changes, and the patient may require psychotherapy or counseling.

Resources

BOOKS

American Psychiatric Association. *Diagnostic and Statistical Manual of Mental Disorders.* 4th ed. Washington, DC: American Psychiatric Press, Inc., 1994.

Israel, Gianna E. and Donald E. Tarver. *Transgender Care: Recommended Guidelines, Practical Information and Personal Accounts.* Philadelphia: Temple University Press, 1997.

Maxmen, Jerrold S., and Nicholas G. Ward. "Sexual and Gender Identity Disorders." In *Essential Psychopathology and Its Treatment,* 2nd ed. New York: W.W. Norton, 1995, pp. 532-38.

PERIODICALS

Dickey, Robert. "Diagnosing and Treating Gender Identity Disorder in Women." *Medscape Mental Health* 2, no. 9 (1997). http://www.medscape.com.

ORGANIZATIONS

American Academy of Child and Adolescent Psychiatry (AACAP). 3615 Wisconsin Ave. NW, Washington, DC 20016. (202) 966-7300. http://www.aacap.org/.

OTHER

The National Transgender Guide. http://www.tgguide.com/.

Paula Anne Ford-Martin

General anesthesia *see* **Anesthesia, general**

Gene therapy

Definition

In its narrowest meaning, gene therapy refers to replacing or fixing a defective gene. In a broader sense, the term is used to denote the use of genes to treat diseases.

KEY TERMS

Achondroplasia—A genetic disorder in which normal growth of cartilage is disturbed, resulting in a form of dwarfism.

Adenosine deaminase deficiency—A deficiency of an important enzyme that helps convert adenosine to inosine.

Deoxyribonucleic acid (DNA)—Often referred to as the "building block of life," DNA is a large, double-helixed molecule that carries genetic information.

Gaucher's disease—A rare metabolic disorder that runs in families and is caused by an enzyme deficiency.

Multifactorial—A condition or disorder resulting from the interaction of several genes, often influenced by environmental factors.

Neurofibromatosis—Also known as von Recklinghausen's disease, this congenital disorder is characterized by tissue and bone deformities, brown spots on the skin, and tumors of the nerves and skin.

Oncogenes—Genes that normally control the growth of cells and may become cancer spreaders when altered by a cancer-causing agent.

Polygenes—A number of genes that interact together to produce a resulting cumulative trait, such as skin color or height.

Tumor suppressor genes—A gene that is able to undo mutations in certain other genes.

Purpose

As of the late 1990s, the field of gene therapy is still considered to be in the experimental stages. There are relatively few cases where gene therapy has been tried on humans, and the vast majority of those have been seriously ill patients. The greatest potential for gene therapy is in the future.

There are at least 4,000 diseases known to be directly caused by a single, faulty gene. These range from **sickle cell anemia** and **cystic fibrosis,** to **achondroplasia** (a disorder in which normal growth of cartilage is disturbed, resulting in a form of dwarfism) and **neurofibromatosis** (a disorder characterized by tissue and bone deformities, brown spots on the skin, and tumors). Correcting illness by substituting a normal gene for an abnormal one is probably the most familiar concept of gene therapy. Yet, in 1995, less than one quarter of all clinical trials involving gene therapy funded by the National Institutes of Health were directed at this type of genetic disease.

Many disorders and conditions are caused by the interaction of several genes. Scientists believe that environmental agents such as viruses or chemicals may act on certain genes to produce these multifactorial diseases. **Diabetes mellitus** and **multiple sclerosis** are two conditions thought to be the result of an interaction between an individual's genes and outside factors. **Cancer** is the most well-known example of this type of illness. A large proportion of the clinical trials using gene therapy involve attempts to stop or at least slow the abnormal growth of cancer cells. This is one of the most promising areas for the use of gene therapy.

A number of ailments are attributed to polygenic causes. This means the interaction of two or more genes is responsible for the disease. Sometimes a whole group of genes may be the culprit, as in **Down syndrome,** where an entire extra chromosome 21 is present in the G group. There is little direct research on correcting the genes responsible for polygenic conditions, however, much has been done regarding detection of and testing for some of these disorders.

As more knowledge is acquired, the role of genes in many human maladies is becoming more apparent. For example, the development of **schizophrenia** and **alcoholism** is now thought to be due, in part, to an inherited predisposition toward these conditions. Direct gene therapy for these types of cases is not at the forefront of research, but may be investigated in the future.

Precautions

There are many valid concerns regarding the potential misuse of gene therapy and related technologies such

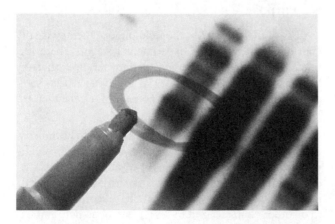

Early detection of cancer. The researcher's pen marks a band on a DNA sequencing autoradiogram confirming a bladder cancer. *(Custom Medical Stock Photo. Reproduced by permission.)*

as **genetic testing.** The potential for discrimination based on genetic makeup is an obvious example. Legislative guarantees regarding confidentiality are one way these issues are being addressed.

Perhaps even more complex issues surrounding gene therapy are not as publicly debated. There is concern among researchers that there is excessive pressure for quick results from genetic treatment. This may be encouraging some investigators to skip over the essentials of basic scientific experimentation. The drive for speed may be further exacerbated by the large numbers of private companies participating in genetic research. They have a primary interest in the business rather than scientific aspects of this field.

As information regarding human genetics grows, other questions will inevitably arise. Where is the line between curing disease and simply enhancing an individual's genetic potential? Should treatments be available to everyone, or just those able to afford them? If genes for intelligence are discovered, should anyone be able to get an ''IQ lift,'' as individuals now are free to enhance their appearance with a face lift? The list is endless and illustrates the issues to be worked out as knowledge increases.

Description

Before discussing the current methods gene therapy employs, a brief review of very basic genetics will be helpful. A gene is the basic unit of heredity. Genes are the biologic substances that cause us to have specific traits, such as blue eyes, brown hair, and AB negative blood. It is most likely that groups of genes, in conjunction with environmental factors like nutrition, are responsible for our height, our skin color, and perhaps our hot temper or keen sense of humor. Genes are made up of segments of a chemical called deoxyribonucleic acid (DNA).

DNA has a unique structure, which allows it to act like a blueprint that instructs the cells to produce specific proteins. These proteins, in turn, direct all of the cell's functions. If the DNA of a particular gene is abnormal, it is as if the blueprint is blurry or unreadable. The protein it is supposed to make may not function properly, or may not be manufactured at all. The abnormal or absent protein then upsets the normal functioning of the cells, which produces the symptoms of disease.

Humans have approximately 100,000 genes. These genes are lined up on structures called chromosomes, somewhat like beads on a string. Every cell in the human body, except red blood cells, contains the same genetic information. But a brain cell will act very differently than a skin cell, because different genes will be used, or ''expressed'' in each.

In principle, gene therapy should be able to insert a normal gene so it can physically replace a flawed one. In practice, scientists are most often working to compensate in some way for the impaired gene. The therapy is more likely to deal with the protein produced by that gene rather than replacing the defective gene with a "normal" version.

The methods being explored to use gene therapy are varied. Approximately half of the experimental therapies involve cancer. Many investigations attempt to stimulate the natural immune system of the body to attack the cancer cells. Others seek to administer a gene which may affect the tumor cell directly. The gene will theoretically cause the tumor itself to secrete a substance which makes the cancer more vulnerable to treatment. In a similar experimental therapy, a gene causes the cancer to make something toxic to itself, virtually a "suicide gene."

Oncogenes are part of the body's normal mechanisms to regulate growth. These genes stimulate the production of proteins which encourage cells to grow. Some cancers are thought to be caused by oncogenes which don't "turn off." Humans also have tumor-suppressor genes. It is thought that these genes don't "turn on" appropriately, allowing cancers to grow unchecked. Manipulating these types of genes is a promising aspect of gene therapy.

Genetic therapies for many other conditions are also being actively investigated. These ailments include acquired immunodeficiency syndrome (**AIDS**), cystic fibrosis, and **muscular dystrophy.** Adenosine deaminase deficiency, the first condition treated with authorized human gene therapy in 1990 continues to be studied, as are several other rare diseases such as **Gaucher disease.**

One of the biggest obstacles to gene therapy is physically placing the therapeutic agent in the right place. Controlling its behavior is another hurdle. The structures involved are smaller than microscopic and not easy to manipulate. Finding an appropriate agent, called a vector, to get the beneficial gene or other material into the target cells at the desired location is a challenge. The body's defense systems cannot distinguish a healing intruder from a harmful one and may attempt to reject the potentially helpful agent. The most common vectors that have been tried are inactivated viruses.

Preparation

Unknown.

Aftercare

Unknown.

Risks

The risks of gene therapy are largely unknown. Some agents have produced undesired inflammatory or immune responses in patients during experimental trials.

Normal results

Successful gene therapy would cure the disease being treated.

Resources

BOOKS

Clark, William. *The New Healers.* New York: Oxford University Press, 1997.

Lyon, Jeff and Peter Gorner. *Altered Fates.* New York: W.W. Norton & Co., 1995.

PERIODICALS

Blaese, R. Michael. "Gene Therapy for Cancer." *Scientific American* (June 1997): 111-115.

Friedmann, Theodore. "Overcoming the Obstacles to Gene Therapy." *Scientific American* (June, 1997): 96-101.

Grace, Eric S. "Better Health Through Gene Therapy." *The Futurist* 32 (Jan.-Feb. 1998): 39-42.

Haseltine, William A. "Discovering Genes for New Medicines." *Scientific American* (March 1997): 92-97.

ORGANIZATIONS

Alliance of Genetic Support Groups. 4301 Connecticut Ave., NW, Suite 404, Washington, DC 20008-2304. (800) 336-GENE (4363). http://medhelp.org/www/agsg.html.

American Cancer Society. 1599 Clifton Rd., NE, Atlanta, GA 30329-4251. (800) 227-2345. http://www.cancer.org.

Office of Rare Diseases (ORD) at National Institutes of Health, Bldg. 31,1BO3, Bethesda, MD 20892-2082, (301) 402-4336. http://rarediseases.info.nih.gov/ord.

Ellen S. Weber

General surgery

Definition

General surgery is the treatment of injury, deformity, and disease using operative procedures.

Purpose

General surgery is frequently performed to alleviate suffering when a cure is unlikely through medication alone. It can be used for routine procedures performed in a physician's office, such as vasectomy, or for more complicated operations requiring a medical team in a hospital setting, such as laparoscopic cholecystectomy (removal of the gallbladder). Areas of the body treated by general surgery include the stomach, liver, intestines, appendix, breasts, thyroid gland, salivary glands, some arteries and veins, and the skin. The brain, heart, eyes,

KEY TERMS

Appendectomy—Removal of the appendix.

Endoscope—Instrument for examining visually the inside of a body canal or a hollow organ such as the stomach, colon, or bladder.

Hysterectomy—Surgical removal of part or all of the uterus.

Laparoscopic cholecystectomy—Removal of the gallbladder using a laparoscope, a fiberoptical instrument inserted through the abdomen.

Microsurgery—Surgery on small body structures or cells performed with the aid of a microscope and other specialized instruments.

Portal—An entrance or a means of entrance.

and feet, to name only a few, are areas that require specialized surgical repair.

New methods and techniques are less invasive than previous practices, permitting procedures that were considered impossible in the past. For example, microsurgery has been used in reattaching severed body parts by successfully reconnecting small blood vessels and nerves.

NUMBER OF INPATIENT SURGERIES PERFORMED ANNUALLY IN THE U.S. (1995)	
Obstetrical Procedures	6.4 million
Digestive System	5.1 million
Cardiovascular System	4.84 million
Musculoskeletal System	3.1 million
Integumentary System	1.3 million
Urinary System	1.1 million
Respiratory System	1,041,000
Nervous System	954,000
Hemic/Lymphatic System	363,000
Nose, Mouth, Pharynx	353,000
Eye	269,000
Endocrine System	85,000
Ear	68,000

Source: "Statistical Rolodex: Inpatient Surgery." NCHS Fastats. Http://www.cdc.gov/nchswww/fastats/insurg.htm

Precautions

Patients who are obese, smoke, have bleeding tendencies, or are over 60, need to follow special precautions, as do patients who have recently experienced an illness such as **pneumonia** or a **heart attack.** Patients on medications such as heart and blood pressure medicine, blood thinners, **muscle relaxants,** tranquilizers, insulin, or sedatives, may require special lab tests prior to surgery and special monitoring during surgery. Special precautions may be necessary for patients using mind-altering drugs such as narcotics, psychedelics, hallucinogens, marijuana, sedatives, or cocaine since these drugs may interact with the anesthetic agents used during surgery.

Description

In earlier times, surgery was a dangerous and dirty practice. Until the middle of the 19th century, as many patients died of surgery as were cured. With the discovery and development of general anesthesia in the mid-1800s, surgery became more humane. And as knowledge about infections grew, surgery became more successful as sterile practices were introduced into the operating room. The last 50 years of the 20th century have seen continued advancements.

Types of General Surgery

General surgery experienced major advances with the introduction of the endoscope. This is an instrument for visualizing the interior of a body canal or a hollow organ. Endoscopic surgery relies on this pencil-thin instrument, capable of its own lighting system and small video camera. The endoscope is inserted through tiny incisions called portals. While viewing the procedure on a video screen, the surgeon then operates with various other small, precise instruments inserted through one or more of the portals. The specific area of the body treated determines the type of endoscopic surgery performed. For example, **colonoscopy** uses an endoscope, which can be equipped with a device for obtaining tissue samples for visual examination of the colon. Gastroscopy uses an endoscope inserted through the mouth to examine the interior of the stomach. **Arthroscopy** refers to joint surgery, and abdominal procedures are called laparoscopies.

Endoscopy is used in both treatment and diagnosis especially involving the digestive and female reproductive systems. Endoscopy has advantages over many other surgical procedures, resulting in a quicker recovery and shorter hospital stay. This non-invasive technique is being used for appendectomies, gallbladder surgery, hysterectomies and the repair of shoulder and knee ligaments. However, endoscopy does not come without limitations such as complications and high operating expense. Also, endoscopy doesn't offer advantages over conventional surgery in all procedures. Some literature states that as general surgeons become more experienced in their prospective fields, additional non-invasive surgery will be a more common option to patients.

ONE-DAY SURGERY

One-day surgery is also termed same-day, or outpatient surgery. Surgical procedures usually take two hours or less and involve minimal blood loss and a short recovery time. In the majority of surgical cases, oral medications control postoperative **pain.** Cataract removal, **laparoscopy,** tonsillectomy, repair of broken bones, **hernia repair,** and a wide range of cosmetic procedures are common same-day surgical procedures. Many individuals prefer the convenience and atmosphere of one-day surgery centers, as there is less competition for attention with more serious surgical cases. These centers are accredited by the Joint Commission on Accreditation of Healthcare Organizations or the Accreditation Association for Ambulatory Health Care.

Preparation

The preparation of patients has advanced significantly with improved diagnostic techniques and procedures. Before surgery the patient may be asked to undergo a series of tests including blood and urine studies, x rays and specific heart studies if the patient's past medical history and/or physical exam warrants this testing. Before any general surgery the physician will explain the nature of the surgery needed, the reason for the procedure, and the anticipated outcome. The risks involved will be discussed along with the types of anesthesia utilized. The expected length of recovery and limitations imposed during the recovery period are also explained in detail before any general surgical procedure.

Surgical procedures most often require some type of anesthetic. Some procedures require only local anesthesia, produced by injecting the anesthetic agent into the skin near the site of the operation. The patient remains awake with this form of medication. Injecting anesthetic agents into a primary nerve located near the surgical site produces block anesthesia (also known as regional anesthesia), which is a more extensive local anesthesia. The patient remains conscious, but is usually sedated. General anesthesia involves injecting anesthetic agents into the blood stream and/or inhaling medicines through a mask placed over the patient's face. During general anesthesia, the patient is asleep and an airway tube is usually placed into the windpipe to help keep the airway open.

As part of the preoperative preparation, the patient will receive printed educational material and may be asked to review audio or videotapes. The patient will be instructed to shower or bathe the evening before or morning of surgery and may be asked to scrub the operative site with a special antibacterial soap. Instructions will also be given to the patient to ingest nothing by mouth for a determined period of time prior to the surgical procedure.

Aftercare

After surgery, blood studies and a laboratory examination of removed fluid or tissue are often performed especially in the case of **cancer** surgery. After the operation, the patient is brought to a recovery room and vital signs, fluid status, dressings and surgical drains are monitored. Pain medications are offered and used as necessary. Breathing exercises are encouraged to maximize respiratory function and leg exercises are encouraged to promote adequate circulation and prevent pooling of blood in the lower extremities. Patients must have a responsible adult accompany them home if leaving the same day as the surgery was performed.

Risks

One of the risks involved with general surgery is the potential for postoperative complications. These complications include—but are not limited to—pneumonia, internal bleeding, and wound infection as well as adverse reactions to anesthesia.

Normal results

Advances in diagnostic and surgical techniques have increased the success rate of general surgery by many times compared to the past. Today's less invasive surgical procedures have reduced the length of hospital stays, shortened recovery time, decreased postoperative pain and decreased the size of surgical incision. On the average, a conventional abdominal surgery requires a three to six-day hospital stay and three to six-week recovery time.

Abnormal results

Abnormal results from general surgery include persistent pain, swelling, redness, drainage or bleeding in the surgical area and surgical wound infection resulting in slow healing.

Resources

BOOKS

Dawson, Dawn P., et al., eds. *Magill's Medical Guide: Health and Illness Supplement.* Pasadena, CA: Salem Press, Inc., 1996.

Larson, David E., ed. *Mayo Clinic Family Health Book,* 2nd edition. New York: William Morrow, 1996.

ORGANIZATIONS

American Medical Association. Washington office: 1101 Vermont Avenue NW Washington, D.C. 20005. 202-789-7400.

OTHER

1997 thrive@ the healthy living experience. General surgery. http://www.thriveonline.com (5/27/98).

Jeffrey Peter Larson

Generalized anxiety disorder

Definition

Generalized anxiety disorder is a condition characterized by "free floating" **anxiety** or apprehension not linked to a specific cause or situation.

Description

Some degree of fear and anxiety is perfectly normal. In the face of real danger, fear makes people more alert and also prepares the body to fight or flee (the so-called "fight or flight" response). When people are afraid, their hearts beat faster and they breathe faster in anticipation of the physical activity that will be required of them. However, sometimes people can become anxious even when there is no identifiable cause, and this anxiety can become overwhelming and very unpleasant, interfering with their daily lives. People with debilitating anxiety are said to be suffering from **anxiety disorders,** such as **phobias, panic disorders,** and generalized anxiety disorder. The person with generalized anxiety disorder generally has chronic (officially, having more days with anxiety than not for at least six months), recurrent episodes of anxiety that can last days, weeks, or even months.

Causes & symptoms

Generalized anxiety disorder afflicts between 2–3% of the general population, and is slightly more common in women than in men. It accounts for almost one-third of cases referred to psychiatrists by general practitioners.

Generalized anxiety disorder may result from a combination of causes. Some people are genetically predisposed to developing it. Psychological traumas that occur during childhood, such as prolonged separation from parents, may make people more vulnerable as well. Stressful life events, such as a move, a major job change, the loss of a loved one, or a divorce, can trigger or contribute to the anxiety.

Psychologically, the person with generalized anxiety disorder may develop a sense of dread for no apparent reason—the irrational feeling that some nameless catastrophe is about to happen. Physical symptoms similar to those found with panic disorder may be present, although

---

not as severe. They may include trembling, sweating, heart **palpitations** (the feeling of the heart pounding in the chest), nausea, and "butterflies in the stomach."

According to the *Diagnostic and Statistical Manual of Mental Disorders,* 4th edition, a person must have at least three of the following symptoms, with some being present more days than not for at least six months, in order to be diagnosed with generalized anxiety disorder:

* Restlessness or feeling on edge
* Being easily fatigued
* Difficulty concentrating
* Irritability
* Muscle tension
* Sleep disturbance.

While generalized anxiety disorder is not completely debilitating, it can compromise a person's effectiveness and quality of life.

Diagnosis

Anyone with chronic anxiety for no apparent reason should see a physician. The physician may diagnose the condition based on the patient's description of the physical and emotional symptoms. The doctor will also try to rule out other medical conditions that may be causing the symptoms, such as excessive **caffeine** use, thyroid disease, **hypoglycemia,** cardiac problems, or drug or alcohol withdrawal. Psychological conditions, such as depressive disorder with anxiety, will also need to be ruled out.

Since generalized anxiety disorder often co-occurs with **mood disorders** and substance abuse, the clinician may have to treat these conditions as well, and therefore must consider them in making the diagnosis.

Treatment

Over the short term, a group of tranquilizers called **benzodiazepines,** such as clonazepam (Klonipin) may help ease the symptoms of generalized anxiety disorder. Sometimes **antidepressant drugs,** such as amitryptiline (Elavil), or **selective serotonin reuptake inhibitors** (SSRIs), such as fluoxetine (Prozac) or sertraline (Zoloft), are also used.

Psychotherapy can be effective in treating generalized anxiety disorder. The therapy may take many forms. In some cases, psychodynamically-oriented psychotherapy can help patients work through this anxiety and solve problems in their lives. Cognitive behavioral therapy aims to reshape the way people perceive and react to potential stressors in their lives. Relaxation techniques have also been used in treatment, as well as in prevention efforts.

Prognosis

When properly treated, most patients with generalized anxiety disorder experience improvement in their symptoms.

Prevention

While preventive measures have not been established, a number of techniques may help manage anxiety, such as relaxation techniques, breathing **exercises,** and distraction—putting the anxiety out of one's mind by focusing thoughts on something else.

Resources

BOOKS

Diagnostic and Statistical Manual of Mental Disorders, 4th edition. Washington, D.C.: American Psychiatric Association, 1994.

Hallowell, Edward M. *Worry: Controlling It and Using It Wisely.* New York: Pantheon Books, 1997.

PERIODICALS

Hale, Anthony S. "ABC of Mental Health." *British Medical Journal* 314 (June 28, 1997): 1886-89.

ORGANIZATIONS

American Psychiatric Association, 1400 K Street NW, Washington DC 20005. (202) 682-6000. http://www.psych.org.

Anxiety Disorders Association of America, 11900 Park Lawn Drive, Ste. 100, Rockville, MD 20852. (301) 231-9350. (800) 545-7367. http://www.adaa.org.

National Institute of Mental Health. Mental Health Public Inquiries, 5600 Fishers Lane, Room 15C-05, Rockville, MD 20857. (301) 443-4513. (888) 826-9438. http://www.nimh.nih.gov/anxiety/index.htm.

Robert Scott Dinsmoor

Genetic counseling

Definition

Genetic counseling aims to facilitate the exchange of information regarding a person's genetic legacy. It attempts to:

- Accurately diagnose a disorder

- Assess the risk of recurrence in the concerned family members and their relatives

- Provide alternatives for decision-making

- Provide support groups that will help family members cope with the recurrence of a disorder.

Purpose

Genetic counselors work with people concerned about the risk of an inherited disease. The counselor does not prevent the incidence of a disease in a family, but can help family members assess the risk for certain hereditary diseases and offer guidance. Many couples seek genetic counseling because there is a family history of known genetic disorders, **infertility, miscarriage,** still births, or early infant mortality. Other reasons for participating in genetic counseling may be the influences of a job or lifestyle that exposes a potential parent to health risks such as radiation, chemicals, or drugs. Any family history of **mental retardation** can be of concern as is a strong

---

KEY TERMS

Sickle-cell anemia—A chronic, inherited blood disorder characterized by crescent-shaped red blood cells. It occurs primarily in people of African descent, and produces symptoms including episodic pain in the joints, fever, leg ulcers, and jaundice.

Tay-Sachs disease—A hereditary disease affecting young children of eastern European Jewish descent. This disease is caused by an enzyme deficiency leading to the accumulation of gangliosides (galactose-containing cerebrosides) found in the surface membranes of nerve cells in the brain and nerve tissue. This deficiency results in mental retardation, convulsions, blindness, and, finally, death.

Thalassemia—An inherited group of anemias occurring primarily among people of Mediterranean descent. It is caused by defective formation of part of the hemoglobin molecule.

family history of heart disease at an early age. Recent statistics show a 3% chance of delivering a baby with **birth defects.** An additional 2% chance of having a baby with **Down syndrome** is present for women in their late thirties and older.

Precautions

Amniocentesis, one of the specific tests used to gather information for genetic counseling, is best performed between weeks 15 and 17 of a **pregnancy** and an additional one to four weeks may be required to culture skin cells and analyze them. Thus, these test data are not available to assist prospective parents in decision-making until the second trimester of the pregnancy. Individuals who participate in genetic counseling and associated testing also must be aware that there are no cures or treatments for some of the disorders that may be identified.

Description

With approximately 2,000 genes identified and approximately 5,000 disorders caused by genetic defects, genetic counseling is important in the medical discipline of obstetrics. Genetic counselors, educated in the medical and the psychosocial aspects of genetic diseases, convey complex information to help people make life decisions. There are limitations to the power of genetic counseling, though, since many of the diseases that have been shown to have a genetic basis currently offer no cure (for example, Down syndrome or **Huntington's disease**). Although a genetic counselor cannot predict the future unequivocally, he or she can discuss the occurrence of a disease in terms of probability.

A genetic counselor, with the aid of the patient or family, creates a detailed family pedigree that includes the incidence of disease in first-degree (parents, siblings, and children) and second-degree (aunts, uncles, and grandparents) relatives. Before or after this pedigree is completed, certain genetic tests are performed using DNA analysis, x ray, ultrasound, urine analysis, **skin biopsy,** and physical evaluation. For a pregnant woman, prenatal diagnosis can be made using amniocentesis or **chorionic villus sampling.**

Family pedigree

An important aspect of the genetic counseling session is the compilation of a family pedigree or medical history. To accurately assess the risk of inherited diseases, information on three generations, including health status and/or cause of **death,** is usually needed. If the family history is complicated information from more distant relatives may be helpful, and medical records may be requested for any family members who have had a genetic disorder. Through an examination of the family history a counselor may be able to discuss the probability

of future occurrence of genetic disorders. In all cases, the counselor provides information in a non-directive way that leaves the decision-making up to the client.

Screening tests

Screening blood tests help identify individuals who carry genes for recessive genetic disorders. Screening tests are usually only done if:

• The disease is lethal or causes severe handicaps or disabilities

• The person is likely to be a carrier due to family pedigree or membership in an at-risk ethnic, geographic or racial group

• The disorder can be treated or reproductive options exist

• A reliable test is available.

Genetic disorders such as **Tay-Sachs disease,** sickle-cell anemia, and **thalassemia** meet these criteria, and screening tests are commonly done to identify carriers of these diseases. In addition, screening tests may be done for individuals with family histories of Huntington's disease (a degenerative neurological disease) or **hemophilia** (a bleeding disorder). Such screening tests can eliminate the need for more invasive tests during a pregnancy.

Another screening test commonly used in the United States in the alpha-fetoprotein (AFP) test. This test is done on a sample of maternal blood around week 16 of a pregnancy. An elevation in the serum AFP level indicates that the fetus may have certain birth defects such as neural tube defects (including **spina bifida** and anencephaly). If the test yields an elevated result, it may be run again after seven days. If the level is still elevated after repeat testing, additional diagnostic tests (e.g. ultrasound and/or amniocentesis) are done in an attempt to identify the specific birth defect present.

Ultrasound

Ultrasound is a noninvasive procedure which uses sound waves to produce a reflected image of the fetus upon a screen. It is used to determine the age and position of the fetus, and the location of the placenta. Ultrasound is also useful in detecting visible birth defects such as spina bifida (a defect in the development of the vertebrae of the spinal column and/or the spinal cord). It is also useful for detecting heart defects, and malformations of the head, face, body, and limbs. This procedure, however, cannot detect biochemical or chromosomal alterations in the fetus.

Amniocentesis

Amniocentesis is useful in determining genetic and developmental disorders not detectable by ultrasound. This procedure involves the insertion of a needle through the abdomen and into the uterus of a pregnant woman. A sample of amniotic fluid is withdrawn containing skin cells that have been shed by the fetus. The sample is sent to a laboratory where fetal cells contained in the fluid are isolated and grown in order to provide enough genetic material for testing. This takes about 7–14 days. The material is then extracted and treated so that visual examination for defects can be made. For some disorders, like Tay-Sachs disease, the simple presence of a telltale chemical compound in the amniotic fluid is enough to confirm a diagnosis.

Chorionic villus sampling

Chorionic villus sampling involves the removal of a small amount of tissue directly from the chorionic villi (minute vascular projections of the fetal chorion that combine with maternal uterine tissue to form the placenta). In the laboratory, the chromosomes of the fetal cells are analyzed for number and type. Extra chromosomes, such as are present in Down syndrome, can be identified. Additional laboratory tests can be performed to look for specific disorders and the results are usually available within a week after the sample is taken. The primary benefit of this procedure is that it is usually performed between weeks 10 and 12 of a pregnancy, allowing earlier detection of fetal disorders.

Preparation

Genetic diagnosis requires that a couple share information about inherited disorders in their background with the genetic counselor, including details of any genetic diseases in either family. A couple undergoing genetic counseling also reports any past miscarriages and discusses the possibility of exposure to chemicals, radiation (including x rays), or other occupational environmental hazards. The couple also needs to disclose information about personal habits before or during pregnancy such as drug or alcohol abuse and the use of prescription or over-the-counter drugs taken by the mother since the beginning of pregnancy. The genetic counselor explains the procedures used in any testing that will be done and describes what each test can and cannot reveal.

Aftercare

Genetic counseling provides couples with information that can help them make decisions about future pregnancies. It also gives couples additional time to emotionally prepare if a disorder is detected in the fetus. The counselor discusses the results of any testing and informs the couple if a problem is apparent. The doctor or genetic counselor also discusses the treatment options available. Genetic counseling is done in a non-directive way, so that any treatment selected remains the personal choice of the individuals involved. Genetic counseling can provide information essential for family planning and pregnancy management, thus maximizing the chances of a positive outcome.

Risks

Because prenatal testing, such as amniocentesis and chorionic villus sampling, is invasive and carries a 1% risk of miscarriage it should never be considered routine.

Normal results

Screening tests and/or prenatal tests reveal no birth defects or genetic abnormalities.

Abnormal results

A birth defect or genetic disorder is detected. The early diagnosis of birth defects and genetic disorders allows a greater number of treatment options. Some disorders can be treated in utero (before birth while the fetus is still in the uterus), while others may require early delivery, immediate surgery, or **cesarean section** to minimize fetal trauma. Prior warning of fetal difficulties allows parents time to prepare emotionally for the birth of the child. In some instances, termination of the pregnancy may be chosen. Whatever the test results, this information is essential for family planning and pregnancy management.

Resources

BOOKS

Banasik, Jacquelyn L. "Genetic and Developmental Disorders." In *Perspectives on Pathophysiology,* by Lee-Ellen C. Copstead. Philadelphia: W.B. Saunders, 1994.

Milunsky, Aubrey. *Choices Not Chances: An Essential Guide to Your Heredity and Health.* Boston: Little Brown, 1989.

Pierce, Benjamin A. *The Family Genetic Sourcebook.* New York: John Wiley & Sons, 1990.

ORGANIZATIONS

American Medical Association. Washington Office: 1101 Vermont Avenue, NW, Washington, DC 20005. (202) 789-7400.

American Society of Human Genetics. 9650 Rockville Pike, Bethesda, MD 20814-3998. (301) 571-1825.

March of Dimes Birth Defects Foundation. National Office: 1275 Mamaroneck Avenue, White Plains, NY 10605. (914) 428-7100.

OTHER

"Genetic Screening Before or During Pregnancy." http:// www.intelihealth.com (June 19, 1998).

Jeffrey Peter Larson

Genetic studies *see* **Genetic testing**

Genetic testing

Definition

Genetic testing examines the genetic information contained inside a person's cells to determine if that person has or will develop a certain disease or could pass a disease to his or her offspring.

Purpose

Some families or ethnic groups have a higher incidence of a certain disease than does the population as a whole. Before having a child, a couple from such a family or ethnic group may want to know if their child would be at risk of having that disease.

Early in **pregnancy,** the baby's cells can be studied for certain defects that could result in physical abnormalities or **mental retardation.** This testing is most common when the mother is over the age of 35 or there is a family history of physical or mental abnormalities.

A genetic disease may be apparent when the child is born or may appear later as the child develops. Genetic testing can help diagnose these diseases. Couples who are having difficulty conceiving a child or who have suffered multiple **miscarriages** may be tested to see if a genetic cause can be identified.

Huntington's disease is an example of a genetic disease that doesn't appear until adulthood. If this disease or another late-onset disease is in a person's family, genetic testing may be able to predict if that person will develop the disease.

Some genetic defects may make a person more susceptible to certain types of **cancer.** Testing for these defects can help predict a person's risk. Other types of genetic tests help diagnose and predict and monitor the course of certain kinds of cancer, particularly leukemia and lymphoma.

Precautions

A person usually meets with a genetic counselor, a person with a master's degree in **genetic counseling** or a

---

KEY TERMS

Autosomal disease—A disease caused by a gene located on chromosomes 1–22.

Carrier—A person who has a disease-causing gene.

Chromosome—The structures made up of DNA, on which are located the genes.

DNA (Deoxyribonucleic acid)—A long molecule made up of two strands of material coiled around each other in unique double helix. DNA contains the blueprint for a person's traits.

Dominant gene—A gene, whose presence as a single copy, controls the expression of a trait.

Gene—A grouping of base pairs that give instruction for a specific trait.

Karyotype—Visual comparison of chromosomes arranged side-by-side with their partner in ascending numerical order, from largest to smallest.

Mutation—Any change in the sequence of DNA.

Positive predictive value (PPV)—The probability that a person with a positive test result has, or will get, the disease.

Recessive gene—A gene that must be present in both copies of the gene pair to control the expression of a trait.

Sensitivity—The likelihood that a negative test means the person will not have the disease or a mutation.

Sex-linked disorder—A disorder caused by a gene located on a sex chromosome, usually the X chromosome.

---

physician specializing and board certified in genetics (a medical geneticist), before most genetic tests.

The counselor should review the person's family history and medical records and the reason for the test. The counselor should explain the likelihood that the test will detect all possible causes of the disease in question (known as the sensitivity of the test), and the likelihood that the disease will develop if the test is positive (known as the positive predictive value of the test).

Learning about the disease in question, the benefits and risks of both a positive and a negative result, and what treatment choices are available if the result is positive, will help prepare the person undergoing testing. The counselor should make sure the person understands how the test results will affect his or her life, family, and future decisions.

After this discussion, the person should have the opportunity to indicate in writing that he or she gave informed consent to the test, verifying that the counselor provided complete and understandable test information.

Description

Genes and chromosomes

Deoxyribonucleic acid (DNA) is a long molecule made up of two strands of material coiled around each other in a unique double helix structure. This structure was discovered in 1953 by Francis Crick and James Watson.

DNA is found in the nucleus, or center, of most cells (Some cells, such as a red blood cell, don't have a nucleus). Each person's DNA is a unique blueprint, giving instructions for a person's physical traits, such as eye color, hair texture, height, and susceptibility to disease. DNA is organized into structures called chromosomes.

The instructions are contained in DNA's long strands as a code spelled out by pairs of bases, which are four chemicals that make up DNA. The bases occur as pairs because a base on one strand lines up with and is bound to a corresponding base on the other strand. The order of these bases form DNA's code. In each cell, there are 3 billion base pairs.

A grouping of base pairs that give instruction for a specific trait is called a gene. Each gene has an assigned place on a specific chromosome. Each normal cell has 46 chromosomes arranged into 23 pairs. Each parent contributes one chromosome to each pair. The first 22 pairs, called autosomal chromosomes, are assigned a number from 1–22. The last pair are the sex chromosomes and include the X and the Y chromosomes. If a child receives an X chromosome from each parent, the child is female.

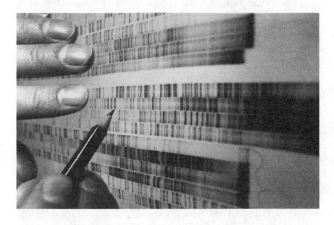

A scientist examines a DNA sequencing autoradiogram on a light box. *(Photo Researchers, Inc. Reproduced by permission.)*

If a child receives an X from the mother, and a Y from the father, the child is male.

Just as each parent contributes one chromosome to each pair, so each parent contributes one gene to each pair. The pair of genes produces a specific trait in the child. Usually one gene has a stronger influence on the trait than the other gene. The stronger gene is called dominant; the weaker gene, recessive. Two copies of a recessive gene are needed to control a trait while only one copy of a dominant gene is needed.

Types of tests

Genetic disease results from a change, or mutation, in a chromosome or in one or several base pairs in a gene. Several types of genetic tests are available to look for the mutations in genes and chromosomes associated with certain diseases. The cost of genetic tests vary: chromosome studies can cost hundreds of dollars and certain gene studies, thousands. Insurance coverage also varies with the company and the policy. It may take several days or weeks to complete a test.

DIRECT DNA MUTATION ANALYSIS

Direct DNA mutation analysis examines DNA for specific gene mutations. Some genes contain more than 100,000 bases and a mutation of any one base can make the gene nonfunctional and cause disease. The more mutations possible, the less likely it is for a test to detect all of them. This test is usually done on white blood cells from a person's blood. The test begins by using chemicals to separate DNA from the rest of the cell. Next, the two strands of DNA are separated by heating. Special enzymes (called restriction enzymes) are added to the single strands of DNA and then act like scissors and cut the strands in specific places. The DNA fragments are then sorted by size through a process called electrophoresis. A special piece of DNA, called a probe, is added to the fragments. The probe is designed to bind to specific mutated portions of the gene. When bound to the probe, the mutated portions appear on x-ray film with a distinct banding pattern.

FAMILY LINKAGE STUDIES

Family linkage studies are done to study a disease when a mutated gene's general location on a chromosome is known but its identity is not. These studies are possible when a chromosome marker has been found associated with a disease. Chromosomes contain certain regions that vary in appearance between individuals. These regions are called polymorphisms. If a polymorphism is always present in family members with the same genetic disease, and absent in family members without the disease, it is likely that the gene responsible for the disease is near that polymorphism. The gene mutation can be indirectly detected in family members by looking for the polymorphism.

To look for the polymorphism, DNA is isolated from cells in the same way it is for direct DNA mutation analysis. A probe is added that will detect the large polymorphism on the chromosome. When bound to the probe, this region will appear on x-ray film with a distinct banding pattern. The pattern of banding of a person being tested for the disease is compared to the pattern from a family member affected by the disease.

Linkage studies have disadvantages not found in direct DNA mutation analysis. These studies require multiple family members to participate in the testing. If key family members choose not to participate, the incomplete family history may make testing other members useless. The indirect method of detecting a mutated gene also causes more opportunity for error.

CHROMOSOME ANALYSIS

Many genetic diseases and syndromes are caused by structural chromosome abnormalities. To analyze a person's chromosomes, his or her cells are allowed to grow and multiply in the laboratory until they reach a certain stage of growth. The length of growing time varies with the type of cells. Cells from blood and bone marrow take 1–2 days; fetal cells from amniotic fluid take 7–10 days.

When the cells are ready, they are placed on a microscope slide using a technique to make them burst open, spreading their chromosomes. The slides are stained: the stain creates a banding pattern unique to each chromosome. Under a microscope, the chromosomes are counted, identified, and analyzed based on their size, shape, and stained appearance.

Karyotypes of the chromosomes are prepared for further study and to document the results. First, a photograph is taken of the chromosomes from one or more cells as seen through the microscope. Then the chromosomes are cut out and arranged side-by-side with their partner in ascending numerical order, from largest to smallest. The karyotype is done either manually or using a computer attached to the microscope. Chromosome analysis is also called cytogenetics.

Applications

CARRIER TESTING

A person who has a mutated gene associated with a disease is called a carrier. A carrier is a person who is not affected by the mutated gene he or she possesses, but can pass the gene to an offspring. Genetic tests have been developed that tell prospective parents whether or not they are carriers of certain diseases. If one or both of the parents is a carrier, the risk of passing the disease to a child can be predicted.

To predict the risk, it is necessary to know if the gene in question is autosomal or sex-linked. If the gene is carried on any one of chromosomes 1–22, the resulting disease is called an autosomal disease. If the gene is carried on the X or Y chromosome, it is called a sex-linked disease.

Sex-linked diseases, such as the bleeding condition **hemophilia,** are usually carried on the X (or female) chromosome. A woman who carries a disease-associated mutated gene on one of her X chromosomes, has a 50% chance of passing that gene to her son. A son who inherits that gene will develop the disease because he does not have another normal copy of the gene on a second X chromosome to compensate for the mutated copy.

The risk of passing an autosomal disease to a child depends on whether the gene is dominant or recessive. A prospective parent carrying a dominant gene, has a 50% chance of passing the gene to a child. A child needs to receive only one copy of the mutated gene to be affected by the disease.

If the gene is recessive, a child needs to receive two copies of the mutated gene, one from each parent, to be affected by the disease. When both prospective parents are carriers, their child has a 25% chance of inheriting two copies of the mutated gene and being affected by the disease; a 50% chance of inheriting one copy of the mutated gene, and being a carrier of the disease but not affected; and a 25% chance of inheriting two normal genes. When only one prospective parent is a carrier, a child has a 50% chance of inheriting one mutated gene and being an unaffected carrier of the disease, and a 50% chance of inheriting two normal genes.

Cystic fibrosis is a disease that affects the lungs and pancreas and is discovered in early childhood. It is the most common autosomal recessive genetic disease found in the caucasian population: 1 in 25 people of Northern European ancestry are carriers of a mutated cystic fibrosis gene. The gene, located on chromosome 7, was identified in 1989.

The gene mutation for cystic fibrosis is detected by a direct DNA test. Over 600 mutations of the cystic fibrosis gene have been found; each of these mutations cause the same disease. Tests are available for the most common mutations. Tests that check for the six most common mutations will detect 85% of carriers for cystic fibrosis. If a person tests negative, it is likely, but not guaranteed that he or she does not have the gene. Both prospective parents must be carriers of the gene to have a child with cystic fibrosis.

Tay-Sachs disease, also autosomal recessive, affects children primarily of Ashkenazi Jewish descent. Children with this disease die between the ages of two and five. This disease was previously detected by looking for a missing enzyme. The mutated gene has now been identified and can be detected using direct DNA mutation analysis.

PRESYMPTOMATIC TESTING

Not all genetic diseases show their effect immediately at birth or early in childhood. Although the gene mutation is present at birth, some diseases don't appear until adulthood. If a specific mutated gene responsible for a late-onset disease has been identified, a person from an affected family can be tested before symptoms appear.

Huntington's disease is a fatal autosomal dominant disease. Its symptoms of mental confusion and abnormal body movements don't appear until middle to late adulthood. The chromosome location of the gene responsible for Huntington's chorea was located in 1983 after studying the DNA from a large Venezuelan family affected by the disease. Ten years later the gene was identified. A test is now available to detect the presence of the mutated gene in a person. The presence of the mutated dominant gene means the person will develop the disease.

The specific genetic cause of **Alzheimer's disease** is not as clear. Although many cases appear to be inherited in an autosomal dominant pattern, many cases exist as single incidents in a family. Like Huntington's, symptoms of mental deterioration first appear in adulthood. Genetic research has found an association between this disease and genes on four different chromosomes. The validity of looking for these genes in a person without symptoms or without family history of the disease is still being studied.

CANCER SUSCEPTIBILITY TESTING

Cancer can result from an inherited mutated gene or a gene that mutated sometime during a person's lifetime. Some genes, called tumor suppressor genes, produce proteins that protect the body from cancer. If one of these genes develops a mutation, it can't produce the protective protein. If the second copy of the gene is normal, its action may be sufficient to continue production, but if that gene later also develops a mutation, the person is vulnerable to cancer. Other genes, called oncogenes, are involved in the normal growth of cells. A mutation in an oncogene can cause too much growth, the beginning of cancer.

Direct DNA tests are currently available to look for gene mutations identified and linked to several kinds of cancer. People with a family history of these cancers are those most likely to be tested. If one of these mutated genes is found, the person is more susceptible to developing the cancer. The likelihood that the person will develop the cancer, even with the mutated gene, is not always known because other genetic and environmental factors are also involved in the development of cancer.

Cancer susceptibility tests are most useful when a positive test result can be followed with clear treatment options. In families with **familial polyposis** of the colon, testing a child for a mutated APC gene can reveal whether or not the child needs frequent monitoring for the disease. In families with potentially fatal familial medullary **thyroid cancer** or multiple endocrine neoplasia type 2, finding a mutated RET gene in a child provides the opportunity for that child to have preventive removal of the thyroid gland. In the same way, MSH1 and MSH2 mutations can reveal which members in an affected family are vulnerable to familiar **colorectal cancer** and would benefit from aggressive monitoring.

In 1994, a mutation linked to early-onset familial breast and **ovarian cancer** was identified. BRCA1 is located on chromosome 17. Women with a mutated form of this gene have an increased risk of developing breast and ovarian cancer. A second related gene, BRCA2, was later discovered. Located on chromosome 13, it also carries increased risk of breast and ovarian cancer. Although both genes are rare in the general population, they are slightly more common in women of Ashkenazi Jewish descent.

When a woman is found to have a mutation of one of these genes, the likelihood that she will get breast or ovarian cancer increases, but not to 100%. Other genetic and environmental factors influence the outcome.

Testing for these genes is most valuable in families where a mutation has already been found. BRCA1 and BRCA2 are large genes; BRCA1 includes 100,000 bases. More than 120 mutations to this gene have been discovered, but a mutation could occur in any one of the bases. Studies show tests for these genes may miss 30% of existing mutations. The rate of missed mutations, the unknown disease likelihood in spite of a positive result, and the lack of a clear preventive response to a positive result, make the value of this test for the general population uncertain.

PRENATAL AND POSTNATAL CHROMOSOME ANALYSIS

Chromosome analysis is done on fetal cells primarily when the mother is over the age of 35, has had multiple miscarriages, or a family history of a genetic abnormality. Prenatal testing is done on the fetal cells in amniotic fluid (the fluid surrounding the baby) at 14–16 weeks of pregnancy or from a **chorionic villus sampling** (from the baby's placenta) at 8–12 weeks. Cells from amniotic fluid grow for 7–10 days before they are ready to be analyzed. Biopsy cells grow faster and can be analyzed sooner.

Chromosome analysis using blood cells is done on a child who is born with or later develops signs of mental retardation or physical malformation. In the older child, chromosome analysis may be done to investigate developmental delays.

Extra or missing chromosomes cause mental and physical abnormalities. A child born with an extra chromosome 21 (trisomy 21) has **Down syndrome.** An extra chromosome 13 or 18 also produce well known syndromes. A missing X chromosome causes **Turner syndrome** and an extra X in a male causes **Klinefelter syndrome.** Other abnormalities are caused by extra or missing pieces of chromosomes. **Fragile X syndrome** is a sex-linked disease, causing mental retardation in males. The abnormality is recognized by a fragile-looking area at the bottom of the X chromosome.

Chromosome material may also be rearranged, such as the end of chromosome 1 moved to the end of chromosome 3. If no material is added or deleted in the exchange, the person may not be affected. Such an exchange, however, can cause **infertility** or abnormalities if passed to children.

Evaluation of a man and woman's infertility or repeated miscarriages will include blood studies of both to check for a chromosome structural rearrangement. Many chromosome abnormalities are incompatible with life; babies with these abnormalities often miscarrry during the first trimester. Cells from a baby that died before birth can be studied to look for chromosome abnormalities that may have caused the **death.**

CANCER DIAGNOSIS AND PROGNOSIS

Certain cancers, particularly leukemia and lymphoma, are associated with changes in chromosomes: extra or missing complete chromosomes, extra or missing portions of chromosomes, or exchanges of material (called translocations) between chromosomes. Studies show that the locations of the chromosome breaks are at locations of tumor suppressor genes or oncogenes.

Chromosome analysis on cells from blood, bone marrow, or solid tumor helps diagnose certain kinds of leukemia and lymphoma and often helps predict how well the person will respond to treatment. After treatment has begun, periodic monitoring of these chromosome changes in the blood and bone marrow gives the physician information as to the effectiveness of the treatment.

A well-known chromosome rearrangement is found in chronic myelogenous leukemia. This leukemia is associated with an exchange of material between chromosomes 9 and 22. The resulting smaller chromosome 22 is called the Philadelphia chromosome.

Preparation

Most tests for genetic diseases of children and adults are done on blood. To collect the 5–10 mL of blood needed, a healthcare worker draws blood from a vein in the inner elbow region. Collection of the sample takes only a few minutes.

Prenatal testing is done either on amniotic fluid or a chorionic villus biopsy. To collect amniotic fluid, a physician performs a procedure called **amniocentesis.** An ultrasound is done to find the baby's position and an area filled with amniotic fluid. The physician inserts a needle through the woman's skin and the wall of her uterus and withdraws 5–10 mL of amniotic fluid. Placental tissue for a chorionic villus biopsy is taken through the cervix. Each procedures take approximately 30 minutes.

Bone marrow is used for chromosome analysis in a person with leukemia or lymphoma. The person is given **local anesthesia.** Then the physician inserts a needle through the skin and into the bone (usually the sternum or hip bone). One-half to 2 mL of bone marrow is withdrawn. This procedure takes approximately 30 minutes.

Aftercare

After blood collection the person can feel discomfort or bruising at the puncture site or may become dizzy or faint. Pressure to the puncture site until the bleeding stops reduces bruising. Warm packs to the puncture site relieve discomfort.

Collection of amniotic fluid, chorionic villus biopsy, and bone marrow are all done under a physician's supervision. The person is asked to rest after the procedure and is watched for weakness and signs of bleeding.

Risks

Collection of amniotic fluid and chorionic villus biopsy have the risk of miscarriage, infection, and bleeding; the risks are higher for the biopsy. A woman should tell her physician immediately if she has cramping, bleeding, fluid loss, an increased temperature, or a change in the baby's movement following either of these procedures.

After bone marrow collection, the puncture site may become tender and the person's temperature may rise. These are signs of a possible infection.

Genetic testing involves other nonphysical risks. Many people fear the possible loss of privacy about personal health information. Results of genetic tests may be reported to insurance companies and affect a person's insurability. Some people pay out-of-pocket for genetic tests to avoid this possibility. Laws have been proposed to deal with this problem. Other family members may be affected by the results of a person's genetic test. Privacy of the person tested and the family members affected is a consideration when deciding to have a test and to share the results.

A positive result carries a psychological burden, especially if the test indicates the person will develop a disease, such as Huntington's chorea. The news that a person may be susceptible to a specific kind of cancer, while it may encourage positive preventive measures, may also negatively shadow many decisions and activities.

Normal results

A normal result for chromosome analysis is 46, XX or 46, XY. This means there are 46 chromosomes (including two X chromosomes for a female or one X and one Y for a male) with no structural abnormalities. A normal result for a direct DNA mutation analysis or linkage study is no gene mutation found.

The person should learn from the genetic counselor the likelihood that the test could miss a mutation or abnormality.

Abnormal results

An abnormal chromosome analysis report will include the total number of chromosomes and will identify the abnormality found. Tests for gene mutations will report the mutations found.

Before making decisions based on an abnormal test result, the person should meet again with a genetic counselor to fully understand the meaning of the results, learn what options are available based on the test result, and what are the risks and benefits of each of those options.

Resources

BOOKS

Berg, Paul, and Maxine Singer. *Dealing with Genes: The Language of Heredity.* Mill Valley, CA: University Science Books, 1992.

Farkas, Daniel H. *DNA Simplified: The Hitchhiker's Guide to DNA.* Washington, DC: American Association of Clinical Chemistry Press, 1996.

Gelehrter, Thomas D. and Francis S. Collins, and David Ginsburg. *Principles of Medical Genetics.* 2nd ed. Baltimore: Williams and Wilkins, 1998.

Grody, Wayne W., and Walter W. Noll. "Molecular Diagnosis of Genetic Diseases. In *Clinical Diagnosis and Management by Laboratory Methods,* edited by John B. Henry. 19th ed. Philadelphia: W. B. Saunders Company, 1996, pp. 1374-1389.

Motulsky, Arno G., Richard A. King, and Jerome I. Rotter. *The Genetic Basis of Common Diseases.* New York: Oxford University Press, 1992.

Mueller, Robert F. and Ian D. Young. *Emery's Elements of Medical Genetics* 9th ed. Churchill Livingstone, New York and Edinburgh: 1995.

Watson, James D. *The Double Helix.* New York: Atheneum, 1968.

PERIODICALS

Auxter, Sue. "Genetic Information—What Should be Regulated?" *Clinical Laboratory News.* (December, 1997): 9-11.

Biesecker, Barbara Bowles. "Genetic Susceptibility Testing for Breast and Ovarian Cancer: A Progress Report." *Journal of the American Medical Women's Association.* (Winter, 1997): 22-27.

Fink, Leslie and Francis S. Collins. "The Human Genome Project: View From the National Institutes of Health." *Journal of the American Medical Women's Association.* (Winter, 1997): 4-7, 15.

Holtzman, Neil A., and Michael S. Watson, eds. *Promoting Safe and Effective Genetic Testing in the United States. Final Report of the Task Force on Genetic Testing.* National Institutes of Health-Department of Energy Working Group on Ethical, Legal, and Social Implications of Human Genome Research, 1997.

Holtzman, Neil A., Patricia D. Murphy, Michael S. Watson, and Patricia A. Barr. "Predictive Genetic Testing: From Basic Research to Clinical Practice." *Science.* (October 24, 1997): 602-605.

Karnes, Pamela S. "Ordering and Interpreting DNA tests." *Mayo Clinical Proceedings.* (December, 1996): 1192-1195.

Malone, Kathleen E, Janet R. Daling, Jennifer D. Thompson, Cecilia A. O'Brien, Leigh V. Francisco, and Elaine A. Ostrander. "BRCA1 Mutations and Breast Cancer in the General Population." *Journal of the American Medical Association.* (March 25, 1998): 922-929.

McKinnon, Wendy C., Bonnie J. Baty, Robin L. Bennett, Monica Magee, Whitney A. Neufeld-Kaiser, Kathyrn F. Peters, Jill C. Sawyer, and Katherine A. Schneider. "Predisposition Genetic Testing for Late-Onset Disorders in Adults: A Position Paper of the National Society of Genetic Counselors." *Journal of the American Medical Association.* (October 15, 1997): 1217-1221.

Newman, Beth, Hua Mu, Lesley M. Butler, Robert C. Millikan, Patricia G. Moorman, and Mary-Claire King. "Frequency of Breast Cancer Attributable to BRCA1 in a Population-Based Series of American Women." *Journal of the American Medical Association.* (March 25, 1998): 915-921.

Ponder, Bruce. "Genetic Testing for Cancer Risk." *Science.* (November 7, 1997): 1050-1054.

Roses, Allen. "Genetic Testing for Alzheimer Disease. Practical and Ethical Issues." *Archives of Neurology.* (October, 1997): 1226-1229.

Whittaker, Lori. "Clinical Applications of Genetic Testing: Implications for the Family Physician." *American Family Physician.* (May, 1996): 2077-2084.

Wisecarver, James. "The ABCs of DNA." *Laboratory Medicine.* (January, 1997): 48-52.

Yablonsky, Terri. "Genetic Testing Helps Patients and Researchers Predict the Future." *Laboratory Medicine.* (May, 1997): 316-321.

Yablonsky, Terri. "Unlocking the Secrets to Disease. Genetic Tests Usher in a New Era in Medicine." *Laboratory Medicine.* (April, 1997): 252-256.

ORGANIZATIONS

Alliance of Genetic Support Groups. 4301 Connecticut Avenue NW, Ste. 404, Washington, DC. 20008-2304. http://204.141.0.149/geneticalliance/.

American College of Medical Genetics. 9650 Rockville Pike, Bethesda, MD 20814-3998. (301) 571-1825. http://www.faseb.org/genetics/acmg/acmgmenu.htm.

American Society of Human Genetics. 9650 Rockville Pike, Bethesda, MD 20814. (301) 571-1825. http://www.faseb.org/genetics/ashg/ashgmenu.htm.

Centers for Disease Control. Office of Genetics and Disease Prevention. 4770 Buford Highway NE, Atlanta, GA. 30341-3724. (770) 488-3235. http://www.cdc.gov/genetics/.

The March of Dimes. 1275 Manaroneck Ave., White Plains, NY 10605. (914) 428-7100. http://www.modimes.org.

The National Human Genome Research Institute.The National Institutes of Health. 9000 Rockville Pike, Bethesda, MD 20892. (301) 496-2433. http://www.nhgri.nih.gov.

The National Society of Genetic Counselors. 233 Canterbury Dr., Wallingford, PA 19086-6617. (610) 872-7608. http://members.aol.com/nsgcweb/nsgchome.htm.

OTHER

Blazing a Genetic Trail. Online genetic tutorial. http://www.hhmi.org/GeneticTrail/.

The Gene Letter. Online newsletter. http://www.geneletter.org.

Online Mendelian Inheritance in Man. Online genetic testing information sponsored by National Center for Biotechnology Information. http://www.ncbi.nlm.nih.gov/Omim/.

Understanding Gene Testing. Online brochure produced by the U.S. Department of Health and Human Services. http://www.gene.com/ae/AE/AEPC/NIH/index.html.

Nancy J. Nordenson

Genital herpes

Definition

Genital herpes is a sexually transmitted disease caused by a herpes virus. The disease is characterized by the formation of fluid-filled, painful blisters in the genital area.

Description

Genital herpes (herpes genitalis, herpes progenitalis) is characterized by the formation of fluid-filled blisters on the genital organs of men and women. The word ''herpes'' comes from the Greek adjective *herpestes,* meaning *creeping,* which refers to the serpent-like pattern that the blisters may form. Genital herpes is a sexually transmitted disease which means that it is spread from person-to-person only by sexual contact. Herpes

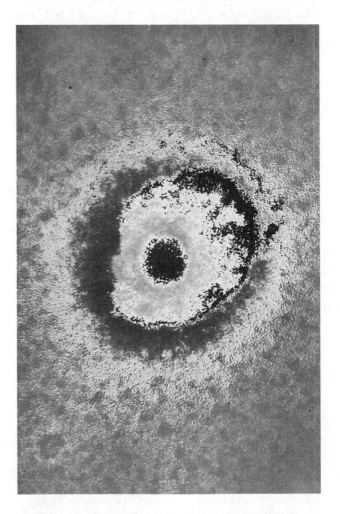

A **false-color transmission electron microscopy (TEM) image of a herpes simplex virus.** *(Custom Medical Stock Photo. Reproduced by permission.)*

may be spread by vaginal, anal, and oral sexual activity. It is not spread by objects (such as a toilet seat or doorknob), swimming pools, hot tubs, or through the air.

Genital herpes is a disease resulting from an infection by a herpes simplex virus. There are eight different kinds of human herpes viruses. Only two of these, herpes simplex types 1 and 2, can cause genital herpes. It has been commonly believed that herpes simplex virus type 1 infects above the waist (causing **cold sores**) and herpes simplex virus type 2 infects below the waist (causing genital sores). This is not completely true. Both herpes virus type 1 and type 2 can cause herpes lesions on the lips or genitals, but recurrent cold sores are almost always type 1. The two viruses seem to have evolved to infect better at one site or the other, especially with regard to recurrent disease.

To determine the occurrence of herpes type 2 infection in the United States, the Centers for Disease Control and Prevention (CDC) used information from a survey called the National Health and Nutrition Examination Survey III (1988–1994). This survey of 40,000 noninstitutionalized people found that 21.9% of persons age 12 or older had antibodies to herpes type 2. This means that 45 million Americans have been exposed at some point in their lives to herpes simplex virus type 2. More women (25.6%) than men (17.8%) had antibodies. The racial differences for herpes type 2 antibodies were whites, 17.6%; blacks, 45.9%; and Mexican Americans, 22.3%. Interestingly, only 2.6% of adults reported that they have had genital herpes. Over half (50% to 60%) of the white adults in the United States have antibodies to herpes simplex virus type 1. The occurrence of antibodies to herpes type 1 is higher in blacks.

Viruses are different from bacteria. While bacteria are independent and can reproduce on their own, viruses cannot reproduce without the help of a cell. Viruses enter human cells and force them to make more virus. A human cell infected with herpes virus releases thousands of new viruses before it is killed. The cell death and resulting tissue damage causes the actual sores. The highest risk for spreading the virus is the time period beginning with the appearance of blisters and ending with scab formation.

Herpes virus can also infect a cell and instead of making the cell produce new viruses, it hides inside the cell and waits. Herpes virus hides in cells of the nervous system called "neurons." This is called "latency." A latent virus can wait inside neurons for days, months, or even years. At some future time, the virus "awakens" and causes the cell to produce thousands of new viruses which causes an active infection. Sometimes an active infection occurs without visible sores. Therefore, an infected person can spread herpes virus to other people even in the absence of sores.

This process of latency and active infection is best understood by considering the genital sore cycle. An active infection is obvious because sores are present. The first infection is called the "primary" infection. This active infection is then controlled by the body's immune system and the sores heal. In between active infections, the virus is latent. At some point in the future latent viruses become activated and once again cause sores. These are called "recurrent infections" or "outbreaks." Genital sores caused by herpes type 1 recur much less frequently than sores caused by herpes type 2.

Although it is unknown what triggers latent viruses to activate, several conditions seem to bring on infections. These include illness, tiredness, exposure to sunlight, menstruation, skin damage, food allergy and hot or cold temperatures. Although many people believe that **stress** can bring on their genital herpes outbreaks, there is no scientific evidence that there is a link between stress and recurrences. However, at least one clinical study has shown a connection between how well people cope with stress and their belief that stress and recurrent infections are linked.

Newborn babies who are infected with herpes virus experience a very severe, and possibly fatal disease. This is called "neonatal herpes infection." In the United States, one in 3,000–5,000 babies born will be infected with herpes virus. Babies can become infected during passage through the birth canal, but can become infected during the **pregnancy** if the membranes rupture early. Doctors will perform a **Cesarean section** on women who go into labor with active genital herpes.

Causes & symptoms

While anyone can be infected by herpes virus, not everyone will show symptoms. Risk factors for genital herpes include: early age at first sexual activity, multiple sexual partners, and a medical history of other sexually-transmitted diseases.

Most patients with genital herpes experience a prodrome (symptoms of oncoming disease) of **pain,** burning, **itching,** or tingling at the site where blisters will form. This prodrome stage may last anywhere from a few hours, to one to two days. The herpes infection prodrome can occur for both the primary infection and recurrent infections. The prodrome for recurrent infections may be severe and cause a severe burning or stabbing pain in the genital area, legs, or buttocks.

Primary genital herpes

The first symptoms of herpes usually occur within two to seven days after contact with an infected person but may take up to two weeks. Symptoms of the primary infection are usually more severe than those of recurrent infections. For up to 70% of the patients, the primary

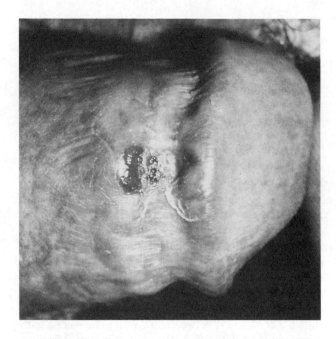

A close-up view of a man's penis with a blister (center of image) caused by the herpes simplex virus. *(Photograph by Dr. P. Marazzi, Custom Medical Stock Photo. Reproduced by permission.)*

infection causes symptoms which affect the whole body (called ''constitutional symptoms'') including tiredness, **headache, fever,** chills, muscle aches, loss of appetite, as well as painful, swollen lymph nodes in the groin. These symptoms are greatest during the first three to four days of the infection and disappear within one week. The primary infection is more severe in women than in men.

Following the prodrome come the herpes blisters, which are similar on men and women. First, small red bumps appear. These bumps quickly become fluid-filled blisters. In dry areas, the blisters become filled with pus and take on a white to gray appearance, become covered with a scab, and heal within two to three weeks. In moist areas, the fluid-filled blisters burst and form painful ulcers which drain before healing. New blisters may appear over a period of one week or longer and may join together to form very large ulcers. The pain is relieved within two weeks and the blisters and ulcers heal without scarring by three to four weeks.

Women can experience a very severe and painful primary infection. Herpes blisters first appear on the labia majora (outer lips), labia minora (inner lips), and entrance to the vagina. Blisters often appear on the clitoris, at the urinary opening, around the anal opening, and on the buttocks and thighs. In addition, women may get herpes blisters on the lips, breasts, fingers, and eyes. The vagina and cervix are almost always involved which causes a watery discharge. Other symptoms that occur in women are: painful or difficult urination (83%), swelling of the urinary tube (85%), **meningitis** (36%), and throat infection (13%). Most women develop painful, swollen lymph nodes (lymphadenopathy) in the groin and pelvis. About one in ten women get a vaginal yeast infection as a complication of the primary herpes infection.

In men, the herpes blisters usually form on the penis but can also appear on the scrotum, thighs, and buttocks. Fewer than half of the men with primary herpes experience the constitutional symptoms. Thirty percent to 40% of men have a discharge from the urinary tube. Some men develop painful swollen lymph nodes (lymphadenopathy) in the groin and pelvis. Although less frequently than women, men too may experience painful or difficult urination (44%), swelling of the urinary tube (27%), meningitis (13%), and throat infection (7%).

Recurrent genital herpes

One or more outbreaks of genital herpes per year occur in 60–90% of those infected with herpes virus. About 40% of the persons infected with herpes simplex virus type 2 will experience six or more outbreaks each year. Genital herpes recurrences are less severe than the primary infection; however, women still experience more severe symptoms and pain than men. Constitutional symptoms are not usually present. Blisters will appear at the same sites during each outbreak. Usually there are fewer blisters, less pain, and the time period from the beginning of symptoms to healing is shorter than the primary infection. One out of every four women experience painful or difficult urination during recurrent infection. Both men and women may develop lymphadenopathy.

Diagnosis

Because genital herpes is so common, it is diagnosed primarily by symptoms. It can be diagnosed and treated by the family doctor, dermatologists (doctors who specialize in skin diseases), urologists (doctors who specialize in the urinary tract diseases of men and women and the genital organs of men), gynecologists (doctors who specialize in the diseases of women's genital organs) and infectious disease specialists. The diagnosis and treatment of this infectious disease should be covered by most insurance providers.

Laboratory tests may be performed to look for the virus. Because healing sores do not shed much virus, a sample from an open sore would be taken for viral culture. A sterile cotton swab would be wiped over open sores and the sample used to infect human cells in culture. Cells which are killed by herpes virus have a certain appearance under microscopic examination. The results of this test are available within two to ten days. Other areas which may be sampled, depending upon the disease symptoms in a particular patient, include the urinary tract, vagina, cervix, throat, eye tissues, and cerebrospinal fluid.

Direct staining and microscopic examination of the lesion sample may also be used. A blood test may be performed to see if the patient has antibodies to herpes virus. The results of blood testing are available within one day. The disadvantage of this blood test is that it usually does not distinguish between herpes type 1 and 2, and only determines that the patient has had a herpes infection at some point in his or her life. Therefore, the viral culture test must be performed to be absolutely certain that the sores are caused by herpes virus.

Because genital sores can be symptoms of many other diseases, the doctor must determine the exact cause of the sores. The above mentioned tests are performed to determine that herpes virus is causing the genital sores. Other diseases which may cause genital sores are **syphilis, chancroid, lymphogranuloma venereum, granuloma inguinale,** herpes zoster, erythema multiform, Behçet's syndrome, inflammatory bowel disease, **contact dermatitis, candidiasis,** and **impetigo.**

Because most newborns who are infected with herpes virus were born to mothers who had no symptoms of infection it is important to check all newborn babies for symptoms. Any skin sore should be sampled to determine if it is caused by herpes simplex. Babies should be checked for sores in their mouth and for signs of herpes infection in their eyes.

Treatment

There is no cure for herpes virus infections. There are **antiviral drugs** available which have some effect in lessening the symptoms and decreasing the length of herpes outbreaks. There is evidence that some may also prevent future outbreaks. These antiviral drugs work by interfering with the replication of the viruses and are most effective when taken as early in the infection process as possible. For the best results, drug treatment should begin during the prodrome stage before blisters are visible. Depending on the length of the outbreak, drug treatment could continue for up to 10 days.

Acyclovir (Zovirax) is the drug of choice for herpes infection and can be given intravenously, taken by mouth (orally), or applied directly to sores as an ointment. Acyclovir has been in use for many years and only five out of 100 patients experience side effects. Side effects of acyclovir treatment include nausea, vomiting, itchy rash, and **hives.** Although acyclovir is the recommended drug for treating herpes infections, other drugs may be used including famciclovir (Famvir), valacyclovir (Valtrex), vidarabine (Vira-A), idoxuridine (Herplex Liquifilm, Stoxil), trifluorothymidine (Viroptic), and penciclovir (Denavir).

Acyclovir is effective in treating both the primary infection and recurrent outbreaks. When taken intravenously or orally, acyclovir reduces the healing time, virus shedding period, and duration of vesicles. The standard oral dose of acyclovir for primary herpes is 200 mg five times daily or 400 mg three times daily for a period of 10 days. Recurrent herpes is treated with the same doses for a period of five days. Intravenous acyclovir is given to patients who require hospitalization because of severe primary infections or herpes complications such as aseptic meningitis or sacral ganglionitis (inflammation of nerve bundles).

Patients with frequent outbreaks (greater than six to eight per year) may benefit from long term use of acyclovir which is called "suppressive therapy." Patients on suppressive therapy have longer periods between herpes outbreaks. The specific dosage used for suppression needs to be determined for each patient and should be reevaluated every few years. Alternatively, patients may use short term suppressive therapy to lessen the chance of developing an active infection during special occasions such as weddings or holidays.

There are several things that a patient may do to lessen the pain of genital sores. Wearing loose fitting clothing and cotton underwear is helpful. Removing clothing or wearing loose pajamas while at home may reduce pain. Soaking in a tub of warm water and using a blow dryer on the "cool" setting to dry the infected area is helpful. Putting an ice pack on the affected area for 10 minutes, followed by 5 minutes off and then repeating this procedure may relieve pain. A zinc sulfate ointment may help to heal the sores. Application of a baking soda compress to sores may be soothing.

Neonatal herpes

Newborn babies with herpes virus infections are treated with intravenous acyclovir or vidarabine for 10 days. These drugs have greatly reduced deaths and increased the number of babies who appear normal at one year of age. However, because neonatal herpes infection is so serious, even with treatment babies may not survive, or may suffer nervous system damage. Infected babies may be treated with long term suppressive therapy.

Alternative treatment

An imbalance in the amino acids lysine and arginine is thought to be one contributing factor in herpes virus outbreaks. A ratio of lysine to arginine that is in balance (that is more lysine than arginine is present) seems to help the immune system work optimally. Thus, a diet that is rich in lysine may help prevent recurrences of genital herpes. Foods that contain high levels of lysine include most vegetables, legumes, fish, turkey, beef, lamb, cheese, and chicken. Patients may take 500 mg of lysine daily and increase to 1,000 mg three times a day during an outbreak. Intake of the amino acid arginine should be reduced. Foods rich in arginine that should be avoided are chocolate, peanuts, almonds, and other nuts and seeds.

Clinical experience indicates a connection between high stress and herpes outbreaks. Some patients respond well to **stress reduction** and relaxation techniques. **Acupressure** and **massage** may relieve tiredness and stress. **Meditation, yoga, tai chi,** and hypnotherapy can also help relieve stress and promote relaxation.

Some herbs, including echinacea (*Echinacea* spp.) and garlic (*Allium sativum*), are believed to strengthen the body's defenses against viral infections. Red marine algae (family Dumontiaceae), both taken internally and applied topically, is thought to be effective in treating herpes type I and type II infections. Other topical treatments may be helpful in inhibiting the growth of the herpes virus, in minimizing the damage it causes, or in helping the sores heal. Zinc sulphate ointment seems to help sores heal and to fight recurrence. Lithium succinate ointment may interfere with viral replication. An ointment made with glycyrrhizinic acid, a component of licorice (*Glycyrrhiza glabra*), seems to inactivate the virus. Topical applications of vitamin E or tea tree oil (*Melaleuca* spp.) help dry up herpes sores. Specific combinations of homeopathic remedies may also be helpful treatments for genital herpes.

Prognosis

Although physically and emotionally painful, genital herpes is usually not a serious disease. The primary infection can be severe and may require hospitalization for treatment. Complications of the primary infection may involve the cervix, urinary system, anal opening, and the nervous system. Persons who have a decreased ability to produce an immune response to infection (called "immunocompromised") due to disease or medication are at risk for a very severe, and possibly fatal, herpes infection. Even with antiviral treatment, neonatal herpes infections can be fatal or cause permanent nervous system damage.

Prevention

The only way to prevent genital herpes is to avoid contact with infected persons. This is not an easy solution because many people aren't aware that they are infected and can easily spread the virus to others. Avoid all sexual contact with an infected person during a herpes outbreak. Because herpes virus can be spread at any time, **condom** use is recommended to prevent the spread of virus to uninfected partners. As of early 1998 there were no herpes vaccines available, although new herpes vaccines are being tested in humans.

Resources

BOOKS

Ebel, Charles. *Managing Herpes: How to Live and Love With a Chronic STD.* American Social Health Association, 1998.

Sacks, Stephen L. *The Truth About Herpes.* Gordon Soules Book Publisher, 1997.

PERIODICALS

Murray, Michael T. "Natural Help for Herpes and Cold Sores." *Let's Live* (April 1997): 68 + .

OTHER

JAMA Women's Health Information Center. 1997. Http://www.ama-assn.org/special/std/std.htm (8 April 1998).

Mayo Health Oasis. 1998. http://www.mayohealth.org (3 March 1998).

Belinda M. Rowland

Genital warts

Definition

Genital warts, which are also called condylomata acuminata or venereal **warts**, are growths in the genital area caused by a sexually transmitted papillomavirus. A papillomavirus is a virus that produces papillomas, or benign growths on the skin and mucous membranes.

Description

Genital warts are the most common sexually transmitted disease (STD) in the general population. It is estimated that 1% of sexually active people between the ages of 18 and 45 have genital warts; however, polymerase chain reaction (PCR) testing indicates that as many as 40% of sexually active adults carry the human papillomavirus (HPV) that causes genital warts.

Genital warts vary somewhat in appearance. They may be either flat or resemble raspberries or cauliflower in appearance. The warts begin as small red or pink growths and grow as large as four inches across, interfering with intercourse and **childbirth.** The warts grow in the moist tissues of the genital areas. In women, they occur on the external genitals and on the walls of the vagina and cervix; in men, they develop in the urethra and on the shaft of the penis. The warts then spread to the area behind the genitals surrounding the anus.

Risk factors for genital warts include:

• Multiple sexual partners

• Infection with another STD

- **Pregnancy**

- Anal intercourse

- Poor personal hygiene

- Heavy perspiration.

Causes & symptoms

There are about 80 types of human papillomavirus. Genital warts are caused by HPV types 1, 2, 6, 11, 16, and 18. HPV is transmitted by sexual contact. The incubation period varies from one to six months.

The symptoms include bleeding, **pain,** and odor as well as the visible warts.

Diagnosis

The diagnosis is usually made by examining scrapings from the warts under a darkfield microscope. If the warts are caused by HPV, they will turn white when a 5% solution of white vinegar is added. If the warts reappear, the doctor may order a biopsy to rule out **cancer.**

Treatment

No treatment for genital warts is completely effective because therapy depends on destroying skin infected by the virus. There are no drugs that will kill the virus directly.

Medications

Genital warts were treated until recently with applications of podophyllum resin, a corrosive substance that cannot be given to pregnant patients. A milder form of podophyllum, podofilox (Condylox), has been introduced. Women are also treated with 5-fluorouracil cream, bichloroacetic acid, or trichloroacetic acid. All of these substances irritate the skin and require weeks of treatment.

Genital warts can also be treated with injections of interferon. Interferon works best in combination with podofilox applications.

Surgery

Surgery may be necessary to remove warts blocking the patient's vagina, urethra, or anus. Surgical techniques include the use of liquid nitrogen, electrosurgery, and **laser surgery.**

Prognosis

Genital warts are benign growths and are not cancerous by themselves. Repeated HPV infection in women, however, appears to increase the risk of later **cervical cancer.** Women infected with HPV types 16 and 18 should have yearly cervical smears. Recurrence is common with all present methods of treatment—including surgery—because HPV can remain latent in apparently normal surrounding skin.

Prevention

The only reliable method of prevention is sexual abstinence. The use of **condoms** minimizes but does not eliminate the risk of HPV transmission. The patient's sexual contacts should be notified and examined.

Resources

BOOKS

Berger, Timothy G. "Skin & Appendages." In *Current Medical Diagnosis & Treatment.* Edited by Lawrence M. Tierney Jr., et al. Stamford, CT: Appleton & Lange, 1998.

Curry, Stephen L. and David L. Barclay. "Benign Disorders of the Vulva & Vagina." In *Current Obstetric & Gynecologic Diagnosis & Treatment.* Edited by Alan H. DeCherney and Martin L. Pernoll. Norwalk, CT: Appleton & Lange, 1994.

Edwards, Libby. "Condylomata Acuminata." In *Conn's Current Therapy.* Edited by Robert E. Rakel. Philadelphia: W. B. Saunders Company, 1998.

Foster, David C. "Vulvar and Vaginal Disease." In *Current Diagnosis.* Edited by Rex B. Conn, et al. Philadelphia: W. B. Saunders Company, 1997.

"Genital Warts." In *Professional Guide to Diseases.* Edited by Stanley Loeb, et al. Springhouse, PA: Springhouse Corporation, 1991.

Hunt, Thomas K. and Reid V. Mueller. "Inflammation, Infection, & Antibiotics." In *Current Surgical Diagnosis & Treatment.* Edited by Lawrence W. Way. Stamford, CT: Appleton & Lange, 1994.

MacKay, H. Trent. "Gynecology." In *Current Medical Diagnosis & Treatment.* Edited by Lawrence M. Tierney Jr., et al. Stamford, CT: Appleton & Lange, 1998.

"Podophyllum Resin." In *Nurses Drug Guide 1995,* edited by Billie Ann Wilson, et al. Norwalk, CT: Appleton & Lange, 1995.

"Sexually Transmitted Diseases: Genital Warts." In *The Merck Manual of Diagnosis and Therapy,* edited by Robert Berkow, et al. Rahway, NJ: Merck Research Laboratories, 1992.

Tyring, Stephen K. "Viral Diseases of the Skin." In *Conn's Current Therapy,* edited by Robert E. Rakel. Philadelphia: W. B. Saunders Company, 1998.

Rebecca J. Frey

Gentamicin *see* **Aminoglycosides**

German measles *see* **Rubella**

Gestalt therapy

Definition

Gestalt therapy is a humanistic therapy technique that focuses on gaining an awareness of emotions and behaviors in the present rather than in the past. The therapist does not interpret experiences for the patient. Instead, the therapist and patient work together to help the patient understand him/herself. This type of therapy focuses on experiencing the present situation rather than talking about what occurred in the past. Patients are encouraged to become aware of immediate needs, meet them, and let them recede into the background. The well-adjusted person is seen as someone who has a constant flow of needs and is able to satisfy those needs.

Purpose

In Gestalt therapy (from the German word meaning *form*), the major goal is self-awareness. Patients work on uncovering and resolving interpersonal issues during therapy. Unresolved issues are unable to fade into the background of consciousness because the needs they represent are never met. In Gestalt therapy, the goal is to discover people connected with a patient's unresolved issues and try to engage those people (or images of those people) in interactions that can lead to a resolution. Gestalt therapy is most useful for patients open to working on self-awareness.

Precautions

The choice of a therapist is crucial. Some people who call themselves "therapists" have limited training in Gestalt therapy. It is important that the therapist be a licensed mental health professional. Additionally, some individuals may not be able to tolerate the intensity of this type of therapy.

Description

Gestalt therapy has developed into a form of therapy that emphasizes medium to large groups, although many Gestalt techniques can be used in one-on-one therapy. Gestalt therapy probably has a greater range of formats than any other therapy technique. It is practiced in individual, couples, and family therapies, as well as in therapy with children.

Ideally, the patient identifies current sensations and emotions, particularly ones that are painful or disruptive. Patients are confronted with their unconscious feelings and needs, and are assisted to accept and assert those repressed parts of themselves.

The most powerful techniques involve role-playing. For example, the patient talks to an empty chair as they imagine that a person associated with an unresolved issue is sitting in the chair. As the patient talks to the "person" in the chair, the patient imagines that the person responds to the expressed feelings. Although this technique may sound artificial and might make some people feel self-conscious, it can be a powerful way to approach buried feelings and gain new insight into them.

Sometimes patients use battacca bats, padded sticks that can be used to hit chairs or sofas. Using a battacca bat can help a patient safely express anger. A patient may also experience a Gestalt therapy marathon, where the participants and one or more facilitators have nonstop **group therapy** over a weekend. The effects of the intense emotion and the lack of sleep can eliminate many psychological defenses and allow significant progress to be made in a short time. This is true only if the patient has adequate psychological strength for a marathon and is carefully monitored by the therapist.

Preparation

Gestalt therapy begins with the first contact. There is no separate diagnostic or assessment period. Instead, assessment and screening are done as part of the ongoing relationship between patient and therapist. This assessment includes determining the patient's willingness and support for work using Gestalt methods, as well as determining the compatibility between the patient and the therapist. Unfortunately, some "encounter groups" led by poorly trained individuals do not provide adequate pre-therapy screening and assessment.

Aftercare

Sessions are usually held once a week. Frequency of sessions held is based on how long the patient can go between sessions without losing the momentum from the previous session. Patients and therapists discuss when to start sessions, when to stop sessions, and what kind of activities to use during a session. However, the patient is encouraged and required to make choices.

Risks

Disturbed people with severe mental illness may not be suitable candidates for Gestalt therapy. Facilities that provide Gestalt therapy and train Gestalt therapists vary. Since there are no national standards for these Gestalt facilities, there are no set national standards for Gestalt therapy or Gestalt therapists.

Normal results

Scientific documentation on the effectiveness of Gestalt therapy is limited. Evidence suggests that this type of therapy may not be reliably effective.

Abnormal results

This approach can be anti-intellectual and can discount thoughts, thought patterns, and beliefs. In the hands of an ineffective therapist, Gestalt procedures can become a series of mechanical **exercises,** allowing the therapist as a person to stay hidden. Moreover, there is a potential for the therapist to manipulate the patient with powerful techniques, especially in therapy marathons where fatigue may make a patient vulnerable.

Resources

BOOKS

Ellis, Willis D. *A Source Book of Gestalt Psychology.* NY: Routledge & Gegan Paul, 1969.

Kendall, Philip C., and Julian D. Norton-Ford. *Clinical Psychology: Scientific and Professional Dimensions.* NY: John Wiley & Sons, 1982.

Kohler, Wolfgang *Gestalt Psychology.* NY: Liveright Publishing Corporation, 1947.

Pursglove, Paul David. *Recognitions in Gestalt Therapy.* New York: Funk & Wagnalls, 1968.

Yontef, Gary. *Awareness, Dialogue, and Process.* Highland, NY: The Gestalt Journal Press, 1993.

ORGANIZATIONS

Association for the Advancement of Gestalt Therapy. 400 East 58th St., New York, NY 10022. (212) 486-1581.

Professional Training, Certification, and Practice. 7424 Greeneville Ave., Suite 113, Dallas, TX 75231. (214) 363-0788.

David James Doermann

Gestational diabetes

Definition

Gestational diabetes is a condition that occurs during **pregnancy.** Like other forms of diabetes, gestational diabetes involves a defect in the way the body processes and uses sugars (glucose) in the diet. Gestational diabetes, however, has a number of characteristics that are different from other forms of diabetes.

Description

Glucose is a form of sugar that is present in many foods, including sweets, potatoes, pasta, and breads. The body uses glucose to provide energy. It is stored in the liver, muscles, and fatty tissue. The pancreas produces a hormone (a chemical produced in one part of the body, which travels to another part of the body in order to exert its effect) called insulin. Insulin is required to allow glucose to enter the liver, muscles, and fatty tissues, thus reducing the amount of glucose in the blood. In diabetes, blood levels of glucose remain abnormally high. In many forms of diabetes, this is because the pancreas does not produce enough insulin.

In gestational diabetes, the pancreas is not at fault. Instead, the problem is in the placenta. During pregnancy, the placenta provides the baby with nourishment. It also produces a number of hormones that interfere with the body's usual response to insulin. This condition is referred to as "insulin resistance." Most pregnant women do not suffer from gestational diabetes, because the pancreas works to produce extra quantities of insulin in order to compensate for insulin resistance. However, when a woman's pancreas cannot produce enough extra insulin, blood levels of glucose stay abnormally high, and the woman is considered to have gestational diabetes.

About 1–3% of all pregnant women develop gestational diabetes. Women at risk for gestational diabetes include those who:

- Are overweight

- Have a family history of diabetes

- Have previously given birth to a very large, heavy baby

- Have previously had a baby who was stillborn, or born with a birth defect

- Have an excess amount of amniotic fluid (the cushioning fluid within the uterus that surrounds the developing fetus)

- Are over 25 years of age

- Belong to an ethnic group known to experience higher rates of gestational diabetes (in the United States, these groups include Mexican-Americans, American Indians,

African-Americans, as well as individuals from Asia, India, or the Pacific Islands)

• Have a previous history of gestational diabetes during a pregnancy.

Causes & symptoms

Most women with gestational diabetes have no recognizable symptoms. However, leaving gestational diabetes undiagnosed and untreated is risky to the developing fetus. Left untreated, a diabetic mother's blood sugar levels will be consistently high. This sugar will cross the placenta and pour into the baby's system through the umbilical cord. The unborn baby's pancreas will respond to this high level of sugar by constantly putting out large amounts of insulin. The insulin will allow the fetus's cells to take in glucose, where it will be converted to fat and stored. A baby who has been exposed to constantly high levels of sugar throughout pregnancy will be abnormally large. Such a baby will often grow so large that he or she cannot be born through the vagina, but will instead need to be born through a surgical procedure (**cesarean section).**

Furthermore, when the baby is born, the baby will still have an abnormally large amount of insulin circulating. After birth, when the mother and baby are no longer attached to each other via the placenta and umbilical cord, the baby will no longer be receiving the mother's high level of sugar. The baby's high level of insulin, however, will very quickly use up the glucose circulating in the baby's bloodstream. The baby is then at risk for having a dangerously low level of blood glucose (a condition called **hypoglycemia).**

Diagnosis

Since gestational diabetes most often exists with no symptoms detectable by the patient, and since its existence puts the developing baby at considerable risk,

screening for the disorder is a routine part of pregnancy care. This screening is usually done between the 24th and 28th week of pregnancy. By this point in the pregnancy, the placental hormones have reached a sufficient level to cause insulin resistance. Screening for gestational diabetes involves the pregnant woman drinking a special solution that contains exactly 50 grams of glucose. An hour later, the woman's blood is drawn and tested for its glucose level. A level less than 140 mg/dl is considered normal.

When the screening glucose level is over 140 mg/dl, a special three-hour glucose tolerance test is performed. This involves following a special diet for three days prior to the test. This diet is set-up to contain at least 150 grams of carbohydrate each day. Just before the test, the patient is instructed to eat and drink nothing (except water) for 10–14 hours. A blood sample is then tested to determine the fasting glucose level. The patient then drinks a special solution containing exactly 100 grams of glucose, and her blood is tested every hour for the next three hours. If two or more of these levels are elevated over normal, then the patient is considered to have gestational diabetes.

Treatment

Treatment for gestational diabetes will depend on the severity of the diabetes. Mild forms can be treated with diet (decreasing the intake of sugars and fats, in particular). Many women are put on strict, detailed **diets,** and are asked to stay within a certain range of calorie intake. **Exercise** is sometimes used to keep blood sugar levels lower. Patients are often asked to regularly measure their blood sugar. This is done by poking a finger with a needle called a lancet, putting a drop of blood on a special type of paper, and feeding the paper into a meter which analyzes and reports the blood sugar level. When diet and exercise do not keep blood glucose levels within an acceptable range, a patient may need to take regular shots of insulin.

Many babies born to women with gestational diabetes are large enough to cause more difficult deliveries, and they may require the use of forceps, suction, or cesarean section. Once the baby is born, it is important to carefully monitor its blood glucose levels. These levels may drop sharply and dangerously once the baby is no longer receiving large quantities of sugar from the mother. When this occurs, it is easily resolved by giving the baby glucose.

Prognosis

Prognosis for women with gestational diabetes, and their babies, is generally good. Almost all such women stop being diabetic after the birth of their baby. However, some research has shown that nearly 50% of these women will develop a permanent form of diabetes within

15 years. The child of a mother with gestational diabetes has a greater-than-normal chance of developing diabetes sometime in adulthood, also. A woman who has had gestational diabetes during one pregnancy has about a 66% chance of having it again during any subsequent pregnancies. Women who had gestational diabetes usually are tested for diabetes at the post-partum checkup or after stopping breastfeeding.

Prevention

There is no known way to actually prevent diabetes, particularly since gestational diabetes is due to the effects of normal hormones of pregnancy. However, the effects of insulin resistance can be best handled through careful attention to diet, avoiding becoming overweight throughout life, and participating in reasonable exercise.

Resources

BOOKS

Ferris, Thomas F. "Gestational Diabetes." In *Harrison's Principles of Internal Medicine,* edited by Anthony S. Fauci, et al. New York: McGraw-Hill, 1998.

Lowe, Ernest and Gary Arsham. *Diabetes: A Guide to Living Well.* Minneapolis: Chronimed Publishing, 1997.

PERIODICALS

Bartholomew, Sallie P. "Make Way for Baby." *Diabetes Forecast* 50, no.12 (December 1997): 20 + .

Morrison, John C. "Prediction of Continued Glucose Intolerance in Women with Gestational Diabetes." *Clinical Diabetes* 14, no. 6 (November/December 1996): 156.

Pasui, Kristine and Kay F. McFarland. "Management of Diabetes in Pregnancy." *American Family Physician* 55, no.8 (June 1997): 2731 +

Weller, Kenneth A. "Diagnosis and Management of Gestational Diabetes." *American Family Physician* 53, no. 6 (May 1, 1996): 2053 + .

ORGANIZATIONS

American Diabetes Association, 1660 Duke Street, Alexandria, VA 22314. (800)DIABETES (800/342-2383).

Rosalyn S. Carson-DeWitt

GI bleeding studies

Definition

GI bleeding studies uses radioactive materials in the investigation of bleeding from the gastrointestinal (GI) tract. These studies go under various names such as "GI bleeding scans" or "Tagged red blood cell scans." They

are performed and interpreted by radiologists (physicians who specialize in diagnosis and treatment of diseases by means of x rays or related substances).

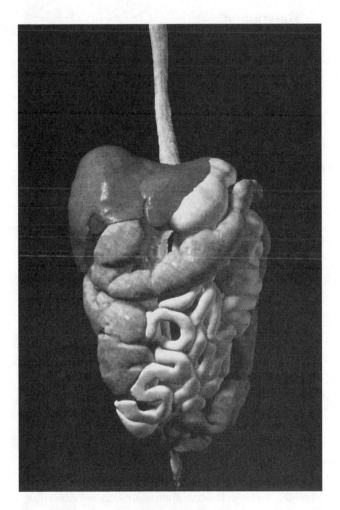

A clay model of the human digestive system. *(Custom Medical Stock Photo. Reproduced by permission.)*

Purpose

These studies are designed to find the source of blood loss from the GI tract; that is the stomach, small bowel, or colon. They work best when bleeding is either too slow, intermittent, or too rapid to be identified by other means, such as endoscopy, upper GI series, or barium enema.

They are particularly useful when other methods have not been able to determine the site or cause of bleeding.

Precautions

Because of the use of radioactive materials, these studies are best avoided in pregnant patients. Another important relates to the interpretation of these tests, whether normal or abnormal. Since these studies are far from perfect, they can only be used as "guides" as to the cause or site of bleeding. In most instances, further studies must be performed to confirm their findings.

Description

Bleeding scans are based on the accumulation of radioactive material as it exits from the vessels during a bleeding episode. Blood is first withdrawn from the patient. Then, the blood, along with a radioactive substance is injected into a vein and over several hours scans measuring radioactivity are performed. The studies were initially reported to be very sensitive and accurate; however, critical evaluation of these tests have shown them to be less accurate than originally believed.

Preparation

No preparation is needed for these tests. They are often done on an "emergency" basis.

Aftercare

No special care is needed after the exam.

Risks

Bleeding scans are free of any risks or side-effects, aside from the fact that they should best be avoided in **pregnancy.**

Normal results

A normal exam would fail to show any evidence of accumulation of radioactive material on the scan. However, scans may be normal in as many as 70% of patients who later turn out to have significant causes of bleeding. This is known as a false-negative result. A patient must be bleeding at the same time the scan is performed for it to be seen. Therefore, not finding evidence of a bleeding source during the study, can be misleading.

Abnormal results

The accumulation of radioactive material indicating a "leakage" of blood from the vessels is abnormal. The scan gives a rough, though not exact, guide as to the location of the bleeding. It can tell where the bleeding may be, but usually not the cause. Thus, extreme caution and skill is needed in interpreting these scans, and decisions involving surgery or other treatment should await more definitive tests.

Resources

BOOKS

Lane, Loren. "Radionuclide Scanning." In *Sleisenger & Fordtran's Gastrointestinal and Liver Disease,* edited by Mark Feldman, et al. Philadelphia: W.B. Saunders Company, 1997, p. 202.

PERIODICALS

Mujica, Victor R. and Barkin, Jamie S. "Occult Gastrointestinal Bleeding." *Gastrointestinal Endoscopy Clinics of North America* (October 1996): 833-845

Shapiro, Marcelle J. "Radionuclide Scans." *Gastroenterology Clinics of North America* (March 1994): 125-128

David S Kaminstein

Giant-cell arteritis *see* **Temporal arteritis**

Giardia lamblia infection *see* **Giardiasis**

Giardiasis

Definition

Giardiasis is a common intestinal infection spread by eating contaminated food, drinking contaminated water, or through direct contact with the organism that causes the disease, *Giardia lamblia*. Giardiasis is found throughout the world and is a common cause of traveller's **diarrhea.** In the United States it is a growing problem, especially among children in childcare centers.

Description

Giardia is one of the most common intestinal parasites in the world, infecting as much as 20% of the entire population of the earth. It is common in overcrowded developing countries with poor sanitation and a lack of

Giardiasis is becoming a growing problem in the United States, where it affects three times more children than adults. In recent years, giardiasis outbreaks have been common among people in schools or daycare centers and at catered affairs and large public picnic areas. Children can easily pass on the infection by touching contaminated toys, changing tables, utensils, or their own feces, and then touching other people. For this reason, infection spreads quickly through a daycare center or institution for the developmentally disabled.

Unfiltered streams or lakes that may be contaminated by human or animal wastes are a common source of infection. Outbreaks can occur among campers and hikers who drink untreated water from mountain streams. While 20 million Americans drink unfiltered city water from streams or rivers, giardiasis outbreaks from tainted city water have been rare. Most of these problems have occurred not due to the absence of filters, but because of malfunctions in city water treatment plants, such as a temporary drop in chlorine levels. It is possible to become infected in a public swimming pool, however, since *Giardia* can survive in chlorinated water for about 15 minutes. During that time, it is possible for an individual to swallow contaminated pool water and become infected.

clean water. Recent tests have found *Giardia* in 7% of all stool samples tested nationwide, indicating that this disease is much more widespread than was originally believed. It has been found not only in humans, but also in wild and domestic animals.

Causes and symptoms

Giardiasis is spread by food or water contaminated by the *Giardia lamblia* protozoan organism found in the human intestinal tract and feces. When the cysts are ingested, the stomach acid degrades the cysts and releases the active parasite into the body. Once within the body, the parasites cling to the lining of the small intestine, reproduce, and are swept into the fecal stream. As the liquid content of the bowel dries up, the parasites form cysts, which are then passed in the feces. Once excreted, the cysts can survive in water for more than three months. The parasite is spread further by direct fecal-oral contamination, such as can occur if food is prepared without adequate hand-washing, or by ingesting the cysts in water or food.

Giardiasis is not fatal, and about two-thirds of infected people exhibit no symptoms. Symptoms will not occur until between one and two weeks after infection. When present, symptoms include explosive, watery diarrhea that can last for a week or more and, in chronic cases, may persist for months. Because the infection interferes with the body's ability to absorb fats from the intestinal tract, the stool is filled with fat. Other symptoms include foul-smelling and greasy feces, stomach **pains,** gas and bloating, loss of appetite, **nausea and vomiting.** In cases in which the infection becomes chronic, lasting for months or years, symptoms might include poor digestion, problems digesting milk, inter-

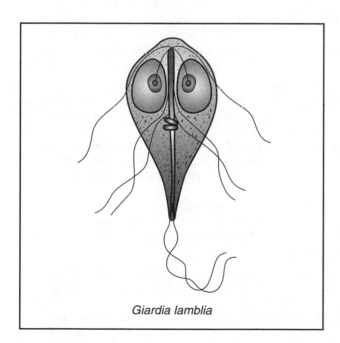

Giardia lamblia

Infection with the protozoan *Giardia lamblia*, shown above, causes diarrhea in humans. *(Illustration by Electronic Illustrators Group).*

mittent diarrhea, fatigue, weakness, and significant weight loss.

Diagnosis

Diagnosis can be difficult because it can be easy to overlook the presence of the giardia cysts during a routine inspection of a stool specimen. In the past, the condition has been diagnosed by examining three stool samples for the presence of the parasites. However, because the organism is shed in some stool samples and not others, the infection may not be discovered using this method.

A newer, more accurate method of diagnosing the condition is the enzyme-linked immunosorbent assay (ELISA) that detects cysts and antigen in stool, and is approximately 90% accurate. While slightly more expensive, it only needs to be done once and is therefore less expensive overall than the earlier test.

Treatment

Acute giardiasis can usually be allowed to run its natural course and tends to clear up on its own. **Antibiotics** are helpful, however, in easing symptoms and preventing the spread of infection. Medications include metronidazole, furazolidone and paromomycin. Healthy carriers with no symptoms do not need antibiotic treatment. If treatment should fail, the patient should wait two weeks and repeat the drug course. Anyone with an impaired immune system (immunocompromised), such as a person with **AIDS,** may need to be treated with a combination of medications.

Prognosis

Giardiasis is rarely fatal, and when treated promptly, antibiotics usually cure the infection. While most people respond quickly to treatment, some have lingering symptoms and suffer with diarrhea and cramps for long periods, losing weight and not growing well. Those most at-risk for a course like this are the elderly, people with a weakened immune system, malnourished children, and anyone with low stomach acid.

Prevention

The best way to avoid giardiasis is to avoid drinking untreated surface water, especially from mountain streams. The condition also can be minimized by practicing the following preventive measures:

• Thoroughly washing hands before handling food

• Maintaining good personal cleanliness

• Boiling any untreated water for at least three minutes

• Properly disposing of fecal material.

Children with severe diarrhea (and others who are unable to control their bowel habits) should be kept at home until the stool returns to normal. If an outbreak occurs in a daycare center, the director should notify the local health department. Some local health departments require a follow-up stool testing to confirm that the person is no longer contagious. People not in high-risk settings can return to their routine activities after recovery.

Resources

BOOKS

Bannister, Barbara A., Norman T. Begg, and Stephen H. Gillespie. *Infectious Disease.* Oxford, England: Blackwell Scientific, Inc., 1996.

Turkington, Carol A. *Infectious Diseases A to Z.* New York: Facts on File, 1998.

Van De Graaff, Kent. *Survey of Infectious and Parasitic Diseases.* New York: McGraw Hill, 1996.

Wilks, David, Mark Farrington, and David Rubenstein. *The Infectious Diseases Manual.* Oxford, England: Blackwell Scientific, Inc., 1995.

PERIODICALS

Hunter, Beatrice Trum. "Giardiasis: The Most Common Parasitic Infection." *Consumers' Research Magazine,* 76 (4)(April 1993): 8-9.

Moser, Penny Ward. "Danger in Diaperland." *In Health,* 5 (5)(Sept.-Oct. 1991).

Pediatrics for Parents editors. "Diarrhea and Day Care Centers." *Pediatrics for Parents,* (June 1991): 6.

Springer, Ilene. "The Summer Vacation Health Guide." *Ladies Home Journal,* 109 (7)(July 1992): 54-57.

Tufts editors. "A Backwoods Parasite Heads for Town." *Tufts University Health & Nutrition Letter,* 15 (6)(August 1997): 3.

ORGANIZATIONS

Centers for Disease Control and Prevention. 1600 Clifton Rd., NE, Atlanta, GA 30333. (404) 639-3311. http://www.cdc.gov/travel/travel.html.

National Institute of Allergies and Infectious Diseases, Division of Microbiology and Infectious Diseases, Bldg. 31, Rm. 7A-50, 31 Center Drive MSC 2520, Bethesda, MD 20892.

World Health Organization, Division of Emerging and Other Communicable Diseases Surveillance and Control. 1211 Geneva 27, Switzerland. http://www.who.ch.

OTHER

Emerging Infectious Diseases Journal, National Center for Infectious Diseases. http://www.cdc.gov/ncidod/EID/eidtext.htm.

International Society of Travel Medicine. http:www.istm.org.

Carol A. Turkington

GIFT *see* Infertility therapies

Gigantism see **Acromegaly and gigantism**

Gilchrist's disease see **Blastomycosis**

Gilles de la Tourette's syndrome see
Tourette syndrome

Gingivitis see **Periodontal disease**

Glaucoma

Definition

Glaucoma is a condition where the optic nerve is subject to damage—usually, but not always, because of excessively high intraocular pressure (pressure within the eye—also called IOP). If untreated, the optic nerve damage results in progressive, permanent vision loss, starting with unnoticeable blind spots at the edges of the field of vision, progressing to tunnel vision, and then to blindness.

Description

Over two million people in the United States have glaucoma, and 80,000 of those are legally blind as a result. It is the leading cause of preventable blindness in the United States and the most frequent cause of blindness in African-Americans, who are at about a three-fold higher risk of glaucoma than the rest of the population. The risk of glaucoma increases dramatically with age, but it can strike any age group, even newborn infants and fetuses.

Glaucoma is actually a class of diseases—there are at least twenty different forms that can be divided into two categories: open-angle glaucoma and narrow-angle glaucoma. To understand what glaucoma is and what these terms mean, it is useful to understand eye structure.

Eyes are sphere-shaped. A tough, non-leaky protective sheath (the sclera) covers the entire eye, except for the clear cornea at the front and the optic nerve at the back. Light comes into the eye through the cornea, then passes through the lens, which focuses it onto the retina (the innermost surface at the back of the eye). The rods and cones of the retina transform the light energy into electrical messages, which are transmitted to the brain by the bundle of nerves known as the optic nerve.

The iris, the colored part of the eye shaped like a round picture frame, is between the dome-shaped cornea and the lens. It controls the amount of light that enters the eye by opening and closing its central hole (pupil) like the diaphragm in a camera. The iris, cornea, and lens are bathed in a liquid called the aqueous humor, which is somewhat similar to plasma. This liquid is continually produced by nearby ciliary tissues and moved out of the eye into the bloodstream by a system of drainage canals (called the trabecular meshwork). The drainage area is located in front of the iris, in the angle formed between the iris and the point at which the iris appears to meet the inside of the cornea.

Glaucoma occurs if the aqueous humor is not removed rapidly enough or if it is made too rapidly, causing pressure to build-up. The high pressure distorts the shape of the optic nerve and destroys the nerve. Destroyed nerve cells result in blind spots in places where the image from the retina is not being transmitted to the brain.

Open-angle glaucoma accounts for over 90% of all cases. It is called "open-angle" because the angle between the iris and the cornea is open, allowing drainage of the aqueous humor. It is usually chronic and progresses slowly. In narrow-angle glaucoma, the angle where aqueous fluid drainage occurs is narrow, and therefore may drain slowly or may be at risk of becoming closed. A closed-angle glaucoma attack is usually acute, occurring when the drainage area is blocked. This can occur, for example, if the iris and lens suddenly adhere to each other and the iris is pushed forward. In patients with very narrow angles, this can occur when the eyes dilate (e.g., when entering a dark room, or if taking certain medications).

One rare form of open-angle glaucoma is different. People with normal-tension glaucoma have optic nerve damage in the presence of normal IOP. As of 1998, the mechanism of this disease is a mystery.

Glaucoma is also a secondary condition of over 60 widely diverse diseases and can also result from injury.

Causes & symptoms

Causes

The cause of vision loss in all forms of glaucoma is optic nerve damage. There are many underlying causes and forms of glaucoma. Most causes of glaucoma are not known, but it is clear that a number of different processes are involved, and a malfunction in any one of them could cause glaucoma. For example, trauma to the eye could result in the angle becoming blocked, or, as a person ages, the lens becomes larger and may push the iris forward. The cause of optic nerve damage in normal-tension glaucoma is also unknown, but there is speculation that the optic nerves of these patients are susceptible to damage at lower pressures than what is usually considered to be abnormally high.

KEY TERMS

Agonist—A drug that mimics one of the body's own molecules.

Alpha-2 agonist (alpha-2 adrenergic receptor agonist)—A class of drugs that bind to and stimulate alpha-2 adrenergic receptors, causing responses similar to those of adrenaline and noradrenaline. They inhibit aqueous humor production and a have a wide variety of effects, including dry mouth, fatigue, and drowsiness.

Aqueous humor—A transparent liquid, contained within the eye, that is composed of water, sugars, vitamins, proteins, and other nutrients.

Betablocker (beta-adrenergic blocker)—A class of drugs that bind beta-adrenergic receptors and thereby decrease the ability of the body's own natural epinephrine to bind to those receptors, leading to inhibition of various processes in the body's sympathetic system. Betablockers can slow the heart rate, constrict airways in the lungs, lower blood pressure, and reduce aqueous secretion by ciliary tissues in the eye.

Carbonic anhydrase inhibitor—A class of diuretic drugs that inhibit the enzyme carbonic anhydrase, an enzyme involved in producing bicarbonate, which is required for aqueous humor production by the ciliary tissues in the eye. Thus, inhibitors of this enzyme inhibit aqueous humor production. Some side effects are urinary frequency, kidney stones, loss of the sense of taste, depression, and anemia.

Cornea—Clear, bowl-shaped structure at the front of the eye. It is located in front of the colored part of the eye (iris). The cornea lets light into the eye and partially focuses it.

Gonioscope—An instrument used to examine the trabecular meshwork; consists of a magnifier and a lens equipped with mirrors, which sits on the patient's cornea.

Hyperosmotic drugs—Refers to a class of drugs for glaucoma that increase the osmotic pressure in the blood, which then pulls water from the eye into the blood.

Iris—The colored part of the eye just behind the cornea and in front of the lens that controls the amount of light sent to the retina.

Lens (the crystalline lens)—A transparent structure in the eye that focuses light onto the retina.

Miotic—A drug that causes pupils to contract.

Ophthalmoscope—An instrument, with special lighting, designed to view structures in the back of the eye.

Optic nerve—The nerve that carries visual messages from the retina to the brain.

Prostaglandin—A group of molecules that exert local effects on a variety of processes including fluid balance, blood flow, and gastrointestinal function.

Prostaglandin analogue—A class of drugs that are similar in structure and function to prostaglandin.

Retina—The inner, light-sensitive layer of the eye containing rods and cones.

Sclera—The tough, fibrous, white outer protective covering that surrounds the eye.

Tonometry—The measurement of pressure.

Trabecular meshwork—A sponge-like tissue located near the cornea and iris that functions to drain the aqueous humor from the eye into the blood.

It is probable that most glaucoma is inherited. At least ten defective genes that cause glaucoma have been identified.

Symptoms

At first, chronic open-angle glaucoma is without noticeable symptoms. The pressure build-up is gradual and there is no discomfort. Moreover, the vision loss is too gradual to be noticed and each eye fills-in the image where its partner has a blind spot. However, if it's not treated, vision loss becomes evident, and the condition can be very painful.

On the other hand, acute closed-angle glaucoma is obvious from the beginning of an attack. The symptoms are blurred vision, severe pain, sensitivity to light, nausea, and halos around lights. The normally clear corneas may be hazy. This is an ocular emergency and needs to be treated immediately.

Similarly, congenital glaucoma is evident at birth. Symptoms are bulging eyes, cloudy corneas, excessive tearing, and sensitivity to light.

Diagnosis

Intraocular pressure, visual field defects, and the appearance of the optic nerve are all considered in the diagnosis of glaucoma. IOP is measured with an instrument known as a tonometer. One type of tonometer involves numbing the eye with an eyedrop that has a

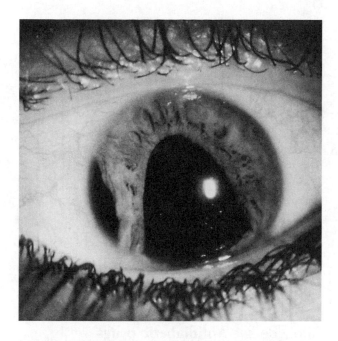

A close-up view of an inflamed eye with acute glaucoma and an irregularly enlarged pupil. *(Custom Medical Stock Photo. Reproduced by permission.)*

yellow coloring in it and touching the cornea with a small probe. This quick test is a routine part of an **eye examination** and is usually included without extra charge in the cost of a visit to an ophthalmologist or optometrist.

Ophthalmoscopes, hand-held instruments with a light source, are used to detect optic nerve damage by looking through the pupil. The optic nerve is examined for changes; the remainder of the back of the eye can be examined as well. Other types of lenses that can be used to examine the back of the eye may also be used. A slit lamp will allow the doctor to examine the front of the eye (i.e., cornea, iris, and lens).

Visual field tests (perimetry) can detect blind spots in a patient's field of vision before the patient is aware of them. Certain defects may indicate glaucoma.

Another test, gonioscopy, can distinguish between narrow-angle and open-angle glaucoma. A gonioscope, which is a hand-held contact lens with a mirror, allows visualization of the angle between the iris and the cornea.

Intraocular pressure can vary throughout the day. For that reason, the doctor may have a patient return for several visits to measure the IOP at different times of the day.

Treatment

Medications

When glaucoma is diagnosed, drugs, typically given as eye drops, are usually tried before surgery. Several classes of medications are effective at lowering IOP and thus preventing optic nerve damage in chronic and neonatal glaucoma. **Beta blockers,** like Timoptic; carbonic anhydrase inhibitors, like acetazolamide; and alpha-2 agonists, such as Alphagan, inhibit the production of aqueous humor. Miotics, like pilocarpine, and prostaglandin analogues, like Xalatan, increase the outflow of aqueous humor.

It is important for patients to tell their doctors about any conditions they have or medications they are taking. Certain drugs used to treat glaucoma would not be prescribed for patients with pre-existing conditions. All of these drugs mentioned above have side effects, some of which are rare but serious and potentially life-threatening, so patients taking them should be monitored closely, especially for cardiovascular, pulmonary, and behavioral symptoms. Different medications lower IOP different amounts, and a combination of medications may be necessary. It is important that patients take their medications and be monitored, to be sure that the IOP is lowered sufficiently. IOP should be measured three to four times per year.

As of 1998, normal-tension glaucoma is treated in the same way as chronic high-intraocular-pressure glaucoma. This reduces IOP to less-than-normal levels, on the theory that overly susceptible optic nerves are less likely to be damaged at lower pressures. Research underway may point to better treatments for this form of glaucoma.

Attacks of acute closed-angle glaucoma are medical emergencies. IOP is rapidly lowered by successive deployment of acetazolamide, hyperosmotic agents, a topical beta-blocker, and pilocarpine. Epinephrine should not be used because it exacerbates angle closure.

Surgery

Laser surgery or microsurgery to open-up the drainage canals or make an opening in the iris can be effective in increasing the outflow of aqueous humor. These surgeries are usually successful, but the effects often last less than a year. Nevertheless, they are an effective treatment for patients whose IOP is not sufficiently lowered by drugs and for those who can't tolerate the drugs. Because all surgeries have risks, patients should speak to their doctors about the procedure being performed.

Sight lost due to glaucoma cannot be restored.

Alternative treatment

Vitamin C, vitamin B_1 (thiamine), chromium, zinc, and rutin may reduce IOP.

There is evidence that marijuana lowers IOP, too. However, marijuana has serious side effects and contains carcinogens, and any IOP-lowering medication must be taken continually to avoid optic nerve damage. Although the Food and Drug Administration (FDA) and National Institutes of Health (NIH) currently recommend against treating glaucoma with marijuana, they are supporting research to learn more about it and to determine the feasibility of separating the components that lower IOP from components that produce side effects and carcinogens.

Any glaucoma patient using alternative methods to attempt to prevent optic nerve damage should also be under the care of a traditionally trained ophthalmologist or optometrist who is licensed to treat glaucoma, so that IOP and optic nerve damage can be monitored.

Prognosis

About half of the people stricken by glaucoma are not aware of it. For them, the prognosis is not good, and many of them will become blind. On the other hand, the prognosis for treated glaucoma is excellent.

Prevention

Because glaucoma may not initially result in symptoms, the best form of prevention is to have regular eye exams.

Patients with narrow angles should avoid certain medications (even over-the-counter medications, such as some cold or allergy medications). Any person who is glaucoma-susceptible (i.e. narrow angles and borderline IOPs) should read the warning labels on over-the-counter medicines and inform their physicians of products they are considering taking. Steroids may also raise IOP, so patients may need to be monitored more frequently if it is necessary to use steroids.

Not enough is known about the underlying mechanisms of glaucoma to prevent the disease itself. However, prevention of optic nerve damage from glaucoma is essential and can be effectively accomplished when the condition is diagnosed and treated. As more is learned about the genes that cause glaucoma, it will become possible to test DNA and identify potential glaucoma victims, so they can be treated even before their IOP becomes elevated.

Resources

BOOKS

Epstein, David L., R. Rand Allingham, and Joel S. Schuman. *Chandler and Grant's Glaucoma,* 4th ed. Baltimore: Williams & Wilkins, 1997.

Marks, Edith and Rita Montauredes. *Coping with Glaucoma.* Garden City Park, NY: Avery, 1997.

ORGANIZATIONS

American Academy of Ophthalmology. P.O. Box 7424, San Francisco, CA 94120-7424. (415) 561-8500. http://www.eyenet.org/aao_index.html.

Glaucoma Research Foundation. 490 Post Street, Suite 830, San Francisco, CA 94102. (415) 986-3162, (800) 826-6693. info@glaucoma.org. http://www.glaucoma.org/.

Prevent Blindness America. 500 East Remington Road, Schaumburg, IL 60173. (800) 331-2020. http://www.prevent-blindness.org.

OTHER

Titcomb, Lucy. "Treatment of Glaucoma." *Pharmacy Magazine.* http://www.pharmacymag.co.uk/glau.htm (29 April 1998).

Lorraine Lica

Glaucoma surgery *see* **Trabeculectomy**

Glioblastoma *see* **Brain tumor**

Glioma *see* **Brain tumor**

Glipizide *see* **Antidiabetic drugs**

Glomerulonephritis

Definition

Acute glomerulonephritis is an inflammatory disease of both kidneys predominantly affecting children from ages 2–12. Chronic glomerulonephritis can develop over a period of 10–20 years and is most often associated with other systemic disease, including diabetes, **malaria,** hepatitis, or **systemic lupus erythematosus.**

Description

Acute glomerulonephritis is an inflammation of the glomeruli, bundles of tiny vessels inside the kidneys. The damaged glomeruli cannot effectively filter waste products and excess water from the bloodstream to make urine. The kidneys appear enlarged, fatty, and congested.

Causes & symptoms

Acute glomerulonephritis most often follows a streptococcal infection of the throat or skin. In children, it is most often associated with an upper respiratory infection, **tonsillitis,** or **scarlet fever.** Kidney symptoms usually begin two to three weeks after the initial infection. Exposure to certain paints, glue or other organic solvents may also be the causative agent. It is thought that the kidney is damaged with exposure to the toxins that are excreted into the urine.

Mild glomerulonephritis may produce no symptoms, and diagnosis is made with laboratory studies of the urine and blood. Individuals with more severe cases of the disease may exhibit:

- Fatigue
- **Nausea and vomiting**
- **Shortness of breath**
- Disturbed vision
- High blood pressure
- Swelling, especially noted in the face, hands, feet, and ankles

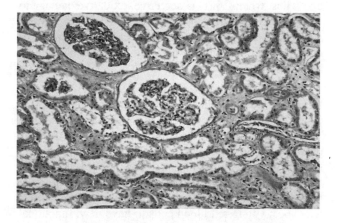

A close-up view of glomerulonephritis affecting the kidney. (*Custom Medical Stock Photo. Reproduced by permission.*)

- Blood and protein in the urine, resulting in a smoky or slightly red appearance.

The individual with chronic glomerulonephritis may discover their condition with a routine physical exam revealing high blood pressure, or an eye exam showing vascular or hemorrhagic changes. The kidneys may be reduced to as little as one-fifth their normal size, consisting largely of fibrous tissues.

Diagnosis

Diagnosis of glomerulonephritis is established based on medical history, combined with laboratory studies. A "dipstick" test of urine will reveal increased protein levels. A 24 hour urine collection allows measurement of the excretion of proteins and creatinine. Creatinine clearance from the bloodstream by the kidneys is considered an index of the glomerular filtration rate. Blood studies may reveal a low **blood count,** and may also be checked for the presence of a streptococcal antibody titer(a sophisticated blood test indicating presence of streptococcal infection). A **kidney biopsy** may also be performed, using ultrasound to guide the needle for obtaining the specimen.

Treatment

The main objectives in the treatment of acute glomerulonephritis are to:

- Decrease the damage to the glomeruli
- Decrease the metabolic demands on the kidneys
- Improve kidney function.

Bedrest helps in maintaining adequate blood flow to the kidney. If residual infection is suspected, antibiotic therapy may be needed. In the presence of fluid overload, **diuretics** may be used to increase output with urination. Iron and vitamin supplements may be ordered if anemia develops, and antihypertensives, if high blood pressure accompanies the illness. In order to rest the kidney during the acute phase, decreased sodium and protein intake may be recommended. The amount of protein allowed is dependent upon the amount lost in the urine, and the requirements of the individual patient. Sodium limitations depend on the amount of **edema** present. Fluid restrictions are adjusted according to the patient's urinary output and body weight.

An accurate daily record of the patient's weight, fluid intake and urinary output assist in estimating kidney function. The patient must be watched for signs of complications and recurrent infection. As edema is reduced and the urine becomes free of protein and red blood cells, the patient is allowed to increase activity. A woman who has had glomerulonephritis requires special medical attention during **pregnancy.**

Prognosis

In acute glomerulonephritis, symptoms usually subside in two weeks to several months, with 90% of children recovering without complications and adults recovering more slowly. Chronic glomerulonephritis is a disease that tends to progress slowly, so that there are no symptoms until the kidneys can no longer function. The resultant renal failure may require dialysis or kidney transplant.

Prevention

Prevention of glomerulonephritis is best accomplished by avoiding upper respiratory infections, as well as other acute and chronic infections, especially those of a streptococcal origin. Cultures of the infection site, usually the throat, should be obtained and antibiotic sensibility of the offending organism determined. Prompt medical assessment for necessary antibiotic therapy should be sought when infection is suspected. The use of prophylactic immunizations is recommended as appropriate.

Resources

BOOKS

Branch, William. *Office Practice of Medicine*. Philadelphia: W. B. Saunders, 1982.

Brunner, Lillian & Doris Suddarth. *Textbook of Medical-Surgical Nursing*. Philadelphia: J. B. Lippincott, 1975.

ORGANIZATIONS

American Association of Kidney Patients. 100 S. Ashley Dr., #280, Tampa, FL 33602. (800)749-2257 or (813)223-7099.

American Kidney Fund. 6110 Executive Blvd. #1010, Rockville, MD 20852. (800)638-8299, or (301)881-3052.

National Kidney Foundation. 30 E. 33rd St., New York, NY 10016. (800)652-9010 or (212)889-2210.

National Kidney Foundation and Urologic Diseases Information Clearinghouse. 3 Information Way, Bethesda, MD 20892-3580. (301)654-4415.

OTHER

Glomerulonephritis www.healthtouch.com (29March1998).

Glomerulonephritis www.thriveonline.com (29March1998)

Kathleen Dredge Wright

Glossopharyngeal neuralgia *see* **Neuralgia**

Glucose loading test *see* **Growth hormone tests**

Glucose-6-phosphate dehydrogenase deficiency

Definition

Glucose-6-phosphate dehydrogenase deficiency is an inherited condition caused by a defect or defects in the gene that codes for the enzyme, glucose-6-phosphate dehydrogenase (G6PD). It can cause **hemolytic anemia,** varying in severity from life-long anemia, to rare bouts of anemia to total unawareness of the condition. The episodes of hemolytic anemia are usually triggered by oxidants, infection, or by eating fava beans.

Description

G6PD deficiency is the most common enzyme deficiency in the world, with about 400 million people living with it. It is most prevalent in people of African, Mediterranean, and Asian ancestry. The incidence in different populations varies from zero in South American Indians to less than 0.1% of Northern Europeans to about 50% of Kurdish males. In the United States, it is most common among African American males; about 11 to 14% are G6PD-deficient.

G6PD deficiency is a recessive sex-linked trait. Thus, males have only one copy of the G6PD gene, but females have two copies. Recessive genes are masked in the presence of a gene that encodes normal G6PD. Accordingly, females with one copy of the gene for G6PD deficiency are usually normal, while males with one copy have the trait.

G6PD is present in all human cells but is particularly important to red blood cells. It is required to make NADPH in red blood cells but not in other cells. It is also required to make glutathione. Glutathione and NADPH both help protect red blood cells against oxidative damage. Thus, when G6PD is defective, oxidative damage to red blood cells readily occurs, and they break open as a result. This event is called hemolysis, and multiple hemolyses in a short time span constitute an episode of hemolytic anemia.

As of 1998, there are almost 100 different known forms of G6PD enzyme molecules encoded by defective G6PD genes, yet not one of them is completely inactive. This suggests that G6PD is indispensable. Many G6PD defective enzymes are deficient in their stability rather than their initial ability to function. Since red blood cells lack nuclei, they, unlike other cells, cannot synthesize new enzyme molecules to replace defective ones. Hence, we expect young red blood cells to have new, functional G6PD and older cells to have non-functioning G6PD. This explains why episodes of hemolytic anemia are frequently self-limiting; new red blood cells are gener-

KEY TERMS

Bilirubin—A breakdown product derived from hemoglobin; removed from the blood by the liver.

Enzyme—A protein catalyst; one of the two kinds of biological catalysts, which are exceedingly specific; each different enzyme only catalyzes one or two specific reactions.

Enzyme activity—A measure of the ability of an enzyme to catalyze a specific reaction.

Glutathione—A molecule that acts as a co-enzyme in cellular oxidation-reduction reactions.

Hemolysis—Lysis (opening) of red blood cells, with concomitant leakage of cell contents from the cells.

Hemolytic anemia—Anemia due to hemolysis.

Jaundice—Yellowish skin color due to liver disease.

Neonatal—Describes babies just after they are born.

Recessive trait—An inherited trait that is outwardly obvious only when two copies of the gene for that trait are present—as opposed to a dominant trait where one copy of the gene for the dominant trait is sufficient to display the trait. The recessive condition is said to be masked by the presence of the dominant gene when both are present; i.e., the recessive condition is seen only in the absence of the dominant gene.

Sex-linked—Refers to genes or traits carried on one of the sex chromosomes, usually the X.

X chromosome—One of the two types of sex chromosomes, present twice in female cells and once in male cells.

ated with enzymes able to afford protection from oxidation.

The geographic distribution of G6PD deficiency, allowing for migration, coincides with the geographic distribution of **malaria.** This fact and survival statistics suggest that G6PD deficiency protects against malaria.

Glucose-6-phosphate dehydrogenase deficiency is also known as G6PD deficiency, favism, and primaquine sensitivity.

Causes & symptoms

Causes

G6PD deficiency is caused by one copy of a defective G6PD gene in males or two copies of a defective G6PD gene in females. Hemolytic anemic attacks can be caused by oxidants, infection, and or by eating fava beans.

Symptoms

The most significant consequence of this disorder is hemolytic anemia, which is usually episodic, but the vast majority of people with G6PD deficiency have no symptoms.

The many different forms of G6PD deficiency have been divided into five classes according to severity.

* Class 1—enzyme deficiency with chronic hemolytic anemia

* Class 2—severe enzyme deficiency with less than 10% of normal activity

* Class 3—moderate to mild enzyme deficiency with 10–60% of normal activity

* Class 4—very mild or no enzyme deficiency

* Class 5—increased enzyme activity Fortunately, only a small number of people fall into Class 1.

The major symptoms of hemolytic anemia are **jaundice,** dark urine, abdominal **pain,** back pain, lowered red blood cell count, and elevated bilirubin. People who suffer from severe and chronic forms of G6PD deficiency in addition may have **gallstones,** enlarged spleens, defective white blood cells, and **cataracts.**

Attacks of hemolytic anemia are serious for infants. Brain damage and **death** are possible but preventable outcomes. Newborns with G6PD deficiency are about 1.5 times as likely to get **neonatal jaundice** than newborns without G6PD deficiency.

Diagnosis

Blood tests can detect G6PD deficiency, either by measuring the G6PD enzyme activity between episodes or by measuring bilirubin during an episode. Such tests cost about $50.00. Family histories are helpful, too.

Treatment

In a typical attack of hemolytic anemia, no treatment is needed; the patient will recover in about eight days. However, blood **transfusions** are necessary in severe cases. Recent success treating elevated bilirubin in newborns by exposing them to bright light has decreased the need for neonatal transfusions.

Alternative treatment

Vitamin E and folic acid (both anti-oxidants) may help decrease hemolysis in G6PD-deficient individuals.

Prognosis

The prognosis for almost everyone with G6PD deficiency is excellent. Large studies have shown that G6PD-deficient individuals do not acquire any illnesses more frequently than the rest of the population. In fact the opposite may be true for some diseases like ischemic heart disease and cerebrovascular disease.

Prevention

Most episodes of hemolytic anemia can be prevented by avoiding fava beans, oxidant drugs, and oxidant chemicals. All of the following oxidants can trigger attacks: acetanilid, dapsone, doxorubicin, furazolidone, methylene blue, nalidixic acid, napthalene, niridazole, nitrofurantoin, phenazopyridine, phenylhydrazine, primaquine, quinidine, quinine, sulfacetamide, sulfamethoxazole, sulfonamide, sulfapyridine, thiazolesulfone, toluidine blue, and trinitrotoluene. Since infections also trigger hemolytic attacks and have other dire consequences, sometimes it is advisable to use one of the listed drugs.

It is especially important to screen newborns who are likely to have G6PD deficiency to ensure that G6PD-deficient babies won't be subjected to any of the triggers of hemolytic anemia. Pregnant women, especially in areas where G6PD deficiency is prevalent, should avoid eating fava beans.

Resources

BOOKS

Luzzatto, Lucio and Atul Mehta. ''Glucose 6-Phosphate Dehydrogenase Deficiency.'' In *The Metabolic and Molecular Bases of Inherited Disease,* 7th ed. Edited by Scriver, Charles R., Arthur L. Beaudet, William S. Sly, and David Valle. New York: McGraw-Hill, 1995.

ORGANIZATIONS

Alliance of Genetic Support Groups (AGSG). 4301 Connecticut Avenue, NW, Suite 404; Washington, DC 20008. (202)966-5557; (800)336-4363. http://www.geneticalliance.org.

OTHER

Favism Home Page. http://rialto.com/favism/index.htm.

Gene Card for G6PD. http://bioinfo.weizmann.ac.il/cgi-bin/lvrebhan/carddisp?G6PD&search = G6PD + deficiency.

Lorraine Lica

Glucosylcerebroside lipidosis *see* **Gaucher disease**

Gluten enteropathy *see* **Celiac disease**

Gluten-free diet *see* **Diets**

Glyburide *see* **Antidiabetic drugs**

Glycogen storage diseases

Definition

Glycogen serves as the primary fuel reserve for the body's energy needs. Glycogen storage diseases, also known as glycogenoses, are genetically linked metabolic disorders that involve the enzymes regulating glycogen metabolism. Symptoms vary by the glycogen storage disease (GSD) type and can include muscle cramps and wasting, enlarged liver, and low blood sugar. Disruption of glycogen metabolism also affects other biochemical pathways as the body seeks alternative fuel sources. Accumulation of abnormal metabolic by-products can damage the kidneys and other organs. GSD can be fatal, but the risk hinges on the type of GSD.

Description

Most of the body's cells rely on glucose as an energy source. Glucose levels in the blood are very stringently controlled within a range or 70–100 mg/dL, primarily by hormones such as insulin and glucagon. Immediately after a meal, blood glucose levels rise and exceed the body's immediate energy requirements. In a process analogous to putting money in the bank, the body bundles up the extra glucose and stores it as glycogen in the liver and muscles. Later, as the blood glucose levels begin to dip, the body makes a withdrawal from its glycogen savings.

The system for glycogen metabolism relies on a complex system of enzymes. These enzymes are responsible for creating glycogen from glucose, transporting the glycogen to and from storage areas within cells, and extracting glucose from the glycogen as needed. Both creating and tearing down the glycogen macromolecule are multistep processes requiring a different enzyme at each step. If one of these enzymes is defective and fails to complete its step, the process halts. Such enzyme defects are the underlying cause of GSDs.

The enzyme defect arises from an error in its gene. Since the error is in the genetic code, GSDs can be passed down from generation-to-generation. However, all but one GSD are linked to autosomal genes, which means a person inherits one copy of the gene from each parent. Following a Mendelian inheritance pattern, the normal

KEY TERMS

Amniocentesis—A medical test done during pregnancy in which a small sample of the amniotic fluid is taken from around the fetus. The fluid contains fetal cells that can be examined for genetic abnormalities.

Autosomal gene—A gene found on one of the 22 autosomal chromosome pairs; i.e., not on a sex (X or Y) chromosome.

Chorionic villus sampling—A medical test done during pregnancy in which a sample of the membrane surrounding the fetus is removed for examination. This examination can reveal genetic fetal abnormalities.

Glucose—A form of sugar that serves as the body's main energy source.

Glycogen—A macromolecule composed mainly of glucose that serves as the storage form of glucose that is not immediately needed by the body.

Glycogenolysis—The process of tearing-down a glycogen molecule to free up glucose.

Glycogenosis—An alternate term for glycogen storage disease. The plural form is glycogenoses.

Gout—A painful condition in which uric acid precipitates from the blood and accumulates in joints and connective tissues.

Mendelian inheritance—An inheritance pattern for autosomal gene pairs. The genetic trait displayed results from one parent's gene dominating over the gene inherited from the other parent.

Osteoporosis—A disease in which the bones become weak and brittle.

Renal disease—Kidney disease.

Transgenic animal—Animals that have had genes from other species inserted into their genetic code.

gene is dominant and the defective gene is recessive. As long as a child receives at least one normal gene, there is no risk for a GSD. GSDs appear only if a person inherits a defective gene from both parents.

The most common forms of GSD are Types I, II, III, and IV, which may account for more than 90% of all cases. The most common form is Type I, or von Gierke's disease, which occurs in one out of every 100,000 births. Other forms, such as Types VI and IX, are so rare that reliable statistics are not available. The overall frequency of all forms of glycogen storage disease is approximately one in 20,000–25,000 live births.

Causes & symptoms

GSD symptoms depend on the enzyme affected. Since glycogen storage occurs mainly in muscles and the liver, those sites display the most prominent symptoms.

There are at least 10 different types of GSDs which are classified according to the enzyme affected:

- Type Ia, or von Gierke's disease, is caused by glucose-6-phosphatase deficiency in the liver, kidney, and small intestine. The last step in glycogenolysis, the breaking down of glycogen to glucose, is the transformation of glucose-6-phosphate to glucose. In GSD I, that step does not occur. As a result, the liver is clogged with excess glycogen and becomes enlarged and fatty. Other symptoms include low blood sugar and elevated levels of lactate, lipids, and uric acid in the blood. Growth is impaired, **puberty** is often delayed, and bones may be weakened by **osteoporosis.** Blood platelets are also affected and frequent **nosebleeds** and easy bruising are common. Primary symptoms improve with age, but after age 20–30, liver tumors, **liver cancer,** chronic renal disease, and **gout** may appear.

- Type Ib is caused by glucose-6-phosphatase translocase deficiency. In order to carry out the final step of glycogenolysis, glucose-6-phosphate has to be transported into a cell's endoplasmic reticulum. If translocase, the enzyme responsible for that movement, is missing or defective, the same symptoms occur as in Type Ia. Additionally, the immune system is weakened and victims are susceptible to bacterial infections, such as **pneumonia,** mouth and gum infections, and inflammatory bowel disease. Types Ic and Id are also caused by defects in the translocase system.

- Type II, or Pompe's disease or acid maltase deficiency, is caused by lysosomal alpha-D-glucosidase deficiency in skeletal and heart muscles. GSD II is subdivided according to the age of onset. In the infantile form, infants seem normal at birth, but within a few months they develop muscle weakness, trouble breathing, and an enlarged heart. Cardiac failure and **death** usually occur before age 2, despite medical treatment. The juvenile and adult forms of GSD II affect mainly the skeletal muscles in the body's limbs and torso. Unlike the infantile form, treatment can extend life, but there is no cure. **Respiratory failure** is the primary cause of death.

- Type III, or Cori's disease, is caused by glycogen debrancher enzyme deficiency in the liver, muscles, and some blood cells, such as leukocytes and erythrocytes. About 15% of GSD III cases only involve the liver. The glycogen molecule is not a simple straight chain of linked glucose molecules, but rather an intricate network of short chains that branch off from one another.

In glycogenolysis, a particular enzyme is required to unlink the branch points. When that enzyme fails, symptoms similar to GSD I occur; in childhood, it may be difficult to distinguish the two GSDs by symptoms alone. In addition to the low blood sugar, retarded growth, and enlarged liver causing a swollen abdomen, GSD III also causes muscles prone to wasting, an enlarged heart, and heightened levels of lipids in the blood. The muscle wasting increases with age, but the other symptoms become less severe.

• Type IV, or Andersen's disease, is caused by glycogen brancher enzyme deficiency in the liver, brain, heart, skeletal muscles, and skin fibroblasts. The glycogen constructed in GSD IV is abnormal and insoluble. As it accumulates in the cells, cell death leads to organ damage. Infants born with GSD IV appear normal at birth, but are diagnosed with enlarged livers and **failure to thrive** within their first year. Infants who survive beyond their first birthday develop **cirrhosis** of the liver by age 3–5 and die as a result of chronic liver failure.

• Type V, or McArdle's disease, is caused by glycogen phosphorylase deficiency in skeletal muscles. Under normal circumstances, muscles cells rely on oxidation of fatty acids during rest or light activity. More demanding activity requires that they draw on their glycogen stockpile. In GSD V, this form of glycogenolysis is disabled and glucose is not available. The main symptoms are muscle weakness and cramping brought on by **exercise,** as well as burgundy-colored urine after exercise due to myoglobin (a breakdown product of muscle) in the urine.

• Type VI, or Hers' disease, is caused by liver phosphorylase deficiency, which blocks the first step of glycogenolysis. In contrast to other GSDs, Type VI seems to be linked to the X chromosome. Low blood sugar is one of the key symptoms, but it is not as severe as in some other forms of GSD. An enlarged liver and mildly retarded growth also occur.

• Type VII, or Tarui's disease, is caused by muscle phosphofructokinase deficiency. Although glucose may be available as a fuel in muscles, the cells cannot metabolize it. Therefore, abnormally high levels of glycogen are stockpiled in the muscle cells. The symptoms are similar to GSD V, but also include anemia and increased levels of uric acid.

• Types VIII and XI are caused by defects of enzymes in the liver phosphorylase activating-deactivating cascade and have symptoms similar to GSD VI.

• Type IX is caused by liver glycogen phosphorylase kinase deficiency and, symptom-wise, is very similar to GSD VI. The main differences are that the symptoms may not be as severe and may also include exercise-related problems in the muscles, such as **pain** and cramps. The symptoms abate after puberty with proper treatment. Most cases of GSD IX are linked to the X chromosome and therefore affect males.

• Type X is caused by a defect in the cyclic adenosine monophosphate-dependent (AMP) kinase enzyme and presents symptoms similar to GSDs VI and IX.

Diagnosis

Diagnosis usually occurs in infancy or childhood, although some milder types of GSD go unnoticed well into adulthood and old age. It is even conceivable that some of the milder GSDs are never diagnosed.

The four major symptoms that typically lead a doctor to suspect GSDs are low blood sugar, enlarged liver, retarded growth, and an abnormal blood biochemistry profile. A definitive diagnosis is obtained by biopsy of the affected organ or organs. The biopsy sample is tested for its glycogen content and assayed for enzyme activity. There are DNA-based techniques for diagnosing some GSDs from more easily available samples, such as blood or skin. These DNA techniques can also be used for prenatal testing.

Treatment

Some GSD types cannot be treated, while others are relatively easy to control through symptom management. In more severe cases, receiving an organ transplant is the only option. In the most severe cases, there are no available treatments and the victim dies within the first few years of life.

Of the treatable types of GSD, many are treated by manipulating the diet. The key to managing GSD I is to maintain consistent levels of blood glucose through a combination of nocturnal intragastric feeding (usually for infants and children), frequent high-carbohydrate meals during the day, and regular oral doses of cornstarch (people over age 2). Juvenile and adult forms of GSD II can be managed somewhat by a high protein diet, which also helps in cases of GSD III, GSD VI, and GSD IX. GSD V and GSD VII can also be managed with a high protein diet and by avoiding strenuous exercise.

For GSD cases in which dietary therapy is ineffective, organ transplantation may be the only viable alternative. Liver transplants have been effective in reversing the symptoms of GSD IV.

Advances in genetic therapy offer hope for effective treatment in the future. This therapy involves using viruses to deliver a correct form of the gene to affected cells. Another potential therapy utilizes transgenic animals to produce correct copies of the defective enzyme in their milk. In late 1997, a Dutch pharmaceutical company, Pharming Health Care Products, began clinical trials to treat GSD II with human alpha-glucosidase derived from the milk of transgenic rabbits. Researchers at Duke University in North Carolina are also focusing on a treatment for Pompe's disease and, aided by Synpac Pharmaceuticals Limited of the United Kingdom, plan to begin clinical trials of a recombinant form of the enzyme in 1998.

Prognosis

People with well-managed, treatable types of GSD can lead long, relatively normal lives. This goal is accomplished with the milder types of GSD, such as Types VI, IX, and X. As the GSD type becomes more severe, a greater level of vigilance against infections and other complications is required. Given current treatment options, complications such as liver disease, **heart failure,** and respiratory failure may not be warded-off indefinitely. Quality of life and life expectancy are substantially decreased.

Prevention

Because GSD is an inherited condition, it is not preventable. If both parents carry the defective gene, there is a one-in-four chance that their offspring will inherit the disorder. Other children may be carriers or they may miss inheriting the gene altogether.

Through chorionic villi sampling and **amniocentesis,** the disorder can be detected prior to birth. Some types of GSD can be detected even before conception occurs, if both parents are tested for the presence of the defective gene. Before undergoing such testing, the prospective parents should meet with a genetic counselor and other professionals in order to make an informed decision.

Resources

BOOKS

Chen, Yuan-Tsong, and Ann Burchell. "Glycogen Storage Diseases." In *The Metabolic and Molecular Bases of Inherited Disease,* 7th Edition, edited by Charles R. Scriver, et al. New York: McGraw-Hill, Health Professions Division, 1995.

PERIODICALS

Goldberg, Teresia, and Alfred Slonim. "Nutrition Therapy for Hepatic Glycogen Storage Diseases." *Journal of the American Dietetic Association* 93 (12)(December 1993): 1423.

Talente, Gregg M., Rosalind A. Coleman, Craig Alter, et al. "Glycogen Storage Disease in Adults." *Annals of Internal Medicine* 120 (1994): 218.

Triomphe, Teeny J. "Glycogen Storage Disease: A Basic Understanding and Guide to Nursing Care." *Journal of Pediatric Nursing* 12 (4)(August 1997): 238.

ORGANIZATIONS

Acid Maltase Deficiency Association. P.O. Box 700248, San Antonio, TX 78270-0248. (210) 494-6144 or (210) 490-7161. http://members.aol.com/amdapage/index.htm.

American Liver Foundation. 1425 Pompton Avenue, Cedar Grove, NJ 07009. (800) GO LIVER (465-4837). http://www.liverfoundation.org/.

Association for Glycogen Storage Disease. P.O. Box 896, Durant, Iowa 52747-9769. (319) 785-6038.

Julia Barrett

Glycosylated hemoglobin test

Definition

Glycosylated hemoglobin is a test that indicates how much sugar has been in a person's blood during the past two to four months. It is used to monitor the effectiveness of diabetes treatment.

Purpose

Diabetes is a disease in which a person cannot effectively use sugar in the blood. Left untreated, blood sugar levels can be very high. High sugar levels increase risk of complications, such as damage to eyes, kidneys, heart, nerves, blood vessels, and other organs.

A routine blood sugar test reveals how close to normal a sugar level is at the time of the test. The glycosylated hemoglobin test reveals how close to normal it has been during the past several months.

This information helps a physician evaluate how well a person is responding to diabetes treatment and to determine how long sugar levels have been high in a person newly diagnosed with diabetes.

Description

The Diabetes Control and Complications Trial (DCCT) demonstrated that persons with diabetes who maintained blood glucose (sugar) and total fasting hemoglobin levels at or close to a normal range decreased their risk of complications by 50–75%. Based on results of this study, the American Diabetes Association (ADA) recommends routine glycosylated hemoglobin testing to measure long-term control of blood sugar.

Glycosylated hemoglobin measures the percentage of hemoglobin bound to glucose. Hemoglobin is a protein found in every red blood cell. As hemoglobin and glucose are together in the red blood cell, the glucose gradually binds to the A1c form of hemoglobin in a process called glycosylation. The amount bound reflects how much glu-

KEY TERMS

Diabetes mellitus—A disease in which a person can't effectively use sugar in the blood to meet the needs of the body. It is caused by a lack of the hormone insulin.

Glucose—The main form of sugar used by the body for energy.

Glycosylated hemoglobin—A test that measures the amount of hemoglobin bound to glucose. It is a measure of how much glucose has been in the blood during the past two to four months.

cose has been in the blood during the past average 120-day lifespan of red cells.

Several methods are used to measure the amount of bound hemoglobin and glucose. They are electrophoresis, chromatography, and immunoassay. All are based on the separation of hemoglobin bound to glucose from that without glucose.

The ADA recommends glycosylated hemoglobin be done during a person's first diabetes evaluation, again after treatment is begun and sugar levels are stabilized, then repeated semiannually. If the person does not meet treatment goals or sugar levels have not stabilized, the test should be repeated quarterly.

Other names for the test include: Hemoglobin A1c, Diabetic control index, GHb, glycosylated hemoglobin, and glycated hemoglobin. The test is covered by insurance. Results are usually available the following day.

Preparation

A person does not need to fast before this test. A healthcare worker ties a tourniquet on the person's upper arm, locates a vein in the inner elbow region, and inserts a needle into that vein. Vacuum action draws the blood through the needle into an attached tube. Collection of the sample takes only a few minutes. This test requires 5 mL of blood.

Aftercare

Discomfort or bruising may occur at the puncture site, or the person may feel dizzy or faint. Pressure to the puncture site until bleeding stops reduces bruising. Warm packs relieve discomfort.

Normal results

Diabetes treatment should achieve glycosylated hemoglobin levels of less than 7.0%. Normal values for a non-diabetic person is 4.0–6.0%.

Because laboratories use different methods, results from different laboratories can not always be compared. The National Glycosylation Standardization Program gives a certification to laboratories using tests standardized to those used in the DCCT study.

Abnormal results

Results require interpretation by a physician with knowledge of the person's clinical condition, as well as the test method used. Some methods give false high or low results if the person has an abnormal hemoglobin, such as hemoglobin S or F.

Conditions that increase the lifespan of red cells, such as a **splenectomy** (removal of the spleen), falsely increase levels. Conditions that decrease the lifespan, such as hemolysis (disruption of the red blood cell membrane), falsely decrease levels.

Resources

PERIODICALS

American Diabetes Association. ''Position Statement: Standards of Medical Care for Patients with Diabetes Mellitus.'' *Diabetes Care* (January, 1998): S23-31.

American Diabetes Association. ''Position Statement: Tests of Glycemia in Diabetes.'' *Diabetes Care* (January, 1998): S69-71.

American Diabetes Association. ''Report of the Expert Committee on the Diagnosis and Classification of Diabetes Mellitus.'' *Diabetes Care* (July, 1997): 1183-1197.

The DCCT Research Group. ''The Effects of Intensive Treatment of Diabetes on the Development and Progression of Long-Term Complications in Insulin-Dependent Diabetes Mellitus.'' *New England Journal of Medicine* (September, 1993): 977-986.

ORGANIZATIONS

American Diabetes Association (ADA). National Service Center. 1660 Duke Street, Alexandria, VA 22314. 703-549-1500. http://www.diabetes.org.

Centers for Disease Control and Prevention (CDC). Division of Diabetes Translation. National Center for Chronic Disease Prevention and Health Promotion. TISB Mail Stop K-13, 4770 Buford Highway NE, Atlanta, GA 30341-3724. 770-488-5080. http://www.cdc.gov/diabetes.

National Diabetes Information Clearinghouse (NDIC). One Information Way, Bethesda, MD 20892-3560. 301-907-8906. http://www.niddk.nih.gov/health/diabetes/ndic.htm.

National Institute of Diabetes and Digestive and Kidney Diseases (NIDDK). National Institutes of Health. Building 31, Rm. 9A04, 31 Center Drive, MSC 2560, Bethesda, MD 208792-2560. (301) 496-3583. http://www/niddk.nih.gov.

Nancy J. Nordenson

Goiter

Definition

Goiter refers to any visible enlargement of the thyroid gland.

Description

The thyroid gland sits astride the trachea (windpipe) and is shaped like a butterfly. It makes thyroxin, a hormone that regulates the metabolic activity of the body, rather like the gas pedal on a car. Too much thyroxin increases the metabolism, causing weight loss, temperature elevation, nervousness, and irritability. Too little thyroxin slows the metabolism down, deepens the voice, causes weight gain and water retention, and retards growth and mental development in children. Both conditions also alter hair and skin growth, bowel function, and menstrual flow.

Curiously, the thyroid gland is often enlarged whether it is making too much hormone, too little, or sometimes even when it is functioning normally. The thyroid is controlled by the pituitary gland, which secretes thyroid stimulating hormone (TSH) in response to the amount of thyroxin it finds in the blood. TSH increases the amount of thyroxin secreted by the thyroid and also causes the thyroid gland to grow.

- Hyperthyroid goiter—If the amount of stimulating hormone is excessive, the thyroid will both enlarge and secrete too much thyroxin. The result—**hyperthyroidism** with a goiter. Graves' disease is the most common form of this disorder.

- Euthyroid goiter—The thyroid is the only organ in the body to use iodine. If dietary iodine is slightly inadequate, too little thyroxin will be secreted, and the pituitary will sense the deficiency and produce more TSH. The thyroid gland will enlarge enough to make sufficient thyroxin.

- Hypothyroid goiter—If dietary iodine is severely reduced, even an enlarged gland will not be able to make enough thyroxin. The gland will keep growing under the influence of TSH, but it may never be able to make enough thyroxin.

Causes & symptoms

Excess TSH (or similar hormones), cysts, and tumors will enlarge the thyroid gland. Of these, TSH enlarges the entire gland while cysts and tumors enlarge only a part of it.

The only symptom from a goiter is the large swelling just above the breast bone. Rarely, it may constrict the trachea (windpipe) or esophagus and cause difficulty breathing or swallowing. The rest of the symptoms come from thyroxin or the lack of it.

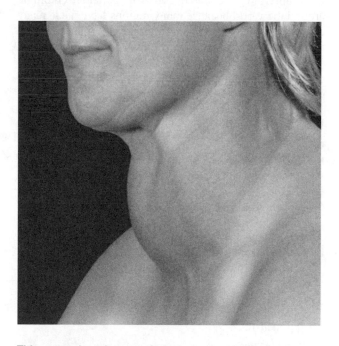

This woman's goiter may have been caused by an insufficient intake of iodine. (*Custom Medical Stock Photo. Reproduced by permission.*)

Diagnosis

The size, shape, and texture of the thyroid gland help the physician determine the cause. A battery of blood tests are required to verify the specific thyroid disease. Functional imaging studies using radioactive iodine determine how active the gland is and what it looks like.

Treatment

Goiters of all types will regress with treatment of the underlying condition. Dietary iodine may be all that is needed. However, if an iodine deficient thyroid that has grown in size to accommodate its deficiency is suddenly supplied an adequate amount of iodine, it could suddenly make large amounts of thyroxin and cause a thyroid storm, the equivalent of racing your car motor at top speed.

Hyperthyroidism can be treated with medications, therapeutic doses of radioactive iodine, or surgical reduction. Surgery is much less common now than it used to be because of progress in drugs and radiotherapy.

Prognosis

Although goiters diminish in size, the thyroid may not return to normal. Sometimes thyroid function does not return after treatment, but thyroxin is easy to take as a pill.

Prevention

Euthyroid goiter and hypothyroid goiter are common around the world because many regions have inadequate dietary iodine, including some places in the United States. International relief groups are providing iodized salt to many of these populations. Because **mental retardation** is a common result of **hypothyroidism** in children, this is an extremely important project.

Resources

BOOKS

Bennett, J. Claude and Fred Plum, ed. *Cecil Textbook of Medicine.* Philadelphia: W. B. Saunders, 1996, pp.1241-1242.

Gregerman, Robert I. "Thyroid disorders" In *Principles of Ambulatory Medicine.* Edited by L. Randol Barker, et al. Baltimore: Williams & Wilkins, 1995, pp.1039-41.

Isselbacher, Kurt, et al., ed. *Harrison's Principles of Internal Medicine.* New York: McGraw-Hill, 1997, pp.1938-1940.

Tierney, Lawrence M., ed. *Current Medical Diagnosis and Treatment* Stamford, CT: Appleton & Lange, 1998, pp.1046-1047.

ORGANIZATIONS

International Council for the Control of Iodine Deficiency Disorders. http://www.tulane.edu/~icec/icciddhome.htm.

The Micronutrient Initiative (c/o International Development Research Centre). 250 Albert Street, Ottawa, Ontario, Canada K1G 3H9. (613) 236-6163, ext. 2050. mi@idrc.ca. http://www.idrc.ca/mi/index.html.

J. Ricker Polsdorfer

Gonadal dysgenesis *see* **Turner syndrome**

. . . .

Gonorrhea

Definition

Gonorrhea is a highly contagious sexually transmitted disease that is caused by the bacterium *Neisseria gonorrhoeae*. The mucous membranes of the genital region may become inflamed without the development of any other symptoms. When symptoms do occur, they are different in men and women. In men, gonorrhea usually begins as an infection of the vessel that carries urine and sperm (urethra). In women, it will most likely infect the narrow part of the uterus (cervix). If untreated, gonorrhea can result in serious medical complications.

Description

Gonorrhea is commonly referred to as "the clap." The incidence of gonorrhea has steadily declined since the 1980s, largely due to increased public awareness campaigns and the risk of contracting other **sexually transmitted diseases,** such as **AIDS.** Still, current estimates range from 400,000 to as many as one million projected cases of gonorrhea in the United States each year. These estimates vary due to the private nature of the disease and the consequent underreporting that occurs. The majority of reported cases of gonorrhea come from public health clinics.

The disease affects people of all ages, races, and socioeconomic levels, but some individuals are more at-risk than others. Adolescents and young adults are the highest risk group, with more than 80% of the reported cases each year occurring in the 15–29 age group. Those individuals with multiple sexual partners and who use no barrier **contraception,** such as **condoms,** are most at-risk. Reported rates vary among racial and ethnic groups.

The risk factors for gonorrhea are not unlike those for all sexually transmitted diseases. Both men and women can become infected through a variety of sexual contact behaviors, including oral, anal, or vaginal intercourse. The disease is transmitted very efficiently. In fact, women run a 60–90% chance of contracting the disease after just one sexual encounter with an infected male. The

KEY TERMS

Cervix—The narrow part or neck of the uterus.

Chlamydia—The most common bacterial sexually transmitted disease in the United States that often accompanies gonorrhea and is known for its lack of evident symptoms in the majority of women.

Ectopic pregnancy—A pregnancy that occurs outside the uterus, such as in the fallopian tubes. Although the fetus will not survive, in some cases, ectopic pregnancy can also result in the death of the mother.

ELISA—Enzyme-linked immunosorbent assay. This test has been used a screening test for AIDS for many years and has also been used to detect gonorrhea bacteria.

HIV—Human immunodeficiency virus, the virus that causes AIDS. The risk of acquiring AIDS is increased by the presence of gonorrhea or other sexually transmitted diseases.

Neisseria gonorrhoeae—The bacterium that causes gonorrhea. It cannot survive for any length of time outside the human body.

Pelvic inflammatory disease (PID)—An infection of the upper genital tract that is the most serious threat to a woman's ability to reproduce. At least 25% of women who contract the disease, which can be a complication of gonorrhea, will experience long-term consequences such as infertility or ectopic pregnancy.

Sexually transmitted diseases (STDs)—A group of diseases which are transmitted by sexual contact. In addition to gonorrhea, this groups generally includes chlamydia, HIV (AIDS), herpes, syphilis, and genital warts.

Sterile—Unable to conceive a child.

Urethra—The canal leading from the bladder, and in men, also a path for sperm fluid.

Urethritis—Inflammation of the urethra.

disease can also be transmitted from an infected mother to her infant during delivery.

Causes and symptoms

If treated early, gonorrhea can be cured. Unfortunately, many individuals with gonorrhea, particularly women, will experience no symptoms to alert them to the possibility that they have contracted gonorrhea, and therefore, many do not seek treatment. When present, the symptoms and complications of gonorrhea are primarily limited to the genital, urinary, and gastrointestinal systems and usually begin between one day and two weeks following infection. If left untreated, serious complications can result if the disease spreads to the bloodstream and infects the brain, heart valves, and joints. Untreated gonorrhea can also result in severe damage to the reproductive system, making an individual unable to conceive a child (sterile).

Symptoms of gonorrhea in women

As many as 80% of women with gonorrhea show no symptoms. If present, symptoms may include the following:

- Bleeding between menstrual periods

- Chronic abdominal **pain**

- Painful urination

- Vaginal discharge, often cloudy and yellow

- In the case of oral infection, there may be no symptoms or only a **sore throat**

- Anal infection may cause rectal **itching** or discharge.

Because women often do not show any symptoms, complications are more likely to occur as the disease progresses. The most common complication is **pelvic inflammatory disease** (PID). PID can occur in up to 40% of women with gonorrhea and may result in damage to the fallopian tubes, a **pregnancy** developing outside the uterus (**ectopic pregnancy**), or sterility. If an infected woman is pregnant, gonorrhea can be passed on to her newborn through the birth canal during delivery. These infants may experience eye infections that could lead to blindness.

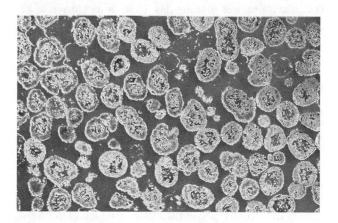

A transmission electron microscopy (TEM) image of
Neisseria gonorrhoeae. (Custom Medical Stock Photo. Reproduced by permission.)

Symptoms of gonorrhea in men

Men are more likely to experience the following symptoms:

• Thick and cloudy discharge from the penis

• Burning or pain during urination

• More frequent urination

• In the case of oral infection, there may be no symptoms or only a sore throat.

• Anal infection may cause rectal itching or discharge.

In men, complications can affect the prostate, testicles, and surrounding glands. Inflammation, tissue death and pus formation (**abscesses**), and scarring can occur and result in sterility.

Diagnosis

The diagnosis of gonorrhea can be made at a public health clinic or a family physician office. First, the doctor will discuss symptoms and the patient's known contact or at-risk behavior. There are three methods available to test for the presence of *Neisseria gonorrhoeae*. These include a culture, a Gram stain, and an ELISA test. Culture of secretions from the infected area is the preferred method for gonorrhea screening in patients with or without symptoms. A cotton swab can be used to collect enough sample for a culture. The sample is incubated for up to two days, providing enough time for the bacteria to multiply and be accurately identified. This test is nearly 100% accurate.

Gram stains are more accurate in the diagnosis of gonorrhea in men than in women. To perform this test, a small amount of discharge from the infected area will be placed on a slide, stained with a special dye, and examined under a microscope for the presence of the gonococcus bacteria. The advantage to this test is that results can be obtained very quickly at the initial visit. Because it requires that the physician or technician to be able to recognize and accurately identify the bacteria simply by looking at it under a microscope, however, this test is only approximately 70% accurate. As a result, one of the other methods will also probably be used to confirm the diagnosis.

ELISA, or enzyme-linked immunosorbent assay, has emerged as a rapid and sensitive test for gonorrhea. It is much more sensitive than the gram stain and is more convenient than the culture test, which involves the transport and storage of samples. As of late 1997, several other diagnostic tests were being researched with the goal of providing a cost-effective method of screening for a variety of sexually transmitted diseases. One of the most interesting of these is a home test that can be taken by the patient themselves, allowing for a degree of privacy and confidentiality.

When a patient suspects exposure to or experiences symptoms of gonorrhea, he or she may see a public health provider or family practice physician. Physicians trained in obstetrics or gynecology may also be involved, particularly if gynecological complications occur. Men who experience complications may be referred to a urologist. There are also infectious disease doctors who specialize in the treatment and research of all infectious diseases, including those transmitted sexually. All doctors must report this highly contagious disease to public health officials, and patients are asked to provide the names of sex partners during the suspected period of infection so that they can be notified of the risk.

Treatment

Gonorrhea has become more difficult and expensive to treat since the 1970s, due to the increased resistance of gonorrhea to certain **antibiotics.** In fact, according to projections from the Centers for Disease Control and Prevention, 30% of the strains of gonorrhea were resistant to routine antibiotics in 1994, and resistance has been increasing steadily. The following antibiotics may be given orally or by injection:

• Ciprofloxacin (Cipro)

• Ofloxacin (Floxin)

• Azithromycin (Zithromax)

• Amoxicillin

• Doxycycline (Doxy)

• Ceftriaxone (Rocephin).

If the patient is allergic to penicillin (or pregnant), erythromycin may be substituted. The most important consideration is to make sure that all of the prescribed medication is taken. If a course of antibiotics is not completed, the medication will only kill those organisms that are susceptible to the antibiotic, allowing those that are resistant to the effects of that particular antibiotic to multiply and possibly cause a new infection that will be more difficult to treat. Patients should refrain from sexual intercourse until treatment is complete and return for follow-up testing. Since another sexually transmitted disease, called chlamydia, often occurs with gonorrhea, patients may be treated for both infections. Any sexual partners during the time of infection, even if those partners do not show symptoms, should be notified and treated when any sexually transmitted disease is involved.

Alternative treatment

Although there is no known alternative to antibiotics in the treatment of gonorrhea, there are herbs and **minerals** that may be used to supplement antibiotic treatment:

- *Lactobacillus acidophilus* or live-culture yogurts are helpful, while taking antibiotics, to replenish gastrointestinal flora.

- The following supplements may be used to improve the body's immune function: zinc, multivitamins and mineral complexes, vitamin C, and garlic (*Allium sativum*).

- Several herbs may reduce some symptoms or help speed healing: kelp has balanced **vitamins** and minerals. Calendula (*Calendula officinalis*), myrrh (*Commiphora molmol*), and thuja (*Thuja occidentalis*) may help reduce discharge and inflammation when used as a tea or douche.

- Hot baths may also help reduce pain and inflammation.

- A variety of herbs may help with symptoms of the reproductive and urinary systems.

- If a physician approves, **fasting,** combined with certain juices, may help cleanse the urinary and gastrointestinal systems.

- There may be **acupressure** and **acupuncture** points that will help with system cleansing. These exact pressure points can be provided and treated by an acupressurist or acupuncturist.

Prognosis

The prognosis for patients with gonorrhea varies based on how early the disease is detected and treated. If treated early and properly, patients can be entirely cured of the disease. Up to 40% of female patients who are not treated early may develop pelvic inflammatory disease (PID) and the possibility of resulting sterility. Although the risk of **infertility** is higher in women than in men, men may also become sterile if the urethra becomes inflamed (**urethritis**) as a result of an untreated gonorrhea infection. Following an episode of PID, a woman is 6–10 times more likely, should a pregnancy occur, to have a pregnancy develop outside the uterus (ectopic pregnancy), which can result in **death.** Liver infection may also occur in untreated women. In approximately 2% of patients with untreated gonorrhea, the gonococcal infection may spread throughout the body and can cause **fever,** arthritis-like joint pain, and **skin lesions.**

Prevention

Currently, there is no vaccine for gonorrhea, but several are under development. The best prevention is to abstain from having sex or to engage in sex only when in a mutually monogamous relationship in which both partners have been tested for gonorrhea, AIDS, and other sexually transmitted diseases. The next line of defense is the use of condoms, which have been shown to be highly effective in preventing disease (and unwanted pregnancies). To be 100% effective, condoms must be used properly. A female birth-control device that blocks the entry of sperm into the cervix (diaphragm) can also reduce the risk of infection. The risk of contracting gonorrhea increases with the number of sexual partners. Any man or woman who has sexual contact with more than one partner is advised to be tested regularly for gonorrhea and other sexually transmitted diseases.

Resources

BOOKS

Balch, James F. *Prescription for Nutritional Healing.* Garden City Park, NY: Avery Publishing Group, 1997.

Committee on Prevention and Control of Sexually Transmitted Diseases. *The Hidden Epidemic: Confronting Sexually Transmitted Diseases.* Edited by Thomas R. England and William T. Butler. Washington, DC: National Academy Press, 1997.

Ross, Linda A. *Sexually Transmitted Diseases Sourcebook: Basic Information About Herpes, Chlamydia, Gonorrhea, Hepatitis, Nongonococcal Urethritis, Pelvic Inflammatory Disease, Syphilis, AIDS, and More, Along with Current Data on Treatments and Preventions.* Detroit, MI: Omnigraphics, 1997.

PERIODICALS

Centers for Disease Control and Prevention. ''Gonorrhea Among Men Who Have Sex With Men: Selected Sexually Transmitted Diseases Clinics, 1993-1996.'' *Journal of the American Medical Association,* 278 (October 15, 1997): 1228-1229.

Newland, Jamesetta A. ''Gonorrhea in Women.'' *American Journal of Nursing,* 97 (August 1997): 16AA.

Newland, Jamesetta A. ''Urethritis in Men.'' *American Journal of Nursing,* 97 (August 1997): 16BB.

''Tips from Other Journals: Trends in Antibiotic Resistance of Gonorrhea.'' *American Family Physician,* 56 (October 1, 1997): 5.

ORGANIZATIONS

American Foundation for the Prevention of Venereal Disease, Inc. 799 Broadway, Suite 638, New York, NY 10003. (212) 759-2069.

American Social Health Association. P.O. Box 13827, Research Triangle Park, NC 27709. (800) 227-8922 (National STD Hotline) or voice line at (919) 361-8400. http://sunsite.unc.edu/ASHA/.

National Center for HIV, STD, and TB Prevention. Centers for Disease Control and Prevention, 1600 Clifton NE, Atlanta, GA 30333. http://www.cdc.gov/nchstp/od/nchstp.html. NCHST@cpsod1.em.cdc.gov.

National Institute of Allergy and Infectious Diseases. National Institutes of Health, Bethesda, MD 20892.

Teresa G. Norris

Goodpasture's syndrome

Definition

An uncommon and life-threatening hypersensitivity disorder believed to be an autoimmune process related to antibody formation in the body. Goodpasture's syndrome is characterized by renal (kidney) disease and lung hemorrhage.

Description

The disorder is characterized by deposits of antibodies in the membranes of both the lung and kidneys, causing both inflammation of kidney glomerulus (**glomerulonephritis**) and lung bleeding. It is typically a disease of young males.

Causes & symptoms

The exact cause is unknown. It is an autoimmune disorder; that is, the immune system is fighting the body's own normal tissues. Sometimes the disorder is triggered by a viral infection, or by the inhalation of gasoline or other hydrocarbon solvents. An association also exists between cigarette smoking and the syndrome.

Symptoms include foamy, bloody, or dark colored urine, decreased urine output, **cough** with bloody sputum, difficulty breathing after exertion, weakness, fatigue, nausea or vomiting, weight loss, nonspecific chest **pain** and/or pale skin.

Diagnosis

The clinician will perform a battery of tests to confirm a diagnosis. These tests include a complete **blood count** (CBC) to confirm anemia, iron levels to check for blood loss and blood urea nitrogen (BUN) and creatinine levels to test the kidney function. A **urinalysis** will be done to check for damage to the kidneys. A sputum test will be done to look for antibodies. A **chest x ray** will be done to assess the amount of fluid in the lung tissues. A lung needle biopsy and a **kidney biopsy** will show immune system deposits.

Treatment

Treatment is focused on slowing the progression of the disease. Treatment is most effective when begun early, before kidney function has deteriorated to a point where the kidney is permanently damaged, and dialysis is necessary. **Corticosteroids,** such as prednisone, or other anti-inflammatory medications may be used to reduce the immune response. Immune suppressants such as cyclo-

phosphamide or azathioprine are used aggressively to reduce immune system effects.

A procedure whereby blood plasma, which contains antibodies, is removed from the body and replaced with fluids or donated plasma (**plasmapheresis**) may be performed daily for two or more weeks to remove circulating antibodies. It is fairly effective in slowing or reversing the disorder. Dialysis to clean the blood of wastes may be required if kidney function is poor. A kidney transplant may be successful, especially if performed after circulating antibodies have been absent for several months.

Prognosis

The probable outcome is variable. Most cases progress to severe renal failure and end-stage renal disease within months. Early diagnosis and treatment makes the probable outcome more favorable.

Prevention

No known prevention of Goodpasture's syndrome exists. People should avoid glue sniffing and the siphoning gasoline. Stopping smoking, if a family history of renal failure exists, may prevent some cases. Early diagnosis and treatment may slow progression of the disorder.

KEY TERMS

Antibody—A protein molecule produced by the immune system in response to a protein that is not recognized as belonging in the body.

Autoimmune disorder—An abnormality within the body whereby the immune system incorrectly attacks the body's normal tissues, thereby causing disease or organ dysfunction.

Blood urea nitrogen (BUN)—A test used to measure the blood level of urea nitrogen, a waste that is normally filtered from the kidneys.

Creatinine—A test used to measure the blood level of creatinine, a waste product filtered out of the blood by the kidneys. Higher than usual levels of this substance may indicate kidney disease.

Glomerulus (glomeruli)—A small tuft of blood capillaries in the kidney, responsible for filtering out waste products.

Resources

BOOKS

Couser, William G. ''Glomerular Disorders.'' In *Cecil Textbook of Medicine,* edited by James B. Wyngaarden, et al. Philadelphia: W. B. Saunders Company, 1992.

Ron Gasbarro

Gout

Definition

Gout is a form of acute arthritis that causes severe **pain** and swelling in the joints. It most commonly affects the big toe, but may also affect the heel, ankle, hand, wrist, or elbow. Gout usually comes on suddenly, goes away after 5–10 days, and can keep recurring. Gout is different from other forms of arthritis because it occurs when there are high levels of uric acid circulating in the blood, which can cause urate crystals to settle in the tissues of the joints.

Description

Uric acid, which is found naturally in the blood stream, is formed as the body breaks down waste products, mainly those containing purine, a substance that is produced by the body and is also found in high concentrations in some foods, including brains, liver, sardines, anchovies, and dried peas and beans. Normally, the kidneys filter uric acid out of the blood and excrete it in the urine. Sometimes, however, the body produces too much uric acid or the kidneys aren't efficient enough at filtering it from the blood, and it builds up in the blood stream, a condition known as hyperuricemia. A person's susceptibility to gout may increase because of the inheritance of certain genes or from being overweight and eating a rich diet. In some cases, another disease (such as lymphoma, leukemia, or **hemolytic anemia**) may be the underlying cause of the uric acid buildup that results in gout.

Hyperuricemia doesn't always cause gout. However, over the course of years, sharp urate crystals build up in the synovial fluid of the joints. Often, some precipitating event, such as an infection, surgery, a stubbed toe, or even a heavy drinking binge can cause inflammation. White blood cells, mistaking the urate crystals for a foreign invader, flood into the joint and surround the crystals, causing inflammation—in other words, the redness, swelling, and pain that are the hallmarks of a gout attack.

Causes & symptoms

As a result of high levels of uric acid in the blood, needle-like urate crystals gradually accumulate in the joints. Urate crystals may be present in the joint for a long time without causing symptoms. Infection, injury to the joint, surgery, drinking too much, or eating the wrong kinds of foods may suddenly bring on the symptoms, which include pain, tenderness, redness, warmth, and swelling of the joint. In many cases, the gout attack begins in the middle of the night. The pain is often so excruciating that the sufferer cannot bear weight on the joint or tolerate the pressure of bedcovers. The inflamed skin over the joint may be red, shiny, and dry, and the inflammation may be accompanied by a mild **fever.** These symptoms may go away in about a week and disappear for months or years at a time. However, over the course of time, attacks of gout recur more and more frequently, last longer, and affect more joints. Eventually, stone-like deposits known as tophi may build up in the joints, ligaments, and tendons, leading to permanent joint deformity and decreased motion. (In addition to causing the tophi associated with gout, hyperuricemia can also cause **kidney stones,** also called renal calculi or uroliths.)

Gout affects an estimated one million Americans. It most commonly afflicts men (800,000 men versus 200,000 women). Uric-acid levels tend to increase in men at **puberty,** and, because it takes 20 years of hyperuricemia to cause gout symptoms, men commonly develop gout in their late 30s or early 40s. Women more typically develop gout later in life, starting in their 60s. According to some medical experts, estrogen protects against hyperuricemia, and when estrogen levels fall during **menopause,** urate crystals can begin to build up in the joints. Excess body weight, regular excessive alcohol intake, the use of blood pressure medications called **diuretics,** and high levels of certain fatty substances in the blood (serum triglycerides) associated with an increased risk of heart disease can all increase a person's risk of developing gout.

Diagnosis

Usually, physicians can diagnose gout based on the **physical examination** and medical history (the patient's description of symptoms and other information). Doctors can also administer a test that measures the level of uric acid in the blood. While normal uric acid levels don't necessarily rule out gout and high levels don't confirm it, the presence of hyperuricemia increases the likelihood of gout. The development of a tophus can confirm the diagnosis of gout. The most definitive way to diagnose gout is

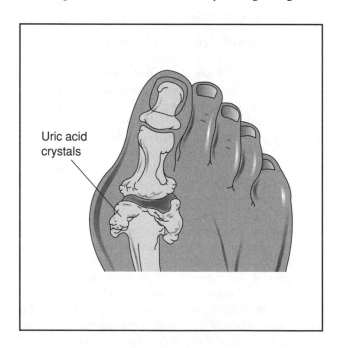

Uric acid crystals

Gout, a form of acute arthritis, most commonly occurs in the big toe. It is caused by high levels of uric acid in the blood, in which urate crystals settle in the tissues of the joints and produce severe pain and swelling. *(Illustration by Electronic Illustrators Group.)*

to take a sample of fluid from the joint and test it for urate crystals.

Treatment

The goals of treatment for gout consist of alleviating pain, avoiding severe attacks in the future, and preventing long-term joint damage. In addition to taking pain medications as prescribed by their doctors, people having gout attacks are encouraged to rest and to increase the amount of fluids that they drink.

Acute attacks of gout can be treated with nonaspirin, **nonsteroidal anti-inflammatory drugs** (NSAIDs) such as naproxen sodium (Aleve), ibuprofen (Advil), or indomethacin (Indocin). In some cases, these drugs can aggravate a peptic ulcer or existing kidney disease and cannot be used. Doctors sometimes also use colchicine (Colbenemid), especially in cases where nonsteroidal anti-inflammatory drugs cannot be used. Colchicine may cause **diarrhea,** which tends to go away once the patient stops taking it. **Corticosteroids** such as prednisone (Deltasone) and adrenocorticotropic hormone (Acthar) may be given orally or may be injected directly into the joint for a more concentrated effect. While all of these drugs have the potential to cause side effects, they are used for only about 48 hours and are not likely to cause major problems. However, **aspirin** and closely related drugs (salicylates) should be avoided because they can ultimately worsen gout.

Once an acute attack has been successfully treated, doctors try to prevent future attacks of gout and long-term joint damage by lowering uric acid levels in the blood. There are two types of drugs for correcting hyperuricemia. Uricosuric drugs, such as probenecid (Benemid) and sulfinpyrazone (Anturane), lower the levels of urate in the blood by increasing its removal from the body (excretion) through the urine. These drugs may promote the formation of kidney stones, and they may not work for all patients, especially those with kidney disease. Allopurinol (Zyloprim), a type of drug called a xanthine-oxidase inhibitor, blocks the production of urate in the body, and can dissolve kidney stones as well as treating gout. The potential side effects of allopurinol include rash, a skin condition known as **dermatitis,** and liver dysfunction. Once people begin taking these medications, they must take them for life or the gout will continue to return.

Alternative treatment

The alternative medicine approach to gout focuses on correcting hyperuricemia by losing weight and limiting the intake of alcohol and purine-rich foods. In addition, consuming garlic (*Allium sativum*) has been recommended to help prevent gout. Increasing fluid intake, especially by drinking water, is also recommended.

During an acute attack, contrast **hydrotherapy** (alternating three-minute hot compresses with 30–second cold compresses) can help dissolve the crystals and resolve the pain faster.

Prognosis

Gout cannot be cured but usually it can be managed successfully. As tophi dissolve, joint mobility generally improves. (In some cases, however, medicines alone do not dissolve the tophi and they must be removed surgically.) Lowering uric acid in the blood also helps to prevent or improve the kidney problems that may accompany gout.

Prevention

For centuries, gout has been known as a "rich man's disease" or a disease of overindulgence in food and drink. While this view is perhaps a little overstated and oversimplified, lifestyle factors clearly influence a person's risk of developing gout. Since **obesity** and excessive alcohol intake are associated with hyperuricemia and gout, losing weight and limiting alcohol intake can help ward off gout. **Dehydration** may also promote the formation of urate crystals, so people taking diuretics or "water pills" may be better off switching to another type of blood pressure medication, and everyone should be sure to drink at least six to eight glasses of water each day. Since purine is broken down in the body into urate, it may also be helpful to avoid foods high in purine, such as organ meats, sardines, anchovies, red meat, gravies, beans, beer, and wine.

Resources

BOOKS

The Burton Goldberg Group. *Alternative Medicine: The Definitive Guide.* Fife, WA: Future Medicine Publishing, 1995.

PERIODICALS

Conos, Juan J. and Robert A. Kalish, "Gout: Effective drug therapy for acute attacks and for the long term." *Consultant* (August 1996): 1752-55.

Emmerson, Bryan T. "The management of gout." *New England Journal of Medicine* (February 15, 1996): 445-51.

Flieger, Ken. "Getting to know gout." *FDA Consultant* (March 1995): 19-22.

Sauber, Colleen M. "Still painful after all these years." *Harvard Health Letter* (June 1995): 6-8.

Smith, Michael L. "Gout, hyperuricemia, and crystal arthritis." *British Medical Journal* (February 25, 1995): 521-24.

ORGANIZATIONS

Arthritis Foundation. 1330 W. Peachtreee Street, P.O. Box 7669, Atlanta, GA 30357-0669. (800) 283-7800. http://www.arthritis.org.

Robert Scott Dinsmoor

Gout drugs

Definition

Gout drugs are medicines that prevent or relieve the symptoms of **gout,** a disease that affects the joints and kidneys.

Purpose

Gout is a disease in which uric acid, a waste product that normally passes out of the body in urine, collects and forms crystals in the joints and the kidneys. When uric acid crystals build up in the joints, the tissue around the joint becomes inflamed, and nerve endings in the area become irritated, causing extreme **pain.** Uric acid crystals in the kidneys can lead to **kidney stones** and eventually to kidney failure.

The symptoms of gout—severe pain, usually in the hand or foot (often at the base of the big toe), but sometimes in the elbow or knee—should be reported to a health care professional. If not treated, gout can lead to high blood pressure, deformed joints, and even **death** from kidney failure. Fortunately, the condition is easily treated. For patients who have just had their first attack, physicians may prescribe only medicine to reduce the pain and inflammation, such as **nonsteroidal anti-inflammatory drugs, corticosteroids,** or colchicine. Patients may also be advised to change their eating and drinking habits, avoiding organ meats and other protein-rich foods, cutting out alcoholic beverages, and drinking more water. Some people never have another gout attack after the first. For those who do, physicians may prescribe additional drugs that either help the body get rid of uric acid or reduce the amount of uric acid the body produces. These drugs will not relieve gout attacks that already have started, but will help prevent attacks when taken regularly.

Description

Three main types of drugs are used in treating gout. Colchicine helps relieve the symptoms of gout by reducing inflammation. Allopurinol (Lopurin, Zyloprim) reduces the amount of uric acid produced in the body. Probenecid (Benemid, Probalan) and sulfinpyrazone

(Anturane) help the body get rid of excess uric acid. Physicians may recommend that patients take more than one type of gout drug at the same time. Some of these medicines may also be prescribed for other medical conditions that are caused by too much uric acid in the body.

Recommended dosage

The recommended dosage depends on the type of gout drug. Check with the physician who prescribed the drug or the pharmacist who filled the prescription for the correct dosage.

Always take gout drugs exactly as directed. Never take larger or more frequent doses than recommended. Patients who are told to take more than one gout drug should carefully follow the physician's directions for taking all medicines.

Gout drugs such as allopurinol, probenecid, and sulfinpyrazone must be taken regularly to prevent gout attacks. The medicine may take some time to begin working, so gout attacks may continue for awhile after starting to take the drug. Continuing to take the drug is important, even if it does not seem to be working at first.

Colchicine may be taken regularly in low doses to help prevent gout attacks or in high doses for only a few hours at a time to relieve an attack. The chance of serious side effects is greater when this medicine is taken in high doses for short periods.

Precautions

Seeing a physician regularly while taking gout drugs is important. The physician will check to make sure the medicine is working as it should and will watch for unwanted side effects. Blood tests may be ordered to help the physician monitor how well the drug is working.

Drinking alcohol, including beer and wine, may increase the amount of uric acid in the body and may interfere with the effects of gout medicine. People with gout (or other conditions that result from excess uric acid) may need to limit the amount of alcohol they drink or stop drinking alcohol altogether.

Some people feel drowsy or less alert when taking gout drugs. Anyone who takes this type of medicine should not drive, use machines or do anything else that might be dangerous until they have found out how the drugs affect them.

Some gout drugs may change the results of certain medical tests. Before having medical tests, anyone taking this medicine should alert the health care professional in charge.

Older people may be especially sensitive to the effects of colchicine. The drug may also stay in their bodies longer than it does in younger people. Both the increased sensitivity to the drug and the longer time for the drug to leave the body may increase the chance of side effects.

Special conditions

People who have certain medical conditions or who are taking certain other medicines can have problems if they take gout drugs. Before taking these drugs, be sure to let the physician know about any of these conditions:

ALLERGIES

Anyone who has ever had unusual reactions to gout drugs or to medicines used to relieve pain or inflammation should let his or her physician know before taking gout drugs. The physician should also be told about any **allergies** to foods, dyes, preservatives, or other substances.

DIABETES

Some gout drugs may cause false results on certain urine sugar tests, but not on others. Diabetic patients who take gout drugs should check with their physicians to find out if their medicine will affect the results of their urine sugar tests.

PREGNANCY

The effects of taking gout drugs during **pregnancy** are not fully understood. Women who are pregnant or who may become pregnant should check with their physicians before using gout drugs.

BREASTFEEDING

Gout drugs may pass into breast milk. Women who are taking this medicine and want to breastfeed their babies should check with their physicians.

OTHER MEDICAL CONDITIONS

Gout drugs may cause problems for people with certain medical conditions. For example, the risk of severe allergic reactions or other serious side effects is greater when people with these medical conditions take certain gout drugs:

- Congestive heart disease
- High blood pressure
- Blood disease
- **Diabetes**
- Kidney disease or kidney stones
- **Cancer** being treated with drugs or radiation
- Stomach or intestinal problems, including stomach ulcer (now or in the past).

Before using gout drugs, people with any of medical problems listed above should make sure their physicians are aware of their conditions.

USE OF CERTAIN MEDICINES

Taking gout drugs with certain other drugs may affect the way the drugs work or may increase the chance of side effects.

Side effects

A skin rash that develops during treatment with gout drugs may be a sign of a serious and possibly life-threatening reaction. If any of these symptoms occur, stop taking the medicine and check with a physician immediately:

- Skin rash, **itching,** or **hives**
- Scaly or peeling skin
- Chills, **fever, sore throat, nausea and vomiting,** yellow skin or eyes, joint pain, muscle aches or pains—especially if these symptoms occur at the same time or shortly after a skin rash.

Patients taking colchicine should stop taking it immediately if they have **diarrhea,** stomach pain, nausea, or vomiting. If these symptoms continue for 3 hours or more after the medicine is stopped, check with a physician.

Other side effects of may also need medical attention. If any of the following symptoms occur while taking gout drugs, check with the physician who prescribed the medicine as soon as possible:

- Pain in the side or lower back
- Painful urination
- Blood in the urine.

Less serious side effects, such as **headache,** loss of appetite, and joint pain and inflammation usually go away as the body adjusts to the drug and do not need medical treatment.

Other side effects may occur. Anyone who has unusual symptoms while taking gout drugs should get in touch with his or her physician.

Interactions

Gout drugs may interact with other medicines. When this happens, the effects of one or both of the drugs may change or the risk of side effects may be greater. Anyone who takes gout drugs should let the physician know all other medicines he or she is taking. Among the drugs that may interact with gout drugs are:

- **Aspirin** or other salicylates. These drugs may keep gout drugs from working properly.
- Nonsteroidal anti-inflammatory drugs such as indomethacin (Indocin) and ketoprofen (Orudis). Taking these medicines with probenecid may increase the chance of side effects from the nonsteroidal anti-inflammatory drugs.
- Blood thinners. When taken with blood thinners, such as warfarin (Coumadin), gout drugs may increase the chance of bleeding. A lower blood thinner dose may be necessary.
- Blood viscosity reducing medicines such as pentoxifylline (Trental). Taking this medicine with blood thinners may increase the chance of bleeding.
- Medicine for infections. Probenecid may increase the levels of these medicines in the blood. This may make the other medicine work better, but may also increase the risk of side effects.
- The immunosuppressant drug azathioprine (Imuran), used to prevent organ rejection in transplant patients and to treat **rheumatoid arthritis.** Taking this medicine with allopurinol can increase the risk of side effects from the azathioprine.
- **Anticancer drugs** such as mercaptopurine (Purinethol), plicamycin (Mithracin), and methotrexate (Rheumatrex). Taking this medicine with gout drugs may increase the risk of side effects from the anticancer drug.
- **Antiretroviral drugs** such as zidovudine (Retrovir). Probenecid may increase the level of this medicine in the blood. This may make side effects more likely.
- Antiseizure medicines such as Depakote (divalproex) and Depakene (valproic acid). Using these medicines with sulfinpyrazone may increase the chance of bleeding.

The list above does not include every drug that may interact with gout drugs. Be sure to check with a physician or pharmacist before combining gout drugs with any other prescription or nonprescription (over-the-counter) medicine.

Nancy Ross-Flanigan

Gouty arthritis *see* **Gout**

Grafts and grafting *see* **Bone grafting; Coronary artery bypass graft surgery; Graft-vs.-host disease; Skin grafting**

Graft-vs.-host disease

Definition

Graft-vs.-host disease is an immune attack on the recipient by cells from a donor.

Description

The main problem with transplanting organs and tissues is that the recipient host does not recognize the new tissue as its own. Instead, it attacks it as foreign in the same way it attacks germs, to destroy it.

If immunogenic cells from the donor are transplanted along with the organ or tissue, they will attack the host, causing graft vs. host disease.

The only transplanted tissues that house enough immune cells to cause graft vs. host disease are the blood and the bone marrow. Blood **transfusions** are used every day in hospitals for many reasons. Bone marrow transplants are used to replace blood forming cells and immune cells. This is necessary for patients whose **cancer** treatment has destroyed their own bone marrow. Because bone marrow cells are among the most sensitive to radiation and **chemotherapy,** it often must be destroyed along with the cancer. This is true primarily of leukemias, but some other cancers have also been treated this way.

Causes & symptoms

Even if the donor and recipient are well matched, graft-vs.-host disease can still occur. There are many different elements involved in generating immune reactions, and each person is different, unless they are identical twins. Testing can often find donors who match all the major elements, but there are many minor ones that will always be different. How good a match is found also depends upon the urgency of the need and some good luck.

Blood transfusion graft-vs.-host disease affects mostly the blood. Blood cells perform three functions: carrying oxygen, fighting infections, and clotting. All of these cell types are decreased in a transfusion graft-vs.-host reaction, leading to anemia (lack of red blood cells in the blood), a decrease in resistance to infections, and an increase in bleeding. The reaction occurs between 4–30 days after the transfusion.

The tissues most affected by bone marrow graft-vs.-host disease are the skin, the liver, and the intestines. One form or the other occurs in close to half of the patients who receive bone marrow transplants.

Bone marrow graft-vs.-host disease comes in an acute and a chronic form. The acute form appears within two months of the transplant; the chronic form usually appears within three months. The acute disease produces a skin rash, liver abnormalities, and **diarrhea** that can be bloody. The skin rash is primarily a patchy thickening of the skin. Chronic disease can produce a similar skin rash, a tightening or an inflammation of the skin, lesions in the mouth, drying of the eyes and mouth, hair loss, liver damage, lung damage, and **indigestion.** The symptoms are similar to an autoimmune disease called **scleroderma.**

Both forms of graft-vs.-host disease bring with them an increased risk of infections, either because of the process itself or its treatment with cortisone-like drugs and immunosuppressives. Patients can die of liver failure, infection, or other severe disturbances of their system.

Treatment

Both the acute and the chronic disease are treated with cortisone-like drugs, immunosuppressive agents like cyclosporine, or with **antibiotics** and immune chemicals from donated blood (gamma globulin). Infection with one particular virus, called cytomegalovirus (CMV) is so likely a complication that some experts recommend treating it ahead of time.

Prognosis

Children with **acute leukemias** have greatly benefited from the treatment made possible by **bone marrow transplantation.** Survival rates have climbed by 15–50%. It is an interesting observation that patients who develop graft-vs.-host disease are less likely to have a recurrence of the leukemia that was being treated. This phenomenon is called graft-vs.-leukemia.

Bone marrow transplant patients who do not have a graft-vs.-host reaction gradually return to normal immune function in a year. A graft-vs.-host reaction may prolong the diminished immune capacity indefinitely, requiring supplemental treatment with immunoglobulins (gamma globulin).

Somehow the grafted cells develop a tolerance to their new home after 6–12 months, and the medications can be gradually withdrawn. Graft-vs.-host disease is not the only complication of blood transfusion or bone marrow transplantation. Host-vs.-graft or rejection is also common and may require a repeat transplant with another donor organ. Infections are a constant threat in bone marrow transplant because of the disease being treated, the prior radiation or chemotherapy and the medications used to treat the transplant.

Prevention

For recipients of blood transfusions who are especially likely to have graft-vs.-host reactions, the red blood cells can safely be irradiated (using x rays) to kill all the immune cells. The red blood cells are less sensitive to radiation and are not harmed by this treatment.

Much current research is directed towards solving the problem of graft-vs.-host disease. There are efforts to remove the immunogenic cells from the donor tissue, and there are also attempts to extract and purify bone marrow cells from the patient before treating the cancer. These cells are then given back to the patient after treatment has destroyed all that were left behind.

Resources

BOOKS

Armitage, James O. ''Bone Marrow Transplantation.'' In *Harrison's Principles of Internal Medicine.* Edited by Kurt Isselbacher, et al. New York: McGraw-Hill, 1998, pp.726-727.

Menitove, Jay E. ''Blood Transfusion.'' In *Cecil Textbook of Medicine.* Edited by J. Claude Bennett and Fred Plum. Philadelphia: W. B. Saunders, 1996, p. 896.

Rappeport, Joel. ''Bone Marrow Transplantation.'' In *Cecil Textbook of Medicine.* Edited by J. Claude Bennett and Fred Plum. Philadelphia: W. B. Saunders, 1996, p. 975.

Ruscetti, Francis W., Jonathan R. Keller, and Dan L. Longo. ''Hematopoiesis.'' In *Harrison's Principles of Internal Medicine.* Edited by Kurt Isselbacher, et al. New York: McGraw-Hill, 1998, p. 637.

J. Ricker Polsdorfer

Granular conjunctivitis *see* **Trachoma**

Granulocytic ehrlichiosis *see* **Ehrlichiosis**

Granulocytopenia *see* **Neutropenia**

Granuloma inguinale

Definition

Granuloma inguinale is a sexually transmitted infection that affects the skin and mucous membranes of the anal and genital areas. Its name is derived from granuloma, a medical term for a mass or growth of granulation tissue, and *inguinale,* a Latin word that means located in the groin. Granulation tissue is tissue formed during wound healing that is rich in blood capillaries and has a rough or lumpy surface.

Description

Granuloma inguinale is a chronic infection with frequent relapses caused by a rod-shaped bacterium. It occurs worldwide but is most common in tropical or subtropical countries, where it is associated with poverty and poor hygiene. As many as 20% of male patients with **sexually transmitted diseases** (STDs) in tropical countries have granuloma inguinale. The disease is less common in the United States, with fewer than 100 reported cases per year. Most patients are between the ages of 20 and 40 years, with a 2:1 male-to-female ratio.

Although granuloma inguinale is relatively uncommon in the United States in comparison with other STDs, it is still a significant public health problem. It can be acquired through casual sexual contacts when traveling abroad. Moreover, patients with granuloma inguinale are vulnerable to superinfection (infection by other disease agents) with other STDs, especially **syphilis.** Patients with granuloma inguinale are also a high-risk group for Acquired Immune Deficiency Syndrome (**AIDS**) transmission, because the disease causes open genital ulcers that can be easily invaded by the AIDS virus.

Granuloma inguinale is spread primarily through heterosexual and male homosexual contact; however, its occurrence in children and sexually inactive adults indicates that it may also be spread by contact with human feces. Granuloma inguinale is not highly contagious; however, persons with weakened immune systems are at greater risk of infection.

Causes & symptoms

Granuloma inguinale, which is sometimes called donovanosis, is caused by *Calymmatobacterium granulomatis*, a rod-shaped bacterium formerly called *Donovania granulomatis*. The bacterium has an incubation period ranging from eight days to 12 weeks, with an average of two to four weeks. The disease has a slow and gradual onset, beginning with an inconspicuous pimple or lumpy eruption on the skin. In 90% of patients, the initial sign of infection is in the genital region, but a minority of patients will develop the sore in their mouth or anal area if their sexual contact involved those parts of the body. Many patients do not notice the sore because it is small and not usually painful. In some women, the first symptom of granuloma inguinale is bleeding from the genitals.

The initial pimple or sore is typically followed by three stages of disease. In the first stage, the patient develops a mass of pink or dull red granulation tissue in the area around the anus. In the second stage, the bacteria erode the skin to form shallow, foul-smelling ulcers which spread from the genital and anal areas to the thighs and lower abdomen. The edges of the ulcers are marked by granulation tissue. In the third stage, the ulcerated areas form deep masses of keloid or scar tissue that may spread slowly for many years.

Patients with long-term infections are at risk for serious complications. The ulcers in second-stage granuloma inguinale often become superinfected with syphilis or other STD organisms. Superinfected ulcers become painful to touch, filled with pus and dead tissue, and are much more difficult to treat. There may be sizable areas of tissue destruction in superinfected patients. In addition, the scar tissue produced by third-stage infection can grow until it closes off parts of the patient's urinary tract. It is also associated with a higher risk of genital **cancer.**

Diagnosis

The most important aspect of diagnosis is distinguishing between granuloma inguinale and other STDs, particularly since many patients will be infected with more than one STD. Public health officials recommend that patients tested for granuloma inguinale be given a blood test for syphilis as well. In addition, the doctor will need to distinguish between granuloma inguinale and certain types of skin cancer, **amebiasis,** fungal infections, and other bacterial ulcers. The most significant distinguishing characteristic of granuloma inguinale is the skin ulcer, which is larger than in most other diseases, painless, irregular in shape, and likely to bleed when touched.

The diagnosis of granuloma inguinale is made by finding Donovan bodies in samples of the patient's skin tissue. Donovan bodies are oval rod-shaped organisms that appear inside infected tissue cells under a microscope. The doctor obtains a tissue sample either by cutting a piece of tissue from the edge of an skin ulcer with a scalpel or by taking a punch biopsy. To make a punch biopsy, the doctor will inject a local anesthetic into an ulcerated area and remove a piece of skin about 1/16 of an inch in size with a surgical skin punch. The tissue sample is then air-dried and stained with Wright's stain, a chemical that will cause the Donovan bodies to show up as dark purple safety pin-shaped objects inside lighter-staining capsules.

Treatment

Granuloma inguinale is treated with oral **antibiotics.** Three weeks of treatment with erythromycin, streptomycin, or tetracycline, or 12 weeks of treatment with ampicillin are standard forms of therapy. Although the skin ulcers will start to show signs of healing in about a week, the patient must take the full course of medication to minimize the possibility of relapse.

Prognosis

Most patients with granuloma inguinale recover completely, although superinfected ulcers may require lengthy courses of medication. Early treatment prevents the complications associated with second- and third-stage infection.

Prevention

Prevention of granuloma inguinale has three important aspects:

• Avoidance of casual sexual contacts, particularly among homosexual males, in countries with high rates of the disease

• Tracing and examination of an infected person's recent sexual contacts

• Monitoring the patient's ulcers or scar tissue for signs of reinfection for a period of six months after antibiotic treatment.

Resources

BOOKS

Chambers, Henry F. "Infectious Diseases: Bacterial & Chlamydial." In *Current Medical Diagnosis & Treatment 1998,* edited by Lawrence M. Tierney, Jr. et al. Stamford, CT: Appleton & Lange, 1998.

Goens, Jean L., et al. "Granuloma Inguinale." In *Current Diagnosis 9,* edited by Rex B. Conn, et al. Philadelphia: W. B. Saunders Company, 1997.

Hunt, Thomas K. and Reid V. Mueller. "Inflammation, Infection, and Antibiotics." In *Current Surgical Diagnosis & Treatment,* edited by Lawrence W. Way. Stamford, CT: Appleton & Lange, 1994.

"Infectious Disease: Sexually Transmitted Diseases." In *The Merck Manual of Diagnosis and Therapy,* vol. I, edited by Robert Berkow, et al. Rahway, NJ: Merck Research Laboratories, 1992.

Rebecca J. Frey

Granulomatous ileitis *see* **Crohn's disease**

Granulomatous uveitis *see* **Uveitis**

Graves' disease *see* **Hyperthyroidism**

Grippe *see* **Influenza**

Griseofulvin *see* **Systemic antifungal drugs**

Group A streptococcus infection *see* **Streptococcal infections**

Group B streptococcus infection *see* **Streptococcal infections**

Group C streptococcus infection *see* **Streptococcal infections**

Group F streptococcus infection *see* **Streptococcal infections**

. . . .

Group therapy

Definition

Group therapy is a form of psychosocial treatment where a small group of patients meet regularly to talk, interact, and discuss problems with each other and the group leader (therapist).

Purpose

Group therapy attempts to give individuals a safe and comfortable place where they can work out problems and emotional issues. Patients gain insight into their own thoughts and behavior, and offer suggestions and support to others. In addition, patients who have a difficult time with interpersonal relationships can benefit from the social interactions that are a basic part of the group therapy experience.

Precautions

Patients who are suicidal, homicidal, psychotic, or in the midst of a major acute crisis are typically not referred for group therapy until their behavior and emotional state have stabilized. Depending on their level of functioning, cognitively impaired patients (like patients with organic brain disease or a traumatic brain injury) may also be unsuitable for group therapy intervention. Some patients with sociopathic traits are not suitable for most groups.

Description

A psychologist, psychiatrist, social worker, or other healthcare professional typically arranges and conducts group therapy sessions. In some therapy groups, two cotherapists share the responsibility of group leadership. Patients are selected on the basis of what they might gain from group therapy interaction and what they can contribute to the group as a whole.

KEY TERMS

Cognitive-behavioral—A therapy technique that focuses on changing beliefs, images, and thoughts in order to change maladjusted behaviors.

Gestalt—A humanistic therapy technique that focuses on gaining an awareness of emotions and behaviors in the present rather than in the past.

Psychodynamic—A therapy technique that assumes improper or unwanted behavior is caused by unconscious, internal conflicts and focuses on gaining insight into these motivations.

Therapy groups may be homogeneous or heterogeneous. Homogeneous groups have members with similar diagnostic backgrounds (for example, they may all suffer from depression). Heterogeneous groups have a mix of individuals with different emotional issues. The number of group members varies widely, but is typically no more than 12. Groups may be time limited (with a predetermined number of sessions) or indefinite (where the group determines when therapy ends). Membership may be closed or open to new members once sessions begin.

The number of sessions in group therapy depends on the makeup, goals, and setting of the group. For example, a therapy group that is part of a substance abuse program to rehabilitate inpatients would be called short-term group therapy. This term is used because, as patients, the group members will only be in the hospital for a relatively short period of time. Long-term therapy groups may meet for six months, a year, or longer. The therapeutic approach used in therapy depends on the focus of the group and the psychological training of the therapist. Some common techniques include psychodynamic, cognitive-behavioral, and **Gestalt therapy.**

In a group therapy session, group members are encouraged to openly and honestly discuss the issues that brought them to therapy. They try to help other group members by offering their own suggestions, insights, and empathy regarding their problems. There are no definite rules for group therapy, only that members participate to the best of their ability. However, most therapy groups do have some basic ground rules that are usually discussed during the first session. Patients are asked not to share what goes on in therapy sessions with anyone outside of the group. This protects the confidentiality of the other members. They may also be asked not to see other group members socially outside of therapy because of the harmful effect it might have on the dynamics of the group.

The therapist's main task is to guide the group in self-discovery. Depending on the goals of the group and the training and style of the therapist, he or she may lead the group interaction or allow the group to take their own direction. Typically, the group leader does some of both, providing direction when the group gets off track while letting them set their own agenda. The therapist may guide the group by simply reinforcing the positive behaviors they engage in. For example, if a group member shows empathy to another member, or offers a constructive suggestion, the therapist will point this out and explain the value of these actions to the group. In almost all group therapy situations, the therapist will attempt to emphasize the common traits among group members so that members can gain a sense of group identity. Group members realize that others share the same issues they do.

The main benefit group therapy may have over individual psychotherapy is that some patients behave and react more like themselves in a group setting than they would one-on-one with a therapist. The group therapy patient gains a certain sense of identity and social acceptance from their membership in the group. Suddenly, they are not alone. They are surrounded by others who have the same anxieties and emotional issues that they have. Seeing how others deal with these issues may give them new solutions to their problems. Feedback from group members also offers them a unique insight into their own behavior, and the group provides a safe forum in which to practice new behaviors. Lastly, by helping others in the group work through their problems, group therapy members can gain more self-esteem. Group therapy may also simulate family experiences of patients and will allow family dynamic issues to emerge.

Self-help groups like Alcoholics Anonymous and Weight Watchers fall outside of the psychotherapy realm. These self-help groups do offer many of the same benefits of social support, identity, and belonging that make group therapy effective for many. Self-help group members meet to discuss a common area of concern (like **alcoholism,** eating disorders, bereavement, parenting). Group sessions are not run by a therapist, but by a nonprofessional leader, group member, or the group as a whole. Self-help groups are sometimes used in addition to psychotherapy or regular group therapy.

Preparation

Patients are typically referred for group therapy by a psychologist or psychiatrist. Some patients may need individual therapy first. Before group sessions begin, the therapist leading the session may conduct a short intake interview with the patient to determine if the group is right for the patient. This interview will also allow the therapist to determine if the addition of the patient will benefit the group. The patient may be given some preliminary information on the group before sessions begin.

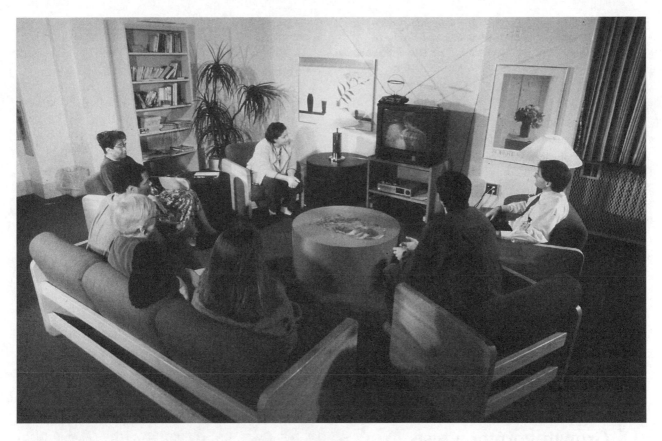

Group therapy is practiced in a variety of settings, including both inpatient and outpatient facilities, and is used to treat anxiety, mood, and personality disorders as well as psychoses. *(Photo Researchers, Inc. Reproduced by permission.)*

This may include guidelines for success (like being open, listening to others, taking risks), rules of the group (like maintaining confidentiality), and educational information on what group therapy is about.

Aftercare

The end of long-term group therapy may cause feelings of grief, loss, abandonment, anger, or rejection in some members. The group therapist will attempt to foster a sense of closure by encouraging members to explore their feelings and use newly acquired coping techniques to deal with them. Working through this termination phase of group therapy is an important part of the treatment process.

Risks

Some very fragile patients may not be able to tolerate aggressive or hostile comments from group members. Patients who have trouble communicating in group situations may be at risk for dropping out of group therapy. If no one comments on their silence or makes an attempt to interact with them, they may begin to feel even more isolated and alone instead of identifying with the group. Therefore, the therapist usually attempts to encourage silent members to participate early on in treatment.

Normal results

Studies have shown that both group and individual psychotherapy benefit about 85% of the patients that participate in them. Optimally, patients gain a better understanding of themselves, and perhaps a stronger set of interpersonal and coping skills through the group therapy process. Some patients may continue therapy after group therapy ends, either individually or in another group setting.

Resources

BOOKS

Bernard, Harold S., and K. Roy MacKenzie, eds. *Basics of Group Psychotherapy.* New York: The Guilford Press, 1994.

Flores, Philip J. *Group Psychotherapy with Addicted Populations: An Integration of Twelve-Step and Psychodynamic Theory*, 2nd ed. New York: The Haworth Press, 1997.

ORGANIZATIONS

American Psychiatric Association (APA), Office of Public Affairs. 1400 K St. NW, Washington, DC 20005. (202) 682-6119. http://www.psych.org.

American Psychological Association (APA), Office of Public Affairs. 750 First St. NE, Washington, DC 20002-4242. (202) 336-5700. http://www.apa.org.

Paula Anne Ford-Martin

Growth hormone stimulation test *see* **Growth hormone tests**

Growth hormone suppression test *see* **Growth hormone tests**

Growth hormone tests

Definition

Growth hormone (hGH), or somatotropin, is a hormone responsible for normal body growth and development by stimulating protein production in muscle cells and energy release from the breakdown of fats. Tests for growth hormone include Somatotropin hormone test, Somatomedin C, Growth hormone suppression test (glucose loading test), and Growth hormone stimulation test (Arginine test or Insulin tolerance test).

Purpose

Growth hormone tests are ordered for the following reasons:

- To identify growth deficiencies, including delayed puberty and small stature in adolescents which can result from pituitary or thyroid malfunction

- To aid in the diagnosis of hyperpituitarism that is evident in gigantism or acromegaly

- To screen for inadequate or reduced pituitary gland function

- To assist in the diagnosis of **pituitary tumors** or tumors related to the hypothalamus, an area of the brain

- To evaluate hGH therapy.

KEY TERMS

Acromegaly—A rare disease resulting from excessive growth hormone caused by a benign tumor. If such a tumor develops within the first ten years of life, the result is gigantism (in which growth is accelerated) and not acromegaly. Symptoms include coarsening of the facial features, enlargement of the hands, feet, ears, and nose, jutting of the jaw, and a long face.

Dwarfism, pituitary—Short stature. When caused by inadequate amounts of growth hormone (as opposed to late growth spurt or genetics), hGH deficiency results in abnormally slow growth and short stature with normal proportions.

Gigantism—Excessive growth, especially in height, resulting from overproduction during childhood or adolescence of growth hormone by a pituitary tumor. Untreated, the tumor eventually destroys the pituitary gland, resulting in death during early adulthood. If the tumor develops after growth has stopped, the result is acromegaly, not gigantism.

Pituitary gland—The pituitary is the most important of the endocrine glands (glands that release hormones directly into the bloodstream). Sometimes referred to as the "master gland," the pituitary regulates and controls the activities of other endocrine glands and many body processes.

Precautions

Taking certain drugs such as amphetamines, dopamine, **corticosteroids,** and phenothiazines may increase and decrease growth hormone secretion, respectively. Other factors influencing hGH secretion include **stress, exercise,** diet, and abnormal glucose levels. These tests should not be done within a week of any radioactive scan.

Description

Several hormones play important roles in human growth. The major human growth hormone (hGH), or somatotropin, is a protein made up of 191 amino acids which is secreted by the anterior pituitary gland and coordinates normal growth and development. Human growth is characterized by two spurts, one at birth and the other at **puberty.** hGH plays an important role at both of these times. Normal individuals have measurable levels of hGH throughtout life. Yet levels of hGH fluctuate during the day and are affected by eating and exercise. Receptors which respond to hGH exist on cells and tissues throughout the body. The most obvious effect of hGH is on linear skeletal development. But the metabolic effects of hGH on muscle, the liver, and fat cells are critical to its function. Humans have two forms of hGH, and the functional difference between the two is unclear. They are both formed from the same gene, but one lacks the amino acids in positions 32–46.

hGH is produced in the anterior portion of the pituitary gland by somatotrophs under the control of hormonal signals in the hypothalamus. Two hypothalamic hormones regulate hGH; they are growth hormone-releasing hormone (GHRH) and growth hormone—inhibiting hormone (GHIH). When blood glucose levels fall, GHRH triggers the secretion of stored hGH. As blood glucose levels rise, GHRH release is turned off. Increases in blood protein levels trigger a similar response. As a result of this hypothalamic feedback loop, hGH levels fluctuate throughout the day. Normal plasma hGH levels 1 to 3 ng/ML with peaks as high as 60 ng/ML. In addition, plasma glucose and amino acid availability for growth is also regulated by the hormones adrenaline, glucagon, and insulin.

Most hGH is released at night. Peak spikes of hGH release occur around 10 p.m., midnight, and 2 a.m. The logic behind this night-time release is that most of hGH's effects are mediated by other hormones, including the somatomedins, IGH-I and IGH-II. As a result, the effects of hGH are spread out more evenly during the day.

A number of hormonal conditions can lead to excessive or diminished growth. Because of its critical role in producing hGH and other hormones, an aberrant pituitary gland will often yield altered growth. Dwarfism (very small stature) can be due to underproduction of hGH, lack of IGH-I, or a flaw in target tissue response to either of these growth hormones. Overproduction of hGH or IGH-I, or an exaggerated response to these hormones can lead to gigantism or acromegaly, both of which are characterized by a very large stature.

Gigantism is the result of hGH overproduction in early childhood leading to a skeletal height up to 8 feet (2.5m) or more. Acromegaly results when hGH is overproduced after the onset of puberty. In this condition, the epiphyseal plates of the long bone of the body do not close, and they remain responsive to additional stimulated growth by hGH. This disorder is characterized by an enlarged skull, hands and feet, nose, neck, and tongue.

Somatrotropin

Somatrotropin is used to identify hGH deficiency in adolescents with short stature, delayed sexual maturity, and other growth deficiencies. It also aids in documenting excess hGH production that is responsible for gigantism or acromegaly, and confirms underactivity or overproduction of the pituitary gland (**hypopituitarism** or hy-

perpituitarism). However, due to the episodic secretion of hGH, as well as hGH production in response to stress, exercise, or other factors, random assays are not an adequate determination of hGH deficiency. To negate these variables and obtain more accurate readings, a blood sample can be drawn 1 to 1.5 hours after sleep (hGH levels increase during sleep), or strenuous exercise can be performed for 30 minutes before blood is drawn (hGH levels increase after exercise). The hGH levels at the end of an exercise period are expected to be maximal.

Somatomedin C

The somatomedin C test is usually ordered to detect pituitary abnormalities, hGH deficiency, and acromegaly. Also called insulin-like growth factor (IGF-1), somatomedin C is considered a more accurate reflection of the blood concentration of hGH because such variables as time of day, activity levels, or diet does not influence the results. Somatomedin C is part of a group of peptides, called somatomedins, through which hGH exerts its effects. Because it circulates in the bloodstream bound to long-lasting proteins, it is more stable than hGH. Levels of somatomedin C do depend on hGH levels, however. As a result, somatomedin C levels are low when hGH levels are deficient. Abnormally low test results of somatomedin C require an abnormally reduced or absent hGH during an hGH stimulation test in order to diagnose hGH deficiency. Nonpituitary causes of reduced somatomedin C include **malnutrition,** severe chronic illness, severe liver disease, **hypothyroidism,** and Laron's dwarfism.

Growth hormone stimulation test

The hGH stimulation test, also called hGH Provocation test, Insulin Tolerance, or Arginine test, is performed to test the body's ability to produce human growth hormone, and to identify suspected hGH deficiency. A normal patient can have low hGH levels, but if hGH is still low after stimulation, a diagnosis can be more accurately made.

Insulin-induced hypoglycemia (via intravenous injection of insulin) stimulates hGH and corticotropin secretion as well. If such stimulation is unsuccessful, then there is a malfunction of the anterior pituitary gland. Blood samples may be obtained following an energetic exercise session lasting 20 minutes.

A substance called hGH-releasing factor has recently been used for hGH stimulation. This approach promises to be more accurate and specific for hGH deficiency caused by the pituitary. Growth hormone deficiency is also suspected when x ray determination of bone age indicates retarded growth in comparison to chronologic age. At present, the best method to identify hGH-deficient patients is a positive stimulation test followed by a positive response to a therapeutic trial of hGH.

Growth hormone suppression test

Also called the glucose loading test, this procedure is used to evaluate excessive baseline levels of human growth hormone, and to confirm diagnosis of gigantism in children and acromegaly in adults. The procedure requires two different blood samples, one drawn before the administration of 100 g of glucose (by mouth), and a second sample two hours after glucose ingestion.

Normally, a glucose load suppresses hGH secretion. In a patient with excessive hGH levels, failure of suppression indicates anterior pituitary dysfunction and confirms a diagnosis of **acromegaly and gigantism.**

Preparation

Somatotropin: This test requires a blood sample. The patient should be **fasting** (nothing to eat or drink from midnight the night before the test). Stress and/or exercise increases hGH levels, so the patient should be at complete rest for 30 minutes before the blood sample is drawn. If the physician has requested two samples, they should be drawn on consecutive days at approximately the same time on both days, preferably between 6 am and 8 am.

Somatomedin C: This test requires a blood sample. The patient should have nothing to eat or drink from midnight the night before the test.

Growth hormone stimulation: This test requires intravenous administration of medications and the withdrawal of frequent blood samples, which are obtained at 0, 60, and 90 minutes after injection of arginine and/or insulin. The patient should have nothing to eat or drink after midnight the night before the test.

Growth hormone suppression: This test requires two blood samples, one before the test and another two hours after administration of 100 g of glucose solution by mouth. The patient should have nothing to eat or drink after midnight, and physical activity should be limited for 10–12 hours before the test.

Risks

Growth hormone stimulation: Only minor discomfort is associated with this test, and results from the insertion of the IV line and the low blood sugar (hypoglycemia) induced by the insulin injection. Some patients may experience sleepiness, sweating and/or nervousness, all of which can be corrected after the test by ingestion of cookies, juice, or a glucose infusion. Severe cases of hypoglycemia may cause ketosis (excessive amounts of fatty acid byproducts in the body), acidosis (a disturbance

of the body's acid-base balance), or **shock.** With the close observation required for the test, these are unlikely.

Growth hormone suppression: Some patients experience nausea after the administration of this amount of glucose. Ice chips can alleviate this symptom.

Normal results

Normal results may vary from laboratory to laboratory but are usually within the following ranges:

Somatotropin:

- Men: 5 ng/ml
- Women: less than 10 ng/ml
- Children: 0–10 ng/ml
- Newborn: 10–40 ng/ml.

Somatomedin C:

- Adult: 42–110 ng/ml
- Child:
- 0–8 years: Girls 7–110 ng/ml; Boys 4–87 ng/ml
- 9–10 years: Girls 39–186 ng/ml; Boys 26–98 ng/ml
- 11–13 years: Girls 66–215 ng/ml; Boys 44–207 ng/ml
- 14–16 years: Girls 96–256 ng/ml; Boys 48 255 ng/ml.

Growth hormone stimulation: greater than 10 ng/ml.

Growth hormone suppression: Normally, glucose suppresses hGH to levels of undetectable to 3 ng/ml in 30 minutes to two hours. In children, rebound stimulation may occur after 2–5 hours.

Abnormal results

Somatotropin hormone: Excess hGH is responsible for the syndromes of gigantism and acromegaly. Excess secretion is stimulated by **anorexia nervosa,** stress, hypoglycemia, and exercise. Decreased levels are seen in hGH deficiency, dwarfism, hyperglycemia, **failure to thrive,** and delayed sexual maturity.

Somatomedin C: Increased levels contribute to the syndromes of gigantism and acromegaly. Stress, major surgery, hypoglycemia, **starvation,** and exercise stimulate hGH secretion, which in turn stimulates somatomedin C.

Growth hormone stimulation: Decreased levels are seen in pituitary deficiency and hGH deficiency. Diseases of the pituitary can result in failure of the pituitary to secrete hGH and/or all the pituitary hormones. As a result, the hGH stimulation test will fail to stimulate hGH secretion.

Growth hormone suppression: The acromegaly syndrome elevates base hGH levels to 75 ng/ml, which in turn are not suppressed to less than 5 ng/ml during the test. Excess hGH secretion may cause unchanged or rising hGH levels in response to glucose loading, confirming a diagnosis of acromegaly or gigantism. In such cases, verification of results is required by repeating the test after a one-day rest.

Resources

BOOKS

Cahill, Mathew. *Handbook of Diagnostic Tests.* Springhouse Corporation, 1995.

Jacobs, David S. *Laboratory Test Handbook,* Fourth Edition. Lexi-Comp Inc., 1996.

Pagana, Kathleen Deska. *Mosby's Manual of Diagnostic and Laboratory Tests.* Mosby, Inc., 1998.

Janis O. Flores

Guaifenesin *see* **Expectorants**

Guided imagery

Definition

The technique of guided imagery focuses the power of the mind on some aspect of the workings of the body in order to cause a real, positive physical response.

Purpose

Once learned, this self-help technique is used to relieve **stress,** explore psychological conflicts, and manage **pain.** Used as an effective means of self-care as well as in various medical settings, it can be applied to any medical situation in which relaxation, symptom relief, and a feeling of personal empowerment is useful.

Precautions

In cases of a serious disease or condition, guided imagery should not be used in place of conventional medicine or surgery. It is not recommended for psychotic patients who often cannot distinguish the difference between suggested images and reality.

Description

Guided imagery has been described by one magazine writer as a kind of "directed daydreaming." It is based on the generally accepted idea that the mind can influence the body. A typical example used by many to make this point is the suggestion that the reader relax and think about a juicy, fresh lemon. The further suggestion that the reader slice it and slowly raise the dripping, pale yellow sections to his or her waiting lips and then suck on it,

---

KEY TERMS

Adjunct—Something joined or added to another thing but not essentially part of it.

Anecdotal—Pertaining to a specific unusual or interesting event or incident.

Brain waves—The electric currents generated by the activity of the brain, especially the cerebral cortex.

Cerebral cortex—The front part of the brain that directs voluntary activities and is associated with the higher function of intelligence.

Gastrointestinal—Relating to the stomach and intestines.

Hormone—A chemical secretion produced by the body's glands that is carried in the bloodstream to effect a change in another organ.

Involuntary functions—Those functions of the nervous system of vertebrates that operate independently of control.

Neurological—Pertaining to the nervous system.

Proponent—One who proposes or advocates something.

Psychotic—Severely mentally ill and characterized by delusions and loss of contact with reality.

Secretion—The substance produced by a gland or cell.

---

almost always results in a standard physiological response: most readers salivate. Proponents of this technique argue that people possess a remarkable degree of self-regulation that generally goes unknown, unexplored, and unused.

It is a known fact, and one to which every adult who has ever been sexually aroused by a thought can testify, that a thought or "image" can affect heart and breathing rate, as well as other involuntary functions like hormone levels, gastrointestinal secretions, and brain wave patterns. Proponents of guided imagery therefore stress the importance of the image (thought) which, they say, does not have to be real to have a actual, physical effect. Guided Imagery then takes the next step and asks why can't the mind be used to cause good things to happen within the body. Also called Visualization, Creative Visualization, or Creative Imagery, this technique teaches how to consciously create positive images to accomplish a desired goal. One neurological explanation of what might go on in the brain during Guided Imagery is that the image or message is sent from the higher centers of the brain (cerebral cortex) to the lower or more primitive centers that regulate a person's involuntary functions, like breathing and heart rate. Whether or not these images are real, the lower part of the brain apparently responds accordingly as long as there is no contradictory information.

In a typical session with a practitioner, the patient or client is placed in a relaxed state by the verbal guidance of the practitioner. Once the patient is relaxed, this calm, receptive state is deepened through breathing **exercises.** This allows the patient to give real focus and direction to his or her imagination. Once truly deep relaxation is achieved, the practitioner encourages the patient to choose a safe place, which is a very personal, truly serene site that may or may not actually exist, in which the patient feels perfect emotional security. It is at this point that the practitioner begins to implement the particular goal of therapy, whether it is to reduce stress or **anxiety,** manage the constant pain of a chronic condition, or assist in the healing process. The skilled practitioner will ask leading questions that encourage patients to describe concretely and in great detail all the particular impressions they are receiving from their image, and also allows them to explore their unconscious, gaining insights into themselves and others. Following several successful sessions with a practitioner, the patient is usually able to do the same on their own, often using written instructions or special tapes.

Risks

As a totally non-invasive therapy that involves no manipulation or even touching, the only risk in Guided Imagery would be in viewing it as a cure-all rather than as an adjunct to conventional medicine.

Normal results

Although there is only anecdotal information about Guided Imagery curing **cancer,** boosting an immune system, or insulating the patient from all pain, it has proven helpful in learning to manage chronic pain, accelerating the recovery and healing process, and reducing stress and anxiety.

Resources

BOOKS

Burton Goldberg Group. *Alternative Medicine: The Definitive Guide.* Puyallup, WA: Future Medicine Publishing, Inc., 1993.

Castleman, Michael. *Nature's Cures.* Emmaus, PA: Rodale Press, Inc., 1996.

Kastner, Mark and Hugh Burroughs. *Alternative Healing.* New York: Henry Holt and Company, 1996.

Naparstek, Belleruth. *Staying Well With Guided Imagery.* New York: Warner Books, 1994.

PERIODICALS

Crane, Tricia. "Guided Imagery: Thinking Yourself Well." *Harper's Bazaar* (April 1988): 161, 223.

Milk, Leslie. "Guided Imagery: Picture Yourself Relaxed." *The Washingtonian* (February 1989): 126.

Shames, Karilee Halo. "Harness the Power of Guided Imagery." *RN* (August 1996): 49-50.

ORGANIZATIONS

The Academy for Guided Imagery. P.O. Box 2070, Mill Valley, CA 94942. (800) 726-2070.

Leonard C. Bruno

Guillain-Barré syndrome

Definition

Guillain-Barré syndrome (GBS) causes progressive muscle weakness and **paralysis** (the complete inability to use a particular muscle or muscle group), which develops over days or up to four weeks, and lasts several weeks or even months.

Description

The classic scenario in GBS involves a patient who has just recovered from a typical, seemingly uncomplicated viral infection. Symptoms of muscle weakness appear one to four weeks later. The most common preceding infections are cytomegalovirus, herpes, Epstein-Barr virus, and viral hepatitis. A gastrointestinal infection with the bacteria *Campylobacter jejuni* is also common and may cause a severe type of GBS from which it is particularly difficult to recover. About 5% of GBS patients have a surgical procedure as a preceding event. Patients with lymphoma, **systemic lupus erythematosus,** or **AIDS** have a higher than normal risk of GBS. Other GBS patients have recently received an immunization, while still others have no known preceding event. In 1976–77, there was a vastly increased number of GBS cases among people who had been recently vaccinated against the Swine flu. The reason for this phenomenon has never been identified, and no other flu vaccine has caused such an increase in GBS cases.

Causes & symptoms

The cause of the weakness and paralysis of GBS is the loss of myelin, which is the material that coats nerve cells (the loss of myelin is called demyelination). Myelin is an insulating substance which is wrapped around nerves in the body, serving to speed conduction of nerve impulses. Without myelin, nerve conduction slows or

KEY TERMS

Autoimmune—The body's immune system directed against the body itself.

Demyelination—Disruption or destruction of the myelin sheath, leaving a bare nerve. Results in a slowing or stopping of impulses traveling along that nerve.

Inflammatory—Having to do with inflammation, the body's response to either invading foreign substances (such as viruses or bacteria) or to direct injury of body tissue.

Myelin—The substance that is wrapped around nerves, and which is responsible for speed and efficiency of impulses traveling through those nerves.

stops. GBS has a short, severe course. It causes inflammation and destruction of the myelin sheath, and it disturbs multiple nerves. Therefore, it is considered an acute inflammatory demyelinating polyneuropathy.

The reason for the destruction of myelin in GBS is unknown, although it is thought that the underlying problem is autoimmune in nature. An autoimmune disorder is one in which the body's immune system, trained to fight against such foreign invaders as viruses and bacteria, somehow becomes improperly programmed. The immune system becomes confused, and is not able to distinguish between foreign invaders and the body itself. Elements of the immune system are unleashed against areas of the body, resulting in damage and destruction. For some reason, in the case of GBS, the myelin sheath appears to become a target for the body's own immune system.

The first symptoms of GBS consist of muscle weakness (legs first, then arms, then face), accompanied by prickly, tingling sensations (paresthesias). Symptoms affect both sides of the body simultaneously, a characteristic that helps distinguish GBS from other causes of weakness and paresthesias. Normal reflexes are first diminished, then lost. The weakness eventually affects all the voluntary muscles, resulting in paralysis. When those muscles necessary for breathing become paralyzed, the patient must be placed on a mechanical ventilator which takes over the function of breathing. This occurs about 30% of the time. Very severely ill GBS patients may have complications stemming from other nervous system abnormalities which can result in problems with fluid balance in the body, severely fluctuating blood pressure, and heart rhythm irregularities.

Diagnosis

Diagnosis of GBS is made by looking for a particular cluster of symptoms (progressively worse muscle weakness and then paralysis), and by examining the fluid that bathes the brain and spinal canal through **cerebrospinal fluid (CSF) analysis.** This fluid is obtained by inserting a needle into the lower back (lumbar region). When examined in a laboratory, the CSF of a GBS patient will reveal a greater-than-normal quantity of protein, with normal numbers of white blood cells and a normal amount of sugar. Electrodiagnostic studies may show slowing or block of conduction in nerve endings in parts of the body other than the brain. Minor abnormalities will be present in 90% of patients.

Treatment

There is no direct treatment for GBS. Instead, treatments are used that support the patient with the disabilities caused by the disease. The progress of paralysis must be carefully monitored, in order to provide mechanical assistance for breathing if it becomes necessary. Careful attention must also be paid to the amount of fluid the patient is taking in by drinking and eliminating by urinating. Blood pressure, heart rate, and heart rhythm also must be monitored.

A procedure called **plasmapheresis,** performed early in the course of GBS, has been shown to shorten the course and severity of GBS. Plasmapheresis consists of withdrawing the patient's blood, passing it through an instrument that separates the different types of blood cells, and returning all the cellular components (red and white blood cells and platelets) along with either donor plasma or a manufactured replacement solution. This is thought to rid the blood of the substances that are attacking the patient's myelin.

It has also been shown that the use of high doses of immunoglobulin given intravenously (by drip through a needle in a vein) may be just as helpful as plasmapheresis. Immunoglobulin is a substance naturally manufactured by the body's immune system in response to various threats. It is interesting to note that corticosteroid medications (such as prednisone), often the mainstay of anti-autoimmune disease treatment, are not only unhelpful, but may in fact be harmful to patients with GBS.

Prognosis

About 85% of GBS patients make reasonably good recoveries. However, 30% of adult patients, and a greater percentage of children, never fully regain their previous level of muscle strength. Some of these patients suffer from residual weakness, others from permanent paralysis. About 10% of GBS patients begin to improve, then suffer a relapse. These patients suffer chronic GBS symptoms. About 5% of all GBS patients die, most from cardiac rhythm disturbances.

Patients with certain characteristics tend to have a worse outcome. These include people of older age, those who required breathing support with a mechanical ventilator, and those who had their worst symptoms within the first seven days.

Prevention

Because so little is known about what causes GBS to develop, there are no known methods of prevention.

Resources

BOOKS

Bosch, E. P. and H. Mitsumoto. ''Disorders of Peripheral Nerves.'' In *Neurology in Clinical Practice: The Neurological Disorders,* edited by Walter G. Bradley, et al. Boston: Butterworth-Heinemann, 1996.

Griffin, J. W. ''Immune-Mediated Neuropathies.'' In *Cecil Essentials of Medicine.* Philadelphia: W.B. Saunders, 1996.

Guberman, A. *An Introduction to Clinical Neurology.* Boston: Little, Brown and Company, 1994.

PERIODICALS

Fulgham, J. R. ''Guillain-Barré syndrome.'' *Critical Care Clinics* (January 1997): 1-15.

Rees, J.H. ''Campylobacter jejuni infection and Guillain-Barré syndrome.'' *New England Journal of Medicine* (November 23, 1995): 1374-79.

Stern, V. ''Terror of the Unknown.'' *The Guardian* (February 13, 1996): T10 + .

Walling, A. D. ''Comparisons of Treatments for Guillain-Barré Syndrome.'' *American Family Physician* (May 15, 1997): 2510 + .

ORGANIZATIONS

American Academy of Neurology. 1080 Montreal Avenue, St. Paul, MN 55116. (612)695-1940. http://www.aan.com.

Guillain-Barré Syndrome Foundation International. P.O. Box 262, Wynnewood, PA 19096. (610)667-0131. http://www.adsnet.com/jsteinhi/html/gbs/gbsfi.html.

Rosalyn S. Carson-DeWitt

Guinea worm infection

Definition

Infection occurs when the parasitic guinea worm resides within the body. Infection is not apparent until a

pregnant female worm prepares to expel embryos. The infection is rarely fatal, but the latter stage is painful. The infection is also referred to as dracunculiasis, and less commonly as dracontiasis.

Description

Before the early 1980s, guinea worms infected 10–15 million people annually in central Africa and parts of Asia. By 1996, worldwide incidence of infection fell to fewer than 153,000 cases per year. Complete eradication of guinea worm infection is a goal of international water safety programs.

To survive, guinea worms require three things: water during the embryo stage, an intermediate host during early maturation, and a human host during adulthood. In bodies of water, such as ponds, guinea worm embryos are eaten by tiny, lobster-like water fleas. Once ingested, the embryos mature into larvae.

Humans become hosts by consuming water containing infected water fleas. Once in the human intestine, larvae burrow into surrounding tissue. After 3–4 months, the worms mate. Males die soon after, but pregnant females continue to grow. As adults, each threadlike worm can be three feet long and harbor three million embryos. More than one guinea worm can infect a person at the same time.

About eight months later, the female prepares to expel mature embryos by migrating toward the skin surface. Until this point, most people are unaware that they are infected. Extreme pain occurs as the worm emerges from under the skin, often around the infected person's ankle. The pain is temporarily relieved by immersing the area in water, an act that contaminates the water and starts the cycle again.

Causes & symptoms

Dracunculus medinensis, or guinea worm, causes infection. Symptoms are commonly absent until a pregnant worm prepares to expel embryos. By secreting an irritating chemical, the worm causes a blister to form on the skin surface. This chemical also causes nausea, vomiting, **dizziness,** and **diarrhea.** The blister is accompanied by a burning, stabbing pain and can form anywhere on the body; but, the usual site is the lower leg or foot. Once the blister breaks, an open sore remains until the worm has expelled all the embryos.

Diagnosis

Guinea worm infection is identified by the symptoms.

Treatment

Most people infected with guinea worm rely on traditional medicine. The worm is extracted by gently and gradually pulling the worm out and winding it around a small strip of wood. Surgical removal is possible, but rarely done in rural areas. Extraction is complemented by herbs and oils to treat the wound site. Such treatment can ease extraction and may help prevent secondary infections.

Modern medicine offers safe surgical removal of the guinea worm, and drug therapy can prevent infection and pain. Using drugs to combat the worms has had mixed results.

Prognosis

If the worm is completely removed, the wound heals in approximately 2–4 weeks. However, if a worm emerges from a sensitive area, such as the sole of a foot, or if several worms are involved, healing requires more time. Recovery is also complicated if the worm breaks during extraction. Serious secondary infections frequently occur in such situations. There is the risk of permanent disability in some cases, and having one guinea worm infection does not confer immunity against future infections.

Prevention

Guinea worn infection is prevented by disrupting transmission. Wells and other protected water sources are usually safe from being contaminated with worm embryos. In open water sources, poisons may be used to kill water fleas. Otherwise, water must be boiled or filtered.

Resources

PERIODICALS

Hunter, John M. "An Introduction to Guinea Worm on the Eve of Its Departure: Dracunculiasis Transmission, Health Effects, Ecology and Control." *Social Science and Medicine* 43 (9)(1996): 1399.

OTHER

The World Health Organization, Division of Control of Tropical Diseases. http://www.who.ch/ctd/html/homepage.html.

Julia Barrett

Gulf War syndrome

Definition

Soliders returning from the Persian Gulf War in 1991 are experiencing a wide variety of symptoms from **asthma** to **sexual dysfunction.** The collected wisdom of the medical world is hard at work to solve the dilemma. They have taken the necessary first step, which is to identify the problem in all its various forms, give it a name, and collect as much information as possible. The next step is well under way—to analyze the data. While the cause and a cure are being pursued, victims are receiving the best treatment currently available. The Department of Defense (DOD) and the Department of Veterans Affairs vows to "leave no stone unturned" in its investigation of this illness.

Description

Warfare is unlike any other human experience. Those who have not lived it first hand cannot comprehend the magnitude of deviation from everything that comes before or follows after. Soldiers returning from war are forever changed. They reliably bring back with them symptoms that have a similarity stretching at least as far back as the Civil War. They are tired; they have trouble breathing; they have headaches; they sleep poorly; they are forgetful; they cannot concentrate. Such is the situation with veterans of Operation Desert Storm, the Persian Gulf War.

Causes & symptoms

There is much current debate over a possible causative agent for Gulf War Syndrome other than the **stress** of warfare. Intensive efforts by the Veterans Administration and other public and private institutions have investigated a wide range of potential factors. These include chemical and biological weapons, the immunizations and

KEY TERMS

Ataxia—Lack of coordination.

Caloric testing—Flushing warm and cold water into the ear stimulates the labyrinth and causes vertigo and nystagmus if all the nerve pathways are intact.

Endemic—Always there.

Paresthesia—An altered sensation often described as burning, tingling, or pin pricks.

Syndrome—Common features of a disease or features that appear together often enough to suggest they may represent a single, as yet unknown, disease entity. When a syndrome is first identified, an attempt is made to define it as strictly as possible, even to the exclusion of some cases, in order to separate out a pure enough sample to study. This process is most likely to identify a cause, a positive method of diagnosis, and a treatment. Later on, less typical cases can be considered.

preventive treatments used to protect against them, and diseases endemic to the Arabian peninsula. So far investigators have not approached a consensus. They even disagree on the likelihood that a specific agent is responsible. There is, however, a likelihood that sarin and/or cyclosarin (nerve gases) were released during the destruction of Iraqi munitions at Kharnisiyah, Iraq.

Statistical analysis tells us that the following symptoms are about twice as likely to appear in Gulf War veterans than in their non-combat peers: depression, post-traumatic stress disorder (PTSD), chronic fatigue, cognitive dysfunction (diminished ability to calculate, order thoughts, evaluate, learn, and remember), **bronchitis,** asthma, **fibromyalgia,** alcohol abuse, **anxiety,** and sexual discomfort. PTSD is the modern equivalent of shell shock (World War I) and battle fatigue (World War II). It encompasses most of the psychological symptoms of war veterans, not excluding nightmares, panic at sudden loud noises, and inability to adjust to peacetime living. **Chronic fatigue syndrome** has a specific medical definition that attempts to separate out common fatigue from a more disabling illness in hope of finding a specific cause. Fibromyalgia is another newly defined syndrome, and as such it has arbitrarily rigid defining characteristics. These include a certain duration of illness, a specified minimum number of tender areas located in designated areas of the body, sleep disturbances, and other associated symptoms and signs.

Researchers have identified three distinct syndromes and several variations in Gulf War veterans. Type One patients suffer primarily from impaired thinking. Type Two patients have a greater degree of confusion and ataxia (loss of coordination). Type Three patients were the most affected by joint **pains,** muscle pains, and extremity paresthesias (unnatural sensations like burning or tingling in the arms and legs). In each of the three types, researchers found different but measurable impairments on objective testing of neurological function. The business of the nervous system is much more complex and subtle than other body functions. Measuring it requires equally complex effort. The tests used in this study carefully measured and compared localized nerve performance at several different tasks against the same values in normal subjects. Brain wave response to noise and touch, eye muscle response to spinning, and caloric testing (stimulation of the ear with warm and cold water, which causes vertigo) were clearly different between the normal and the test subjects. The researchers concluded that there was ''a generalized injury to the nervous system.'' Another research group concluded their study by stating that there was ''a spectrum of neurologic injury involving the central, peripheral, and autonomic nervous systems.''

Diagnosis

Until there is a clear definition of the disease, diagnosis is primarily an **exercise** in identifying those Gulf War veterans who have undefined illness in an effort to learn more about them and their symptoms. The Veterans Administration currently has a program devoted to this problem, which is gathering data and analyzing it intensively and continuously.

Treatment

Specific treatment awaits specific diagnosis and identification of a causative agent. Meanwhile, veterans can benefit from the wide variety of supportive and non-specific approaches to this and similar problems. There are many drugs available for symptomatic relief. Psychological counseling by those specializing in this area can be immensely beneficial, even life-saving for those contemplating suicide. Veterans' benefits are available for those who are impaired by their symptoms.

Alternative treatment

The symptoms can be worked with using many modalities of alternative health care. The key to working successfully with people living their lives with Gulf War syndrome is long-term, ongoing care, whether it be hypnotherapy, **acupuncture,** homeopathy, nutrition, vitamin/mineral therapy, or bodywork.

Prognosis

The outlook for war veterans spans the spectrum. Gradual return to a functioning life may take many years of work and much help. Even in the absence of an identifiable and curable cause, recovery is possible.

Resources

BOOKS

Foa, Edna B. "Posttraumatic stress disorder." *Treatments of Psychiatric Disorders.* Edited by Glen O Garbbard. Washington, DC: American Psychiatric Press Inc., 1995, pp. 1499-1520.

Isselbacher, Kurt, et al., ed. *Harrison's Principles of Internal Medicine.* New York: McGraw-Hill, 1998, pp. 1955-1957.

Lowenstein, Richard J. "Dissociative amnesia and dissociative fugue." *Treatments of Psychiatric Disorders.* Edited by Glen O. Garbbard. Washington, DC: American Psychiatric Press Inc., 1995, pp. 1569-1597.

Spigel, David. "Acute Stress Disorder." *Treatments of Psychiatric Disorders.* Edited by Glen O. Garbbard. Washington, DC: American Psychiatric Press Inc., 1995, pp. 1521-1536.

PERIODICALS

Coker, W.J. "A review of Gulf War illness." *Journal of the Royal Naval Medical Service* 82 (Summer 1996): 141-146.

Ficarra, B.J. "Medical mystery: Gulf war syndrome." *Journal of Medicine* 26(1995): 87-94.

Gulf War News. Office of the Special Assistant for Gulf War Illnesses, 5113 Leesburg Pike, Suite 901, Falls Church, Virginia 22041. 703-578-8518. cdipaolo@gwillness.osd.mil.

Haley, R.W., et al. "Evaluation of neurologic function in Gulf War veterans. A blinded case-control study." *JAMA* 277 (January 15, 1997): 223-230.

Haley, R.W., T.L. Kurt, and J. Hom. "Is there a Gulf War Syndrome? Searching for syndromes by factor analysis of symptoms." *JAMA* 277 (January 15, 1997): 215-222.

Hyams, K.C., F.S. Wignall, and R. Roswell. "War syndromes and their evaluation: from the U.S. Civil War to the Persian Gulf War." *Annals of Internal Medicine* 125 (September 1996): 398-405.

Jamal, G.A. "The 'Gulf War syndrome': Is there evidence of dysfunction in the nervous system?" *Journal of Neurology, Neurosurgery & Psychiatry* 60 (April 1996): 449-451.

"Self-reported illness and health status among Gulf War veterans. A population-based study. The Iowa Persian Gulf Study Group." *JAMA* 277 (January 15, 1997): 238-245.

Wittich, A.C. "Gynecologic evaluation of the first female soldiers enrolled in the Gulf War Comprehensive Clinical Evaluation Program at Tripler Army Medical Center." *Military Medicine* 161 (November 1996): 635-637.

ORGANIZATIONS

Office of the Special Assistant for Gulf War Illnesses. 5113 Leesburg Pike, Suite 901, Falls Church, Virginia, 22041. 703 578-8518. brostker@gwillness.osd.mil. http://www.gulflink.osd.mil.

U.S. Department of Defense. Comprehensive Clinical Evaluation Program (CCEP). 800-796-9699.

Veterans Administration. Persian Gulf Medical Information Helpline. 400 South 18th Street, St. Louis, Missouri 63103-2271. 800-749-8387.

Veterans Administration. Persian Gulf Registry. 800-PGW-VETS (800-749-8387). http://www.va.gov/.

J. Ricker Polsdorfer

Gum disease *see* **Periodontal disease**

Günther's disease *see* **Porphyrias**

Gynecomastia

Definition

Gyne refers to female, and mastia refers to the breast. Gynecomastia is strictly a male disease and is any growth of the adipose (fatty) and glandular tissue in a male breast. Not all breast growth in men is considered abnormal, just excess growth.

Causes & symptoms

Breast growth is directed exclusively by female hormones—estrogens. Although men have some estrogen in their system, it is usually insufficient to cause much breast enlargement because it is counterbalanced by male

---

KEY TERMS

Androgen—Male sex hormone.

Cirrhosis—Diffuse scarring caused by alcohol or chronic hepatitis often leading to liver failure.

Estrogen—Sex hormone responsible for stimulating female sexual characteristics.

Klinefelter syndrome—A condition in a male characterized by having an extra X (female) chromosome and suffering from infertility and gynecomastia.

Thyroid—A gland in the neck that makes thyroxin. Thyroxin regulates the speed of metabolism.

---

hormones—androgens. Upsetting the balance, either by more of one or less of the other, results in the male developing female characteristics, breast growth being foremost.

At birth both male and female infants will have little breast buds from their mother's hormones. These recede until adolescence, when girls always, and boys sometimes, have breast growth. At this time, the boy's breast growth is minimal, often one-sided and temporary.

Extra or altered sex chromosomes can produce intersex problems of several kinds. Breast growth along with male genital development is seen in **Klinefelter syndrome**—the condition of having an extra X (female) chromosome—and a few other chromosomal anomalies. One of the several glands that produce hormones can malfunction for reasons other than chromosomes. Failure of androgen production is as likely to produce gynecomastia as overabundant estrogen production. Testicular failure and castration can also be a cause. Some **cancers** and some benign tumors can make estrogens. **Lung cancer** is known to increase estrogens.

If the hormone manufacturing organs are functioning properly, problems can still arise elsewhere. The liver is the principle chemical factory in the body. Other organs like the thyroid and kidneys also effect chemical processes. If any of these organs are diseased, a chemical imbalance can result that alters the manufacturing process. Men with **cirrhosis** of the liver will often develop gynecomastia from increased production of estrogens.

Finally, drugs can also cause breast enlargement. Estrogens are given to men to treat **prostate cancer** and a few other diseases. Marijuana and heroin, along with some prescription drugs, have estrogen effects in some men. On the list are methyldopa (for blood pressure), cimetidine (for peptic **ulcers**), diazepam (Valium), antidepressants, and spironolactone (a diuretic).

Diagnosis

Carefully feeling the area beneath the nipple of an adolescent boy with breast enlargement will reveal a discreet and sometimes tender lump the size of a fat nickel or quarter. For more serious gynecomastia, the underlying disease will require evaluation, if it is not already well understood.

Treatment

This condition is usually not treated. If it is the result of endocrine disease, hormone manipulations may reduce the effects of the imbalance. There are a number of medical and surgical interventions possible. Radiation of misbehaving organs and cancers is considered an effective treatment.

Prognosis

The progress of gynecomastia is determined by its cause.

Resources

BOOKS

Bennett, J. Claude and Fred Plum, ed. *Cecil Textbook of Medicine*. Philadelphia: W. B. Saunders, 1996, pp. 1332-1333.

Fitzgerald, Paul A. ''Endocrinology.'' In *Current Medical Diagnosis and Treatment*. Edited by Lawrence M. Tierney Jr., et al. Stamford, CT: Appleton & Lange, 1998, p. 1032.

Wilson, Jean D. ''Endocrine disorders of the breast.'' In *Harrison's Principles of Internal Medicine*. Edited by Kurt Isselbacher, et al. New York: McGraw-Hill, 1997, pp. 111-115.

J. Ricker Polsdorfer

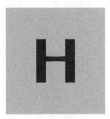

Hair transplantation

Definition

Hair transplantation is a surgical procedure used to treat baldness or hair loss. Typically, tiny patches of scalp are removed from the back and sides of the head and implanted in the bald spots in the front and top of the head.

Purpose

Hair transplantation is a cosmetic procedure performed on men (and occasionally on women) who have significant hair loss, thinning hair, or bald spots where hair no longer grows. In men, hair loss and baldness are most commonly due to genetic factors (a tendency passed on in families) and age. Male pattern baldness, in which the hairline gradually recedes to expose more and more of the forehead, is the most common form. Men may also experience a gradual thinning of hair at the crown or very top of the skull. For women, hair loss is more commonly due to hormonal changes and is more likely to be a thinning of hair from the entire head. An estimated 50,000 men get transplants each year. Transplants can also be done to replace hair lost due to **burns,** injury, or diseases of the scalp.

Precautions

Although hair transplantation is a fairly simple procedure, some risks are associated with any surgery. It is important to inform the physician about any medications currently being used and about previous allergic reactions to drugs or anesthetic agents. Patients with blood clotting disorders also need to inform their physician before the procedure is performed.

Description

Hair transplantation surgery is performed by a physician in an office, clinic, or hospital setting. Each surgery

lasts 2–3 hours during which approximately 250 grafts will be transplanted. A moderately balding man may require up to 1,000 grafts to get good coverage of a bald area, so a series of surgeries scheduled 3–4 months apart is usually required. The patient may be completely awake during the procedure with just a local anesthetic drug applied to numb the areas of the scalp. Some patients may be given a drug to help them relax or may be given an anesthetic drug that puts them to sleep.

The most common transplant procedure uses a thin strip of hair and scalp from the back of the head. This strip is cut into smaller clumps of five or six hairs. Tiny cuts are made in the balding area of the scalp and a clump is implanted into each slit. The doctor performing the surgery will attempt to recreate a natural looking hairline along the forehead. Minigrafts, micrografts, or implants of single hair follicles can be used to fill in between larger implant sites and can provide a more natural-looking hairline. The implants will also be arranged so that thick and thin hairs are interspersed and the hair will grow in the same direction.

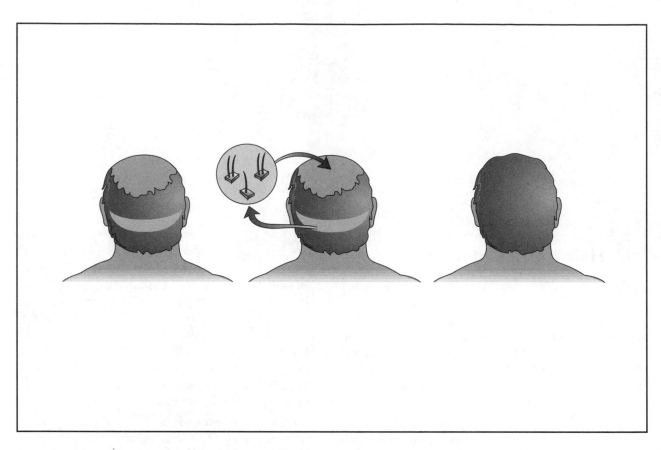

The most common hair transplant procedure involves taking small strips of scalp containing hair follicles from the donor area, usually at the sides or back of the head. These strips are then divided into several hundred smaller grafts. The surgeon relocates these grafts containing skin, follicle, and hair to tiny holes in the balding area by using microsurgical instruments or lasers. *(Illustration by Electronic Illustrators Group.)*

Another type of hair replacement surgery is called scalp reduction. This involves removing some of the skin from the hairless area and ''stretching'' some of the nearby hair-covered scalp over the cut-away area.

Health insurance will not pay for hair transplants that are done for cosmetic reasons. Insurance may pay for hair replacement surgery to correct hair loss due to accident, burn, or disease.

It is important to be realistic about what the final result of a hair transplant will look like. This procedure does not create new hair, it simply redistributes the hair that the patient still has. Some research has been conducted where chest hair has been transplanted to the balding scalp, but this procedure is not widely practiced.

Preparation

It is important to find a respected, well-established, experienced surgeon and discuss the expected results prior to the surgery. The patient may need blood tests to check for bleeding or clotting problems and may be asked not to take **aspirin** products before the surgery. The type of anesthesia used will depend on how extensive the surgery will be and where it will be performed. The patient may be awake during the procedure, but may be given medication to help them relax. A local anesthetic drug which numbs the area will be applied or injected into the skin at the surgery sites.

Aftercare

The area may need to be bandaged overnight. The patient can return to normal activities; however, strenuous activities should be avoided in the first few days after the surgery. On rare occasions, the implants can be ''ejected'' from the scalp during vigorous **exercise.** There may be some swelling, bruising, **headache,** and discomfort around the graft areas and around the eyes. These symptoms can usually be controlled with a mild **pain** reliever like aspirin. Scabs may form at the graft sites and should not be scraped off. There may be some numbness at the sites, but it will diminish within 2–3 months.

Risks

Although there are rare cases of infection or scarring, the major risk is probably that the grafted area does not look the way the patient expected it to look.

Normal results

The transplanted hair will fall out within a few weeks, however, new hair will start to grow in the graft sites within about 3 months. A normal rate of hair growth is about 0.25–0.5 in (6–13 mm) per month.

Abnormal results

Major complications as a result of hair transplantation are extremely rare. Occasionally, a patient may have problems with delayed healing, infection, scarring, or rejection of the graft; but this is uncommon.

Resources

BOOKS

Strough, Dow B. amd Robert S. Hamber, eds. *Hair Replacement-Surgical and Medical.* St. Louis, MO: Mosby-Yearbook, 1996.

Unger, Walter P., ed. *Hair Transplantation*, 3rd ed. New York: Marcel Dekker, 1995.

PERIODICALS

Bernstein, R. M. and W. R. Rassman. "The Aesthetics of Follicular Transplantation." *Dermatologic Surgery (B2S)* 23 no. 9 (Sep 1997): 785-799.

Bernstein, R. M. and W. R. Rassman. "Follicular Transplantation: Patient Evaluation and Surgical Planning." *Dermatologic Surgery (B2S)* 23 no. 9 (Sep 1997): 771-784, 801-805.

Brady, D. A. "Chest Hair Used As Donor Material in Hair Restoration Surgery." *Dermatologic Surgery* 23 no. 9 (Sep 1997): 841-844.

Byron, C. "Hair Raising." *Men's Health* 10 no. 6 (Jul-Aug 1995): 72-77, 112, 114.

Chang, L. Y., et. al. "Use of the Scalp as a Donor Site for Large Burn Wound Coverage: Review of 150 Patients." *World Journal of Surgery* 22 no. 3 (Mar 1998): 296-300.

Fischer, David. "The Bald Truth." *U.S. News & World Report* (Aug 4, 1997): 44-50.

Hitzig, G. S., J. P. Schwinning, and S. L. Handler. "Linear Grafting Using a Modified Slot Method: Introducing the Linear Punch." *Dermatologic Surgery (B2S)* 23 no. 9 (Sep 1997): 788-792.

ORGANIZATIONS

American Academy of Cosmetic Surgery. 401 N. Michigan Avenue, Chicago, IL 60611-4267. (313)527-6713. http://www.cosmeticsurgeryonline.com/.

American Academy of Facial Plastic and Reconstructive Surgery. 1110 Vermont Avenue NW, Suite 220, Washington, DC 20005. 800-332-3223.

OTHER

"Hair Transplant." In *The Body Electric*. http://www.surgery.com/topics/hatra/hatraread.html.

"Transplants," "Flap Surgery," "The Perfect Candidate." In *Transplant Network*. http://www.hair-transplants.net/.

Altha Roberts Edgren

Hairy cell leukemia

Definition

Hairy cell leukemia is a disease in which the cells that are present in the blood and bone marrow turn abnormal or cancerous. It is called "hairy cell leukemia" because the cells have tiny "hairy" projections when examined under the microscope.

Description

Hairy cell leukemia is a rare cancer. There are approximately 600 new cases diagnosed every year in the United States. The disease commonly affects older people, with the average age at diagnosis being 50 years. The disease is four times more common in men.

There are three types of cells found in the blood: red blood cells that carry oxygen to all the parts of the body; the white blood cells which are responsible for fighting infection and protecting the body from diseases; and platelets which help in the clotting of blood. Hairy cell leukemia affects the white blood cells called lymphocytes. The lymphocytes are made in the bone marrow, spleen, and the lymph nodes.

When hairy cell leukemia develops, the white blood cells become abnormal and accumulate in the spleen, causing it to become enlarged. The cells may also collect in the bone marrow and stop it from producing blood cells. As a result there may not be enough normal white blood cells in the blood to fight infections.

Causes & symptoms

The cause of hairy cell leukemia is not known. It is a slowly progressing disease and the patients may not show any symptoms for many years. As the disease advances, the patients may have an enlarged spleen, because of the accumulation of the abnormal cells in the spleen. The liver may at times become enlarged. The blood tests may show abnormal counts of all the different types of cells. This happens because the cancerous cells invade the bone marrow as well and prevent it from producing normal

KEY TERMS

Anemia—A condition where there is low iron in the blood due to a deficiency of red blood cells.

Bone marrow—The spongy tissue inside the large bones in the body which is responsible for making the red blood cells, white blood cells and the platelets.

Bone marrow biopsy—A procedure where a needle is inserted into the large bones of the hip or spine and a small piece of marrow is removed for microscopic examination.

Immunotherapy—A mode of cancer treatment where the immune system is stimulated to fight the cancer.

Leukemia—A disease in which the cells that constitute the blood become cancerous or abnormal.

Lymph nodes—Oval shaped organs that are the size of peas. They are located throughout the body and contain clusters of cells called lymphocytes. They filter out and destroy the bacteria, foreign particles and cancerous cells from the blood.

Spleen—An organ that lies next to the stomach. Its function is to remove the worn out blood cells and foreign materials from the blood stream.

Splenectomy—A surgical procedure which involves removal of the spleen.

blood cells. Because of the low white cell count in the blood, the patient may have frequent infections. **Fever** accompanies the infections. There may also be other symptoms such as unexplained weight loss, fatigue, and night sweats. The low red cell count may cause **anemia,** and the low **platelet count** may cause the person to bruise easily.

Diagnosis

If a patient complains of fatigue and has recurrent infections, and if the spleen is enlarged, the doctor may order several blood tests. In these tests, the total numbers of each of the different types of blood cells (CBC) are reported. If the blood tests are abnormal, the doctor may order a "bone marrow biopsy". During this procedure, a needle is inserted into the bone and a small amount of marrow is withdrawn for microscopic examination. This test will help the physician in identifying the type of leukemia and planning the treatment.

Treatment

Some people with hairy cell leukemia have very few or no symptoms at all and may not need any treatment. If the spleen is enlarged, it may be removed in a surgical procedure known as **splenectomy.** This usually causes a remission of the disease.

Chemotherapy and bone marrow transplantation are rarely used in the treatment of hairy cell leukemia. Modern therapy relies heavily on the use of 2CDA (cladribine, pentastatin, fludarabine, interferon).

Biological therapy or immunotherapy, where the body's own immune cells are used to fight cancer is also being investigated in clinical trials for hairy cell leukemia. A substance called interferon that is produced by the white blood cells of the body has shown some promise in treating the disease and is being investigated further.

Prognosis

Most patients have excellent prognosis and can expect to live ten years or longer. The disease may remain silent for years with treatment.

Prevention

Since the cause for the disease is unknown and there are no specific risk factors, there is no known prevention.

Resources

BOOKS

Dollinger, Malin. *Everyone's Guide to Cancer Therapy.* Somerville House Books Limited, 1994.

Morra, Marion E. *Choices.* Avon Books, October 1994.

Murphy, Gerald P. *Informed Decisions: The Complete book of Cancer Diagnosis, Treatment and Recovery.* American Cancer Society, 1997.

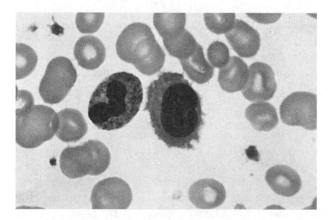

A magnified image of white blood cells with "hairy" projections. (Photograph by M. Abbey, Photo Researchers, Inc. Reproduced by permission.)

ORGANIZATIONS

American Cancer Society (National Headquarters). 1599 Clifton Road, N.E. Atlanta, Georgia 30329. (800) 227-2345; http://www.cancer.org.

Cancer Research Institute (National Headquarters). 681, Fifth Avenue, New York, N.Y. 10022. (800) 992-2623. http://www.cancerresearch.org.

Hairy Cell Leukemia Research Foundation. 2345 County Farm Lane, Schaumburg, IL 60194. (800) 693-6173.

Leukemia Society of America, Inc. National Office, 600 Third Avenue, 4th Floor, New York, NY 10016. (800) 955-4LSA.

National Cancer Institute. 9000 Rockville Pike, Building 31, room 10A16, Bethesda, Maryland, 20892. (800) 422-6237. http://wwwicic.nci.nih.gov.

Oncolink. University of Pennsylvania Cancer Center. Website: http://cancer.med.upenn.edu.

OTHER

NCI/PDQ Patient Statement, "Hairy cell leukemia." National Cancer Institute.

Lata Cherath

Halitosis *see* **Bad breath**

Hallucinations

Definition

Hallucinations are false or distorted sensory experiences that appear to be real perceptions. These sensory impressions are generated by the mind rather than by any external stimuli, and may be seen, heard, felt, and even smelled or tasted.

Description

A hallucination occurs when environmental, emotional, or physical factors such as **stress,** medication, extreme fatigue, or mental illness cause the mechanism within the brain that helps to distinguish conscious perceptions from internal, memory-based perceptions to misfire. As a result, hallucinations occur during periods of consciousness. They can appear in the form of visions, voices or sounds, tactile feelings (known as haptic hallucinations), smells, or tastes.

Patients suffering from **dementia** and psychotic disorders such as **schizophrenia** frequently experience hallucinations. Hallucinations can also occur in patients who are not mentally ill as a result of stress overload or exhaustion, or may be intentionally induced through the use of drugs, **meditation,** or sensory deprivation. A 1996

KEY TERMS

Aura—A subjective sensation or motor phenomenon that precedes and indicates the onset of a neurological episode, such as a migraine or an epileptic seizure.

Hypnogogic hallucination—A hallucination, such as the sensation of falling, that occurs at the onset of sleep.

Hypnopompic hallucination—A hallucination that occurs as a person is waking from sleep.

Sensory deprivation—A situation where an individual finds himself in an environment without sensory cues. Also, (used here) the act of shutting one's senses off to outside sensory stimuli to achieve hallucinatory experiences and/or to observe the psychological results.

---

report, published in the *British Journal of Psychiatry,* noted that 37% of 4,972 people surveyed experienced hypnagogic hallucinations (hallucinations that occur as a person is falling to sleep). Hypnopomic hallucinations (hallucinations that occur just upon waking) were reported by 12% of the sample.

Causes & symptoms

Common causes of hallucinations include:

- Drugs. Hallucinogenics such as ecstasy (3,4-methylenedioxymethamphetamine, or MDMA), LSD (lysergic acid diethylamide, or acid), mescaline (3,4,5-trimethoxyphenethylamine, or peyote), and psilocybin (4-phosphoryloxy-N, N-dimethyltryptamine, or mushrooms) trigger hallucinations. Other drugs such as marijuana and PCP have hallucinatory effects. Certain prescription medications may also cause hallucinations. In addition, drug withdrawal may induce tactile and visual hallucinations; as in an alcoholic suffering from delirium tremens (DTs).

- Stress. Prolonged or extreme stress can impede thought processes and trigger hallucinations.

- Sleep deprivation and/or exhaustion. Physical and emotional exhaustion can induce hallucinations by blurring the line between sleep and wakefulness.

- Meditation and/or sensory deprivation. When the brain lacks external stimulation to form perceptions, it may compensate by referencing the memory and form hallucinatory perceptions. This condition is commonly found in blind and deaf individuals.

- Electrical or neurochemical activity in the brain. A hallucinatory sensation—usually involving touch—called an aura, often appears before, and gives warning of, a migraine. Also, auras involving smell and touch (tactile) are known to warn of the onset of an epileptic attack.

- Mental illness. Up to 75% of schizophrenic patients admitted for treatment report hallucinations.

- Brain damage or disease. Lesions or injuries to the brain may alter brain function and produce hallucinations.

Diagnosis

Aside from hypnogogic and hypnopompic hallucinations, more than one event suggests a person should seek evaluation. A general physician, psychologist, or psychiatrist will try to rule out possible organic, environmental, or psychological causes through a detailed medical examination and social history. If a psychological cause such as schizophrenia is suspected, a psychologist will typically conduct an interview with the patient and his family and administer one of several clinical inventories, or tests, to evaluate the mental status of the patient.

Occasionally, people who are in good mental health will experience a hallucination. If hallucinations are infrequent and transitory, and can be accounted for by short-term environmental factors such as sleep deprivation or meditation, no treatment may be necessary. However, if hallucinations are hampering an individual's ability to function, a general physician, psychologist, or psychiatrist should be consulted to pinpoint their source and recommend a treatment plan.

Treatment

Hallucinations that are symptomatic of a mental illness such as schizophrenia should be treated by a psychologist or psychiatrist. Antipsychotic medication such as thioridazine (Mellaril), haloperidol (Haldol), chlorpromazine (Thorazine), clozapine (Clozaril), or risperidone (Risperdal) may be prescribed.

Prognosis

In many cases, chronic hallucinations caused by schizophrenia or some other mental illness can be controlled by medication. If hallucinations persist, psychosocial therapy can be helpful in teaching the patient the coping skills to deal with them. Hallucinations due to sleep deprivation or extreme stress generally stop after the cause is removed.

Resources

BOOKS

American Psychiatric Association. *Diagnostic and Statistical Manual of Mental Disorders, 4th ed.* (DSMV-IV) Washington, DC: American Psychiatric Press, Inc., 1994.

Siegel, Ronald K. *Fire in the Brain: Clinical Tales of Hallucination.* New York: Dutton, 1992.

PERIODICALS

Bental, R.P. "The Illusion of Reality: A Review and Integration of Psychological Research on Hallucinations." *Psychological Bulletin* 107, no. 1 (Jan 1990): 82-95.

Beyerstein, Barry L. "Believing is Seeing: Organic and Psychological Reasons for Hallucinations and Other Anomalous Psychiatric Symptoms." *Medscape Mental Health* 1, no. 11 (1996). http://www.medscape.com.

Ohayon, M.M., et al. "Hypnagogic and Hypnopompic Hallucinations: Pathological Phenomena?" *The British Journal of Psychiatry* 169 no. 4 (October 1996): 459-67.

ORGANIZATIONS

American Psychological Association (APA). Office of Public Affairs. 750 First St. NE, Washington, DC 20002-4242. (202) 336-5700. http://www.apa.org/.

National Alliance for the Mentally Ill (NAMI). 200 North Glebe Road, Suite 1015, Arlington, VA 22203-3754. (800) 950-6264. http://www.nami.org.

Paula Anne Ford-Martin

Hallux valgus *see* **Bunion**

Haloperidol *see* **Antipsychotic drugs**

Hammertoe

Definition

Hammertoe is a condition in which the toe is bent in a claw-like position. It can be present in more than one toe but is most common in the second toe.

Description

Hammertoe is described as a deformity in which the toes bend downward with the toe joint usually enlarged. Over time, the joint enlarges and stiffens as it rubs against shoes. Other foot structures involved include the overlying skin and blood vessels and nerves connected to the involved toes.

Causes & symptoms

The shortening of tendons responsible for the control and movement of the affected toe or toes cause hammertoe. Top portions of the toes become callused from the friction produced against the inside of shoes. This common foot problem often results from improper fit of footwear. This is especially the case with high-heeled shoes placing pressure on the front part of the foot that compresses the smaller toes tightly together. The condition frequently stems from muscle imbalance, and usually leaves the affected individual with impaired balance.

Diagnosis

A thorough medical history and physical exam by a physician is always necessary for the proper diagnosis of hammertoe and other foot conditions. Because the condition involves bony deformity, x rays can help to confirm the diagnosis.

Treatment

Conservative

Wearing proper footwear and stockings with plenty of room in the toe region can provide treatment for hammertoe. Stretching exercises may be helpful in lengthening the excessively tight tendons.

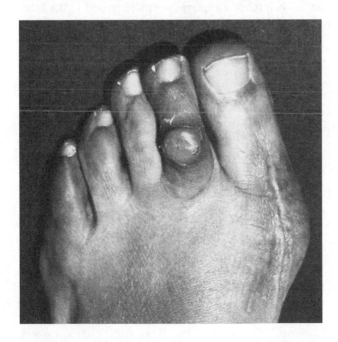

Hammertoe most commonly affects the second toe, which, as shown, often develops a corn over the deformity.
(Photograph by Dr. H.C. Robinson, Custom Medical Stock Photo. Reproduced by permission.)

Surgery

In advanced cases, where conservative treatment is unsuccessful, surgery may be recommended. The tendons that attach to the involved toes are located and an incision is made to free the connective tissue to the foot bones. Additional incisions are made so the toes no longer bend in a downward fashion. The middle joints of the affected toes are connected together permanently with surgical hardware such as pins and wire sutures. The incision is then closed with fine sutures. These sutures are removed approximately seven to ten days after surgery.

Alternative treatment

Various soft tissue and joint treatments offered by **chiropractic** and **massage** therapy may be useful to decrease the tightness of the affected structures.

Prognosis

If detected early, hammertoe can be treated nonsurgically. If surgery becomes necessary, surgical risks are minimal with the overall outcome providing good results.

Prevention

Wearing comfortable shoes that fit well can prevent many foot ailments. Foot width may increase with age. Feet should always be measured before buying shoes. The upper part of the shoes should be made of a soft, flexible material to match the shape of the foot. Shoes made of leather can reduce the possibility of skin irritations. Soles should provide solid footing and not be slippery. Thick soles lessen pressure when walking on hard surfaces. Low-heeled shoes are more comfortable, safer, and less damaging than high-heeled shoes.

Resources

BOOKS

Scully, Rosemary M. and Marylou R. Barnes. *Physical Therapy.* Philadelphia, PA: J. B. Lippincott, 1989.

ORGANIZATIONS

American Orthopedic Foot and Ankle Society. 222 South Prospect, Park Ridge, IL 60068.

American Podiatry Medical Association. 9312 Old Georgetown Road, Bethesda, MD 20814.

OTHER

Thriveonline. Hammertoe Correction. http://www.thriveonline.com. (4/23/98).

Jeffrey Peter Larson

Hand-foot-mouth disease

Definition

Hand-foot-mouth disease is an infection of young children in which characteristic fluid-filled blisters appear on the hands, feet, and inside the mouth.

Description

Coxsackie viruses belong to a family of viruses called Enteroviruses. These viruses live in the gastrointestinal tract, and are therefore present in feces. They can be spread easily from one person to another when poor hygiene allows the virus within the feces to be passed from person to person. After exposure to the virus, development of symptoms takes only four to six days. Hand-foot-mouth disease can occur year-round, although the largest number of cases are in summer and fall months.

Causes & symptoms

Hand-foot-mouth disease is very common among young children, and often occurs in clusters of children who are in daycare together. It is spread when poor hand-washing after a diaper change or contact with saliva (drool) allows the virus to be passed from one child to another.

Within about four to six days of acquiring the virus, an infected child may develop a relatively low-grade **fever,** ranging from 99–102°F (37.2–38.9°C). Other symptoms include fatigue, loss of energy, decreased appetite, and a sore sensation in the mouth, which may interfere with feeding. After one to two days, fluid-filled bumps (vesicles) appear on the inside of the mouth, along the surface of the tongue, on the roof of the mouth, and on the insides of the cheeks. These are tiny blisters, about 3–7 mm in diameter. Eventually, they may appear on the palms of the hands and on the soles of the feet. Occasionally, these vesicles may occur in the diaper region.

The vesicles in the mouth cause the majority of discomfort, and the child may refuse to eat or drink due to **pain.** This phase usually lasts for an average of a week. As long as the bumps have clear fluid within them, the disease is at its most contagious. The fluid within the vesicles contains large quantities of the causative viruses. Extra care should be taken to avoid contact with this fluid.

Diagnosis

Diagnosis is made by most practitioners solely on the basis of the unique appearance of blisters of the mouth, hands, and feet, in a child not appearing very ill.

Treatment

There are no treatments available to cure or decrease the duration of the disease. Medications like **acetaminophen** or ibuprofen may be helpful for decreasing pain, and allowing the child to eat and drink. It is important to try to encourage the child to take in adequate amounts of fluids, in the form of ice chips or popsicles if other foods or liquids are too uncomfortable.

Prognosis

The prognosis for a child with hand-foot-mouth disease is excellent. The child is usually completely better within about a week of the start of the illness.

Prevention

Prevention involves careful attention to hygiene. Thorough, consistent hand-washing practices, and discouraging the sharing of clothes, towels, and stuffed toys are all helpful. Virus continues to be passed in the feces for several weeks after infection, so good hygiene should be practiced long after all signs of infection have passed.

Resources

BOOKS

Morag, Abraham, and Pearay L. Ogra. "Viral Infections." In *Nelson Textbook of Pediatrics,* edited by Richard Behrman. Philadelphia: W.B. Saunders Co., 1996.

Ray, C. George. "Enteroviruses." In *Sherris Medical Microbiology: An Introduction to Infectious Diseases,* edited by Kenneth J. Ryan. Norwalk, CT: Appleton and Lange, 1994.

Stoffman, Phyllis.*The Family Guide to Preventing and Treating 100 Infectious Diseases.* New York: John Wiley and Sons, Inc., 1995.

PERIODICALS

Huerter, Christopher, et al. "Helpful Clues to Common Rashes." *Patient Care* 31, 8 (April 30, 1997): 9+.

Rosalyn S. Carson-DeWitt

Hand-Schüller-Christian syndrome *see* **Histiocytosis X**

Hantavirus infections

Definition

The hantaviruses are a group of viruses which can infect humans with two serious illnesses: hemorrhagic **fever** with renal syndrome (HFRS), and Hantavirus pulmonary syndrome (HPS).

Description

Hantaviruses live without causing symptoms within various species of rodents, and are passed to humans by exposure to the urine, feces, or saliva of those infected rodents. Five different hantaviruses have thus far been identified as important in humans. Each is found in specific geographic regions, and therefore is spread by different rodent carriers. Further, each type of virus causes a slightly different form of illness in its human hosts:

- Hantaan virus is carried by the striped field mouse, and exists in Korea, China, Eastern Russia, and the Balkans. Hantaan virus causes a severe form of hemorrhagic fever with renal syndrome (HFRS).

- Puumula virus is carried by bank voles, and exists in Scandinavia, western Russia, and Europe. Puumula virus causes a milder form of HFRS, usually termed *nephropathia epidemica*.

- Seoul virus is carried by a type of rat called the Norway rat, and exists worldwide, but causes disease almost exclusively in Asia. Seoul virus causes a form of HFRS which is slightly more mild than that caused by Hantaan virus, but resulting in more problems with the liver.

- Prospect Hill virus is carried by meadow voles, and exists in the United States, but has not been found to cause human disease.

- Sin Nombre virus, perhaps the most recently identified hantavirus, is carried by the deer mouse. This virus was responsible for severe cases of HPS which occurred in the Southwestern United States in 1993.

Causes & symptoms

Hemorrhagic fever with renal syndrome (HFRS)

Hantaviruses which produce forms of hemorrhagic fever with renal syndrome (HFRS) cause a classic group of symptoms, including fever, malfunction of the kidneys, and low **platelet count.** Because platelets are the

blood cells which are important in proper clotting, low numbers of circulating platelets can result in spontaneous heavy bleeding, or hemorrhage.

Patients with HFRS have **pain** in the head, abdomen, and lower back, and may report bloodshot eyes and blurry vision. Tiny pinpoint hemorrhages, called petechiae, may appear on the upper body and the soft palate in the mouth. The patient's face, chest, abdomen, and back often appear flushed and red, as if sunburned.

After about five days, the patient may have a sudden drop in blood pressure; often it drops low enough to cause the clinical syndrome called **shock.** Shock is a state in which blood circulation throughout the body is insufficient to deliver proper quantities of oxygen. Lengthy shock can result in permanent damage to the body's organs, particularly the brain, which is very sensitive to oxygen deprivation.

Around day eight of HFRS, kidney involvement results in multiple derangements of the body chemistry. Simultaneously, the hemorrhagic features of the illness begin to cause spontaneous bleeding, as demonstrated by bloody urine, bloody vomit, and in very serious cases, brain hemorrhages with resulting changes in consciousness.

Day eleven often brings further chemical derangements, with associated confusion, **hallucinations,** seizures, and lung complications. Those who survive this final phase usually begin to turn the corner towards recovery at this time, although recovery takes approximately six weeks.

Hantavirus pulmonary syndrome (HPS)

Hantavirus pulmonary syndrome (HPS) begins with a fever, followed by a drop in blood pressure, shock, and leakiness of the blood vessels of the lungs, which results in fluid accumulation in the lungs, and subsequent **shortness of breath.** The fluid accumulation can be so rapid and so severe as to put the patient in **respiratory failure** within only a few hours.

Diagnosis

The diagnosis of infection by a hantavirus uses serologic techniques. The patient's blood is drawn, and various reactions are measured in a laboratory which identify the presence of specific immune substances (antibodies), substances which an individual's body would only produce in response to the hantavirus.

It is very difficult to demonstrate the actual virus in human tissue, or to grow cultures of the virus within the laboratory, so the majority of diagnostic tests use indirect means to demonstrate the presence of the virus.

Treatment

Treatment of hantavirus infections is primarily supportive, because there are no agents available to kill the viruses and interrupt the infection. Supportive care, then, consists of providing treatment in response to the patient's symptoms. Because both HFRS and HPS progress so very rapidly, patients must be very closely monitored, so that treatment may be started at the first sign of a particular problem. Low blood pressure is treated with medications (pressors), blood **transfusions** are given for both hemorrhage and shock states, hemodialysis is used in kidney failure. (Hemodialysis involves mechanically cleansing the blood outside of the body, to replace the kidney's normal function of removing various toxins form the blood.)

The anti-viral agent ribavirin is being studied to determine whether it has any use in treating hantavirus infections. Its use is currently in the experimental stage.

Prognosis

The diseases caused by hantaviruses are extraordinarily lethal. About 6–15% of people who contract HFRS have died. Almost half of all people who contract HPS will die. It is essential that people living in areas where the hantaviruses exists seek quick medical treatment, should they begin to develop an illness which might be due to a hantavirus.

Prevention

There are no immunizations currently available against any of the hantaviruses. The only forms of prevention involve rodent control within the community, and within individual households. Avoiding areas known to be infested by rodents is essential.

Resources

BOOKS

Ray, C. George. "Hantaviruses." In *Sherris Medical Microbiology: An Introduction to Infectious Diseases,* edited by Kenneth J. Ryan. Norwalk, CT: Appleton and Lange, 1994.

Stoffman, Phyllis. *The Family Guide to Preventing and Treating 100 Infectious Diseases.* New York: John Wiley and Sons, Inc., 1995.

PERIODICALS

Chisolm, Saundra. "Common Questions About Hantavirus Pulmonary Syndrome." *American Journal of Nursing* 97 no. 4 (April 1997): 68+.

"Hantavirus Pulmonary Syndrome" *The Journal of the American Medical Association* 275 no. 18 (May 8, 1996): 1395+.

"Outbreak of Hantavirus is Unusual." *The New York Times* 146 (June 17, 1997): C4+.

ORGANIZATIONS

Centers for Disease Control and Prevention. (404) 332-4559. http://www.cdc.gov/travel/travel.html.

Rosalyn S. Carson-DeWitt

Haptoglobin test

Definition

This test is done to help evaluate a person for hemolytic anemia.

Purpose

Haptoglobin is a blood protein made by the liver. The haptoglobin levels decrease in **hemolytic anemia.** Hemolytic anemias include a variety of conditions that result in hemolyzed, or burst, red blood cells.

Decreased values can also indicate a slower type of red cell destruction unrelated to anemia. For example, destruction can be caused by mechanical heart valves or abnormal hemoglobin, such as sickle cell disease or **thalassemia.**

Haptoglobin is known as an acute phase reactant. Its level increases during acute conditions such as infection, injury, tissue destruction, some **cancers, burns,** surgery, or trauma. Its purpose is to remove damaged cells and debris and rescue important material such as iron.

KEY TERMS

Acute phase reactant—A substance in the blood that increases as a response to an acute condition such as infection, injury, tissue destruction, some cancers, burns, surgery, or trauma.

Haptoglobin—A blood protein made by the liver. Its main role is to save iron by attaching itself to any hemoglobin released from a red cell.

Hemoglobin—The protein in the red blood cell that carries oxygen.

Hemolytic anemia—A variety of conditions that result in hemolyzed, or burst, red blood cells.

Haptoglobin levels can be used to monitor the course of these conditions.

Description

Hemoglobin is the protein in the red blood cell that carries oxygen throughout the body. Iron is an essential part of hemoglobin; without iron, hemoglobin can not function. Haptoglobin's main role is to save iron by attaching itself to any hemoglobin released from a red cell.

When red blood cells are destroyed, the hemoglobin is released. Haptoglobin is always present in the blood waiting to bind to released hemoglobin. White blood cells (called macrophages) bring the haptoglobin-hemoglobin complex to the liver, where the haptoglobin and hemoglobin are separated and the iron is recycled.

In hemolytic anemia, so many red cells are destroyed that most of the available haptoglobin is needed to bind the released hemoglobin. The more severe the hemolysis, the less haptoglobin remains in the blood.

Haptoglobin is measured in several different ways. One way is called rate nephelometry. A person's serum is mixed with a substance that will bind to haptoglobin. The amount of bound haptoglobin is measured using a rate nephelometer, which measures the amount of light scattered by the bound haptoglobin. Another way of measuring haptoglobin is to measure it according to how much hemoglobin it can bind.

Preparation

This test requires 5 mL of blood. The person being tested should avoid taking **oral contraceptives** or androgens before this test. A healthcare worker ties a tourniquet on the person's upper arm, locates a vein in the inner elbow region, and inserts a needle into that vein. Vacuum action draws the blood through the needle into an attached tube. Collection of the sample takes only a few minutes.

Aftercare

Discomfort or bruising may occur at the puncture site or the person may feel dizzy or faint. Pressure to the puncture site until the bleeding stops reduces bruising. Warm packs to the puncture site relieve discomfort.

Normal results

Normal results vary based on the laboratory and test method used. Haptoglobin is not present in newborns at birth, but develop adult levels by 6 months.

Abnormal results

Decreased haptoglobin levels usually indicates hemolytic anemia. Other causes of red cell destruction also decrease haptoglobin: a blood **transfusion** reaction; mechanical heart valve; abnormally shaped red cells; or abnormal hemoglobin, such as thalassemia or **sickle cell anemia.**

Haptoglobin levels are low in liver disease, because the liver can not manufacture normal amounts of haptoglobin. Low levels may also indicate an inherited lack of haptoglobin, a condition found particularly in African Americans.

Haptoglobin increases as a reaction to illness, trauma, or rheumatoid disease. High haptoglobin values should be followed-up with additional tests. Drugs can also effect haptoglobin levels.

Normal results vary widely from person to person. Unless the level is very high or very low, haptoglobin levels are most valuable when the results of several tests done on different days are compared.

Nancy J. Nordenson

Hardening of the arteries *see*
Atherosclerosis

Harelip *see* **Cleft lip and palate**

Harri-Drummond instrumentation *see*
Spinal instrumentation

Harrington rod *see* **Spinal instrumentation**

Hartnup disease

Definition

Hartnup disease is an inherited nutritional disorder with primary symptoms including a red, scaly rash and sensitivity to sunlight.

Description

Hartnup disease was first identified in the 1950s in the Hartnup family in London. A defect in intestines and kidneys makes it difficult to break down and absorb protein in the diet. This causes a condition very similar to pellegra (niacin deficiency). The condition occurs in about one of every 26,000 live births.

Causes & symptoms

Hartnup disease is an in-born error of metabolism, that is, a condition where certain nutrients cannot be digested and absorbed properly. The condition is passed on genetically in families. It occurs when a person inherits two recessive genes for the disease, one from each parent. People with Hartnup disease are not able to absorb some of the amino acids (the smaller building blocks that make up proteins) in their intestines. One of the amino acids that is not well absorbed is tryptophan, which the body uses to make its own form of niacin.

The majority of people with this disorder do not show any symptoms. About 10–20% of people with Hartnup disease do have symptoms. The most prominent symptom is a red, scaly rash that gets worse when the patient is exposed to sunlight. **Headache, fainting,** and **diarrhea** may also occur. **Mental retardation,** cerebral ataxia (muscle weakness), and **delirium** (a confused, agitated, delusional state) are some of the more serious complications that can occur. Short stature has also been noted in some patients. Although this is an inherited disease, the development of symptoms depends on a variety of factors including diet, environment, and other genetic traits controlling amino acid levels in the body. Symptoms can be brought on by exposure to sunlight, **fever,** drugs, or other **stresses.** Poor nutrition frequently precedes an attack of symptoms. The frequency of attacks usually decreases as the patient gets older.

Diagnosis

The symptoms of this disease suggest a deficiency of a B vitamin called niacin. A detailed diet history can be used to assess if there is adequate protein and **vitamins** in the diet. The diagnosis of Hartnup disease is confirmed by a laboratory test of the urine which will contain an abnormally high amount of amino acids (aminoaciduria).

Treatment

The vitamin niacin is given as a treatment for Hartnup disease. The typical dosage ranges from 40–200 mg of nicotinamide (a form of niacin) per day to prevent pellagra-like symptoms. Some patients may require dietary supplements of tryptophan.

Eating a healthy, high protein diet can relieve the symptoms and prevent them from recurring.

Prognosis

The prognosis for a healthy life is good once the condition has been identified and treated.

Prevention

Hartnup disease is an inherited condition. Parents may not have the disease themselves, but may pass the genes responsible for it on to their children. **Genetic testing** can be used to identify carriers of the genes. Symptoms can usually be controlled with a high protein diet, vitamin supplements of niacin, and by avoiding the stresses that contribute to attacks of symptoms.

Resources

BOOKS

''Hartnup disease.'' In *Cecil Textbook of Medicine,* 20th ed., Vol. 1, edited by J. Claude Bennett and Fred Plum. Philadelphia, PA: W.B. Saunders Company, 1996.

"Hartnup disease." In *The Merck Manual of Diagnosis and Therapy,* edited by Robert Berkow. Rahway, NJ: Merck Research Laboratories, 1992.

"Neutral aminoaciduria: Hartnup disease." In *Internal Medicine,* 5th ed., edited by Jay H. Stein. St. Louis, MO: Mosby, 1998.

"Selected disorders of amino acid transport." In *Harrison's Principles of Internal Medicine,* 14th ed., Vol. 2, edited by Anthony S. Fauci, et al. New York, NY: McGraw-Hill, 1998.

ORGANIZATIONS

The National Organization for Rare Disorders, Inc. P.O. Box 8923, New Fairfield, CT 06812-8923. (203) 746-6518. (800) 999-6673. http://www.nord-rdb.com/~orphan.

NIH/National Institute of Diabetes, Digestive and Kidney Diseases. Building 31, Room 9A04, 31 Center Drive, Bethesda MD 20892-2560. (301) 496-3583.

OTHER

Hartnup disorder.http://www.ncbi.nlm.nih.gov.

Nephrology: Hartnup disease. http://www.medstudents.com.br/nefro/nefro3.htm.

Altha Roberts Edgren

Hashimoto's disease *see* **Thyroiditis**

Hay fever *see* **Allergic rhinitis**

HBF test *see* **Fetal hemoglobin test**

HCG *see* **Infertility drugs**

Head and neck cancer

Definition

The term head and neck cancers refers to a group of **cancers** found in the head and neck region. This includes tumors found in:

- The oral cavity (mouth). The lips, the tongue, the teeth, the gums, the lining inside the lips and cheeks, the floor of the mouth (under the tongue), the roof of the mouth and the small area behind the wisdom teeth are all included in the oral cavity.

- The oropharynx (which includes the back one-third of the tongue, the back of the throat and the tonsils).

- Nasopharynx (which includes the area behind the nose).

- Hypopharynx (lower part of the throat).

- The larynx (voice box, located in front of the neck, in the region of the Adam's apple). In the larynx, the cancer can occur in any of the three regions: the glottis (where the vocal cords are); the supraglottis (the area above the glottis), and the subglottis (the area that connects the glottis to the windpipe).

KEY TERMS

Biopsy—The surgical removal and microscopic examination of living tissue for diagnostic purposes.

Chemotherapy—Treatment of cancer with synthetic drugs that destroy the tumor either by inhibiting the growth of the cancerous cells or by killing the cancer cells.

Clinical trials—Highly regulated and carefully controlled patient studies, where either new drugs to treat cancer or novel methods of treatment are investigated.

Computerized tomography scan (CT scan)—A medical procedure where a series of X-rays are taken and put together by a computer in order to form detailed pictures of areas inside the body.

Laryngoscopy—A medical procedure that uses flexible, lighted, narrow tubes inserted through the mouth or nose to examine the larynx and other areas deep inside the neck.

Magnetic resonance imaging (MRI)—A medical procedure used for diagnostic purposes where pictures of areas inside the body can be created using a magnet linked to a computer.

Radiation therapy—Treatment using high energy radiation from x-ray machines, cobalt, radium, or other sources.

Stoma—When the entire larynx must be surgically removed, an opening is surgically created in the neck so that the windpipe can be brought out to the neck. This opening is called the stoma.

Ultrasonogram—A procedure where high-frequency sound waves that cannot be heard by human ears are bounced off internal organs and tissues. These sound waves produce a pattern of echoes which are then used by the computer to create sonograms, or pictures of areas inside the body.

X rays—High energy radiation used in high doses, either to diagnose or treat disease.

The most frequently occurring cancers of the head and neck area are oral cancers and laryngeal cancers. Almost half of all the head and neck cancers occur in the oral cavity, and a third of the cancers are found in the larynx. By definition, the term "head and neck cancers" usually excludes tumors that occur in the brain.

Description

Head and neck cancers involve the respiratory tract and the digestive tract; and they interfere with the functions of eating and breathing. Laryngeal cancers affect speech. Loss of any of these functions is significant. Hence, early detection and appropriate treatment of head and neck cancers is of utmost importance.

Roughly 10% of all cancers are related to the head and the neck. It is estimated that more than 55,000 Americans will develop cancer of the head and neck in 1998, and nearly 13,000 will die from the disease. The American Cancer Society estimates that in 1998, approx-

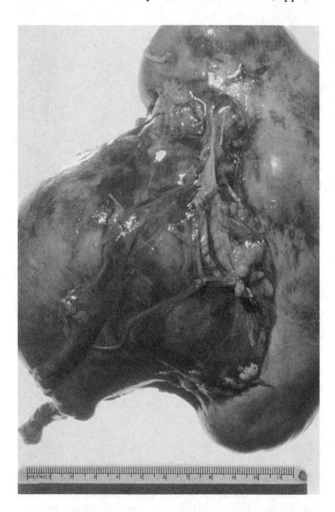

A specimen of a squamous cell carcinoma of the tongue and jaw. (Custom Medical Stock Photo. Reproduced by permission.)

imately, 11,100 new cases of laryngeal cancer alone will be diagnosed and 4,300 people will die of this disease. Oral cancer is the sixth most common cancer in the United States. Approximately 40,000 new cases are diagnosed each year and it causes at least 8,000 **deaths.** Among the major cancers, the survival rate for head and neck cancers is one of the poorest. Less than 50% of the patients survive five years or more after initial diagnosis. This is because the early signs of head and neck cancers are frequently ignored. Hence, when it is first diagnosed, it is often in an advanced stage and not very amenable to treatment.

The risk for both oral cancer and laryngeal cancer seems to increase with age. Most of the cases occur in individuals over 40 years of age, the average age at diagnosis being 60. While oral cancer strikes men twice as often as it does women, laryngeal cancer is four times more common in men than in women. Both diseases are more common in black Americans than among whites.

Causes & symptoms

Although the exact cause for these cancers is unknown, tobacco is regarded as the single greatest risk factor: 75–80% of the oral and laryngeal cancer cases occur among smokers. Heavy alcohol use has also been included as a risk factor. A combination of tobacco and alcohol use increases the risk for oral cancer by 6–15 times more than for users of either substance alone. In rare cases, irritation to the lining of the mouth, due to jagged teeth or ill-fitting dentures, has been known to cause oral cancer. Exposure to asbestos appears to increase the risk of developing laryngeal cancer.

In the case of lip cancer, just like skin cancer, exposure to sun over a prolonged period has been shown to increase the risk. In the Southeast Asian countries (India and Sri Lanka), chewing of betel nut has been associated with cancer of the lining of the cheek. An increased incidence of nasal cavity cancer has been observed among furniture workers, probably due to the inhalation of wood dust. A virus (Epstein-Barr) has been shown to cause nasopharyngeal cancer.

Head and neck cancers are one of the easiest to detect. The early signs can be both seen and felt. The signs and symptoms depend on the location of the cancer:

- Mouth and oral cavity: a sore that does not heal within two weeks, unusual bleeding from the teeth or gums, a white or red patch in the mouth, a lump or thickening in the mouth, throat, or tongue.

- Larynx: persistent hoarseness or **sore throat,** difficulty breathing, or **pain.**

- Hypopharynx and oropharynx: difficulty in swallowing or chewing food, ear pain.

• Nose, sinuses, and nasopharyngeal cavity: pain, bloody discharges from the nose, blocked nose, and frequent sinus infections that do not respond to standard **antibiotics.**

When detected early and treated appropriately, head and neck cancers have an excellent chance of being cured completely.

Diagnosis

Specific diagnostic tests used depend on the location of the cancer. The standard tests are:

Physical examination

The first step in diagnosis is a complete and thorough examination of the oral and nasal cavity, using mirrors and other visual aids. The tongue and the back of the throat are examined as well. Any suspicious looking lumps or lesions are examined with fingers (palpation). In order to look inside the larynx, the doctor may sometimes perform a procedure known as **laryngoscopy.** In indirect laryngoscopy, the doctor looks down the throat with a small, long handled mirror. Sometimes the doctor inserts a lighted tube (laryngoscope or a fiberoptic scope) through the patient's nose or mouth. As the tube goes down the throat, the doctor can observe areas that cannot be seen by a simple mirror. This procedure is called a direct laryngoscopy. Sometimes patients may be given a mild sedative to help them relax, and a local anesthetic to ease any discomfort.

Blood tests

The doctor may order blood or other immunological tests. These tests are aimed at detecting antibodies to the Epstein-Barr virus, which has been known to cause cancer of the nasopharynx.

Imaging tests

X rays of the mouth, the sinuses, the skull, and the chest region may be required. A **computed tomography scan** (CT scan), a procedure in which a computer takes a series of x ray pictures of areas inside the body, may be done. Ultrasonograms (images generated using sound waves) or an MRI (**magnetic resonance imaging**) a procedure in which a picture is created using magnets linked to a computer), are alternate procedures which a doctor may have done to get detailed pictures of the areas inside the body.

Biopsy

When a sore does not heal or a suspicious patch or lump is seen in the mouth, larynx, nasopharynx, or throat, a biopsy may be performed to rule out the possibility of cancer. The biopsy is the most definitive diagnostic tool for detecting the cancer. If cancerous cells are detected in the biopsied sample, the doctor may perform more extensive tests in order to find whether, and to where, the cancer may have spread.

Treatment

The cancers can be treated successfully if diagnosed early. The choice of treatment depends on the size of the tumor, its location, and whether it has spread to other parts of the body.

In the case of lip and mouth cancers, sometimes surgery is performed to remove the cancer. **Radiation therapy,** which destroys the cancerous cells, is also one of the primary modes of treatment, and may be used alone or in combination with surgery. If lip surgery is drastic, **rehabilitation** cosmetic or **reconstructive surgery** may have to be considered,.

Cancers of the nasal cavity are often diagnosed late because they have no specific symptoms in their early stages, or the symptoms may just resemble chronic **sinusitis.** Hence, treatment is often complex, involving a combination of radiotherapy and surgery. Surgery is generally recommended for small tumors. If the cancer cannot be removed by surgery, radiotherapy is used alone.

Treatment of oropharynx cancers (cancers that are either in the back of the tongue, the throat, or the tonsils) generally involves radiation therapy and/or surgery. After aggressive surgery and radiation, rehabilitation is often necessary and is an essential part of the treatment. The patient may experience difficulties with swallowing, chewing, and speech and may require a team of health care workers, including speech therapists, prosthodontists, occupational therapists etc.

Cancers of the nasopharynx are different from the other head and neck cancers in that there does not appear to be any association between alcohol and tobacco use and the development of the cancer. In addition, the incidence is seen primarily in two age groups: young adults and 50–70 year-olds. The Epstein-Barr virus has been implicated as the causative agent in most patients. While 80–90% of small tumors are curable by radiation therapy, advanced tumors that have spread to the bone and cranial nerves are difficult to control. Surgery is not very helpful and, hence, is rarely attempted. Radiation remains the only treatment of choice to treat the cancer that has metastasized (traveled) to the lymph nodes in the neck.

In the case of cancer of the larynx, radiotherapy is the first choice to treat small lesions. This is done in an attempt to preserve the voice. If the cancer recurs later, surgery may be attempted. If the cancer is limited to one of the two vocal cords, laser excision surgery is used. In order to treat advanced cancers, a combination of surgery and radiation therapy is often used. Because the chances of a cure in the case of advanced laryngeal cancers are rather low with current therapies, the patient may be advised to participate in clinical trials so they may get access to new experimental drugs and procedures, such as **chemotherapy,** that are being evaluated.

When only part of the larynx is removed, a relatively slight change in the voice may occur—the patient may sound slightly hoarse. However, in a total **laryngectomy,** the entire voice box is removed. The patients then have to re-learn to speak using different approaches, such as esophageal speech, tracheo-esophageal (TE) speech, or by means of an artificial larynx.

In esophageal speech, the patients are taught how to create a new type of voice by forcing air through the esophagus (food pipe) into the mouth. This method has a high success rate of approximately 65% and patients are even able to go back to jobs that require a high level of verbal communication, such as telephone operators and salespersons.

In the second approach, TE speech, a small opening, called a fistula, is created surgically between the trachea (breathing tube to the lungs) and the esophagus (tube into the stomach) to carry air into the throat. A small tube, known as the "voice prosthesis," is placed in the opening of the fistula to keep it open and to prevent food and liquid from going down into the trachea. In order to talk, the stoma (or the opening made at the base of the neck) must be covered with one's thumb during exhalation. As the air is forced out from the trachea into the esophagus, it vibrates the walls of the esophagus. This produces a sound that is then modified by the lips and tongue to produce normal sounding speech.

In the third approach, an artificial larynx, a battery driven vibrator, is placed on the outside of the throat. Sound is created as air passes through the stoma (opening made at the base of the neck) and the mouth forms words.

Prognosis

Oral Cavity

With early detection and immediate treatment, survival rates can be dramatically improved. For lip and oral cancer, if detected at its early stages, almost 80% of the patients survive five years or more. However, when diagnosed at the advanced stages, the five year survival rate drops to a mere 18%.

Nose and sinuses

Cancers of the nasal cavity often go undetected until they reach an advanced stage. If diagnosed at the early stages, the five-year survival rates are 60–70%. However, if cancers are more advanced, only 10–30% of the patients survive five years or more.

Oropharynx

In cancer of the oropharynx, 60–80% of the patients survive five years or more if the cancer is detected in the early stages. As the cancer advances, the survival rate drops to 15–30%.

Nasopharynx

Patients who are diagnosed with early stage cancers that have originated in the nasopharynx have an excellent chance of a complete cure (almost 95%). Unfortunately, most of the time, the patients are in an advanced stage at the time of initial diagnosis. With the new chemotherapy drugs, the five year survival rate has improved and 5–40% of the patients survive five years or longer.

Larynx

Small cancers of the larynx have an excellent five-year survival rate of 75–95%. However, as with most of the head and neck cancers, the survival rates drop dramatically as the cancer advances. Only 15–25% of the patients survive five years or more after being initially diagnosed with advanced laryngeal cancer.

Prevention

Refraining from the use of all tobacco products (cigarettes, cigars, pipe tobacco, chewing tobacco), consuming alcohol in moderation, and practicing good **oral hygiene** are some of the measures that one can take to prevent head and neck cancers. Since there is an association between excessive exposure to the sun and lip cancer, people who spend a lot of time outdoors in the sun should protect themselves from the sun's harmful rays. Regular **physical examinations,** or mouth examination by the patient himself, or by the patient's doctor or dentist, can help detect oral cancer in its very early stages.

Since working with asbestos has been shown to increase one's risk of getting cancer of the larynx, asbestos workers should follow safety rules to avoid inhaling asbestos fibers. Also, **malnutrition** and vitamin deficiencies have been shown to have some association with an increased incidence of head and neck cancers. The American Cancer Society, therefore, recommends eating a healthy diet, consisting of at least five servings of fruits and vegetables every day, and six servings of food from other plant sources such as cereals, breads, grain products, rice, pasta and beans. Reducing one's intake of high-fat food from animal sources is advised.

Resources

BOOKS

Berkow, Robert, et al., eds. *Merck Manual of Diagnosis and Therapy, 16th edition.* Rahway, NJ: Merck Research Laboratories, 1992.

Dollinger, Malin. *Everyone's Guide to Cancer Therapy.* Kansas City, MO: Somerville House Books Limited, 1994.

Morra, Marion E. *Choices.* New York: Avon Books, 1994.

ORGANIZATIONS

American Association of Oral and Maxillofacial Surgeons. 9700 W. Bryn Mawr; Rosemont, IL 60018. (800) 467-5268.

International Association of Laryngectomees (IAL). 7440 North Shadeland Avenue, Suite 100, Indianapolis, IN 46250.

National Cancer Institute (National Institutes of Health). 9000 Rockville Pike, Bethesda, MD 20892. (800) 422-6237.

National Oral Health Information ClearingHouse; 1 NOHIC Way, Bethesda, MD 20892-3500. (301)-402-7364.

Oral Health Education Foundation, Inc. 5865 Colonist Drive, P.O. Box 396, Fairburn, GA 30213. (770) 969-7400.

Lata Cherath

Head injury

Definition

Injury to the head may damage the scalp, skull or brain. The most important consequence of head trauma is traumatic brain injury. Head injury may occur either as a closed head injury, such as the head hitting a car's windshield, or as a penetrating head injury, as when a bullet pierces the skull. Both may cause damage that ranges from mild to profound. Very severe injury can be fatal because of profound brain damage.

Description

External trauma to the head is capable of damaging the brain, even if there is no external evidence of damage. More serious injuries can cause skull fracture, blood clots between the skull and the brain, or bruising and tearing of the brain tissue itself.

Injuries to the head can be caused by traffic accidents, **sports injuries,** falls, workplace accidents, assaults, or bullets. Most people have had some type of head injury at least once in their lives, but rarely do they require a hospital visit.

However, each year about two million people suffer from a more serious head injury, and up to 750,000 of them are severe enough to require hospitalization. Brain injury is most likely to occur in males between ages 15 and 24, usually as a result of car and motorcycle accidents. About 70% of all accidental **deaths** are due to head

injuries, as are most of the disabilities that occur after trauma.

A person who has had a head injury and who is experiencing the following symptoms should seek medical care immediately:

• Serious bleeding from the head or face

• Loss of consciousness, however brief

• Confusion and lethargy

• Lack of pulse or breathing

• Clear fluid drainage from the nose or ear.

Causes & symptoms

A head injury may cause damage both from the direct physical injury to the brain and from secondary factors, such as lack of oxygen, brain swelling, and disturbance of blood flow. Both closed and penetrating head injuries can cause swirling movements throughout the brain, tearing nerve fibers and causing widespread bleeding or a blood clot in or around the brain. Swelling may raise pressure within the skull (intracranial pressure) and may block the flow of oxygen to the brain.

Head trauma may cause a concussion, in which there is a brief loss of consciousness without visible structural damage to the brain. In addition to loss of consciousness, initial symptoms of brain injury may include:

- Memory loss and confusion

- Vomiting

- **Dizziness**

- Partial **paralysis** or numbness

- **Shock**

- **Anxiety.**

After a head injury, there may be a period of impaired consciousness followed by a period of confusion and impaired memory with disorientation and a breakdown in the ability to store and retrieve new information. Others experience temporary **amnesia** following head injury that begins with memory loss over a period of weeks, months, or years before the injury (retrograde amnesia). As the patient recovers, memory slowly returns. Post-traumatic amnesia refers to loss of memory for events during and after the accident.

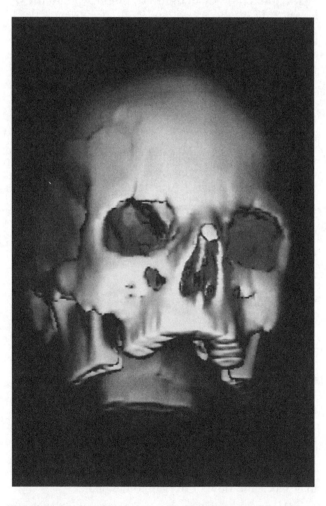

A three-dimensional computed tomography scan (CT) of a human skull showing a depressed skull fracture above the right eye. *(Custom Medical Stock Photo. Reproduced by permission.)*

Epilepsy occurs in 2–5% of those who have had a head injury; it is much more common in people who have had severe or penetrating injuries. Most cases of epilepsy appear right after the accident or within the first year, and become less likely with increased time following the accident.

Closed head injury

Closed head injury refers to brain injury without any penetrating injury to the brain. It may be the result of a direct blow to the head; of the moving head being rapidly stopped, such as when a person's head hits a windshield in a car accident; or by the sudden deceleration of the head without its striking another object. The kind of injury the brain receives in a closed head injury is determined by whether or not the head was unrestrained upon impact and the direction, force, and velocity of the blow. If the head is resting on impact, the maximum damage will be found at the impact site. A moving head will cause a ''contrecoup injury'' where the brain damage occurs on the side opposite the point of impact, as a result of the brain slamming into that side of the skull. A closed head injury also may occur without the head being struck, such as when a person experiences **whiplash.** This type of injury occurs because the brain is of a different density than the skull, and can be injured when delicate brain tissues hit against the rough, jagged inner surface of the skull.

Penetrating head injury

If the skull is fractured, bone fragments may be driven into the brain. Any object that penetrates the skull may implant foreign material and dirt into the brain, leading to an infection.

Skull fracture

A skull fracture is a medical emergency that must be treated promptly to prevent possible brain damage. Such an injury may be obvious if blood or bone fragments are visible, but it's possible for a fracture to have occurred without any apparent damage. A skull fracture should be suspected if there is:

- Blood or clear fluid leaking from nose or ears

- Unequal pupil size

- **Bruises** or discoloration around the eyes or behind the ears

- Swelling or depression of the part of the head.

Intracranial hemorrhage

Bleeding (hemorrhage) inside the skull may accompany a head injury and cause additional damage to the brain. A blood clot (hematoma) may occur if a blood vessel between the skull and the brain ruptures; when the blood leaks out and forms a clot, it can press against brain tissue, causing symptoms from a few hours to a few weeks after the injury. If the clot is located between the bones of the skull and the covering of the brain (dura), it is called an epidural hematoma. If the clot is between the dura and the brain tissue itself, the condition is called a **subdural** hematoma. In other cases, bleeding may occur deeper inside the brain. This condition is called intracerebral hemorrhage or intracerebral contusion (from the word for bruising).

In any case, if the blood flow is not stopped, it can lead to unconsciousness and death. The symptoms of bleeding within the skull include:

- **Nausea and vomiting**
- **Headache**
- Loss of consciousness
- Unequal pupil size
- Lethargy.

Postconcussion syndrome

If the head injury is mild, there may be no symptoms other than a slight headache, or there also may be confusion, dizziness, and blurred vision. While the head injury may seem to have been quite mild, in many cases symptoms persist for days or weeks. Up to 60% of patients who sustain a mild brain injury continue to experience a range of symptoms called ''postconcussion syndrome,'' as long as six months or a year after the injury.

The symptoms of postconcussion syndrome can result in a puzzling interplay of behavioral, cognitive, and emotional complaints that can be difficult to diagnose, including:

- Headache
- Dizziness
- Mental confusion
- Behavior changes
- Memory loss
- Cognitive deficits
- Depression
- Emotional outbursts.

Diagnosis

The extent of damage in a severe head injury can be assessed with **computed tomography scan** (CT scan), **magnetic resonance imaging** (MRI), **positron emission tomography (PET)** scans, electroencephalograms (EEG), and routine neurological and neuropsychological evaluations.

Doctors use the Glasgow Coma Scale to evaluate the extent of brain damage based on observing a patient's ability to open his or her eyes, respond verbally, and respond to stimulation by moving (motor response). Patients can score from 3 to 15 points on this scale. People who score below 8 when they are admitted usually have suffered a severe brain injury and will need rehabilitative therapy as they recover. In general, higher scores on the Glasgow Coma Scale indicate less severe brain injury and a better prognosis for recovery.

Patients with a mild head injury who experience symptoms are advised to seek out the care of a specialist; unless a family physician is thoroughly familiar with medical literature in this newly emerging area, experts warn that there is a good chance that patient complaints after a mild head injury will be downplayed or dismissed. In the case of mild head injury or postconcussion syndrome, CT and MRI scans, electroencephalograms (EEG), and routine neurological evaluations all may be normal because the damage is so subtle. In many cases, these tests can't detect the microscopic damage that occurs when fibers are stretched in a mild, diffuse injury. In this type of injury, the axons lose some of their covering and become less efficient. This mild injury to the white matter reduces the quality of communication between different parts or the brain. A PET scan, which evaluates cerebral blood flow and brain metabolism, may be of help in diagnosing mild head injury, although this is still largely considered to be an experimental procedure.

Patients with continuing symptoms after a mild head injury should call a local chapter of a head-injury foundation that can refer patients to the best nearby expert.

Treatment

If a **concussion,** bleeding inside the skull, or skull fracture is suspected, the patient should be kept quiet in a darkened room, with head and shoulders raised slightly on pillow or blanket.

After initial emergency treatment, a team of specialists may be needed to evaluate and treat the problems that result. A penetrating wound may require surgery. Those with severe injuries or with a deteriorating level of consciousness may be kept hospitalized for observation. If there is bleeding inside the skull, the blood may need to be surgically drained; if a clot has formed, it may need to be removed. Severe skull **fractures** also require surgery. Supportive care and specific treatments may be required if the patient experiences further complications. People who experience seizures, for example, may be given **anticonvulsant drugs,** and people who develop fluid on the brain (**hydrocephalus**) may have a shunt inserted to drain the fluid.

In the event of long-term disability as a result of head injury, there are a variety of treatment programs available, including long-term **rehabilitation,** coma treatment centers, transitional living programs, behavior management programs, life-long residential or day treatment programs and independent living programs.

Prognosis

Prompt, proper diagnosis and treatment can help alleviate some of the problems after a head injury. However, it is usually difficult to predict the outcome of a brain injury in the first few hours or days; a patient's prognosis may not be known for many months or even years.

The outlook for someone with a minor head injury is generally good, although recovery may be delayed and symptoms such as headache, dizziness, and cognitive problems can persist for up to a year or longer after an accident. This can limit a person's ability to work and cause strain in personal relationships.

Serious head injuries can be devastating, producing permanent mental and physical disability. Epileptic seizures may occur after a severe head injury, especially a penetrating brain injury, a severe skull fracture, or a serious brain hemorrhage. Recovery from a severe head injury can be very slow, and it may take five years or longer to heal completely. Risk factors associated with an increased likelihood of memory problems or seizures after head injury include age, length and depth of coma, duration of post-traumatic and retrograde amnesia, presence of focal brain injuries, and initial Glasgow Coma Scale score.

Prevention

Many severe head injuries could be prevented by wearing protective helmets during certain sports, or when riding a bike or motorcycle. Seat belts and airbags can prevent many head injuries as a result of car accidents. Appropriate protective headgear should always be worn on the job where head injuries are a possibility.

Resources

BOOKS

Greenberg, David A. *Clinical Neurology,* 2nd ed. Norwalk, CT: Appleton & Lange, 1993.

Weiner, William J. *Neurology for the Non-Neurologist,* 3rd ed. Philadelphia: J.B. Lippincott, 1994.

PERIODICALS

Mild Traumatic Brain Injury Committee. "Definition of Mild Traumatic Brain Injury." *Journal of Head Trauma Rehabilitation.* 8 (1993):86-87.

Soren, S. and Kraus, J.F. "Occurrence, Severity and Outcomes of Brain Injury" *Journal of Head Trauma Rehabilitation.* 6 (1991):1-10.

ORGANIZATIONS

American Epilepsy Society. 638 Prospect Ave., Hartford, CT 06105. (203) 232-4825.

Brain Injury Association. 1776 Massachusetts Ave. NW, Ste. 100, Washington, DC 20036. (800) 444-6443.

Family Caregiver Alliance. 425 Bush St., Ste. 500, San Francisco, CA 94108. (800) 445-8106. http://www.caregiver.org.

Head Injury Hotline. PO Box 84151, Seattle, WA 98124. (206) 621-8558.

Head Trauma Support Project, Inc. 2500 Marconi Ave., Ste. 203, Sacramento, CA 95821. (916) 482-5770.

National Head Injury Foundation. 333 Turnpike Rd., Southboro, MA 01722. (617) 485-9950.

Carol A. Turkington

Head lice *see* **Lice infestation**

Head trauma *see* **Head injury**

. . . .

Headache

Definition

A headache involves **pain** in the head which can arise from many disorders or may be a disorder in and of itself.

Description

There are three types of primary headaches: tension-type (muscular contraction headache), migraine (vascular headaches), and cluster. Virtually everyone experiences a tension-type headache at some point. An estimated 18% of American women suffer migraines, compared to 6% of men. **Cluster headaches** affect fewer than 0.5% of the population, and men account for approximately 80% of all cases. Headaches caused by illness are secondary headaches and are not included in these numbers.

Approximately 40–45 million people in the United States suffer chronic headaches. Headaches have an enormous impact on society due to missed workdays and productivity losses.

Causes & symptoms

Traditional theories about headaches link tension-type headaches to muscle contraction, and migraine and cluster headaches to blood vessel dilation (swelling). Pain-sensitive structures in the head include blood vessel walls, membranous coverings of the brain, and scalp and neck muscles. Brain tissue itself has no sensitivity to

KEY TERMS

Abortive—Referring to treatment which relieves symptoms of a disorder.

Analgesics—A class of pain-relieving medicines, including aspirin and Tylenol.

Biofeedback—A technique in which a person is taught to consciously control the body's response to a stimulus.

Chronic—Referring to a condition that occurs frequently or continuously or on a regular basis.

Prophylactic—Referring to treatment which prevents symptoms of a disorder from appearing.

Transcutaneous electrical nerve stimulation—A method that electrically stimulates nerve and blocks the transmission of pain signals, called TENS.

pain. Therefore, headaches may result from contraction of the muscles of the scalp, face or neck; dilation of the blood vessels in the head; or brain swelling that stretches the brain's coverings. Involvement of specific nerves of the face and head may also cause characteristic headaches. Sinus inflammation is a common cause of headache. Keeping a headache diary may help link headaches to stressful occurrences, menstrual phases, food triggers, or medication.

Tension-type headaches are often brought on by stress, overexertion, loud noise, and other external factors. The typical tension-type headache is described as a tightening around the head and neck, and an accompanying dull ache.

Migraines are intense throbbing headaches occurring on one or both sides of the head. The pain is accompanied by other symptoms such as nausea, vomiting, blurred vision, and aversion to light, sound, and movement. Migraines are often triggered by food items, such as red wine, chocolate, and aged cheeses. For women, a hormonal connection is likely, since headaches occur at specific points in the menstrual cycle, with use of **oral contraceptives,** or the use of **hormone replacement therapy** after **menopause.**

Cluster headaches cause excruciating pain. The severe, stabbing pain centers around one eye, and eye tearing and nasal congestion occur on the same side. The headache lasts from 15 minutes to 4 hours and may recur several times in a day. Heavy smokers are more likely to suffer cluster headaches, which are also associated with alcohol consumption.

Diagnosis

Since headaches arise from many causes, a physical exam assesses general health and a neurologic exam evaluates the possibility of neurologic disease that is causing the headache. If the headache is the primary illness, a doctor elicits a thorough history of the headache. Questions revolve around its frequency and duration, when it occurs, pain intensity and location, possible triggers, and any prior symptoms. This information aids in classifying the headache.

Warning signs that should point out the need for prompt medical intervention include:

• "Worst headache of my life." This may indicate **subarachnoid hemorrhage** from a ruptured aneurysm (swollen blood vessel) in the head or other neurological emergency.

• Headache accompanied by one-sided weakness, numbness, visual loss, speech difficulty, or other signs. This may indicate a **stroke.** Migraines may include neurological symptoms.

• Headache that becomes worse over a period of 6 months, especially if most prominent in the morning or if accompanied by neurological symptoms. This may indicate a **brain tumor.**

• Sudden onset of headache. If accompanied by **fever** and stiff neck, this can indicate **meningitis.**

Headache diagnosis may include neurological imaging tests such as **computed tomography scan** (CT scan) or **magnetic resonance imaging** (MRI).

Treatment

Headache treatment is divided into two forms: abortive and prophylactic. Abortive treatment addresses a headache in progress, and prophylactic treatment prevents headache occurrence.

Tension-type and **migraine headaches** can be treated with **aspirin, acetaminophen,** ibuprofen, or naproxen. In early 1998, the FDA approved extra-strength Excedrin, which includes **caffeine,** for mild to moderate migraines. Prescription medications such as antidepressants and **muscle relaxants** can address tension-type headaches, and ergotamine tartrate or sumatriptan can relieve or prevent migraines. Cluster headaches may also be treated with ergotamine and sumatriptan, as well as by inhaling pure oxygen. Prophylactic treatments include prednisone, **calcium channel blockers,** and methysergide.

Alternative treatment

Alternative headache treatments include:

• **Acupuncture** or **acupressure**

- **Biofeedback**

- **Chiropractic**

- Herbal remedies using feverfew (*Chrysanthemum parthenium*), valerian (*Valeriana officinalis*), white willow (*Salix alba*), or skullcap (*Scutellaria lateriflora*), among others

- Homeopathic remedies chosen specifically for the individual and his/her type of headache

- Hydrotherapy

- **Massage**

- Magnesium supplements

- Regular physical **exercise**

- Relaxation techniques, such as **meditation** and **yoga**

- **Transcutaneous electrical nerve stimulation** (TENS). A test that electrically stimulates nerves and blocks the signals of pain transmission.

Prognosis

Headaches are typically resolved through the use of **analgesics** and other treatments.

Prevention

Some headaches may be prevented by avoiding triggering substances and situations, or by employing alternative therapies, such as yoga and regular exercise. Since food allergies are often linked with headaches, especially cluster headaches and migraines, identification and elimination of the allergy-causing food(s) from the diet can be an important preventive measure.

Resources

BOOKS

Rapoport, Alan M., and Fred D. Sheftell. *Headache Disorders: A Management Guide for Practitioners.* Philadelphia: W.B. Saunders Company, 1996.

PERIODICALS

Chaballa, Mark, and Karen J. Tietze. "Headache." *American Druggist,* 213 no. 6 (1996): 42.

ORGANIZATIONS

American Council for Headache Education. 19 Mantua Road, Mt. Royal, NJ 08061. (609) 423-0043 or (800) 255-2243. http://www.achenet.org/.

National Headache Foundation. 428 West St. James Place, Chicago, IL 60614. (773) 388-6399 or (800) 843-2256. http://www.headaches.org/.

Julia Barrett

Hearing aids

Definition

A hearing aid is a device that can amplify sound waves in order to help a deaf or hard-of-hearing person hear sounds more clearly.

Purpose

Recent technology can help most people with **hearing loss** understand speech better and achieve better communication.

Precautions

It's important that a person being fitted for a hearing aid understand what an aid can and can't do. An aid can help a person hear better, but it won't return hearing to normal levels. Hearing aids boost all sounds, not just those the person wishes to hear. Especially when the source of sound is far away (such as up on a stage), environmental noise can interfere with good speech perception. And while the aid amplifies sound, it doesn't necessarily improve the clarity of the sound. A hearing aid is a machine, and can never duplicate the true sound that people with normal hearing experience, but it will help the person take advantage of the hearing that remains.

Description

More than 1,000 different models are available in the United States. All of them include a microphone (to pick up sound), amplifier (to boost sound strength), a receiver or speaker (to deliver sound to the ear), and are powered by a battery. Depending on the style, it's possible to add features to filter or block out background noise, minimize feedback, lower sound in noisy settings, or boost power when needed.

Hearing aids are either "monaural" (a hearing aid for one ear), or "binaural" (for two ears); more than 65% of all users have binaural aids. Hearing aids are divided into several different types:

- Digital

- In-the-ear

- In-the-canal

- Behind-the-ear

- On-the-body.

Digital aids are sophisticated, very expensive aids that borrow computer technology to allow a person to tailor an aid to a specific hearing loss pattern. Using miniature computer chips, the aids can selectively boost

KEY TERMS

Audiologist—A person with a degree and/or certification in the areas of identification and measurement of hearing impairments and rehabilitation of those with hearing problems.

Eardrum—A paper-thin covering stretching across the ear canal that separates the middle and outer ears.

Middle ear—The small cavity between the eardrum and the oval window that houses the three tiny bones of hearing.

Oval window—A tiny opening at the entrance to the inner ear.

certain frequencies while leaving others alone. This means a person could wear such an aid to a loud party, and screen out unwanted background noise, while tuning in on one-on-one conversations. The aid is programmed by the dealer to conform to the patient's specific hearing loss. Some models can be programmed to allow the wearer to choose different settings depending on the noise of the environment.

In-the-ear aids are lightweight devices whose custom-made housings contain all the components; this device fits into the ear canal with no visible wires or tubes. It's possible to control tone but not volume with these aids, so they are helpful only for people with mild hearing loss. Some people find these aids are easier to put on and take off than behind-the-ear aids. However, because they are custom-fit to a person's ear, it is not possible to try on before ordering. Some people find them uncomfortable in hot weather.

In-the-canal aids fit far into the ear canal, with only a small bit extending into the external ear. The smallest is the MicroCanal, which fits out of sight down next to the eardrum and is removed with a small transparent wire. These are extremely expensive, but they are not visible, offer better acoustics, and are easier to maintain. They can more closely mimic natural sound because of the position of the microphone; this position also cuts down on wind noise. But their small size makes them harder to handle, and their battery is especially small and difficult to insert. Adjusting the volume may be hard, since a person must stick a finger down into the ear to adjust volume, and this very tiny aid doesn't have the power of other, larger, aids.

Behind-the-ear aids include a microphone, amplifier and receiver inside a small curved case worn behind the ear; the case is connected to the earmold by a short plastic tube. The earmold extends into the ear canal. Some

models have both tone and volume control, plus a telephone pickup device. However, many users, think them unattractive and out of date; and people who wear glasses find that the glasses interfere with the aid's fit. Others don't have space behind the ear for the mold to fit comfortably. However, they do offer a few advantages.

Behind-the-ear aids:

• Don't require as much maintenance
• Are easily interchangeable if they need to be serviced
• Are more powerful
• Are easier to handle than smaller aids
• Can provide better sound quality
• Tend to be more reliable.

Eyeglass models are the same as behind-the-ear devices, except that the case fits into an eyeglass frame instead of resting behind the ears. Not many people buy this type of aid, but those who do believe it's less obvious, although there is a tube that travels from the temple of the glasses to the earmold. But it can be hard to fit this type of aid, and repairs can be problematic. Also, if the aid breaks, the person also loses the benefit of the glasses.

CROS or the crossover system type of hearing aid is often used in conjunction with the eyeglass model. The CROS (contralateral routing of signal) system features a microphone behind the ear that feeds the amplified signal to the better ear, eliminating "head shadow," which occurs when the head blocks sound from the better ear. This type may help make speech easier to understand for people with a high-frequency loss in both ears.

A BI-CROS system uses two microphones (one above each ear) that send signals to a single amplifier. Sound then travels to a single receiver, which transfers it to the better ear via a conventional earmold.

On-the-body aids feature a larger microphone, amplifier, and power supply inside a case carried inside the pocket, or attached to clothing. The receiver attaches directly to the earmold; its power comes through a flexible wire from the amplifier. Although larger than other aids, the on-the-body aids are more powerful and easier to adjust than other devices. While not popular for everyone, they are often used by those with a profound hearing loss, or by very young children. Some people who are almost totally deaf find they need the extra power boost available only from a body aid.

The latest aids on the market may eliminate the amplifier and speaker in favor of a tiny magnet mounted on a silicone disk, similar to a contact lens, which rests right on the eardrum. Called the Earlens, it is designed to be held in place by a thin film of oil. Users wear a wireless microphone, either in the ear or on a necklace, that picks up sounds and converts them into magnetic signals, making the magnet vibrate. As the Earlens vi-

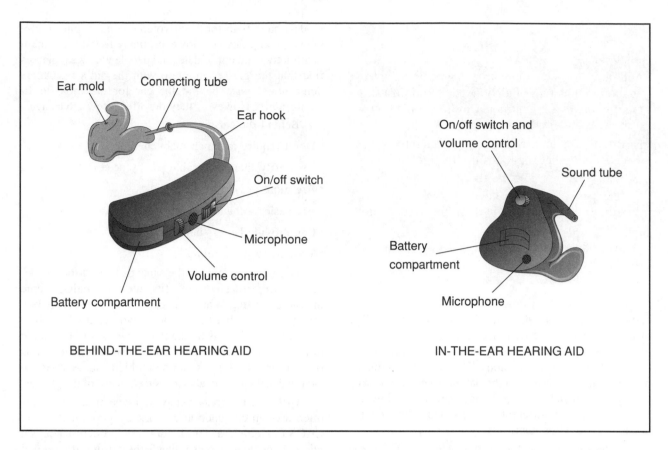

Ear mold   Connecting tube

Ear hook

On/off switch

Microphone

Volume control

Battery compartment

BEHIND-THE-EAR HEARING AID

On/off switch and
volume control

Sound tube

Battery
compartment

Microphone

IN-THE-EAR HEARING AID

Hearing aids are devices that can amplify sound waves to help a deaf or hard-of-hearing person hear sounds more clearly. *(Illustration by Electronic Illustrators Group.)*

brates, so does the eardrum, transmitting normal-sounding tones to the middle and inner ears.

Other researchers are bypassing the middle ear completely; they surgically implant a tiny magnet in the inner ear. By attaching a magnet to the round window, they open a second pathway to the inner ear. An electromagnetic coil implanted in bone behind the ear vibrates the implanted magnet. Unlike the Earlens, this magnetic implant would not block the normal hearing pathway.

Preparation

The fist step in getting a hearing aid is to have a medical exam and a hearing evaluation. (Most states prohibit anyone selling a hearing aid until the patient has been examined by a physician to rule out medical problems.) After performing a hearing evaluation, an audiologist should be able to determine whether a hearing aid will help, and which one will do the most good. This is especially important because aids can be very expensive (between $500 and $4,000), and are often not covered by health insurance. Hearing aids come in a wide range of styles and types, requiring careful testing to make sure the aid is the best choice for a particular hearing loss.

Some audiologists sell aids; others can make a recommendation, or give one a list of competent dealers in one's area. Patients should shop around and compare prices. In all but three states, hearing aids must be fitted and sold only by licensed specialists called dealers, specialists, dispensers, or dispensing audiologists.

The hearing aid dealer will make an impression of the consumer's ears using a putty-like material, from which a personalized earmold will be created. It's the dealer's job to make sure the aid fits properly. The person may need several visits to find the right hearing aid and learn how to use it. The dealer will help the consumer learn how to put the aid on, adjust the controls, and maintain the device. The dealer should be willing to service the aid and provide information about what to do if sensitivity to the earmold develops. (Some people are allergic to the materials in the mold.)

Aftercare

Within several weeks, the wearer should return to the dealer to have the aid checked, and to discuss the progress in wearing the aid. About 40% of all aids need some modification or adjustment in the beginning.

Within the first month of getting an aid, the patient should make an appointment for a full hearing examination to determine if the aid is functioning properly.

Risks

While there are no medical risks to hearing aids, there is a risk associated with hearing aids: many people end up not wearing their aids because they say everything seems loud when wearing them. This is because they have lived for so long with a hearing problem that they have forgotten how loud ''normal'' sound can be. Other potential problems with hearing aids include earmold discomfort, and a build up of excess ear wax after getting a hearing aid.

Normal results

A hearing aid will boost the loudness of sound, which can improve a person's ability to understand speech.

Resources

BOOKS

Carmen, Richard. *The Consumer Handbook on Hearing Loss and Hearing Aids.* New York: Auricle Ink Publishers, 1997.

Turkington, Carol A. *The Hearing Loss Sourcebook.* New York: Penguin, 1997.

PERIODICALS

Dickinson, Ben. ''30/40/50: Listen Up While You Still Can.'' *Esquire* 129 (Jan. 1, 1998): 101.

Young, Leslie A. ''Sonic Boomers: Clinton's Hearing Aid Catches His Generation's Ear.'' *Rocky Mountain News* (Oct. 14, 1997): 3D.

ORGANIZATIONS

American Academy of Otolaryngology-Head and Neck Surgery. One Prince St., Alexandria, VA 22316. (703) 836-4444.

Better Hearing Institute. PO Box 1840, Washington, DC 20013. (800) EAR WELL. http://www.betterhearing.org.

Hear Now. 9745 E. Hampden Ave., Ste. 300, Denver, CO 80231. (800) 648-HEAR. (202) 651-5258.

Hearing Industries Association. 1800 M St. NW, Washington, DC 20036. (202) 651-5258.

National Hearing Aid Society. 20361 Middlebelt, Livonia, MI 48152. (800) 521-5247 or (313) 478-2610.

National Information Center on Deafness. Gallaudet College, 800 Florida Ave. NE, Washington, DC 20002. (202) 651-5051; (202) 651-5052 (TDD).

Carol A. Turkington

Hearing loss

Definition

Hearing loss is any degree of impairment of the ability to apprehend sound.

Description

Sound can be measured accurately. The term decibel (dB) refers to an amount of energy moving sound from its source to our ears or to a microphone. A drop of more than 10 dB in the level of sound a person can hear is significant.

Sound travels through a medium like air or water as waves of compression and rarefaction. These waves are collected by the external ear and cause the tympanic membrane (ear drum) to vibrate. The chain of ossicles connected to the ear drum—the incus, malleus, and stapes—carries the vibration to the oval window, increasing its amplitude twenty times on the way. There the energy causes a standing wave in the watery liquid (endolymph) inside the Organ of Corti. (A standing wave is one that does not move. A vibrating cup of coffee will demonstrate standing waves.) The configuration of the standing wave is determined by the frequency of the sound. Many thousands of tiny nerve fibers detect the highs and lows of the standing wave and transmit their findings to the brain, which interprets the signals as sound.

To summarize, sound energy passes through the air of the external ear, the bones of the middle ear and the liquid of the inner ear. It is then translated into nerve impulses, sent to the brain through nerves and understood there as sound. It follows that there are five steps in the hearing process:

- Air conduction through the external ear to the ear drum

- Bone conduction through the middle ear to the inner ear

- Water conduction to the Organ of Corti

- Nerve conduction into the brain

- Interpretation by the brain.

Hearing can be interrupted in several ways at each of the five steps.

The external ear canal can be blocked with ear wax, **foreign objects,** infection, and tumors. Overgrowth of the bone, a condition that occurs when the ear canal has been flushed with cold water repeatedly for years, can also narrow the passageway, making blockage and infection more likely. This condition occurs often in Northern Californian surfers and is therefore called ''surfer's ear.''

The ear drum is so thin a physician can see through it into the middle ear. Sharp objects, pressure from an infection in the middle ear, even a firm cuffing or slapping of the ear, can rupture it. It is also susceptible to pressure changes during scuba diving.

Several conditions can diminish the mobility of the ossicles (small bones) in the middle ear. **Otitis media** (an infection in the middle ear) occurs when fluid cannot escape into the throat because of blockage of the eustachian tube. The fluid that accumulates, whether it be pus or just mucus, dampens the motion of the ossicles. A disease called **otosclerosis** can bind the stapes in the oval window and thereby cause deafness.

All the conditions mentioned so far, those that occur in the external and middle ear, are causes of conductive hearing loss. The second category, sensory hearing loss, refers to damage to the Organ or Corti and the acoustic nerve. Prolonged exposure to loud noise is the leading cause of sensory hearing loss. A million people have this condition, many identified during the military draft and rejected as being unfit for duty. The cause is often believed to be prolonged exposure to rock music. Occupational noise exposure is the other leading cause of noise induced hearing loss (NIHL) and is ample reason for wearing ear protection on the job. A third of people over 65 have presbycusis—sensory hearing loss due to aging. Both NIHL and presbycusis are primarily high frequency losses. In most languages, it is the high frequency sounds that define speech, so these people hear plenty of noise,

they just cannot easily make out what it means. They have particular trouble selecting out speech from background noise. Brain infections like **meningitis,** drugs such as the aminoglycoside **antibiotics** (streptomycin, gentamycin, kanamycin, tobramycin), and **Meniere's disease** also cause permanent sensory hearing loss. Meniere's disease combines attacks of hearing loss with attacks of vertigo. The symptoms may occur together or separately. High doses of salicylates like **aspirin** and quinine can cause a temporary high-frequency loss. Prolonged high doses can lead to permanent deafness. There is an hereditary form of sensory deafness and a congenital form most often caused by **rubella** (German **measles**).

Sudden hearing loss—at least 30dB in less than three days—is most commonly caused by cochleitis, a mysterious viral infection.

The final category of hearing loss is neural. Damage to the acoustic nerve and the parts of the brain that perform hearing are the most likely to produce permanent hearing loss. **Strokes, multiple sclerosis,** and **acoustic neuromas** are all possible causes of neural hearing loss.

Hearing can also be diminished by extra sounds generated by the ear, most of them from the same kinds of disorders that cause diminished hearing. These sounds are referred to as **tinnitus** and can be ringing, blowing, clicking, or anything else that no one but the patient hears.

Diagnosis

An examination of the ears and nose combined with simple hearing tests done in the physician's office can detect many common causes of hearing loss. An audiogram often concludes the evaluation, since these simple means often produce a diagnosis. If the defect is in the brain or the acoustic nerve, further neurological testing and imaging will be required.

The audiogram has many uses in diagnosing hearing deficits. The pattern of hearing loss across the audible frequencies gives clues to the cause. Several alterations in the testing procedure can give additional information. For example, speech is perceived differently than pure tones. Adequate perception of sound combined with inability to recognize words points to a brain problem rather than a sensory or conductive deficit. Loudness perception is distorted by disease in certain areas but not in others. Acoustic neuromas often distort the perception of loudness.

Treatment

Conductive hearing loss can almost always be restored to some degree, if not completely.

• Matter in the ear canal can be easily removed with a dramatic improvement in hearing.

DECIBEL RATINGS AND HAZARDOUS LEVELS OF NOISE	
Decibel Level	**Example Of Sounds**
30	Soft whisper
35	Noise may prevent the listener from falling asleep
40	Quiet office noise level
50	Quiet conversation
60	Average television volume, sewing machine, lively conversation
70	Busy traffic, noisy restaurant
80	Heavy city traffic, factory noise, alarm clock
90	Cocktail party, lawn mower
100	Pneumatic drill
120	Sandblasting, thunder
140	Jet airplane
180	Rocket launching pad
Above 110 decibels, hearing may become painful	
Above 120 decibels is considered deafening	
Above 135 decibels, hearing will become extremely painful and hearing loss may result if exposure is prolonged	
Above 180 decibels, hearing loss is almost certain with any exposure	

Source: *FDA Consumer, Gale Encyclopedia of Psychology,* 1996.

- Surfer's ear gradually regresses if cold water is avoided or a special ear plug is used. In advanced cases, surgeons can grind away the excess bone.

- Middle ear infection with fluid is also simple to treat. If medications do not work, surgical drainage of the ear is accomplished through the ear drum, which heals completely after treatment.

- Traumatically damaged ear drums can be repaired with a tiny skin graft.

- Surgical repair of otosclerosis through an operating microscope is one of the most intricate of procedures, substituting tiny artificial parts for the original ossicles.

Sensory and neural hearing loss, on the other hand, cannot readily be cured. Fortunately it is not often complete, so that **hearing aids** can fill the deficit.

In-the-ear hearing aids can boost the volume of sound by up to 70 dB. (Normal speech is about 60 dB.) Federal law now requires that they be dispensed only upon a physician's prescription. For complete conduction hearing loss there are now available bone conduction hearing aids and even devices that can be surgically implanted in the cochlea.

Tinnitus can sometimes be relieved by adding white noise (like the sound of wind or waves crashing on the shore) to the environment.

Decreased hearing is such a common problem that there are legions of organizations to provide assistance. Special language training, both in lip reading and signing, special schools and special camps for children are all available in most regions of the United States.

Alternative treatment

Conductive hearing loss can be treated with alternative therapies that are specific to the particular condition. Sensory hearing loss may be helped by homeopathic therapies. Oral supplementation with essential fatty acids such as flax oil and omega 3 oil can help alleviate the accumulation of wax in the ear.

Prevention

Prompt treatment and attentive follow-up of middle ear infections in children will prevent this cause of conductive hearing loss. Control of infectious childhood diseases such as measles has greatly reduced sensory hearing loss as a complication of epidemic diseases. Laws that require protection from loud noise in the work-

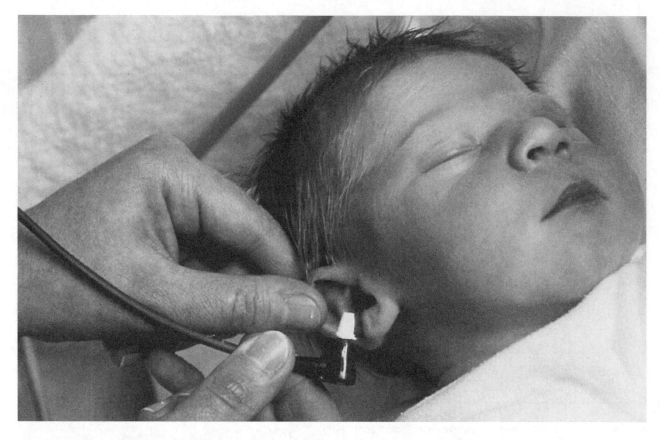

An Oto-Acoustic Emission (OAE) hearing test being performed on a newborn baby. The probe emits harmless sound into the baby's ear, and the response of the inner ear is detected and registered on a computer. Early diagnosis of a hearing disorder is important in young children, who may experience difficulties in speech and language development. *(Photograph by James King-Holmes, Photo Researchers, Inc. Reproduced by permission.)*

place have achieved substantial reduction in noise-induced hearing loss. Surfers should use the right kind of ear plugs.

Resources

BOOKS

Alberti, R.W. "Occupational hearing loss." In *Disorders of the nose, throat, ear, head, and neck.* Edited by John Jacob Ballenger. Philadelphia: Lea & Febiger, 1991, pp. 1053-68.

Austin, David F. "Non-inflammatory diseases of the labyrinth." In *Disorders of the nose, throat, ear, head, and neck.* Edited by John Jacob Ballenger. Philadelphia: Lea & Febiger, 1991, pp. 1209-13.

Bennett, J. Claude and Fred Plum, ed. *Cecil Textbook of Medicine* Philadelphia: W. B. Saunders, 1996, pp. 2021-24.

Niparko, John K. "Hearing loss and associated problems." In *Principles of Ambulatory Medicine.* Edited by L. Randol Barker, et al. Baltimore: Williams & Wilkins, 1995, pp. 1403-15.

Rakel, Robert E., ed. *Current Therapy.* Philadelphia: W. B. Saunders, 1998, pp. 459-460.

Tierney, Lawrence M., et al., ed. *Current Medical Diagnosis and Treatment.* Stamford, CT: Appleton & Lange, 1998, pp. 215.

PERIODICALS

Cohen, N. and S. Waltzman. "The Department of Veterans Affairs Cochlear Implant Study Group." *New England Journal of Medicine* 328 (1993): 233.

Nadol, J.B. "Hearing loss." *New England Journal of Medicine* 329 (1993): 092.

ORGANIZATIONS

Alexander Graham Bell Association for the Deaf. 3417 Volta Place NW, Washington, DC 20007-2778. (202)337-5220. http:/www.agbell.org.

Auditory-Verbal International. 2121 Eisenhower Avenue, Suite 402, Alexandria, VA 22314. (703)739-1049, (703)739-0874. avi@auditory-verbal.org. http://www.auditory-verbal.org/contact.htm.

Better Hearing Institute. Washington, DC. 800-EAR-WELL. mail@betterhearing.org. http://www.betterhearing.org.

Central Institute for the Deaf. Washington University. St. Louis, Missouri. http://cidmac.wustl.edu.

The League for the Hard of Hearing. 71 West 23rd Street, New York, New York 10010-4162. (212)741-7650. http://www.lhh.org.

National Association of the Deaf. NADHQ@juno.com. http://www.nad.org.

National Institute on Deafness and Other Communication Disorders. National Institutes of Health, Bethesda, Maryland 20892. webmaster@ms.nidcd.nih.gov. http://www.nih.gov/nidcd.

Self Help for Hard of Hearing People, Inc. 79 O Woodmon Avenue, Suite 120C, Bethesda, MD 20814. (301)657-2248. http://www.shhh.org.

The Sight & Hearing Association (SHA). http://www.sightandhearing.org.

The World Recreation Association of the Deaf (WRAD). http://www.wrad.org.

OTHER

Vessel, B. "Deaf Source." http://home.earthlink.net/~drblood (April 26, 1998).

J. Ricker Polsdorfer

Hearing test with an audiometer *see*
Audiometry

....

Hearing tests with a tuning fork

Definition

A tuning fork is a metal instrument with a handle and two prongs or tines. Tuning forks, made of steel, aluminum, or magnesium-alloy will vibrate at a set frequency to produce a musical tone when struck. The vibrations produced can be used to assess a person's ability to hear various sound frequencies.

Purpose

A vibrating tuning fork held next to the ear or placed against the skull will stimulate the inner ear to vibrate, and can help determine if there is **hearing loss.**

Precautions

No special precautions are necessary when tuning forks are used to conduct a hearing test.

KEY TERMS

Mastoid process—The protrusions of bone behind the ears at the base of the skull.

Rinne test—A hearing test using a vibrating tuning fork which is held near the ear and held at the back of the skull.

Weber test—A hearing test using a vibrating tuning fork which is held at various points along the midline of the skull and face.

Description

Two types of hearing tests with tuning forks are typically conducted. In the Rinne test, the vibrating tuning fork is held against the skull, usually on the bone behind the ear (mastoid process) to cause vibrations through the bones of the skull and inner ear. It is also held next to, but not touching, the ear, to cause vibrations in the air next to the ear. The patient is asked to determine which sound is louder, the sound heard through the bone or through the air. A second hearing test using a tuning fork is the Weber test. For this test, the stem or handle of the vibrating tuning fork is placed at various points along the midline of the skull and face. The patient is then asked to identify which ear hears the sound created by the vibrations. Tuning forks of different sizes produce different frequencies of vibrations and can be used to establish the range of hearing for an individual patient.

Preparation

No special preparation is required for a hearing test with tuning forks.

Aftercare

No special aftercare is required. If hearing loss is revealed during testing with tuning forks, the patient may require further testing to determine the extent of the hearing loss.

Risks

There are no risks associated with the use of tuning forks to screen for hearing loss.

Normal results

With the Rinne test, a person will hear the tone of the vibration longer and louder when the tuning fork is held next to the ear, rather than when it is held against the mastoid bone. For the Weber test, the tone produced when the tuning fork is placed along the center of the skull, or face, sounds about the same volume in each ear.

Abnormal results

The Rinne test detects a hearing loss when a patient hears a louder and longer tone when the vibrating tuning fork is held against the mastoid bone than when it is held next to the ear. The volume of sound vibrations conducted through parts of the skull and face in the Weber test can indicate which ear may have a hearing loss.

Resources

BOOKS

"Clinical Evaluation of Complaints Referable to the Ears." In *The Merck Manual.* 16th ed., edited by Robert Berkow. Rahway, NJ: Merck & Co. Inc., 1992, pp 2318-2319.

Stedman's Medical Dictionary 26th ed., edited by Marjory Spraycar. Baltimore, MD: Williams & Wilkins, 1995.

PERIODICALS

Abdulrazzak, A. "Office Screening for Age-Related Hearing and Vision Loss." *Geriatrics* 52 no. 6 (June 1997): 45-57.

ORGANIZATIONS

American Academy of Otolaryngology-Head and Neck Surgery. One Prince Street, Alexandria, VA 22314. (703) 836-4444.

Ear Foundation. 2000 Church Street, Box 111, Nashville, TN 37236. (615) 329-7807, (800) 545-HEAR.

Altha Roberts Edgren

Heart arrest *see* **Sudden cardiac death**

Heart arrhythmias *see* **Arrhythmias**

Heart attack

Definition

A heart attack is the death of, or damage to, part of the heart muscle because the supply of blood to the heart muscle is severely reduced or stopped.

Description

Heart attack is the leading cause of death in the United States. More than 1.5 million Americans suffer a heart attack every year, and almost half a million die, according to the American Heart Association. Most heart attacks are the end result of years of silent but progressive

---

coronary artery disease, which can be prevented in many people. A heart attack is often the first symptom of coronary artery disease. According to the American Heart Association, 63% of women and 48% of men who died suddenly of coronary artery disease had no previous symptoms. Heart attacks are also called myocardial infarctions (MIs).

A heart attack occurs when one or more of the coronary arteries that supply blood to the heart are completely blocked and blood to the heart muscle is cut off. The blockage is usually caused by **atherosclerosis,** the build-up of plaque in the artery walls, and/or by a blood clot in a coronary artery. Sometimes, a healthy or atherosclerotic coronary artery has a spasm and the blood flow to part of the heart decreases or stops. Why this happens is unclear, but it can result in a heart attack.

About half of all heart attack victims wait at least two hours before seeking help. This increases their chance of sudden death or being disabled. The longer the artery remains blocked during a heart attack, the more damage will be done to the heart. If the blood supply is cut-off severely or for a long time, muscle cells suffer irreversible injury and die. The patient can die. That is why it is important to recognize the signs of a heart attack and seek prompt medical attention at the nearest hospital with 24-hour emergency cardiac care.

About one fifth of all heart attacks are silent, that is, the victim does not know one has occurred. Although the victim feels no **pain,** silent heart attacks can still damage the heart.

The outcome of a heart attack also depends on where the blockage is, whether the heart rhythm is disturbed, and whether another coronary artery supplies blood to that part of the heart. Blockages in the left coronary artery are usually more serious than in the right coronary artery. Blockages that cause an arrhythmia, an irregular heartbeat, can cause sudden death.

Causes & symptoms

Heart attacks are generally caused by severe coronary artery disease. Most heart attacks are caused by blood clots that form on atherosclerotic plaque. This blocks a coronary artery from supplying oxygen-rich blood to part of the heart. A number of major and contributing risk factors increase the risk of developing coronary artery disease. Some of these can be changed and some cannot. People with more risk factors are more likely to develop coronary artery disease.

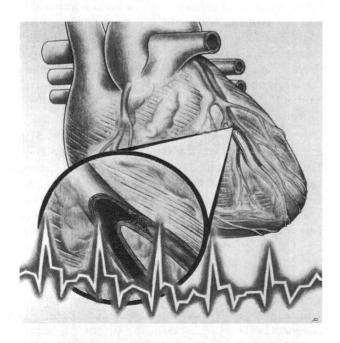

Heart attacks are generally caused by severe coronary artery disease. Most heart attacks are caused by blood clots that form on atherosclerotic plaque, which blocks a coronary artery from supplying oxygen-rich blood to part of the heart, as highlighted in the illustration above.
(Illustration by Andrew Bezear, Photo Researchers, Inc. Reproduced by permission.)

Major risk factors

Major risk factors significantly increase the risk of coronary artery disease. Those which cannot be changed are:

- Heredity. People whose parents have coronary artery disease are more likely to develop it. African Americans are also at increased risk, due to their higher rate of severe **hypertension** than whites.

- Sex. Men under the age of 60 years of age are more likely to have heart attacks than women of the same age.

- Age. Men over the age of 45 and women over the age of 55 are considered at risk. Older people (those over 65) are more likely to die of a heart attack. Older women are twice as likely to die within a few weeks of a heart attack as a man. This may be because of their other co-existing medical problems.

Major risk factors which can be changed are:

- Smoking. Smoking greatly increases both the chance of developing coronary artery disease and the change of dying from it. Smokers have two to four times the risk of non-smokers of **sudden cardiac death** and are more than twice as likely to have a heart attack. They are also more likely to die within an hour of a heart attack. Second-hand smoke may also increase risk.

- High cholesterol. Cholesterol is a soft, waxy substance that is produced by the body, as well as obtained from eating foods such as meat, eggs, and other animal products. Cholesterol level is affected by age, sex, heredity, and diet. Risk of developing coronary artery disease increases as blood cholesterol levels increase. When combined with other factors, the risk is even greater. Total cholesterol of 240 mg/dL and over poses a high risk, and 200–239 mg/dL a borderline high risk. In LDL cholesterol, high risk starts at 130–159 mg/dL, depending on other risk factors. HDL (healthy cholesterol) can lower or raise the coronary risk also.

- High blood pressure. High blood pressure makes the heart work harder, and over time, weakens it. It increases the risk of heart attack, **stroke,** kidney failure, and congestive **heart failure.** A blood pressure of 140 over 90 or above is considered high. As the numbers increase, high blood pressure goes from Stage 1 (mild) to Stage 4 (very severe). When combined with **obesity,** smoking, high cholesterol, or diabetes, the risk of heart attack or stroke increases several times.

- Lack of physical activity. This increases the risk of coronary artery disease. Even modest physical activity is beneficial if done regularly.

Contributing risk factors

Contributing risk factors have been linked to coronary artery disease, but their significance and prevalence are not known yet. Contributing risk factors are:

• **Diabetes mellitus.** The risk of developing coronary artery disease is seriously increased for diabetics. More than 80% of diabetics die of some type of heart or blood vessel disease.

• Obesity. Excess weight increases the strain on the heart and increases the risk of developing coronary artery disease, even if no other risk factors are present. Obesity increases both blood pressure and blood cholesterol, and can lead to diabetes.

• **Stress** and anger. Some scientists believe that stress and anger can contribute to the development of coronary artery disease. Stress, the mental and physical reaction to life's irritations and challenges, increases the heart rate and blood pressure, and can injure the lining of the arteries. Evidence shows that anger increases the risk of dying from heart disease and more than doubles the risk of having a heart attack right after an episode of anger.

More than 60% of heart attack victims experience symptoms before the heart attack occurs. These sometimes occur days or weeks before the heart attack. Sometimes, people do not recognize the symptoms of a heart attack or are in denial that they are having one. Symptoms are:

• Uncomfortable pressure, fullness, squeezing, or pain in the center of the chest. This lasts more than a few minutes, or may go away and return.

• Pain that spreads to the shoulders, neck, or arms.

• Chest discomfort accompanied by lightheadedness, fainting, sweating, nausea, or **shortness of breath.**

All of these symptoms do not occur with every heart attack. Sometimes, symptoms disappear and then reappear. A person with any of these symptoms should immediately call an emergency rescue service or be driven to the nearest hospital with a 24-hour cardiac care unit, whichever is quicker.

Diagnosis

Experienced emergency care personnel can usually diagnose a heart attack simply by looking at the patient. To confirm this diagnosis, they talk with the patient, check heart rate and blood pressure, perform an electrocardiogram, and take a blood sample. The electrocardiogram shows which coronary artery is blocked. Electrodes covered with conducting jelly are placed on the patient's chest, arms, and legs. They send impulses of the heart's activity through an oscilloscope (a monitor) to a recorder, which traces them on paper. The blood test shows the leak of enzymes or other biochemical markers from damaged cells in the heart muscle.

Treatment

Heart attacks are treated with **cardiopulmonary resuscitation (CPR)** when necessary to start and keep the patient breathing and his heart beating. Additional treatment can include close monitoring, electric shock, drug therapy, re-vascularization procedures, percutaneous transluminal coronary **angioplasty** and coronary artery bypass surgery. Upon arrival at the hospital, the patient is closely monitored. An electrical-shock device, a defibrillator, may be used to restore a normal rhythm if the heartbeat is fluttering uncontrollably. Oxygen is often used to ease the heart's workload or to help victims of severe heart attack breath easier. If oxygen is used within hours of the heart attack, it may help limit damage to the heart.

Drugs to stabilize the patient and limit damage to the heart include thrombolytics, **aspirin,** anticoagulants, painkillers and tranquilizers, beta-blockers, ace-inhibitors, nitrates, rhythm-stabilizing drugs, and **diuretics.** Drugs that limit damage to the heart work only if given within a few hours of the heart attack. Thrombolytic drugs that break up blood clots and enable oxygen-rich blood to flow through the blocked artery increase the patient's chance of survival if given as soon as possible after the heart attack. Thrombolytics given within a few hours after a heart attack are the most effective. Injected intravenously, these include anisoylated plasminogen streptokinase activator complex (APSAC) or anistreplase (Eminase), recombinant tissue-type plasminogen activator (r-tPA, Retevase, or Activase), and streptokinase (Streptase, Kabikinase).

To prevent additional heart attacks, aspirin and an anticoagulant drug often follow the thrombolytic drug. These prevent new blood clots from forming and existing blood clots from growing. Anticoagulant drugs help prevent the blood from clotting. The most common anticoagulants are heparin and warfarin. Heparin is given intravenously while the patient is in the hospital; warfarin, taken orally, is often given later. Aspirin helps to prevent the dissolved blood clots from reforming.

To relieve pain, a nitroglycerine tablet taken under the tongue may be given. If the pain continues, morphine sulfate may be prescribed. Tranquilizers such as diazepam (Valium) and alprazolam (Ativan) may be prescribed to lessen the trauma of a heart attack.

To slow down the heart rate and give the heart a chance to heal, beta-blockers are often given intravenously right after the heart attack. These can also help prevent the sometimes fatal **ventricular fibrillation.** Beta-blockers include atenolol (Tenormin), metoprolol

(Lopressor), nadolol, pindolol (Visken), propranolol (Inderal), and timolol (Blocadren).

Nitrates, a type of vasodilator, are also given right after a heart attack to help improve the delivery of blood to the heart and ease heart failure symptoms. Nitrates include isosorbide mononitrate (Imdur), isosorbide dinitrate (Isordil, Sorbitrate), and nitroglycerin (Nitrostat).

When a heart attack causes an abnormal heartbeat, arrhythmia drugs may be given to restore the heart's normal rhythm. These include: amiodarone (Cordarone), atropine, bretylium, disopyramide (Norpace), lidocaine (Xylocaine), procainamide (Procan), propafenone (Rythmol), propranolol (Inderal), quinidine, and sotalol (Betapace). Angiotensin-converting enzyme (ACE) inhibitors reduce the resistance against which the heart beats and are used to manage and prevent heart failure. They are used to treat heart attack patients whose hearts do not pump well or who have symptoms of heart failure. Taken orally, they include Altace, Capoten, Lotensin, Monopril, Prinivil, Vasotec, and Zestril. Angiotensin receptor blockers, such as losartan (Cozaar) may substitute. Diuretics can help get rid of excess fluids that sometimes accumulate when the heart is not pumping effectively. Usually taken orally, they cause the body to dispose of fluids through urination. Common diuretics include: bumetanide (Bumex), chlorthalidone (Hygroton), chlorothiazide (Diuril), furosemide (Lasix), hydrochlorothiazide (HydroDIRUIL, Esidrix), spironolactone (Aldactone), and triamterene (Dyrenium).

Percutaneous transluminal coronary angioplasty and coronary artery bypass surgery are invasive revascularization procedures which open blocked coronary arteries and improve blood flow. They are usually performed only on patients for whom clot-dissolving drugs do not work, or who have poor exercise **stress tests,** poor left ventricular function, or **ischemia.** Generally, angioplasty is performed before coronary artery bypass surgery.

Percutaneous transluminal coronary angioplasty, usually called coronary angioplasty, is a non-surgical procedure in which a catheter (a tiny plastic tube) tipped with a balloon is threaded from a blood vessel in the thigh or arm into the blocked artery. The balloon is inflated and compresses the plaque to enlarge the blood vessel and open the blocked artery. The balloon is then deflated and the catheter is removed. Coronary angioplasty is performed by a cardiologist in a hospital and generally requires a two-day stay. It is successful about 90% of the time. For one third of patients, the artery narrows again within six months after the procedure. The procedure can be repeated. It is less invasive and less expensive than coronary artery bypass surgery.

In coronary artery bypass surgery, called bypass surgery, a detour is built around the coronary artery blockage with a healthy leg or chest wall artery or vein. The healthy vein then supplies oxygen-rich blood to the heart. Bypass surgery is major surgery appropriate for patients with blockages in two or three major coronary arteries or severely narrowed left main coronary arteries, as well as those who have not responded to other treatments. It is performed in a hospital under general anesthesia using a heart-lung machine to support the patient while the healthy vein is attached to the coronary artery. About 70% of patients who have bypass surgery experience full relief from **angina;** about 20% experience partial relief. Long term, symptoms recur in only about three or four percent of patients per year. Five years after bypass surgery, survival expectancy is 90%, at 10 years it is about 80%, at 15 years it is about 55%, and at 20 years it is about 40%.

There are three experimental surgical procedures for unblocking coronary arteries which are currently being studied: **atherectomy,** where the surgeon shaves off and removes strips of plaque from the blocked artery; laser angioplasty, where a catheter with a laser tip is inserted to burn or break down the plaque; and insertion of a metal coil called a stent that can be implanted permanently to keep a blocked artery open.

Prognosis

The aftermath of a heart attack is often severe. Two-thirds of heart attack patients never recover fully. Within one year, 27% of men and 44% of women die. Within six years, 23% of men and 31% of women have another heart attack, 13% of men and 6% of women experience sudden death, and about 20% have heart failure. People who survive a heart attack have a chance of sudden death that is four to six times greater than others and a chance of illness and death that is two to nine times greater. Older women are more likely than men to die within a few weeks of a heart attack.

Prevention

Many heart attacks can be prevented through a healthy lifestyle, which can reduce the risk of developing coronary artery disease. For patients who have already had a heart attack, a healthy lifestyle and carefully following doctor's orders can prevent another heart attack. A heart healthy lifestyle includes eating right, regular exercise, maintaining a healthy weight, no smoking, moderate drinking, no illegal drugs, controlling hypertension, and managing stress.

A healthy diet includes a variety of foods that are low in fat (especially saturated fat), low in cholesterol, and high in fiber; plenty of fruits and vegetables; and limited sodium. Some foods are low in fat but high in cholesterol, and some are low in cholesterol but high in fat. Saturated fat raises cholesterol, and, in excessive amounts, it increases the amount of the proteins in blood that form blood clots. Polyunsaturated and monounsaturated fats are relatively good for the heart. Fat should comprise no more than 30 percent of total daily calories.

Cholesterol, a waxy, lipid-like substance, comes from eating foods such as meat, eggs, and other animal products. It is also produced in the liver. Soluble fiber can help lower cholesterol. Cholesterol should be limited to about 300 mg per day. Many popular lipid-lowering drugs can reduce LDL-cholesterol by an average of 25–30% when combined with a low-fat, low-cholesterol diet. Fruits and vegetables are rich in fiber, **vitamins,** and **minerals.** They are also low calorie and nearly fat free. Vitamin C and beta-carotene, found in many fruits and vegetables, keep LDL-cholesterol from turning into a form that damages coronary arteries. Excess sodium can increase the risk of high blood pressure. Many processed foods contain large amounts of sodium. Limit daily intake to about 2,400 mg—about the amount in a teaspoon of salt.

The "Food Guide" Pyramid developed by the U.S. Departments of Agriculture and Health and Human Services provides easy to follow guidelines for daily heart-healthy eating: 6–11 servings of bread, cereal, rice, and pasta; 3–5 servings of vegetables; 2–4 servings of fruit; 2–3 servings of milk, yogurt, and cheese; and 2–3 servings of meat, poultry, fish, dry beans, eggs, and nuts. Fats, oils, and sweets should be used sparingly.

Regular aerobic exercise can lower blood pressure, help control weight, and increase HDL ("good") cholesterol. It may keep the blood vessels more flexible. Moderate intensity aerobic exercise lasting about 30 minutes four or more times per week is recommended for maximum heart health, according to the Centers for Disease Control and Prevention and the American College of Sports Medicine. Three 10-minute exercise periods are also beneficial. Aerobic exercise—activities such as walking, jogging, and cycling—uses the large muscle groups and forces the body to use oxygen more efficiently. It can also include everyday activities such as active gardening, climbing stairs, or brisk housework.

Maintaining a desirable body weight is also important. About one quarter of all Americans are overweight, and nearly one-tenth are obese, according to the Surgeon General's Report on Nutrition and Health. People who are 20% or more over their ideal body weight have an increased risk of developing coronary artery disease. Losing weight can help reduce total and LDL cholesterol, reduce triglycerides, and boost relative levels of HDL cholesterol. It may also reduce blood pressure.

Smoking has many adverse effects on the heart. It increases the heart rate, constricts major arteries, and can create irregular heartbeats. It also raises blood pressure, contributes to the development of plaque, increases the formation of blood clots, and causes blood platelets to cluster and impede blood flow. Heart damage caused by smoking can be repaired by quitting—even heavy smokers can return to heart health. Several studies have shown that ex-smokers face the same risk of heart disease as non-smokers within 5 to 10 years of quitting.

Drinking should be done in moderation. Modest consumption of alcohol can actually protect against coronary artery disease. This is believed to be because alcohol raises HDL ("good") cholesterol levels. The American Heart Association defines moderate consumption as one ounce of alcohol per day—roughly one cocktail, one 8-ounce glass of wine, or two 12-ounce glasses of beer. In some people, however, moderate drinking can increase risk factors for heart disease, such as raising blood pressure. Excessive drinking is always bad for the heart. It usually raises blood pressure, and can poison the heart and cause abnormal heart rhythms or even heart failure. Illegal drugs, like cocaine, can seriously harm the heart and should never be used.

High blood pressure, one of the most common and serious risk factors for coronary artery disease, can be completely controlled through lifestyle changes and medication. People with moderate hypertension may be able to control it through lifestyle changes such as reducing sodium and fat, exercising regularly, managing stress, quitting smoking, and drinking alcohol in moderation. If these changes do not work, and for people with severe hypertension, there are eight types of drugs that provide effective treatment.

Stress management means controlling mental and physical reactions to life's irritations and challenges. Techniques for controlling stress include: taking life more slowly, spending time with family and friends, thinking positively, getting enough sleep, exercising, and practicing relaxation techniques.

Daily aspirin therapy has been proven to help prevent blood clots associated with atherosclerosis. It can also prevent heart attacks from recurring, prevent heart attacks from being fatal, and lower the risk of strokes.

Resources

BOOKS

American Heart Association. *Guide to Heart Attack Treatment, Recovery, Prevention.* New York: Time Books, 1996.

DeBakey, Michael E., and Antonio M. Gotto Jr. *The New Living Heart.* Holbrook, MA: Adams Media Corporation, 1997.

Notelovitz, Morris, and Diana Tonnessen. *The Essential Heart Book for Women.* New York: St. Martin's Press, 1996.

Texas Heart Institute. ''Coronary Artery Disease, Angina, and Heart Attacks.'' In *Texas Heart Institute Heart Owner's Handbook.* New York: John Wiley & Sons, 1996.

PERIODICALS

''Drugs or Angioplasty After a Heart Attack?'' *Harvard Health Letter* 22, no. 10(August 1997): 8.

Marble, Michelle. ''FDA Urged to Expand Uses for Aspirin, Benefits for Women.'' *Women's Health Weekly* (February 10, 1997).

''More on Anger and Heart Disease.'' *Harvard Heart Letter* (May 1997): 6-7.

ORGANIZATIONS

American Heart Association. National Center. 7272 Greenville Avenue, Dallas, TX 75231-4596. (214) 373-6300. http://www.medsearch.com/pf/profiles/amerh/.

National Heart, Lung, and Blood Institute Information Center. P.O. Box 30105, Bethesda, MD 20824-0105. http://www.nhlbi.gov/nhlbi/nhbli.htm.

Texas Heart Institute Heart Information Service. P.O. Box 20345, Houston, TX 77225-0345. 1-800-292-2221. Http://www.tmc.edu/thi/his.html.

Lori De Milto

Heart block

Definition

Heart block refers to a delay in the normal flow of electrical impulses that cause the heart to beat. They are further classified as first-, second-, or third-degree block.

Description

The muscles of the heart contract in a rhythmic order for each heart beat, because electrical impulses travel along a specific route called the conduction system. The main junction of this system is called the atrioventricular node (AV node). Just as on a highway, there are occasionally some delays getting the impulse from one point to another. These delays are classified according to their severity.

In first-degree heart block, the signal is just slowed down a little as it travels along the defective part of the conduction system so that it arrives late traveling from the atrium to the ventricle.

In second-degree heart block, not every impulse reaches its destination. The block may affect every other beat, every second or third beat, or be very rare. If the blockage is frequent, it results in an overall slowing of the heart called bradycardia.

Third-degree block, also called complete heart block, is the most serious. When no signals can travel through the AV node, the heart uses its backup impulse generator in the lower portion of the heart. Though this impulse usually keeps the heart from stopping entirely, it is too slow to be an effective pump.

Causes & symptoms

First-degree heart block is fairly common. It is seen in teenagers, young adults and in well-trained athletes. The condition may be caused by **rheumatic fever,** some types of heart disease and by some drugs. First-degree heart block produces no symptoms.

Some cases of second-degree heart block may benefit from an artificial pace-maker. Second-degree block can occasionally progress to third-degree.

Third-degree heart block is a serious condition that affects the heart's ability to pump blood effectively. Symptoms include **fainting, dizziness** and sudden **heart failure.** If the ventricles beat more than 40 times per minute, symptoms are not as severe, but include tiredness, low blood pressure on standing, and **shortness of breath.**

Young children who have received a forceful blunt chest injury, can experience first-, or second-degree heart block.

Diagnosis

Diagnosis of first-, and second-degree heart block is made by observing it on an electrocardiograph (ECG).

Third-degree heart block usually results in symptoms such as fainting, dizziness and sudden heart failure, which require immediate medical care. A physical exam and ECG confirm the presence of heart block.

Treatment

Some second- and almost all third-degree heart blocks require an artificial pacemaker. In an emergency, a temporary pacemaker can be used until an implanted device is advisable. Most people need the pacemaker for the rest of their lives.

Prognosis

Most people with first- and second-degree heart block don't even know they have it. For people with third-degree block, once the heart has been restored to its normal, dependable rhythm, most people, most people live full and comfortable lives.

Resources

BOOKS

McGoon, Michael D., Editor-in-Chief. *Mayo Clinic Heart Book: The Ultimate Guide to Heart Health.* New York: William Morrow and Company, Inc., 1993

PERIODICALS

Grady, Thomas A. et al. "Prognostic Significance of Exercise-induced Left Bundle-branch Block." *Journal of the American Medical Association* 279(2)(January 14, 1998): 153(4).

ORGANIZATIONS

American Heart Association. 7320 Greenville Avenue, Dallas, TX 75231. 1-800-889-7943.

Dorothy Elinor Stonely

Heart catheterization *see* **Cardiac catheterization**

Heart failure

Definition

Heart failure is a condition in which the heart has lost the ability to pump enough blood to the body's tissues. With too little blood being delivered, the organs and other tissues do not receive enough oxygen and nutrients to function properly.

Description

According to the American Heart Association, about 4.9 million Americans are living with congestive heart failure. Of these, 2.5 million are males and 2.4 million are females. Ten people out of every 1,000 people over age 65 have this condition. There are about 400,000 new cases each year.

Heart failure happens when a disease affects the heart's ability to deliver enough blood to the body's tissues. Often, a person with heart failure may have a buildup of fluid in the tissues, called **edema.** Heart failure with this kind of fluid buildup is called congestive heart failure. Where edema occurs in the body depends on the part of the heart that is affected by heart failure. Heart failure caused by abnormality of the lower left chamber of the heart (left ventricle) means that the left ventricle cannot pump blood out to the body as fast as it returns from the lungs. Because blood cannot get back to the heart, it begins to back up in the blood vessels of the lungs. Some of the fluid in the blood is forced into the breathing space of the lungs, causing **pulmonary edema.** A person with pulmonary edema has **shortness of breath,** which may be acute and severe and life threatening. A person with congestive heart failure feels tired because not enough blood circulates to supply the body's tissues with the oxygen and nutrients they need. Abnormalities of the heart structure and rhythm can also be responsible for left ventricular congestive heart failure.

In right-sided heart failure, the lower right chamber of the heart (right ventricle) cannot pump blood to the lungs as fast as it returns from the body through the veins. Blood then engorges the right side of the heart and the veins. Fluid backed up in the veins is forced out into the tissues, causing swelling (edema), usually in the feet and legs. Congestive heart failure of the right ventricle is often caused by abnormalities of the heart valves and lung disorders.

When the heart cannot pump enough blood, it tries to make up for this by becoming larger. By becoming enlarged (hypertrophic) the ventricle can contract more strongly and pump more blood. When this happens, the heart chamber becomes larger and the muscle in the heart wall becomes thicker. The heart also compensates by pumping more often to improve blood output and circulation. The kidneys try to compensate for a failing heart by retaining more salt and water to increase the volume of blood. This extra fluid can also cause edema. Eventually, as the condition worsens over time these measures are not enough to keep the heart pumping enough blood needed by the body. Kidneys often weaken under these circumstances, further aggravating the situation and making therapy more difficult.

For most people, heart failure is a chronic disease with no cure. However, it can be managed and treated with medicines and changes in diet, **exercise,** and lifestyle habits. **Heart transplantation** is considered in some cases.

Causes & symptoms

The most common causes of heart failure are:

• **Coronary artery disease** and **heart attack** (which may be "silent")

• Cardiomyopathy

• High blood pressure (**hypertension**)

• Heart valve disease

KEY TERMS

Angioplasty—A technique for treating blocked coronary arteries by inserting a catheter with a tiny balloon at the tip into the artery and inflating it.

Angiotensin-converting enzyme (ACE) inhibitor—A drug that relaxes blood vessel walls and lowers blood pressure.

Arrhythmias—Abnormal heartbeat.

Atherosclerosis—Buildup of a fatty substance called a plaque inside blood vessels.

Calcium channel blocker—A drug that relaxes blood vessels and lowers blood pressure.

Cardiac catheterization—A diagnostic test for evaluating heart disease; a catheter is inserted into an artery and passed into the heart.

Cardiomyopathy—Disease of the heart muscle.

Catheter—A thin, hollow tube.

Congenital heart defects—Abnormal formation of structures of the heart or of its major blood vessels present at birth.

Congestive heart failure—A condition in which the heart cannot pump enough blood to supply the body's tissues with sufficient oxygen and nutrients; back up of blood in vessels and the lungs causes build up of fluid (congestion) in the tissues.

Coronary arteries—Arteries that supply blood to the heart muscle.

Coronary artery bypass—Surgical procedure to reroute blood around a blocked coronary artery.

Coronary artery disease—Narrowing or blockage of coronary arteries by atherosclerosis.

Digitalis—A drug that helps the heart muscle to have stronger pumping action.

Diuretic—A type of drug that helps the kidneys eliminate excess salt and water.

Edema—Swelling caused by fluid buildup in tissues.

Ejection fraction—A measure of the portion of blood that is pumped out of a filled ventricle.

Heart valves—Valves that regulate blood flow into and out of the heart chambers.

Hypertension—High blood pressure.

Hypertrophic—Enlarged.

Idiopathic cardiomyopathy—Cardiomyopathy without a known cause.

Pulmonary edema—Buildup of fluid in the tissue of the lungs.

Vasodilator—Any drug that relaxes blood vessel walls.

Ventricles—The two lower chambers of the heart.

• **Congenital heart disease**

• **Alcoholism** and drug abuse.

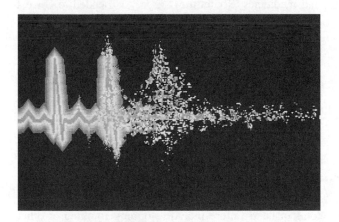

A computer-generated image of a fading electrocardiogram (ECG) trace, a record of the electrical activity within the heart as it beats. The "normal" trace at the left degenerates into fragments at the right.
(Photograph by Mehau Kulyk, Custom Medical Stock Photo. Reproduced by permission.)

The most common cause of heart failure is coronary artery disease. In coronary artery disease, the arteries supplying blood to the heart become narrowed or blocked. When blood flow to an area of the heart is completely blocked, the person has a heart attack. Some heart attacks go unrecognized. The heart muscle suffers damage when its blood supply is reduced or blocked. If the damage affects the heart's ability to pump blood, heart failure develops.

Cardiomyopathy is a general term for disease of the heart muscle. Cardiomyopathy may be caused by coronary artery disease and various other heart problems. Sometimes the cause of cardiomyopathy cannot be found. In these cases the heart muscle disease is called idiopathic cardiomyopathy. Whatever the cause, cardiomyopathy can weaken the heart, leading to heart failure.

High blood pressure is another common cause of heart failure. High blood pressure makes the heart work harder to pump blood. After a while, the heart cannot keep up and the symptoms of heart failure develop.

Defects of the heart valves, congenital heart diseases, alcoholism, and drug abuse cause damage to the heart that can all lead to heart failure.

A person with heart failure may experience the following:

• Shortness of breath

• Frequent coughing, especially when lying down

• Swollen feet, ankles, and legs

• Abdominal swelling and **pain**

• Fatigue

• **Dizziness** or **fainting**

• Sudden **death.**

A person with left-sided heart failure may have shortness of breath and coughing caused by the fluid buildup in the lungs. Pulmonary edema may cause the person to cough up bubbly phlegm that contains blood. With right-sided heart failure, fluid build-up in the veins and body tissues causes swelling in the feet, legs, and abdomen. When body tissues, such as organs and muscles, do not receive enough oxygen and nutrients they cannot function as well, leading to tiredness and dizziness.

Diagnosis

Diagnosis of heart failure is based on:

• Symptoms

• Medical history

• **Physical examination**

• **Chest x ray**

• Electrocardiogram (ECG; also called EKG)

• Other imaging tests

• **Cardiac catheterization.**

A person's symptoms can provide important clues to the presence of heart failure. Shortness of breath while engaging in activities and episodes of shortness of breath that wake a person from sleep are classic symptoms of heart failure. During the physical examination, the physician listens to the heart and lungs with a stethoscope for telltale signs of heart failure. Irregular heart sounds, ''gallops,'' a rapid heart rate, and murmurs of the heart valves may be heard. If there is fluid in the lungs a crackling sound may be heard. Rapid breathing or other changes in breathing may also be present. Patients with heart failure may also have a rapid pulse.

By pressing on the abdomen, the physician can feel if the liver is enlarged. The skin of the fingers and toes may have a bluish tint and feel cool if not enough oxygen is reaching them.

A chest x ray can show if there is fluid in the lungs and if the heart is enlarged. Abnormalities of heart valves and other structures may also be seen on chest x ray.

An electrocardiogram gives information on the heart rhythm and the size of the heart. It can show if the heart chamber is enlarged and if there is damage to the heart muscle from blocked arteries.

Besides chest x ray, other imaging tests may help make a diagnosis. **Echocardiography** uses sound waves to make images of the heart. These images can show if the heart wall or chambers are enlarged and if there are any abnormalities of the heart valves. An echocardiogram can also be used to find out how much blood the heart is pumping. It determines the amount of blood in the ventricle (ventricular volume) and the amount of blood the ventricle pumps each time it beats (called the ejection fraction). A healthy heart pumps at least one-half the amount of blood in the left ventricle with each heartbeat. Radionuclide ventriculography also measures the ejection fraction by imaging with very low doses of an injected radioactive substance as it travels through the heart.

Cardiac catheterization involves using a small tube (catheter) that is inserted through a blood vessel into the heart. It is used to measure pressure in the heart and amount of blood pumped by the heart. This test can help find abnormalities of the coronary arteries, heart valves, and heart muscle, and other blood vessels. Combined with echocardiography and other tests, cardiac catheterization can help find the cause of heart failure. It is not always necessary, however.

Treatment

Heart failure usually is treated with lifestyle changes and medicines. Sometimes surgery is needed to correct abnormalities of the heart or heart valves. Heart transplantation is a last resort to be considered in certain cases.

Dietary changes to maintain proper weight and reduce salt intake may be needed. Reducing salt intake helps to lessen swelling in the legs, feet, and abdomen. Appropriate exercise may also be recommended, but it is important that heart failure patients only begin an exercise program with the advice of their doctors. Walking, bicycling, swimming, or low-impact aerobic exercises may be recommended. There are good heart **rehabilitation** programs at most larger hospitals.

Other lifestyle changes that may reduce the symptoms of heart failure include stopping smoking or other tobacco use, eliminating or reducing alcohol consumption, and not using harmful drugs.

One or more of the following types of medicines may be prescribed for heart failure:

• **Diuretics**

- Digitalis
- **Vasodilators**
- **Beta blockers**
- Angiotensin converting enzyme inhibitors (ACE inhibitors)
- Angiotensin receptor blockers (ARBs)
- **Calcium channel blockers.**

Diuretics help eliminate excess salt and water from the kidneys by making patients urinate more often. This helps reduce the swelling caused by fluid buildup in the tissues. Digitalis helps the heart muscle to have stronger pumping action. Vasodilators, ACE inhibitors, ARBs, and calcium channel blockers lower blood pressure and expand the blood vessels so blood can move more easily through them. This action makes it easier for the heart to pump blood through the vessels.

Surgery is used to correct certain heart conditions that cause heart failure. Congenital heart defects and abnormal heart valves can be repaired with surgery. Blocked coronary arteries can usually be treated with **angioplasty** or coronary artery bypass surgery.

With severe heart failure, the heart muscle may become so damaged that available treatments do not help. Patients with this stage of heart failure are said to have end-stage heart failure. Heart transplant is usually considered for patients with end-stage heart failure when all other treatments have stopped working.

Prognosis

Most patients with mild or moderate heart failure can be successfully treated with dietary and exercise programs and the right medications. Many people are able to participate in normal daily activities and lead relatively active lives.

Patients with severe heart failure may eventually have to consider heart transplantation. Approximately 50% of patients diagnosed with congestive heart failure live for five years with the condition. Women with heart failure usually live longer than men with heart failure.

Prevention

Heart failure is usually caused by the effects of some type of heart disease. The best way to try to prevent heart failure is to eat a healthy diet and get regular exercise, but many causes of heart failure cannot be prevented. People with risk factors for coronary disease (such as high blood pressure and high cholesterol levels) should work closely with their physician to reduce their likelihood of heart attack and heart failure.

Heart failure sometimes can be avoided by identifying and treating any conditions that might lead to heart disease. These include high blood pressure, alcoholism, and coronary artery disease. Regular blood pressure checks and obtaining immediate medical care for symptoms of coronary artery disease, such as chest pain, will help to get these conditions found and treated early, before they can damage the heart muscle.

Finally, diagnosing and treating heart failure before the heart becomes severely damaged can improve the prognosis. With proper treatment, many patients may continue to lead active lives for a number of years.

Resources

BOOKS

Bellenir, Karen and Peter D. Dresser, editors. *Cardiovascular Diseases and Disorders Sourcebook.* Detroit: Omnigraphics, 1995.

Texas Heart Institute. *Heart Owner's Handbook.* New York: John Wiley and Sons, 1996.

ORGANIZATIONS

American Heart Association. 7272 Greenview Avenue, Dallas, TX 75231-4596. (800) AHS-USA1. http://www.amhrt.org/.

National Heart, Lung, and Blood Institute. Information Center, PO Box 30105, Bethesda, MD 20824-0105. (301) 251-1222.

Texas Heart Institute. Heart Information Service, PO Box 20345, Houston, TX 77225-0345. (800) 292-2221.

Toni Rizzo

Heart murmurs

Definition

A heart murmur is an abnormal, extra sound during the heartbeat cycle made by blood moving through the heart and its valves. It is detected by the physician's examination using a stethoscope.

Description

A heart which is beating normal makes two sounds, "lubb" when the valves between the atria and ventricles close, and "dupp" when the valves between the ventricles and the major arteries close. A heart murmur is a series of vibratory sounds made by turbulent blood flow. The sounds are longer than normal heart sounds and can be heard between the normal sounds of the heart.

Heart murmurs are common in children and can also result from heart or valve defects. Nearly two thirds of heart murmurs in children are produced by a normal heart and are harmless. This type of heart murmur is usually called an ''innocent'' heart murmur. It can also be called ''functional'' or ''physiologic.'' Innocent heart murmurs are usually very faint, intermittent, and occur in a small area of the chest. Pathologic heart murmurs may indicate the presence of a serious heart defect. They are louder, continual, and may be accompanied by a click or gallop.

Some heart murmurs are continually present; others happen only when the heart is working harder than usual, including during **exercise** or certain types of illness. Heart murmurs can be diastolic or systolic. Those which occur during relaxation of the heart between beats are called diastolic murmurs. Those which occur during contraction of the heart muscle are called systolic murmurs. The characteristics of the murmur may suggest specific alterations in the heart or its valves.

Causes & symptoms

Innocent heart murmurs are caused by blood flowing through the chambers and valves of the heart or the blood vessels near the heart. Sometimes **anxiety, stress, fever,** anemia, overactive thyroid, and **pregnancy** will cause innocent murmurs that can be heard by a physician using a stethoscope. Pathologic heart murmurs, however, are caused by structural abnormalities of the heart. These include defective heart valves or holes in the walls of the heart. Valve problems are more common. Valves that do not open completely cause blood to flow through a smaller opening than normal, while those that do not close properly may cause blood to go back through the valve. A hole in the wall between the left and right sides of the heart, called a septal defect, can cause heart murmurs. Some septal defects close on their own; others

require surgery to prevent progressive damage to the heart.

The symptoms of heart murmurs differ depending on the cause of the heart murmur. Innocent heart murmurs and those which do not impair the function of the heart have no symptoms. Murmurs that are due to severe abnormalities of a heart valve may cause **shortness of breath, dizziness,** chest **pains, palpitations,** and lung congestion.

Diagnosis

Heart murmurs can be heard when a physician listens to the heart through a stethoscope during a regular checkup. Very loud heart murmurs and those with clicks or extra heart sounds should be evaluated further. Infants with heart murmurs who do not thrive, eat, or breath properly and older children who lose consciousness suddenly or are intolerance to exercise should also be evaluated. If the murmur sounds suspicious, the physician may order a **chest x ray,** an electrocardiogram, and an echocardiogram.

An electrocardiogram (ECG) shows the heart's activity and may reveal muscle thickening, damage, or a lack of oxygen. Electrodes covered with conducting jelly are placed on the patient's chest, arms, and legs. They send impulses of the heart's activity through a monitor (oscilloscope) to a recorder which traces them on paper. The test takes about 10 minutes and is commonly performed in a physician's office. An exercise ECG can reveal additional information.

An echocardiogram (cardiac ultrasound), may be ordered to identify a structural problem that is causing the heart murmur. An echocardiogram uses sound waves to create an image of the heart's chambers and valves. The technician applies gel to a hand-held transducer then presses it against the patient's chest. The sound waves are converted into an image that can be displayed on a monitor. Performed in a cardiology outpatient diagnostic laboratory, the test takes 30 minutes to an hour.

Treatment

Innocent heart murmurs do not affect the patient's health and require no treatment. Heart murmurs due to septal defects may require surgery. Those due to valvular defects may require **antibiotics** to prevent infection during certain surgical or dental procedures. Severely damaged or diseased valves can be repaired or replaced through surgery.

Alternative treatment

If a heart murmur requires surgical treatment, there are no alternative treatments, although there are alternative therapies that are helpful for pre- and post-surgical support of the patient. If the heart murmur is innocent, heart activity can be support using the herb hawthorn (*Crataegus laevigata* or *C. oxyacantha*) or coenzyme Q10. These remedies improve heart contractility and the heart's ability to use oxygen. If the murmur is valvular in origin, herbs that act like antibiotics as well as options that build resistance to infection in the valve areas may be considered.

Prognosis

Most children with innocent heart murmurs grow out of them by the time they reach adulthood. Severe causes of heart murmurs may progress to severe symptoms and **death.**

Resources

PERIODICALS

Gutgesell, Howard P., et al. "Common Cardiovascular Problems in the Young: Part I. Murmurs, Chest Pain, Syncope and Irregular Rhythms." *American Family Physician* 56, no. 7(November 1, 1997): 1825-1827.

Sapin, Samuel. "Recognizing Normal Heart Murmurs: A Logic-Based Mnemonic." *Pediatrics* 99, no. 4(April 1, 1997): 616.

Smith, Karen M. "The Innocent Heart Murmur in Children." *Journal of Pediatric Health Care* 11, no. 5(September/October 1997): 207-214.

ORGANIZATIONS

American Heart Association. National Center. 7272 Greenville Avenue, Dallas, TX 75231-4596. (214) 373-6300. http://www.medsearch.com/pf/profiles/amerh/.

Texas Heart Institute Heart Information Service. P.O. Box 20345, Houston, TX 77225-0345. 1-800-292-2221. http://www.tmc.edu/thi/his.html.

OTHER

"Heart Murmurs in Infants: Not Always Cause for Alarm." *Mayo Health Oasis.* 26 February 1998. http://www.mayohealth.org/ (4 March 1998).

"When Your Child's Doctor Hears a Heart Murmur." *Children's National Medical Center.* 1998. http://www.cnmc.org/heart.htm (6 March 1998).

Lori De Milto

Heart muscle infection *see* **Myocarditis**

Heart pacemakers *see* **Pacemakers**

Heart scan *see* **Echocardiography**

Heart septal defect *see* **Atrial septal defect**

Heart sonogram *see* **Echocardiography**

Heart surgery for congenital defects

Definition

A variety of surgical procedures that are performed to repair the many types of heart defects that may be present at birth.

Purpose

Heart surgery for congenital defects is performed to repair a defect as much as possible and improve the flow of blood and oxygen to the body. While congenital heart defects vary in their severity, most require surgery. Surgery is recommended for congenital heart defects that result in a lack of oxygen, a poor quality of life, or a patient who does not thrive. Some types of congenital heart defects that don't cause symptoms are treated surgically because they can lead to serious complications.

Precautions

There are many types of surgery for congenital heart defects and many considerations in the decision to operate. The patient's cardiologist or surgeon will discuss these issues on an individual basis.

Description

There are many types of congenital heart defects. Most obstruct the flow of blood in the heart, or the vessels near it, or cause an abnormal flow of blood through the heart. Rarer types include newborns born with one ventricle, one side of the heart that is not completely formed, or the pulmonary artery and the aorta coming out of the same ventricle. Most congenital heart defects require surgery during infancy or childhood. Recommended ages for surgery for the most common congenital heart defects are:

- Atrial septal defects: during the preschool years

- Patent ductus arteriosus: between ages one and two

- Coarctation of the aorta: in infancy, if it's symptomatic, at age four otherwise

- Tetralogy of Fallot: age varies, depending on the patient's signs and symptoms

- Transposition of the great arteries: often in the first weeks after birth, but before the patient is 12 months old.

Surgical procedures seek to repair the defect as much as possible and restore circulation to as close to normal as possible. Sometimes, multiple, serial, surgical procedures are necessary. Smaller congenital heart defects can now be repaired in a **cardiac catheterization** lab instead of

KEY TERMS

Atresia—A congenital defect in which the blood pumped through the body has too little oxygen. In tricuspid atresia, the baby lacks a triscupid valve. In pulmonary atresia, a pulmonary valve is missing.

Coarctation of the aorta—A congenital defect in which severe narrowing or constriction of the aorta obstructs the flow of blood.

Congenital heart defects—Congenital means conditions which are present at birth. Congenital heart disease includes a variety of defects that babies are born with.

Patent ductus arteriosus—A congenital defect in which the temporary blood vessel connecting the left pulmonary artery to the aorta in the fetus doesn't close in the newborn.

Septal defects—These are holes in the septum, the muscle wall separating the right and left sides of the heart. Atrial septal defects are openings between the two upper heart chambers and ventricular septal defects are openings between the two lower heart chambers.

Stenosis—A narrowing of the heart's valves. This congenital defect can occur in the pulmonary (lung) or aortic (the main heart artery) valve.

Tetralogy of Fallot—A cyanotic defect in which the blood pumped through the body has too little oxygen. Tetralogy of Fallot includes four defects: a large hole between the ventricles, narrowing at or beneath the pulmonary valve, an overly muscular right ventricle, and an aorta over the large hole.

Transposition of the great arteries—A cyanotic defect in which the blood pumped through the body has too little oxygen. The pulmonary artery and the aorta are reversed.

an operating room. Catheterization procedures include balloon atrial septostomy and **balloon valvuloplasty.** Surgical procedures include arterial switch, Damus-Kaye-Stansel procedure, Fontan procedure, Ross procedure, shunt procedure, and venous switch or intra-atrial baffle.

Catheterization procedures

Balloon atrial septostomy and balloon valvuloplasty are cardiac catheterization procedures. Cardiac catheterization procedures can save the lives of critically ill neonates and in some cases eliminate or delay more

invasive surgical procedures. It is expected that catheterization procedures will continue to replace more types of surgery for congenital heart defects in the future. A thin tube called a catheter is inserted into an artery or vein in the leg, groin, or arm and threaded into the area of the heart which needs repair. The patient receives a local anesthetic at the insertion site and is awake but sedated during the procedure.

BALLOON ATRIAL SEPTOSTOMY

Balloon atrial septostomy is the standard procedure for correcting transposition of the great arteries; it is sometimes used in patients with mitral, pulmonary, or tricupsid atresia (atresia is a defect that causes the blood to carry too little oxygen to the body). Balloon atrial septostomy enlarges the atrial opening. A special balloon-tipped catheter is inserted into the right atrium and inflated to create a large opening in the atrial septum.

BALLOON VALVULOPLASTY

Balloon valvuloplasty uses a balloon-tipped catheter to open a narrowed heart valve, improving the flow of blood. It is the procedure of choice in pulmonary stenosis and is sometimes used in aortic stenosis. Balloons made of plastic polymers are placed at the end of the catheter and inflated to relieve the obstruction in the heart valve. Long-terms results are excellent in most cases. The operative death rate is 2–4%.

Surgical procedures

These procedures are performed under general anesthesia. Some require the use of a heart-lung machine, which cools the body to reduce the need for oxygen and takes over for the heart and lungs during the procedure.

ARTERIAL SWITCH

Arterial switch is performed to correct transposition of the great arteries, where the position of the pulmonary artery and the aorta are reversed. The procedure involves connecting the aorta to the left ventricle and the pulmonary artery to the right ventricle.

DAMUS-KAYE-STANSEL PROCEDURE

Transposition of the great arteries can also be corrected by the Damus-Kaye-Stansel procedure, in which the pulmonary artery is cut in two and connected to the ascending aorta and right ventricle.

FONTAN PROCEDURE

For tricuspid atresia and pulmonary atresia, the Fontan procedure connects the right atrium to the pulmonary artery directly or with a conduit, and the atrial defect is closed. Survival is over 90%.

PULMONARY ARTERY BANDING

Pulmonary artery banding is narrowing the pulmonary artery with a band to reduce blood flow and pressure in the lungs. It is used for **ventricular septal defect,** atrioventricular canal defect, and tricuspid atresia. Later, the band can be removed and the defect corrected with open heart surgery.

ROSS PROCEDURE

To correct aortic stenosis, the Ross procedure grafts the pulmonary artery to the aorta.

SHUNT PROCEDURE

For **Tetralogy of Fallot,** tricuspid atresia, or pulmonary atresia, the shunt procedure creates a passage between blood vessels, sending blood into parts of the body that need it.

VENOUS SWITCH

For transposition of the great arteries, venous switch creates a tunnel inside the atria to re-direct oxygen-rich blood to the right ventricle and aorta and venous blood to the left ventricle and pulmonary artery.

OTHER TYPES OF SURGERY

These surgical procedures are also used to treat common congenital heart defects. A medium to large ventricular or atrial septal defect can be closed by suturing it or covering it with a Dacron patch. For patent ductus arteriosus, surgery consists of dividing the ductus into two and tying off the ends. If performed within the patient's first few years, there is practically no risk associated with this operation. Surgery for coarctation of the aorta involves opening the chest wall, removing the defect, and reconnecting the ends of the aorta. If the defect is too long to be reconnected, a Dacron graft is used to replace the missing piece. In uncomplicated cases, the risk of the operation is 1–2%.

Preparation

Before surgery for congenital heart defects, the patient will receive a complete evaluation, which includes a physical exam, a detailed family history, a **chest x ray,** an electrocardiogram, an echocardiogram, and usually cardiac catheterization. For six to eight hours before the surgery, the patient cannot eat or drink anything. An electrocardiogram shows the heart's activity and may reveal a lack of oxygen. Electrodes covered with conducting jelly are placed on the patient's chest, arms, and legs and the heart's impulses are traced on paper. An echocardiogram uses sound waves to create an image of the heart's chambers and valves. Gel is applied to a handheld transducer and then pressed against the patient's chest. Cardiac catheterization is an invasive diagnostic technique used to evaluate the heart in which a long tube is inserted into a blood vessel and guided into the heart. A contrast solution is injected to make the heart visible on x rays.

Aftercare

After heart surgery for congenital defects, the patient goes to an intensive care ward where he or she is connected to a variety of tubes and monitors, including a ventilator. Patients are monitored every 15 minutes until vital signs are stable. Heart sounds, oxygenation, and the electrocardiogram are monitored. Chest tubes will be checked to ensure that they're draining properly and there is no hemorrhage. **Pain** medications will be administered. Complications such as **stroke,** lung blood clots, and reduced blood flow to the kidneys will be watched for. After the ventilator and breathing tube are removed, **chest physical therapy** and exercises to improve circulation will be started.

Risks

Complications from heart surgery for congenital defects can be severe. They include **shock,** congestive **heart failure,** lack of oxygen or too much carbon dioxide in the blood, irregular heartbeat, stroke, infection, kidney damage, lung blood clot, low blood pressure, hemorrhage, cardiac arrest, and death.

Resources

BOOKS

"Congenital Heart Disease." In *Current Medical Diagnosis & Treatment,* 36th ed., edited by Lawrence Tierney, et al. Stamford, CT: Appleton & Lange, 1997.

DeBakey, Michael E. and Antonio M. Gotto, Jr. "Congenital Abnormalities of the Heart." In *The New Living Heart.* Holbrook, MA: Adams Media Corporation, 1997.

Park, Myung K. *Pediatric Cardiology for Practitioners,* 3rd ed. St. Louis, MO: Mosby, 1996.

Texas Heart Institute. "Congenital Heart Disease." In *Texas Heart Institute Heart Owners Handbook.* New York: John Wiley & Sons, 1996.

PERIODICALS

Hicks, George L. "Cardiac Surgery." *Journal of the American College of Surgeons* 186, no. 2(February 1998): 129-132.

Rao, P. S. "Interventional Pediatric Cardiology: State of the Art and Future Directions." *Pediatric Cardiology* 19 (1998): 107-124.

ORGANIZATIONS

American Heart Association. National Center. 7272 Greenville Avenue, Dallas, TX 75231-4596. (214) 373-6300. http://www.medsearch.com/pf/profiles/amerh/.

Congenital Heart Anomalies Support, Education & Resources, Inc. 2112 North Wilkins Road, Swanton, OH 43558. (419) 825-5575. http://www.csun.edu/~hfmthoo6/chaser/.

Congenital Heart Disease Information and Resources. 1561 Clark Drive, Yardley, PA 19067. http://www.tchin.org/.

Texas Heart Institute Heart Information Service. P.O. Box 20345, Houston, TX 77225-0345. 1-800-292-2221. http://www.tmc.edu/thi/his.html.

Lori De Milto

Heart transplantation

Definition

Heart transplantation, also called cardiac transplantation, is the replacement of a patient's diseased or injured heart with a healthy donor heart.

Purpose

Heart transplantation is performed on patients with end-stage **heart failure** or some other life-threatening heart disease. Before a doctor recommends heart transplantation for a patient, all other possible treatments for his or her disease must have been tried. The purpose of heart transplantation is to extend and improve the life of a person who would otherwise die from heart failure. Most patients who receive a new heart were so sick before transplantation that they could not live a normal life. Replacing a patient's diseased heart with a healthy, functioning donor heart often allows the recipient to return to normal daily activities.

Precautions

Because healthy donor hearts are in short supply, strict rules dictate who should or should not get a heart transplant. Patients who have conditions that might cause the new heart to fail should not have a heart transplant. Similarly, patients who may be too sick to survive the surgery or the side effects of the drugs they must take to keep their new heart working would not be good transplant candidates.

Patients who have any of the following conditions may not be eligible for heart transplantation:

- Active infection

- **Pulmonary hypertension**

- Chronic lung disease with loss of more than 40% of lung function

- Untreatable liver or kidney disease

- Diabetes that has caused serious damage to vital organs

- Disease of the blood vessels in the brain, such as a **stroke**

- Serious disease of the arteries

- Mental illness or any condition that would make a patient unable to take the necessary medicines on schedule

- Continuing alcohol or drug abuse.

KEY TERMS

Anesthesia—Loss of the ability to feel pain, caused by administration of an anesthetic drug.

Angina—Characteristic chest pain which occurs during exercise or stress in certain kinds of heart disease.

Cardiopulmonary bypass—Mechanically circulating the blood with a heart/lung machine that bypasses the heart and lungs.

Cardiovascular—Having to do with the heart and blood vessels.

Complete blood count (CBC)—A blood test to check the numbers of red blood cells, white blood cells, and platelets in the blood.

Coronary artery disease—Blockage of the arteries leading to the heart.

Crossmatch—A test to determine if patient and donor tissues are compatible.

Donor—A person who donates an organ for transplantation.

Echocardiogram—A test that visualizes and records the position and motion of the walls of the heart using ultrasound waves.

Electrocardiogram (ECG)—A test that measures electrical conduction of the heart.

End-stage heart failure—Severe heart disease that does not respond adequately to medical or surgical treatment.

Endomyocardial biopsy—Removal of a small sample of heart tissue to check it for signs of damage caused by organ rejection.

Fatigue—Loss of energy; tiredness.

Graft—A transplanted organ or other tissue.

Immunosuppressive drug—Medication used to suppress the immune system.

Inotropic drugs—Medications used to stimulate the heart beat.

Pulmonary hypertension—An increase in the pressure in the blood vessels of the lungs.

Recipient—A person who receives an organ transplant.

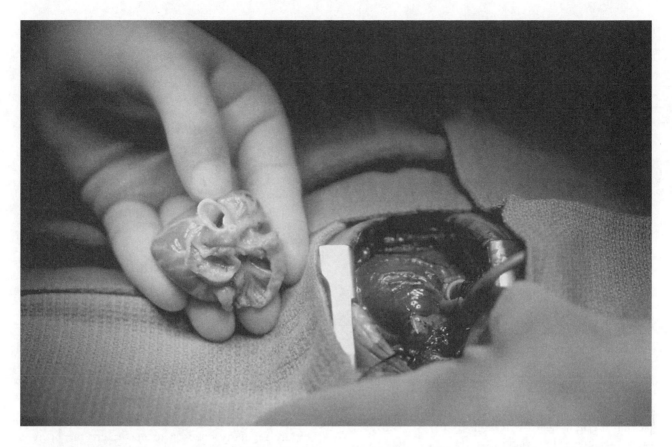

A comparison of the old and new hearts of Dylan Stork, the smallest heart transplant recipient in the world. Dylan was 7 weeks old and weighed 5.5 pounds (2.5 kg) at the time of the operation. *(Photograph by Alexander Tsiaras, Photo Researchers, Inc. Reproduced by permission.)*

Description

Patients with end-stage heart disease that threatens their life even after medical treatment may be considered for heart transplantation. Potential candidates must have a complete medical examination before they can be put on the transplant waiting list. Many types of tests are done, including blood tests, x rays, and tests of heart, lung, and other organ function. The results of these tests indicate to doctors how serious the heart disease is and whether or not a patient is healthy enough to survive the transplant surgery.

Organ waiting list

A person approved for heart transplantation is placed on the heart transplant waiting list of a heart transplant center. All patients on a waiting list are registered with the United Network for Organ Sharing (UNOS). UNOS has organ transplant specialists who run a national computer network that connects all the transplant centers and organ-donation organizations.

When a donor heart becomes available, information about it is entered into the UNOS computer and compared to information from patients on the waiting list. The computer program produces a list of patients ranked according to blood type, size of the heart, and how urgently they need a heart. Because the heart must be transplanted as quickly as possible, the list of local patients is checked first for a good match. After that, a regional list, and then a national list, are checked. The patient's transplant team of heart and transplant specialists makes the final decision as to whether a donor heart is suitable for the patient.

The transplant procedure

When a heart becomes available and is approved for a patient, it is packed in a sterile cold solution and rushed to the hospital where the recipient is waiting.

Heart transplant surgery involves the following basic steps:

- A specialist in cardiovascular anesthesia gives the patient general anesthesia.

- Intravenous **antibiotics** are usually given to prevent bacterial wound infections.

- The patient is put on a heart/lung machine, which performs the functions of the heart and lungs and pumps the blood to the rest of the body during surgery. This procedure is called cardiopulmonary bypass.

- After adequate blood circulation is established, the patient's diseased heart is removed.

- The donor heart is attached to the patient's blood vessels.

- After the blood vessels are connected, the new heart is warmed up and begins beating. If the heart does not begin to beat immediately, the surgeon may start it with an electrical shock.

- The patient is taken off the heart/lung machine.

- The new heart is stimulated to maintain a regular beat with medications for two to five days after surgery, until the new heart functions normally on its own.

Heart transplant recipients are given immunosuppressive drugs to prevent the body from rejecting the new heart. These drugs are usually started before or during the heart transplant surgery. Immunosuppressive drugs keep the body's immune system from recognizing and attacking the new heart as foreign tissue. Normally, immune system cells recognize and attack foreign or abnormal cells, such as bacteria, **cancer** cells, and cells from a transplanted organ. The drugs suppress the immune cells and allow the new heart to function properly. However, they can also allow infections and other adverse effects to occur to the patient.

Because the chance of rejection is highest during the first few months after the transplantation, recipients are usually given a combination of three or four immunosuppressive drugs in high doses during this time. Afterwards, they must take maintenance doses of immunosuppressive drugs for the rest of their lives.

Cost and insurance coverage

The total cost for heart transplantation varies, depending on where it is performed, whether transportation and lodging are needed, and on whether there are any complications. The costs for the surgery and first year of care are estimated to be about $250,000. The medical tests and medications after the first year cost about $21,000 per year.

Insurance coverage for heart transplantation varies depending on the policy. Most commercial insurance companies pay a certain percentage of heart transplant costs. Medicare pays for heart transplants if the surgery is performed at Medicare-approved centers. Medicaid pays for heart transplants in 33 states and in the District of Colombia.

Preparation

Before patients are put on the transplant waiting list, their blood type is determined so a compatible donor heart can be found. The heart must come from a person with the same blood type as the patient, unless it is blood type O. A blood type O heart can be transplanted into a person with any type of blood.

A panel reactive antibodies (PRA) test is also done before heart transplantation. This test tells doctors whether or not the patient is at high risk for having a hyperacute reaction against a donor heart. A hyperacute reaction is a strong immune response against the new heart that happens within minutes to hours after the new heart is transplanted. If the PRA shows that a patient has a high risk for this kind of reaction, then a crossmatch is done between a patient and a donor heart before transplant surgery. A crossmatch checks how close the match is between the patient's tissue type and the tissue type of the donor heart.

Most people are not high risk and a crossmatch usually is not done before the transplant because the surgery must be done as quickly as possible after a donor heart is found.

While waiting for heart transplantation, patients are given treatment to keep the heart as healthy as possible. They are regularly checked to make sure the heart is pumping enough blood. Intravenous medications may be used to improve cardiac output. If these drugs are not effective, a mechanical pump can help keep the heart functioning until a donor heart becomes available. Inserted through an artery into the aorta, the pump assists the heart in pumping blood.

Aftercare

Immediately following surgery, patients are monitored closely in the intensive care unit (ICU) of the hospital for 24–72 hours. Most patients need to receive oxygen for 4–24 hours following surgery. Blood pressure, heart function, and other organ functions are carefully monitored during this time.

Heart transplant patients start taking immunosuppressive drugs before or during surgery to prevent immune rejection of the heart. High doses of immunosuppressive drugs are given at this time, because rejection is most likely to happen within the first few months after the surgery. A few months after surgery, lower doses of immunosuppressive drugs usually are given and must be taken for the rest of the patient's life.

For 6–8 weeks after the transplant surgery, patients usually come back to the transplant center twice a week for **physical examinations** and medical tests. These tests check for any signs of infection, rejection of the new heart, or other complications.

In addition to physical examination, the following tests may be done during these visits:

- Laboratory tests to check for infection

- **Chest x ray** to check for early signs of lung infection

- Electrocardiogram (ECG) to check heart function

- Echocardiogram to check the function of the ventricles in the heart

- Blood tests to check liver and kidney function

- Complete **blood counts** (CBC) to check the numbers of blood cells

- Taking of a small tissue sample from the donor heart (endomyocardial biopsy) to check for signs of rejection.

During the physical examination, the blood pressure is checked and the heart sounds are listened to with a stethoscope to determine if the heart is beating properly and pumping enough blood. Kidney and liver function are checked because these organs may lose function if the heart is being rejected.

An endomyocardial biopsy is the removal of a small sample of the heart muscle. This is done with a very small instrument that is inserted through an artery or vein and into the heart. The heart muscle tissue is examined under a microscope for signs that the heart is being rejected. Endomyocardial biopsy is usually done weekly for the first 4–8 weeks after transplant surgery and then at longer intervals after that.

Risks

The most common and dangerous complications of heart transplant surgery are organ rejection and infection. Immunosuppressive drugs are given to prevent rejection of the heart. Most heart transplant patients have a rejection episode soon after transplantation, but doctors usually diagnose it immediately when it will respond readily to treatment. Rejection is treated with combinations of immunosuppressive drugs given in higher doses than maintenance immunosuppression. Most of these rejection situations are successfully treated.

Infection can result from the surgery, but most infections are a side effect of the immunosuppressive drugs. Immunosuppressive drugs keep the immune system from attacking the foreign cells of the donor heart. However, the suppressed immune cells are also unable to adequately fight bacteria, viruses, and other microorganisms. Microorganisms that normally do not affect persons with healthy immune systems can cause dangerous infections in transplant patients taking immunosuppressive drugs.

Patients are given antibiotics during surgery to prevent bacterial infection. Patients may also be given an antiviral drug to prevent virus infections. Patients who develop infections may need to have their immunosuppressive drugs changed or the dose adjusted. Infections are treated with antibiotics or other drugs, depending on the type of infection.

Other complications that can happen immediately after surgery are:

- Bleeding

- Pressure on the heart caused by fluid in the space surrounding the heart (pericardial tamponade)

- Irregular heart beats

- Reduced cardiac output

- Increased amount of blood in the circulatory system

- Decreased amount of blood in the circulatory system.

About half of all heart transplant patients develop **coronary artery disease** 1–5 years after the transplant. The coronary arteries supply blood to the heart. Patients with this problem develop chest **pains** called **angina.** Other names for this complication are coronary allograft vascular disease and chronic rejection.

Outcomes

Heart transplantation is an appropriate treatment for many patients with end-stage heart failure. The outcomes of heart transplantation depend on the patient's age, health, and other factors. About 73% of heart transplant patients are alive four years after surgery.

After transplant, most patients regain normal heart function, meaning the heart pumps a normal amount of blood. A transplanted heart usually beats slightly faster than normal because the heart nerves are cut during surgery. The new heart also does not increase its rate as quickly during **exercise.** Even so, most patients feel much better and their capacity for exercise is dramatically improved from before they received the new heart. About 85% of patients return to work and other daily activities. Many are able to participate in sports.

Resources

BOOKS

Bellenir, Karen and Peter D. Dresser, eds. *Cardiovascular Diseases and Disorders Sourcebook.* Detroit: Omnigraphics, 1995.

Texas Heart Institute. *Heart Owner's Handbook.* New York: John Wiley and Sons, 1996.

ORGANIZATIONS

American Council on Transplantation. P.O. Box 1709, Alexandria, VA 22313. 1-800-ACT-GIVE.

Health Services and Resources Administration, Division of Organ Transplantation. Room 11A-22, 5600 Fishers Lane, Rockville, MD 20857.

United Network for Organ Sharing (UNOS). 1-800-24-DO-NOR.

OTHER

Craven, John and Susan Farrow. *Surviving Transplantation.* SupportNET Publications, 1996-1997. http://www.stjosephs.london.on.ca/SJHC/about/programs/mental/survive/frmain.htm

National Institutes of Health. *"Facts About Heart and Heart/Lung Transplants."* gopher://fido.nhlbi.nih.gov/00/educprog/other/pubs/public/hrtlung.txt.

United Network for Organ Sharing (UNOS) *"What Every Patient Needs to Know."* http://www.unos.org/frame_Default.asp?Category = Patients.

Toni Rizzo

Heart tumors *see* **Myxoma**

Heart valve repair

Definition

Heart valve repair is a surgical procedure used to correct a malfunctioning heart valve. Repair usually involves separating the valve leaflets (the one-way "doors" of the heart valve which open and close to pump blood through the heart) or forcing them open with a balloon catheter, a technique known as *balloon valvuloplasty.*

Purpose

To correct damage to the mitral, aortic, pulmonary, or tricuspid heart valves caused by a systemic infection, **endocarditis,** rheumatic heart disease, a congenital heart defect, or mitral and/or aortic valve disease. Damaged valves may not open properly (stenosis) or they may not close adequately (valve regurgitation, insufficiency, or incompetence).

Precautions

Patients who have a diseased heart valve that is badly scarred or calcified may be better candidates for valve replacement surgery.

Description

Heart valve repair is performed in a hospital setting by a cardiac surgeon. During valve repair surgery, the patient's heart is stopped, and his/her blood is circulated outside of the body through an *extracorporeal bypass circuit,* also called heart-lung machine or just "the pump." The extracorporeal circuit consists of tubing and medical devices that take over the function of the patient's heart and lungs during the procedure. As blood

---

KEY TERMS

Angiogram—An angiogram uses a radiopaque substance, or dye, to make the blood vessels or arteries visible under x-ray.

Calcified—Hardened by calcium deposits.

Catheter—A long, thin, flexible tube used in valvuloplasty to widen the valve opening.

Echocardiogram—Ultrasound of the heart; generates a picture of the heart through the use of soundwaves.

Edema—Fluid accumulation in the body.

Scintigram—A nuclear angiogram; a scintigram involves injection of a radioactive substance into the patient's circulatory system. As the substance travels through the body, a special scanning camera takes pictures.

Stenosis—Narrowing of the heart valve opening.

---

passes through the circuit, carbon dioxide is removed from the bloodstream and replaced with oxygen. The oxygenated blood is then returned to the body. Other components may also be added to the circuit to filter fluids from the blood or concentrate red blood cells.

In cases of valve disease where the leaflets have become fused together, a procedure known as a valvulotomy is performed. In valvulotomy, the leaflets of the valves are surgically separated, or partially resected, with an incision to increase the size of the valve opening. The surgeon may also make adjustments to the chordae, the cord-like tissue that connects the valve leaflets to the ventricle muscles, to improve valve function.

Another valve repair technique, **balloon valvuloplasty,** is used in patients with pulmonary, aortic, and **mitral valve stenosis** to force open the valve. Valvuloplasty is similar to a cardiac **angioplasty** procedure in that it involves the placement of a balloon-tipped catheter into the heart. Once inserted into the valve, the balloon is inflated and the valve dilates, or opens. Valvuloplasty does not require a bypass circuit.

Preparation

A number of diagnostic tests may be administered prior to valve repair surgery. **Magnetic resonance imaging** (MRI), echocardiogram, angiogram, and/or scintigram are used to help the surgeon get an accurate picture of the extent of damage to the heart valve and the status of the coronary arteries.

Aftercare

The patient's blood pressure and vital signs will be carefully monitored following a valve repair procedure, and he or she watched closely for signs of **edema** or congestive **heart failure.**

Echocardiography or other diagnostic tests are ordered for the patient at some point during or after surgery to evaluate valvular function. A **cardiac rehabilitation** program may also be recommended to assist the patient in improving **exercise** tolerance after the procedure.

Risks

As with any invasive surgical procedure, hemorrhage, infarction, stroke, heart attach, and infection are all possible complications of heart valve repair. The overall risks involved with the surgery depend largely on the complexity of the procedure and physical condition of the patient.

Normal results

Ideally, a successful heart valve repair procedure will return heart function to age-appropriate levels. If valvuloplasty is performed, a follow-up valve repair or replacement surgery may be necessary at a later date.

Resources

BOOKS

DeBakey, Michael E. and Antonio Gotto, Jr. *The New Living Heart* Holbrook, MA: Adams Media Corporation, 1997.

Paula Anne Ford-Martin

. . . .
Heart valve replacement

Definition

Heart valve replacement is a surgical procedure during which surgeons remove a damaged valve from the heart and substitute a healthy one.

Purpose

Four valves direct blood to and from the body through the heart: the aortic valve, the pulmonic valve, the tricuspid valve, and the mitral valve. Any of these valves may malfunction because of a birth defect, infection, disease, or trauma. When the malfunction is so severe that it interferes with blood flow, an individual will have heart **palpitations, fainting** spells, and/or difficulty breathing. These symptoms will progressively

---

KEY TERMS
. . . .

Anticoagulants—Drugs that prevent blood clots from forming.

Aortic valve—A fold in the channel leading from the aorta to the left ventricle of the heart. The aortic valve directs blood flow that has received oxygen from the lungs to the aorta which transmits blood to the rest of the body.

Cardiac catheterization—A thin tube called a catheter is inserted into an artery or vein in the leg, groin or arm. The catheter tube is carefully threaded into the area of the heart needing surgical repair. A local anaesthesia is used at the insertion sites.

Cardiopulmonary bypass machine—A mechanical instrument that takes over the circulation of the body while heart surgery is taking place.

Echocardiography—A diagnostic instrument that assesses the structure of the heart using sound waves.

Electrocardiography—A diagnostic instrument that evaluates the function of the heart by measuring the electrical activity generated by the beating of the heart.

Mitral valve—A fold in between the left atrium and the left ventricle of the heart that directs blood that has received oxygen from the lungs to the aortic valve and the aorta.

Pulmonic valve—A fold in the pulmonary artery that directs blood to the lungs. It may be transferred to replace a severely diseased aortic valve during heart valve replacement surgery for aortic stenosis.

Tricuspid valve—A fold in between the right atrium and the right ventricle of the heart that directs blood that needs oxygen to the lungs.

---

worsen and cause **death** unless the damaged valve is replaced surgically.

Precautions

Abnormal tricuspid valves usually are not replaced because they do not cause serious symptoms. Mildly or even moderately diseased mitral valves may not need to be replaced because their symptoms are tolerable or they can be treated with such drugs as **beta blockers** or calcium antagonists, which slow the heart rate. However, a severely diseased mitral valve should be repaired or re-

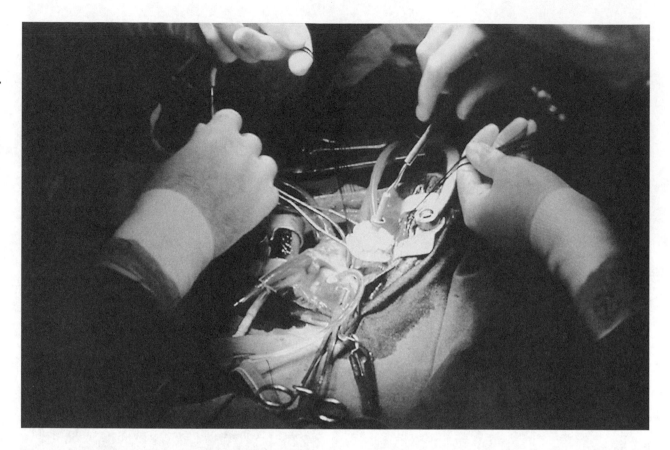

Open heart surgery to replace the mitral heart valve. The replacement valve, made from the tissue of a porcupine pericardium, is being held by sutures in the center of the photo. The tubes carrying blood are connected to a heart-lung machine. *(Photograph by Martin Dohm, Photo Researchers, Inc. Reproduced by permission.)*

placed unless the person is too ill to tolerate the operation because of another condition or illness.

Description

After cutting through and separating the breastbone and ribs, surgeons place the patient on a cardiopulmonary bypass machine, which will perform the functions of the heart and lungs during the operation. They then open the heart and locate the faulty valve. Slicing around the edges of the valve, they loosen it from the tendons that connect it to the rest of the heart and withdraw it. The new valve is inserted and sutured into place. The patient is then taken off the bypass machine and the chest is closed. The surgery takes three to five hours and is covered by most insurance plans.

There are three types of replacement valves. One class is made from animal tissue, usually a pig's aortic valve. Another is mechanical and is made of metal and plastic. The third, includes human valves that have been removed from an organ donor or that, rarely, are the patient's own pulmonic valve.

There is no single ideal replacement valve. The choice between an animal valve or a mechanical valve depends largely on the age of the patient. Because valves obtained from animals have a life expectancy of 7–15 years, they usually are given to older patients. Mechanical valves are used in younger patients because they are more durable. Because mechanical valves are made of foreign material, however, blood clots can form on their surface. Therefore, patients who receive these valves must take anticoagulants the rest of their lives.

Donor or pulmonic valves are given only to those patients who will deteriorate rapidly because of a narrowing of the passageway between the aorta and the left ventrical (aortic stenosis). These valves are limited in their use because of the small supply available from donors and the strain that could be caused by removing and transferring a patient's own pulmonic valve.

Preparation

Before patients undergo heart valve replacement, they must be evaluated carefully for any signs that they may not tolerate the surgery.

Preoperative tests include:

• **Electrocardiography,** which assesses the electrical activity of the heart

• **Echocardiography,** which uses sound waves to show the extent of the obstruction of blood flow through the heart and determine the degree of loss of heart function due to the malfunctioning valve

• **Chest x ray,** which provides an overall view of the anatomy of the heart and the lungs.

Cardiac catheterization may also be performed to further asses the valve and to determine if coronary bypass surgery should also be done.

Aftercare

A patient usually spends 1–3 days in the hospital intensive care unit (ICU) after heart valve replacement so that the working of his or her heart and circulation can be monitored closely. When first brought to the ICU after surgery, the patient undergoes a neurological examination to be sure he or she has not suffered a **stroke.** The patient continues to breathe by means of a tube inserted in the trachea at the time of surgery. This mechanical ventilation is not withdrawn until the patient is fully awake from anesthesia, shows signs that he or she can breathe satisfactorily without mechanical support, and has steadfast circulation.

Once stablilized, the patient is transferred to a standard medical/surgical unit where he or she receives drugs that will prevent excess fluid from building up around the heart. As soon as possible, the patient begins walking and exercising to regain strength. He or she is also placed on a diet that is low in salt and cholesterol.

After being released from the hospital, the patient continues a daily **exercise** program that includes vigorous walking, and he or she may also join a recommended **cardiac rehabilitation** program. He or she usually can return to work or other normal activities within two months of the surgery.

Risks

Complications following heart valve replacement are not common, but can be serious. All valves made from animal tissue will develop calcium deposits over time. If these deposits hamper the function of the valve, it must be replaced. Valves may become dislodged. Blood clots may form on the surface of the substitute valve, break off into the general circulation, and become wedged in an artery supplying blood to the brain, kidneys, or legs. These blood clots may cause fainting spells, stroke, kidney failure, or loss of circulation to the legs. These blood clots can be treated with drugs or surgery.

Infection of heart muscle affects up to 2% of patients who have heart valve replacement. Such an infection is treated with intravenous **antibiotics.** If the infection persists, the new valve may have to be replaced.

Normal results

Few patients die as a result of the surgery. Approximately 3% of all patients die during or immediately after heart valve replacement, and less than 1% of patients below the age of 65 die because of the operation. The vast majority of patients who have heart valve replacement return to normal activity after the surgery. Depending on the type of valve they receive, these patients will have no symptoms of valve abnormality for at least seven years. Also, their quality of life will improve because they may no longer will have difficulty breathing, fainting spells, or palpitations.

Resources

BOOKS

American Heart Association. *American Heart Association's Your Heart: An Owner's Manual.* Englewood Cliffs, NJ: Prentice Hall, 1991.

Schlant, Robert C. and Alexander, R. Wayne, eds. *The Heart, Arteries and Veins,* 18th edition. New York: McGraw-Hill, Inc., 1994.

Texas Heart Institute. *Texas Heart Institute Heart Owner's Handbook.* New York: John Wiley and Sons, 1996.

Youngson, Robert M. *The Surgery Book.* New York: St. Martin's Press, 1993.

ORGANIZATIONS

The American College of Cardiology. 9111 Old Georgetown Road, Bethesda, MD 20814. (800)253-4636. http://www.acc.org.

American College of Surgeons. 55 E. Erie Street, Chicago, IL 60611. (312) 202-5000. http://www.facs.org.

American Heart Association. 7320 Greenville Avenue, Dallas, TX 75321. (214) 373-6300. http://wwwamhrt.org.

Karen Marie Sandrick

KEY TERMS

Barrett's syndrome—Also called Barrett's esophagus or Barrett's epithelia, this is a condition where the squamous epithelial cells that normally line the esophagus are replaced by thicker columnar epithelial cells.

Digestive enzymes—Molecules that catalyze the breakdown of large molecules (usually food) into smaller molecules.

Esophagitis—Inflamation of the esophagus.

Fundoplication—A surgical procedure that increases pressure on the LES by stretching and wrapping the upper part of the stomach around the sphincter.

Gastroesophageal reflux—The flow of stomach contents into the esophagus.

Hiatus hernia—A protrusion of part of the stomach through the diaphragm to a position next to the esophagus.

Metabolic—Refers to the chemical reactions in living things.

Mucus—Thick, viscous, gel-like material that functions to moisten and protect inner body surfaces.

Peristalsis—A sequence of muscle contractions that progressively squeeze one small section of the digestive tract and then the next to push food along the tract, something like pushing toothpaste out of its tube.

Scleroderma—An autoimmune disease with many consequences, including esophageal wall thickening.

Squamous epithelial cells—Thin, flat cells found in layers or sheets covering surfaces such as skin and the linings of blood vessels and esophagus.

Ulceration—An open break in surface tissue.

Heartburn

Definition

Heartburn is a burning sensation in the chest that can extend to the neck, throat, and face; it is worsened by bending or lying down. It is the primary symptom of gastroesophageal reflux, which is the movement of stom-ach acid into the esophagus. On rare occasions, it is due to **gastritis** (stomach lining inflammation).

Description

More than one third of the population is afflicted by heartburn, with about one tenth afflicted daily. Infrequent heartburn is usually without serious consequences, but chronic or frequent heartburn (recurring more than twice per week) can have severe consequences. Accordingly, early management is important.

Understanding heartburn depends on understanding the structure and action of the esophagus. The esophagus is a tube connecting the throat to the stomach. It is about 10 in long in adults, lined with squamous (plate-like) epithelial cells, coated with mucus, and surrounded by muscles that push food to the stomach by sequential waves of contraction (peristalsis). The lower esophageal sphincter (LES) is a thick band of muscles that encircles the esophagus just above the uppermost part of the stom-ach. This sphincter is usually tightly closed and normally opens only when food passes from the esophagus into the stomach. Thus, the contents of the stomach are normally kept from moving back into the esophagus.

The stomach has a thick mucous coating that protects it from the strong acid it secretes into its interior when food is present, but the much thinner esophageal coating doesn't provide protection against acid. Thus, if the LES opens inappropriately or fails to close completely, and stomach contents leak into the esophagus, the esophagus can be burned by acid. The resulting burning sensation is called heartburn.

Occasional heartburn has no serious long-lasting ef-fects, but repeated episodes of gastroesophageal reflux can ultimately lead to esophageal inflammation (esopha-

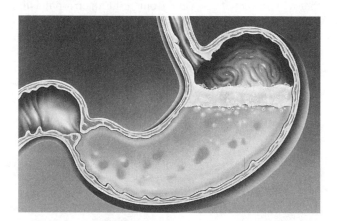

An illustration of foaming antacid on top of the contents of a human stomach. Heartburn is caused by a backflow of the stomach's acidic contents into the esophagus, causing inflammation and a sense of pain that can rise to the throat. *(Illustration by John Bavosi, Custom Medical Stock Photo. Reproduced by permission.)*

gitis) and other damage. If episodes occur more frequently than twice a week, and the esophagus is repeatedly subjected to acid and digestive enzymes from the stomach, ulcerations, scarring, and thickening of the esophagus walls can result. This thickening of the esophagus wall causes a narrowing of the interior of the esophagus. Such narrowing affects swallowing and peristaltic movements. Repeated irritation can also result in changes in the types of cells that line the esophagus. The condition associated with these changes is termed Barrett's syndrome and can lead to **esophageal cancer.**

Causes & symptoms

Causes

A number of different factors may contribute to LES malfunction with its consequent gastroesophageal acid reflux:

- The eating of large meals that distend the stomach can cause the LES to open inappropriately.

- Lying down within two to three hours of eating can cause the LES to open.

- **Obesity, pregnancy,** and tight clothing can impair the ability of the LES to stay closed by putting pressure on the abdomen.

- Certain drugs, notably nicotine, alcohol, diazepam (Valium), meperidine (Demerol), theophylline, morphine, prostaglandins, **calcium channel blockers,** nitrate heart medications, anticholinergic and adrenergic drugs (drugs that limit nerve reactions), including dopamine, can relax the LES.

- Progesterone is thought to relax the LES.

- Greasy foods and some other foods such as chocolate, coffee, and peppermint can relax the LES.

- **Paralysis** and **scleroderma** can cause the LES to malfunction.

- Hiatus **hernia** may also cause heartburn according to some gastroenterologists. (Hiatus hernia is a protrusion of part of the stomach through the diaphragm to a position next to the esophagus.).

Symptoms

Heartburn itself is a symptom. Other symptoms also caused by gastroesophageal reflux can be associated with heartburn. Often heartburn sufferers salivate excessively or regurgitate stomach contents into their mouths, leaving a sour or bitter taste. Frequent gastroesophageal reflux leads to additional complications including difficult or painful swallowing, **sore throat,** hoarseness, coughing, **laryngitis, wheezing, asthma, pneumonia,** gingivitis, **bad breath,** and earache.

Diagnosis

Gastroenterologists and internists are best equipped to diagnose and treat gastroesophageal reflux. Diagnosis is usually based solely on patient histories that report heartburn and other related symptoms. Additional diagnostic procedures can confirm the diagnosis and assess damage to the esophagus, as well as monitor healing progress. The following diagnostic procedures are appropriate for anyone who has frequent, chronic, or difficult-to-treat heartburn or any of the complicating symptoms noted in the previous paragraph.

X rays taken after a patient swallows a barium suspension can reveal esophageal narrowing, ulcerations or a reflux episode as it occurs. However, this procedure cannot detect the structural changes associated with different degrees of esophagitis. This diagnostic procedure has traditionally been called the "upper GI series" or "barium swallow" and costs about $250.00.

Esophagoscopy is a newer procedure that uses a thin flexible tube to view the inside of the esophagus directly. It should be done by a gastroenterologist or gastrointestinal endoscopist and costs about $700. It gives an accurate picture of any damage present and gives the physician the ability to distinguish between different degrees of esophagitis.

Other tests may also be used. They include pressure measurements of the LES; measurements of esophageal acidity (pH), usually throughout a 24-hour period; and microscopic examination of biopsied tissue from the esophageal wall (to inspect esophageal cell structure for Barrett's syndrome and malignancies).

Note: A burning sensation in the chest is usually heartburn and is not associated with the heart. However, chest pain that radiates into the arms and is not accompanied by regurgitation is a warning of a possible serious heart problem. Anyone with these symptoms should contact a doctor immediately.

Treatment

Drugs

Occasional heartburn is probably best treated with over-the-counter **antacids.** These products go straight to the esophagus and immediately begin to decrease acidity. However, they should not be used as the sole treatment for heartburn sufferers who either have two or more episodes per week or who suffer for periods of over three weeks. There is a risk of kidney damage and other metabolic changes.

H2 blockers (histamine receptor blockers, such as Pepsid AC, Zantac, Tagamet) decrease stomach acid production and are effective against heartburn. H2 blocker treatment also allows healing of esophageal damage but is not very effective when there is a high degree of damage. It takes 30–45 minutes for these drugs to take effect, so they must be taken prior to an episode. Thus, they should be taken daily, usually two to four times per day for several weeks. Six to twelve weeks of standard-dose treatment relieves symptoms in about half the patients. Higher doses relieve symptoms in a greater fraction of the population, but at least 25% of heartburn sufferers are not helped by H2 blockers.

Proton-pump inhibitors also inhibit acid production by the stomach, but are much more effective than H2 blockers for some people. They are also more effective in aiding the healing process. Esophagitis is healed in about 90% of the patients undergoing proton-pump inhibitor treatment.

The long-term effects of inhibiting stomach acid production are unknown. Without the antiseptic effects of a consistently very acidic stomach environment, users of H2 blockers or proton-pump inhibitors may become more susceptible to bacterial and viral infection. Absorption of some drugs is also lowered by this less-acidic environment.

Prokinetic agents (also known as motility drugs) act on the LES, stimulating it to close more tightly, thereby keeping stomach contents out of the esophagus. It is not known how effectively these drugs promote healing. Some of the early motility drugs had serious neurological side effects, but a new drug, cisapride, seems to act only on digestive system nerve connections.

Surgery

Fundoplication, a surgical procedure to increase pressure on the LES by stretching and wrapping the upper part of the stomach around the sphincter, is a treatment of last resort. About 10% of heartburn sufferers undergo this procedure. It is not always effective and its effectiveness may decrease over time, especially several years after surgery. Dr. Robert Marks and his colleagues at the University of Alabama reported in 1997 on the long-term outcome of this procedure. They found that 64% of the patients in their study who had fundoplication between 1992 and 1995 still suffered from heartburn and reported an impaired quality of life after the surgery.

However, **laparoscopy** (an examination of the interior of the abdomen by means of the laparoscope) now provides hope for better outcomes. Fundoplication performed with a laparoscope is less invasive. Five small incisions are required instead of one large incision. Patients recover faster, and it is likely that studies will show they suffer from fewer surgical complications.

Alternative treatment

Prevention, as outlined below, is a primary feature for heartburn management in alternative medicine and traditional medicine. Dietary adjustments can eliminate many causes of heartburn.

Herbal remedies include bananas, aloe vera gel, chamomile (*Matricaria recutita*), ginger (*Zingiber officinale*), and citrus juices, but there is little agreement here. For example, ginger, which seems to help some people, is claimed by other practitioners to *cause* heartburn and is thought to relax the LES. There are also many recommendations to *avoid* citrus juices, which are themselves acidic. Licorice (*Glycyrrhiza uralensis*) can help relieve the symptoms of heartburn by reestablishing balance in the acid output of the stomach.

Several homeopathic remedies are useful in treating heartburn symptoms. Among those most often recommended are *Nux vomica, Carbo vegetabilis*, and *Arsenicum album*. **Acupressure** and **acupuncture** may also be helpful in treating heartburn.

Sodium bicarbonate (baking soda) is an inexpensive alternative to use as an antacid. It reduces esophageal acidity immediately, but its affect is not long-lasting and should not be used by people on sodium-restricted **diets.**

Prognosis

The prognosis for people who get heartburn only occasionally or people without esophageal damage is excellent. The prognosis for people with esophageal damage who become involved in a treatment program that promotes healing is also excellent. The prognosis for anyone with esophageal cancer is very poor. There is a strong likelihood of a painful illness and a less than 5% chance of surviving more than five years.

Prevention

Given the lack of completely satisfactory treatments for heartburn or its consequences and the lack of a cure for esophageal cancer, prevention is of the utmost importance. Proponents of traditional *and* alternative medicine agree that people disposed to heartburn should:

• Avoid eating large meals.

• Avoid alcohol, **caffeine,** fatty foods, fried foods, hot or spicy foods, chocolate, peppermint, and nicotine.

• Avoid drugs known to contribute to heartburn, such as nitrates (heart medications like Isonate and Nitrocap), calcium channel blockers (e.g., Cardizem and Procardia), and anticholinergic drugs (e.g., Probanthine and Bentyl), and check with their doctors about any drugs they are taking.

• Avoid clothing that fits tightly around the abdomen.

• Control body weight.

• Wait about three hours after eating before going to bed or lying down.

- Elevate the head of their bed six to nine inches to alleviate heartburn at night. This can be done with bricks under the bed or with a wedge designed for this purpose.

Resources

BOOKS

Castell, Donald O. *The Esophagus.* Boston: Little, Brown, 1995.

Wolfe, M. Michael, and Thomas Nesi. *The Fire Inside: Extinguishing Heartburn and Related Symptoms.* New York: Norton, 1996.

PERIODICALS

"Acid blockers: How You Can Head Off Heartburn Before it Starts." *Mayo Clinic Health Letter* (November, 1997).

Mittal, Ravinder K. and David H. Balaban. "Mechanisms of Disease: The Esophagogastric Junction." *New England Journal of Medicine* 336 (March 27, 1997): 924-932.

Vaezi, Michael F., and Joel E. Richter. "Gastroesophageal Reflux Disease." *Current Opinion in Gastroenterology* 13 (July, 1997): 327-332.

ORGANIZATIONS

The American College of Gastroenterology (ACG). P.O. Box 3099, Alexandria, VA 22302. (703) 820-7400; (800) HRT-BURN. http://www.healthtouch.com.

The American Gastroenterological Association (AGA). 7910 Woodmont Ave., 7th Floor, Bethesda, MD 20814. (310) 654-2055. http://www.gastro.org/index.html. aga001@aol.com.

American Society for Gastrointestinal Endoscopy. 13 Elm St., Manchester, MA 01944. (508) 526-8330. http://www.asge.org/doc/201.

National Digestive Diseases Information Clearinghouse. 2 Information Way, Bethesda, MD 20892-3570. (E-mail: nddic@aerie.com) http://www.niddk.nih.gov/Brochures/NDDIC.htm.

Lorraine Lica

Heat cramps *see* **Heat disorders**

Heat disorders

Definition

Heat disorders are a group of physically related illnesses caused by prolonged exposure to hot temperatures, restricted fluid intake, or failure of temperature regulation mechanisms of the body. Disorders of heat exposure include heat cramps, heat exhaustion, and heat **stroke** (also called sunstroke). Hyperthermia is the gen-

---

> **KEY TERMS**
>
> **Convulsions**—Also termed seizures; a sudden violent contraction of a group of muscles.
>
> **Electrolytes**—An element or compound that when melted or dissolved in water dissociates into ions and is able to conduct an electrical current. Careful and regular monitoring of electrolytes and intravenous replacement of fluid and electrolytes are part of the acute care in many illnesses.
>
> **Rehydration**—The restoration of water or fluid to a body that has become dehydrated.

eral name given to heat-related illnesses. The two most common forms of hyperthermia are heat exhaustion and heat stroke, which is especially dangerous and requires immediate medical attention.

Description

Heat disorders are harmful to people of all ages, but their severity is likely to increase as people age. Heat cramps in a 16-year-old may be heat exhaustion in a 45-year-old and heat stroke in a 65-year-old. The body's temperature regulating mechanisms rely on the thermal regulating centers in the brain. Through these complex centers, the body tries to adapt to high temperatures by adjusting the amount of salt in the perspiration. Salt helps the cells in body tissues retain water. In hot weather, a healthy body will lose enough water to cool the body while creating the lowest level of chemical imbalance. Regardless of extreme weather conditions, the healthy human body keeps a steady temperature of approximately 98.6°F (37°C). In hot weather, or during vigorous activity, the body perspires. As perspiration evaporates from the skin, the body is cooled. If the body loses too much salt and fluids, the symptoms of **dehydration** can occur.

Heat cramps

Heat cramps are the least severe of the heat-related illnesses. This heat disorder is often the first signal that the body is having difficulty with increased temperature. Individuals exposed to excessive heat should think of heat cramps as a warning sign to a potential heat-related emergency.

Heat exhaustion

Heat exhaustion is a more serious and complex condition than heat cramps. Heat exhaustion can result from prolonged exposure to hot temperatures, restricted fluid intake, or failure of temperature regulation mechanisms of the body. It often affects athletes, firefighters, construction workers, factory workers, and anyone who wears heavy clothing in hot humid weather.

Heat stroke

Heat exhaustion can develop rapidly into heat stroke. Heat stroke can be life threatening and because the percentage of victims dying from heat stroke is very high, immediate medical attention is critical when problems first begin. Heat stroke, like heat exhaustion, is also a result of prolonged exposure to hot temperatures, restricted fluid intake, or failure of temperature regulation mechanisms of the body. However, the severity of impact on the body is much greater with heat stroke.

Causes & symptoms

Heat cramps

Heat cramps are painful muscle spasms caused by the excessive loss of salts (electrolytes), due to heavy perspiration. The muscle tissue becomes less flexible, causing pain, difficult movement, and involuntary tightness. Heavy exertion in extreme heat, restricted fluid intake, or failure of temperature regulation mechanisms of the body may lead to heat cramps. This disorder occurs more often in the legs and abdomen than in other areas of the body. Individuals at higher risk are those working in extreme heat, elderly people, young children, people with health problems, and those who are unable to naturally and properly cool their bodies. Individuals with poor circulation and who take medications to reduce excess body fluids can be at risk when conditions are hot and humid.

Heat exhaustion

Heat exhaustion is caused by exposure to high heat and humidity for many hours, resulting in excessive loss of fluids and salts through heavy perspiration. The skin may appear cool, moist, and pale. The individual may complain of **headache** and nausea with a feeling of overall weakness and exhaustion. **Dizziness,** faintness, and mental confusion are often present, as is rapid and weak pulse. Breathing becomes fast and shallow. Fluid loss reduces blood volume and lowers blood pressure. Yellow or orange urine often is a result of inadequate fluid intake, along with associated intense thirst. Insufficient water and salt intake or a deficiency in the production of sweat place an individual at high risk for heat exhaustion.

Heat stroke

Heat stroke is caused by overexposure to extreme heat, resulting in a breakdown in the body's heat regulating mechanisms. The body's temperature reaches a dangerous level, as high as 106°F (41.1°C). An individual with heat stroke has a body temperature higher than 104°F (40°C). Other symptoms include mental confusion with possible combativeness and bizarre behavior, staggering, and faintness.

The pulse becomes strong and rapid (160–180 beats per minute) with the skin taking on a dry and flushed appearance. There is often very little perspiration. The individual can quickly lose consciousness or have convulsions. Before heatstroke, an individual suffers from heat exhaustion and the associated symptoms. When the body can no longer maintain a normal temperature, heat exhaustion becomes heatstroke. Heat stroke is a life-threatening medical emergency that requires immediate initiation of life-saving measures.

Diagnosis

The diagnosis of heat cramps usually involves the observation of individual symptoms such as muscle cramping and thirst. Diagnosis of heat exhaustion or heat stroke, however, may require a physician to review the medical history, document symptoms, and obtain a blood pressure and temperature reading. The physician may also take blood and urine samples for further laboratory testing. A test to measure the body's electrolytes can also give valuable information about chemical imbalances caused by the heat-related illness.

Treatment

Heat cramps

The care of heat cramps includes placing the individual at rest in a cool environment, while giving cool water with a teaspoon of salt per quart, or a commercial sports drink. Usually rest and liquids are all that is needed for the patient to recover. Mild stretching and massaging of the muscle area follows once the condition improves. The individual should not take salt tablets, since this may actually worsen the condition. When the cramps stop, the person can usually start activity again if there are no other signs of illness. The individual needs to continue drinking fluids and should be watched carefully for further signs of heat-related illnesses.

Heat exhaustion

The individual suffering from heat exhaustion should stop all physical activity and move immediately to a cool place out of the sun, preferably a cool, air-conditioned location. She or he should then lay down with feet slightly elevated, remove or loosen clothing, and drink cold (but not iced), slightly salty water or commercial sports drink. Rest and replacement of fluids and salt is usually all the treatment that is needed, and hospitalization is rarely required. Following rehydration, the person usually recovers rapidly.

Heat stroke

Simply moving the individual afflicted with heat stroke to a cooler place is not enough to reverse the internal overheating. Emergency medical assistance should be called immediately. While waiting for help to arrive, quick action to lower body temperature must take place. Treatment involves getting the victim to a cool place, loosening clothes or undressing the heat stroke victim, and allowing air to circulate around the body. The next important step is wrapping the individual in wet towels or clothing, and placing ice packs in areas with the greatest blood supply. These areas include the neck, under the arm and knees, and in the groin. Once the patient is under medical care, **cooling treatments** may continue as appropriate. The victim's body temperature will be monitored constantly to guard against overcooling. Breathing and heart rate will be monitored closely, and fluids and electrolytes will be replaced intravenously. Anti-convulsant drugs may be given. After severe heat stroke, bed rest may be recommended for several days.

Prognosis

Prompt treatment for heat cramps is usually very effective with the individual returning to activity thereafter. Treatment of heat exhaustion usually brings full recovery in one to two days. Heatstroke is a very serious condition and its outcome depends upon general health and age. Due to the high internal temperature of heat stroke, permanent damage to internal organs is possible.

Prevention

Because heat cramps, heat exhaustion, and heat stroke have a cascade effect on each other, the prevention of the onset of all heat disorders is similar. Avoid strenuous **exercise** when it is very hot. Individuals exposed to extreme heat conditions should drink plenty of fluids. Wearing light and loose-fitting clothing in hot weather is important, regardless of the activity. It is important to consume water often and not to wait until thirst develops. If perspiration is excessive, fluid intake should be increased. When urine output decreases, fluid intake should also increase. Eating lightly salted foods can help replace salts lost through perspiration. Ventilation in any working areas in warm weather must be adequate. This can be achieved as simply as opening a window or using an electric fan. Proper ventilation will promote adequate sweat evaporation to cool the skin. Sunblocks and **sunscreens** with a protection factor of 15 (SPF 15) can be very helpful when one is exposed to extreme direct sunlight.

Resources

BOOKS

American Red Cross. *Standard First Aid.* St. Louis, MO: Mosby Year Book, 1993.

Larson, David E., ed. *Mayo Clinic Family Health Book,* 2nd ed. New York: William Morrow, 1996.

Morris, M., M. Walsh, and Shelton G. Walsh. *The Team Physicians Hand Book.* Philadelphia: Hanley & Belfus, 1990.

OTHER

Griffith, H. "Complete Guide to Symptoms, Illness & Surgery." The Putnam Berkley Group, Inc., 1995 http://www.thriveonline.com.

Jeffrey Peter Larson

Heat exhaustion *see* **Heat disorders**

Heat treatments

Definition

Heat treatments are applications of therapeutic thermal agents to specific body areas experiencing injury or dysfunction.

Purpose

The general purpose of a heat treatment is to increase the extensibility of soft tissues, remove toxins from cells, enhance blood flow, increase function of the tissue cells, encourage muscle relaxation, and help relieve **pain.** There are two types of heat treatments: superficial and deep. Superficial heat treatments apply heat to the outside of the body. Deep heat treatments direct heat toward specific inner tissues through ultrasound or by electric current. Heat treatments are beneficial prior to **exercise,** providing a warm-up effect to the soft tissues involved.

Precautions

Heat treatments should not be used on individuals with circulation problems, heat intolerance, or lack of sensation in the affected area. Low blood circulation may contribute to heat-related injuries. Heat treatments also should not be used on individuals afflicted with heart, lung, or kidney diseases. Deep heat treatments should not be used on areas above the eye, heart, or on a pregnant patient. Deep heat treatments over areas with metal surgical implants should be avoided in case of rapid temperature increase and subsequent injury.

Description

There are four different ways to convey heat:

• Conduction is the transfer of heat between two objects in direct contact with each other.

• Conversion is the transition of one form of energy to heat.

• Radiation involves the transmission and absorption of electromagnetic waves to produce a heating effect.

• Convection occurs when a liquid or gas moves past a body part creating heat.

Hot packs, water bottles, and heating pads

Hot packs are a very common form of heat treatment utilizing conduction as a form of heat transfer. Moist heat packs are readily available in most hospitals, physical therapy centers, and athletic training rooms. Treatment temperature should not exceed 131°F (55°C). The pack is used over multiple layers of toweling to achieve a comfortable warming effect for approximately 30 minutes. More recently, several manufacturers have developed packs that may be warmed in a microwave over a specified amount of time prior to use.

Hot-water bottles are another form of superficial heat treatment. The bottles are filled half way with hot water between 115–125°F (46.1–52°C). Covered by a protective toweling, the hot-water bottle is placed on the treatment area and left until the water has cooled off.

Electrical heating pads continue to be used, however because of the need for an electrical outlet, safety and convenience become an issue.

Paraffin

Paraffin, a conductive form of superficial heat, is often used for heating uneven surface of the body such as the hands. It consists of melted paraffin wax and mineral oil. Paraffin placed in a small bath unit, becomes solid at room temperature and is used as a liquid heat treatment when heated at 126–127.4°F (52–53°C). The most common form of paraffin application is called the dip and wax method. In this technique, the patient will dip 8–12 times and then the extremity will be covered with a plastic bag and a towel for insulation. Most treatment sessions are about 20 minutes.

Hydrotherapy

Hydrotherapy is used in a form of heat treatment for many musculoskeletal disorders. The hydrotherapy tanks and pools are all generally set at warm temperatures, never exceeding 150°F (65.6°C). Because the patient often performs resistance exercises while in the water, higher water temperatures become a concern as the treatment becomes more physically draining. Because of this, many hydrotherapy baths are now being set at 95–110°F (35–43.3°C). There are also units available with moveable turbine jets, which provide a light massage effect. Hydrotherapy is helpful as a warm-up prior to exercise.

Fluidotherapy

Fluidotherapy is a form of heat treatment developed in the 1970s. It is a dry heat modality consisting of cellulose particles suspended in air. Units come in different sizes and some are restricted to only treating a hand or foot. The turbulence of the gas-solid mixture provides thermal contact with objects that are immersed in the medium. Temperatures of this treatment range from 110–123°F (43.3–50.5°C). Fluidotherapy allows the patient to exercise the limb during the treatment, and also massages the limb, increasing blood flow.

Ultrasound

Ultrasound heat treatments penetrate the body to provide relief to inner tissue. Ultrasound energy comes from the acoustic or sound spectrum and is undetectable to the human ear. By using conducting agents such as gel or mineral oil, the ultrasound transducer warms areas of the musculoskeletal system. Some areas of the musculoskeletal system absorb ultrasound better that others. Muscle tissue and other connective tissue such as ligaments and tendons absorb this form of energy very well, however fat absorbs to a much lesser degree. Ultrasound has a relatively longlasting effect, continuing up to one hour.

Diathermy

Diathermy is another deep heat treatment. An electrode drum is used to apply heat to an affected area. It consists of a wire coil surrounded by dead space and other insulators such as a plastic housing. Plenty of toweling must be layered between the unit and the patient. This device is unique in that it utilizes the basis of a magnetic field on connective tissues. One advantage of diathermy over various other heat treatments is that fat does resist an electrical field, which is not the case with a magnetic field. It is found to be helpful with those experiencing chronic **low back pain** and muscle spasms. Prior to ultrasound technology, diathermy was a popular heat therapy of the 1940s–1960s.

Preparation

Before administering any form of heat treatment, heat sensitivity is accessed and the skin over the affected area is cleansed. When a patient is undergoing any form of heat treatment, supervision should always be present especially in the treatment of hydrotherapy.

Aftercare

Once the heat treatment has been completed, any symptoms of **dizziness** and nausea should be noted and documented along with any skin irritations or discoloring not present prior to the heat treatment. A one hour interval between treatments should be adhered to in order to avoid restriction of blood flow.

Risks

All heat treatments have the potential of tissue damage resulting from excessive temperatures. Proper insulation and treatment duration should be carefully administered for each method. Overexposure during a superficial heat treatment may result in redness, blisters, burns, or reduced blood circulation. During ultrasound therapy, excessive treatment over bony areas with little soft tissue (such as hand, feet, and elbow) can cause excessive heat resulting in pain and possible tissue damage. Exposure to the electrode drum during diathermy may produce hot spots.

Resources

BOOKS

Scully, Rosemary M. and Marylou R. Barnes. *Physical Therapy.* Philadelphia: J.B. Lippincott Co., 1989.

PERIODICALS

Mclaughlin, Christine. "Hot Packs in the Clinic: Are They Overutilized?"*Advance Magazine for Physical Therapists* (April 29,1996): 6.

Roland, Pamela. "Some Like It Hot and Cold." *Advance Magazine for Physical Therapists* (May 22,1995): 6.

ORGANIZATIONS

American Physical Therapy Association. 1111 North Fairfax Street. Alexandria, VA 22314. (703) 684-APTA.

Jeffrey Peter Larson

Heatstroke *see* **Heat disorders**

Heavy menstruation *see* **Dysfunctional uterine bleeding**

Heavy metal poisoning

Definition

Heavy metal poisoning is the toxic accumulation of heavy metals in the soft tissues of the body.

> ## KEY TERMS
>
> **Chelation**—The process by which a molecule encircles and binds to a metal and removes it from tissue.
>
> **Heavy metal**—One of 23 chemical elements that has a specific gravity (a measure of density) at least five times that of water.

Description

Heavy metals are chemical elements that have a specific gravity (a measure of density) at least five times that of water. The heavy metals most often implicated in human poisoning are lead, mercury, arsenic, and cadmium. Some heavy metals, such as zinc, copper, chromium, iron, and manganese, are required by the body in small amounts, but these same elements can be toxic in larger quantities.

Heavy metals may enter the body in food, water, or air, or by absorption through the skin. Once in the body, they compete with and displace essential **minerals** such as zinc, copper, magnesium, and calcium, and interfere with organ system function. People may come in contact with heavy metals in industrial work, pharmaceutical manufacturing, and agriculture. Children may be poisoned as a result of playing in contaminated soil.

Causes & symptoms

Symptoms will vary, depending on the nature and the quantity of the heavy metal ingested. Patients may complain of nausea, vomiting, **diarrhea,** stomach **pain, headache,** sweating, and a metallic taste in the mouth. Depending on the metal, there may be blue-black lines in the gum tissues. In severe cases, patients exhibit obvious impairment of cognitive, motor, and language skills. The expression "mad as a hatter" comes from the mercury **poisoning** prevalent in 17th century France among hatmakers who soaked animal hides in a solution of mercuric nitrate to soften the hair.

Diagnosis

Heavy metal poisoning may be detected using blood and urine tests, hair and tissue analysis, or x ray.

In childhood, blood lead levels above 80 μg/dL generally indicate lead poisoning, however, significantly lower levels (>30 μg/dL) can cause mental retardation and other cognitive and behavioral problems in affected children. The Centers for Disease Control and Pevention considers a blood lead level of 10 μg/dL or higher in children a cause for concern. In adults, symptoms of lead poisoning are usually seen when blood lead levels exceed 80 μg/dL for a number of weeks.

Blood levels of mercury should not exceed 3.6 μg/dL, while urine levels should not exceed 15 μg/dL. Symptoms of mercury poisoning may be seen when mercury levels exceed 20 μg/dL in blood and 60 μg/dL in urine. Mercury levels in hair may be used to gauge the severity of chronic mercury exposure.

Since arsenic is rapidly cleared from the blood, blood arsenic levels may not be very useful in diagnosis. Arsenic in the urine (measured in a 24-hour collection following 48 hours without eating seafood) may exceed 50 μg/dL in people with arsenic poisoning. If acute arsenic poisoning is suspected, an x ray may reveal ingested arsenic in the abdomen (since arsenic is opaque to x rays). Arsenic may also be detected in the hair and nails for months following exposure.

Cadmium toxicity is generally indicated when urine levels exceed 10 μg/dL of creatinine and blood levels exceed 5 μg/dL.

Treatment

The treatment for most heavy metal poisoning is **chelation therapy.** A chelating agent specific to the metal involved is given either orally, intramuscularly, or intravenously. The three most common chelating agents are calcium disodium edetate, dimercaprol (BAL), and penicillamine. The chelating agent encircles and binds to the metal in the body's tissues, forming a complex; that complex is then released from the tissue to travel in the bloodstream. The complex is filtered out of the blood by the kidneys and excreted in the urine. This process may be lengthy and painful, and typically requires hospitalization. Chelation therapy is effective in treating lead, mercury, and arsenic poisoning, but is not useful in treating cadmium poisoning. To date, no treatment has been proven effective for cadmium poisoning.

In cases of acute mercury or arsenic ingestion, vomiting may be induced. Washing out the stomach (gastric lavage) may also be useful. The patient may also require treatment such as intravenous fluids for complications of poisoning such as **shock,** anemia, and kidney failure.

Prognosis

The chelation process can only halt further effects of the poisoning; it cannot reverse neurological damage already sustained.

Prevention

Because exposure to heavy metals is often an occupational hazard, protective clothing and respirators should be provided and worn on the job. Protective clothing should then be left at the work site and not worn

home, where it could carry toxic dust to family members. Industries are urged to reduce or replace the heavy metals in their processes wherever possible. Exposure to environmental sources of lead, including lead-based paints, plumbing fixtures, vehicle exhaust, and contaminated soil, should be reduced or eliminated.

Resources

BOOKS

Fauci, Anthony S., ed. *Harrison's Principles of Internal Medicine.* 14th ed. New York: McGraw-Hill, 1998.

ORGANIZATIONS

Food and Drug Administration. Office of Inquiry and Consumer Information. 5600 Fisher Lane, Room 12-A-40, Rockville, MD 20857. (301) 827-4420. http://www.fda.gov/fdahomepage.html.

National Institutes of Health. National Institute of Environmental Health Sciences Clearinghouse. EnviroHealth, 2605 Meridian Parkway, Suite 115, Durham, NC 27713. (919) 361-9408.

National Organization for Rare Disorders. PO Box 8923, New Fairfield, CT 06812-8923. (203) 746-6481 or (800) 999-6673. http://www.nord-rdb.com/~orphan.

Bethany Thivierge

Heel spurs

Definition

A heel spur is a bony projection on the sole (plantar) region of the heel bone (also known as the calcaneous). This condition may accompany or result from severe cases of inflammation to the structure called plantar fascia. This associated plantar fascia is a fibrous band of connective tissue on the sole of the foot, extending from the heel to the toes.

Description

Heel spurs are a common foot problem resulting from excess bone growth on the heel bone. The bone growth is usually located on the underside of the heel bone, extending forward to the toes. One explanation for this excess production of bone is a painful tearing of the plantar fascia connected between the toes and heel. This can result in either a heel spur or an inflammation of the plantar fascia, medically termed plantar fascitis. Because this condition is often correlated to a decrease in the arch of the foot, it is more prevalent after the age of six to eight years, when the arch is fully developed.

KEY TERMS

Calcaneous—The heel bone.

Genu valgus—Deformity in which the legs are curved inward so that the knees are close together, nearly or actually knocking as a person walks with ankles widely apart of each other.

Plantar fascia—A tough fibrous band of tissue surrounding the muscles of the sole of the foot. Also called plantar aponeurosis.

Pronation—The lowering or descending of the inner edge of the foot by turning the entire foot outwards.

Causes & symptoms

One frequent cause of heel spurs is an abnormal motion and mal-alignment of the foot called pronation. For the foot to function properly, a certain degree of pronation is required. This motion is defined as an inward action of the foot, with dropping of the inside arch as one plants the heel and advances the weight distribution to the toes during walking. When foot pronation becomes extreme from the foot turning in and dropping beyond the normal limit, a condition known as excessive pronation creates a mechanical problem in the foot. In some cases the sole or bottom of the foot flattens and becomes unstable because of this excess pronation, especially during critical times of walking and athletic activities. The portion of the plantar fascia attached into the heel bone or calcaneous begins to stretch and pull away from the heel bone.

At the onset of this condition, pain and swelling become present, with discomfort particularly noted as pushing off with the toes occurs during walking. This movement of the foot stretches the fascia that is already irritated and inflamed. If this condition is allowed to continue, pain is noticed around the heel region because of the newly formed bone, in response to the stress. This results in the development of the heel spur. It is common among athletes and others who run and jump a significant amount.

An individual with the lower legs angulating inward, a condition called genu valgus or ''knock knees,'' can have a tendency toward excessive pronation. As a result, this too can lead to a fallen arch resulting in plantar fasciitis and heel spurs. Women tend to have more genu valgus than men do. Heel spurs can also result from an abnormally high arch.

Other factors leading to heel spurs include a sudden increase in daily activities, an increase in weight, or a change of shoes. Dramatic increase in training intensity or duration may cause plantar fasciitis. Shoes that are too flexible in the middle of the arch or shoes that bend before the toe joints will cause an increase in tension in the plantar fascia and possibly lead to heel spurs.

The pain this condition causes forces an individual to attempt walking on his or her toes or ball of the foot to avoid pressure on the heel spur. This can lead to other compensations during walking or running that in turn cause additional problems to the ankle, knee, hip, or back.

Diagnosis

A thorough medical history and physical exam by a physician is always necessary for the proper diagnosis of heel spurs and other foot conditions. X rays of the heel area are helpful, as excess bone production will be visible.

Treatment

Conservative

Heel spurs and plantar fasciitis are usually controlled with conservative treatment. Early intervention includes stretching the calf muscles while avoiding re-injuring the plantar fascia. Decreasing or changing activities, losing excess weight, and improving the proper fitting of shoes are all important measures to decrease this common source of foot pain. Modification of footwear includes shoes with a raised heel and better arch support. Shoe orthotics recommended by a healthcare professional are often very helpful in conjunction with **exercises** to increase strength of the foot muscles and arch. The orthotic prevents excess pronation and lengthening of the plantar fascia and continued tearing of this structure. To aid in this reduction of inflammation, applying ice for 10–15 minutes after activities and use of anti-inflammatory medication can be helpful. Physical therapy can be beneficial with the use of heat modalities, such as ultrasound that creates a deep heat and reduces inflammation. If the pain caused by inflammation is constant, keeping the foot raised above the heart and/or compressed by wrapping with an ace bandage will help.

Corticosteroid injections are also frequently used to reduce pain and inflammation. Taping can help speed the healing process by protecting the fascia from reinjury, especially during stretching and walking.

Heel surgery

When chronic heel pain fails to respond to conservative treatment, surgical treatment may be necessary. Heel surgery can provide relief of pain and restore mobility. The type of procedure used is based on examination and usually consists of releasing the excessive tightness of the plantar fascia, called a plantar fascia release. Depending on the presence of excess bony build up, the procedure may or may not include removal of heel spurs. Similar to other surgical interventions, there are various modifications and surgical enhancements regarding surgery of the heel.

Alternative treatment

Acupuncture and accupressure have been used to address the pain of heel spurs, in addition to using friction **massage** to help break up scar tissue and delay onset of bony formations.

Prognosis

Usually, heel spurs are curable with conservative treatment. If not, heel spurs are curable with surgery. About 10% of those that continue to see a physician for plantar fascitis have it for more than a year. If there is limited success after approximately one year of conservative treatment, patients are often advised to have surgery.

Prevention

To prevent this condition, wearing shoes with proper arches and support is very important. Proper stretching is always a necessity, especially when there is an increase in activities or a change in running technique. It is not recommended to attempt working through the pain, as this can change a mild case of heel spurs and plantar fascitis into a long lasting and painful episode of this condition.

Resources

BOOKS

Perkins, Kenneth E. "Lower Extremity Orthotics in Geriatric Rehabilitation." In *Geriatric Physical Therapy,* edited by Andrew Guccione. St. Louis, MO: Mosby Year Book Inc, 1993.

PERIODICALS

Feeny, Tracy. "If The Shoe Fits." *Advance Magazine for Physical Therapists.* (July 1997): 7.

ORGANIZATIONS

American Orthopedic Foot and Ankle Society. 222 South Prospect, Park Ridge, IL 60068.

American Podiatry Medical Association. 9312 Old Georgetown Road, Bethesda, MD 20814.

OTHER

Roberts. *"Plantar Fascitis".* 1998. www.heelspurs.com. (4-9-98).

Jeffrey Peter Larson

Heimlich maneuver

Definition

The Heimlich maneuver is an emergency procedure for removing a foreign object lodged in the airway that is preventing a person from breathing.

Purpose

Every year about 3,000 adults die because they accidentally inhale rather than swallow food. The food gets stuck and blocks their trachea, making breathing impossible. **Death** follows rapidly unless the food or other foreign material can be displaced from the airway. This condition is so common it has been nicknamed the "cafe coronary."

In 1974 Dr. Henry Heimlich first described an emergency technique for expelling foreign material blocking the trachea. This technique, now called the Heimlich maneuver or abdominal thrusts, is simple enough that it can be performed immediately by anyone trained in the maneuver. The Heimlich maneuver is a standard part of all first aid courses.

The theory behind the Heimlich maneuver is that by compressing the abdomen below the level of the diaphragm, air is forced under pressure out of the lungs dislodging the obstruction in the trachea and bringing the foreign material back up into the mouth.

The Heimlich maneuver is used mainly when solid material like food, coins, vomit, or small toys are blocking the airway. There has been some controversy about whether the Heimlich maneuver is appropriate to use routinely on **near-drowning** victims. After several studies of the effectiveness of the Heimlich maneuver on reestablishing breathing in near-drowning victims, the American Red Cross and the American Heart Association both recommend that the Heimlich maneuver be used only as a last resort after traditional airway clearance techniques and cardiopulmonary resuscitation (CPR) have been tried repeatedly and failed or if it is clear that a solid foreign object is blocking the airway.

Precautions

Incorrect application of the Heimlich maneuver can damage the chest, ribs, and internal organs of the person on whom it is performed. People may also vomit after being treated with the Heimlich maneuver.

Description

The Heimlich maneuver can be performed on all people. Modifications are necessary if the **choking** victim is very obese, pregnant, a child, or an infant.

KEY TERMS

Diaphragm—The thin layer of muscle that separates the chest cavity containing the lungs and heart from the abdominal cavity containing the intestines and digestive organs.

Trachea—The windpipe. A tube extending from below the voice box into the chest where it splits into two branches, the bronchi, that lead to each lung.

Indications that a person's airway is blocked include:

• The person can not speak or cry out.

• The person's face turns blue from lack of oxygen.

• The person desperately grabs at his or her throat.

• The person has a weak **cough,** and labored breathing produces a high-pitched noise.

• The person does all of the above, then becomes unconscious.

Performing the Heimlich maneuver on adults

To perform the Heimlich maneuver on a conscious adult, the rescuer stands behind the victim. The victim may either be sitting or standing. The rescuer makes a fist with one hand, and places it, thumb toward the victim, below the rib cage and above the waist. The rescuer encircles the victim's waist, placing his other hand on top of the fist.

In a series of 6–10 sharp and distinct thrusts upward and inward, the rescuer attempts to develop enough pressure to force the foreign object back up the trachea. If the maneuver fails, it is repeated. It is important not to give up if the first attempt fails. As the victim is deprived of oxygen, the muscles of the trachea relax slightly. Because of this loosening, it is possible that the foreign object may be expelled on a second or third attempt.

If the victim is unconscious, the rescuer should lay him or her on the floor, bend the chin forward, make sure the tongue is not blocking the airway, and feel in the mouth for **foreign objects,** being careful not to push any farther into the airway. The rescuer kneels astride the victim's thighs and places his fists between the bottom of the victim's breastbone and the navel. The rescuer then executes a series of 6–10 sharp compressions by pushing inward and upward.

After the abdominal thrusts, the rescuer repeats the process of lifting the chin, moving the tongue, feeling for and possibly removing the foreign material. If the airway is not clear, the rescuer repeats the abdominal thrusts as

often as necessary. If the foreign object has been removed, but the victim is not breathing, the rescuer starts CPR.

Performing the Heimlich maneuver under special circumstances

OBVIOUSLY PREGNANT AND VERY OBESE PEOPLE

The main difference in performing the Heimlich maneuver on this group of people is in the placement of the fists. Instead of using abdominal thrusts, chest thrusts are used. The fists are placed against the middle of the breastbone, and the motion of the chest thrust is in and downward, rather than upward. If the victim is unconscious, the chest thrusts are similar to those used in CPR.

CHILDREN

The technique in children over one year of age is the same as in adults, except that the amount of force used is less than that used with adults in order to avoid damaging the child's ribs, breastbone, and internal organs.

INFANTS UNDER ONE YEAR OLD

The rescuer sits down and lays the infant along his or her forearm with the infant's face pointed toward the floor. The rescuer's hand supports the infant's head, and his or her forearm rests on his or her own thigh for additional support. Using the heel of the other hand, the rescuer administers four or five rapid blows to the infant's back between the shoulder blades.

After administering the back blows, the rescuer sandwiches the infant between his or her arms, and turns the infant over so that the infant is lying face up supported by the opposite arm. Using the free hand, the rescuer places the index and middle finger on the center of the breastbone and makes four sharp chest thrusts. This series of back blows and chest thrusts is alternated until the foreign object is expelled.

SELF-ADMINISTRATION OF THE HEIMLICH MANEUVER

To apply the Heimlich maneuver to oneself, one should make a fist with one hand and place it in the middle of the body at a spot above the navel and below the breastbone, then grasp the fist with the other hand and push sharply inward and upward. If this fails, the victim should press the upper abdomen over the back of a chair, edge of a table, porch railing or something similar, and thrust up and inward until the object is dislodged.

Preparation

Any lay person can be trained to perform the Heimlich maneuver. Knowing how may save someone's life. Before doing the maneuver, it is important to determine if the airway is completely blocked. If the person choking can talk or cry, Heimlich maneuver is not appropriate. If the airway is not completely blocked, the choking victim should be allowed to try to cough up the foreign object on his or her own.

Aftercare

Many people vomit after being treated with the Heimlich maneuver. Depending on the length and severity of the choking episode, the choking victim may need to be taken to a hospital emergency room.

Risks

Incorrectly applied, the Heimlich maneuver can break bones or damage internal organs. In infants, the rescuer should never attempt to sweep the baby's mouth

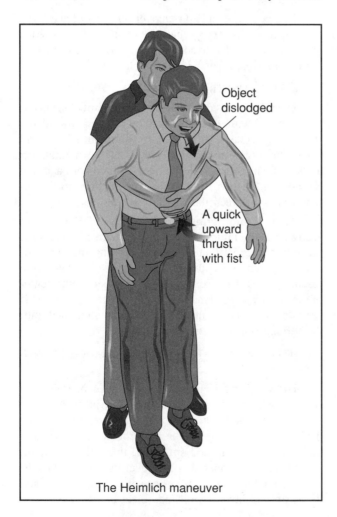

Object dislodged

A quick upward thrust with fist

The Heimlich maneuver

To perform the Heimlich maneuver on a conscious adult (as illustrated above), the rescuer stands behind the victim and encircles his waist. The rescuer makes a fist with one hand and places the other hand on top, positioned below the rib cage and above the waist. The rescuer then applies pressure by a series of upward and inward thrusts to force the foreign object back up the victim's trachea. *(Illustration by Electronic Illustrators Group.)*

without looking to remove foreign material. This is likely to push the material farther down the trachea.

Normal results

In many cases the foreign material is dislodged from the throat, and the choking victim suffers no permanent effects of the episode. If the foreign material is not removed, the person dies from lack of oxygen.

Resources

BOOKS

"Heimlich Maneuver." In *Everything You Need to Know About Medical Treatments.* Springhouse, PA: Springhouse Corp., 1996.

PERIODICALS

Dworkin, Gerald "The Heimlich Maneuver Controversy in Near-Drowning Resuscitation. In*Parks and Recreation* (Nov 1997) v32, n11 p16.

ORGANIZATIONS

American Heart Association. (800) 242-8721. http://www.amhrt.org.

Tish Davidson

Heliobacter pylori infection *see* **Helicobacteriosis**

. . . .

Helicobacteriosis

Definition

Helicobacteriosis refers to infection of the gastrointestinal tract with the bacteria, *Helicobacter pylori* (*H. pylori*). While there are other rarer strains of *Helicobacter* species that can infect humans, only *H. pylori* has been convincingly shown to be a cause of disease in humans. The organism was first documented to cause injury to the stomach in 1983, by two researchers in Australia, who ingested the organism to prove their theory. Since then, this bacteria has been shown to be the main cause of ulcer disease, and has revolutionized the treatment of peptic ulcer disease. It is also believed to be a cause of various cancers of the stomach.

Description

H. pylori is a gram-negative, spiral shaped organism, that contains flagella (tail-like structure) and other properties that allow it to survive in the acidic environment of the stomach. In addition to flagella, which allow the

KEY TERMS

Antibiotic—A medication that is designed to kill or weaken bacteria.

Endoscope, Endoscopy—An Endoscope as used in the field of Gastroenterology is a thin flexible tube which uses a lens or miniature camera to view various areas of the gastrointestinal tract. When the procedure is performed to examine certain organs such as the bile ducts or pancreas, the organs are not viewed directly, but rather indirectly through the injection of x-ray. The performance of an exam using an endoscope is referred by the general term Endoscopy. Diagnosis through biopsies or other means and therapeutic procedures can be done with these instruments.

Gram-negative—Refers to the property of many bacteria in which they do not take or color with Gram's stain, a method which is used to identify bacteria. Gram-positive bacteria which take up the stain turn purple, while Gram-negative bacteria which do not take up the stain turn red.

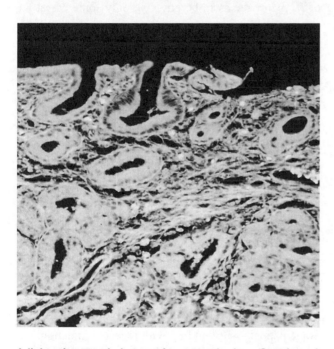

A light microscopic image of a stomach ulcer. Gastric and duodenal ulcers are usually caused by infection with the bacteria *Helicobacter pylori*. This bacterium is also believed to be a cause of various cancers of the stomach. *(Photograph by J.L. Carson, Custom Medical Stock Photo. Reproduced by permission.)*

organism to move around in the liquid mucous layer of the stomach, *H. pylori* also produces an enzyme called "urease," that protects it from harm by gastric acid. As the production of this enzyme is relatively unusual, new diagnostic tests have enabled rapid identification of the bacteria.

H. pylori also produces two other chemicals; a cytotoxin called VacA, and a protein known as CagA. Patients with ulcer disease are more likely to produce the cytotoxin (VacA). The CagA protein not only occurs frequently in ulcer disease but also in **cancer.** It is still not known how these substances enable *H. pylori* to cause disease.

Causes & symptoms

Infection with *H. pylori* is largely dependent on two factors; age and income status. The bacteria is acquired mainly in childhood, especially in areas of poor hygiene or overcrowding. *H. pylori* is 2–3 times more prevalent in developing, non-industrialized countries. In the United States for example, the organism is believed to be present in about onethird of the population.

The exact way in which *H. pylori* gets passed from one individual to another is uncertain, but person to person transmission is most likely. In most cases, children are felt to be the source of spread. Reinfection of those who have been cured has been documented, especially in areas of overcrowding.

The bacteria is well adapted to survival within the stomach. Not only does it survive there for years, but once infection begins, a form of chronic inflammation (chronic **gastritis**) always develops. In most individuals, initial infection causes little or no symptoms; however, some individuals such as the original researchers who ingested the bacteria, wind up with abdominal **pain** and nausea.

In about 15% of infected persons, ulcer disease develops either in the stomach or duodenum. Why some develop ulcer disease and others do not, remains unclear. Ulcer symptoms are characterized by upper abdominal pain that is typically of a burning or "gnawing" type, and usually is rapidly relieved by **antacids** or food.

Acid secretion increases in most patients with duodenal **ulcers.** This increase returns to normal once *H. pylori* is eliminated. It is now known that elimination of the bacteria will decrease substantially the risk of recurrent bouts of ulcer disease in the far majority (85% or so) of patients.

In the last decade it has been shown that *H. pylori* is not only the prime cause of ulcer disease of the stomach and duodenum, but is also strongly associated with various tumors of the stomach. Bacterial infection is 9 times more common in patients with cancer of the stomach, and 7 times more common in those with lymphoma of the stomach (tumor of the lymphatic tissue), called a MALT tumor. It is believed that the prolonged inflammation leads to changes in cell growth and tumors. Eliminating *H. pylori* can lead to regression of some tumors.

In addition to the above damage caused by *H. pylori*, some individuals lose normal gastric function, such as the ability to absorb vitamin B-12.

Diagnosis

There are basically two types of tests to identify infection; one group is "invasive" in that it involves the use of endoscopy to obtain biopsy specimens for evaluation, while the other "noninvasive" methods depend on blood or breath samples. None of these tests are 100% perfect. Invasive tests can be less accurate because of technical limits; for example the biopsy may miss the area where the bacteria hides. As of 1997, there was no agreement on a "gold standard" test.

Invasive studies make use of tissue obtained by endoscopic biopsy to identify the organism. The bacteria can be searched for in pieces of biopsy tissue or grown (cultured) from the specimen. *H. pylori* though is not easy to culture. Another method uses the bacteria's production of the enzyme urease. Biopsy specimens are placed on a card which changes color if urease is present. Results are often available within a few minutes, but can take up to 24 hours.

Non-invasive tests are of two types; blood tests and breath test. Blood tests measure antibodies to make a diagnosis accurately within minutes. This can be done immediately in the doctor's office. In addition, antibody levels can be measured several months after treatment, to see if *H. pylori* has been eradicated.

The breath test uses radioactive or non-radioactive forms of a compound called urea, which the patient drinks. The method that uses a radioactive form urea is easier to perform, as the equipment is commonly available in x-ray departments. Radiation exposure is less than that of a chest x-ray. The test that uses non-radioactive urea is safer for children. The breath test is the best way to be sure of elimination of *H. pylori*. The test can be used within 30 days after treatment. This is a big advantage over following antibody levels which take 6 months or longer to diminish.

Treatment

For years the treatment of ulcer disease was based on decreasing acid secretion by the stomach. This worked, but ulcers almost always recurred once treatment was stopped. In the 1990s, it was clearly shown that the bacteria *H. pylori* and not acid, was the cause of most ulcers.

It is now known that the "cure" of ulcer disease is possible if the bacterial infection is eliminated. Several different strategies have been developed and as of 1997 the FDA approved five of these. Many more are available in Europe and newer regimens continue to be developed. Furthermore, a decrease in size and possible cure of some tumors of the stomach have been reported.

All treatments have in common the use of at least one antibiotic to eliminate infection, combined with other antibacterial drugs. Some therapies use two drugs while others use three. Infection fails to be cured in 10% of patients even with the most aggressive treatments.

The drawbacks of medications are their side effects and the need to take these for up to two weeks or more. The main symptoms are gastrointestinal, and include nausea, vomiting, and **diarrhea.** In some instances, side effects are severe enough to discontinue treatment. Some of the newer therapeutic combinations produce fewer side effects, and require less length of treatment.

It is now clear that those with documented ulcer disease should be treated and all attempts to eliminate the bacteria be made, even if repeated courses of medication is necessary.

For patients with tumors of the stomach, elimination of *H. pylori* seems to be effective only some cases.

Other controversies are;

• What to do with patients who have a family history of cancer of the stomach and are infected. It is still not proven that they should be treated, but many authorities do suggest this. Further studies will be needed.

• Another difficult problem concerns a syndrome called "Non Ulcer **Dyspepsia"** or NUD. This is characterized by symptoms of dyspepsia (**indigestion**), without ulcer disease. Treatment of this group of patients remains controversial and further study is needed in this area.

Prognosis

As noted above, the elimination of *H. pylori* and cure of ulcer disease and is now possible in more than 80% of those infected. The finding that most ulcers are due to an infectious agent has brought a dramatic change in treatment and outlook for those suffering from that disease. Some patients will wind up with repeated infection, but this is most common in overcrowded areas.

Prevention

Attempts to develop a vaccine to protect against infection may be worthwhile in areas where the *H. pylori* infection rate and occurrence of cancer of the stomach is quite high, such as in Japan.

Resources

BOOKS

Atherton, John C., and Blaser, Martin J. "Helicobacter Infections." In *Harrison's Principles of Internal Medicine,* edited by Anthony S. Fauci, et al. New York: McGraw-Hill, 1998, pp. 941-943.

Peterson, Walter L., and Graham, David Y. "Helicobacter pylori." In *Sleisenger & Fordtran's Gastrointestinal and Liver Disease,* edited by Mark Feldman, et al. Philadelphia: W.B. Saunders Company. 1997, pp. 604-619.

PERIODICALS

Hunt, Richard H. "Peptic Ulcer Disease: Defining the Treatment Strategies in the Era of Helicobacter pylori." *American Journal of Gastroenterology* 92 no. 4 Supplement(1997): 36S.

Lee, Adrian. "The Helicobacter pylori Genome—New Insights into Pathogenesis and Therapeutics." *New England Journal of Medicine* 338 no. 12(1998): 832.

Parsonnet, Julie. "Helicobacter pylori in the Stomach—A Paradox Unmasked." *New England Journal of Medicine* 335 no. 4(1996): 278.

Rabeneck, Linda and Graham, David Y. "Helicobacter pylori: When to Test, When to Treat." *Annals of Internal Medicine* 126 no. 4(1997): 315.

Walsh, John H. and Peterson, Walter L. "Drug Therapy: The Treatment of Helicobacter pylori Infection in the Management of Peptic Ulcer Disease." *New England Journal of Medicine* 333 no. 15(1995): 984.

ORGANIZATIONS

The Helicobacter Foundation. http://www.helico.com/.

OTHER

Barry Marshall's Home Page. http://jimi.vianet.net.au/~bjmrshll/.

GI Focus-Helicobacter pylori. http://www.acg.gi.org/phyforum/gifocus/2ei.html.

H. Pylori and Peptic Ulcer. http://www.niddk.nih.gov/health/digest/pubs/hpylori/hpylori.htm.

Management Strategies for Helicobacter pyloriSeropositive Patients with Dyspepsia. http://www.acponline.org/journals/annals/15feb97/treatcounsel.htm.

Moving closer to an ulcer vaccine. http://www.msnbc.com/news/161712.asp.

Treating Stomach Ulcers and H. pylori Infection. http://www.aafp.org/patientinfo/ulcers.html.

Ulcers and Bacteria-The Role of H. pylori. http://www.aafp.org/patientinfo/hpylori.html.

What Is Helicobacter pylori Infection?. http://www.cdc.gov/ncidod/aip/aip_a2b.htm.

David S. Kaminstein

Hellerwork

Definition

Hellerwork is a type of bodywork that combines deep tissue **massage** with movement education and guided verbal dialog.

Purpose

This technique is aimed at preventing illness and achieving vitality by realigning the body and releasing physical and emotional tensions.

Precautions

Hellerwork does not treat disease. It is safe for most people, although it should not be used in cases of **cancer** where tissue manipulation could speed the progress of the disease.

Description

Hellerwork is named after its founder, Joseph Heller, an engineer and former disciple of **Rolfing.** Rolfing was created in the 1930s by Dr. Ida P. Rolf, and consists of the manipulation or massage of the body's connective tissue and muscles in order to realign and balance the body's structure and therefore improve posture and overall physical and emotional health. In the 1970s, Heller left his position as president of the Rolf Institute in Colorado to create his own variation of deep tissue massage therapy. Heller believed that manipulation alone was insufficient, since he felt it did not provide long-term or lasting results. He therefore added educational aspects, as well as a process that involves the patient in a dialog or discussion. In addition to actual bodywork therefore, he provided education and guidance on how to move properly so as to release tensions, and supplemented that with a dialog in which the practitioner engages the client in a discussion designed to reveal the important role our habits and emotions play in our health. In order to bring about lasting, beneficial changes in the body, Heller designed a structured, thematic approach consisting of eleven sessions that realign the body and reeducate the mind.

The physical goals that Hellerwork seeks to achieve are essentially the same as those of Rolfing. Basically, its manipulation technique is a systems approach to putting the entire body back into its original balance in which a person's nervous system, organs, mind, and natural healing systems function efficiently.

The complete Hellerwork program consists of eleven 90-minute sessions, the first of which includes three photographs—back, side, and front views—to document the participant's starting posture and overall appearance.

The first three sessions consist of gentle or superficial bodywork, in which the practitioner applies pressure with his or her hands, fingers, or sometimes elbows, and works on realigning the chest area to permit fuller and more natural breathing. To this strictly physical aspect of therapy, Hellerwork adds a psychological content such as engaging the client in a discussion that suggests to him or her how certain emotional states or attitudes can affect breathing.

The next series of four sessions are called the core sessions and involve such muscles as those of the inside leg, pelvis, and spine, as well as those of the head and neck. Often, these muscles are tight and not very flexible, and once the practitioner manipulates and loosens them, the client is instructed in how to move them more harmoniously.

The final series is called the integrative sessions, since they work toward integrating the physical realignments and the instruction received into the client's everyday life. Thus, by the program's end, clients will have not only been instructed on how to sit, stand, walk, and run in a manner that is most natural with their particular makeup, but also they will have become more aware of the importance of proper movement, as well as how they can maintain what they have learned and achieved. Photographs taken at the last session are compared with those taken at the beginning.

Overall, Hellerwork can be beneficial for those with muscular problems that are caused by poor posture and movement. It also can serve to make individuals more aware of any emotional or situational problems that could be contributing to their physical difficulties.

Risks

Although safe for most people, Hellerwork could aggravate cases of inflammatory nerve, muscle, or joint conditions. It is also not recommended for those with an organic disease.

Normal results

The goal of Hellerwork is to promote overall health through the prevention of disease by keeping the body and mind in perfect balance. It is also employed to help people with everyday aches and **pains,** as well as those who have neck or back pain, or **headache.**

Resources

BOOKS

Bradford, Nikki, ed. *Alternative Healthcare.* San Diego, CA: Thunder Bay Press, 1996.

Burton Goldberg Group. *Alternative Medicine: The Definitive Guide.* Puyallup, WA: Future Medicine Publishing Group, 1993.

Nash, Barbara. *From Acupressure to Zen: An Encyclopedia of Natural Therapies.* Almeda, CA: Hunter House, Inc., 1996.

PERIODICALS

Chipkin, Harvey. "Hellerwork." *Health* (September 1984): 13.

ORGANIZATIONS

The Body of Knowledge/Hellerwork. 406 Berry St. Mt. Shasta, CA 96067. (916) 926-2500.

Leonard C. Bruno

Hemangiomas *see* **Birthmarks**

Hematocrit

Definition

The hematocrit measures how much space in the blood is occupied by red blood cells. It is useful when evaluating a person for anemia.

Purpose

Blood is made up of red and white blood cells, and plasma. A decrease in the number or size of red cells also decreases the amount of space they occupy, resulting in a lower hematocrit. An increase in the number or size of red cells increases the amount of space they occupy, resulting in a higher hematocrit. Thalassemia is a condition which can cause an increased number of red blood cells but a decreased size and hematocrit.

The hematocrit is usually done on a person with symptoms of anemia. An anemic person has fewer or smaller than normal red cells. A low hematocrit, combined with other abnormal blood tests, confirms the diagnosis.

Some conditions, such as polycythemia, cause an overproduction of red blood cells, resulting in an increased hematocrit.

Transfusion decisions are based on the results of laboratory tests, including hematocrit. Transfusion is not considered if the hematocrit level is reasonable. The level differs for each person, depending on his or her clinical condition.

Description

Blood drawn from a fingerstick is often used for hematocrit testing. The blood fills a small tube, which is then spun in a small centrifuge. As the tube spins, the red blood cells go to the bottom of the tube, the white blood cells cover the red in a thin layer called the buffy coat, and the liquid plasma rises to the top. The spun tube is examined for the line that divides the red cells from the buffy coat and plasma. The height of the red cell column is measured as a percent of the total blood column. The higher the column of red cells, the higher the hematocrit.

The hematocrit test can also be done on an automated instrument as part of a complete **blood count.** It is also called Packed Red Cell Volume or Packed Cell Volume, or abbreviated as Hct or Crit. The test is covered by insurance when medically necessary. Results are usually available the same or following day.

Preparation

To collect the blood by fingerstick, a healthcare worker punctures a finger with a lancet and allows the blood to fill a small tube held to the puncture site.

Tests done on an automated instrument require 5–7 mL of blood. A healthcare worker ties a tourniquet on the person's upper arm, locates a vein in the inner elbow region, and inserts a needle into that vein. Vacuum action draws the blood through the needle into an attached tube. Collection of the sample takes only a few minutes.

Aftercare

Discomfort or bruising may occur at the puncture site or the person may feel dizzy or faint. Pressure to the puncture site until the bleeding stops reduces bruising. Warm packs to the puncture site relieve discomfort.

Normal results

Normal values vary with age and sex. Adult male 42–52% Adult female 36–48%

Abnormal results

Hematocrit values decrease when the size or number of red cells decrease. This is most common in anemia, but other conditions have similar effects: excessive bleeding, damaged cells due to a mechanical heart valve, liver disease, and **cancers** affecting the bone marrow. Additional tests, and the person's symptoms and medical history help distinguish these conditions or diagnose a specific type of anemia. Hematocrit values increase when the size or number of red cells increase, such as in polycythemia.

Fluid volume in the blood affects the hematocrit. Pregnant women have extra fluid, which dilutes the blood, decreasing the hematocrit. **Dehydration** concentrates the blood, increasing the hematocrit.

Nancy J. Nordenson

Hemiballismus *see* **Movement disorders**

Hemiplegia *see* **Paralysis**

Hemochromatosis

Definition

Hemochromatosis is an inherited blood disorder that causes the body to retain excessive amounts of iron. This iron overload can lead to serious health consequences, most notably **cirrhosis** of the liver.

Description

Hemochromatosis is also known as iron overload, bronze diabetes, hereditary hemochromatosis and familial hemochromatosis. The inherited disorder causes increased absorption of intestinal iron, well beyond that needed to replace the body's loss of iron. Iron overload diseases afflict as many as 1.5 million persons in the United States. The most common of these, as well as one of the most common genetic disorders in the United States, is hereditary hemochromatosis. Men and women are equally affected by hemochromatosis, but women are diagnosed later in life because of blood loss from menstruation and childbirth. It most commonly appears in patients between the ages of 40–60, since it takes many years for the body to accumulate excessive iron.

Hemochromatosis causes excess iron storage in several organs of the body including the liver, pancreas, endocrine glands, heart, skin, and intestinal lining. The buildup of iron in these organs can lead to serious complications, including **heart failure,** liver cancer, and cirrhosis of the liver. It is estimated that about 5% of cirrhosis cases are caused by hereditary hemochromatosis.

Idiopathic pulmonary hemosiderosis, a disorder afflicting children and young adults, is a similar overload disorder characterized by abnormal accumulation of hemosiderin. Hemosiderin is a protein found in most tissues, especially the liver. It is produced by digestion of hematin, an iron-related substance.

Causes & symptoms

Hereditary hemochromatosis is passed by an autosomal recessive trait on the genes. (Scientists have recently identified the precise gene.) Because of its hereditary nature, as many as 25% of the siblings of hemochromatosis patients will also develop the disorder.

The symptoms of hemochromatosis include fatigue, weight loss, weakness, **shortness of breath,** heart **palpitations,** chronic abdominal **pain,** and impaired sexual performance. The patient may also show symptoms commonly connected with heart failure, diabetes or cirrhosis of the liver. Changes in the pigment of the skin may appear, such as grayness in certain areas, or a tanned or yellow (**jaundice**) appearance.

Idiopathic pulmonary hemosiderosis may first, and only, appear as paleness of the skin. Sometimes, the patient will experience spitting of blood from the lungs or bronchial tubes.

Diagnosis

The most common diagnostic methods for hemochromatosis are blood tests and **computed tomography scan** (CT scan). In recent years, CT scans with quantitative assessment of iron concentration has almost eliminated the need for **liver biopsy.** Blood tests will measure excessive iron levels. Concentrations of transferrin, a protein that transports iron and liver enzymes will also be measured. Serum ferritin and iron saturation are the best screening tests. Another test that measures an iron protein complex. In some cases, DNA testing for certain indications that young siblings will develop the disease will be conducted. X-ray studies of the liver, pituitary gland, and other iron absorbing organs may reveal abnormal iron deposits. CT scans, or **magnetic resonance imaging** (MRI) are the exams of choice for these studies.

Once a physician has identified signs of hemochromatosis with blood tests, a liver biopsy may be necessary. This involves insertion of a thin needle into the liver while the patient is under local anesthesia. The needle will extract a small amount of liver tissue, which can be analyzed microscopically to measure its iron content and other signs of hemochromatosis. Diagnosis of idiopathic pulmonary hemosiderosis begins with blood tests and x-ray studies of the chest.

Treatment

Patients who show signs of iron overload will often be treated with **phlebotomy.** Phlebotomy is a procedure that involves drawing blood from the patient, much like blood donation. Its purpose as a treatment is to rid the body of excess iron storage. Patients may need these procedures one or two times a week for a year or more. Less frequent phlebotomy may be continued in subsequent years to keep excess iron from accumulating. Patients who cannot tolerate phlebotomy due to other medical problems can be treated with Desferal (desferrioxamine). Diet restrictions may also be prescribed to limit the amount of iron ingested. Individuals who know they have the genetic makeup for hemochromatosis may postpone its onset by limiting iron intake and avoiding iron supplements. Complications from hemochromatosis, such as cirrhosis or diabetes, may also require treatment. Treatment for idiopathic pulmonary hemosiderosis is based on symptoms.

Alternative treatment

Diet restrictions may help lower the amount of iron in the body, but may not be enough to prevent or treat hemochromatosis. Patients who know they have the hereditary markers for the disease may limit iron-rich foods such as liver, red meat and iron-fortified cereals help keep iron levels down.

Prognosis

With early detection, the prognosis is usually good, particularly if the patient has worked aggressively to deplete iron before symptoms began. However, if left untreated, complications may arise which can be fatal. These include liver cancer, liver cirrhosis, **diabetes mellitus,** and failure to achieve iron depletion through phlebotomy. The prognosis for patients with idiopathic pulmonary hemosiderosis is fair, depending on detection and complications.

Prevention

Screening for hemochromatosis has become more cost effective, particularly for certain groups of people. Relatives, especially siblings, of patients with hemochromatosis should be tested for genes that indicate predisposition to the disease. Those relatives can begin to take measures to reduce iron intake or deplete iron stores prior to onset of symptoms.

Resources

PERIODICALS

Chazin, Suzanne. "Is Iron Making You Sick?" *Readers Digest,* (October 1995).

Wolfe, Yun Lee. "Case of the Ceaselss Fatigue" *Prevention Magazine,* (July 1997):88.

ORGANIZATIONS

American Hemochromatosis Society, Inc. 777 E. Atlantic Ave., Z-363, Delray Beach, FL 33483-5352. http://www.americanhs.org.

Hemochromatosis Foundation, Inc. P.O. Box 8569, Albany, NY 12208-0569. (518)489-0972.

Iron Overload Diseases Association, Inc. 433 Westwind Drive, North Palm Beach, FL 33408. (407)840-8512.

Teresa G. Norris

Hemodialysis *see* **Kidney dialysis**

Hemoglobin electrophoresis

Definition

Hemoglobin electrophoresis (also called Hgb electrophoresis), is a test that measures the different types of hemoglobin in the blood. The method used is called electrophoresis, a process that causes movement of particles in an electric field, resulting in formation of "bands" that separate toward one end or the other in the field.

Purpose

Hgb electrophoresis is performed when a disorder associated with abnormal hemoglobin (hemoglobinopathy) is suspected. The test is used primarily to diagnose diseases involving these abnormal forms of hemoglobin, such as **sickle cell anemia** and thalassemia.

Precautions

Blood **transfusions** within the previous 12 weeks may alter test results.

Description

Hemoglobin (Hgb) is comprised of many different types, the most common being A_1, A_2, F, S, and C.

Hgb A_1 is the major component of hemoglobin in the normal red blood cell. Hgb A_2 is a minor component of normal hemoglobin, comprising approximately 2–3% of the total.

Hgb F is the major hemoglobin component in the fetus, but usually exists only in minimal quantities in the normal adult. Levels of Hgb F greater than 2% in patients over three years of age are considered abnormal.

Hgb S is an abnormal form of hemoglobin associated with the disease of sickle cell anemia, which occurs predominantly in African-Americans. A distinguishing characteristic of sickle cell disease is the crescent-shaped red blood cell. Because the survival rate of this type of cell is limited, patients with sickle cell disease also have anemia.

Hgb C is another hemoglobin variant found in African Americans. Red blood cells containing Hgb C have a decreased life span and are more readily destroyed than normal red blood cells, resulting in mild to severe **hemolytic anemia.**

Each of the major hemoglobin types has an electrical charge of a different degree, so the most useful method for separating and measuring normal and abnormal hemoglobins is electrophoresis. This process involves subjecting hemoglobin components from dissolved red blood cells to an electric field. The components then move away from each other at different rates, and when

KEY TERMS

Hemoglobin C disease—A disease of abnormal hemoglobin, occurring in 2–3% of African-Americans. Only those who have two genes for the disease develop anemia, which varies in severity. Symptoms include episodes of abdominal and joint pain, an enlarged spleen and mild jaundice.

Hemoglobin H disease—A thalassemia-like syndrome causing moderate anemia and red blood cell abnormalities.

Heterozygous—Two different genes controlling a specified inherited trait.

Homozygous—Identical genes controlling a specified inherited trait.

Thalassemias—The name for a group of inherited disorders resulting from an imbalance in the production of one of the four chains of amino acids that make up hemoglobin. Thalassemias are categorized according to the amino acid chain affected. The two main types are alpha-thalassemia and beta-thalassemia. The disorders are further characterized by the presence of one defective gene (thalassemia minor) or two defective genes (thalassemia major). Symptoms vary, but include anemia, jaundice, skin ulcers, gallstones, and an enlarged spleen.

separated form a series of distinctly pigmented bands. The bands are then compared with those of a normal sample. Each band can be further assessed as a percentage of the total hemoglobin, thus indicating the severity of any abnormality.

Preparation

This test requires a blood sample. No special preparation is needed before the test.

Risks

Risks for this test are minimal, but may include slight bleeding from the blood-drawing site, **fainting** or feeling lightheaded after venipuncture, or hematoma (blood accumulating under the puncture site).

Normal results

Normal reference values can vary by laboratory, but are generally within the following ranges.

Adults:

- Hgb A_1: 95–98%
- Hgb A_2: 2–3%
- Hgb F: 0.8–2.0%
- Hgb S: 0%
- Hgb C: 0%.

    Child (Hgb F):

- 6 months: 8%
- Greater than 6 months: 1–2%
- Newborn (Hgb F): 50–80%.

Abnormal results

Abnormal reference values can vary by laboratory, but when they appear within these ranges, results are usually associated with the conditions that follow in parentheses.

Hgb A_2:

- 4–5.8% (β-**thalassemia** minor)
- Under 2% (Hgb H disease).

    Hgb F:

- 2–5% (β-thalassemia minor)
- 10–90% (β-thalassemia major)
- 5–35% (Heterozygous hereditary persistence of fetal hemoglobin, or HPFH)
- 100% (Homozygous HPFH)
- 15% (Homozygous Hgb S).

    Homozygous Hgb S:

- 70–98% (Sickle cell disease).

    Homozygous Hgb C:

- 90–98%(Hgb C disease).

Resources

BOOKS

Cahill, Mathew. *Handbook of Diagnostic Tests.* Springhouse, PA: Springhouse Corporation, 1995.

Jacobs, David S. *Laboratory Test Handbook,* 4th ed. Hudson, OH: Lexi-Comp Inc., 1996.

Pagana, Kathleen Deska. *Mosby's Manual of Diagnostic and Laboratory Tests.* St. Louis: Mosby, Inc., 1998.

Janis O. Flores

Hemoglobin F test *see* **Fetal hemoglobin test**

Hemoglobin test

Definition

Hemoglobin is a protein inside red blood cells that carries oxygen throughout the body. A hemoglobin test reveals how much hemoglobin is in a person's blood, helping to diagnose and monitor anemia and **polycythemia vera.**

Purpose

A hemoglobin test is done when a person is ill or during a general physical examination. Good health requires an adequate amount of hemoglobin. The amount of oxygen in the body tissues depends on how much hemoglobin is in the red cells. Without enough hemoglobin, the tissues lack oxygen and the heart and lungs must work harder to try to compensate.

If the test indicates a "less than" or "greater than" normal amount of hemoglobin, the cause of the decrease or increase must be discovered. A low hemoglobin usually means the person has anemia. Anemia results from conditions that decrease the number or size of red cells, such as excessive bleeding, a dietary deficiency, destruction of cells because of a **transfusion** reaction or mechanical heart valve, or an abnormally formed hemoglobin.

A high hemoglobin may be caused by polycythemia vera, a disease in which too many red blood cells are made.

Hemoglobin levels also help determine if a person needs a blood transfusion. Usually a person's hemoglobin must be below 8 gm/dl before a transfusion is considered.

Description

Hemoglobin is made of heme, an iron compound, and globin, a protein. The iron gives blood its red color. Hemoglobin tests make use of this red color. A chemical is added to a sample of blood to make the red blood cells burst. When they burst, the red cells release hemoglobin into the surrounding fluid, coloring it clear red. By mea-

suring the color using an instrument called a spectrophotometer, the amount of hemoglobin is determined.

Hemoglobin is often ordered as part of a complete **blood count** (CBC), a test that includes other blood cell measurements.

Some people inherit hemoglobin with an abnormal structure. These abnormal hemoglobins cause diseases, such as sickle cell or Hemoglobin C disease. Special tests, using a process called **hemoglobin electrophoresis,** identify abnormal hemoglobins.

Preparation

This test requires 5 mL of blood. A healthcare worker ties a tourniquet on the person's upper arm, locates a vein in the inner elbow region, and inserts a needle into that vein. Vacuum action draws the blood through the needle into an attached tube. Collection of the sample takes only a few minutes.

The person should avoid smoking before this test as smoking can increase hemoglobin levels.

Aftercare

Discomfort or bruising may occur at the puncture site or the person may feel dizzy or faint. Pressure to the puncture site until the bleeding stops reduces bruising. Warm packs to the puncture site relieve discomfort.

Normal results

Normal values vary with age and sex. Women generally have lower hemoglobin values than men. Men 14.0–18.0 g/dL Women 12.0–16.0 g/dL

Abnormal results

A low hemoglobin usually indicates the person has anemia. Further tests are done to discover the cause and type of anemia. Dangerously low hemoglobin levels put a person at risk of a **heart attack,** congestive **heart failure,** or **stroke.**

A high hemoglobin indicates the body is making too many red cells. Further tests are done to see if this is caused by polycythemia vera, or as a reaction to illness, high altitudes, heart failure, or lung disease.

Fluid volume in the blood affects hemoglobin values. Pregnant women and people with **cirrhosis** have extra fluid, which dilutes the blood, decreasing the hemoglobin. **Dehydration** concentrates the blood, increasing the hemoglobin.

Resources

PERIODICALS

Hsia, Connie C. W. "Respiratory Function of Hemoglobin." *New England Journal of Medicine.* 338 (January 98): 239-247.

Nancy J. Nordenson

Hemolytic anemia

Definition

Red blood cells have a normal life span of approximately 90–120 days, at which time the old cells are destroyed and replaced by the body's natural processes. Hemolytic anemia is a disorder in which the red blood cells are destroyed prematurely. The cells are broken down at a faster rate than the bone marrow can produce new cells. Hemoglobin, the component of red blood cells that carries oxygen, is released when these cells are destroyed.

Description

As a group, **anemias** (conditions in which the number of red blood cells or the amount of hemoglobin in them is below normal) are the most common blood disorders. Hemolytic anemias, which result from the increased destruction of red blood cells, are less common than anemias caused by excessive blood loss or by decreased hemoglobin or red cell production.

Since a number of factors can increase red blood cell destruction, hemolytic anemias are generally identified by the disorder that brings about the premature destruction. Those disorders are classified as either inherited or acquired. Inherited hemolytic anemias are caused by inborn defects in components of the red blood cells—the cell membrane, the enzymes, or the hemoglobin. Acquired hemolytic anemias are those that result from various other causes. With this type, red cells are produced normally, but are prematurely destroyed because of damage that occurs to them in the circulation.

Causes & symptoms

Inherited hemolytic anemias involve conditions that interfere with normal red blood cell production. Disorders that affect the red blood cell membrane include hereditary spherocytosis, in which the normally disk-shaped red cells become spherical, and hereditary elliptocytosis, in which the cells are oval, rather than disk-shaped. Other hereditary conditions that cause hemolytic anemia include disorders of the hemoglobin, such as

KEY TERMS

Antibody—Antibodies are parts of the immune system which counteract or eliminate foreign substances or antigens.

Erythrocyte—The name for red blood cells or red blood corpuscles. These components of the blood are responsible for carrying oxygen to tissues and removing carbon dioxide from tissues.

Hemolysis—The process of breaking down of red blood cells. As the cells are destroyed, hemoglobin, the component of red blood cells which carries the oxygen, is liberated.

Thalassemia—One of a group of inherited blood disorders characterized by a defect in the metabolism of hemoglobin, or the portion of the red blood cells that transports oxygen throughout the blood stream.

sickle cell anemia and **thalassemia,** and red blood cell enzyme deficiencies, such as G6PD deficiency.

The causes of acquired hemolytic anemias vary, but the most common are responses to certain medications and infections. Medications may cause the body to develop antibodies that bind to the red blood cells and cause their destruction in the spleen. Immune hemolytic anemia most commonly involves antibodies that react against the red blood cells at body temperature (warm—antibody hemolytic anemia), which can cause premature destruction of the cells. About 20% of hemolytic anemias caused by warm antibodies come from diseases such as lymphocytic leukemia, 10% from an autoimmune disease, and others are drug-induced. Cold-antibody hemolytic anemia is a condition in which the antibodies react with the red blood cells at a temperature below that of normal body temperature. Red blood cells can also receive mechanical damage as they circulate through the blood vessels. Aneurysms, artificial heart valves, or very high blood pressure can cause the red cells to break up and release their contents. In addition, hemolytic anemia may be caused by a condition called **hypersplenism,** in which a large, overactive spleen rapidly destroys red blood cells.

Major symptoms of hemolytic anemias are similar to those for all anemias, including **shortness of breath;** noticeable increase in heart rate; especially with exertion; fatigue; pale appearance; and dark urine. A yellow tint, or **jaundice,** may be seen in the skin or eyes of hemolytic anemia patients. Examination may also show an enlarged spleen. A more emergent symptom of hemolytic anemia is **pain** in the upper abdomen. Severe anemia is indicated if there are signs of **heart failure** or an enlarged liver.

Diagnosis

In order to differentiate hemolytic anemia from others, physicians will examine the blood for the number of young red blood cells, since the number of young cells is increased in hemolytic anemia. The physician will also examine the abdominal area to check for spleen or liver enlargement. If the physician knows the duration of hemolysis, it may also help differentiate between types of anemia. There are a number of other indications that can be obtained from blood samples that will help a physician screen for hemolytic anemia. An antiglobulin (Coomb's) test may be performed as the initial screening exam after determining hemolysis. In the case of immune hemolytic anemia, a direct Coomb's test is almost always positive.

Treatment

Treatment will depend on the cause of the anemia, and may involve treatment of the underlying cause. If the hemolytic anemia was brought on by hereditary spherocytosis, the spleen may be removed. Corticosteroid medications, or adrenal steroids, may be effective, especially in hemolytic anemia due to antibodies. If the cause of the disorder is a medication, the medication should be stopped. When anemia is severe in conditions such as sickle cell anemia and thalassemia, blood **transfusions** may be indicated.

Prognosis

Hemolytic anemias are seldom fatal. However, if left untreated, hemolytic anemia can lead to heart failure or liver complications.

Prevention

Hemolytic anemia due to inherited disorders can not be prevented. Acquired hemolytic anemia may be prevented if the underlying disorder is managed properly.

Resources

PERIODICALS

American Autoimmune Related Diseases Association, Inc. *In. Focus: A quarterly newsletter of the AARDA.* Detroit, MI. (313)371-8600. http://www.aarda.org.

ORGANIZATIONS

The American Society of Hematology. 1200 19th Street NW, Suite 300, Washington, DC 20036-2422. (202)857-1118. http://www.hematology.org.

National Heart, Lung and Blood Institute. Building 31, Room 4A21, Bethesda, MD 20892. (301)496-4236. http://www.nhlbi.nih.gov.

OTHER

National Organization for Rare Disorders, Inc. website.http://www.pcnet.com/~orphan/.

Teresa G. Norris

. . . .

Hemophilia

Definition

Hemophilia is a genetic disorder—usually inherited—of the mechanism of blood clotting. Depending on the degree of the disorder present in an individual, excess bleeding may occur only after specific, predictable events (such as surgery, dental procedures, or injury), or may occur spontaneously, with no known initiating event.

Description

The normal mechanism for blood clotting is a complex series of events involving the interaction of the injured blood vessel, blood cells (called platelets), and over 20 different proteins which also circulate in the blood.

When a blood vessel is injured in a way that causes bleeding, platelets collect over the injured area, and form a temporary plug to prevent further bleeding. This temporary plug, however, is too disorganized to serve as a long-term solution, so a series of chemical events occur, resulting in the formation of a more reliable plug. The final plug involves tightly woven fibers of a material called fibrin. The production of fibrin requires the interaction of several chemicals, in particular a series of proteins called clotting factors. At least thirteen different clotting factors have been identified.

The clotting cascade, as it is usually called, is the series of events required to form the final fibrin clot. The cascade uses a technique called amplification to rapidly produce the proper sized fibrin clot from the small number of molecules initially activated by the injury.

In hemophilia, certain clotting factors are either decreased in quantity, absent, or improperly formed. Because the clotting cascade uses amplification to rapidly plug up a bleeding area, absence or inactivity of just one clotting factor can greatly increase **bleeding time.**

Hemophilia A is the most common type of bleeding disorder and involves decreased activity of factor VIII. There are three levels of factor VIII deficiency: severe, moderate and mild. This classification is based on the percentage of normal factor VIII activity present:

KEY TERMS

Amplification—A process by which something is made larger. In clotting, only a very few chemicals are released by the initial injury; they result in a cascade of chemical reactions which produces increasingly larger quantities of different chemicals, resulting in an appropriately-sized, strong fibrin clot.

Factors—Coagulation factors are substances in the blood, such as proteins and minerals, that are necessary for clotting. Each clotting substance is designated with roman numerals I through XIII.

Fibrin—The final substance created through the clotting cascade, which provides a strong, reliable plug to prevent further bleeding from the initial injury.

Hemorrhage—Very severe, massive bleeding which is difficult to control. Hemorrhage can occur in hemophiliacs after what would be a relatively minor injury to a person with normal clotting factors.

Mutation—In genetic inheritance, a permanent change in part of a chromosome.

Platelets—Blood cells involved in the clotting process.

Trauma—Injury.

• Individuals with less than 1% of normal factor VIII activity level have severe hemophilia. Half of all people with hemophilia A fall into this category. Such individuals frequently experience spontaneous bleeding, most frequently into their joints, skin, and muscles. Surgery or trauma can result in life-threatening hemorrhage, and must be carefully managed.

• Individuals with 1–5% of normal factor VIII activity level have moderate hemophilia, and are at risk for heavy bleeding after seemingly minor traumatic injury.

• Individuals with 5–40% of normal factor VIII activity level have mild hemophilia, and must prepare carefully for any surgery or dental procedures.

Individuals with hemophilia B have symptoms very similar to those of hemophilia A, but the deficient factor is factor IX. This type of hemophilia is also known as Christmas disease.

Hemophilia C is very rare, and much more mild than hemophilia A or B; it involves factor XI.

Causes & symptoms

How hemophilia is inherited

Hemophilia A and B are both caused by a genetic defect present on the X chromosome. (Hemophilia C is inherited in a different fashion.) About 70% of all people with hemophilia A or B inherited the disease. The other thirty percent have hemophilia because of a spontaneous genetic mutation.

The following concepts are important to understanding the inheritance of these diseases. All humans have two chromosomes which determine their gender: females have XX, males have XY. Because the trait is carried only on the X chromosome, it is called ''sex-linked.'' The chromosome's flawed unit is referred to as the gene.

Since both factors VIII and IX are produced by a genetic defect of the X chromosome, hemophilia A and B are both sex-linked diseases. Because a female child always receives two X chromosomes, she nearly always will receive at least one normal X chromosome. Therefore, even if she receives one flawed X chromosome, she will still be capable of producing a sufficient quantity of factors VIII and IX to avoid the symptoms of hemophilia. Such a person who has one flawed chromosome, but does not actually suffer from the disease, is called a carrier. She carries the flaw which causes hemophilia and can pass it on to her offspring. If, however, she has a son who receives her flawed X chromosome, he will be unable to produce the right quantity of factors VIII or IX, and he will suffer some degree of hemophilia. (Males inherit one X and one Y chromosome, and therefore have only one X chromosome.)

In rare cases, a hemophiliac father and a carrier mother can pass on the right combination of parental chromosomes to result in a hemophiliac female child. This situation, however, is extraordinarily rare. The vast majority of people with either hemophilia A or B are male.

About 30% of all people with hemophilia A or B are the first member of their family to ever have the disease. These individuals have had the unfortunate occurrence of a spontaneous mutation; meaning that in their early development, some random genetic accident befell their X chromosome, resulting in the defect causing hemophilia A or B. Once such a spontaneous genetic mutation takes place, offspring of the affected person can inherit the newly-created, flawed chromosome.

Symptoms of hemophilia

In the case of severe hemophilia, the first bleeding event usually occurs prior to eighteen months of age. In some babies, hemophilia is suspected immediately, when a routine **circumcision** (removal of the foreskin of the penis) results in unusually heavy bleeding. Toddlers are

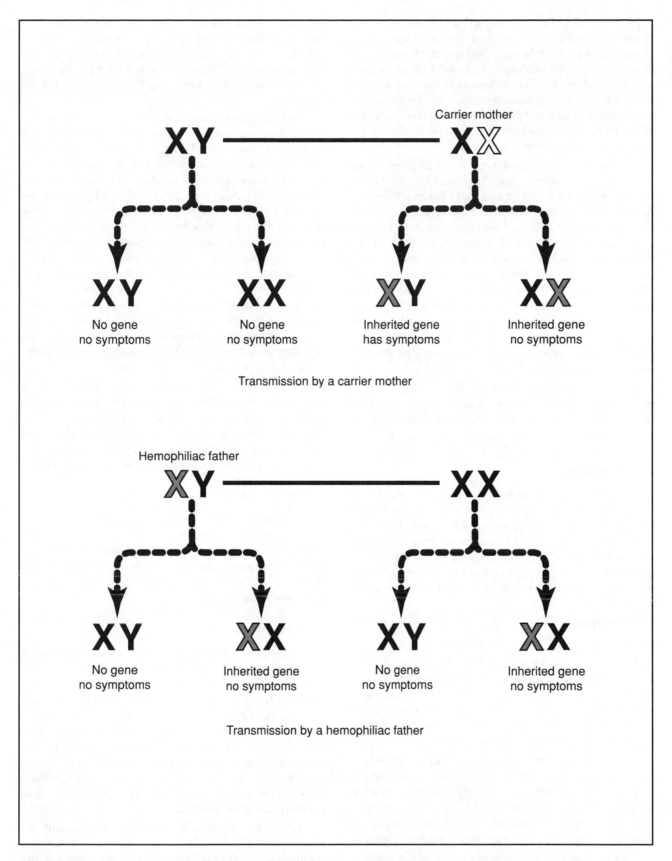

Hemophilia A and B are both caused by a genetic defect present on the X chromosome. Approximately 70% of people with hemophilia A or B inherited the disease, while the remaining 30% develop hemophilia due to a spontaneous genetic mutation. *(Illustration by Electronic Illustrators Group.)*

at particular risk, because they fall frequently, and may bleed into the soft tissue of their arms and legs. These small bleeds result in bruising and noticeable lumps, but don't usually need treatment. As a child becomes more active, bleeding may occur into the muscles; a much more painful and debilitating problem. These muscle bleeds result in pain and pressure on the nerves in the area of the bleed. Damage to nerves can cause numbness and decreased ability to use the injured limb.

Some of the most problematic and frequent bleeds occur into the joints, particularly into the knees and elbows. Repeated bleeding into joints can result in scarring within the joints and permanent deformities. Individuals may develop arthritis in joints which have suffered continued irritation from the presence of blood. Mouth injuries can result in compression of the airway, and, therefore, can be life-threatening. A blow to the head, which might be totally insignificant in a normal individual, can result in bleeding into the skull and brain. Because the skull has no room for expansion, the hemophiliac individual is at risk for brain damage due to blood taking up space and exerting pressure on the delicate brain tissue.

People with hemophilia are at very high risk of hemorrhage (severe, heavy, uncontrollable bleeding) from injuries (such as motor vehicle accidents) and also from surgery.

Diagnosis

Various tests are available to measure, under very carefully controlled conditions, the length of time it takes to produce certain components of the final fibrin clot. Tests (called assays) can also determine the percentage of factors VIII and IX present compared to known normal percentages. This information can help in demonstrating the type of hemophilia present, as well as the severity.

Treatment

Various types of factors VIII and IX are available to replace a patient's missing factors. These are administered intravenously (directly into the patient's veins by needle). These factor preparations may be obtained from a single donor, by pooling the donations of as many as thousands of donors, or by laboratory creation through highly advanced genetic techniques.

The frequency of treatment with factors depends on the severity of the individual patient's disease. Patients with relatively mild disease will only require treatment in the event of injury, or to prepare for scheduled surgical or dental procedures. Patients with more severe disease will require regular treatment to avoid spontaneous bleeding.

While appropriate treatment of hemophilia can both decrease suffering and be life-saving, complications associated with treatment can also be quite serious. About 20% of all patients with hemophilia A begin to produce chemicals within their bodies which rapidly destroy infused factor VIII. The presence of such a chemical may greatly hamper efforts to prevent or stop a major hemorrhage.

Individuals who receive factor prepared from pooled donor blood are at risk for serious infections which may be passed through blood. Hepatitis, a severe and potentially fatal viral liver infection, may be contracted from pooled factor preparations. Recently, a good deal of concern has been raised about the possibility of hemophiliacs contracting a fatal slow virus infection of the brain (**Creutzfeldt-Jakob disease**) from blood products. Unfortunately, pooled factor preparations in the early 1980s were almost all contaminated with human **immunodeficiency** virus (HIV), the virus which causes **AIDS.** Currently, careful methods of donor testing, as well as methods of inactivating viruses present in donated blood, have greatly lowered this risk. But a large number of hemophiliacs were infected with HIV. In fact, some statistics show that HIV is still the leading cause of **death** among hemophiliacs.

The most exciting new treatments currently being researched involve efforts to transfer new genes to hemophiliacs. These new genes would have the ability to produce the missing factors. As yet, these techniques are not being performed on humans, but there is great hope that eventually this type of **gene therapy** will be available.

Prognosis

Prognosis is very difficult to generalize. Because there are so many variations in the severity of hemophilia, and because much of what befalls a hemophiliac patient will depend on issues such as physical activity level and accidental injuries, statistics on prognosis are not generally available.

Prevention

Prevention is two pronged: one involves prevention of complications in the already-diagnosed hemophiliac patient; the other involves preventing the disease in subsequent offspring. The most important thing an individual with hemophilia can do to prevent complications of his disease is to avoid injury. Those individuals who require dental work or any surgery may need to be pretreated with an infusion of factor to avoid hemorrhage. Also, hepatitis vaccines should be given to hemophiliacs. Medications or drugs which promote bleeding (such as **aspirin**) should be avoided.

Certainly, people who know that their family includes hemophiliacs should receive careful **genetic counseling** before deciding to have a baby. Families with a positive history of hemophilia can also have tests done during a **pregnancy** to determine whether the fetus is a hemophiliac.

Resources

BOOKS

Corrigan, James J. "Hemorrhagic and Thrombotic Diseases." In *Nelson Textbook of Pediatrics,* edited by Richard Behrman, et al. Philadelphia: W.B. Saunders Co., 1996.

Hay, William W., et al. *Current Pediatric Diagnosis and Treatment.* Norwalk, CT: Appleton & Lange, 1995.

PERIODICALS

Berntorp, E., et al. "Modern Treatment of Haemophilia." *Bulletin of the World Health Organization.* 73, 5 (September-October 1995): 691 +.

ORGANIZATIONS

National Hemophilia Foundation, 116 West 32nd Street, 11th Floor, New York, NY 10001. (800) 42-HANDI. http://www.info@hemophilia.org.

Rosalyn S. Carson-DeWitt

Hemophilus ducreyi infection *see* **Chancroid**

Hemophilus infections

Definition

Hemophilus infections, most of which are due to *Haemophilus influenzae* infections, are a group of contagious diseases that are caused by a gram-negative bacterium, and affect only humans. Some hemophilus infections are potentially fatal.

Description

H. influenzae is a common organism worldwide; it has been found in the nasal secretions of as many as 90% of healthy individuals in the general population. Hemophilus infections are characterized by acute inflammation with a discharge (exudate). They may affect almost any organ system, but are most common in the respiratory tract. The organism can be transmitted by person-to-person contact, or by contact with nasal discharges and other body fluids. Hemophilus infections in the United States are most likely to spread in the late winter or early spring.

The primary factor influencing the rate of infection is age; children between the ages of six months and four years are most vulnerable to *H. influenzae.* In previous years, about 50% of children would acquire a hemophilus

---

KEY TERMS

Bacterium—A microscopic one-celled organism. *Haemophilus influenzae* is a specific bacterium.

Epiglottitis—Inflammation of the epiglottis. The epiglottis is a piece of cartilage behind the tongue that closes the opening to the windpipe when a person swallows. An inflamed epiglottis can swell and close off the windpipe, thus causing the patient to suffocate.

Exudate—A discharge produced by the body. Some exudates are caused by infections.

Gram-negative—A term that means that a bacterium will not retain the violet color when stained with Gram's dye. *Haemophilus influenzae* is a gram-negative bacterium.

Intubation—The insertion of a tube into the patient's airway to protect the airway from collapsing. Intubation is sometimes done as an emergency procedure for patients with epiglottitis.

Nosocomial—Contracted in a hospital. Pneumonia caused by *H. influenzae* is an example of a nosocomial infection.

Sepsis—Invasion of body tissues by disease organisms or their toxins. Sepsis may be either localized or generalized. *Haemophilus influenzae* can cause bacterial sepsis in newborns.

Stridor—A harsh or crowing breath sound caused by partial blockage of the patient's upper airway.

Tracheotomy—An emergency procedure in which the surgeon cuts directly through the patient's neck into the windpipe in order to keep the airway open.

---

infection before reaching one year of age; almost all children would develop one before age three. These figures are declining, however, as a result of the increasing use of hemophilus vaccines for children.

Adults are also susceptible to hemophilus diseases. *H. influenzae* **pneumonia** is a common nosocomial infection (illnesses contracted in hospitals). The rate of hemophilus infections in the adult population has increased over the past 40 years. The reasons for this change are unclear, but some researchers speculate that the overuse of **antibiotics** has led to the development of drug-resistant strains of *H. influenzae.* The risk factors for hemophilus infections among adults include:

• Smoking

• **Alcoholism**

- Chronic lung disease

- Old age

- Living in a city or institutional housing with a large group of people

- Poor nutrition and hygiene

- HIV infection, or other immune system disorder.

Causes & symptoms

Hemophilus infections are primarily caused by *Haemophilus influenzae*, a gram-negative bacterium that is capable of spreading from the nasal tissues and upper airway, where it is usually found, to the chest, throat, or middle ear. The organism sometimes invades localized areas of tissue, producing **meningitis, infectious arthritis, conjunctivitis, cellulitis, epiglottitis,** or inflammation of the membrane surrounding the heart. The most serious infections are caused by a strain called *H. influenzae* b (Hib). Before routine **vaccination,** Hib was the most common cause of bacterial meningitis, and responsible for most of the cases of acquired **mental retardation** in the United States.

Hemophilus infections in children

BACTERIAL SEPSIS IN THE NEWBORN

Bacterial **sepsis** (sepsis is the presence of illness-causing microorganisms, or their poisons, in the blood) is a potentially fatal illness in newborn infants. The child may acquire the disease organisms as it passes through the mother's birth canal, or from the hospital environment. *H. influenzae* can also produce inflammations of the eye (conjunctivitis) in newborn children. The signs of sepsis may include **fever,** crankiness, feeding problems, breathing difficulties, pale or mottled skin, or drowsiness. Premature birth is the most significant risk factor for hemophilus infections in newborns.

EPIGLOTTITIS

Epiglottitis is a potentially fatal hemophilus infection. Although children are more likely to develop epiglottitis, it can occur in adults as well. When the epiglottis (a piece of cartilage behind the tongue which protects the opening to the windpipe by opening and closing) is infected, it can swell to the point where it blocks the windpipe. The symptoms of epiglottitis include a sudden high fever, drooling, the feeling of an object stuck in the throat, and **stridor.** The epiglottis will look swollen and bright red if the doctor examines the patient's throat with a laryngoscope (a viewing device).

MENINGITIS

Meningitis caused by Hib is most common in children between nine months and four years of age. The child usually develops upper respiratory symptoms fol-lowed by fever, loss of appetite, vomiting, **headache,** and a stiff or sore neck or back. In severe cases, the child may have convulsions or go into **shock** or **coma.**

OTHER INFECTIONS

Hib is the second most common cause of middle ear infection and **sinusitis** in children. The symptoms of sinusitis include fever, **pain, bad breath,** and coughing. Children may also develop infectious arthritis from Hib. The joints most frequently affected are the large weight-bearing joints.

Hemophilus infections in adults

PNEUMONIA

Hib pneumonia is the most common hemophilus infection in adults. The symptoms include **empyema** (sputum containing pus), and fever. The hemophilus organism can usually be identified from sputum samples. Hib pneumonia is increasingly common in the elderly.

MENINGITIS

Meningitis caused by Hib can develop in adults as a complication of an ear infection or sinusitis. The symptoms are similar to those in children but are usually less severe in adults.

Diagnosis

The diagnosis is usually based on a combination of the patient's symptoms and the results of **blood counts,** cultures, or antigen detection tests.

Laboratory tests

Laboratory tests can be used to confirm the diagnosis of hemophilus infections. The bacterium can be grown on chocolate agar, or identified by **blood cultures** or Gram stain of body fluids. Antigen detection tests can be used to identify hemophilus infections in children. These tests include latex agglutination and electrophoresis.

Other laboratory findings that are associated with hemophilus infections include anemia (low red blood cell count), and a drop in the number of white blood cells in children with severe infections. Adults often show an abnormally high level of white blood cells; cell counts of 15,000 to 30,000/mm3 are not unusual.

Treatment

Because some hemophilus infections are potentially fatal, treatment is started without waiting for the results of laboratory tests.

Medications

Hemophilus infections are treated with antibiotics. Patients who are severely ill are given ampicillin or a third-generation cephalosporin, such as cefotaxime or ceftriaxone, intravenously. Patients with milder infections are given oral antibiotics, including amoxicillin, cefaclor, erythromycin, or trimethoprim-sulfamethoxazole. Patients who are allergic to penicillin are usually given cefaclor or trimethoprim-sulfamethoxazole.

Patients with Hib strains that are resistant to ampicillin may be given chloramphenicol. Chloramphenicol is not a first-choice drug because of its side effects, including interference with bone marrow production of blood cells.

The duration of antibiotic treatment depends on the location and severity of the hemophilus infection. Adults with respiratory tract infections, or Hib pneumonia, are usually given a 10–14 day course of antibiotics. Meningitis is usually treated for 10–14 days, but a seven-day course of treatment with ceftriaxone appears to be sufficient for infants and children. Ear infections are treated for 7–10 days.

Supportive care

Patients with serious hemophilus infections require bed rest and a humidified environment (such as a **croup** tent) if the respiratory tract is affected. Patients with epiglottitis frequently require intubation (insertion of a breathing tube) or a **tracheotomy** to keep the airway open. Patients with inflammation of the heart membrane, pneumonia, or arthritis may need surgical treatment to drain infected fluid from the chest cavity or inflamed joints.

Supportive care also includes monitoring of blood cell counts for patients using chloramphenicol, ampicillin, or other drugs that may affect production of blood cells by the bone marrow.

Prognosis

The most important factors in the prognosis are the severity of the infection and promptness of treatment. Untreated hemophilus infections—particularly meningitis, sepsis, and epiglottitis—have a high mortality rate. Bacterial sepsis of the newborn has a mortality rate between 13–50%. The prognosis is usually good for patients with mild infections who are treated without delay. Children who develop Hib arthritis sometimes have lasting problems with joint function.

Prevention

Hemophilus vaccines

There are three different vaccines for hemophilus infections used to immunize children in the United States: PRP-D, HBOC, and PRP-OMP. PRP-D is used only in children older than 15 months. HBOC is administered to infants at two, four, and six months after birth, with a booster dose at 15–18 months. PRP-OMP is administered to infants at two and four months, with the third dose at the child's first birthday. All three vaccines are given by intramuscular injection. About 5% of children may develop fever or soreness in the area of the injection.

Other measures

Other preventive measures include isolating patients with respiratory hemophilus infections; treating appropriate contacts of infected patients with rifampin; maintaining careful standards of cleanliness in hospitals, including proper disposal of soiled tissues; and washing hands properly.

Resources

BOOKS

Abzug, Mark J., "Infectious Diseases: Bacterial, Spirochetal, Protozoal, Metazoal, & Mycotic." In *Handbook of Pediatrics,* edited by Gerald B. Merenstein, et al. Norwalk, CT: Appleton & Lange, 1994.

Apicella, Michael A., and Timothy F. Murphy. "*Haemophilus*, Infection and Immunity." In *Encyclopedia of Immunology,* vol. II, edited by Ivan M. Roitt and Peter J. Delves. London: Academic Press, 1992.

Chambers, Henry F., "Infectious Diseases: Bacterial & Chlamydial." In *Current Medical Diagnosis & Treatment 1998,* edited by Lawrence M. Tierney, Jr., et al. Stamford, CT: Appleton & Lange, 1997.

Feigin, Ralph D., and Frederick M. Murphy. "*Haemophilus* Infections." In *Harrison's Principles of Internal Medicine,* edited by Eugene Braunwald, et al. New York: McGraw Hill Book Company, 1987.

"*Hemophilus influenzae* Infection." In *Professional Guide to Diseases,* edited by Stanley Loeb, et al. Springhouse, PA: Springhouse Corporation, 1991.

"Infectious Disease: Bacterial Diseases." In *The Merck Manual of Diagnosis and Therapy,* vol. II, edited by Robert Berkow, et al. Rahway, NJ: Merck Research Laboratories, 1992.

"Infectious Diseases: Neonatal Sepsis." In *Neonatology: Management, Procedures, On-Call Problems, Diseases and Drugs,* edited by Tricia Lacy Gomella, et al. Norwalk, CT: Appleton & Lange, 1994.

Ogle, John W., "Immunization Procedures, Vaccines, Antisera & Skin Tests." In *Handbook of Pediatrics,* edited by Gerald B. Merenstein, et al. Norwalk, CT: Appleton & Lange, 1994.

Rebecca J. Frey

Hemophilus influenzae infections *see*
Hemophilus infections

Hemoptysis

Definition

Hemoptysis is the coughing up of blood or bloody sputum from the lungs or airway. It may be either self-limiting or recurrent. Massive hemoptysis is defined as 200–600 mL of blood coughed up within a period of 24 hours or less.

Description

Hemoptysis can range from small quantities of bloody sputum to life-threatening amounts of blood. The patient may or may not have chest **pain.**

Causes & symptoms

Hemoptysis can be caused by a range of disorders:

- Infections. These include **pneumonia; tuberculosis; aspergillosis;** and parasitic diseases, including ascariasis, **amebiasis,** and paragonimiasis.
- Tumors that erode blood vessel walls.
- Drug abuse. Cocaine can cause massive hemoptysis.
- Trauma. Chest injuries can cause bleeding into the lungs.
- Vascular disorders, including aneurysms, **pulmonary embolism,** and malformations of the blood vessels.
- **Bronchitis.** Its most common cause is long-term smoking.
- Foreign object(s) in the airway.
- Blood clotting disorders.
- Bleeding following such surgical procedures as bronchial biopsies and heart catheterization.

Diagnosis

The diagnosis of hemoptysis is complicated by the number of possible causes.

Patient history

It is important for the doctor to distinguish between blood from the lungs and blood coming from the nose, mouth, or digestive tract. Patients may aspirate, or breathe, blood from the nose or stomach into their lungs and cough it up. They may also swallow blood from the chest area and then vomit. The doctor will ask about stomach **ulcers,** repeated vomiting, liver disease, **alcoholism,** smoking, tuberculosis, mitral valve disease, or treatment with anticoagulant medications.

Physical examination

The doctor will examine the patient's nose, throat, mouth, and chest for bleeding from these areas and for signs of chest trauma. The doctor also listens to the patient's breathing and heartbeat for indications of heart abnormalities or lung disease.

Laboratory tests

Laboratory tests include blood tests to rule out clotting disorders, and to look for food particles or other evidence of blood from the stomach. Sputum can be tested for fungi, bacteria, or parasites.

X-ray and bronchoscopy

Chest x-rays and **bronchoscopy** are the most important studies for evaluating hemoptysis. They are used to evaluate the cause, location, and extent of the bleeding. The bronchoscope is a long, flexible tube used to identify tumors or remove **foreign objects.**

Imaging and other tests

Computed tomography scans (CT scans) are used to detect aneurysms and to confirm x-ray results. Ventilation-perfusion scanning is used to rule out pulmonary embolism. The doctor may also order an angiogram to rule out pulmonary embolism, or to locate a source of bleeding that could not be seen with the bronchoscope.

In spite of the number of diagnostic tests, the cause of hemoptysis cannot be determined in 20–30% of cases.

Treatment

Massive hemoptysis is a life-threatening emergency that requires treatment in an intensive care unit. The patient will be intubated (the insertion of a tube to help breathing) to protect the airway, and to allow evaluation of the source of the bleeding. Patients with **lung cancer,** bleeding from an aneurysm (blood clot), or persistent traumatic bleeding require chest surgery.

Patients with tuberculosis, aspergillosis, or bacterial pneumonia are given **antibiotics.**

Foreign objects are removed with a bronchoscope.

If the cause cannot be determined, the patient is monitored for further developments.

Prognosis

The prognosis depends on the underlying cause. In cases of massive hemoptysis, the mortality rate is about 15%. The rate of bleeding, however, is not a useful predictor of the patient's chances for recovery.

Resources

BOOKS

Idell, Steven. ''Hemoptysis.'' In *Current Diagnosis 9,* edited by Rex B. Conn, et al. Philadelphia: W. B. Saunders Company, 1997.

''On-Call Problems: Hemoptysis.'' In *Surgery On Call,* edited by Leonard G. Gomella and Alan T. Lefor. Stamford, CT: Appleton & Lange, 1996.

''Pulmonary Disorders: Hemoptysis.'' In *The Merck Manual of Diagnosis and Therapy,* vol. II, edited by Robert Berkow, et al. Rahway, NJ: Merck Research Laboratories, 1992.

Stauffer, John L. ''Lung.'' In *Current Medical Diagnosis & Treatment 1998,* edited by Lawrence M. Tierney, Jr., et al. Stamford, CT: Appleton & Lange, 1997.

Rebecca J. Frey

Hemorrhagic colitis *see E. coli* **0157:H7 infection**

Hemorrhagic fever with renal syndrome *see* **Hantavirus infections**

Hemorrhagic fevers

Definition

Hemorrhagic fevers are caused by viruses that exist throughout the world. However, they are most common in tropical areas. Early symptoms, such as muscle aches and **fever,** can progress to a mild illness or to a more debilitating, potentially fatal disease. In severe cases, a prominent symptom is bleeding, or hemorrhaging, from orifices and internal organs.

Description

Although hemorrhagic fevers are regarded as emerging diseases, they probably have existed for many years. This designation isn't meant to imply that they are newly developing, but rather that human exposure to the causative viruses is increasing to the point of concern.

These viruses are maintained in nature in insect, arthropod (insects, spiders and other invertebrates with external hard skeletons), or animal populations—so-called disease reservoirs. Individuals within these populations become infected with a virus but do not die from it. In many cases, they don't even develop symptoms. Then the viruses are transmitted from a reservoir population to humans by vectors—either members of the reservoir population or an intervening species, such as mosquitoes.

KEY TERMS

Antibody—A molecule created by the body's immune system to combat a specific infectious agent, such as a virus or bacteria.

Antigen—A specific feature, such as a protein, on an infectious agent. Antibodies use this feature as a means of identifying infectious intruders.

Coagulating factors—Components within the blood that help form clots.

Endemic—Referring to a specific geographic area in which a disease may occur.

Hemorrhage—As a noun, this refers to the point at which blood is released. As a verb, this refers to bleeding.

Incubation—The time period between exposure to an infectious agent, such as a virus or bacteria, and the appearance of symptoms of illness.

Petechiae—Pinpoint hemorrhages that appear as reddish dots beneath the surface of the skin.

Reservoir—A population in which a virus is maintained without causing serious illness to the infected individuals.

Ribavirin—A drug that is used to combat viral infections.

Vector—A member of the reservoir population or an intervening species that can transmit a virus to a susceptible victim. Mosquitoes are common vectors, as are ticks and rodents.

Hemorrhagic fevers are generally endemic, or linked to specific locations. If many people reside in an endemic area, the number of cases may soar. For example, **dengue fever,** a type of hemorrhagic fever, affects approximately 100 million people annually. A large percentage of those infected live in densely populated southeast Asia; an area in which the disease vector, a mosquito, thrives. Some hemorrhagic fevers are exceedingly rare, because people very infrequently encounter the virus. Marburg hemorrhagic fever, which has affected fewer than 40 people since its discovery in 1967, provides one such example. Fatality rates are also variable. In cases of dengue hemorrhagic fever-dengue **shock** syndrome, 1–5% of the victims perish. On the other end of the spectrum is Ebola, an African hemorrhagic fever, that kills 30–90% of those infected.

The onset of hemorrhagic fevers may be sudden or gradual, but all of them are linked by the potential for hemorrhaging. However, not all cases progress to this very serious symptom. Hemorrhaging may be attributable to the destruction of blood coagulating factors or to increased permeability of body tissues. The severity of bleeding ranges from petechiae, which are pinpoint hemorrhages under the skin surface, to distinct bleeding from body orifices such as the nose or vagina.

Causes & symptoms

The viruses that cause hemorrhagic fevers are found most commonly in tropical locations; however, some are found in cooler climates. Typical disease vectors include rodents, ticks, or mosquitoes, but person-to-person transmission in health care settings or through sexual contact can also occur.

Filoviruses

Ebola is the most famous of the Filoviridae, a virus family that also includes the Marburg virus. Ebola is endemic to Africa, particularly the Republic of the Congo and Sudan; the Marburg virus is found in sub-Saharan Africa. The natural reservoir of filoviruses is unknown. The incubation period, or time between infection and appearance of symptoms, is thought to last three to eight days, possibly longer.

Symptoms appear suddenly, and include severe **headache,** fever, chills, muscle aches, malaise, and appetite loss. These symptoms may be accompanied by nausea, vomiting, **diarrhea,** and abdominal **pain.** Victims become apathetic and disoriented. Severe bleeding commonly occurs from the gastrointestinal tract, nose and throat, and vagina. Other bleeding symptoms include petechiae and oozing from injection sites. Ebola is fatal in 30–90% of cases.

Arenaviruses

Viruses of the Arenaviridae family cause the Argentinian, Brazilian, Bolivian, and Venezuelan hemorrhagic fevers. Lassa fever, which occurs in west Africa, also arises from an arenavirus. Infected rodents, the natural reservoir, shed virus particles in their urine and saliva, which humans may inhale or otherwise come in contact with.

Fever, muscle aches, malaise, and appetite loss gradually appear one to two weeks after infection with the South American viruses. Initial symptoms are followed by headache, back pain, **dizziness,** and gastrointestinal upset. The face and chest appear flushed and the gums begin to bleed. In about 30% of cases, the disease progresses to bleeding under the skin and from the mucous membranes, and/or to effects on the nervous system, such as **delirium, coma,** and convulsions. Untreated, South American hemorrhagic fevers have a 10–30% fatality rate.

Lassa fever also begins gradually, following an 8–14 day incubation. Initial symptoms resemble those of the South American hemorrhagic fevers, followed by a **sore throat,** muscle and joint pain, severe headache, pain above the stomach, and a dry **cough.** The face and neck become swollen, and fluid may accumulate in the lungs. Bleeding occurs in 15–20% of infected individuals, mostly from the gums and nose. Overall, the fatality rate is lower than 2%, but hospitals may encounter 20% fatality rates, treating typically the most serious of cases.

Flaviviruses

The Flaviviridae family includes the viruses that cause yellow and dengue fevers.

Yellow fever occurs in tropical areas of the Americas and Africa and is transmitted from monkeys to humans by mosquitoes. The virus may produce a mild, possibly unnoticed illness, but some individuals are suddenly stricken with a fever, weakness, **low back pain,** muscle pain, nausea, and vomiting. This phase lasts one to seven days, after which the symptoms recede for one to two days. Symptoms then return with greater intensity, along with **jaundice,** delirium, seizures, stupor, and coma. Bleeding occurs from the mucous membranes and under the skin surface, and dark blood appears in stools and vomit.

Mosquitoes also transmit the dengue virus. Dengue fever is endemic in southeast Asia and areas of the Americas. Cases have also been reported in the Caribbean, Saudi Arabia, and northern Australia. This virus causes either the mild dengue fever or the more serious dengue hemorrhagic fever-dengue shock syndrome (DHF-DSS).

In children, dengue fever is characterized by a sore throat, runny nose, slight cough, and a fever lasting for a week or less. Older children and adults experience more severe symptoms: fever, headache, muscle and joint pain, loss of appetite, and a rash. The skin appears flushed, and intense pain occurs in the bones and limbs. After nearly a week, the fever subsides for one to two days before returning. Minor hemorrhaging, such as from the gums, or more serious gastrointestinal bleeding may occur.

DHF-DSS primarily affects children younger than 15 years. The symptoms initially resemble those of dengue fever in adults, without the bone and limb pain. As the fever begins to abate, the individual's condition worsens and hemorrhaging occurs from the nose, gums, and injection sites. Bleeding is also seen from the gastro-intestinal, genitourinary, and respiratory tracts.

Bunyaviruses

The Bunyaviridae family includes several hundred viruses but only a few are responsible for hemorrhagic fevers in humans.

Rift Valley fever is caused by the phlebovirus, found in sub-Saharan Africa and the Nile delta. Natural reservoirs are wild and domestic animals, and transmission occurs through contact with infected animals or through mosquito bites. The incubation period lasts 3–12 days. Most cases of Rift Valley fever are mild and may be symptomless. If symptoms develop, they include fever, backache, muscle and joint pain, and headache. Hemor-rhagic symptoms occur rarely; while **death,** which occurs in fewer than 3% of cases, is attributable to massive liver damage.

Crimean-Congo hemorrhagic fever is caused by nairovirus and occurs in central and southern Africa, Asia, Eurasia, and the Middle East. The virus is found in hares, birds, ticks, and domestic animals and may be transmitted by ticks or by contact with infected animals. The nairovirus incubation period is 3–12 days; after which an individual experiences fever, chills, headache, severe muscle pain, pain above the stomach, nausea, vomiting, and appetite loss. Bleeding under the skin and gastrointestinal and vaginal bleeding may develop in the most severe cases. Death rates range from 10% in southern Russia to 50% in parts of Asia.

Hemorrhagic fever with renal (kidney) syndrome is caused by the hantaviruses: Hantaan, Seoul, Puumala, and Dobrava. Hantaan virus occurs in northern Asia, the Far East, and the Balkans; Seoul virus is found world-wide; Puumala virus is found in Scandinavia and north-ern Europe; while Dobrava virus occurs in the Balkans. Wild rodents are the natural reservoirs and transmit the virus via their excrement or body fluids or through direct contact. Initial symptoms develop within 10–40 days and include fever, headache, muscle pain, and dizziness.

Other symptoms are blurry vision, abdominal and back pain, nausea, and vomiting. High levels of protein in the urine signal kidney damage; hemorrhaging may also oc-cur. Death rates range from 0–10%.

Diagnosis

Since the hemorrhagic fevers share symptoms with many other diseases, positive identification of the disease relies on evidence of the viruses in the bloodstream—such as detection of antigens and antibodies—or **isolation** of the virus from the body. Disruptions in the normal levels of bloodstream components may be helpful in determining some, but not all, hemorrhagic fevers.

Treatment

Lassa fever, and possibly other hemorrhagic fevers, respond to ribavirin, an antiviral medication. However, most of the hemorrhagic fever viruses can only be treated with supportive care. Such care centers around maintain-ing correct fluid and electrolyte balances in the body and protecting the patient against secondary infections. Hepa-rin and vitamin K administration, coagulation factor re-placement, and blood **transfusions** may be effective in lessening or stopping hemorrhage in some cases.

Prognosis

Recovery from some hemorrhagic fevers is more certain than from others. The filoviruses are among the most lethal; fatality rates for Ebola range from 30–90%, while DHF-DSS cases result in a 1–5% fatality rate. Whether a case occurs during an epidemic or as an iso-lated case also has a bearing on the outcome. For exam-ple, isolated cases of yellow fever have a 5% mortality rate, but 20–50% of epidemic cases may be fatal.

Permanent disability can occur with some types of hemorrhagic fever. About 10% of severely ill Rift Valley fever victims suffer retina damage and may be perma-nently blind, and 25% of South American hemorrhagic fever victims suffer potentially permanent deafness.

Proper treatment is vital. In cases of DHF-DSS, fa-tality can be reduced from 40–50% to less than 2% with adequate medical care. For individuals who survive hem-orrhagic fevers, prolonged convalescence is usually inev-itable. However, survivors seem to gain lifelong immunity against the virus that made them ill.

Prevention

Hemorrhagic fevers can be prevented through vector control and personal protection measures. Attempts have been made in urban and settled areas to destroy mosquito and rodent populations. In areas where such measures are impossible, individuals can use insect repellents, mos-quito netting, and other methods to minimize exposure.

Vaccines have been developed against yellow fever, Argentinian hemorrhagic fever, and Crimean-Congo hemorrhagic fever. Vaccines against other hemorrhagic fevers are being researched.

Resources

BOOKS

Garrett, Laurie. *The Coming Plague: Newly Emerging Diseases in a World Out of Balance.* New York: Farrar, Straus, and Giroux, 1994.

Gorbach, Sherwood L., John G. Bartlett, and Neil R. Blacklow, editors. Chapters 266, 267, and 269 in *Infectious Diseases.* 2nd ed. Philadelphia: W.B. Saunders Company, 1998.

PERIODICALS

Lacy, Mark D., and Raymond A. Smego. "Viral Hemorrhagic Fevers." *Advances in Pediatric Infectious Diseases* 12 (1997): 21.

Le Guenno, Bernard. "Emerging Viruses." *Scientific American* October (1995): 56.

OTHER

Outbreak. (An on-line information service about emerging diseases.) http://www.outbreak.org/.

Julia Barrett

Hemorrhoids

Definition

Hemorrhoids are enlarged veins in the anus or lower rectum. They often go unnoticed and usually clear up after a few days, but can cause long-lasting discomfort, bleeding and be excruciatingly painful. Effective medical treatments are available, however.

Description

Hemorrhoids (also called piles) can be divided into two kinds, internal and external. Internal hemorrhoids lie inside the anus or lower rectum, beneath the anal or rectal lining. External hemorrhoids lie outside the anal opening. Both kinds can be present at the same time.

Hemorrhoids are a very common medical complaint. More than 75% of Americans have hemorrhoids at some point in their lives, typically after age 30. Pregnant women often develop hemorrhoids, but the condition usually clears up after **childbirth.** Men are more likely than women to suffer from hemorrhoids that require professional medical treatment.

Causes & symptoms

Precisely why hemorrhoids develop is unknown. Researchers have identified a number of reasons to explain hemorrhoidal swelling, including the simple fact that people's upright posture places a lot of pressure on the

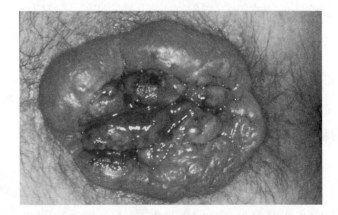

Clinical photo of a thrombosed external hemorrhoid.
(Custom Medical Stock Photo. Reproduced by permission.)

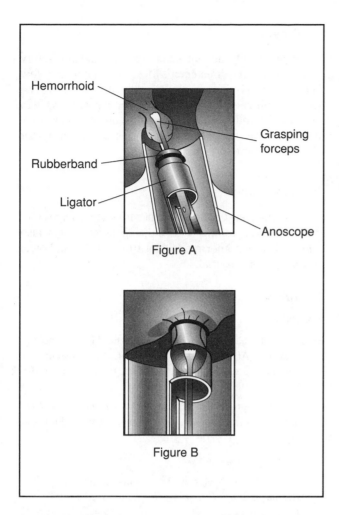

Hemorrhoid

Grasping forceps

Rubberband

Ligator

Anoscope

Figure A

Figure B

Rubber band ligation is probably the most widely used treatment for internal hemorrhoids. An applicator is used to place one or two small rubber bands around the base of the hemorrhoid, cutting off its blood supply (figures A and B). After 3-10 days, the rubber bands and the hemorrhoid fall off, leaving a scab which disappears within a week or two. *(Illustration by Electronic Illustrators Group.)*

anal and rectal veins. Aging, **obesity, pregnancy,** chronic **constipation** or **diarrhea,** excessive use of **enemas** or **laxatives,** straining during bowel movements, and spending too much time on the toilet are considered contributing factors. Heredity may also play a part in some cases. There is no reason to believe that hemorrhoids are caused by jobs requiring, for instance, heavy lifting or long hours of sitting, although activities of that kind may make existing hemorrhoids worse.

The commonest symptom of internal hemorrhoids is bright red blood in the toilet bowl or on one's feces or toilet paper. When hemorrhoids remain inside the anus they are almost never painful, but they can prolapse (protrude outside the anus) and become irritated and sore.

Sometimes, prolapsed hemorrhoids move back into the anal canal on their own or can be pushed back in, but at other times they remain permanently outside the anus until treated by a doctor.

Small external hemorrhoids usually do not produce symptoms. Larger ones, however, can be painful and interfere with cleaning the anal area after a bowel movement. When, as sometimes happens, a blood clot forms in an external hemorrhoid (creating what is called a thrombosed hemorrhoid), the skin around the anus becomes inflamed and a very painful lump develops. On rare occasions the clot will begin to bleed after a few days and leave blood on the underwear. A thrombosed hemorrhoid will not cause an **embolism.**

Diagnosis

Diagnosis begins with a visual examination of the anus, followed by an internal examination during which the doctor carefully inserts a gloved and lubricated finger into the anus. The doctor may also use an anoscope, a small tube that allows him or her to see into the anal canal. Under some circumstances the doctor may wish to check for other problems by using a sigmoidoscope or colonoscope, a flexible instrument that allows inspection of the lower colon (in the case of the sigmoidoscope) or the entire colon (in the case of the colonoscope).

Treatment

Hemorrhoids can often be effectively dealt with by dietary and lifestyle changes. Softening the feces and avoiding constipation by adding fiber to one's diet is important, because hard feces lead to straining during defecation. Fruit, leafy vegetables, and whole-grain breads and cereals are good sources of fiber, as are bulk laxatives and fiber supplements such as Metamucil or Citrucel. Exercising, losing excess weight, and drinking six to eight glasses a day of water or another liquid (not alcohol) also helps. Soap or toilet paper that is perfumed may irritate the anal area and should be avoided, as should excessive cleaning, rubbing, or wiping of that area. Reading in the bathroom is also considered a bad idea, because it adds to the time one spends on the toilet and may increase the strain placed on the anal and rectal veins. After each bowel movement, wiping with a moistened tissue or pad sold for that purpose helps lessen irritation. Hemorrhoid pain is often eased by sitting in a tub of warm water for about 10 or 15 minutes two to four times a day (**sitz bath**). A cool compress or ice pack to reduce swelling is also recommended (the ice pack should be wrapped in a cloth or towel to prevent direct contact with the skin). Many people find that over-the-counter hemorrhoid creams and foams bring relief, but these medications do not make hemorrhoids disappear.

When painful hemorrhoids do not respond to home-based remedies, professional medical treatment is necessary. The choice of treatment depends on the type of hemorrhoid, what medical equipment is available, and other considerations.

Rubber band ligation is probably the most widely used of the many treatments for internal hemorrhoids (and the least costly for the patient). This procedure is performed in the office of a family doctor or specialist, or in a hospital on an outpatient basis. An applicator is used to place one or two small rubber bands around the base of the hemorrhoid, cutting off its blood supply. After 3 to 10 days the bands, the hemorrhoid falls off, leaving a sore that heals in a week or two. Because internal hemorrhoids are located in a part of the anus that does not sense pain, anesthetic is unnecessary and the procedure is painless in most cases. Although there can be minor discomfort and bleeding for a few days after the bands are applied, complications are rare and most people are soon able to return to work and other activities. If more than one hemorrhoid exists or if banding is not entirely effective the first time (as occasionally happens), the procedure may need to be repeated a few weeks later. After five years, 15–20% of patients experience a recurrence of internal hemorrhoids, but in most cases all that is needed is another banding.

External hemorrhoids, and some prolapsed internal hemorrhoids, are removed by conventional surgery in a hospital. Depending on the circumstances, this requires a local, regional, or general anesthetic. Surgery does cause a fair amount of discomfort, but an overnight hospital stay is usually not necessary. Full healing takes two to four weeks, but most people are able to resume normal activities at the end of a week. Hemorrhoids rarely return after surgery.

Alternative treatment

Like mainstream practitioners, alternative practitioners stress the importance of a high-fiber diet. To prevent hemorrhoids by strengthening the veins of the anus, rectum, and colon, they recommend blackberries, blueberries, cherries, vitamin C, butcher's broom (*Ruscus aculeatus*), and flavonoids (plant pigments found in fruit and fruit products, tea, and soy). Herbal teas, ointments, and suppositories, and other kinds of herbal preparations, are suggested for reducing discomfort and eliminating hemorrhoids. In particular, pilewort (*Ranunculus ficaria*), applied in an ointment or taken as a tea, can reduce the pain of external hemorrhoids. **Acupuncture, acupressure, aromatherapy,** and homeopathy are also used to treat hemorrhoids.

Prognosis

Hemorrhoids do not cause **cancer** and are rarely dangerous or life threatening. Most clear up after a few days without professional medical treatment. However, because **colorectal cancer** and other digestive system diseases can cause anal bleeding and other hemorrhoid-like symptoms, people should always consult a doctor when those symptoms occur.

Prevention

A high-fiber diet and the other lifestyle changes recommended for coping with existing hemorrhoids also help to prevent hemorrhoids. Not straining during bowel movements is essential.

Resources

BOOKS

Billingham, Richard P. "Hemorrhoids, Anal Fissure, and Anorectal Abscess and Fistula." In *Conn's Current Therapy,* edited by Robert E. Rakel. Philadelphia: W.B. Saunders, 1998.

The Burton Goldberg Group. *Alternative Medicine: The Definitive Guide.* Puyallup, WA: Future Medicine Publishing, 1993.

PERIODICALS

Pfenninger, John L. "Modern Treatments for Internal Haemorrhoids." *British Medical Journal* 314 (1997): 1211+.

Surrell, James. "Nonsurgical Treatment Options for Internal Hemorrhoids." *American Family Physician* (September 1995): 821+.

ORGANIZATIONS

National Digestive Diseases Information Clearinghouse. 2 Information Way, Bethesda, MD 20892-3570. http://www.niddk.nih.gov/health/digest/nddic.htm.

Howard Baker

Henoch-Schönlein purpura *see* **Allergic purpura**

Heparin *see* **Anticoagulant and antiplatelet drugs**

Hepatic carcinoma *see* **Liver cancer**

Hepatic coma *see* **Liver encephalopathy**

Hepatitis A

Definition

Hepatitis A is an inflammation of the liver caused by a virus, the hepatitis A virus (HAV). It is usually not very severe and runs an acute course, generally starting within two to six weeks after contact with the virus, and lasting no longer than two months. HAV may occur in single cases after contact with an infected relative or sex partner. Alternately, epidemics may develop when food or drinking water is contaminated by the feces of an infected person.

Description

Hepatitis A is commonly known as infectious hepatitis because it spreads relatively easily from those infected to close contacts. Once the infection ends, there is no lasting, chronic phase of illness. However it is not uncommon to have a second episode of symptoms about a month after the first; this is called a relapse, but it is not clear that the virus persists when symptoms recur. Some patients have multiple relapses. Both children and adults may be infected by HAV. Children are the chief victims, but very often have no more than a flu-like illness or no symptoms at all, whereas adults are far likelier to have more severe symptoms.

KEY TERMS

Antibody—A substance made by the body in response to a foreign body, such as a virus, which is able to attack and destroy the invading virus.

Contamination—The process by which an object or body part becomes exposed to an infectious agent such as a virus.

Epidemic—A situation where a large number of infections by a particular agent—such as a virus— develops in a short time. The agent is rapidly transmitted to many individuals.

Incubation period—The interval from initial exposure to an infectious agent, such as a virus, and the first symptoms of illness.

Jaundice—Yellowing of the skin (and whites of the eyes) when pigments normally eliminated by the liver collect in high amounts in the blood.

Vaccine—A substance prepared from a weakened or killed virus which, when injected, helps the body to form antibodies that will prevent infection by the natural virus.

Epidemics of HAV infection can infect dozens and even hundreds (or, on rare occasions, thousands) of persons. In the public's mind, outbreaks of hepatitis A usually are linked with the eating of contaminated food at a restaurant. It is true that food handlers—who may themselves have no symptoms—can start an alarming, widespread epidemic. Many types of food can be infected by sewage containing HAV, but shellfish, such as clams, are a common culprit.

Apart from contaminated food and water, certain groups are at increased risk of getting infectious hepatitis:

- Children at day care centers make up an estimated 14–40% of all cases of HAV infection in the United States. Changing diapers transmits infection through fecal-oral contact. Toys and other objects may remain contaminated for some time. Often a child without symptoms brings the infection home to siblings and parents.

- Troops living under crowded conditions at military camps or in the field. During World War II there were an estimated five million cases in German soldiers and civilians.

- Anyone living in heavily populated and squalid conditions, such as the very poor and those placed in refugee or prisoner-of-war camps.

- Homosexual men are increasingly at risk of HAV infection from oral-anal sexual contact.

- Tourists visiting an area where hepatitis A is common are at risk of becoming ill.

Causes & symptoms

The time from exposure to HAV and the onset of symptoms ranges from two to seven weeks and averages about a month. The virus is passed in the feces, especially late during this incubation period, before symptoms first appear. It can live for several hours on the skin surface, and during this time may be transmitted to others. Infected persons are most contagious starting a week or so before symptoms develop, and remain so up until the time jaundice (yellowing of the skin) is noted.

Often the first symptoms to appear are fatigue, aching all over, nausea, and a loss of appetite. Those who like drinking coffee and smoking cigarettes may lose their taste for them. Mild fever is common; it seldom is higher than 101°F (38.3°C). The liver often enlarges, causing pain or tenderness in the right upper part of the abdomen. Jaundice then develops, typically lasting seven to ten days. Many patients do not visit the doctor until their skin turns yellow. As many as three out of four children have no symptoms of HAV infection, but about 85% of adults will have symptoms. Besides jaundice, the commonest are abdominal pain, loss of appetite, and feeling generally poorly.

Special situations

An occasional patient with hepatitis A will remain jaundiced for a month, two months or even longer—but eventually the jaundice will pass. Very rarely, a patient will develop such severe hepatitis that the liver fails. HAV infection causes about 100 **deaths** each year in the United States. Rare complications include arthritis and inflammation of small blood vessels (**vasculitis**). In developed countries, a pregnant woman who contracts hepatitis A can be expected to do well. In developing countries, however, the infection may prove fatal, probably because nutrition is not adequate.

Diagnosis

The early, flu-like symptoms and jaundice, as well as rapid recovery, suggest infectious hepatitis without special tests being done. If there is any question, a specialist in gastrointestinal disorders or infectious diseases can confirm the diagnosis. This is done by detecting a specific antibody, called hepatitis A IgM antibody, that develops when HAV is present in the body. This test always registers positive when a patient has symptoms, and should continue to register positive for four to six months. However, hepatitis A IgM antibody will persist lifelong in the blood and is protective against reinfection.

Treatment

Once symptoms appear, no **antibiotics** or other medicines will shorten the course of infectious hepatitis. Patients should rest in bed as needed, take a healthy diet, and avoid drinking alcohol and/or any medications that could further damage the liver. If a patient feels well it is all right to return to school or work even if some jaundice remains.

Prognosis

Most patients with acute hepatitis, even when severe, begin feeling better in two to three weeks, and recover completely in four to eight weeks. After recovering from hepatitis A, a person no longer carries the virus and remains immune for life. In the United States, serious complications are infrequent and deaths are very rare. In the U.S., as many as 75% of adults over 50 years of age will have blood test evidence of previous hepatitis A.

Prevention

The single best way to keep from spreading hepatitis A infection is to wash the hands carefully after using the toilet. Those who are infected should not share items that might carry infection. Special care should be taken to avoid transmitting infection to a sex partner. Travelers should avoid water and ice if unsure of their purity, or they can boil water for one minute before drinking it. All foods eaten should be packaged, well cooked or, in the case of fresh fruit, peeled.

If exposure is a possibility, infection may be prevented by an injection of a serum fraction containing antibody against HAV. This material, called immune serum globulin (ISG), is 90% protective even when injected after exposure—providing it is given within two weeks. Anyone living with an infected patient should receive ISG. For long-term protection, a killed virus hepatitis A vaccine became available in 1995. More than 95% of those vaccinated will develop an adequate amount of anti-HAV antibody. Those who should consider being vaccinated include healthcare professionals, those working at day care and similar facilities, frequent travelers to areas with poor sanitation, those with any form of chronic liver disease, and those who are very sexually active.

Resources

BOOKS

Johnson, A. *Liver Disease & Gallstones.* Oxford Academic Trade, 1993.

Rosenthal, M. Sara. *The Gastrointestinal Sourcebook.* Los Angeles, CA: Lowell House, 1997.

ORGANIZATIONS

American Liver Foundation. 1425 Pompton Ave., Cedar Grove, NJ 07009. (800) 223-0179. http://sadieo.ucsf.edu/alf/alffinal/homepagealf.html.

OTHER

HepNet: The Hepatitis Information Network. Feb. 2, 1998. http://www.hepnet.com.

David A. Cramer

Hepatic encephalopathy *see* **Liver encephalopathy**

Hepatitis, alcoholic

Definition

Alcoholic hepatitis is an inflammation of the liver caused by alcohol.

Description

Irritation, be it from toxins or infections, causes a similar response in body organs. The response is known as inflammation and consists of:

• An increase in the blood to the affected organ

• Redness and swelling of the organ

KEY TERMS

Cirrhosis—Disruption of normal liver structure and function caused by any type of chronic disease such as hepatitis and alcohol abuse.

Fatty liver—An abnormal amount of fat tissue in the liver caused by alcohol abuse.

Hemolysis—Disintegration of read blood cells.

Protozoa—One celled microscopic organisms like amoeba.

* Influx of immune agents like white blood cells and their arsenal of chemical weapons

* **Pain.**

As the acute process subsides, there is either healing or lingering activity. Lingering activity—chronic disease—has a milder presentation with similar ingredients. Healing often takes the form of scarring, wherein normal functioning tissue is replaced by tough, fibrous, and nonproductive scar. Both chronic disease and healing can happen simultaneously, so that scar tissue progressively replaces normal tissue. This leads to **cirrhosis,** a liver so scarred it is unable to do its job adequately.

Alcohol can cause either an acute or a chronic disease in the liver. The acute disease can be severe, even fatal, and can bring with it hemolysis—blood cell destruction. Alcohol can also cause a third type of liver disease—**fatty liver,** in which the continuous action of alcohol turns the liver to useless fat. This condition eventually progresses to cirrhosis if the poisoning continues.

Causes & symptoms

Inflammation of the liver can be caused by a great variety of agents—poisons, drugs, viruses, bacteria, protozoa, and even larger organisms like worms. Alcohol is a poison if taken in more than modest amounts. It favors destroying stomach lining, liver, heart muscle, and brain tissue. The liver is a primary target because alcohol travels to the liver after leaving the intestines. Those who drink enough to get alcohol poisoning have a tendency to be undernourished, since alcohol provides ample calories but little nutrition. It is suspected that both the alcohol and the poor nutrition produce alcoholic hepatitis.

Diagnosis

Hepatitis of all kinds causes notable discomfort, loss of appetite, nausea, pain in the liver, and usually **jaundice** (turning yellow). Blood test abnormalities are unmistakably those of hepatitis, but selecting from so many the precise cause may take additional diagnostic work.

Treatment

As with all poisonings, removal of the offending agent is primary. There is no specific treatment for alcohol poisoning. General supportive measures must see the patient through until the liver has healed by itself. In the case of fulminant (sudden and severe) disease, the liver may be completely destroyed and have to be replaced by a transplant.

Prognosis

The liver is robust. It can heal without scarring after one or a few episodes of hepatitis that resolve without lingering. It can, moreover, regrow from a fragment of its former self, provided there is not disease or poison still inhibiting it.

Prevention

Alcohol is lethal in many ways when ingested in excess. Research suggests that the maximum healthy dose of alcohol per day is roughly one pure ounce—the amount in two cocktails, two glasses of wine, or two beers.

Resources

BOOKS

Boyd, William. *Textbook of Pathology.* Philadelphia, PA: Lea & Febiger, 1970, p. 875.

Friedman, Scott L. "Cirrhosis of the liver and its major sequelae." In *Cecil Textbook of Medicine,* edited by J. Claude Bennett and Fred Plum. Philadelphia: W. B. Saunders, 1996, pp. 789-791.

Lidofsky, Steven D. and Bruce F. Scharschmidt. "Jaundice." In *Sleisenger & Fordtran's Gastrointestinal and Liver Disease,* edited by Mark Feldman, et al. Philadelphia: W. B. Saunders, 1998, p. 1767.

McQuaid, Kenneth R. "Alimentary tract." In *Current Medical Diagnosis and Treatment,* edited by Lawrence M. Tierney Jr., et al. Stamford, CT: Appleton & Lange, 1996, pp. 566-568.

Podolsky, Daniel K. and Kurt J. Isselbacher. "Cirrhosis and alcoholic liver disease." In *Harrison's Principles of Internal Medicine,* edited by Kurt Isselbacher, et al. New York: McGraw-Hill, 1998, pp. 1704-1710.

ORGANIZATIONS

American Liver Foundation. 1425 Pompton Avenue, Cedar Grove, New Jersey 07009. 800-223-0179.

Local chapters of Alcoholics Anonymous.

J. Ricker Polsdorfer

Hepatitis, autoimmune

Definition

A form of liver inflammation in which the body's immune system attacks liver cells.

Description

Autoimmunity causes the body's defense mechanisms to turn against itself. Many of the tissues in the body can be the target of such an attack. While one tissue type predominates, others may be involved in a general misdirection of immune activity, perhaps because the specific target antigen is present in differing quantities in each of the affected tissues. There seem to be hereditary causes for autoimmunity, since these diseases tend to run in families and have genetic markers. Among the more common diseases believed to fall within this category are **rheumatoid arthritis, systemic lupus erythematosus, multiple sclerosis,** and **psoriasis.**

The process of autoimmune disease is very similar to infectious disease and allergy, so that great caution is observed in placing a disorder in this class. Germs were found to cause several diseases originally thought to be autoimmune. Allergens cause others. Many more may be uncovered. Autoimmunity is often believed to originate with a virus infection. A chemical in the virus resembles a body chemical so closely that the immune system attacks both.

Autoimmune hepatitis is similiar to viral hepatitis, a disease of the liver. It can be an acute disease that kills over a third of its victims within six months, it can persist for years, or it can return periodically. Some patients develop cirrhosis of the liver which, over time, causes the liver to cease functioning.

Causes & symptoms

Symptoms of autoimmune hepatitis resemble those of other types of hepatitis. Patients who develop autoimmune hepatitis experience **pain** under the right ribs, fatigue and general discomfort, loss of appetite, nausea, sometimes vomiting and **jaundice.** In addition, other parts of the body may be involved and contribute their own symptoms.

Diagnosis

Extensive laboratory testing may be required to differentiate this disease from viral hepatitis. The distinction may not even be made during the initial episode. There are certain markers of autoimmune disease in the blood that can lead to the correct diagnosis if they are sought. In advanced or chronic cases a **liver biopsy** may be necessary.

KEY TERMS

Allergen—Any chemical that causes an immune reaction only in people sensitive to it.

Antigen—Any chemical that can be the target of an immune response.

Biopsy—Surgical removal of a piece of tissue for examination.

Jaundice—A yellow color to the skin from bile that backs up into the circulation.

Treatment

Autoimmune hepatitis is among the few types of hepatitis that can be treated effectively. Since treatment itself introduces problems in at least 20% of patients, it is reserved for the more severe cases. Up to 80% of patients improve with cortisone treatment, although a cure is unlikely. Another drug—azathioprine—is sometimes used concurrently. Treatment continues for over a year and may be restarted during a relapse. At least half the patients relapse at some point, and most will still continue to have progressive liver scarring.

If the liver fails, transplant is the only recourse.

Prognosis

In spite of treatment autoimmune hepatitis can re-erupt at any time, and may continue to damage and scar the liver. The rate of progression varies considerably from patient to patient.

Resources

BOOKS

Dienstag, Jules L. Isselbacher, Kurt J. ''Chronic hepatitis.'' *Harrison's Principles of Internal Medicine,* 14th edition, edited by Kurt Isselbacher et al. New York: McGraw-Hill, 1998, 1701-3.

McQuaid, Kenneth R. ''Alimentary tract.'' *Current Medical Diagnosis and Treatment,* edited by Lawrence M. Tierney, Jr., et al. Stamford, CT: Appleton & Lange, 1996, pp. 584-5.

Ockner, Robert K. ''Chronic hepatitis.'' *Cecil Textbook of Medicine,* edited by J. Claude Bennett and Fred Plum. Philadelphia, PA: W. B. Saunders, 1996, pp. 777-8.

ORGANIZATIONS

American Liver Foundation. 1425 Pompton Avenue, Cedar Grove, New Jersey 07009. 800 223-0179.

J. Ricker Polsdorfer

Hepatitis B

Definition

Hepatitis B is a potentially serious form of liver inflammation due to infection by the hepatitis B virus (HBV). It occurs in both rapidly developing (acute) and long-lasting (chronic) forms, and is one of the commonest chronic infectious diseases worldwide. An effective vaccine is available which will prevent the disease in those who are later exposed.

Description

Commonly called "serum hepatitis," hepatitis B ranges from mild to very severe. Some people who are infected by HBV develop no symptoms and are totally unaware of the fact, but they may carry HBV in their blood and pass the infection on to others. In its chronic form, HBV infection may destroy the liver through a scarring process, called **cirrhosis,** or it may lead to **cancer** of the liver.

When a person is infected by HBV, the virus enters the bloodstream and body fluids, and is able to pass through tiny breaks in the skin, mouth, or the male or female genital area. There are several ways of getting the infection:

- During birth, a mother with hepatitis B may pass HBV on to her infant.
- Contact with infected blood is a common means of transmitting hepatitis B. One way this may happen is by being stuck with a needle. Both healthcare workers and those who inject drugs into their veins are at risk in this way.
- Having sex with a person infected by HBV is an important risk factor (especially anal sex).

Although there are many ways of passing on HBV, the virus actually is not very easily transmitted. There is no need to worry that casual contact, such as shaking hands, will expose one to hepatitis B. There is no reason not to share a workplace or even a bathroom with an infected person.

More than 300 million persons throughout the world are infected by HBV. While most who become chronic carriers of the virus live in Asia and Africa, there are no fewer than 1.5 million carriers in the United States. Because carriers represent a constant threat of transmitting the infection, the risk of hepatitis B is always highest where there are many carriers. Such areas are said to be endemic for hepatitis B. When infants or young children living in an endemic area are infected, their chance of becoming a chronic hepatitis B carrier is at least 90%. This probably is because their bodies are not able to make

the substances (antibodies) that destroy the virus. In contrast, no more than 5% of infected teenagers and adults develop chronic infection.

Causes & symptoms

With the exception of HBV, all the common viruses that cause hepatitis are known as RNA viruses because they contain ribonucleic acid or RNA as their genetic material. HBV is the only deoxyribonucleic acid or DNA virus that is a major cause of hepatitis. HBV is made up of several fragments, called antigens, that stimulate the body's immune system to produce the antibodies that can neutralize or even destroy the infecting virus. It is, in fact, the immune reaction, not the virus, that seems to cause the liver inflammation.

Acute hepatitis B

In the United States, a majority of acute HBV infections occur in teenagers and young adults. Half of these youth never develop symptoms, and only about 20%—or one in five infected patients—develop severe symptoms and yellowing of the skin (**jaundice**). Jaundice occurs when the infected liver is unable to get rid of certain colored substances, or pigments, as it normally does. The remaining 30% of patients have only "flu-like" symptoms and will probably not even be diagnosed as having hepatitis unless certain tests are done.

The commonest symptoms of acute hepatitis B are loss of appetite, nausea, generally feeling poorly, and **pain** or tenderness in the right upper part of the abdomen (where the liver is located). Compared to patients with

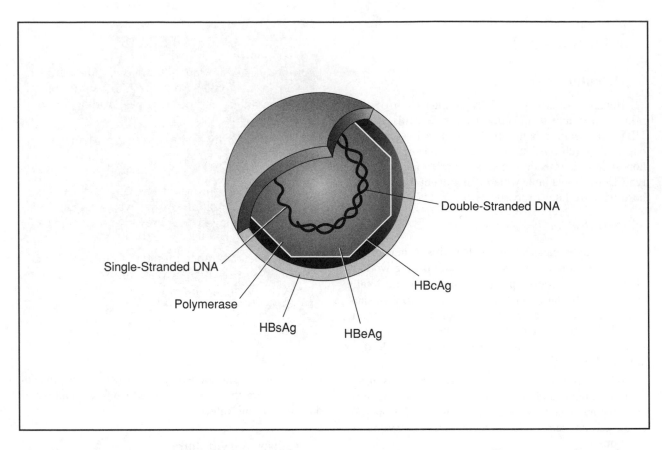

Hepatitis B virus (HBV) is composed of an inner protein core and an outer protein capsule. The outer capsule contains the hepatitis B surface antigen (HBsAg). The inner core contains HBV core antigen (HBcAg) and hepatitus B e-antigen (HBeAg). This cell also contains polymerase, which catalyzes the formation of the cell's DNA. HBV is the only hepatitis-causing virus that has DNA, instead of RNA. *(Illustration by Electronic Illustrators Group.)*

hepatitis A or C, those with HBV infection are less able to continue their usual activities and require more time resting in bed.

Occasionally patients with HBV infection will develop joint swelling and pain (arthritis) as well as **hives** or a skin rash before jaundice appears. The joint symptoms usually last no longer than three to seven days.

Typically the symptoms of acute hepatitis B do not persist longer than two or three months. If they continue for four months, the patient has an abnormally long-lasting acute infection. In a small number of patients—probably fewer than 3%—the infection keeps getting worse as the liver cells die off. Jaundice deepens, and patients may bleed easily when the levels of coagulation factors (normally made by the liver) decrease. Large amounts of fluid collect in the abdomen and beneath the skin (**edema**). The least common outcome of acute HBV infection, seen in fewer than 1% of patients, is fulminant hepatitis, when the liver fails entirely. Only about half of these patients can be expected to live.

Chronic hepatitis B

HBV infection lasting longer than six months is said to be chronic. After this time it is much less likely for the infection to disappear. Not all carriers of the virus develop chronic liver disease; in fact, a majority have no symptoms. But, about one in every four HBV carriers do develop liver disease which gets worse over time, as the liver becomes more and more scarred and less able to carry out its normal functions. A badly scarred liver is called cirrhosis. Patients are likely to have an enlarged liver and spleen, as well as tiny clusters of abnormal blood vessels in the skin that resemble spiders.

The most serious complication of chronic HBV infection is **liver cancer.** Worldwide this is the commonest cancer to occur in men. Nevertheless, the overall chance that liver cancer will develop at any time in a patient's life is probably much lower than 10%. Patients with chronic hepatitis B who drink or smoke are more likely to develop liver cancer. It is not unusual for a person to simultaneously have both HBV infection and infection by

HIV (human **immunodeficiency** virus, the cause of **AIDS**).

Diagnosis

Hepatitis B is diagnosed by detecting one of the viral antigens—called hepatitis B surface antigen (HBsAg)—in the blood. Later in the acute disease, HBsAg may no longer be present, in which case a test for antibodies to a different antigen—hepatitis B core antigen—is used. If HBsAg can be detected in the blood for longer than six months, chronic hepatitis B is diagnosed. A number of tests can be done to learn how well, or poorly, the liver is working. They include blood clotting tests and tests for enzymes which are found in abnormally high amounts when any form of hepatitis is present.

Treatment

There are no specific treatments for acute hepatitis B. Patients should rest in bed as needed, continue to eat a healthy diet, and avoid alcohol. Any non-critical surgery should be postponed.

Prognosis

Each year an estimated 150,000 persons in the United States get hepatitis B. More than 10,000 will require hospital care, and as many as 5,000 will die from complications of the infection. About 90% of all those infected will have acute disease only. A very large majority of these patients will recover within three months. It is the remaining 10%, with chronic infection, who account for most serious complications and **deaths** from HBV infection. In the United States, perhaps only 2% of all those who are infected will become chronically ill. The course of chronic HBV infection in any particular patient is unpredictable. Some patients who do well at first may later develop serious complications. Even when no symptoms of liver disease develop, chronic carriers remain a threat to others by serving as a source of infection.

Prevention

The best way to prevent any form of viral hepatitis is to avoid contact with blood and other body fluids of infected individuals. The use of **condoms** during sex is also advisable.

If a person is exposed to hepatitis B, a serum preparation containing a high level of antibody against HBV may prevent infection if given within three to seven days of exposure. Babies born of a mother with HBV should receive the vaccine within 24 hours. An effective and very safe vaccine is available that reliably prevents hepatitis B. **Vaccination** is suggested for most infants and for children aged 10 and younger whose parents are from a place where hepatitis B is common. Teenagers not vacci-

nated as children and all adults at risk of exposure also should be vaccinated against hepatitis B. Three doses are recommended.

Those at increased risk of getting hepatitis B, and who therefore should be vaccinated, include:

- Household contacts of a person carrying HBV
- Healthcare workers who often come in contact with patients' blood or other body fluids
- Patients with kidney disease who periodically undergo hemodialysis
- Homosexual men who are sexually active, and heterosexuals who have multiple sex partners
- Persons coming from areas where HBV infection is a major problem
- Prisoners and others living in crowded institutions
- Drug abusers who use needles to inject drugs into their veins.

Resources

BOOKS

Johnson, A. *Liver Disease & Gallstones.* Oxford Academic Trade, 1993.

ORGANIZATIONS

Hepatitis B Foundation. 101 Greenwood Ave., Suite 570, Jenkintown, PA 19046. (215) 884-8786. E-mail: info@hepb.org.

OTHER

HepNet: The Hepatitis Information Network. Feb. 2, 1998. http://www.hepnet.com.

David A. Cramer

Hepatitis C

Definition

Hepatitis C is a form of liver inflammation that causes rapidly developing (acute), and very often long-lasting (chronic) disease. Spread mainly by contact with infected blood, the hepatitis C virus (HCV) causes most cases of viral liver infection not due to the A and B hepatitis viruses. In fact, before other viral types were found, hepatitis C was referred to as ''non-A, non-B hepatitis.''

Description

HCV is a blood-borne virus that is the major cause of ''**transfusion** hepatitis,'' which can develop in patients

KEY TERMS

Antibody—A substance formed in the body in response to a foreign body, such as a virus, which can attack and destroy the invading foreign body or virus.

Carrier—A person who, after recovering from a viral infection, continues to "carry" the virus in the blood and can pass it on to others who then may develop infection.

Contamination—Passage of an infectious organism, such as a virus, from an infected person to an object such as a needle, which then, when used, may pass infection to another person.

Hepatocellular carcinoma—A dangerous cancer of the liver that may develop in patients who have had hepatitis, sometimes as long as 20 or 30 years earlier.

Porphyria—Any of a group of disturbances of porphyrin metabolism characterized by excess pophyrins (various biologially active compounds with a distinct structure) in the urine and by exterme sensitivity to light.

who are given blood. The existence of a third hepatitis virus (besides the A and B viruses) became clear in 1974, but HCV was first identified in 1989. Thereafter, tests were devised to detect the virus in blood units before transfusing them. As a result, since the early 1990s transfused blood is less commonly the cause of hepatitis C.

The hepatitis C form of hepatitis is generally mild in its early, acute stage, but it is much likelier than **hepatitis B** to produce chronic liver disease. About two of every three persons who are infected by HCV may continue to have the virus in their blood and so become carriers, who can transmit the infection to others.

The most common way of transmitting hepatitis C is when blood containing the virus enters another person's circulation through a break in the skin or the mucosa (inner lining) of the mouth or genitals. HCV also can be passed from an infected mother to the infant she is carrying. (The risk of infection from breast milk is very low.) Also, HCV can be spread through sexual intercourse, especially if one partner is acutely infected at the time.

Those at increased risk of developing hepatitis C include:

• Healthcare workers who come in contact with infected blood from a cut or bruise, or from a device or instrument that has been infected ("contaminated").

• Persons who inject illicit drugs into their veins—especially if they share needles and syringes with other users.

• Anyone who gets a tattoo or has his or her skin pierced with an infected needle.

• Persons with **hemophilia** (who because they bleed very easily may require large amounts of blood and blood products over time).

• Patients with kidney disease who have periodic dialysis—a treatment that rids their blood of toxic substances—and often requires the patient to have blood transfusions.

About one-fourth of patients with hepatitis C do not belong to any of these high-risk groups. Although blood transfusion is a much less common cause of HCV infection than in earlier years, cases still occur. Also, sexual transmission is possible, and may take place with either heterosexual or homosexual behavior.

Causes & symptoms

More than half of all patients who develop hepatitis C have no symptoms or signs of liver disease. Some, however, may have a minor illness with flu-like symptoms. Any form of hepatitis may keep the liver from eliminating certain colored (pigmented) substances as it normally does. These pigments collect in the skin, turning it yellow, and also may cause yellowing of the whites of the eyes. About one in four patients with hepatitis C will develop this yellowing of the skin called **jaundice** (or yellow jaundice). Some patients lose their appetite and frequently feel tired. Patients may also feel nauseous or even vomit.

In most patients, HCV can still be found in the blood six months after the start of acute infection, and these patients are considered to be carriers. If the virus persists for one year, it is very unlikely to disappear. About 20% of chronic carriers develop **cirrhosis** (scarring) of the liver when the virus damages or destroys large numbers of liver cells, which are then replaced by scar tissue. Cirrhosis may develop only after a long period of time—as long as 20 years—has passed. Many patients will not develop cirrhosis and instead have a mild, chronic form of infection called chronic persistent hepatitis.

Patients with chronic HCV infection are at risk of developing certain very serious complications:

• Patients with hepatitis C who develop cirrhosis may go on to have liver cancer—called hepatocellular carcinoma. Patients with liver cancer have a average life expectancy measured in months unless the tumor is totally removed.

• Patients also are at risk of developing a combination of joint **pain,** weakness, and areas of bleeding into the skin. The kidneys and brain also may be affected. Perhaps 5% of patients with chronic HCV infection develop this condition, called cryoglobulinemia.

- Patients with porphyria (metabolic disturbances characterized by extreme sensitivity to light) develop blisters in areas of their skin that are exposed to sunlight. The skin also may be easily bruised, and, in time, can become discolored.

Diagnosis

Hepatitis C should be suspected if a patient develops jaundice and reports recent contact with the blood of a person who may have been infected. There is a blood test to detect HCV IgG antibody, a substance that the body makes to combat HCV. Care is required, as the test often does not show positive for up to two to three months after infection. Also, the test only shows whether a person has ever been infected by HCV, not whether the virus is still present. There is another test that can detect carriers, but it requires a special laboratory and it is expensive. Simpler blood tests can be done to show how much jaundice-causing pigment is in a patient's blood, or to measure the levels of certain proteins made by the liver. High levels of these "liver enzymes" indicate that the liver is inflamed and is not performing its work properly. Rising levels suggest that the infection is getting worse.

Treatment

Patients who fail to recover promptly may be advised to see a specialist in gastrointestinal disorders (which include liver disease) or infectious diseases. A balanced diet with little fat is best, and patients should limit their alcohol intake, or, better, avoid alcohol altogether. Any medication that can cause liver damage should be avoided. The amount of time in bed depends on how poorly a particular patient feels.

A natural body protein, interferon alpha, now can be made in large amounts by genetic engineering, and improves the outlook for many patients who have chronic hepatitis C. The protein can lessen the symptoms of infection and improve liver function. Not all patients respond, however, and others get less benefit the longer they take interferon. **Fever** and flu-like symptoms are frequent side effects of this treatment. Using a high dose for six months, nearly half of patients have responded positively. Half the patients who do respond well will relapse after the drug is stopped. Newer medications that work alone or with interferon are being studied.

When hepatitis destroys most or all of the liver, the only hope may be a liver transplant. Unfortunately the new liver usually becomes infected by HCV. On the other hand, total liver failure is less frequent than in patients with hepatitis B.

Prognosis

In roughly one-fifth of patients who develop hepatitis C, the acute infection will subside, and they will recover completely within four to eight weeks and have no later problems. Other patients face two risks: they themselves may develop chronic liver infection and possibly serious complications such as liver cancer, and, also, they will continue carrying the virus and may pass it on to others. The overall risk of developing cirrhosis, or liver scarring, is about 15% of all patients infected by HCV. Liver failure is less frequent in patients with chronic hepatitis C than in those with other forms of hepatitis.

Prevention

No vaccine has yet been developed to prevent hepatitis C in persons exposed to the virus. There are, however, many ways in which infection may be avoided:

- Those who inject drugs should never share needles, syringes, swabs, spoons, or anything else that comes in contact with bodily fluids. They should always use clean equipment.

- Hands should be washed before and after contact with another person's blood or if the skin is penetrated.

- The sharing of personal items should be avoided, particularly those that can puncture the skin or inside of the mouth, such as razors, nail files and scissors, and even toothbrushes.

- **Condoms** should be used for either vaginal or oral sex.

If a person does develop hepatitis C, its spread may be prevented by:

- Not donating blood

- Not sharing personal items with others

- Wiping up any spilled blood while using gloves, household bleach, and disposable paper towels

- Carefully covering any cut or wound with a bandaid or dressing

- Practicing safe sex; especially during the acute phase of the infection.

Resources

BOOKS

Everson, Gregory T., and Hedy Weinberg. *Living with Hepatitis C: Survivor's Guide.* New York: Hatherleigh Press, 1998.

Roybal, Beth Ann Petro. *Hepatitis C: A Personal Guide to Good health.* Berkeley, CA: Ulysses Press, 1997.

ORGANIZATIONS

American Liver Foundation. 1425 Pompton Ave., Cedar Grove, NJ 07009. (800) 223-0179. http://sadieo.ucsf.edu/alf/alffinal/homepagealf.html.

OTHER

HepNet: The Hepatitis Information Network. Feb. 2, 1998.
http://www.hepnet.com.

David A. Cramer

Hepatitis D

Definition

Hepatitis D (or delta, the Greek letter "D"), is a form of liver inflammation that occurs only in patients who also are infected by the **hepatitis B** virus. Infection by the hepatitis delta virus (HDV) either occurs at the same time as hepatitis B develops, or develops later when infection by hepatitis B virus (HBV) has entered the chronic (long-lasting) stage.

Description

Delta hepatitis can be quite severe, but it is seen only in patients already infected by HBV. In the late 1970s, Italian physicians discovered that some patients with hepatitis B had another type of infectious agent in their liver cells. Later the new virus—HDV—was confirmed by experimentally infecting chimpanzees. When both viruses are present, acute infection tends to be more severe. Furthermore, patients with both infections are likelier than those with HBV alone to develop chronic liver disease, and, when it occurs, it is more severe.

About 300 million persons worldwide carry HBV. Of them, at least 5% probably also have delta hepatitis. In North America HDV infection appears to be less frequent: 4% of all patients with acute hepatitis B have HDV infection. The delta virus causes an estimated 2% of all cases of acute viral hepatitis in the United States. The rate of HDV infection varies widely in different parts of the world; it is a very serious infection in some countries and quite mild in others. Chronic delta hepatitis is a more serious disease than either chronic hepatitis B alone or hepatitis C.

Certain individuals—the same ones who are at increased risk of developing hepatitis B—are the prime candidates to be infected by HDV. For example:

- Not infrequently, HDV infection occurs in patients with chronic HBV infection who also have **hemophilia,** a bleeding disease. These patients are at risk because they require large amounts of transfused blood and blood products that may contain HDV.

- In some areas, one-fourth to one-half of patients with chronic HBV infection who inject themselves with il-

licit drugs become infected by HDV as well. Drug abusers who share contaminated needles are likely to infect one another.

- Patients who get HBV infection by sexual contact may also be infected by HDV, although the delta virus is less often spread in this way than is HBV itself. Between 10–25% of homosexual men with chronic HBV infection harbor the delta virus.

- Like hepatitis B, HDV infection may develop in healthcare workers who are victims of a needle stick, and it also can be spread within households when personal items such as a razor or toothbrush are shared.

Causes & symptoms

The delta virus is a small and incomplete viral particle. Perhaps this is why it cannot cause infection on its own. Its companion virus, HBV, actually forms a covering over the HDV particle. In chronically ill patients (those whose virus persists longer than six months), the combined viruses cause inflammation throughout the liver and eventually destroy the liver cells, which are then replaced by scar tissue. This scarring is called **cirrhosis.**

When HBV and HDV infections develop at the same time, a condition called coinfection, recovery is the rule. Only 2–5% of patients become chronic carriers (have the virus remain in their blood more than six months after infection). It may be that HDV actually keeps HBV from reproducing as rapidly as it would if it were alone, so chronic infection is less likely.

KEY TERMS

Alpha-interferon—A natural body substance that now can be made in large quantities and is an effective treatment for some types of viral inflammatory disease, including hepatitis C.

Antibody—A substance formed in the body in response to an invading microorganism, such as a virus, which can attack and destroy the invading virus.

Coinfection—Invasion of the body by two viruses at about the same time.

Hemophilia—A bleeding disease that may call for the transfusion of large amounts of blood and blood products.

Superinfection—Infection by a second virus after a previous infection by a different virus has become well established.

When HBV infection occurs first and is followed by HDV infection, the condition is called superinfection. This is a more serious situation. Between half and two-thirds of patients with superinfection develop severe acute hepatitis. Once the liver cells contain large numbers of HBV viruses, HDV tends to reproduce more actively. Massive infection and liver failure are more common in superinfection. The risk of **liver cancer,** however, is no greater than from hepatitis B alone.

As with other forms of hepatitis, the earliest symptoms are nausea, loss of appetite, joint **pains,** and tiredness. There may be **fever** (not marked) and an enlarged liver may cause discomfort or actual pain in the right upper part of the abdomen. Later, **jaundice** (a yellowing of the skin and whites of the eyes that occurs when the liver is no longer able to eliminate certain pigmented substances) may develop.

Diagnosis

HDV infection may be diagnosed by detecting the antibody against the virus. Unfortunately this test cannot detect acute coinfection or superinfection as early as when symptoms first develop. Antibody against HDV usually is found no sooner than 30 days after symptoms appear. Until recently, the virus itself could only be identified by testing a small sample of liver tissue. Scientists now are developing a blood test for HDV that should make diagnosis faster and easier. When HDV is present, liver enzymes (proteins made by the liver) are present in abnormally high amounts. In some patients with coinfection, the enzyme levels peak twice, once when HBV infection starts and again at the time of HDV infection.

Treatment

As in any form of hepatitis, patients in the acute stage should rest in bed as needed, eat a balanced diet, and avoid alcohol. Alpha-interferon, the natural body substance which helps control hepatitis C, has generally not been found helpful in treating hepatitis D. If the liver is largely destroyed and has stopped functioning, **liver transplantation** is an option. Even when the procedure is successful, disease often recurs and cirrhosis may actually develop more rapidly than before.

Prognosis

A large majority of patients with coinfection of HBV and HDV recover from an episode of acute hepatitis. However, about two-thirds of patients chronically infected by HDV go on to develop cirrhosis of the liver. In one long-term study, just over half of patients who became carriers of HDV had moderate or severe liver disease, and one-fourth of them died. If very severe liver failure develops, the chance of a patient surviving is no better than 50%. A liver transplant may improve this figure to 70%. When transplantation is done for cirrhosis, rather than for liver failure, nearly 90% of patients live five years or longer. The major concern with transplantation is infection of the transplanted liver; this may occur in as many as 40% of transplant patients.

When a child with viral hepatitis develops cirrhosis, HDV infection is commonly responsible. A woman who develops delta hepatitis while pregnant will do as well as if she were not pregnant; and there is no increased risk that the newborn will be malformed in any way.

Prevention

The vaccine against hepatitis B also prevents delta hepatitis, since it cannot occur unless HBV infection is present. Hopefully, a vaccine can be developed that will keep delta infection from developing in chronic HBV carriers. However, if a person already has HBV infection, any exposure to blood should be strictly avoided. A high level of sexual activity with multiple partners is also a risk factor for delta hepatitis.

Resources

BOOKS

Johnson, A. *Liver Disease & Gallstones.* Oxford Academic Trade, 1993.

PERIODICALS

Tepper, M.L., and P. R. Gully. "Viral Hepatitis: Know Your D, E, F and Gs." *Canadian Medical Association Journal* (1997): 1735.

ORGANIZATIONS

American Liver Foundation. 1425 Pompton Ave., Cedar Grove, NJ 07009. (800) 223 0179. http://sadieo.ucsf.edu/alf/alffinal/homepagealf.html.

David A. Cramer

Hepatitis E

Definition

The hepatitis E virus (HEV) is a common cause of hepatitis that is transmitted via the intestinal tract, and is not caused by the **hepatitis A** virus. Spread most often by contaminated drinking water, HEV infection occurs mainly in developing countries.

Description

Hepatitis E is also known as epidemic non-A, non-B hepatitis. Like hepatitis A, it is an acute and short-lived illness that can sometimes cause liver failure. HEV, discovered in 1987, is spread by the fecal-oral route. It is constantly present (endemic) in countries where human waste is allowed to get into drinking water without first being purified. Large outbreaks (epidemics) have occurred in Asian and South American countries where there is poor sanitation. In the United States and Canada no outbreaks have been reported, but persons traveling to an endemic region may return with HEV.

Causes & symptoms

There are at least two strains of HEV, one found in Asia and another in Mexico. The virus may start dividing in the gastrointestinal tract, but it grows mostly in the liver. After an incubation period (the time from when a person is first infected by a virus until the appearance of the earliest symptoms) of two to eight weeks, infected persons develop **fever,** may feel nauseous, lose their appetite, and often have discomfort or actual **pain** in the right upper part of the abdomen where the liver is located. Some develop yellowing of the skin and the whites of the eyes (**jaundice**). Most often the illness is mild and disappears within a few weeks with no lasting effects. Children younger than 14 years and persons over age 50 seldom have jaundice or show other clinical signs of hepatitis.

Hepatitis E never becomes a chronic (long-lasting) illness, but on rare occasions the acute illness damages and destroys so many liver cells that the liver can no longer function. This is called fulminant liver failure, and may cause **death.** Pregnant women are at much higher risk of dying from fulminant liver failure; this increased risk is not true of any other type of viral hepatitis. The great majority of patients who recover from acute infection do not continue to carry HEV and cannot pass on the infection to others.

Diagnosis

HEV can be found by microscopically examining a stool sample, but this is not a reliable test, as the virus often dies when stored for a short time. Like other hepatitis viruses, HEV stimulates the body's immune system to produce a substance called an antibody, which can swallow up and destroy the virus. Blood tests can determine elevated antibody levels, which indicate the presence of HEV virus in the body. Unfortunately, such antibody blood tests are not widely available.

Treatment

There is no way of effectively treating the symptoms of any acute hepatitis, including hepatitis E. During acute infection, a patient should take a balanced diet and rest in bed as needed.

Prognosis

In the United States hepatitis E is not a fatal illness, but elsewhere about 1–2% of those infected die of advanced liver failure. In pregnant women the death rate is as high as 20%. It is not clear whether having hepatitis E once guarantees against future HEV infection.

Prevention

Most attempts to use blood serum containing HEV antibody to prevent hepatitis in those exposed to HEV have failed. Hopefully, this approach can be made to work so that pregnant women living in endemic areas can be protected. No vaccine is available, though several are being tested. It also is possible that effective anti-viral drugs will be found. The best ways to prevent hepatitis E are to provide safe drinking water and take precautions to use sterilized water and beverages when traveling.

Resources

BOOKS

Rosenthal, M. Sara. *The Gastrointestinal Sourcebook.* Los Angeles, CA: Lowell House, 1997.

PERIODICALS

Mast, E. E., and M. J. Alter. ''Epidemiology of Viral Hepatitis: An Overview.'' *Seminars in Virology* 4 (1993): 273-283.

Tepper, M. L., and P. R. Gully. "Viral Hepatitis: Know Your D, E, F and Gs." *Canadian Medical Association Journal* (1997): 1735.

ORGANIZATIONS

American Liver Foundation. 1425 Pompton Ave., Cedar Grove, NJ 07009. (800) 223-0179. http://sadieo.ucsf.edu/alf/alffinal/homepagealf.html.

OTHER

King, J.W. *Bug Bytes*. Louisiana State University Medical Center, Shreveport LA. http://www.ccm.lsumc.edu/bugbytes/.

David A. Cramer

Hepatitis G

Definition

Hepatitis G is a newly discovered form of liver inflammation caused by hepatitis G virus (HGV), a distant relative of the **hepatitis C** virus.

Description

HGV, also called hepatitis GB virus, was first described early in 1996. Little is known about the frequency of HGV infection, the nature of the illness, or how to prevent it. What is known is that transfused blood containing HGV has caused some cases of hepatitis. For this reason, patients with **hemophilia** and other bleeding conditions who require large amounts of blood or blood products are at risk of hepatitis G. HGV has been identified in between 1–2% of blood donors in the United States. Also at risk are patients with kidney disease who have blood exchange by hemodialysis, and those who inject drugs into their veins. It is possible that an infected mother can pass on the virus to her newborn infant. Sexual transmission also is a possibility.

Often patients with hepatitis G are infected at the same time by the **hepatitis B** or C virus, or both. In about three of every thousand patients with acute viral hepatitis, HGV is the only virus present. There is some indication that patients with hepatitis G may continue to carry the virus in their blood for many years, and so might be a source of infection in others.

Causes & symptoms

Some researchers believe that there may be a group of GB viruses, rather than just one. Others remain doubtful that HGV actually causes illness. If it does, the type of acute or chronic (long-lasting) illness that results is not clear. When diagnosed, acute HGV infection has usually been mild and brief. There is no evidence of serious complications, but it is possible that, like other hepatitis viruses, HGV can cause severe liver damage resulting in liver failure. The virus has been identified in as many as 20% of patients with long-lasting viral hepatitis, some of whom also have hepatitis C.

KEY TERMS

Antibody—A substance made by the body's immune system in response to an invading virus; antibodies then attack and destroy the virus.

Hemophilia—A bleeding disorder that often makes it necessary to give patients dozens or even hundreds of units of blood and blood products over time.

Diagnosis

The only method of detecting HGV is a complex and costly DNA test that is not widely available. Efforts are under way, however, to develop a test for the HGV antibody, which is formed in response to invasion by the virus. Once antibody is present, however, the virus itself generally has disappeared, making the test too late to be of use.

Treatment

There is no specific treatment for any form of acute hepatitis. Patients should rest in bed as needed, avoid alcohol, and be sure to eat a balanced diet.

Prognosis

What little is known about the course of hepatitis G suggests that illness is mild and does not last long. When more patients have been followed up after the acute phase, it will become clear whether HGV can cause severe liver damage.

Prevention

Since hepatitis G is a blood-borne infection, prevention relies on avoiding any possible contact with contaminated blood. Drug users should not share needles, syringes, or other equipment.

Resources

ORGANIZATIONS

American Liver Foundation. 1425 Pompton Ave., Cedar Grove, NJ 07009. (800) 223-0179. http://sadieo.ucsf.edu/alf/alffinal/homepagealf.html.

David A. Cramer

Hepatitis virus studies *see* **Hepatitis virus tests**

Hepatitis virus tests

Definition

Viral hepatitis is any type of liver inflammation caused by a viral infection. The three most common viruses now recognized to cause liver disease are **hepatitis A, hepatitis B,** and hepatitis non-A, non-B (also called **hepatitis C**). Several other types have been recognized: **hepatitis D, hepatitis E,** and the recently identified **hepatitis G.** A seventh type (hepatitis F) is suspected but not yet confirmed.

Purpose

The different types of viral hepatitis produce similar symptoms, but they differ in terms of transmission, course of treatment, prognosis, and carrier status. When the clinical history of a patient is insufficient for differentiation, hepatitis virus tests are used as an aid in diagnosis and in monitoring the course of the disease. These tests are based primarily on antigen-antibody reactions—an antigen being a protein foreign to the body, and an antibody another type of protein manufactured by lymphocytes (a type of white blood cell) to neutralize the antigen.

Description

There are five major types of viral hepatitis. The diseases, along with the antigen-antibody tests available to aid in diagnosis, are described below.

Hepatitis A

Commonly called infectious hepatitis, this is caused by the hepatitis A virus (HAV). It is usually a mild disease, most often spread by food and water contamination, but sometimes through sexual contact. Immunologic tests are not commercially available for the HAV antigen, but two types of antibodies to HAV can be detected. IgM antibody (anti-HAV/IgM), appears approximately three to four weeks after exposure and returns to normal within several months. IgG (anti-HAV/IgG) appears approximately two weeks after the IgM begins to increase and remains positive. Acute hepatitis is suspected if IgM is elevated; conversely, if IgG is elevated without IgM, a convalescent stage of HAV is presumed. IgG antibody can remain detectable for decades after infection.

Hepatitis B

Commonly known as serum hepatitis, this is caused by the hepatitis B virus (HBV). The disease can be mild or severe, and it can be acute (of limited duration) or chronic (ongoing). It is usually spread by sexual contact with another infected person, through contact with infected blood, by intravenous drug use, or from mother to child at birth.

HBV, also called the Dane particle, is composed of an inner protein core surrounded by an outer protein capsule. The outer capsule contains the hepatitis B surface antigen (HBsAg), formerly called the Australia antigen. The inner core contains HBV core antigen (HBcAg), and the hepatitis B e-antigen (HBeAg). Antibodies to these antigens are called anti-HBs, anti-HBc, and anti-HBe. Testing for these antigens and antibodies is as follows:

- Hepatitis B surface antigen (HBsAg). This is the first test for hepatitis B to become abnormal. HBsAg begins to elevate before the onset of clinical symptoms, peaks during the first week of symptoms, and usually disappears by the time the accompanying **jaundice** (yellowing of the skin and other tissues) begins to subside. HBsAg indicates an active HBV infection. A person is considered to be a carrier if this antigen persists in the blood for six or more months.

- Hepatitis B surface antibody (anti-HBs). This appears approximately one month after the disappearance of the HBsAg, signaling the end of the acute infection period. Anti-HBs is the antibody that demonstrates immunity after administration of the hepatitis B vaccine. Its presence also indicates immunity to subsequent infection.

- Hepatitis B core antigen (HBcAg). No tests are commercially available to detect this antigen.

- Hepatitis B core antibody (anti-HBc). This appears just before acute hepatitis develops and remains elevated (although it slowly declines) for years. It is also present in chronic hepatitis. The hepatitis B core antibody is elevated during the time lag between the disappearance of the hepatitis B surface antigen and the appearance of the hepatitis B surface antibody in an interval called the "window." During this time, the hepatitis B core antibody is the only detectable marker of a recent hepatitis B infection.

- Hepatitis B e-antigen (HBeAg). This is more useful as an index of infection than for diagnostic purposes. The presence of this antigen correlates with early and active disease, as well as with high infectivity in patients with acute HBV infection. When HBeAg levels persist in the blood, the development of chronic HBV infection is suspected.

- Hepatitis B e-antibody (anti-HBe). In the bloodstream, this indicates a reduced risk of infectivity in patients who have previously been HBeAg positive. Chronic hepatitis B surface antigen carriers can be positive for either HBeAg or anti-HBe, but are less infectious when anti-HBe is present. Antibody to e antigen can persist for years, but usually disappears earlier than anti-HBs or anti-HBc.

Hepatitis C

Previously known as non-A, non-B hepatitis, this disease is primarily caused by the hepatitis C virus (HCV). It is generally mild, but more likely than hepatitis B to lead to chronic liver disease, possible liver failure, and the eventual need for transplant. Chronic carrier states develop in more than 80% of patients, and chronic liver disease is a major problem. As many as 20% of patients with chronic hepatitis C will develop liver failure or **liver cancer.** HCV is spread through sexual contact, as well as through sharing drug needles, although nearly half of infections can't be traced as to origin.

Hepatitis C is detected by HCV serology (tests on blood sera). A specific type of assay called enzyme-linked immunosorbent assay (ELISA) was developed to detect antibody to hepatitis C for diagnostic purposes, as well as for screening blood donors. Most cases of post-**transfusion** non-A, non-B hepatitis are caused by HCV, but application of this test has virtually eliminated post-transfusion hepatitis. An HCV viral titer to detect HCV RNA in the blood is now available, and recently, IgM anti-HCV core is proving to be a useful acute marker for HCV infection.

Hepatitis D

Also called delta hepatitis, this is caused by the hepatitis D virus (HDV). The disease occurs only in those who have HBV in the blood from a past or simultaneously occurring infection. Experts believe transmission may occur through sexual contact, but further research is needed to confirm that. Most cases occur among those who are frequently exposed to blood and blood products. Many cases also occur among drug users who share contaminated needles. Hepatitis D virus (HDV) antigen can be detected by radioimmunoassay within a few days after infection, together with IgM and total antibodies to HDV.

Hepatitis E

Caused by the hepatitis E virus (HEV), this is actually another type of non-A, non-B hepatitis. The virus is most often spread through fecally contaminated water, but the role of person-to-person transmission is unclear. This form of hepatitis is quite rare in the United States. There are currently no antigen or antibody tests widely available to accurately detect HEV.

Preparation

Hepatitis virus tests require a blood sample. It is not necessary for the patient to withhold food or fluids before any of these tests, unless requested to do so by the physician.

Risks

Risks for these tests are minimal for the patient, but may include slight bleeding from the blood-drawing site, **fainting** or feeling lightheaded after venipuncture, or hematoma (blood accumulating under the puncture site).

Normal results

Reference ranges for the antigen/antibody tests are as follows:

- Hepatitis A antibody, IgM: Negative
- Hepatitis B core antibody: Negative
- Hepatitis B e antibody: Negative
- Hepatitis B e-antigen: Negative
- Hepatitis B surface antibody: Varies with clinical circumstance (Note: As the presence of anti-HBs indicates past infection with resolution of previous hepatitis B infection, or **vaccination** against hepatitis B, additional patient history may be necessary for diagnosis.)
- Hepatitis B surface antigen: Negative
- Hepatitis C serology: Negative
- Hepatitis D serology: Negative.

Abnormal results

Hepatitis A: A single positive anti-HAV test may indicate previous exposure to the virus, but due to the antibody persisting so long in the bloodstream, only evidence of a rising anti-HAV titer confirms hepatitis A. Determining recent infection rests on identifying the antibody as IgM (associated with recent infection). A negative anti-HAV test rules out hepatitis A.

Hepatitis B: High levels of HBsAg that continue for three or more months after onset of acute infection suggest development of chronic hepatitis or carrier status. Detection of anti-HBs signals late convalescence or recovery from infection. This antibody remains in the blood to provide immunity to reinfection.

Hepatitis C (non-A, non-B hepatitis): Anti-HBc develops after exposure to hepatitis B. As an early indicator of acute infection, antibody (IgM) to core antigen (anti-HBc IgM) is rarely detected in chronic infection, so it is useful in distinguishing acute from chronic infection, and hepatitis B from non-A, non-B.

Resources

BOOKS

Cahill, Mathew. *Handbook of Diagnostic Tests.* Springhouse, PA: Springhouse Corporation, 1995.

Jacobs, David S. *Laboratory Test Handbook,* 4th ed. Hudson, OH: Lexi-Comp Inc., 1996.

Pagana, Kathleen Deska. *Mosby's Manual of Diagnostic and Laboratory Tests.* St. Louis: Mosby, Inc., 1998.

Janis O. Flores

Hepatitis-associated antigen (HAA) test *see* **Hepatitis virus tests**

Hepatobiliary scan *see* **Gallbladder nuclear medicine scan**

Hepatoblastoma *see* **Liver cancer**

Hepatocellular carcinoma *see* **Liver cancer**

Hepatoma *see* **Liver cancer**

Herbal medicine *see* **Herbal remedies, western**

Herbal remedies, western

Definition

Herbal remedies involve the use of plants as medicines to restore and maintain health.

Purpose

Herbal remedies are employed in the western world by practitioners of holistic medicine who believe that all individuals possess an inner vital force that is constantly working to maintain physical, emotional, and mental

---

KEY TERMS

Absorption—The taking up of substances by the skin or other tissues.

Alkaloid—A class of nitrogen-containing compounds, found mainly in plants, that have very powerful physiological effects.

Antibiotic—Any substance derived from fungi or bacteria that destroys or inhibits the growth of microorganisms.

Antiseptic—Any substance that checks the growth or action of microorganisms.

Constituent—A component or an element.

Dilute—A weakened solution or substance.

Diuretic—An agent that increases the amount of urine produced and excreted.

Douche—The rinsing of the vagina with a liquid.

Germ theory of disease—The theory that certain diseases are caused by the invasion of the body by microorganisms.

Holistic—That which pertains to the entire person, including the body, mind, and spirit.

Pharmaceutical—Relating to the preparation and dispensation of medicines.

Pharmacology—The branch of science concerned with all aspects of the interactions of drugs and their effect on living organisms.

Poultice—A soft composition, usually heated and spread on a cloth, that is applied to a sore or inflamed part of the body.

Sedative—Any agent that slows down nervous activity.

Suppository—A solid medication designed to be introduced into and dissolved within a body cavity other than the mouth.

Synergism—The coordinated action of two or more substances to produce an effect that none can produce by itself.

Synthetic drugs—Man-made medicines produced entirely from chemical substances.

---

health. Although they do not discount the germ theory of disease held by conventional western medicine, medical herbalists in the western world say that this theory does not fully explain why people become ill. They argue that many diseases and conditions come about because the individual's inner force or natural immune system is weakened or out of balance. Therefore, they prescribe herbal or plant remedies that are found in nature in order to return an individual's natural inner balance, strengthen the resistance to disease, and maintain good health.

Precautions

Herbal remedies can be dangerous and must be treated with respect. Some of the most potent and toxic chemicals come from plants. Simply because something is described as "natural" does not mean that it cannot have serious side effects. While most commonly used herbal remedies are safe, it is best to obtain the advice of a well-trained practitioner before using any plant-based medication that is not well known, especially since herbals may interact with conventional drugs. Further, it is important to use herbal remedies correctly and stick to the prescribed doses. It should also be recognized that the sale of herbals in the United States is largely unregulated, and consumers cannot be certain of their quality.

Description

History

The origins of western herbal remedies are found at least as far back as 3000 B.C. in the ancient civilization of Egypt. Herbal remedies were also used in ancient Greece, Rome, and the Middle East. After the arrival of Columbus, many New World plants became available to Europeans, and by the time of Henry VIII in England (1491-1547), an entire European or western medical system that blended plant use and astrology had developed. For centuries, medicine in the West meant herbal medicine. It is only since World War II that the West relied on anything but natural plants to cure its ills. Since then however, modern medicine with its synthetic drugs and high technology has become so dominant that herbal cures are almost totally eclipsed. At the approach of a new millennium, however, herbal remedies are undergoing a renaissance in the West, and are beginning to be accepted as, at least, complementary to conventional medicine.

Resurgence of practice of herbal medicine

This resurgence in the West of herbal remedies has many understandable causes. First among these may be the impersonal nature of modern medicine as it is often practiced. Many patients feel alienated by their physicians, who do not always seem to treat them as individuals. This alienation is compounded by the often extreme costs of high-tech medicine. Further, many synthetic drugs have adverse side effects, or have been overused to the point of no longer being effective. Increasingly, western herbal medicine offers an attractive alternative to many people. In 1995, herbal products totaled an estimated $2 billion in sales in the United States alone. Much of this popularity is attributable not only to a belief in the effectiveness of herbals, but also because of herbal medicine's holistic emphasis, its respect for the individual, and its emphasis on self-help. The practice of herbal medicine fits in well with the sentiment of people wishing to take charge of their own lives.

Such intangible aspects as these appear to have as much to do with the resurgence in the West of herbalism as the effectiveness of its remedies. The principles upon which herbal medicine is based are therefore important to at least consider. First among these is its great concern for the uniqueness of the individual. As an established value of holistic medicine in general, this notion differs from conventional medicine, which uses a single drug to treat a single disease. On the contrary, herbal medicine tailors the remedy to meet the many and varied needs of the individual, resulting in the possibility that two people with the same medical condition may receive two very different herbal prescriptions. Second, herbalists see a person's symptoms as an indication that his or her body is struggling to restore its natural inner balance, upon which—they argue—all self-healing is based. Herbal remedies are therefore prescribed to restore that natural balance and allow the body to work its own way back to health. Thus the person who takes an herbal remedy should not always expect to see all symptoms disappear immediately, since the natural medicine is intended rather to support the body's systems. The proper functioning body will then remedy the symptoms.

Another aspect of western herbal remedies that makes their practice very different from the conventional pharmacology of modern medicine is the fact that it involves not simply a single, chemical constituent, but, rather, the entire plant. This "whole plant" philosophy can begin to be better understood by considering the notion that a single plant is greater than the sum of its parts. Because any plant is literally made up of hundreds, if not thousands, of different chemicals that interact in a highly complex manner, a herbal medication cannot be reduced to the simple isolation of a certain plant's active constituent or major ingredient. This phenomenon is known as synergism, which means, in this context, the effect produced by all of a plant's constituent parts working and combining together. It is exactly this frustratingly complex phenomenon that makes herbal medicine so difficult for conventionally trained health professionals to accept. The important point here is that an herbal remedy cannot be reduced to a simple list of its active constituents.

Purpose of herbal medicines

Herbalists believe their remedies work in our bodies in the same chemical manner as do the synthetic drugs of conventional medicine, but that is probably the only similarity. Because herbal remedies employ the entire plant or herb rather than just one of the chemicals it might contain, its chemicals enter the bloodstream by an indirect route and sometimes have a much slower effect. However, it is exactly this fact that the entire plant (rather than a single ingredient) is used that makes herbal remedies a more complex pharmaceutical system than synthetic drugs. In addition to the **vitamins** and **minerals** that herbs contain, there are trace elements of tannins, alkaloids, oils, and other less commonly known agents. A good example of how two natural substances that appear similar can be very different is coffee and tea. Both are known to contain significant and roughly equal amounts of **caffeine.** Yet coffee is much more stimulating than tea, since tea leaves contain much more tannin. Tannin is known to reduce the amount of nutrients and drugs that pass from the intestines into the bloodstream, which means that less of the tea's caffeine is absorbed. Comparing a natural antibiotic, like garlic, with a synthetic dose of penicillin reveals that synthetic **antibiotics** work well but also indiscriminately, killing even the good bacteria in the body's gastrointestinal system. Garlic, on the other hand, actually stimulates beneficial bacteria to work better.

In the West, herbal remedies are used to improve the quality of the body's digestion and absorption of nutrients, as well as to encourage the efficiency of its respiratory and circulatory systems. Other remedies work on strengthening the body's nervous and endocrine systems, which contributes to a stronger immune system. Herbs also are used to remove waste and toxins from the body's cells, and to soothe the skin and promote healing.

Herbs and plants are classified according to what action they have or which of the body's systems they affect. For example, some are diuretic, meaning they stimulate the production and elimination of urine. Others have a sedative effect and reduce the level of nervous activity. Still others are antiseptic and protect against infection. A complete list of the effects and actions of medicinal plants is very extensive, and they are capable of treating many conditions.

Administration of herbs

Herbal remedies are administered in many different ways. Some can be drunk, others are applied to the skin as a cream, ointment, or poultice. Certain ones are taken internally in tablet or capsule form, or as suppositories and douches, and others are simply added to pleasant, warm bath water. Herbal remedies must be treated with care, however, especially if combinations are taken. It is essential that a qualified professional herbalist or naturopathic physician be consulted for guidance, since it is still the rare mainstream physician who prescribes herbal remedies. Also, only select insurance companies, such as American Western Life, cover the cost of herbals, and then only when prescribed by a healthcare professional.

A consultation with a medical herbalist or naturopath usually begins with an interview that may take as long as one hour. It is important that the specialist learn about the patient from as many angles as possible. Thus, he or she also may ask non-medical questions concerning the client's worries, or certain personality traits, as well as some value-oriented questions. Describing oneself, as well as one's physical complaints and symptoms, allows the therapist to assess the patient and, in turn, be assessed by the patient. Medical herbalists are also qualified to conduct a routine **physical examination,** such as any doctor might do. The therapist then arrives at some understanding of the total person as well as the patient's medical condition, and eventually discovers the cause of the problem without necessarily being able to give it a name or a diagnosis. By the end of the appointment, the herbalist will have told the patient what he or she believes the problem to be and what is necessary to correct it.

In addition to suggesting dietary and **exercise** changes, the herbalist will prescribe a suitable herbal remedy, telling the patient how and when to take or use the prescription. Follow-up appointments are often suggested. Throughout this process, the herbalist examines and studies a person—not a condition, seeking to prescribe a remedy for that person and not just for his or her specific complaint.

Useful herbs

Often, an herbal remedy will be composed of plants whose names are recognized by few people, yet many of modern medicine's standard pharmaceuticals, in fact, were derived from plants. Most know that **aspirin** came from the bark of the willow tree, and that morphine and codeine are derived from the opium poppy. Chamomile and peppermint are recognized relaxants, and aloe effectively soothes skin problems. The heart drug digoxin comes from the common flower called foxglove. Tubocurarine, the most powerful muscle relaxant known, is derived from a South American plant containing curare. Cocaine comes from the cocoa plant, and the anti-malarial quinine is derived from the cinchona tree. Probably the best known and most popular plant in the world is ginseng, a tonic drug that reputedly builds vital energy. Clinical studies of other, less well-known plants have demonstrated their effective properties. Valerian has been helpful for **insomnia,** garlic has reduced blood pressure and cholesterol levels, and St. John's wort has been shown to have powerful antiviral qualities. In the case of these and hundreds of other "herbals," there is nothing unscientific or unproved about their physical effects. Herbal remedies are indeed chemicals in their natural state and should be regarded as dilute forms of drugs that can produce a biological effect.

New uses for old plants are continuing to be realized. In 1993, the British medical journal *Lancet* reported that in tests conducted in both Germany and Italy, extracts from the ancient Chinese ginkgo tree were successful in treating cerebral insufficiency in older patients. As a remedy that improves the circulation of blood to the head, it is able to help the memory of elderly people. The Latin name for the purple cone flower is *Echinacea,* and its demonstrated ability to stimulate the body's natural immune system makes it a candidate to treat some patients with HIV infection. These and other breakthroughs continually point to the validity of naturally occurring remedies.

Condition of practice of herbal medicine

While herbal remedies in the United States have demonstrated the beginnings of a real renaissance in the late 1990s, no such resurgence was necessary in Europe. There, herbal remedies have never really gone out of fashion. Still, even in countries with a strong herbal tradition, interest and actual use of herbal remedies has increased. The herbal medicine market in Europe had $2.2 billion in sales in 1993 alone, 70% of which was in Germany. Even in England, a sales upswing is obvious, and between 1990 and 1995 herbal sales there climbed by 25%. In 1995 in the United States, the herbal remedy market totaled an estimated $2 billion in sales, not including the sale of vitamins and minerals, which nearly doubled that amount. Along with this sales explosion, there was a related upsurge in the availability of information resources, sparked, in turn, by an increase in professional research interest and activity.

In England, the first undergraduate course in herbal medicine to be established in western Europe was started at Middlesex University in London in 1994. In the United States, research programs have begun at the University of Massachusetts—Amherst, Delaware State College, and at Purdue University. American businesses specializing in herbs are now served by two trade organizations, the American Herbal Products Association of Austin, Texas, and the International Herb Growers and Marketers Association of Mundelein, Illinois. Those specializing in medicinal herbs are represented in the American Botanical Council of Austin, Texas, and the Herb Research Foundation of Boulder, Colorado.

Despite this increase in attention, research, and use, the regulatory situation for herbal remedies in the United States is far from ideal from the consumer's point of view. Herbal products sold in the United States are largely unregulated, since they are considered to be dietary supplements, and, therefore, are regarded as "food" rather than "drugs." For drugs to be sold, the Food and Drug Administration (FDA) requires manufacturers to conduct lengthy studies to prove the safety and efficiency of both prescription and over-the-counter drugs. However, manufacturers of herbal remedies are held to no such rigorous standard. By placing herbal remedies in the same category as dietary supplements, like vitamins and minerals, the FDA effectively exempts them from having to be rigorously tested. Further, the 1994 Dietary Supplement Health and Education Act allows herbal manufacturers to make "limited claims" on their labels as long as they do not claim to "diagnose, prevent, mitigate, treat or cure a specific disease." All of this leads to a situation in the United States where the burden is placed squarely on the consumer, who must either get expert advice or go it alone and be very careful. The United States is virtually alone in the way it treats herbal remedies. Canada and most of the countries in western Europe take a very practical approach. Germany is perhaps most advanced in its regulation, and its consumers receive safe, properly identified and labeled, and quality-controlled herbal products. The extent to which herbal remedies are taken seriously in that country is seen in that all German medical students are required to pass an examination testing their knowledge of the clinical uses of herbals. Once the regulatory situation in the United States is improved, the next problem facing herbal manufacturers and consumers will be that of assuring consistent supplies of high quality herbs and plants.

With few exceptions, the history of herbal remedies in the West is really the history of western medicine. Just as herbs and plants were an essential part of medicine until the post World War II boom in synthetic drugs, so they are becoming once again a valid alternative and effective complement to conventional western medicine. In this way at least, western medicine is becoming more like medicine practiced nearly everywhere else in the world. The World Health Organization (WHO) of the United Nations estimates that as much as 80% of the world population relies on the use of various forms of traditional (herbal) medicine for its primary healthcare.

Risks

The improper use of herbal remedies can bring unwanted and sometimes dangerous results. Some remedies are toxic when taken in high doses, or if taken by pregnant women or small children. Herbal remedies should never be substituted in cases of severe, acute illness when rapid and strong-acting medicines are required, nor in cases of major physical trauma when surgery is necessary. Self-prescribing without consulting an herbal expert can also be dangerous.

Normal results

Herbal remedies can benefit a wide range of conditions and, with the guidance of an experienced practitioner, can be used in some way to treat most illnesses and disorders. Plant or herb remedies have shown to be particularly effective for skin conditions, such as eczema, for problems of digestion, such as **irritable bowel syndrome,** and for urinary conditions, like **cystitis.** What should not be expected, however, is for conditions to respond immediately as is sometimes the case with the synthetic "magic bullet" drugs of conventional western medicine. Further, since herbal remedies attempt to treat the underlying condition or problem rather than the symptoms, individuals who take these natural remedies should not expect the symptoms to disappear until the basic underlying physical problem has responded to the herbal and been resolved.

Resources

BOOKS

Bradford, Nikki, ed. *Alternative Healthcare.* San Diego: Thunder Bay Press, 1997.

Burton Goldberg Group. *Alternative Medicine: The Definitive Guide.* Puyallup, WA: Future Medicine Publishing, Inc., 1993.

Chevallier, Andrew. *The Encyclopedia of Medicinal Plants.* London: Dorling Kindersley Ltd., 1996.

Foster, Steven. *Herbal Renaissance.* Salt Lake City: Gibbs Smith Publisher, 1993.

Griffin, Judy. *Mother Nature's Herbal.* St. Paul: Llewellyn Publications, 1997.

Jacobs, Jennifer. *The Encyclopedia of Alternative Medicine.* Boston: Journey Editions, 1996.

PERIODICALS

Joyce, Christopher. "Western Medicine Men Return to the Field." *BioScience* (June 1992): 399-403.

Land, Thomas. "Herbal Healing." *The New Leader* (November 17, 1986): 3.

Picker, Lauren. "Herbal Medicine Goes Mainstream." *American Health* (May 1996):70-75.

ORGANIZATIONS

American Botanical Council. P.O. Box 201660, Austin, TX 78720. (512) 331-8868.

American Herbalists Guild. 3411 Cunnison Lane, P.O. Box 1683, Soquel, CA 95073. (408) 464-2441.

Leonard C. Bruno

Hereditary cerebral hemorrhage with amyloidosis *see* **Cerebral amyloid angiopathy**

Hereditary chorea *see* **Huntington's disease**

Hereditary fructose intolerance

Definition

Hereditary fructose intolerance is an inherited condition where the body does not produce the chemical needed to break down fructose (fruit sugar).

Description

Fructose is a sugar found naturally in fruits, vegetables, honey, and table sugar. Fructose intolerance is a disorder caused by the body's inability to produce an enzyme called aldolase B (also called fructose 1-phosphate aldolase) that is necessary for absorption of fructose. The undigested fructose collects in the liver and kidneys, eventually causing liver and kidney failure. One person in about 20,000 is born with this disorder. It is reported more frequently in the United States and Northern European countries than in other parts of the world. It occurs with equal frequency in males and females.

Causes & symptoms

Fructose intolerance is an inherited disorder passed on to children through their parents' genes. Both the mother and father have the gene that causes the condition, but may not have symptoms of fructose intolerance themselves. (This is called an autosomal recessive pattern of inheritance.) The disorder will not be apparent until the infant is fed formula, juice, fruits, or baby foods that contain fructose. Initial symptoms include vomiting, **dehydration,** and unexplained **fever.** Other symptoms include extreme thirst and excessive urination and sweating. There will also be a loss of appetite and a failure to grow. **Tremors** and seizures caused by low blood sugar can occur. The liver becomes swollen and the patient becomes jaundiced with yellowing of the eyes and skin. Left untreated, this condition can lead to **coma** and **death.**

Diagnosis

Urine tests can be used to detect fructose sugar in the urine. Blood tests can also be used to detect *hyperbilirubinemia* and high levels of liver enzymes in the blood. A **liver biopsy** may be performed to test for levels of enzymes present and to evaluate the extent of damage to the liver. A fructose-loading test where a dose of fructose is given to the patient in a well-controlled hospital or clinical setting may also be used to confirm fructose intolerance. Both the biopsy and the loading test can be very risky, particularly in infants that are already sick.

Treatment

Once diagnosed, fructose intolerance can be successfully treated by eliminating fructose from the diet. Patients usually respond within three to four weeks and can make a complete recovery if fructose-containing foods are avoided. Early recognition and treatment of the disease is important to avoid damage to the liver, kidneys, and small intestine.

Prognosis

If the condition is not recognized and the diet is not well controlled, death can occur in infants or young children. With a well-controlled diet, the child can develop normally.

Prevention

Carriers of the gene for hereditary fructose intolerance can be identified through DNA analysis. Anyone who is known to carry the disease or who has the disease in his or her family can benefit from genetic counseling. Since this is a hereditary disorder, there is currently no known way to prevent it other than assisting at-risk individuals with family planning and reproductive decisions.

Resources

BOOKS

Greene, Harry L. "Fructose Intolerance." In *Cecil Textbook of Medicine.* 20th ed. Philadelphia: W.B. Saunders, 1996.

"Hereditary Fructose Intolerance." In *Internal Medicine*, edited by Jay H. Stein. 5th ed. St. Louis: Mosby, 1998.

ORGANIZATIONS

National Institutes of Health. National Institute of Diabetes, Digestive and Kidney Diseases. Building 31, Room 9A04, 31 Center Drive, Bethesda, MD 20892-2560. (301) 496-3583.

OTHER

What Is Hereditary Fructose Intolerance? http://bio.bu.edu/~vfunari/.

Altha Roberts Edgren

Hereditary hemorrhagic telangiectasia

Definition

Hereditary hemorrhagic telangiectasia is an inherited condition characterized by abnormal blood vessels which are delicate and prone to bleeding. Hereditary hemorrhagic telangiectasia is also known as Rendu-Osler-Weber disease.

Description

The term telangiectasia refers to a spot formed, usually on the skin, by a dilated capillary or terminal artery. In hereditary hemorrhagic telangiectasia these spots occur because the blood vessel is fragile and bleeds easily. The bleeding may appear as small, red or reddish-violet spots on the face, lips, inside the mouth and nose or the tips of the fingers and toes. Other small telangiectasias may occur in the digestive tract.

Unlike **hemophilia,** where bleeding is caused by an ineffective clotting mechanism in the blood, bleeding in hereditary hemorrhagic telangiectasia is caused by fragile blood vessels. However, like hemophilia, bleeding may be extensive and can occur without warning.

Causes & symptoms

Hereditary hemorrhagic telangiectasia, an autosomal dominant inherited disorder, occurs 1 in 50,000 people.

Recurrent **nosebleeds** are a nearly universal symptom in this condition. Usually the nosebleeds begin in childhood and become worse with age. The skin changes

Hernia

KEY TERMS

Autosomal dominant—A pattern of inheritance in which the dominant gene on any non-sex chromosome carries the defect.

Chromosome—A threadlike structure in the cell which transmits genetic information.

begin at **puberty,** and the condition becomes progressively worse until about 40 years of age, when it stabilizes.

Diagnosis

The physician will look for red spots on all areas of the skin, but especially on the upper half of the body, and in the mouth and nose and under the tongue.

Treatment

There is no specific treatment for hereditary hemorrhagic telangiectasia. The bleeding resulting from the condition can be stopped by applying compresses or direct pressure to the area. If necessary, a laser can be used to destroy the vessel. In severe cases, the leaking artery can be plugged or covered with a graft from normal tissue.

Prognosis

In most people, recurrent bleeding results in an iron deficiency. It is usually necessary to take iron supplements.

Prevention

Hereditary hemorrhagic telangiectasia is an inherited disorder and cannot be prevented.

Resources

ORGANIZATIONS

The American Medical Association, 515 North State Street, Chicago, IL, 60610, 312/464-5000.

Association of Birth Defect Children, 3526 Emerywood Lane, Orlando, FL, 32806,305/859-2821.

Dorothy Elinor Stonely

Hereditary hyperuricemia *see* **Lesch-Nyhan syndrome**

Hereditary spinocerebellar ataxia *see* **Friedreich's ataxia**

Hermaphroditism *see* **Intersex states**

Hernia

Definition

Hernia is a general term used to describe a bulge or protrusion of an organ through the structure or muscle that usually contains it.

Description

There are many different types of hernias. The most familiar type are those that occur in the abdomen, in which part of the intestines protrude through the abdominal wall. This may occur in different areas and, depending on the location, the hernia is given a different name.

An inguinal hernia appears as a bulge in the groin and may come and go depending on the position of the person or their level of physical activity. It can occur with or without **pain.** In men, the protrusion may descend into the scrotum. Inguinal hernias account for 80% of all hernias and are more common in men.

Femoral hernias are similar to inguinal hernias but appear as a bulge slightly lower. They are more common in women due to the strain of **pregnancy.**

A ventral hernia is also called an incisional hernia because it generally occurs as a bulge in the abdomen at the site of an old surgical scar. It is caused by thinning or stretching of the scar tissue, and occurs more frequently in people who are obese or pregnant.

An umbilical hernia appears as a soft bulge at the navel (umbilicus). It is caused by a weakening of the area or an imperfect closure of the area in infants. This type of hernia is more common in women due to pregnancy, and in Chinese and black infants. Some umbilical hernias in infants disappear without treatment within the first year.

A hiatal or diaphragmatic hernia is different from abdominal hernias in that it is not visible on the outside of the body. With a hiatal hernia, the stomach bulges upward through the muscle that separates the chest from the abdomen (the diaphragm). This type of hernia occurs more often in women than in men, and it is treated differently from other types of hernias.

Causes & symptoms

Most hernias result from a weakness in the abdominal wall that either develops or that an infant is born with (congenital). Any increase in pressure in the abdomen, such as coughing, straining, heavy lifting, or pregnancy,

KEY TERMS
. . . .

Endoscopy—A diagnostic procedure in which a tube is inserted through the mouth, into the esophagus and stomach. It is used to visualize various digestive disorders, including hiatal hernias.

Herniorrhaphy—Surgical repair of a hernia.

Incarcerated hernia—A hernia that can not be reduced, or pushed back into place inside the intestinal wall.

Reducible hernia—A hernia that can be gently pushed back into place or that disappears when the person lies down.

Strangulated hernia—A hernia that is so tightly incarcerated outside the abdominal wall that the intestine is blocked and the blood supply to that part of the intestine is cut off.

can be a considered causative factor in developing an abdominal hernia. **Obesity** or recent excessive weight loss, as well as aging and previous surgery, are also risk factors.

Most abdominal hernias appear suddenly when the abdominal muscles are strained. The person may feel tenderness, a slight burning sensation, or a feeling of heaviness in the bulge. It may be possible for the person to push the hernia back into place with gentle pressure, or the hernia may disappear by itself when the person reclines. Being able to push the hernia back is called reducing it. On the other hand, some hernias cannot be pushed back into place, and are termed incarcerated or irreducible.

A hiatal hernia may also be caused by obesity, pregnancy, aging, or previous surgery. About 50% of all people with hiatal hernias do not have any symptoms. If symptoms exist they will include **heartburn**, usually 30–60 minutes following a meal. There may be some mid chest pain due to gastric acid from the stomach being pushed up into the esophagus. The pain and heartburn are usually worse when lying down. Frequent belching and feelings of abdominal fullness may also be present.

Diagnosis

Generally, abdominal hernias need to be seen and felt to be diagnosed. Usually the hernia will increase in size with an increase in abdominal pressure, so the doctor may ask the person to cough while he or she feels the area. Once a diagnosis of an abdominal hernia is made, the doctor will usually send the person to a surgeon for a

consultation. Surgery provides the only cure for a hernia through the abdominal wall.

With a hiatal hernia, the diagnosis is based on the symptoms reported by the person. The doctor may then order tests to confirm the diagnosis. If a barium swallow is ordered, the person drinks a chalky white barium solution, which will help any protrusion through the diaphragm show up on the x ray that follows. Currently, a diagnosis of hiatal hernia is more frequently made by endoscopy. This procedure is done by a gastroenterologist (a specialist in digestive diseases). During an endoscopy the person is given an intravenous sedative and a small tube is inserted through the mouth, then into the esophagus and stomach where the doctor can visualize the hernia. The procedure takes about 30 minutes and

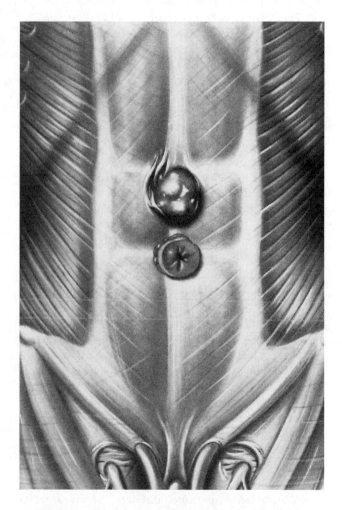

An illustration of an epigastric (abdominal) hernia in an adult male. The torso is shown with its skin removed. Epigastric hernia is usually caused by a congenital weakness in muscles of the central upper abdomen; the intestine bulges out through the muscle at a point between the navel and breastbone. *(Illustration by John Bavosi, Photo Researchers, Inc. Reproduced by permission.)*

usually causes no discomfort. It is done on an outpatient basis.

Treatment

Once an abdominal hernia occurs it tends to increase in size. Some patients with abdominal hernias wait and watch for a while prior to choosing surgery. In these cases, they must avoid strenuous physical activity such as heavy lifting or straining with **constipation.** They may also wear a truss, which is a support worn like a belt to keep a small hernia from protruding. People can tell if their hernia is getting worse if they develop severe constant pain, **nausea and vomiting,** or if the bulge does not return to normal when lying down or when they try to gently push it back in place. In these cases they should consult with their doctor immediately. But, ultimately, surgery is the treatment in almost all cases.

There are risks to not repairing a hernia surgically. Left untreated, a hernia may become incarcerated, which means it can no longer be reduced or pushed back into place. With an incarcerated hernia the intestines become trapped outside the abdomen. This could lead to a blockage in the intestine. If it is severe enough it may cut off the blood supply to the intestine and part of the intestine might actually die.

When the blood supply is cut off, the hernia is termed ''strangulated.'' Because of the risk of tissue death (necrosis) and **gangrene,** and because the hernia can block food from moving through the bowel, a strangulated hernia is a medical emergency requiring immediate surgery. Repairing a hernia before it becomes incarcerated or strangulated is much safer than waiting until complications develop.

Surgical repair of a hernia is called a herniorrhaphy. The surgeon will push the bulging part of the intestine back into place and sew the overlying muscle back together. When the muscle is not strong enough, the surgeon may reinforce it with a synthetic mesh.

Surgery can be done on an outpatient basis. It usually takes 30 minutes in children and 60 minutes in adults. It can be done under either local or general anesthesia and is frequently done with a laparoscope. In this type of surgery, a tube that allows visualization of the abdominal cavity is inserted through a small puncture wound. Several small punctures are made to allow surgical instruments to be inserted. This type of surgery avoids a larger incision.

A hiatal hernia is treated differently. Medical treatment is preferred. Treatments include:

• Avoiding reclining after meals

• Avoiding spicy foods, acidic foods, alcohol, and tobacco

• Eating small, frequent, bland meals

• Eating a high-fiber diet.

There are also several types of medications that help to manage the symptoms of a hiatal hernia. **Antacids** are used to neutralize gastric acid and decrease heartburn. Drugs that reduce the amount of acid produced in the stomach (H2 blockers) are also used. This class of drugs includes famotidine (sold under the name Pepcid), cimetidine (Tagamet), and ranitidine (Zantac). Omeprazole (Prilosec) is not an H2 blocker, but is another drug that suppresses gastric acid secretion and is used for hiatal hernias. Another option may be metoclopramide (Reglan), a drug that increases the tone of the muscle around the esophagus and causes the stomach to empty more quickly.

Alternative treatment

There are alternative therapies for hiatal hernia. Visceral manipulation, done by a trained therapist, can help replace the stomach to its proper positioning. Other options in addition to H2 blockers are available to help regulate stomach acid production and balance. One of them, deglycyrrhizinated licorice (DGL), helps balance stomach acid by improving the protective substances that line the stomach and intestines and by improving blood supply to these tissues. DGL does not interrupt the normal function of stomach acid.

As with traditional therapy, dietary modifications are important. Small, frequent meals will keep pressure down on the esophageal sphincter. Also, raising the head of the bed several inches with blocks or books can help with both the quality and quantity of sleep.

Prognosis

Abdominal hernias generally do not recur in children but can recur in up to 10% of adult patients. Surgery is considered the only cure, and the prognosis is excellent if the hernia is corrected before it becomes strangulated.

Hiatal hernias are treated successfully with medication and diet modifications 85% of the time. The prognosis remains excellent even if surgery is required in adults who are in otherwise good health.

Prevention

Some hernias can be prevented by maintaining a reasonable weight, avoiding heavy lifting and constipation, and following a moderate **exercise** program to maintain good abdominal muscle tone.

Resources

BOOKS

Bare, Brenda G., and Suzanne C. Smeltzer. *Brunner and Suddarth's Textbook of Medical-Surgical Nursing.* 8th edition. Philadelphia: Lippincott-Raven Publishers, 1996.

Polaske, Arlene L., and Suzanne E. Tatro. *Luckmann's Core Principles and Practice of Medical Surgical Nursing.* Philadelphia: W.B. Saunders Company, 1996.

PERIODICALS

Kingsley, A.N., I.L. Lichtenstein, and W.K. Sieber. "Common Hernias In Primary Care." *Patient Care* (April 1990): 98-119.

Leung, A.K.C., W.L. Robson, and A.L. Wong. "Diagnosis At a Glance." *Emergency Medicine* (January 1993): 3536.

Lipsyte, R. "Pig-out Penalty . . . Hiatal Hernia." *American Health: Fitness Of Body And Mind* (November, 1994): 49-50.

Spiro, H.M. "Hiatus Hernia and Reflux Esophagitis." *Hospital Practice* (January, 1994): 51-66.

Joyce Susan Siok

Hernia repair

Definition

Hernia repair is a surgical procedure to return an organ that protrudes through a weak area of muscle to its original position.

Purpose

Hernias occur when a weakness in the wall of the abdomen allows an organ, usually the intestines, to bulge out of place. Hernias may result from a genetic predisposition toward this weakness. They can also be the result of weakening the muscle through improper **exercise** or poor lifting techniques. Both children and adults get hernias. Some are painful, while others are not.

There are three levels of hernias. An uncomplicated hernia is one where the intestines bulge into the peritoneum (the membrane lining the abdomen), but they can still be manipulated back into the body (although they don't stay in place without corrective surgery). This is termed a reducible hernia.

If the intestines bulge through the hernia defect and become trapped, this is called an incarcerated hernia. If the blood supply to an incarcerated hernia is shut off, the

---

> ### KEY TERMS
>
> **Endoscopy**—A procedure in which an instrument containing a camera is inserted into the gastrointestinal tract so that the doctor can visually inspect the gastrointestinal system.
>
> **Gangrene**—Death and decay of body tissue because the blood supply is cut off. Tissues that have died in this way must be surgically removed.
>
> **Peritoneum**—The transparent membrane lining the abdominal cavity that holds organs such as the intestines in place.

hernia is called a strangulated hernia. Strangulated hernias can result in **gangrene.**

Both incarcerated and strangulated hernias are medical emergencies and require emergency surgery to correct. For this reason, doctors generally recommend the repair of an uncomplicated hernia, even if it causes no discomfort to the patient.

Precautions

Hernia repair can be performed under local, regional, or general anesthesia. The choice depends on the age and health of the patient and the type of hernia. Generally hernia repair is very safe surgery, but—as with any surgery—the risk of complications increases if the patient smokes, is obese, is very young or very old, uses alcohol heavily, or uses illicit drugs.

Description

Hernia repairs are performed in a hospital or outpatient surgical facility by a general surgeon. Depending on the patient's age, health, and the type of hernia, patients may be able to go home the same day or may remain hospitalized for up to three to five days.

There are two types of hernia repair. A herniorrhaphy is used for simpler hernias. The intestines are returned to their proper place and the defect in the abdominal wall is mended. A hernioplasty is used for larger hernias. In this procedure, plastic or steel mesh is added to the abdominal wall to repair and reinforce the weak spot.

There are five kinds of common hernia repairs. They are named for the part of the body closest to the hernia, or bulge.

Femoral hernia repair

This procedure repairs a hernia that occurs in the groin where the thigh meets the abdomen. It is called a

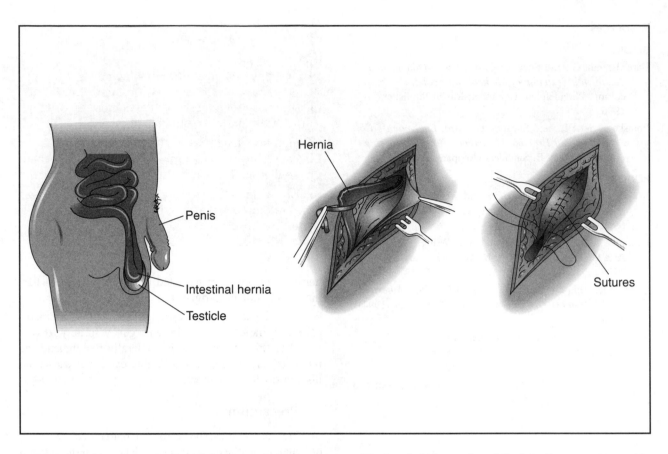

In this inguinal hernia repair, an incision is made in the abdomen. The hernia is located, and the intestines are returned to the abdomen. The abdominal wall is then sutured together to close any space and reinforce the weak area. *(Illustration by Electronic Illustrators Group.)*

femoral hernia repair because it is near the spot where the femoral artery and vein pass from the leg into the trunk of the body. Sometimes this type of hernia creates a noticeable bulge.

An incision is made in the groin area. The tissues are separated from the hernia sac, and the intestines are returned to the abdomen. The area is often reinforced with webbing before it is sewn shut. The skin is closed with sutures or metal clips that can be removed in about one week.

Inguinal hernia repair

Inguinal hernia repair closes a weakness in the abdominal wall that is near the inguinal canal, the spot where the testes descend from the body into the scrotum. This type of hernia occurs in about two percent of adult males.

An incision is made in the abdomen, then the hernia is located and repaired. The surgeon must be alert not to injure the spermatic cord, the testes, or the blood supply to the testes. If the hernia is small, it is simply repaired. If it is large, the area is reinforced with mesh to prevent a recurrence. External skin sutures can be removed in about a week. Patients should not resume sexual activity until being cleared by their doctor.

Umbilical hernia repair

This procedure repairs a hernia that occurs when the intestines bulge through the abdomen wall near the navel. Umbilical hernias are most common in infants.

An incision is made near the navel. The hernia is located and the intestines are returned to the abdomen. The peritoneum is closed, then the large abdominal muscle is pulled over the weak spot in such a way as to reinforce the area. External sutures or skin clips can be removed in about 10 days.

Incisional hernia repair

Incisional hernias occur most frequently at the site of a scar from earlier abdominal surgery. Once again, the abdomen is opened and the intestines returned to their proper place. The area is reinforced with mesh, and the abdominal wall is reconstructed to prevent another hernia from developing. External sutures can be removed in about a week.

Hiatal hernia

A hiatal hernia repair is slightly different from the other hernias described here, because it corrects a weakness or opening in the diaphragm, the muscle that separates the chest cavity from the abdominal cavity. This surgery is done to prevent the stomach from shifting up into the chest cavity and to prevent the stomach from spilling gastric juices into the esophagus, causing pain and scarring.

An incision is made in the abdomen or chest, and the hole or weakness in the diaphragm is located and repaired. The top of the stomach is wrapped around the bottom of the esophagus, and they are sutured together to hold the stomach in place. Sometimes the vagus nerve is cut in order to decrease the amount of acid the stomach produces. External sutures can be removed in about one week. This type of hernia repair often requires a longer hospital stay than the other types, although techniques are being improved that reduce invasiveness of the surgery and the length of the hospital stay.

Preparation

Before the operation, the patient will have blood and urine collected for testing. X rays are taken of the affected area. In a hiatal hernia, an endoscopy (a visual inspection of the organs) is done.

Patients should meet with the anesthesiologist before the operation to discuss any medications or conditions that might affect the administration of anesthesia. Patients may be asked to temporarily discontinue certain medications. The day of the operation, patients should not eat or drink anything. They may be given an enema to clear the bowels.

Aftercare

Patients should eat a clear liquid diet until the gastrointestinal tract begins functioning again. Normally this is a short period of time. After that, they are free to eat a healthy, well-balanced diet of their choice. They may bathe normally, using a gentle, unscented soap. An antibiotic ointment may be prescribed for the incision. After the operation, a hard ridge will form along the incision line. With time, this ridge softens and becomes less noticeable. Patients who remain in the hospital will have blood drawn for follow-up studies.

Patients should begin easy activities, such as walking, as soon as they are comfortable, but should avoid strenuous exercise for four to six weeks, and especially avoid heavy lifting. Learning and practicing proper lifting techniques is an important part of patient education after the operation. Patients may be given a laxative or stool softener so that they will not strain to have bowel movements. They should discuss with their doctor when to resume driving and sexual activity.

Risks

As with any surgery, there exists the possibility of excessive bleeding and infection after the surgery. In inguinal and femoral hernia repair, a slight risk of damage to the testicles or their blood supply exists for male patients. Accidental damage may be caused to the intestinal tract, but generally complications are few.

Normal results

The outcome of surgery depends on the age and health of the patient and on the type of hernia. Although most hernias can be repaired without complications, hernias recur in 10–20% of people who have had hernia surgery.

Resources

BOOKS

Griffith, H. Winter. ''Hernia Repair.'' In *The Complete Guide to Symptoms, Illness and Surgery,* 3rd ed. New York: Berkeley Publishing, 1995, pp. 805-11.

''Hernia Repair.'' In *The Patient's Guide to Medical Tests,* edited by Barry Zaret, et al. New York: Houghton Mifflin, 1997, pp. 148-50.

OTHER

Thrive Online. ''Hernia Repair.'' www.thriveonline.com/health/Library/surgery/surgery148.htm to surgery151.htm.

Tish Davidson

Herniated disk

Definition

Disk herniation is a rupture of fibrocartilagenous material (annulus fibrosis) that surrounds the intervertebral disk. This rupture involves the release of the disk's center portion containing a gelatinous substance called the nucleus pulposus. Pressure from the vertebrae above and below may cause the nucleus pulposus to be forced outward, placing pressure on a spinal nerve and causing considerable **pain** and damage to the nerve. This condition most frequently occurs in the lumbar region and is also commonly called herniated nucleus pulposus, prolapsed disk, ruptured intervertebral disk, or slipped disk.

Description

The spinal column is made up of 26 vertebrae that are joined together and permit forward and backward bending, side bending, and rotation of the spine. Five distinct regions comprise the spinal column, including the cervical (neck) region, thoracic (chest) region, lumbar (low back) region, sacral and coccygeal (tailbone) region. The cervical region consists of seven vertebrae, the thoracic region includes 12 vertebrae, and the lumbar region contains five vertebrae. The sacrum is composed of five fused vertebrae, which are connected to four fused vertebrae forming the coccyx. Intervertebral disks lie between each adjacent vertebra.

Each disk is composed of a gelatinous material in the center, called the nucleus pulposus, surrounded by rings of a fiberous tissue (annulus fibrosus). In disk herniation, an intervertebral disk's central portion herniates or slips through the surrounding annulus fibrosus into the spinal canal, putting pressure on a nerve root. Disk herniation most commonly affects the lumbar region between the fifth lumbar vertebra and the first sacral vertebra. However, disk herniation can also occur in the cervical spine. The incidence of cervical disk herniation is most common between the fifth and sixth cervical vertebrae. The second most common area for cervical disk herniation occurs between the sixth and seventh cervical vertebrae. Disk herniation is less common in the thoracic region.

Predisposing factors associated with disk herniation include age, gender, and work environment. The peak age for occurrence of disk herniation is between 20–45 years of age. Studies have shown that males are more commonly affected than females in lumbar disk herniation by a 3:2 ratio. Prolonged exposure to a bent-forward work posture is correlated with an increased incidence of disk herniation.

There are four classifications of disk pathology:

• A protrusion may occur where a disk bulges without rupturing the annulus fibrosis.

• The disk may prolapse where the nucleus pulposus migrates to the outermost fibers of the annulus fibrosis.

• There may be a disk extrusion, which is the case if the annulus fibrosis perforates and material of the nucleus moves into the epidural space.

• The sequestrated disk may occur as fragments from the annulus fibrosis and nucleus pulposus are outside the disk proper.

Causes & symptoms

Any direct, forceful, and vertical pressure on the lumbar disks can cause the disk to push its fluid contents into the vertebral body. Herniated nucleus pulposus may occur suddenly from lifting, twisting, or direct injury, or it can occur gradually from degenerative changes with episodes of intensifying symptoms. The annulus may also become weakened over time, allowing stretching or tearing and leading to a disk herniation. Depending on the location of the herniation, the herniated material can also press directly on nerve roots or on the spinal cord, causing a shock-like pain (**sciatica**) down the legs, weakness, numbness, or problems with bowels, bladder, or sexual function.

Diagnosis

Several radiographic tests are useful for confirming a diagnosis of disk herniation and locating the source of pain. These tests also help the surgeon indicate the extent of the surgery needed to fully decompress the nerve. X rays show structural changes of the lumbar spine. **Myelography** is a special x ray of the spine in which a dye or air is injected into the patient's spinal canal. The patient lies strapped to a table as the table tilts in various directions and spot x rays are taken. X rays showing a narrowed dye column in the intervertebral disk area indicate possible disk herniation.

Computed tomography scan (CT or CAT scans) exhibit the details of pathology necessary to obtain consistently good surgical results. **Magnetic resonance imaging** (MRI) analysis of the disks can accurately detect the early stages of disk aging and degeneration. Electomyograms (EMGs) measure the electrical activity of the muscle contractions and possibly show evidence of nerve damage. An EMG is a powerful tool for assessing

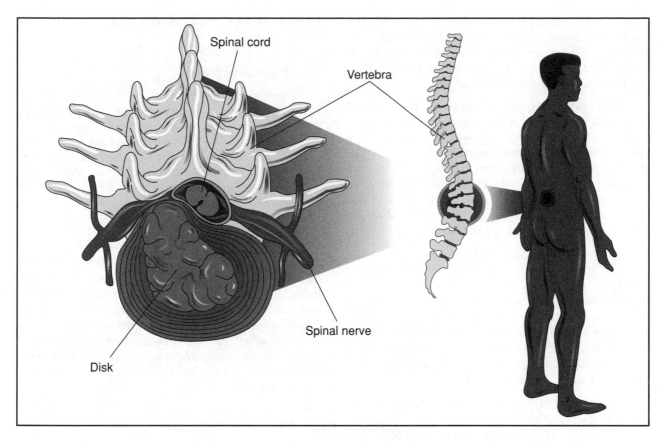

A herniated disk refers to the rupture of fibrocartilagenous material, called the annulus fibrosis, that surrounds the intervertebral disk. When this occurs, pressure from the vertebrae above and below may force the disk's center portion, a gel-like substance, outward, placing additional pressure on the spinal nerve and causing pain and damage. *(Illustration by Electronic Illustrators Group.)*

muscle fatigue associated with muscle impairment with **low back pain.**

Treatment

Drugs

Unless serious neurologic symptoms occur, herniated disks can initially be treated with pain medication and up to 48 hours of bed rest. There is no proven benefit from resting more than 48 hours. Patients are then encouraged to gradually increase their activity. Pain medications, including antiinflammatories, muscle relaxers, or in severe cases, narcotics, may be continued if needed.

Epidural steroid injections have been used to decrease pain by injecting an antiinflammatory drug, usually a corticosteroid, around the nerve root to reduce inflammation and **edema** (swelling). This partly relieves the pressure on the nerve root as well as resolves the inflammation.

Physical therapy

Physical therapists are skilled in treating acute back pain caused by the disk herniation. The physical therapist can provide noninvasive therapies, such as ultrasound or diathermy to project heat deep into the tissues of the back or administer manual therapy, if mobility of the spine is impaired. They may help improve posture and develop an **exercise** program for recovery and long-term protection. Appropriate exercise can help take pressure off inflamed nerve structures, while improving overall posture and flexibility. **Traction** can be used to try to decrease pressure on the disk. A lumbar support can be helpful for a herniated disk at this level as a temporary measure to reduce pain and improve posture.

Surgery

Surgery is often appropriate for conditions that do not improve with the usual treatment. In this event, a strong, flexible spine is important for a quick recovery after surgery. There are several surgical approaches to treating a herniated disk, including the classic disc-ectomy, microdiscectomy, or percutanteous discectomy. The basic differences among these procedures are the size of the incision, how the disk is reached surgically, and how much of the disk is removed.

Discectomy is the surgical removal of the portion of the disk that is putting pressure on a nerve causing the back pain. In the classic disectomy, the surgeon first enters through the skin and then removes a bony portion of the vertebra called the lamina, hence the term lam-inectomy. The surgeon removes the disk material that is pressing on a nerve. Rarely is the entire lamina or disk entirely removed. Often, only one side is removed and the surgical procedure is termed hemi-laminectomy.

In microdiscectomy, through the use of an operating microscope, the surgeon removes the offending bone or disk tissue until the nerve is free from compression or stretch. This procedure is possible using local anesthesia. Microsurgery techniques vary and have several advan-tages over the standard discectomy, such as a smaller incision, less trauma to the musculature and nerves, and easier identification of structures by viewing into the disk space through microscope magnification.

Percutaneous disk excision is performed on an out-patient basis, is less expensive than other surgical proce-dures, and does not require a general anesthesia. The purpose of percutaneous disk excision is to reduce the volume of the affected disk indirectly by partial removal of the nucleus pulposus, leaving all the structures impor-tant to stability practically unaffected. In this procedure, large incisions are avoided by inserting devices that have cutting and suction capability. Suction is applied and the disk is sliced and aspirated.

Athroscopic microdiscectomy is similar to percu-taneous discectomy, however it incorporates modified arthroscopic instruments, including scopes and suction devices. A suction irrigation of saline solution is estab-lished through two entry sites. A video discoscope is introduced from one site and the deflecting instruments from the opposite side. In this way, the surgeon is able to search and extract the nuclear fragments under direct visualization.

Laser disk decompression is performed using similar means as percutaneous excision and arthroscopic mi-crodiscectomy, however laser energy is used to remove the disk tissue. Here, laser energy is percutanteously in-troduced through a needle to vaporize a small volume of nucleus pulposus, thereby dropping the pressure of the disk and decompressing the involved neural tissues. One disadvantage of this procedure is the high initial cost of the laser equipment. It is important to realize that only a very small percentage of people with herniated lumbar disks go on to require surgery. Further, surgery should be followed by appropriate **rehabilitation** to decrease the chance of reinjury.

Chemonucleolysis

Chemonucleolysis is an alternative to surgical exci-sion. Chymopapain, a purified enzyme derived from the papaya plant, is injected percutaneously into the disk space to reduce the size of the herniated disks. It hydroly-ses proteins, thereby decreasing water-binding capacity, when injected into the nucleus pulposus inner disk mate-rial. The reduction in size of the disk relieves pressure on the nerve root.

Spinal fusion

Spinal fusion is the process by which bone grafts harvested from the iliac crest (thick border of the ilium located on the pelvis) are placed between the interverte-bral bodies after the disk material is removed. This ap-proach is used when there is a need to reestablish the normal bony relationship between the vertebrae. A total discectomy may be needed in some cases because lumbar spinal fusion can help prevent recurrent lumbar disk her-niation at a particular level.

Alternative treatment

Acupuncture involves the use of fine needles in-serted along the pathway of the pain to move energy locally and relieve the pain. An acupuncturist determines the location of the nerves affected by the herniated disk and positions the needles appropriately. **Massage** therapists may also provide short-term relief from a her-niated disk. Following manual examination and x-ray diagnosis, chiropractic treatment usually includes manip-ulation to correct muscle and joint malfunctions, while care is taken not to place an additional strain on the injured disk. If a full trial of conservative therapy fails, or if neurologic problems (weakness, bowel or bladder problems, and sensory loss) develop, the next step is usually evaluation by an orthopedic surgeon.

Prognosis

Only 5–10% of patients with unrelenting sciatica and neurological involvement, leading to chronic pain of the lumbar spine, need to have a surgical procedure performed. This strongly suggests that many patients with herniated disks at the lumbar level respond well to conservative treatment. For those patients who do require surgery for lumbar disk herniation, the reviewed proce-dures of nerve root decompression caused by disk hernia-tion is favorable. Results of studies varied from 60–90% success rates. Disk surgery has progressively evolved in the direction of decreasing invasiveness. Each surgical procedure is not without possible complications, which can lead to chronic low back pain and restricted lifestyle.

Prevention

Proper exercises to strengthen the lower back and abdominal muscles are key in preventing excess stress and compressive forces on lumbar disks. Good posture will help prevent problems on cervical, thoracic, and lumbar disks. A good flexibility program is critical for prevention of muscle and spasm that can cause an increase in compressive forces on disks at any level. Proper lifting of heavy objects is important for all muscles and levels of the individual disks. Good posture in sitting, standing, and lying down is helpful for the spine. Losing weight, if needed, can prevent weakness and unnecessary stress on the disks caused by **obesity.** Choosing proper footwear may also be helpful to reduce the impact forces to the lumbar disks while walking on hard surfaces. Wearing special back support devices may be helpful if heavy lifting is required with combinations of twisting.

Resources

BOOKS

Kessler, R.M. *Management of Common Musculoskeletal Disorders: Physical Therapy Principles and Methods.* Philadelphia: J.B. Lippincott Co., 1990.

Magee, G.G. *Orthopedic Assessment.* Philidelphia: W.B. Saunders, 1992.

Tourtellotte, C. *Musculoskeletal Problems.* Springhouse, PA: Springhouse Corp., 1988.

PERIODICALS

Choy, D.S. "Percutaneous Laser Disk Decompression: A New Therapeutic Modality." *Spine* 17 (1992): 949-956.

Frymore, J.W. "Back Pain and Sciatica." *The New England Journal of Medicine* 138 (1988).

OTHER

FreedomQuest Inc. "Acupuncture." 1998. http://acupuncture.com/Acup/AcuInd.htm.

Medical Strategies Inc. (MSI). "Back Pain." 1993-1998. Healthtouch Online http://www.healthtouch.com.

Jeffrey Larson

Hernioplasty *see* **Hernia repair**

Herniorrhaphy *see* **Hernia repair**

Herpes encephalitis *see* **Encephalitis**

Herpes genitalis *see* **Genital herpes**

Herpes simplex *see* **Cold sore**

Herpes simplex type 2 *see* **Genital herpes**

Herpes type 1 *see* **Cold sore**

Herpes type 2 *see* **Genital herpes**

Herpes zoster infection *see* **Shingles**

Herpetic gingivostomatitis *see* **Cold sore**

Hers' disease *see* **Glycogen storage diseases**

Heterotopic transplantation *see* **Liver transplantation**

Heterotropia *see* **Strabismus**

HFRS *see* **Hantavirus infections**

HHV-6 infection *see* **Roseola**

Hiatal hernia *see* **Hernia**

Hiccups

Definition

Hiccups are the result of an involuntary, spasmodic contraction of the diaphragm followed by the closing of the throat.

Description

Hiccups are one of the most common, but thankfully mildest, disorders to which humans are prey. Virtually everyone experiences them at some point, but they rarely last long or require a doctor's care. Occasionally, a bout of hiccups will last longer than two days, earning it the name "persistent hiccups." Very few people will experience intractable hiccups, in which hiccups last longer than one month.

A hiccup involves the coordinated action of the diaphragm and the muscles which close off the windpipe (trachea). The diaphragm is a dome-shaped muscle separating the chest and abdomen, normally responsible for expanding the chest cavity for inhalation. Sensation from the diaphragm travels to the spinal cord through the phrenic nerve and the vagus nerve, which pass through the chest cavity and the neck. Within the spinal cord, nerve fibers from the brain monitor sensory information and adjust the outgoing messages that control contraction. These messages travel along the phrenic nerve.

Irritation of any of the nerves involved in this loop can cause the diaphragm to undergo involuntary contraction, or spasm, pulling air into the lungs. When this occurs, it triggers a reflex in the throat muscles. Less than a tenth of a second afterward, the trachea is closed off, making the characteristic "hic" sound.

Causes & symptoms

Hiccups can be caused by central nervous system disorders, injury or irritation to the phrenic and vagus nerves, and toxic or metabolic disorders affecting the central or peripheral nervous systems. They may be of unknown cause or may be a symptom of psychological stress. Hiccups often occur after drinking carbonated beverages or alcohol. They may also follow overeating or rapid temperature changes. Persistent or intractable hiccups may be caused by any condition which irritates or damages the relevant nerves, including:

- Overstretching of the neck
- **Laryngitis**
- **Heartburn** (gastroesophageal reflux)
- Irritation of the eardrum (which is innervated by the vagus nerve)
- **General anesthesia**
- Surgery
- Bloating
- Tumor
- Infection
- Diabetes.

Diagnosis

Hiccups are diagnosed by observation, and by hearing the characteristic sound. Diagnosing the cause of intractable hiccups may require imaging studies, blood tests, pH monitoring in the esophagus, and other tests.

Treatment

Most cases of hiccups will disappear on their own. Home remedies which interrupt or override the spas-modic nerve circuitry are often effective. Such remedies include:

- Holding one's breath for as long as possible
- Breathing into a paper bag
- Swallowing a spoonful of sugar
- Bending forward from the waist and drinking water from the wrong side of a glass.

Treating any underlying disorder will usually cure the associated hiccups. Chlorpromazine (Thorazine) relieves intractable hiccups in 80% of cases. Metoclopramide (Reglan), carbamazepam, valproic acid (Depakene), and phenobarbital are also used. As a last resort, surgery to block the phrenic nerve may be performed, although it may lead to significant impairment of respiration.

Prognosis

Most cases of hiccups last no longer than several hours, with or without treatment.

Prevention

Some cases of hiccups can be avoided by drinking in moderation, avoiding very hot or very cold food, and avoiding cold showers. Carbonated beverages when drunk through a straw deliver more gas to the stomach than when sipped from a container; therefore, avoid using straws.

Resources

BOOKS

Hurst, J. W. *Medicine for the Practicing Physician, 4th ed.* Appleton & Lange, 1996.

High blood magnesium level *see* **Magnesium imbalance**

High blood phosphate level *see* **Phosphorus imbalance**

High blood pressure *see* **Hypertension; Preeclampsia and eclampsia; Pulmonary hypertension; Renovascular hypertension**

High calcium blood level *see* **Hypercalcemia**

High potassium blood level *see* **Hyperkalemia**

High sodium blood level *see*
Hypernatremia

High-altitude sickness *see* **Altitude sickness**

High-risk pregnancy

Definition

Thousands of women are living successfully with diseases like **asthma,** epilepsy, and **ulcerative colitis.** When these women become pregnant, though, they are often considered to have high-risk pregnancies.

Description

A **pregnancy** can be considered a high-risk pregnancy for a variety of reasons. Twins, triplets, and other multiple pregnancies are always considered high-risk because of the increased chance of **premature labor.** A pregnancy is also considered high-risk when prenatal tests indicate that the baby has a serious health problem (for example, a heart defect). In such cases, the mother will need special tests, and possibly medication, to carry the baby safely through to delivery. Complications caused by pregnancy itself, such as **preeclampsia** or **gestational diabetes,** can also turn a normal pregnancy into a high-risk pregnancy. Finally, many women who have chronic illnesses require special attention when they become pregnant. This entry will discuss the special needs of pregnant women who have chronic illnesses.

When women with chronic illnesses become pregnant, they are often considered to have high-risk pregnancies. It is difficult to predict what will happen to various medical conditions during pregnancy. Of the women who have asthma, for example, 25% will get worse during pregnancy, 50% will have no change due to pregnancy, and 25% will actually get better during pregnancy. No one understands why this is so, and no one can predict the experience a woman might have.

Most women will see one healthcare provider during pregnancy, either an obstetrician, a midwife, or a nurse practitioner. Women who have a medical problem may need to see a medical specialist as well. These women may also need the expert advice and care of a perinatologist. A perinatologist is a medical doctor (obstetrician) who specializes in the care of women who are at high risk for having problems during pregnancy. Perinatologists care for women who have pre-existing medical problems as well as women who develop complications during pregnancy.

Diagnosis

A woman who has a medical problem will have even more tests than the average pregnant woman. These might include tests to monitor the medical problem or blood tests to check the levels of medication. In most medical conditions, pregnancy changes the amount of medication that is necessary to control the problem. Frequent blood tests let the doctor adjust medication as often as needed.

Some medical conditions can increase the risk of **birth defects.** The doctor may suggest an ultrasound to check the baby early in the second trimester (16–18 weeks of pregnancy). At that point, the baby is large enough that the doctor can see the organs and structures clearly.

Other medical conditions may affect the baby's growth. The provider may request ultrasound exams every few weeks to make sure the medical condition is not interfering with the baby's growth and health.

Treatment

Treatment varies widely with the type of disease, the effect that pregnancy has on the disease, and the effect that the disease has on pregnancy. Additional tests may help determine the need for changes in medication or additional treatment.

Prognosis

The prognosis depends in large part on the specific medical condition. Some medical conditions make it difficult to get pregnant and lead to a higher risk of problems in the baby. An example of this type of condition is thyroid disease. In thyroid disease, the thyroid gland (located in the neck) may produce too much or too little thyroid hormone. Abnormal levels of thyroid hormone can cause problems in pregnancy and affect the health of the baby. Fortunately, thyroid disease can be treated with medication. As long as the level of thyroid hormone is controlled throughout pregnancy, there should be no problems for mother or baby.

There is a large group of medical conditions that usually does not interfere with pregnancy, but is affected by pregnancy. This group includes asthma, epilepsy, and ulcerative colitis. For example, some women with ulcerative colitis experience a worsening of their symptoms during pregnancy, while others will have no change or may get better during pregnancy. No one understands why this is so, but each of these women should be monitored very carefully throughout pregnancy.

There is also a group of medical conditions that can have a major impact on pregnancy. Women with lupus (disease caused by alterations in the immune system that result in inflammation of connective tissue and organs) or kidney disease face real risks during pregnancy. Pregnancy can cause their symptoms to worsen significantly and can lead to serious illness. Because these diseases can affect the mother's ability to supply oxygen and nutrients to the baby through the placenta, they can cause problems for the baby as well. These babies may not be able to grow and gain weight properly (**intrauterine growth retardation**). There is also an increased risk of **stillbirth.**

Diabetes is a medical condition that is both affected by pregnancy and affects pregnancy. Diabetes can lead to **miscarriages,** birth defects, and stillbirths. When a woman monitors her blood sugar carefully and treats high levels with insulin, the risk of these negative outcomes drops a great deal. Unfortunately, pregnancy makes diabetes much harder to control. In general, blood sugar and the need for insulin to control it rise throughout pregnancy.

Most medical conditions do not lead to complications in pregnancy. With frequent visits to healthcare providers, and careful attention to medication, women with medical problems usually enjoy healthy, successful pregnancies. There are a few medical conditions that can cause health risks to both mother and baby during pregnancy. Women with these medical problems should consider these risks before deciding to become pregnant. Many of these women will benefit from the care of a perinatologist during pregnancy. Only rarely (in the case of severe heart disease, for example) are the risks to the mother so high that she should not consider pregnancy at all.

Prevention

A pre-pregnancy visit with a healthcare provider is especially important for a woman who has a medical problem. The doctor will discuss how women with this condition usually fare during pregnancy. For some diseases (such as lupus), pregnancy can mean increased risk of health problems for mother and baby.

Sometimes, the medication a woman needs to control a medical condition can cause problems for the baby. There may be another medication available that is safer for use in pregnancy. In some cases there is no other medication, and a woman must weigh the risks to the baby when deciding whether or not to become pregnant.

A woman who has not had a pre-pregnancy visit should contact a healthcare provider as soon as she learns she is pregnant. Often, the provider will schedule the first prenatal visit within a day or two, instead of waiting until 8–10 weeks of pregnancy. This is because certain medical conditions can increase the risk of miscarriage. The provider will want to be sure that any medication is adjusted properly to increase the chance of having a successful pregnancy.

Resources

BOOKS

Carlson, Karen J., and Stephanie A. Eisenstat, eds. "Medical Problems in Pregnancy." In *Primary Care of Women.* St. Louis, MO: Mosby-Year Book, Inc. 1995, 346-383.

Cunningham, Gary, et al. "Medical and Surgical Complications in Pregnancy." In *Williams Obstetrics,* 20th ed. Stamford, CT: Appleton & Lange, 1997, 1045-1316.

Amy B. Tuteur

Hindu medicine *see* **Ayurvedic medicine**

Hip bath *see* **Sitz bath**

Hip replacement *see* **Joint replacement**

. . . .
Hirschsprung's disease

Definition

Hirschsprung's disease, also known as congenital megacolon, is an abnormality in which certain nerve fibers are absent in segments of the bowel, resulting in severe bowel obstruction.

Description

Hirschsprung's disease is caused when cells in the wall of the colon (parasympathetic **ganglion** cells) do not develop before birth. The affected segment of the intes-

KEY TERMS

Anus—The opening into the rectum, through which feces pass.

Barium enema x ray—A procedure that involves the administration of barium into the intestines by a tube inserted into the rectum. Barium is a chalky substance that enhances the visualization of the gastrointestinal tract on x ray.

Colostomy—The creation of an artificial opening into the colon through the skin for the purpose of removing bodily waste. Colostomies are usually required because key portions of the intestine have been removed.

Enterocolitis—Severe inflammation of the intestines that affects the intestinal lining, muscle, nerves, and blood vessels.

Manometry—A balloon study of internal anal sphincter pressure and relaxation.

Meconium—The first waste products to be discharged from the body in a newborn infant, usually greenish in color and consisting of mucus, bile, and so forth.

Megacolon—Dilation of the colon.

Parasympathetic ganglion cell—Type of nerve cell that is normally found in the wall of the colon.

tine lacks the ability to relax and move bowel contents along. As a result of this area of constriction, the bowel proximal (or above the stricture) dilates, producing megacolon (dilation of the colon). The disease affects varying lengths of bowel segment, most often involving the region around the rectum. In 10% of children, the entire colon and part of the small intestine are involved.

The disease occurs once in every 5,000 births, and it is about four times more common in males than females.

Causes & symptoms

Hirschsprung's disease develops in the fetus early in **pregnancy** when, for unknown reasons, nerve cells fail to develop in a segment of bowel. The absence of these nerve fibers, which help control the movement of bowel contents, results in intestinal obstruction and other symptoms. There may be a genetic basis to Hirschsprung's disease, since 4–50% of siblings are also afflicted and about 10% of children with the disease have a genetic condition, such as Down's syndrome.

The initial symptom is usually severe, continuous **constipation.** A newborn may fail to pass meconium

(the first stool) within 24 hours of birth, may repeatedly vomit yellow or green colored bile, and may have a distended (swollen, uncomfortable) abdomen. Occasionally, infants may have only mild or intermittent constipation, often with **diarrhea.**

While two thirds of cases are diagnosed in the first three months of life, Hirschsprung's disease may also be diagnosed later in infancy or childhood. Occasionally, even adults are diagnosed with a variation of the disease. In older infants, symptoms and signs may include anorexia (lack of appetite or inability to eat), lack of the urge to move the bowels, empty rectum on **physical examination,** distended abdomen, and a mass in the colon that can be felt by the physician during examination. It should be suspected in older children with abnormal bowel habits, especially a history of constipation dating back to infancy and ribbon-like stools.

Occasionally, the presenting symptom may be a severe intestinal infection called enterocolitis, which is life threatening. The symptoms are usually explosive, watery stools and **fever** in a very ill-appearing infant. There is a great need to diagnose the condition before the intestinal obstruction causes an overgrowth of bacteria that evolves into a medical emergency. Enterocolitis can lead to severe diarrhea and massive fluid loss, which can cause **death** from **dehydration** unless surgery is done immediately to relieve the obstruction.

Diagnosis

Hirschsprung's disease in the newborn must be distinguished from other causes of intestinal obstruction. The diagnosis is suspected by the child's medical history and physical examination, especially the rectal exam. The diagnosis is confirmed by a **barium enema** x ray, which yields a picture of the bowel. The x ray will indicate if a segment of bowel is constricted, causing dilation and obstruction. A biopsy of rectal tissue will reveal the absence of the nerve fibers. Adults may also undergo manometry, a balloon study of internal anal sphincter pressure and relaxation.

Treatment

Hirschsprung's disease must be treated surgically. The goal is to remove the diseased, nonfunctioning segment of the bowel and restore bowel function. This is often done in two stages. The first stage relieves the intestinal obstruction by performing a **colostomy.** This is the creation of an opening in the abdomen (stoma) through which bowel contents can be discharged into a waste bag. When the child's weight, age, or condition is deemed appropriate, surgeons close the stoma, remove the diseased portion of bowel, and perform a "pull-through" procedure, which repairs the colon by connecting functional bowel to the anus. This usually establishes fairly normal bowel function.

Prognosis

Overall, prognosis is very good. Most infants with Hirschsprung's disease achieve good bowel control after surgery, but a small percentage of children may have lingering problems with soilage or constipation. These infants are also at higher risk for an overgrowth of bacteria in the intestines, including subsequent episodes of enterocolitis, and should be closely followed by a physician.

Prevention

Hirschsprung's disease is a congenital abnormality that has no known means of prevention. It is important to diagnose the condition early in order to prevent the development of enterocolitis.

Resources

BOOKS

Phillips, Sidney F., and John H. Pemberton. "Megacolon: Congenital and Acquired." In *Sleisenger & Fordtran's Gastrointestinal and Liver Disease,* edited by Mark Feldman, et al. Philadelphia: W.B. Saunders Co., 1998.

PERIODICALS

Fortuna, Randall S., et al. "Critical Analysis of the Operative Treatment of Hirschsprung's Disease." *Archives of Surgery* 131 (May 1996): 520.

Swenson, Orvar. "Early History of the Therapy of Hirschsprung's Disease: Facts and Personal Observations Over 50 Years." *Pediatric Surgery* 31 (1997): 1003.

ORGANIZATIONS

American Pseudo-Obstruction & Hirschsprung's Society. 158 Pleasant St., North Andover, MA 01845. (978)685-4477.

Caroline A. Helwick

Hirsutism

Definition

Excessive growth of facial or body hair in women is called hirsutism.

Description

Hirsutism is not a disease. The condition usually develops during **puberty** and becomes more pronounced

as the years go by. However, an inherited tendency, overproduction of male hormones (androgens), medication, or disease, can cause it to appear at any age.

Women who have hirsutism usually have irregular menstrual cycles. They sometimes have small breasts and deep voices, and their muscles and genitals may become larger than women without the condition.

Types of hirsutism

Idiopathic hirsutism is probably hereditary, because there is usually a family history of the disorder. Women with idiopathic hirsutism have normal menstrual cycles and no evidence of any of the conditions associated with secondary hirsutism.

Secondary hirsutism is most often associated with **polycystic ovary syndrome** (an inherited hormonal disorder characterized by menstrual irregularities, biochemical abnormalities, and **obesity**). This type of hirsutism may also be caused by:

• Malfunctions of the pituitary or adrenal glands

• Use of male hormones or minoxidil (Loniten), a drug used to widen blood vessels

• Adrenal or ovarian tumors.

Causes & symptoms

Hirsutism is rarely caused by a serious underlying disorder. **Pregnancy** occasionally stimulates its development. Hirsutism triggered by tumors is very unusual.

Hair follicles usually become enlarged, and the hairs themselves become larger and darker. A woman whose hirsutism is caused by an increase in male hormones has a pattern of hair growth similar to that of a man. A woman whose hirsutism is not hormone-related has long, fine hairs on her face, arms, chest, and back.

Diagnosis

Diagnosis is based on a family history of hirsutism, a personal history of menstrual irregularities, and masculine traits. Laboratory tests are not needed to assess the status of patients whose menstrual cycles are normal and who have mild, gradually progressing hirsutism.

A family physician or endocrinologist may order blood tests to measure hormone levels in women with long-standing menstrual problems or more severe hirsutism. **Computed tomography scans** (CT scans) are sometimes performed to evaluate diseases of the adrenal glands. Additional diagnostic procedures may be used to confirm or rule out underlying diseases or disorders.

Treatment

Primary hirsutism can be treated mechanically. Mechanical treatment involves bleaching or physically removing unwanted hair by:

- Cutting
- Electrolysis
- Shaving
- Tweezing
- Waxing
- Using hair-removing creams (depilatories).

Low-dose dexamethasone (a synthetic adrenocortical steroid), birth-control pills, or medications that suppress male hormones (for example, spironolactone) may be prescribed for patients whose condition stems from high androgen levels.

Treatment of secondary hirsutism is determined by the underlying cause of the condition.

Prognosis

Birth-control pills alone cause this condition to stabilize in one of every two patients and to improve in one of every 10.

When spironolactone (Aldactone) is prescribed to suppress hair growth, 70% of patients experience improvement within six months. When women also take birth-control pills, menstrual cycles become regular and hair growth is suppressed even more.

Resources

BOOKS

Fauci, Anthony S., et al, eds. *Harrison's Principles of Internal Medicine,* 14th ed. New York: McGraw-Hill, 1998.

ORGANIZATIONS

American Society for Reproductive Medicine. 1209 Montgomery Highway, Birmingham, AL 35216-2809. (205) 978-5000. http://www.asrm.com.

OTHER

Hirsutism and Hyperandrogenism in Women. http://www.advancedfertility.com/hirsute.htm. (26 April 1998).

Pathaphysiology and Treatment of Hirsutism. http://www.aafp.org/app/970600ap/tips17.html. (26 April 1998).

Maureen Haggerty

Histamine headache *see* **Cluster headache**

Histamine H$_2$ blockers *see* **Antiulcer drugs**

Histiocytosis X

Definition

Histiocytosis X, or Langerhans cell histiocytosis as it is also referred, is a group of childhood diseases characterized by an overabundance of histiocytes. A histiocyte is a type of immunogenic cell that travels through tissues looking for germs. It is part of the body's defense system, and its job is to consume germs.

Description

Nearly every cell in the body can grow beyond its accustomed limits. If the cell is localized, the result is a tumor, but if the cell exists in many places the result is more like a leukemia, with symptoms showing up in many places. These histiocytosis diseases, and their cousin **mastocytosis,** produce masses of cells in various organs that produce symptoms. The bones are involved 80% of the time, and, along with the bones, often the bone marrow is involved, causing anemia. Bone involvement of the skull can cause growths behind the eyes that bulge them forward. It can also affect the brain in several ways.

These cells also accumulate in the lungs, liver, and spleen. Any of those organs can fail as a result.

Causes & symptoms

One of these diseases is hereditary; it is called familial erythrophagocytic lymphohistiocytosis (FHL). For the others, there is no known cause.

Symptoms range from mild **pain** at the site of cell masses to rapid **death** from lung, liver, or brain failure. The skin may have all kinds of **rashes** and eruptions. The endocrine system may fail altogether because the pituitary is damaged. Gums may swell, teeth fall out, and ears may drain chronic infections.

Diagnosis

Because these diseases are rare and have so many different manifestations, the diagnosis may be unclear at first. A biopsy is necessary to identify the disease, and after that a thorough examination of every suspected organ may be required to determine its extent.

Treatment

If only one organ is involved or the disease seems to be running a benign course, little treatment is needed. However, these diseases are often malignant. When they are very aggressive, they are treated like **cancers** with **chemotherapy**, radiation, and cortisone-like drugs. Treatment is not often successful.

Prognosis

Some cases remit spontaneously with few symptoms and no residual effects from the disease. Others are rapidly fatal.

Resources

BOOKS

Faller, Douglas V. "Diseases of Lymph Nodes and Spleen." In *Cecil Textbook of Medicine,* edited by J. Claude Bennett and Fred Plum. Philadelphia: W. B. Saunders, 1996, p. 907.

Komp, Diane M. "Letterer-Siwe Disease." In *Cecil Textbook of Medicine,* edited by J. Claude Bennett and Fred Plum. Philadelphia: W. B. Saunders, 1996, pp. 955-966.

Ladisch, Stephan. "Histiocytosis Syndromes of Childhood." In *Nelson Textbook of Pediatrics,* edited by Waldo E. Nelson, et al. Philadelphia: W. B. Saunders, 1996, pp. 1997-1999.

Reynolds, Herbert Y. "Interstitial Lung Diseases." In *Harrison's Principles of Internal Medicine,* edited by Kurt Isselbacher, et al. New York: McGraw-Hill, 1998, p. 1465.

Toews, Galen B. "Interstitial Lung Disease." In *Cecil Textbook of Medicine,* edited by J. Claude Bennett and Fred Plum. Philadelphia: W. B. Saunders, 1996, p. 395.

J. Ricker Polsdorfer

Histoplasma capsulatum infection *see* **Histoplasmosis**

Histoplasmosis

Definition

Histoplasmosis is an infectious disease caused by inhaling the microscopic spores of the fungus *Histoplasma capsulatum.* The disease exists in three forms. Acute or primary histoplasmosis causes flu-like symptoms. Most people who are infected recover without medical intervention. Chronic histoplasmosis affects the lungs and can be fatal. Disseminated histoplasmosis affects many organ systems in the body and is often fatal, especially to people with acquired **immunodeficiency** syndrome (**AIDS**).

Description

Histoplasmosis is an airborne infection. The spores that cause this disease are found in soil that has been contaminated with bird or bat droppings. In the United States, the disease is most common in eastern and midwestern states and is widespread in the upper Mississippi, Ohio, Missouri, and St. Lawrence river valleys. Sometimes histoplasmosis is called Ohio Valley disease, Central Mississippi River Valley disease, Appalachian Mountain disease, Darling's disease, or *Histoplasma capsulatum* infection.

Anyone can get histoplasmosis, but people who are come into contact with bird and bat excrement are more likely to be infected. This includes farmers, gardeners, bridge inspectors and painters, roofers, chimney cleaners, demolition and construction workers, people installing or servicing heating and air conditioning units, people restoring old or abandoned buildings, and people who explore caves.

The very young and the elderly, especially if they have a pre-existing lung disease or are heavy smokers, are more likely to develop symptoms that are more severe. People who have a weakened immune system, either from diseases such as AIDS or leukemia, or as the result of medications they take (**corticosteroids,** chemotherapy drugs), are more likely to develop chronic or disseminated histoplasmosis.

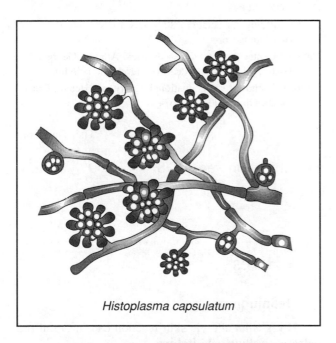

Histoplasma capsulatum

Histoplasma capsulatum. If a person inhales the spores of this fungus, they may contract histoplasmosis, an infectious disease which can exist in three forms: acute or primary histoplasmosis, which causes flu-like symptoms; chronic histoplasmosis, which affects the lungs and can be fatal; and disseminated histoplasmosis, which can affect multiple body systems and is often fatal. *(Illustration by Electronic Illustrators Group.)*

Causes & symptoms

When the spores of *H. capsulatum* are inhaled, they lodge in the lungs where they divide and cause lesions. This is known as acute or primary histoplasmosis. It is not contagious.

Many otherwise healthy people show no symptoms of infection at all. When symptoms do occur, they appear 3–17 days after exposure (average time is 10 days). The symptoms are usually mild and resemble those of a cold or flu; **fever,** dry **cough,** enlarged lymph glands, tiredness, and a general feeling of ill health. A small number of people develop bronchopneumonia. About 95% of people who are infected either experience no symptoms or have symptoms that clear up spontaneously. These people then have partial immunity to re-infection.

In some people, the spores that cause the disease continue to live in the lungs. In about 5% of people who are infected, usually those with chronic lung disease, diabetes mellitus, or weakened immune systems, the disease progresses to chronic histoplasmosis. This can take months or years. Symptoms of chronic histoplasmosis resemble those of **tuberculosis.** Cavities form in the lung tissue, parts of the lung may collapse, and the lungs fill with fluid. Chronic histoplasmosis is a serious disease that can result in **death.**

The rarest form of histoplasmosis is disseminated histoplasmosis. Disseminated histoplasmosis is seen almost exclusively in patients with AIDS or other immune defects. In disseminated histoplasmosis the infection may move to the spleen, liver, bone marrow, or adrenal glands. Symptoms include a worsening of those found in chronic histoplasmosis, as well as weight loss, **diarrhea,** the development of open sores in the mouth and nose, and enlargement of the spleen, liver, and adrenal gland.

Diagnosis

A simple skin test similar to that given for tuberculosis will tell if a person has previously been infected by the fungus *H. capsulatum.* Chest x rays often show lung damage caused by the fungus, but do not lead to a definitive diagnosis because the damage caused by other diseases has a similar appearance on the x ray. Diagnosis of chronic or disseminated histoplasmosis can be made by culturing a sample of sputum or other body fluids in the laboratory to isolate the fungus. The urine, blood serum, washings from the lungs, or cerebrospinal fluid can all be tested for the presence of an antigen produced in response to the infection. Most cases of primary histoplasmosis go undiagnosed.

Treatment

Acute primary histoplasmosis generally requires no treatment other than rest. Non-prescription drugs such as **acetaminophen** (Tylenol) may be used to treat pain and relieve fever. Avoiding smoke and using a cool air humidifier may ease chest pain.

Patients with an intact immune system who develop chronic histoplasmosis are treated with the drug ketoconazole (Nizoral) or amphotericin B (Fungizone). Patients with suppressed immune systems are treated with amphotericin B, which is given intravenously. Because of its potentially toxic side effects, hospitalization is often required. The patient may also receive other drugs to minimize the side effects of the amphotericin B.

Patients with AIDS must continue to take the drug itraconazole (Sporonox) orally for the rest of their lives in order to prevent a relapse. If the patient can not tolerate itraconazole, the drug fluconazole (Diflucan) can be substituted.

Alternative treatment

In non-immunocompromised patients, alternative therapies can be very successful. Alternative treatment for fungal infections focuses on creating an environment where the fungus cannot survive. This is accomplished by maintaining good health and eating a diet low in dairy products, sugars, including honey and fruit juice, and foods like beer that contain yeast. This is complemented by a diet high in raw food. Supplements of antioxidant **vitamins** C, E, and A, along with B complex, may also be added to the diet. *Lactobacillus acidophilus* and *Bifidobacteria* will replenish the good bacteria in the intestines. Antifungal herbs, like garlic, can be consumed in relatively large does and for an extended period of time in order to be most effective.

Prognosis

Most people recover from primary histoplasmosis in a few weeks without medical intervention. Patients with chronic histoplasmosis who are treated with antifungal drugs generally recover rapidly if they do not have an underlying serious disease. When left untreated, or if serious disease is present, histoplasmosis can be fatal.

AIDS patients with disseminated histoplasmosis vary in their response to amphotericin B, depending on their general health and how well they tolerate the side effects of the drug. Treatment often suppresses the infection temporarily, but patients with AIDS are always in danger of a relapse and must continue to take medication for the rest of their lives to keep the infection at bay. New combinations of therapies and new drugs are constantly being evaluated, making hard statistics on prognosis difficult to come by. AIDS patients have problems with multiple opportunistic infections, making it difficult to isolate death rates due to any one particular fungal infection.

Prevention

Since the spores of *H. capsulatum* are so widespread, it is almost impossible to prevent exposure in endemic areas. Dust suppression measures when working with contaminated soil may help limit exposure. Individuals who are at risk of developing the more severe forms of the disease should avoid situations where they will be exposed to bat and bird droppings.

Resources

BOOKS

Griffith, H. Winter. *Complete Guide to Symptoms, Illness & Surgery.* Putnam Berkely Group, 1995.

PERIODICALS

Centers for Disease Control and Prevention. *Histoplasmosis: Protecting Workers at Risk.* (September 1997). http://www.cdc.gov/niosh/97146eng.html.

Medical Mycology Research Center. *Histoplasmosis capsulati and Histoplasmosis duboisii.* University of Texas Medical Branch at Galveston. (May 1997). http://www.fungus.utmb.edu.

ORGANIZATIONS

American Lung Association. 800-LUNG-USA. http://www.lungusa.org.

National Center for Infectious Diseases. Atlanta, Georgia. 404-639-3158. www.cdc.gov/ncidod/ncid/ncid.htm.

National Institute for Occupational Safety and Health. Cincinnati, Ohio. 800-356-4674.

Tish Davidson

HIV infection *see* **AIDS**

Hives

Definition

Hives is an allergic skin reaction causing localized redness, swelling, and **itching.**

Description

Hives is a reaction of the body's immune system that causes areas of the skin to swell, itch, and become reddened (wheals). When the reaction is limited to small areas of the skin, it is called "urticaria." Involvement of larger areas, such as whole sections of a limb, is called ''angioedema.''

Causes & symptoms

Causes

Hives is an allergic reaction. The body's immune system is normally responsible for protection from foreign invaders. When it becomes sensitized to normally harmless substances, the resulting reaction is called an allergy. An attack of hives is set off when such a substance, called an allergen, is ingested, inhaled, or otherwise contacted. It interacts with immune cells called mast cells, which reside in the skin, airways, and digestive system. When mast cells encounter an allergen, they release histamine and other chemicals, both locally and into the bloodstream. These chemicals cause blood vessels to

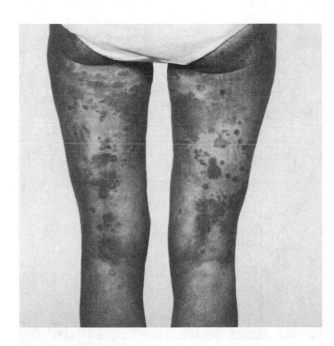

Hives on the back of a young woman's legs. The accompanying inflammation develops as an allergic reaction which ranges in size from small spots to patches measuring several inches across. *(Photograph by John Radcliffe, Custom Medical Stock Photo. Reproduced by permission.)*

become more porous, allowing fluid to accumulate in tissue and leading to the swollen and reddish appearance of hives. Some of the chemicals released sensitize **pain** nerve endings, causing the affected area to become itchy and sensitive.

A wide variety of substances may cause hives in sensitive people, including foods, drugs, and insect bites or stings. Common culprits include:

- Nuts, especially peanuts, walnuts, and Brazil nuts
- Fish, mollusks, and shellfish
- Eggs
- Wheat
- Milk
- Strawberries
- Food additives and preservatives
- Penicillin or other **antibiotics**
- Flu vaccines
- **Tetanus** toxoid vaccine
- Gamma globulin
- Bee, wasp, and hornet stings
- Bites of mosquitoes, fleas, and **scabies.**

Symptoms

Urticaria is characterized by redness, swelling, and itching of small areas of the skin. These patches usually grow and recede in less than a day, but may be replaced by others in other locations. Angioedema is characterized by more diffuse swelling. Swelling of the airways may cause **wheezing** and respiratory distress. In severe cases, airway obstruction may occur.

Diagnosis

Hives are easily diagnosed by visual inspection. The cause of hives is usually apparent, but may require a careful medical history in some cases.

Treatment

Mild cases of hives are treated with **antihistamines,** such as diphenhydramine (Benadryl). More severe cases may require oral **corticosteroids,** such as prednisone. Topical corticosteroids are not effective. Airway swelling may require emergency injection of epinephrine (adrenaline).

Alternative treatment

An alternative practitioner will try to determine what allergic substance is causing the reaction and help the patient eliminate or minimize its effects. To deal with the symptoms of hives, an oatmeal bath may help to relieve itching. Chickweed (*Stellaria media*), applied as a poultice (crushed or chopped herbs applied directly to the skin) or added to bath water, may also help relieve itching. Several homeopathic remedies, including *Urtica urens* and *Apis* (*Apis mellifica*), may help relieve the itch, redness, or swelling associated with hives.

Prognosis

Most cases of hives clear up within one to seven days without treatment, providing the cause (allergen) is found and avoided.

Prevention

Preventing hives depends on avoiding the allergen causing them. Analysis of new items in the diet or new drugs taken may reveal the likely source of the reaction. Chronic hives may be aggravated by **stress, caffeine,** alcohol, or tobacco; avoiding these may reduce the frequency of reactions.

Resources

BOOKS

Lawlor, G. J., Jr., T.J. Fischer, and D.C. Adelman. *Manual of Allergy and Immunology.* Little, Brown and Co., 1995.

Novick, N. L. *You Can Do Something About Your Allergies.* MacMillan, 1994.

HLA test *see* **Human leukocyte antigen test**

HMG-CoA reductase inhibitors *see* **Cholesterol-reducing drugs**

Hodgkin's disease

Definition

Hodgkin's disease is a type of **cancer** involving tissues of the lymphatic system. There are a variety of cancers, called lymphomas, that can affect lymph tissue. Hodgkin's disease represents a specific type of lymphoma. Its cause is unknown, although some interaction between individual genetic makeup, environmental exposures, and infectious agents is suspected.

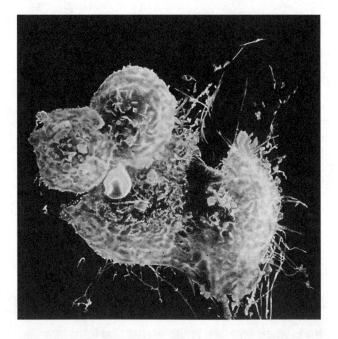

A scanning electron micrograph (SEM) image of dividing Hodgkin's cells from the pleural effusions (abnormal accumulations of fluid in the lungs) of a 55-year-old male patient. *(Photograph by Dr. Andrejs Liepins, Photo Researchers, Inc. Reproduced by permission.)*

Description

Hodgkin's lymphoma can occur at any age, although the majority of these lymphomas occur in people between the ages of 15–34, and after the age of 60. An understanding of the lymphatic system, as well as a general understanding of the nature of cancer, is helpful in making sense out of Hodgkin's disease.

The lymphatic system

The lymphatic system is part of the body's immune system. It consists of a number of elements:

- A network of vessels which serve to drain tissue fluid from all the major organs of the body, including the skin, and from all four limbs. These vessels pass through lymph nodes on their way to empty their contents into major veins at the base of the neck and within the abdomen.

- The lymph nodes are clusters of specialized cells which serve to filter the lymph fluid, trapping foreign substances, including viruses, bacteria, and cancer cells, as well as any other encountered debris. (For example, lymph nodes which receive fluid from the lungs of city dwellers often contain gritty, dark material due to filtering of debris from polluted city air.)

- Lymphocytes are cells of the immune system. They are produced within bone marrow, lymph nodes, and spleen and circulate throughout the body in both blood and lymph fluid. These cells work to identify and rid the body of any invaders that threaten health.

- Clusters of scavenger-like immune cells exist in major organs, and provide immune surveillance on location. These include the tonsils and adenoids (in the throat/pharynx), Kupffer cells (in the liver), Peyer's patches (in the intestine), and other specialized immune cells stationed in the lungs and the brain.

Cancer

Cancer is a condition in which a particular type of cell within the body begins to multiply in an out-of-control fashion. This may mean that cancer cells multiply more quickly, or it may mean that cancer cells take on abnormal characteristics.

For example, at a very early stage in embryonic development (development of a fetus within the uterus), generic body cells begin to differentiate; that is, they acquire specific characteristics which ultimately allow liver cells to function as liver cells, blood cells as blood cells, brain cells as brain cells, etc. Cancer, then, is sometimes considered to be a process of de-differentiation, during which a type of cell loses its individuality and becomes a more embryonic cell. Such cells also lose their sense of organization and no longer position themselves appropriately within their resident tissue.

Cancer cells can also acquire the ability to invade other tissues. Normally, for example, breast cells are found only in breast tissue. However, cancerous breast cells can invade into other tissue spaces, so that **breast cancer** can spread to bone, liver, brain, etc.

Lymphoma is a cancer of the lymph system. Depending on the specific type, a lymphoma can have any or all of the characteristics of cancer: rapid multiplication of cells, abnormal cell types, loss of normal arrangement of cells with respect to each other, and invasive ability.

Causes & symptoms

Hodgkin's lymphoma usually begins in a lymph node. This node enlarges; but may or may not cause any **pain**—as would enlarged lymph nodes due to infectious causes. Hodgkin's lymphoma progresses in a fairly predictable way, traveling from one group of lymph nodes on to the next. More advanced cases of Hodgkin's include involvement of the spleen, the liver, and bone marrow.

Constitutional symptoms—symptoms which affect the whole body—are common. They include **fever,** weight loss, heavy sweating at night, and **itching.** Some patients note pain after drinking alcoholic beverages.

As nodes swell, they may push on other nearby structures, resulting in other symptoms. These symptoms include pain from pressure on nerve roots, as well as loss of function of specific muscle groups served by the compressed nerves. Kidney failure may result from compression of the ureters, the tubes which carry urine from the kidneys to the bladder. The face, neck, or legs may swell due to pressure slowing the flow in veins which should drain blood from those regions (superior vena cava syndrome). Pressure on the spinal cord can result in **paralysis** of the legs. Compression of the trachea and/or bronchi (airways) can cause **wheezing** and **shortness of breath.** Masses in the liver can cause the accumulation of certain chemicals in the blood, resulting in **jaundice** (a yellowish discoloration of the skin and the whites of the eyes).

As Hodgkin's lymphoma progresses, a patient's immune system becomes less and less effective at fighting infection. Thus, patients with Hodgkin's lymphoma become increasingly more susceptible to both common infections caused by bacteria and unusual (opportunistic) infections caused by viruses, fungi, and protozoa.

Diagnosis

As with many forms of cancer, diagnosis of Hodgkin's disease has two important components:

- The identification of Hodgkin's lymphoma as the cause of the patient's disease.

- The staging of the disease. Staging is an attempt to identify the degree of spread of the lymphoma.

Diagnosis of Hodgkin's lymphoma requires removal of a sample of a suspicious lymph node (biopsy) and careful examination of the tissue under a microscope. In Hodgkin's lymphoma, certain very characteristic cells—called Reed-Sternberg cells—must be present in order to confirm the diagnosis. These cells usually contain two or more nuclei. (The nucleus is the oval, centrally-located structure within a cell which houses the genetic material of the cell.). Reed-Sternberg cells also have other unique characteristics which cause them to appear under the microscope as "owl's eyes" or yin-yang cells. In addition to the identification of these Reed-Sternberg cells, other cells in the affected tissue sample are examined. The characteristics of these other cells help to classify the specific subtype of Hodgkin's lymphoma present.

Once Hodgkin's disease has been diagnosed, staging is the next important step. This involves **computed tomography scans** (CT scans) of the abdomen, chest, and pelvis, to identify areas of lymph node involvement. In rare cases, a patient must undergo abdominal surgery so that lymph nodes in the abdominal area can be biopsied (staging laparotomy). Some patients have their spleens removed during this surgery, both to help with staging and to remove a focus of the disease. Bone marrow biopsy is also required unless there is obvious evidence of vital organ involvement. Some physicians also order lymphangiograms (a radiograph of the lymphatic vessels).

Staging is important because it helps to determine what kind of treatment a patient should receive. On the one hand, it is important to understand the stage of the disease so that the treatment chosen is sufficiently strong to provide the patient with a cure. On the other hand, all the available treatments have serious side effects. The goal of staging, then, is to allow the patient to have the type of treatment necessary to achieve a cure, but to minimize the severity of short and long-term side effects from which the patient may suffer.

Treatment

Treatment of Hodgkin's lymphoma has become increasingly effective over the years. The type of treatment used for Hodgkin's depends on the information obtained by staging, and may include **chemotherapy** (treatment with a combination of drugs), and /or radiotherapy (treatment with x rays which kill cancer cells).

Both chemotherapy and radiotherapy have unfortunate side effects. Chemotherapy can result in nausea, vomiting, hair loss, and increased susceptibility to infec-

tion. Radiotherapy can cause **sore throat,** difficulty swallowing, **diarrhea,** and growth abnormalities in children. Both forms of treatment, especially in combination, can result in sterility (the permanent inability to have offspring), as well as heart and lung damage.

The most serious negative result of the currently available treatments for Hodgkin's disease is the possible development in the future of another form of cancer—often called second malignancy. These second cancers might be leukemia (cancer of a blood component), breast cancer, bone cancer, or **thyroid cancer.** A great deal of cancer research is devoted to preventing these second malignancies.

Prognosis

Hodgkin's is one of the most curable forms of cancer. Current treatments are quite effective. Children have a particularly high rate of cure from the disease, with about 75% still living cancer-free 20 years after the original diagnosis. Adults with the most severe form of the disease have about a 50% cure rate.

Resources

BOOKS

Dollinger, Malin, et al. *Everyone's Guide to Cancer Therapy.* Kansas City: Andrews McKeel Publishing, 1997.

Freedman, Arnold S., and Lee M. Nadler. "Hodgkin's Disease." In *Harrison's Principles of Internal Medicine,* edited by Anthony S. Fauci, et al. New York: McGraw-Hill, 1998.

Murphy, Gerald P., et al. *Informed Decisions.* New York: Viking, 1997.

PERIODICALS

Stoval, Ellen. "A Cancer Survivor Discusses Her Experiences." *Washington Post* 118 (February 14, 1995): WH15+.

ORGANIZATIONS

The Lymphoma Research Foundation of America, Inc. 8800 Venice Boulevard, Suite 207, Los Angeles, CA 90034. (310) 204-7040. http://www.lymphoma.org.

Rosalyn S. Carson-DeWitt

Holter monitoring

Definition

Holter monitoring is continuous monitoring of the electrical activity of a patient's heart muscle (**electrocardiography**) for 24 hours, using a special portable

KEY TERMS

Cardiac arrhythmia—An abnormal heart rhythm.

Electrocardiography—Recording of the electrical activity of the heart muscle, used to diagnose certain heart abnormalities.

device called a Holter monitor. Patients wear the Holter monitor while carrying out their usual daily activities.

Purpose

Holter monitoring is used to help determine whether someone has an otherwise undetected heart disease, such as abnormal heart rhythm (cardiac arrhythmia), or inadequate blood flow through the heart. Specifically, it can detect abnormal electrical activity in the heart that may

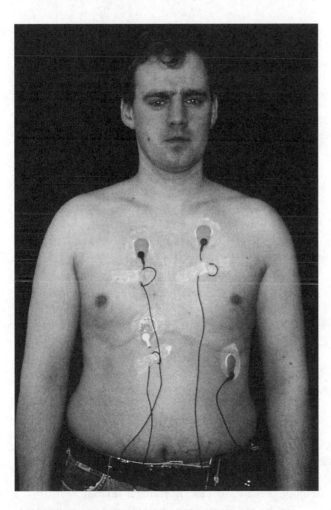

A male patient wears electrodes attached to his chest, which is connected to a Holter monitor at his waist. *(Photograph by Dr. P. Marazzi, Photo Researchers, Inc. Reproduced by permission.)*

occur randomly or only under certain circumstances, such as during sleep or periods of physical activity or **stress,** which may or may not be picked up by standard, short-term electrocardiography performed in a doctor's office.

Traditionally, an exercise **stress test** has been used to screen people for "silent" heart disease (heart disease with none of the usual symptoms). However, an exercise stress test is not completely foolproof, often producing false negative results (indicating no heart disease when heart disease is actually present) and false positives (indicating heart disease when there is none). Furthermore, some people cannot undergo exercise stress testing because of other medical conditions, such as arthritis.

Holter monitoring, also known as ambulatory or 24-hour electrocardiography, offers an alternate means of testing people for heart disease. By monitoring electrocardiographic activity throughout the day, Holter monitoring can uncover heart problems that occur during the patient's everyday activities. It can also help to recognize any activities that may be causing the heart problems. And it can define and correlate symptoms that may be caused by irregularities of the heart.

Precautions

Holter monitoring is an extremely safe procedure and no special precautions are required.

Description

The technician affixes electrodes on the surface of the skin at specific areas of the patient's chest, using adhesive patches with special gel that conducts electrical impulses. Typically, electrodes are placed under each collarbone and each bottom rib, and several electrodes are placed across the chest in a rough outline of the heart. The electrodes are attached to a portable electrocardiographic device called a Holter monitor, which records the electrical activity of the heart over 24–48 hours. The device is worn over the patient's shoulder or attached to a belt around the waist.

The Holter monitor records the continuous electrical activity throughout the course of the day, while the patient carries out his or her daily activities. During this time, the patient also keeps a detailed log or diary, recording his or her various activities, such as exercise, eating, sleeping, straining, breathing too hard (hyperventilating), and any stressful situations. The patient also notes the time and circumstances of any symptoms—especially chest **pain, dizziness, shortness of breath,** heart **palpitations,** and any other signs of heart trouble. Some Holter monitors allow patients to record their symptoms electronically, highlighting the portion of the electrocardiogram recorded while the symptoms are occurring.

After 24–48 hours, the Holter monitor is removed. A computer-assisted analysis is performed on the electrocardiographic recording, and the doctor compares the recording against the patient's log to see if there is any correlation between electrocardiographic abnormalities and any of the patient's activities or symptoms. The physician makes a final interpretation.

Preparation

In the doctor's office, electrodes are attached to the patient's chest. In some cases, the patient's chest hair may have to be shaved to facilitate attaching the electrodes. The patient then begins carrying the monitor on a shoulder harness, in a pocket, or on the belt while carrying out his or her usual daily routine. The patient should inform the doctor of any drugs he or she may be taking, because certain drugs can alter heart rhythms and may affect the results of the test.

Aftercare

The patient returns to the doctor's office to have the monitor and electrodes removed. No special measures need to be taken following Holter monitoring. The test results are usually available within a few days after the monitor is removed.

Risks

There are no known risks associated with Holter monitoring. The main complaint that people have with Holter monitoring is that the monitor may be cumbersome and interfere with certain activities, especially sleeping. Bathing and showering are not allowed during the study.

Normal results

A normal Holter monitoring test shows relatively normal electrical activity in the heart around the clock and no evidence of silent **ischemia** (deprivation of oxygen-rich blood).

Abnormal results

An abnormal result on Holter monitoring may indicate ischemia to the heart muscle or heart rhythm disturbances. Abnormalities are especially likely to show up during periods of stress or heavy activity, but sometimes serious abnormalities are recorded while the patient is sleeping.

Resources

BOOKS

Faculty Members of the Yale University School of Medicine. *The Patient's Book of Medical Tests.* Boston, New York: Houghton Mifflin Company, 1997.

PERIODICALS

''Cardiac Stress Testing: New Variations on an Old Theme.'' *Harvard Men's Health Watch* 1 (March 1997): 1-4.

''Use Cardiac Event Recorders to Evaluate Patients with Palpitations.'' *Modern Medicine* 64 (May 1996): 49.

''Use Holter Studies When Exercise Tests are Nondiagnostic.'' *Modern Medicine* 62 (April 1994): 59.

ORGANIZATIONS

American Heart Association, 7272 Greenville Avenue, Dallas, TX 75231. (214) 373-6300. http://www.amhrt.org.

National Heart, Lung, and Blood Institute, Information Center, P.O. Box 30105, Bethesda, MD 20824-0105. (301) 951-3260. http://www.nhlbi.nih.gov.

Robert Scott Dinsmoor

Holtzman ink blot test

Definition

The Holtzman Inkblot Technique (HIT) is a projective personality assessment test for persons ages five and up.

Purpose

The HIT is used to assess the personality structure of a test subject. It is sometimes used as a diagnostic tool in assessing **schizophrenia,** depression, **addiction,** and character disorders.

Precautions

Psychometric testing requires a clinically trained examiner. The HIT should be administered and interpreted by a trained psychologist, psychiatrist, or appropriately trained mental health professional.

Some consider projective tests to be less reliable than objective personality tests. If the examiner is not well-trained in psychometric evaluation, subjective interpretations may affect the outcome of the test.

Description

The HIT, developed by psychologist Wayne Holtzman and colleagues, was introduced in 1961. The test was designed to overcome some of the deficiencies of its famous predecessor, the Rorschach Inkblot Test.

Unlike the Rorschach, the Holtzman is a standardized measurement with clearly defined objective scoring criteria. The HIT consists of 45 inkblots. The test administrator, or examiner, has a stack of 47 cards with inkblots

(45 test cards and 2 practice cards) face down in front of him or her. The examiner hands each card to the subject and asks the test subject what he or she sees in the inkblot. Only one response per inkblot is requested. Occasionally, the examiner may ask the test subject to clarify or elaborate on a response. The Administration of the HIT typically takes 50–80 minutes. The HIT is then scored against 22 personality-related characteristics.

The HIT can also be administered in a group setting. In group testing, 30–45 inkblots are projected onto a screen and test subjects provide written responses to each inkblot.

The 1997 Medicare reimbursement rate for psychological and neuropsychological testing is $58.35 an hour. Billing time typically includes test administration, scoring and interpretation, and reporting. Many insurance plans cover all or a portion of diagnostic psychological testing.

Normal results

Because of the complexity of the scoring process and the projective nature of the test, results for the HIT should only be interpreted by a clinically trained psychologist, psychiatrist, or appropriately trained mental health professional.

Resources

BOOKS

Maddox, Taddy. *Tests: A Comprehensive Reference for Assessments in Psychology, Education, and Business.* 4th ed. Austin: Pro-ed, 1997.

Shore, Milton. F, Patrick J. Brice, and Barbara G. Love. *When Your Child Needs Testing.* New York: Crossroad Publishing, 1992.

Wodrich, David L. *Children's Psychological Testing: A Guide for Nonpsychologists.* Baltimore: Paul H. Brookes Publishing, 1997.

ORGANIZATIONS

The American Psychological Association. 750 First St., N.E., Washington, DC 20002-4242. (202)336-5500. http://www.apa.org/psychnet.

The ERIC Clearinghouse on Assessment and Evaluation. O'Boyle Hall, Department of Education. The Catholic University of America, Washington, DC 20064. (800)464-3742. http://www.ericae.net.

Paula Anne Ford-Martin

Homeopathic medicine

Definition

Homeopathic medicine, or homeopathy, is a holistic system of treatment that originated in the late eighteenth century. The name homeopathy is derived from two Greek words that mean "like disease" because the system is based on the notion that a medicine capable of curing a disease will mimic or imitate its symptoms. Samuel Hahnemann (1755-1843), the founder of homeopathic medicine, used the Latin phrase *similia similibus curentur*, or "let like be cured with like," to summarize the underlying principle of his system. Homeopaths use the term allopathy, or "other disease," to describe the use of drugs in conventional medicine to oppose or counteract the symptom being treated.

Hahnemann was trained in the standard medical practice of his day and licensed as a physician in 1779. In 1796, he gave up his practice because he was disturbed by the poor results of orthodox medical treatment. He supported himself by working as a translator of medical texts. In the course of translating an English physician's research on a treatment for **malaria,** Hahnemann experimented on himself with small doses of the drug until he responded to it by developing symptoms resembling malaria. He concluded that the curative powers of the substance were derived from its ability to produce symptoms resembling those of its target disease. Hahnemann's reasoning was similar to that of Edward Jenner, who discovered the principle of **vaccination** in 1798 by observing that exposure to a mild form of pox conferred immunity against **smallpox,** a deadly disease with similar symptoms.

Hahnemann followed up his experiment by studying local records of accidental **poisonings** from commonly used medications. He found that when these substances were taken in overdose, they produced symptoms similar to those of the diseases for which they were given. For example, mercury was used to treat **syphilis,** but could cause syphilis-like ulcers in high doses. Hahnemann referred to his discovery as "the law of similars"—that substances that produced specific symptoms when given to healthy people in sufficient quantity could heal sick people of similar symptoms when given in highly diluted

KEY TERMS

Acute prescribing—Homeopathic treatment for disease symptoms resulting from situational stresses in the patient's life.

Allopathy—A word coined by Hahnemann in 1842 to describe conventional medical treatment of symptoms. Allopathic treatment of disease symptoms uses substances or techniques to oppose or suppress the symptoms.

Constitutional homeopathy—Homeopathic treatment directed at a patient's long-term underlying weakness, evaluated on the basis of recurrent symptom patterns.

Materia medica—In homeopathy, reference books compiled from provings of the various natural remedies. The *materia medica* are indexed for the psychological and physical symptoms produced by each substance, as well as for the medicines known to cause a specific symptom.

Modalities—The factors and circumstances that cause a patient's symptoms to improve or worsen.

Mother tincture—The first stage in the preparation of a homeopathic remedy, made by soaking a plant, animal, or mineral product in a solution of alcohol.

Polypharmacy homeopathy—The use of combination remedies in homeopathic treatment, in contrast to single-medicine prescribing.

Potentization—The process of increasing the power of homeopathic preparations by successive dilutions and successions of a mother tincture.

Proving—The method used in homeopathy to evaluate the medicinal applications of a substance. The homeopath doses healthy adults with the substance in question until symptoms are elicited and then documents the results.

Succussion—The act of shaking diluted homeopathic remedies as part of the process of potentization.

Trituration—The process of diluting a nonsoluble substance for homeopathic use by grinding it into a fine powder and mixing it with lactose.

forms. He then began to analyze the remedies available in nature by what he called provings. Provings of homeopathic remedies are still compiled by dosing healthy adults with various substances and documenting the results, in terms of the dose needed to produce the symp-

toms and the length of the dose's effectiveness. The symptoms are then classified in three categories, depending on whether they are produced in all provers, in a majority of provers, or only in a small number. The findings are collected in large homeopathic reference works called *materia medica* or materials of medicine as well as in homeopathic repertories.

Purpose

The purpose of homeopathy is the restoration of the body to homeostasis, or healthy balance, which is considered its natural state. The symptoms of a disease are regarded as the body's own defensive attempt to correct its imbalance, rather than as enemies to be defeated. Because a homeopath regards symptoms as positive evidence of the body's inner intelligence, he or she will prescribe a remedy designed to stimulate this internal curative process rather than suppress the symptoms.

The holistic nature of homeopathic treatment means that practitioners do not focus on isolated symptoms when treating patients. Even if the patient seeks help for only one illness, such as a cold or a skin rash, the homeopath will evaluate the disorder in the context of the patient's overall physical and psychological characteristics. It is thought that a careful assessment of all the patient's symptoms over the course of years will reflect a basic weakness specific to that person's constitution. Constitutional homeopathy is a form of treatment that focuses on recurrent patterns in the patient's medical history. In acute treatment, which is given for colds, vomiting, **fever,** and similar problems, the homeopath selects a remedy on the basis of the patient's symptomatic reactions to recent **stresses** in his or her life.

Precautions

Although a number of practitioners have written books on homeopathic self-care, these writers emphasize the limits of home treatment. The complexity of the case-taking process, and the difficulty involved in the consultation of the repertory or the *materia medica* persuade most patients to consult practitioners for serious illnesses rather than attempting to treat themselves.

Description

Homeopathic practice incorporates several principles besides the law of similars:

Single-medicine prescribing

Classical homeopathy prescribes only one medication at a time for the totality of the patient's symptoms. If the patient has an illness for which several different remedies have been proved, the practitioner will select the remedy that most closely fits the overall symptom profile. For example, two patients might come to the practitioner with a fever; but one might have warm, flushed skin and muscle twitching along with the fever and be given belladonna, while the other patient might have a dry skin and dry **cough** and so be given aconite.

Contemporary homeopaths do not always adhere strictly to the principle of single-medicine prescribing. Combination or polypharmacy homeopathy is increasingly popular in Europe. In addition, combinations of low-potency homeopathic preparations are now sold in pharmacies in the United States for use at home. Most classical homeopaths maintain that the curative powers of these combinations are lower than the single medicine that would be appropriate for the specific patient.

Minimal dosing

Because the goal of homeopathic treatment is the assistance of the body's innate capacity for self-regulation, practitioners do not give patients a second dose of medicine until the first has completed its work. It is believed that the body's ability to heal itself is sufficiently strong that only a small amount of medication is needed to begin the process.

Potentization of medicines

The most controversial aspect of Hahnemann's system is his theory of potentization in the preparation of medicines. Potentization is a process of increasing the potency of a remedy by a process of dilution and succussion, or shaking on a special machine or by hand. A homeopathic medication is formulated by preparing what is called a mother tincture, which is made by soaking plant, animal, or mineral materials in a solution of alcohol. The mother tincture is then diluted with either 10 or 100 parts of alcohol and succussed on the machine. The process of dilution and succussion is repeated many times in order to achieve the desired potency. Homeopaths maintain that succussion is necessary to transfer the energy of the natural substance to the solution. In addition, the potency of the remedy is regarded to increase with each dilution. After the tincture has been diluted to the prescribed potency, the resulting solution is added to a bottle of sucrose/lactose tablets, which are stored in a cool, dark place. If the remedy is not soluble in water, it is ground to a fine powder and mixed with powdered lactose (called trituration) to achieve the desired potency.

Preparation

Case-taking

The first stage in homeopathic treatment is the practitioner's detailed notation of the patient's symptoms. Homeopathic case-taking includes not only the symptoms directly associated with the illness but other physi-

cal complaints that the patient may have and his or her psychological reactions. The reader should note that homeopathy uses the word symptom in a broader sense than mainstream medicine. In homeopathy, symptoms include any physical or emotional change that is observed during the course of an illness. In addition to noting the location and severity of the symptoms, the homeopath will ask about its modalities. The modalities are the circumstances or factors (e.g., weather, time of day, behavior or activity, etc.) that make the symptom either better or worse.

Selection of remedy

The practitioner will choose the medication by matching the patient's symptom profile with the symptoms that the remedy has been proved to cause in healthy people. Dose repetition or change of medication is based on observation of the patient's response. The principle of minimal dosing implies that the dose should not be repeated until the previous dose has ceased to act.

Risks

There are few risks associated with homeopathic treatment in the United States. In terms of training, many homeopaths are licensed graduates of conventional medical schools in many fields. Homeopaths include naturopaths, registered nurses, and physicians. There are also lay practitioners of homeopathy whose practice should be more limited than licensed professionals.

The remedies are safe in terms of their chemical composition and have far fewer side effects than conventional medications. However, a exacerbation of symptoms can occur with initial dosage of a remedy. Because of the extensive and detailed documentation in homeopathic *materia medica*, erroneous prescriptions are relatively uncommon. In addition, the dilution of homeopathic remedies prevents the patient from being harmed by an incorrectly prescribed medication.

Normal results

Normal results of homeopathic treatment are successful treatment and/or the strengthening of the patient's constitution.

Resources

BOOKS

Cummings, Stephen, and Dana Ullmann. *Everybody's Guide to Homeopathic Medicines.* New York: G. P. Putnam's Sons, 1991.

Inglis, Brian, and Ruth West. *The Alternative Health Guide.* New York: Alfred A. Knopf, 1983.

MacEoin, Beth. *Homeopathy.* New York: HarperCollins Publishers, 1994.

Mills, Simon, and Steven J. Finando. *Alternatives in Healing*. New York: New American Library, 1988.

A Visual Encyclopedia of Unconventional Medicine, edited by Ann Hill. New York: Crown Publishers, Inc., 1979.

ORGANIZATIONS

American Institute of Homeopathy, 1585 Glencoe Street #44, Denver, CO 80220.

National Center for Homeopathy, 801 North Fairfax #306, Alexandria, VA 22314.

Rebecca J. Frey

Homeopathic remedies, acute prescribing

Definition

Homeopathy, acute prescribing, is that part of homeopathy that treats short-term illness, which has had an abrupt onset and needs immediate attention.

Homeopathy is an alternative system of medical care based on the notion that a medicine capable of curing a disease will mimic or imitate its symptoms. It is holistic in its emphasis on treating the whole patient rather than focusing on the parts of the body affected by his or her immediate illness. Homeopathic remedies are almost always made from natural materials—plant, animal, or mineral substances—that have been treated to form mother tinctures or nonsoluble powders. Liquid extracts are then potentized, or increased in power, by a series of dilutions and successions, or shakings. It is thought that succussion is necessary to transfer the energy of the natural substance to the solution. In addition, the potency of the remedy is regarded to increase with each dilution. After the tincture has been diluted to the prescribed potency, the resulting solution is added to a bottle of sucrose/lactose tablets, which are stored in a cool, dark place. If the remedy is not soluble in water, it is ground to a fine powder and triturated with powdered lactose to achieve the desired potency.

Purpose

The purpose of acute prescribing in homeopathy is the treatment of short-term illnesses with sudden onset to gain rapid improvement. In **homeopathic medicine,** acute refers primarily to the speed of onset and self-limiting character of the disorder rather than its seriousness. Colds, **influenza, sore throats,** insect stings, cuts, **bruises,** vomiting, **diarrhea, fever,** muscle aches, and short-term **insomnia** are all examples of conditions that are treated by acute prescribing. The remedies given in

KEY TERMS

Acute prescribing—Homeopathic treatment for self-limiting illnesses with abrupt onset.

Allopathy—Conventional medical treatment of disease symptoms that uses substances or techniques to oppose or suppress the symptoms.

Law of similars—The basic principle of homeopathic medicine that governs the selection of a specific remedy. The law of similars holds that a substance of natural origin that produces certain symptoms in a healthy person will cure those symptoms in a sick person.

Modalities—The factors and circumstances that cause a patient's symptoms to improve or worsen.

Mother tincture—The first stage in the preparation of a homeopathic remedy, made by soaking a plant, animal, or mineral product in a solution of alcohol.

Potentization—The process of increasing the power of homeopathic preparations by successive dilutions and succussions of a mother tincture.

Succussion—The act of shaking diluted homeopathic remedies as part of the process of potentization.

Trituration—The process of diluting a nonsoluble substance for homeopathic use by grinding it to a fine powder and mixing it with lactose powder.

acute homeopathic prescribing are intended to stimulate the body's internal ability to heal itself; they do not kill germs or suppress symptoms. Acute prescribing can be done—within limits—by patients at home, as well as by homeopathic practitioners. Study courses, self-treatment guides, and homeopathic home medicine kits are now available by mail order from homeopathic pharmacies and educational services.

Precautions

Homeopathic acute prescribing is not recommended either for the treatment of chronic conditions requiring constitutional prescribing, nor for severe infections requiring antibiotic treatment, nor for conditions requiring major surgery. It is also not recommended for the treatment of mental health problems.

Persons who are treating themselves with homeopathic remedies should follow professional guidelines regarding the limitations of home treatment. Most homeopathic home treatment guides include necessary information regarding symptoms and disorders that require professional attention.

Description

Homeopathic prescribing differs in general from allopathic medicine in its tailoring of remedies to the patient's overall personality type and totality of symptoms, rather than to the disease. Whereas a conventional physician would prescribe the same medication or treatment regimen to all patients with the **common cold,** for example, a homeopathic practitioner would ask detailed questions about each patient's symptoms and the modalities, or factors, that make them better or worse. As a result, the homeopath might prescribe six different remedies for six different patients with the same illness.

Homeopathic classification of symptoms

Homeopathic practitioners use the word symptom in a more inclusive fashion than traditional medicine. In homeopathy, symptoms include any change that the patient experiences during the illness, including changes in emotional or mental patterns.

Homeopaths classify symptoms according to a hierarchy of four categories for purposes of acute prescribing:

- Peculiar symptoms. These are symptoms unique to the individual that do not occur in most persons with the acute disease. Homeopaths make note of peculiar symptoms because they often help to determine the remedy.

- Mental and emotional symptoms. These are important general symptoms that inform the homeopath about the patient's total experience of the disorder.

- Other general symptoms. These are physical symptoms felt throughout the patient's body, such as tiredness, changes in appetite, or restlessness.

- Particular symptoms. Particular symptoms are localized in the body; they include such symptoms as nausea, skin **rashes, headache,** etc.

During homeopathic case-taking, the practitioner will evaluate the intensity of the patient's symptoms, assess their depth within the patient's body, note any peculiar symptoms, evaluate the modalities of each symptom, and make a list of key symptoms to guide the selection of the proper medicine.

Homeopathic remedies

Homeopathic medicines are usually formulated from diluted or triturated natural substances. The most common forms of administration are liquid dilutions and two sizes of pellets, or cylindrical tablets (for triturated remedies). A dose consists of one drop of liquid; 10–20 small pellets; or 1–3 large pellets. Since the remedies are so

dilute, the exact size of the dose is not of primary importance. The frequency of dosing is considered critical, however; patients are advised not to take further doses until the first has completed its effect.

Homeopathic remedies can be kept indefinitely with proper handling. Proper handling includes storing the remedies in the original bottles and discarding them if they become contaminated by sunlight or other intense light; temperatures over 100°F (37.8°C); vapors from camphor, mothballs, or perfume; or from other homeopathic remedies being opened in the same room at the same time.

Preparation

Case-taking

The first step in acute prescribing is a lengthy interview with the patient, known as case-taking. In addition to noting the character, location, and severity of the patient's symptoms, the homeopath will ask about their modalities. The modalities are the circumstances or factors (e.g., weather, time of day, body position, behavior or activity, etc.) that make the symptom either better or worse. Case-taking can be done by the patient or a family member as well as by a homeopath.

Selection and administration of a remedy

The choice of a specific remedy is guided by the patient's total symptom profile rather than by the illness. Homeopathic remedies are prescribed according to the law of similars, which holds that a substance that produces specific symptoms in healthy people cures those symptoms in sick people when given in highly diluted forms. For example, a patient with influenza who is irritable, headachy, and suffering from joint or muscle **pains** is likely to be given *Bryonia* (wild hops), because this plant extract would cause this symptom cluster in a healthy individual.

Patients are instructed to avoid touching homeopathic medicines with their fingers. The dose can be poured onto a piece of white paper or the bottle's cap and tipped directly into the mouth. Homeopathic remedies are not taken with water; patients should not eat or drink anything for 15–20 minutes before or after taking the dose. In addition, it is thought that certain strong-smelling substances, including coffee, mint flavoring, mouthwash, eucalyptus, and camphor, can reverse the effects of homeopathic remedies. Patients are therefore encouraged to avoid using these substances for the duration of their illness.

Aftercare

Aftercare of acute prescribing consists of careful observation and recording of the patient's reactions to the remedy. Close observation is necessary because homeopathic prescribing does not have hard-and-fast rules about dosage intervals. Based on the principle of minimal dosing, homeopathic practice does not give a patient a second dose of medicine until the first has stopped acting, no matter how long the activity is thought to last. If the patient shows marked improvement within an hour or two following administration of the remedy, no further doses are given. If the patient's improvement is not dramatic, the remedy may be repeated on a flexible schedule. The general rule is that the more acute the patient's symptoms, the more frequently the medicine should be repeated. Dosage intervals can range from every 10–15 minutes for high fevers or severe pain to twice a day for mild colds.

The specific remedy is given for no longer than two to three days. Homeopaths maintain that the patient should improve within that time frame if the correct medicine was chosen. If there is no improvement, another remedy may be tried.

Risks

The most common risk associated with homeopathic acute prescribing is ignoring the limitations of self-treatment. The remedies themselves are so highly diluted as to be harmless to patients.

Normal results

Normal results are recovery from the illness being treated.

Resources

BOOKS

Cummings, Stephen, and Dana Ullmann. *Everybody's Guide to Homeopathic Medicines.* New York: G. P. Putnam's Sons, 1991.

Inglis, Brian, and Ruth West. *The Alternative Health Guide.* New York: Alfred A. Knopf, 1983.

MacEoin, Beth. *Homeopathy.* New York: HarperCollins Publishers, 1994.

Mills, Simon, and Steven J. Finando. *Alternatives in Healing.* New York: New American Library, 1988.

A Visual Encyclopedia of Unconventional Medicine, edited by Ann Hill. New York: Crown Publishers, Inc., 1979.

Vithoulkas, George. *Homeopathy: Medicine of the New Man.* New York: Fireside Books (Simon & Schuster), 1992.

ORGANIZATIONS

American Institute of Homeopathy, 1585 Glencoe Street #44, Denver, CO 80220.

International Foundation for the Promotion of Homeopathy. 76 Lee Street, Mill Valley, CA 94941.

National Center for Homeopathy, 801 North Fairfax #306, Alexandria, VA 22314.

Rebecca J. Frey

Homeopathic remedies, constitutional prescribing

Definition

Constitutional prescribing of homeopathic remedies refers to the selection and administration of homeopathic preparations over a period of time for treatment related to what practitioners call miasmic disorders, those caused by a generational predisposition to a disease.

Purpose

The purpose of constitutional prescribing of homeopathic remedies is the treatment of what is known as miasms, or miasmic disorders. The term miasm comes from a Greek word meaning stain or pollution. As in acute prescribing, constitutional prescribing is holistic in that it is intended to treat the patient on the emotional and spiritual levels of his or her being as well as the physical. Constitutional prescribing is also aimed at eventual cure of the patient, not just suppression or relief of immediate symptoms.

Precautions

Constitutional homeopathic prescribing is not appropriate for diseases or health crises requiring emergency treatment, whether medical, surgical, or psychiatric. In addition, constitutional prescribing should not be self-administered. Although home treatment kits of homeopathic remedies are available for acute self-limited disorders, the knowledge of homeopathic theory and practice required for constitutional evaluation is beyond the scope of most patients.

Description

Constitutional prescribing is based on the patient's symptom profile and specific aspects of homeopathic theory.

Homeopathic classification of symptoms

Homeopathic practitioners use the word symptom in a more inclusive fashion than traditional medicine. In homeopathy, symptoms include any change that the patient experiences during the illness, including changes in emotional or mental patterns.

KEY TERMS

Aggravation—Another term used by homeopaths for the healing crisis.

Allopathy—Conventional medical treatment of disease symptoms that uses substances or techniques to oppose or suppress the symptoms.

Constitutional prescribing—Homeopathic treatment for long-term or chronic disorders related to inherited predispositions to certain types of illness.

Healing crisis—A temporary worsening of the patient's symptoms during successive stages of homeopathic treatment.

Law of similars—The basic principle of homeopathic medicine that governs the selection of a specific remedy. The law of similars holds that a substance of natural origin that produces certain symptoms in a healthy person will cure those symptoms in a sick person.

Laws of cure—A set of three rules used by homeopaths to assess the progress of a patient's recovery.

Materia medica—In homeopathy, reference books compiled from provings of the various natural remedies.

Miasm—In homeopathic theory, a general weakness or predisposition to chronic disease that is transmitted down the generational chain.

Modalities—The factors and circumstances that cause a patient's symptoms to improve or worsen. Modalities include weather, time of day, the patient's body position, the effects of foods, and similar factors.

Repertories—Homeopathic reference books consisting of descriptions of symptoms. The process of selecting a homeopathic remedy from the patient's symptom profile is called repertorizing.

Homeopaths classify symptoms according to a hierarchy of four categories:

• Peculiar symptoms. These are symptoms unique to the individual that do not occur in most persons. Homeopaths make note of peculiar symptoms because they often help to determine the remedy.

• Mental and emotional symptoms. These are important general symptoms that inform the homeopath about the patient's total experience of the disorder.

• Other general symptoms. These are physical symptoms felt throughout the patient's body, such as tiredness, changes in appetite, or restlessness.

• Particular symptoms. Particular symptoms are localized in the body; they include such symptoms as nausea, skin **rashes,** or **headaches.**

Miasms

Homeopaths regard the patient's symptom profile as a systemic manifestation of an underlying chronic disorder called a miasm. Miasms are serious disturbances of what homeopaths call the patient's vital force that are inherited from parents at the time of conception. German doctor Samuel Hahnemann, who developed homeopathy in the late 18th century, believed that the parents' basic lifestyle, their emotional condition and habitual diet, and even the atmospheric conditions at the time of conception would affect the number and severity of miasms passed on to the child. Hahnemann himself distinguished three miasms: the psoric, which he considered the most universal source of chronic disease in humans; the syphilitic; and the sycotic, which he attributed to **gonorrhea.** Later homeopaths identified two additional miasms, the cancernic and the tuberculinic. The remaining major source of miasms is allopathic medicine. It is thought that specific allopathic treatments—particularly **smallpox vaccinations,** cortisone preparations, major tranquilizers, and antibiotics—can produce additional layers of miasms in the patient's constitution. Constitutional prescribing evaluates the person's current state or miasmic picture, and selects a remedy intended to correct or balance that state. The homeopath may prescribe a different remedy for each miasmic layer over time, but gives only one remedy at a time directed at the person's current state. The basic principle governing the prescription of each successive remedy is the law of similars, or "like cures like."

Hering's laws of cure

The homeopathic laws of cure were outlined by Constantine Hering, a student of Hahnemann who came to the United States in the 1830s. Hering enunciated three laws or principles of the patterns of healing that are used by homeopaths to evaluate the effectiveness of specific remedies and the overall progress of constitutional prescribing:

• Healing progresses from the deepest parts of the organism to the external parts. Homeopaths consider the person's mental and emotional dimensions, together with the brain, heart, and other vital organs, as a person's deepest parts. The skin, hands, and feet are considered the external parts.

- Symptoms appear or disappear in the reverse of their chronological order of appearance. In terms of constitutional treatment, this law means that miasms acquired later in life will resolve before earlier ones.
- Healing proceeds from the upper to the lower parts of the body.

Healing crises

Homeopaths use Hering's laws to explain the appearance of so-called healing crises or aggravations in the course of homeopathic treatment. It is not unusual for patients to experience temporary worsening of certain symptoms after taking their first doses of homeopathic treatment. For example, a person might notice that arthritic **pains** in the shoulders are better but that the hands feel worse. Hering's third law would indicate that the remedy is working because the symptoms are moving downward in the body. In constitutional prescribing, a remedy that removes one of the patient's miasmic layers will then allow the symptoms of an older miasm to emerge. Thus the patient may find that a physical disease is followed by a different set of physical problems or by emotional symptoms.

Preparation

The most important aspects of preparation for constitutional prescribing are the taking of a complete patient history and careful patient education.

Case-taking

Homeopathic case-taking for constitutional prescribing is similar to that for acute prescribing, but more in-depth. The initial interview generally takes between one and a half to two hours. The practitioner is concerned to record the totality of the patient's symptoms and the modalities that influence their severity. Also included are general characteristics about the patient and their lifestyle choices. For example, a practitioner might ask the patient if he or she likes being outside or if he or she is generally hot or cold. There is also an emphasis on the patient's lifetime medical history, particularly records of allopathic treatments.

Patient education

Homeopaths regard patients as equal partners in the process of recovery. They will take the time to explain the theories underlying constitutional prescribing to the patient as well as taking the history. Patient education is especially important in constitutional prescribing in order to emphasize the need for patience with the slowness of results and length of treatment, and to minimize the possibility of self-treatment with allopathic drugs if the patient has a healing crisis.

Homeopathic remedies

The preparation, selection, administration, and storage of remedies for constitutional prescribing are the same as in acute prescribing. These procedures are described more fully in the article on acute prescribing.

Aftercare

As in acute prescribing, constitutional prescribing of homeopathic remedies is followed by close observation of the patient's responses. Based on the principle of minimal dosing, homeopathic practice does not give a patient a second dose of medicine until the first has stopped acting. In acute prescribing, the patient is expected to show some response to the remedy within hours or at most a few days if the proper substance has been selected. In constitutional prescribing, the homeopath evaluates the activity of remedies over a much longer time frame. This is assessed by a follow-up visit, generally 4–6 weeks after the remedy has been given.

The length of constitutional treatment varies widely, depending on the patient's basic level of health and his or her previous treatment with allopathic medicines. Given the homeopathic emphasis on treating the whole person and tailoring treatment to his or her unique symptom profile, most practitioners are reluctant to define the length of time needed for complete recovery. One rule of thumb that has been offered, however, is that the patient will need one month of treatment for every year that he or she has suffered from a chronic disorder.

Risks

The primary risks to the patient from constitutional homeopathic treatment are the symptoms of the healing crisis and possible limitations in the practitioner's expertise. The complexity of constitutional prescribing requires homeopaths to have detailed knowledge of the *materia medica* and the repertories, and to take careful and extensive case notes.

Normal results

Normal results of homeopathic constitutional prescribing are eventual if slow recovery from chronic disorders, and/or overall improvement of the patient's basic level of energy and functioning.

Resources

BOOKS

Ainsworth, J. B. L. "Homoeopathy." In *The Encyclopedia of Alternative Medicine and Self-Help,* edited by Malcolm Hulke. New York: Schocken Books, 1979.

Cummings, Stephen, and Dana Ullmann. *Everybody's Guide to Homeopathic Medicines.* New York: G. P. Putnam's Sons, 1991.

Inglis, Brian, and Ruth West. *The Alternative Health Guide.* New York: Alfred A. Knopf, 1983.

MacEoin, Beth. *Homeopathy.* New York: HarperCollins Publishers, 1994.

Mills, Simon, and Steven J. Finando. *Alternatives in Healing.* New York: New American Library, 1988.

A Visual Encyclopedia of Unconventional Medicine, edited by Ann Hill. New York: Crown Publishers, Inc., 1979.

Vithoulkas, George. *Homeopathy: Medicine of the New Man.* New York: Fireside Books (Simon & Schuster), 1992.

ORGANIZATIONS

American Institute of Homeopathy. 1585 Glencoe Street #44, Denver, CO 80220.

International Foundation for the Promotion of Homeopathy. 76 Lee Street, Mill Valley, CA 94941.

National Center for Homeopathy. 801 North Fairfax #306, Alexandria, VA 22314.

OTHER

Homeopathy Home Page. http://www.dungeon.com:80/home/cam/homeo.html.

Rebecca J. Frey

Homeopathy *see* **Homeopathic medicine**

Hong Kong flu *see* **Influenza**

Hookworm disease

Definition

Hookworm disease is an illness caused by one of two types of S-shaped worms that infect the intestine of humans (the worm's host).

Description

Two types of hookworm are responsible for hookworm disease in humans. *Necator americanus* and *Ancylostoma duodenale* have similar life cycles and similar methods of causing illness. The adult worm of both *Necator americanus* and *Ancylostoma duodenale* is about 10 mm long, pinkish-white in color, and curved into an S-shape or double hook.

Both types of hookworm have similar life cycles. The females produce about 10,000–20,000 eggs per day. These eggs are passed out of the host's body in feces. The eggs enter the soil, where they incubate. After about 48 hours, the immature larval form hatches out of the eggs. These larvae take about six weeks to develop into the mature larval form that is capable of causing human

infection. If exposed to human skin at this point (usually bare feet walking in the dirt or bare hands digging in the dirt), the larvae will bore through the skin and ride through the lymph circulation to the right side of the heart. The larvae are then pumped into the lungs. There they bore into the tiny air sacs (alveoli) of the lungs. Their presence within the lungs usually causes enough irritation to produce coughing. The larvae are coughed up into the throat and mouth, and are then swallowed and passed into the small intestine. It is within the intestine that they develop into the adult worm, producing illness in their human host.

Ancylostoma duodenale is found primarily in the Mediterranean, the Middle East, and throughout Asia.

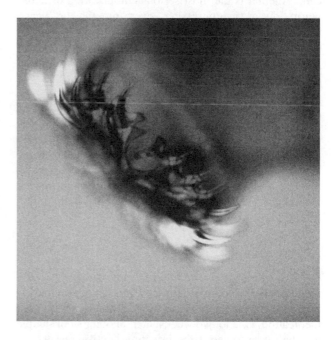

A micrographic image of the head of the hookworm *Ancylostoma spp.* (Photo Researchers, Inc. Reproduced by permission.)

Necator americanus is common in tropical areas including Asia, parts of the Americas, and throughout Africa. Research suggests that at least 25% of all people in the world have hookworm disease. In the United States, 700,000 people are believed to be infected with hookworms at any given time.

Causes & symptoms

Hookworms cause trouble for their human host when the worms attach their mouths to the lining of the small intestine and suck the person's blood.

An itchy, slightly raised rash called "ground itch" may appear around the area where the larvae first bored through the skin. The skin in this area may become red and swollen. This lasts for several days and commonly occurs between the toes.

When the larvae are in the lungs, the patient may have a **fever,** cough, and some **wheezing.** Some people, however, have none of these symptoms.

Once established within the intestine, the adult worms can cause abdominal **pain,** decreased appetite, **diarrhea,** and weight loss. Most importantly, the worms suck between 0.03–0.2 ml of blood per day. When a worm moves from one area of the intestine to another, it detaches its mouth from the intestinal lining, leaving an irritated area that may continue to bleed for some time. This results in even further blood loss. A single adult worm can live for up to 14 years in a patient's intestine. Over time, the patient's blood loss may be very significant. Anemia is the most serious complication of hookworm disease, progressing over months or years. Children are particularly harmed by such anemia, and can suffer from heart problems, **mental retardation,** slowed growth, and delayed sexual development. In infants, hookworm disease can be deadly.

Diagnosis

Diagnosis of hookworm disease involves collecting a stool sample for examination under a microscope. Hookworm eggs have a characteristic appearance. Counting the eggs in a specific amount of feces allows the healthcare provider to estimate the severity of the infection.

Treatment

Minor infections are often left untreated, especially in areas where hookworm is very common. If treatment is required, the doctor will prescribe a three-day dose of medication. One to two weeks later, another stool sample will be taken to see if the infection is still present.

Anemia is treated with iron supplements. In severe cases, blood **transfusion** may be necessary. Two medications, pyrantel pamoate and mebendazole, are frequently used with good results.

Prognosis

The prognosis for patients with hookworm disease is generally good. However, reinfection rates are extremely high in countries with poor sanitation.

Prevention

Prevention of hookworm disease involves improving sanitation and avoiding contact with soil in areas with high rates of hookworm infection. Children should be required to wear shoes when playing outside in such areas, and people who are gardening should wear gloves.

Resources

BOOKS

Plorde, James J. "Hookworms." In *Sherris Medical Microbiology: An Introduction to Infectious Diseases,* edited by Kenneth J. Ryan. Norwalk, CT: Appleton & Lange, 1994.

Stoffman, Phyllis. *The Family Guide to Preventing and Treating 100 Infectious Diseases.* New York: John Wiley and Sons, Inc., 1995.

PERIODICALS

Farley, Dixie. "Treating Tropical Diseases." *FDA Consumer* (January-February 1997): 26 + .

Hotez, P. J., and D. I. Pritchard. "Hookworm Infection." *Scientific American* (June 1995): 68 + .

ORGANIZATIONS

Centers for Disease Control and Prevention. (404) 332-4559. http://www.cdc.gov/ncidod/dpd/hookworm.htm.

Rosalyn S. Carson-DeWitt

Hormone replacement therapy

Definition

Hormone replacement therapy (HRT) is the use of synthetic or natural female hormones to make up for the decline or lack of natural hormones produced in a woman's body. HRT is sometimes referred to as estrogen replacement therapy (ERT), because the first medications that were used in the 1960s for female hormone replacement were estrogen compounds.

KEY TERMS

Dilation and curettage (D & C)—A surgical procedure in which the patient's cervix is widened (dilated) and the endometrium is scraped with a scoop-shaped instrument (curette).

Estrogen—The primary sex hormone that controls normal sexual development in females. During the menstrual cycle, estrogen helps prepare the body for possible pregnancy.

Follicle-stimulating hormone (FSH)—A hormone produced by the pituitary gland that stimulates the follicles in the ovaries to swell and release ripe ova. Doctors sometimes use its levels in a woman's blood to evaluate whether she is in menopause.

Hormone—A substance secreted by an endocrine gland that is carried by blood or other body fluids to its target tissues or organs.

Hot flash—A warm or hot sensation on the face, neck and upper body, sometimes accompanied by flushing and sweating. Some women refer to hot flashes as hot flushes.

Osteoporosis—A bone disorder in which the bones become brittle, porous, and easily broken. It is a major health concern for postmenopausal women.

Ovary—The female sex gland that produces eggs and female reproductive hormones.

Ovulation—The cyclical process of egg maturation and release from the ovary.

Progesterone—A female hormone produced by the ovary. It functions to prepare the lining of the uterus to receive a fertilized ovum.

Progesterone challenge test—A test that is given to see if a woman is still secreting estrogen. It consists of doses of progesterone given over a 10-day period.

Progestin—Synthetic progesterone available as an oral medication.

Testosterone—A male sex hormone that is sometimes given as part of HRT to women whose ovaries have been removed. Testosterone helps with problems of sexual desire.

Uterus—The hollow organ in women in which fertilized eggs develop during pregnancy. The uterus is sometimes called the womb.

Estrogens

In order to understand how HRT works and the controversies surrounding it, women should know that there are different types of estrogen medications commonly prescribed in the United States and Europe. These drugs are given in a variety of prescription strengths and methods of administration. There are at present three estrogen compounds used in Western countries. Only the first two are readily available in the United States.

- Estrone. Estrone is the form of estrogen present in women after **menopause.** It is available as tablets under the brand name Ogen. The most commonly prescribed estrogen in the United States, Premarin, is a so-called conjugated estrogen that is a mixture of estrone and other estrogens.

- Estradiol. This is the form of estrogen naturally present in premenopausal women. It is available as tablets (Estrace), skin patches (Estraderm), or vaginal creams (Estrace).

- Estriol. Estriol is a weaker form of estrogen produced by the breakdown of other forms of estrogen in the body. This is the form of estrogen most commonly given in Europe, under the brand name Estriol. It is the only form that is thought not to cause **cancer.**

In addition to pills taken by mouth, skin patches, and vaginal creams, estrogen preparations can be given by injection or by pellets implanted under the skin. Estrogen implants, however, are used less and less frequently.

Progestins

Most HRT programs as of 1998 include progestin treatment with estrogen compounds. Progestins—which are also sometimes called progestogens—are synthetic forms of progesterone that are given to reduce the possibility that estrogen by itself will cause cancer of the uterus. Progestins are commonly prescribed under the brand names Provera and Depo-Provera. Other common brand names are Norlutate, Norlutin, and Aygestin.

Estrogen/testosterone combinations

Women's ovaries secrete small amounts of a male sex hormone (testosterone) throughout their lives. Women who have had both ovaries removed by surgery are sometimes given testosterone along with estrogen as part of HRT. Combinations of these hormones are available as tablets under the brand name Estratest or as vaginal creams. Women who cannot take estrogens can use 1% testosterone cream by itself for problems with vaginal soreness.

Estrogen/tranquilizer combinations

There are several medications that combine estrogen with a tranquilizer like chlordiazepoxide (sold under the trade name Menrium) or meprobamate (sold under the trade name PMB). Many doctors warn against these combination drugs because the tranquilizers can be habit-forming.

Purpose

HRT has two primary purposes: preventive treatment against **osteoporosis** and heart disease; and relief of physical symptoms associated with menopause.

Menopausal symptoms

Women in midlife enter a stage of development called menopause, when their menstrual periods become irregular and finally stop. The early phase of this transition is called the perimenopause. In the United States, the average age at menopause is presently 50 or 51, but some women begin menopause as early as 40 and others as late as 55. It can take as long as 10 years for a woman to complete the process. Women who have had their ovaries removed surgically are said to have undergone surgical menopause.

Doctors have not always agreed on definitions of the menopause. Some use age as the baseline. Others define menopause as the point at which a woman has had no menstrual periods for a full calendar year. Still others define menopause as the end of ovulation. It is not always clear, however, when a woman has had her last period or when she has stopped ovulating. One study indicates that as many as 10% of women who have not had a period for a year will have another menstrual period after that point. In addition, women who take **oral contraceptives** can have breakthrough bleeding long after they have stopped ovulating. As a result, some doctors now measure the level of follicle-stimulating hormone (FSH) in a woman's blood to estimate whether the woman has entered menopause. During perimenopause, the FSH levels in a woman's blood rise as her body attempts to stimulate the release of ripe ova. An FSH level over 40 is considered an indicator of menopause.

During the menopausal transition, the levels of estrogen in the woman's body drop. The lowered estrogen level is responsible for a group of symptoms that include hot flashes (or flushes), weight gain, changes in skin texture, mood swings, heart **palpitations,** sleep disturbances, a need to urinate more frequently, and loss of sexual desire. The estrogen that is given in HRT can eliminate hot flashes, night sweats, lack of vaginal lubrication, and urinary tract problems. HRT will *not* prevent weight gain or wrinkles. It also does not cure depression in most women.

Preventive care

HRT is recommended by many doctors on the grounds that estrogen replacement helps to protect women against two serious midlife health problems.

OSTEOPOROSIS

Osteoporosis is a disorder in which the bones become more brittle and more easily fractured. It is a particular problem for postmenopausal women because the lower levels of estrogen in the blood lead to weakening of the bone. About 25% of Caucasian women will develop severe osteoporosis; Asian women have a slightly lower risk level; Latina and African American women are least at risk.

In addition to race, there are other factors that put some women at higher risk of developing osteoporosis. Women in any of the following groups should take bone loss into account when considering HRT.

- Family history of osteoporosis
- Menopause before age 40
- Kidney disease and dialysis
- Thin body build or being underweight
- History of colitis, **Crohn's disease,** or chronic **diarrhea**
- Thyroid medications
- Childlessness
- Chronic use of **antacids**
- Lack of **exercise**
- Poor food choices, including high salt intake, lack of vitamin D, high **caffeine** consumption, and low calcium intake
- Smoking and alcohol abuse
- Cortisone therapy.

HEART DISEASE

Heart disease is a major health concern of women in midlife. It is the leading cause of **death** in women over 60. The primary disorders of the circulatory system in postmenopausal women are **stroke, hypertension,** and **coronary artery disease.** Current studies of women on HRT do not yield a completely clear picture. In particular, although estrogen given without progestins has been shown to offer some protection against heart disease, the effect of progestins in offsetting the benefits of estrogen complicates the research findings. It seems likely that estrogen levels are only part of the picture in evaluating a woman's risk of heart disease.

The major factors that are known to increase the risk of heart disease include:

- History of smoking

- Being overweight
- High-fat **diets**
- Alcohol abuse
- Family history of heart disease
- High blood pressure
- High blood cholesterol levels
- Diabetes.

Less important risk factors include being African American, having a sedentary lifestyle, undergoing menopause before age 45, and having high levels of family- or job-related **stress.**

Precautions

Medical conditions

Certain groups of women should not use HRT. They include women with:

- **Breast cancer**
- Cancer of the uterus
- Abnormal vaginal bleeding that has not been diagnosed
- High blood pressure that rises when HRT is used
- Liver disease
- **Gallstones** or diseases of the gallbladder.

Drug interactions

HRT can interact with other prescription medications that a woman may be taking. Women who are taking **corticosteroids,** drugs to slow the clotting of blood (anticoagulants), and rifampin should ask their doctor about possible interactions.

Combining estrogens with certain other medicines can cause liver damage. Among the drugs that may cause liver damage when taken with estrogens are:

- **Acetaminophen** (Tylenol), when used in high doses over long periods
- Anabolic steroids such as nandrolone (Anabolin) or oxymetholone (Anadrol)
- Medicine for infections
- Antiseizure medicines such as divalproex (Depakote), valproic acid (Depakene), or phenytoin (Dilantin)
- **Antianxiety drugs,** including chlorpromazine (Thorazine), prochlorperazine (Compazine), and thioridazine (Mellaril).

In addition, estrogens may interfere with the effects of bromocriptine (Parlodel), used to treat **Parkinson's disease** and other conditions; they may also increase the chance of toxic side effects when taken with cyclosporine (Sandimmune), a drug that helps prevent organ transplant rejection.

Description

As described earlier, HRT medications come in several different forms, including tablets, stick-on patches, injections, and creams or rings that are worn inside the vagina. The form prescribed depends on the purpose of the hormone replacement therapy. Women who want relief from vaginal dryness, for example, would be given a cream or vaginal ring. Women using HRT to relieve hot flashes or to prevent osteoporosis and heart disease often prefer oral medications or patches. All HRT medications used in the United States are available only with a doctor's prescription.

HRT treatment regimens

One of the complications of HRT is the number of treatment options, including combinations of types of estrogen; dosage levels; forms of administration; and whether or not progestins are used with the estrogen to offset the risk of uterine cancer. This variety, however, means that a woman who wants to use HRT while minimizing side effects can try different forms of medication or dosage schedules when she consults her doctor. It is vital, however, for women to follow their doctor's directions exactly and not change dosages themselves.

At present, women who are taking a combination of estrogens and progestins are placed on one of three dosage schedules:

- Estrogen pills taken daily from the first through the 25th day of each month, with a progestin pill taken daily during the last 10–14 days of the cycle. Both drugs are then stopped for the next five to six days to allow the uterus to shed its lining.
- Estrogen pills taken on a daily basis with low-dose progestin pills, also on a daily basis. Both medications are taken continuously with no days off.
- Estrogen pills and low-dose progestins taken on a daily basis for five days each week, with both medications stopped on the last two days of each week.

Controversies over HRT

It is important to know that there is still considerable disagreement over the advantages and disadvantages of HRT. As of June 1998, a major American research team was urging further research into other strategies for health care in menopausal women. In the United Kingdom, the so-called ''Million Women'' study is being conducted to evaluate different types of HRT and the long-term health risks of this treatment.

INCREASED RISK OF BREAST CANCER

The most important controversy over HRT is whether it increases a woman's risk of developing breast cancer. Some studies not only indicate a connection, but suggest that the risk of breast cancer rises with the length of time that a woman has been taking HRT. According to an American study published in June 1998, the risk of breast cancer increases by 2.3% for each year that a woman takes HRT. A Swedish study found that the risk of breast cancer doubled after six years of HRT, which agrees with American findings that risk is connected to length of treatment.

TIMING AND LENGTH OF TREATMENT

One of the disagreements about HRT concerns the best time to begin using it. Some doctors think that women should begin using HRT while they are still in perimenopause. Others think that there is no harm in a woman's waiting to decide. Either way, the question of timing means that a woman should keep track of changes in her periods and other signs of perimenopause so that her doctor can evaluate her readiness for HRT.

The other question of timing concerns length of treatment. Some women use HRT only as long as they need it to relieve the symptoms of menopause. Others regard it as a lifetime commitment because of concerns about osteoporosis. As has already been mentioned, some studies indicate a correlation between length of HRT treatment and an increased risk of breast cancer. As the next section indicates, some women stop using HRT because of side effects. One study found that the average length of time that women stay on HRT is 23 months.

UNWANTED SIDE EFFECTS

Much of the disagreement about unwanted side effects from HRT concerns the role of progestins in the estrogen/progestin combinations that are commonly prescribed. Many women who find that estrogen relieves hot flashes and other symptoms of menopause have the opposite experience with progestin. Progestin frequently causes moodiness, depression, sore breasts, weight gain, and severe **headaches.** A 1992 study reviewed in the *Journal of the American Medical Association* reported on the high rate of HRT "dropouts." Two-thirds of the women who tried HRT stopped because of the side effects of Provera. A Danish study found a 40% "dropout" rate.

FEMINIST ISSUES

Feminist concerns about HRT include the social as well as the medical aspects of menopause. Many women have mixed feelings about HRT because they see it as part of Western society's overemphasis on youth and physical beauty in women, to the neglect of their mental and spiritual capacities. Others raise questions about the long-term wisdom of interfering with a natural part of the human life cycle and treating menopause as a "disease." It is a good idea for women who are considering HRT to look at their health concerns within the context of their value systems and their lives as a whole.

Other treatment approaches

Women who are uncertain about HRT, or who should not take estrogens, should know about other treatment options.

NATURAL PROGESTERONE

Progestins, which are synthetic hormones, were developed because natural progesterone cannot be absorbed in the body when taken in pill form. A new technique called micronization has made it possible for women to take natural progesterone by mouth. Many women prefer this form of hormone because it lacks the side effects of the synthetic progestins even though it is somewhat more expensive. The most common form of natural progesterone is called Prometrium and it is available by prescription only. Another form of natural progesterone consists of the hormone suspended in vitamin E oil. It is absorbed through the skin and is available without a prescription.

ALTERNATIVE THERAPIES

Many mainstream as well as alternative practitioners recommend changes in diet and nutrition as helpful during menopause. Women who limit their intake of fats and salts, increase their use of fresh fruits and vegetables, cut out smoking, and drink only in moderation often find that these dietary changes help them feel better. Naturopaths typically recommend vitamin and mineral supplements for general well-being as well as for relief from hot flashes and leg cramps. In addition, herbal teas and tonics are helpful to some women in treating water retention, **insomnia, constipation,** or moodiness.

Women who find menopause emotionally stressful because of negative social attitudes toward older women are often helped by **meditation, biofeedback,** therapeutic **massage,** and other relaxation techniques. **Yoga** and **tai chi** provide physical exercise as well as **stress reduction.** Exercise is an important safeguard against osteoporosis.

Preparation

Women who are considering HRT should visit their doctor for a series of tests to make sure that they do not have any serious health disorders. They should have a Pap smear and breast examination to rule out cancer. They should also have a **urinalysis,** a **bone density test,** and blood tests to measure their red blood cell level, blood sugar level, cholesterol level, and liver and thyroid function.

In addition to these tests, most doctors will also give a progesterone challenge test. It consists of doses of progesterone given over a 10-day period to see if the woman is still producing her own estrogen. If she bleeds at the end of the test, she is still producing estrogen.

Aftercare

Aftercare is a very important part of HRT. Women who are taking HRT will need to see their doctor more frequently. At a minimum, they should be checked twice a year with a blood pressure test and breast examination. They should have a complete physical on a yearly basis. Any abnormal bleeding must be reported to the doctor as soon as it occurs. The doctor will need to order a tissue biopsy or dilation and curettage (D & C) in order to rule out cancer of the uterus.

Women who are taking HRT and decide to stop should taper their dosage over a period of several months rather than discontinuing abruptly. A gradual reduction minimizes the possibility of hot flashes and other side effects.

Risks

The short-term risks associated with HRT include a range of physical side effects. Common side effects include fluid retention, bloating, weight gain, sore breasts, leg cramps, vaginal discharges, **migraine headaches,** hair loss, **nausea and vomiting, acne,** depression, **shortness of breath,** and **dizziness.** Potentially serious side effects include tissue growths in the uterus (fibroids), gallstones, **thrombophlebitis, hypoglycemia,** abnormal growth (hyperplasia) of uterine tissue, thyroid disorders, high blood pressure, and cancer.

Normal results

Normal results of HRT include relief of hot flashes, night sweats, vaginal dryness, and urinary symptoms associated with menopause. The type of long-term study (called a prospective study) that is necessary to establish the protective or preventive effects of HRT has not yet been done.

Resources

BOOKS

Compton, Madonna Sophia, MA. *Women at the Change: The Intelligent Woman's Guide to Menopause.* St. Paul, MN: Llewellyn Publications, 1998.

Greenwood, Sadja. *Menopause, Naturally: Preparing for the Second Half of Life.* Volcano, CA: Volcano Press, 1992.

Greer, Germaine. *The Change: Women, Aging, and the Menopause.* New York: Fawcett Columbine, 1991.

Nurses Drug Guide 1995, edited by Billie Ann Wilson, et al. Norwalk, CT: Appleton & Lange, 1995.

Sander, Pela. "Natural Healing Therapies." In *Women of the 14th Moon: Writings on Menopause,* edited by Dena Taylor and Amber Coverdale Sumrall. Freedom, CA: The Crossing Press, 1991.

ORGANIZATIONS

American Heart Association. 7320 Greenville Avenue, Dallas, TX 75321. (214)373-6300.

National Women's Health Network. 514 10th Street, NW, Washington, DC 20004. (202)347-1140.

North American Menopause Society (NAMS). 11100 Euclid Avenue, 7th Avenue, McDonald Hospital, Cleveland, OH 44105.

Women's International Pharmacy. 5708 Monona Drive, Madison, WI 53716. (800)279-5708.

OTHER

Menopausal Hormone Replacement Therapy. Fact sheet. National Cancer Institute website: http://rex.nci.nih.gov.

Rebecca J. Frey

Hospital-acquired infections
Definition

A hospital-acquired infection is usually one that first appears three days after a patient is admitted to a hospital or other health-care facility. Infections acquired in a hospital are also called nosocomial infections.

Description

About 5–10% of patients admitted to hospitals in the United States develop a nosocomial infection. Hospital-acquired infections are usually related to a procedure or treatment used to diagnose or treat the patient's illness or injury. About 25% of these infections can be prevented by healthcare workers taking proper precautions when caring for patients.

Hospital-acquired infections can be caused by bacteria, viruses, fungi, or parasites. These microorganisms may already be present in the patient's body or may come from the environment, contaminated hospital equipment, healthcare workers, or other patients. Depending on the causal agents involved, an infection may start in any part of the body. A localized infection is limited to a specific part of the body and has local symptoms. For example, if a surgical wound in the abdomen becomes infected, the area of the wound becomes red, hot, and painful. A generalized infection is one that enters the bloodstream and causes general systemic symptoms such as **fever,** chills, low blood pressure, or mental confusion.

Hospital-acquired infections may develop from surgical procedures, catheters placed in the urinary tract or blood vessels, or from material from the nose or mouth that is inhaled into the lungs. The most common types of hospital-acquired infections are urinary tract infections (UTIs), **pneumonia,** and surgical wound infections.

Causes & symptoms

All hospitalized patients are susceptible to contracting a nosocomial infection. Some patients are at greater risk than others—young children, the elderly, and persons with compromised immune systems are more likely to get an infection. Other risk factors for getting a hospital-acquired infection are a long hospital stay, the use of indwelling catheters, failure of healthcare workers to wash their hands, and overuse of **antibiotics.**

Any type of invasive procedure can expose a patient to the possibility of infection. Common causes of hospital-acquired infections include:

• Urinary bladder catheterization

• Respiratory procedures

• Surgery and **wounds**

• Intravenous (IV) procedures.

Urinary tract infection (UTI) is the most common type of hospital-acquired infection. Most hospital-acquired UTIs happen after **urinary catheterization.** Catheterization is the placement of a catheter through the urethra into the urinary bladder. This procedure is done to empty urine from the bladder, relieve pressure in the bladder, measure urine in the bladder, put medicine into the bladder, or for other medical reasons.

The healthy urinary bladder is sterile, which means it doesn't have any bacteria or other microorganisms in it. There may be bacteria in or around the urethra but they normally cannot enter the bladder. A catheter can pick up bacteria from the urethra and allow them into the bladder, causing an infection to start.

Bacteria from the intestinal tract are the most common type to cause UTIs. Patients with poorly functioning immune systems or who are taking antibiotics are also at risk for infection by a fungus called *Candida.*

Pneumonia is the second most common type of hospital-acquired infection. Bacteria and other microorganisms are easily brought into the throat by respiratory procedures commonly done in the hospital. The microorganisms come from contaminated equipment or the hands of health care workers. Some of these procedures are respiratory intubation, suctioning of material from the throat and mouth, and mechanical ventilation. The introduced microorganisms quickly colonize the throat area. This means that they grow and form a colony, but have not yet caused an infection. Once the throat is colonized, it is easy for a patient to inhale the microorganisms into the lungs.

Patients who cannot **cough** or gag very well are most likely to inhale colonized microorganisms into their lungs. Some respiratory procedures can keep patients from gagging or coughing. Patients who are sedated or who lose consciousness may also be unable to cough or gag. The inhaled microorganisms grow in the lungs and cause an infection that can lead to pneumonia.

Surgical procedures increase a patient's risk of getting an infection in the hospital. Surgery directly invades the patient's body, giving bacteria a way into normally sterile parts of the body. An infection can be acquired from contaminated surgical equipment or from healthcare workers. Following surgery, the surgical wound can become infected. Other wounds from trauma, **burns,** and **ulcers** may also become infected.

Many hospitalized patients need a steady supply of medications or nutrients delivered to their bloodstream. An intravenous (IV) catheter is placed in a vein and the medication or other substance is infused into the vein. Bacteria transmitted from the surroundings, contaminated equipment, or healthcare workers' hands can invade the site where the catheter is inserted. A local infection may develop in the skin around the catheter. The bacteria can also enter the blood through the vein and cause a generalized infection. The longer a catheter is in place, the greater the risk of infection.

Other hospital procedures that put patients at risk for nosocomial infection are gastrointestinal procedures, obstetric procedures, and **kidney dialysis.**

Fever is often the first sign of infection. Other symptoms and signs of infection are rapid breathing, mental confusion, low blood pressure, reduced urine output, and a high white blood cell count.

Patients with a UTI may have pain when urinating and blood in the urine. Symptoms of pneumonia may include difficulty breathing and coughing. A localized infection causes swelling, redness, and tenderness at the site of infection.

Diagnosis

An infection is suspected any time a hospitalized patient develops a fever that cannot be explained by a known illness. Some patients, especially the elderly, may not develop a fever. In these patients, the first signs of infection may be rapid breathing or mental confusion.

Diagnosis of a hospital-acquired infection is based on:

- Symptoms and signs of infection

- Examination of wounds and catheter entry sites

- Review of procedures that might have led to infection

- Laboratory test results.

A complete **physical examination** is conducted in order to locate symptoms and signs of infection. Wounds and the skin where catheters have been placed are examined for redness, swelling, or the presence of pus or an **abscess.** The physician reviews the patient's record of procedures performed in the hospital to determine if any posed a risk for infection.

Laboratory tests are done to look for signs of infection. A complete **blood count** can reveal if the white blood cell count is high. White blood cells are immune system cells that increase in numbers in response to an infection. White blood cells or blood may be present in the urine when there is a UTI.

Cultures of blood, urine, sputum, other body fluids, or tissue are done to look for infectious microorganisms. If an infection is present, it is necessary to identify the microorganism so the patient can be treated with the correct medication. A sample of the fluid or tissue is placed in a special medium that bacteria will grow in. Other tests can also be done on blood and body fluids to look for and identify bacteria, fungi, viruses, or other microorganisms responsible for an infection.

If a patient has symptoms suggestive of pneumonia, a chest x ray is done to look for infiltrates of white blood cells and other inflammatory substances in the lung tissue. Samples of sputum can be studied with a microscope or cultured to look for bacteria or fungi.

Treatment

Once the source of the infection is identified, the patient is treated with antibiotics or other medication that kills the responsible microorganism. Many different anti-biotics are available that are effective against different bacteria. Some common antibiotics are penicillin, **cephalosporins, tetracyclines,** and erythromycin. More and more commonly, some types of bacteria are becoming resistant to the standard antibiotic treatments. When this happens, a different, more powerful antibiotic must be used. Two strong antibiotics that have been effective against resistant bacteria are vancomycin and imipenem, although some bacteria are developing resistance to these antibiotics as well.

Fungal infections are treated with antifungal medications. Examples of these are amphotericin B, nystatin, ketoconazole, itraconazole, and fluconazole.

A number of **antiviral drugs** have been developed that slow the growth or reproduction of viruses. Acyclovir, ganciclovir, foscarnet, and amantadine are examples of antiviral medications.

Prognosis

Hospital-acquired infections are serious illnesses that cause **death** in about 1% of cases. Rapid diagnosis and identification of the responsible microorganism is necessary, so treatment can be started as soon as possible.

Prevention

Hospitals and other healthcare facilities have developed extensive **infection control** programs to prevent nosocomial infections. These programs focus on identifying high risk procedures and other possible sources of infection. High risk procedures such as urinary catheterization should be performed only when necessary and catheters should be left in for as little time as possible. Medical instruments and equipment must be properly sterilized to ensure they are not contaminated. Frequent handwashing by healthcare workers and visitors is necessary to avoid passing infectious microorganisms to hospitalized patients.

Antibiotics should only be used when necessary. Use of antibiotics creates favorable conditions for infection with the fungal organism *Candida*. Overuse of antibiotics is also responsible for the development of bacteria that are resistant to antibiotics.

Resources

BOOKS

Andreoli, T. E., J. C. Bennet, C. C. Carpenter, and F. Plum. *Cecil Essentials of Medicine.* Philadelphia: W.B. Saunders Company, 1997.

Schaffer, S. D. and L. S. Garzon, et al. *Infection Prevention and Safe Practice.* New York: Mosby-Year Book, 1996.

Toni Rizzo

Hot-spot imaging *see* **Technetium heart scan**

HTLV-1 associated myelopathy *see* **Tropical spastic paraparesis**

HTLV-1 infection *see* **Tropical spastic paraparesis**

Human bite infections

Definition

Human bite infections are potentially serious infections caused by rapid growth of bacteria in broken skin.

Description

Bites—animal and human—are responsible for about 1% of visits to emergency rooms. Bite injuries are more common during the summer months.

Closed-fist injury

In adults, the most common form of human bite is the closed-fist injury, sometimes called the "fight bite." These injuries result from the breaking of the skin over the knuckle joint when a person's fist strikes someone's teeth during a fight.

Causes & symptoms

In children, bite infections result either from accidents during play or from fighting. Most infected bites in adults result from fighting.

The infection itself can be caused by a number of bacteria that live in the human mouth. These include streptococci, staphylococci, anaerobic organisms, and *Eikenella corrodens*. Infections that begin less than 24 hours after the injury are usually produced by a mixture of organisms and can cause a necrotizing infection (causing the death of a specific area of tissue), in which tissue is rapidly destroyed. If a bite is infected, the skin will be sore, red, swollen, and warm to the touch.

Diagnosis

In most cases the diagnosis is made by an emergency room doctor on the basis of the patient's history.

Because the human mouth contains a variety of bacteria, the doctor will order a laboratory culture in order to choose the most effective antibiotic.

Treatment

Treatment involves surgical attention as well as medications. Because bites cause puncturing and tearing of skin rather than clean-edged cuts, they must be carefully cleansed. The doctor will wash the wound with water under high pressure and debride it. **Debridement** is the removal of dead tissue and **foreign objects** from a wound to prevent infection. If the bite is a closed-fist injury, the doctor will look for torn tendons or damage to the spaces between the joints. Examination includes x rays to check for bone **fractures** or foreign objects in the wound.

Doctors do not usually suture a bite wound because the connective tissues and other structures in the hand form many small closed spaces that make it easy for infection to spread. Emergency room doctors often consult surgical specialists if a patient has a deep closed-fist injury or one that appears already infected.

The doctor will make sure that the patient is immunized against **tetanus,** which is routine procedure for any open wound. Because of risk of infection, all patients with human bite **wounds** should be given **antibiotics.** Patients with closed-fist injuries may need inpatient treatment in addition to an intravenous antibiotic.

Prognosis

The prognosis depends on the location of the bite and whether it was caused by a child or an adult. Bites caused by children rarely become infected because they are usually shallow. Between 15–30% of bites caused by adults become infected, with a higher rate for closed-fist injuries.

Prevention

Prevention of human bite infections depends upon prompt treatment of any bite caused by a human being, particularly a closed-fist injury.

Resources

BOOKS

Battan, F. Keith. "Pediatric Emergencies: Bites and Stings." In *Handbook of Pediatrics,* edited by Gerald B. Merenstein, et al. Norwalk, CT: Appleton & Lange, 1994.

Battan, F. Keith, et al. "Emergencies, Injuries, & Poisoning." In *Current Pediatric Diagnosis & Treatment,* edited by William W. Hay, Jr. et al. Stamford, CT: Appleton & Lange, 1997.

Hirschmann, Jan V. "Localized Infections and Abscesses." In *Harrison's Principles of Internal Medicine,* edited by Eugene Braunwald, et al. New York: McGraw-Hill Book Company, 1987.

Jacobs, Richard A. "General Problems in Infectious Diseases: Animal & Human Bite Wounds." In *Current Medical Diagnosis & Treatment 1998,* edited by Lawrence M. Tierney, Jr., et al. Stamford, CT: Appleton & Lange, 1997.

Rebecca J. Frey

Human chorionic gonadotropin *see*
Infertility drugs

Human chorionic gonadotropin pregnancy test

Definition

The most common test of **pregnancy** involves the detection of a hormone known as human chorionic gonadotropin (hCG) in a sample of blood or urine.

Purpose

To determine whether or not a woman is pregnant.

Description

Shortly after a woman's egg is fertilized by her male partner's sperm and is implanted in the lining or the womb (uterus), a placenta begins to form. This organ will help nourish the developing new life. The placenta produces hCG, whose presence, along with other hormones, helps maintain the early stages of pregnancy. Because hCG is produced only by placental tissue and the hormone can be found in the blood or urine of a pregnant woman, it has become a convenient chemical test of pregnancy.

After implantation, the level of detectable hCG rises very rapidly, approximately doubling in quantity every two days until a peak is reached between the sixth and eighth week. Over the next ten or more weeks, the quantity of hCG slowly decreases. After this point, a much lower level is sustained for the duration of the pregnancy. Detectable levels of this hormone may even persist for a month or two after delivery.

Blood tests for hCG are the most sensitive and can detect a pregnancy earlier than urine tests. Blood tests for hCG can also distinguish normal pregnancies from impending **miscarriages** or pregnancies that occur outside of the uterus (ectopic pregnancies).

If a woman misses her menstrual period and wants to know if she may be pregnant, she can purchase one of many home pregnancy test kits that are currently available. Although each of these products may look slightly different and provide a different set of directions for use, each one detects the presence of hCG. This indicator contains chemical components called antibodies that are sensitive to a certain quantity of this hormone.

Precautions

Although home pregnancy tests may be advertised as having an accuracy of 97% or better, studies indicate that, in practice, pregnancy tests performed in the home may incorrectly indicate that a woman is not pregnant (a false positive result) between 25–50% of the time. Studies also indicate that the false negative results are usually the result failing to follow the package directions or testing too soon after a missed menstrual period. Waiting a few days after the missed period was expected can increase the accuracy of the test. Blood and urine tests performed by a laboratory are from 97–100% accurate in detecting pregnancy.

Preparation

Generally, no preparation is required for a pregnancy test given in a doctor's office.

Home pregnancy test kits can be divided into two basic types. One type involves the use of a wand-like device that a woman must place into her urine stream for a brief period of time. The other type of kit involves the use of a cup, a dropper, and a wand or stick with a small well. The cup is used to collect the urine, and the dropper is used to transfer a specific number of drops into the well. Results are displayed by a color change. It's important to follow the package directions very carefully (the techniques vary from brand to brand) and to read the results in the time specified.

Aftercare

No special care is required after a urine test for hCG. Women who feel faint or who continue to bleed after a blood test should be observed until the condition goes away.

Risks

Tests for hCG levels pose no direct risk to a woman's health. The main risk with a home pregnancy test is a false negative result, which may be lessened by following the manufacturer's instructions carefully and waiting at least several days after the expected menstrual period to test. A false negative result can cause a delay in seeking for prenatal care, which can pose a risk to both the woman and the baby.

Abnormal results

In most cases, a positive result is an indication of pregnancy. However, false positive results may also occur. If a pregnancy test is performed within a month or two of a recent birth or miscarriage, it is possible to test positive for pregnancy since hCG may still be detected in a woman's urine. Sometimes positive pregnancy tests provide clues of an early miscarriage that might have otherwise gone unrecognized because it occurred before or just after a missed period. An **ectopic pregnancy** (one in which an embryo implants outside the uterus), certain types of masses (such as an ovarian tumor or a **hydatidiform mole**), and the use of some fertility drugs that contain hCG are among other possibilities behind false positive results.

Normal results

A woman should notify her physician immediately if her home pregnancy test is positive. Pregnancy can then be confirmed with hCG urine or blood tests taken in the doctor's office and evaluated by laboratory personnel. If performed accurately, home pregnancy tests have been found to be highly reliable. However, the versions of these tests performed by qualified laboratory technologists are considered to be definitive. Often, such a test will produce positive results before a woman experiences symptoms or before a doctor's exam reveals signs of pregnancy.

Resources

BOOKS

Cunningham, F. Gary, ed. *Williams Obstetrics*, 20th ed. Stanford: Appleton and Lang, 1977.

PERIODICALS

Bastian, L.A., et al. "Is This Patient Pregnant?" *JAMA: The Journal of the American Medical Association* 278 no. 7: 586-591.

Peredy, T.R., and R.D. Powers. "Bedside Diagnostic Testing of Body Fluids." *American Journal of Emergency Medicine* 15 no. 4: 404-405.

"Pregnancy Tests: They Can't Get Much Simpler Than This." *Consumer Reports* (October 1996): 48-49.

OTHER

"Reliable Ways to Find Out if You're Pregnant or Ready to Conceive." Available at Mayo Clinic Health Oasis. (28 Feb. 1996). http://www.mayo.ivi.com.

Betty Mishkin

Human herpes virus, type 6 infection *see* Roseola

Human immunodeficiency virus infection *see* AIDS

Human leukocyte antigen test

Definition

The human leukocyte antigen test, also known as HLA, is a test that detects antigens (genetic markers) on white blood cells. There are four types of human leukocyte antigens: HLA-A, HLA-B, HLA-C, and HLA-D.

Purpose

The HLA test is used to provide evidence of tissue compatibility typing of tissue recipients and donors. It is also an aid in **genetic counseling** and in paternity testing.

Precautions

This test may have to be postponed if the patient has recently undergone a **transfusion.**

Description

Human leukocyte antigen (leukocyte is the name for white blood cell, while antigen refers to a genetic marker) is a substance that is located on the surface of white blood cells. This substance plays an important role in the body's immune response.

Because the HLA antigens are essential to immunity, identification aids in determination of the degree of tissue compatibility between transplant recipients and donors. Testing is done to diminish the likelihood of rejection after transplant, and to avoid graft-versus-host disease (GVHD) following major organ or **bone marrow transplantation.** It should be noted that risk of GVHD exists even when the donor and recipient share major antigens. As an example, it was recently discovered that a

KEY TERMS

Autoimmune disorders—A disorder caused by a reaction of an individual's immune system against the organs or tissues of the body. Autoimmune processes can have different results: slow destruction of a particular type of cell or tissue, stimulation of an organ into excessive growth, or interference in function.

Haplotype—A set of alleles (an alternative form of a gene that can occupy a particular place on a chromosome) of a group of closely linked genes which are usually inherited as a unit.

Phenotype—1) The entire physical, biochemical, and physiologic makeup of an individual, as opposed to genotype. 2) The expression of a single gene or gene pair.

mismatch of HA-1 (a minor antigen) was a cause of GVHD in bone marrow grafts from otherwise HLA-identical donors.

HLA can aid in paternity exclusion testing, a highly specialized area of forensic medicine. To resolve cases of disputed paternity, a man who demonstrates a phenotype (two haplotypes: one from the father and one from the mother) with no haplotype or antigen pair identical to one of the child's is excluded as the father. Conversely, a man who has one haplotype identical to one of the child's may be the father (the probability varies with the appearance of that particular haplotype in the population). Because of the issues involved, this type of testing is referred to experts.

Certain HLA types have been linked to diseases, such as **rheumatoid arthritis, multiple sclerosis,** serum lupus erythematosus, and other **autoimmune disorders.** By themselves, however, none of the HLA types are considered definitive. Because the clinical significance of many of the marker antigens has not yet been well defined, definitive diagnosis of disease is obtained by the use of more specific tests.

Preparation

The HLA test requires a blood sample. There is no need for the patient to be **fasting** (having nothing to eat or drink) before the test.

Risks

Risks for this test are minimal, but may include slight bleeding from the blood-drawing site, **fainting** or feeling lightheaded after venipuncture, or hematoma (blood accumulating under the puncture site).

Normal results

Identification of specific leukocyte antigens, HLA-A, HLA-B, HLA-C and HLA-D.

Abnormal results

Incompatible groups between organ donors and recipients may cause unsuccessful tissue transplantation.

Certain diseases have a strong association with certain types of HLAs, which may aid in genetic counseling. For example, Hashimoto's **thyroiditis** (an autoimmune disorder involving underproduction by the thyroid gland) is associated with HLA-DR5, while B8 and Dw3 are allied with Graves' disease (another autoimmune disorder, but with overproduction by the thyroid gland). Hereditary **hemochromatosis** (too much iron in the blood) is associated with HLA-A3, B7, and B14. HLA-A3 is found in approximately 70% of patients with hemochromatosis, but as is the case with other HLA-associated disorders, the expense of HLA typing favors use of other tests. In cases of suspected hemochromatosis, for example, diagnosis is better aided by two tests called transferrin saturation and serum ferritin.

Resources

BOOKS

Cahill, Mathew. *Handbook of Diagnostic Tests.* Springhouse, PA: Springhouse Corporation, 1995.

Jacobs, David S. *Laboratory Test Handbook, 4th ed.* Cleveland, OH: Lexi-Comp Inc., 1996.

Pagana, Kathleen Deska. *Mosby's Manual of Diagnostic and Laboratory Tests.* St. Louis, MO: Mosby, Inc., 1998.

Janis O. Flores

Humanistic therapy *see* **Gestalt therapy; Human-potential movement**

Human-potential movement

Definition

The human-potential movement is a term used for humanistic psychotherapies that first became popular in the 1960s and early 1970s. The movement emphasized the development of individuals through such techniques as encounter groups, sensitivity training, and primal ther-

KEY TERMS

Encounter group—A form of humanistic therapy in which participants meet with a trained leader to increase self-awareness and social skills through emotional sharing and confrontation.

Humanistic therapy—An approach to psychotherapy that emphasizes human uniqueness, positive qualities, and individual potential. It is sometimes used as a synonym for the human potential movement.

Primal therapy—A form of humanistic therapy that originated in the 1970s. Participants were encouraged to relive painful events and release feelings through screaming or crying rather than analysis.

Sensitivity training—A form of humanistic group therapy that began in the 1950s. Members participated in unstructured discussions in order to improve understanding of themselves and others.

apy. Although the human-potential movement and humanistic therapy are sometimes used as synonyms, in reality, humanistic therapy preceded the human-potential movement and provided the movement's theoretical base. Humanistic therapy flourished in the 1940s and 1950s. Its theorists were mostly psychologists rather than medical doctors. They included Gordon Allport, Abraham Maslow, Everett Shostrom, Carl Rogers, and Fritz Perls.

The human-potential movement and humanistic therapy is distinguished by the following emphases:

* A concern for what is uniquely human rather than what humans share with other animals.

* A focus on each person's open-ended growth rather than reshaping individuals to fit society's demands.

* An interest in the here-and-now rather than in a person's childhood history or supposed unconscious conflicts.

* A holistic approach concerned with all levels of human being and functioning—not just the intellectual—including creative and spiritual functioning.

* A focus on psychological health rather than disturbance.

Purpose

The purpose of humanistic therapy is to allow a person to make full use of his or her personal capacities leading to self-actualization. Self-actualization requires the integration of all the components of one's unique personality. These elements or components of personality include the physical, emotional, intellectual, behavioral, and spiritual. The marks of a self-actualized person are maturity, self-awareness, and authenticity. Humanistic therapists think that most people—not only those with obvious problems—can benefit from opportunities for self-development. Humanistic therapy uses both individual and group approaches.

Precautions

Psychotic patients, substance abusers, and persons with severe **personality disorders** or disorders of impulse control may not be appropriate for treatment with humanistic methods.

Description

Humanistic approaches to individual treatment usually follow the same format as other forms of outpatient counseling. Therapists may be medical doctors, nurses, psychologists, social workers, or clergy. Humanistic group treatment formats are flexible, and a wide range of treatment methods are used, ranging from encounter groups and therapy groups to assertiveness training and consciousness-raising groups. In addition, the humanistic tradition has fostered the publication of self-help books for people interested in psychological self-improvement.

Risks

The chief risks include the reinforcement of self-centered tendencies in some patients and the dangers resulting from encounter groups led by persons without adequate training. Poorly led encounter groups can be traumatic to persons with low tolerance for confrontation or "uncovering" of private issues.

Normal results

The anticipated outcome of humanistic therapy is a greater degree of personal wholeness, self-acceptance, and exploration of one's potential. In group treatment, participants are expected to grow in interpersonal empathy and relationship skills. However, there have been few controlled studies to determine the reasonableness of these expectations.

Resources

BOOKS

Lasch, Christopher. *The Culture of Narcissism: American Life in an Age of Diminishing Expectations.* New York: W. W. Norton & Company, 1978.

Meissner, W. W. "Theories of Personality." In *The New Harvard Guide to Psychiatry,* edited by Armand M. Nicholi, Jr. Cambridge, MA, and London, UK: The Belknap Press of Harvard University Press, 1988.

Rogers, Carl R. *Client-Centered Therapy.* Boston: Houghton Mifflin Company, 1965.

Severin, Frank T. "Humanistic Psychology." In *The Encyclopedia of Psychiatry, Psychology, and Psychoanalysis,* edited by Benjamin B. Wolman. New York: Henry Holt and Company, 1996.

Shostrom, Everett L. *From Manipulator to Master.* New York: Bantam Books, 1983.

Rebecca J. Frey

Humpback *see* **Kyphosis**

Hunchback *see* **Kyphosis**

Hunter's syndrome *see* **Mucopolysaccharidoses**

Huntington's chorea *see* **Huntington's disease**

Huntington's disease

Definition

Huntington's disease is an inherited, progressive, neurodegenerative disease causing uncontrolled physical movements and mental deterioration.

Description

Huntington's disease (HD) is a genetic disorder that causes progressive loss of cells in areas of the brain responsible for some aspects of movement control and mental abilities. A person with HD gradually develops abnormal movements and changes in cognition, behavior, and personality.

The onset of symptoms of HD is usually between the ages of 30 and 50; although in 10% of cases, onset is in late childhood or early adolescence. Approximately 30,000 people in the United States are affected by HD, with another 150,000 at risk for developing it.

Huntington's disease is also called Huntington's chorea, from the Greek word for "dance," referring to the involuntary movements that develop as the disease progresses. It is occasionally referred to as "Woody Guthrie's disease" for the American folk singer who died from it.

KEY TERMS

Cognition—The mental activities associated with thinking, learning, and memory.

Computed tomography (CT) scan—A process which uses x rays taken from many different angles to view a cross-section of the body's tissues.

DNA—Deoxyribonucleic acid; the genetic material that controls heredity.

Heimlich maneuver—An action designed to expel an obstructing piece of food from the throat. It is performed by placing the fist on the abdomen, underneath the breastbone, grasping the fist with the other hand (from behind), and thrusting it inward and upward.

Neurodegenerative—Relating to degeneration of nerve tissues.

Causes & symptoms

Causes

Huntington's disease is caused by a defect in the gene for a protein of unknown function called huntingtin. The defective gene contains 40 or more so-called "CAG repeats," compared to only 30 of these repeats in the normal huntingtin gene. C, A, and G are DNA nucleotides, the building blocks of genes. The extra building blocks in the huntingtin gene cause the protein that is made from it to contain an extra section as well. It is currently thought that this extra protein section interacts with other proteins in brain cells where it occurs, and that this interaction ultimately leads to cell death.

The HD gene is a dominant gene, meaning that only one copy of it is needed to develop the disease. HD affects both males and females. The gene may be inherited from either parent, who will also be affected by the disease. A parent with the HD gene has a 50% chance of passing it on to each offspring. The chances of passing on the HD gene are not affected by the results of previous pregnancies.

Symptoms

The symptoms of HD fall into three categories: motor or movement symptoms, personality and behavioral changes, and cognitive decline. The severity and rate of progression of each type of symptom can vary from person to person.

Early motor symptoms include restlessness, twitching, and a desire to move about. Handwriting may become less controlled, and coordination may decline. Later symptoms include:

- Dystonia, or sustained abnormal postures, including facial grimaces, a twisted neck, or an arched back.

- Chorea, in which involuntary jerking, twisting, or writhing motions become pronounced.

- Slowness of voluntary movements, inability to regulate the speed or force of movements, inability to initiate movement, and slowed reactions.

- Difficulty speaking and swallowing, due to involvement of the muscles of the throat.

- Localized or generalized weakness, and impaired balance ability.

- Rigidity, especially in late-stage disease.

Personality and behavioral changes include depression, irritability, **anxiety,** and apathy. The person with HD may become impulsive, aggressive, or socially withdrawn.

Cognitive changes include loss of ability to plan and execute routine tasks, slowed thought, and impaired or inappropriate judgment. Short-term memory loss usually occurs, although long-term memory is usually spared. The person with late-stage HD usually retains knowledge of his environment and recognizes family members or other loved ones, despite severe cognitive decline.

Diagnosis

Diagnosis of HD begins with a detailed medical history, and a thorough physical and neurological exam. Family medical history is very important, since HD is an inherited disease. **Magnetic resonance imaging** (MRI) or **computed tomography scan** (CT scan) imaging may be performed to look for degeneration in the basal ganglia and cortex, the brain regions most affected in HD.

A genetic test is available for confirmation of the clinical diagnosis. In this test, a small blood sample is taken, and DNA from it is analyzed to determine the CAG repeat number. A person with a repeat number of 30 or below will not develop HD. A person with a repeat number between 35 and 40 may not develop the disease within their normal lifespan. A person with a very high number of repeats (70 or above) is likely to develop the juvenile-onset form.

Prenatal testing is available. A person at risk for HD (a child of an affected person) may obtain fetal testing without determining whether she herself carries the gene. This "nondisclosing" test, also called a linkage test, examines the pattern of DNA near the gene in both parent and fetus, but does not analyze for the triple repeat itself. If the DNA patterns do not match, the fetus can be assumed not to have inherited the HD gene, even if present in the parent. A pattern match indicates the fetus probably has the same genetic makeup of the at-risk parent. It does not indicate whether the parent (or fetus) actually has the defective gene.

Treatment

There is no cure for HD, nor any treatment that can slow the rate of progression. Treatment is aimed at reducing the disability caused by the motor impairments, and treating behavioral and emotional symptoms.

Physical therapy is used to maintain strength and compensate for lost strength and balance. Stretching and range of motion exercises help minimize contracture, or muscle shortening, a result of weakness and disuse. The physical therapist also advises on the use of mobility aids such as walkers or wheelchairs.

Motor symptoms may be treated with drugs, although some studies suggest that anti-chorea treatment rarely improves function. Chorea can be suppressed with drugs that deplete dopamine, an important brain chemical regulating movement. As HD progresses, natural dopamine levels fall, leading to loss of chorea and an increase in rigidity and movement slowness. Treatment with L-dopa (which resupplies dopamine) may help here. Frequent reassessment of the effectiveness and appropriateness of any drug therapy is necessary.

Occupational therapy is used to design compensatory strategies for lost abilities in the activities of daily living, such as eating, dressing, and grooming. The occupational therapist advises on modifications to the home that improve safety, accessibility, and comfort.

Difficulty swallowing may be lessened by preparation of softer foods, blending food in an electric blender, and taking care to eat slowly and carefully. Use of a straw for all liquids can help. The potential for **choking** on food is a concern, especially late in the disease progression. Caregivers should learn the use of the **Heimlich maneuver.** In addition, passage of food into the airways increases the risk for **pneumonia.** A gastric feeding tube may be needed, if swallowing becomes too difficult or dangerous.

Speech difficulties may be partially compensated for through use of picture boards or other augmentative communication devices. Loss of cognitive ability affects both speech production and understanding. A speech-language pathologist can work with the family to develop simplified and more directed communication strategies, including speaking slowly, using simple words, and repeating sentences exactly.

Early behavioral changes, including depression and anxiety, may respond to drug therapy. Maintaining a calm, familiar, and secure environment is useful as the disease progresses. Support groups for both patients and caregivers form an important part of treatment. Information on local support groups is available from the Huntington's Disease Society of America.

Experimental transplant of fetal brain tissue has been attempted in a few HD patients. Early results show some promise, but further trials are needed to establish the effectiveness of this treatment.

Prognosis

The person with Huntington's disease may be able to maintain a job for several years after diagnosis, despite the increase in disability. Loss of cognitive functions and increase in motor and behavioral symptoms eventually prevent the person with HD from continuing employment. Ultimately, severe motor symptoms prevent mobility.

Death usually occurs 15–20 years after disease onset. Progressive weakness of respiratory and swallowing muscles leads to increased respiratory infection, and choking, the most common causes of death.

Prevention

Huntington's disease cannot be prevented in a person with the gene defect.

Resources

BOOKS

Watts R.L., and W.C. Koller, eds. *Movement Disorders.* New York: McGraw-Hill, 1997

ORGANIZATIONS

Huntington's Disease Society of America. 140 W. 22nd St. New York, NY 10011. (800) 345-HDSA.

Hurler's syndrome *see* **Mucopolysaccharidoses**

Hyaline membrane disease *see* **Respiratory distress syndrome**

Hydatid disease *see* **Echinococcosis**

Hydatidiform mole

Definition

A hydatidiform mole is a relatively rare condition in which tissue around a fertilized egg that normally would have developed into the placenta instead develops as an abnormal cluster of cells. (This is also called a molar

pregnancy.) This grapelike mass forms inside of the uterus after fertilization instead of a normal embryo. A hydatidiform mole triggers a positive pregnancy test and in some cases can become cancerous.

Description

A hydatidiform mole ("hydatid" means "drop of water" and "mole" means "spot") occurs in about 1 out of every 1,500 (1/1,500) pregnancies in the United States. In some parts of Asia, however, the incidence may be as high as 1 in 200 (1/200). Molar pregnancies are most likely to occur in younger and older women (especially over age 45) than in those between ages 20–40. About 1–2% of the time a woman who has had a molar pregnancy will have a second one.

A molar pregnancy occurs when cells of the chorionic villi (tiny projections that attach the placenta to the lining of the uterus) don't develop correctly. Instead, they turn into watery clusters that can't support a growing baby. A partial molar pregnancy includes an abnormal embryo (a fertilized egg that has begun to grow) that does not survive. In a compete molar pregnancy there is a small cluster of clear blisters or pouches that don't contain an embryo.

If not removed, about 15% of moles can become cancerous. They burrow into the wall of the uterus and cause serious bleeding. Another 5% will develop into fast-growing cancers called choriocarcinomas. Some of these tumors spread very quickly outside the uterus in other parts of the body. Fortunately, cancer developing from these moles is rare and highly curable.

Causes & symptoms

The cause of hydatidiform mole is unclear; some experts believe it is caused by problems with the chromosomes (the structures inside cells that contain genetic information) in either the egg or sperm, or both. It may be associated with poor nutrition, or a problem with the ovaries or the uterus. A mole sometimes can develop from placental tissue that is left behind in the uterus after a **miscarriage** or **childbirth.**

Women with a hydatidiform mole will have a positive pregnancy test and often believe they have a normal pregnancy for the first three or four months. However, in these cases the uterus will grow abnormally fast. By the end of the third month, if not earlier, the woman will experience vaginal bleeding ranging from scant spotting to excessive bleeding. She may have **hyperthyroidism** (overproduction of **thyroid hormones** causing symptoms such as weight loss, increased appetite, and intolerance to heat). Sometimes, the grapelike cluster of cells itself will be shed with the blood during this time. Other symptoms may include severe **nausea and vomiting** and high blood pressure. As the pregnancy progresses, the fetus will not move and there will be no fetal heartbeat.

Diagnosis

The physician may not suspect a molar pregnancy until after the third month or later, when the absence of a fetal heartbeat together with bleeding and severe nausea and vomiting indicates something is amiss.

First, the physician will examine the woman's abdomen, feeling for any strange lumps or abnormalities in the uterus. A tubal pregnancy, which can be life threatening if not treated, will be ruled out. Then the physician will check the levels of human chorionic gonadotropin (hCG), a hormone that is normally produced by a placenta or a mole. Abnormally high levels of hCG together with the symptoms of vaginal bleeding, lack of fetal heartbeat, and an unusually large uterus all indicate a molar pregnancy. An ultrasound of the uterus to make sure there is no living fetus will confirm the diagnosis.

Treatment

It is extremely important to make sure that all of the mole is removed from the uterus, since it is possible that the tissue is potentially cancerous. Often, the tissue is naturally expelled by the fourth month of pregnancy. In some instances, the physician will give the woman a drug called oxytocin to trigger the release of the mole that is not spontaneously aborted.

If this does not happen, however, a vacuum aspiration can be performed to remove the mole. In a procedure similar to a **dilatation and curettage** (D & C), a woman is given an anesthetic (to deaden feeling during the procedure), her cervix (the structure at the bottom of the uterus) is dilated and the contents of the uterus is gently suctioned out. After the mole has been mostly removed, gentle scraping of the uterus lining is usually performed.

If the woman is older and does not want any more children, the uterus can be surgically removed (**hysterectomy**) instead of a vacuum aspiration because of the higher risk of cancerous moles in this age group.

Because of the cancer risk, the physician will continue to monitor the patient for at least two months after the end of a molar pregnancy. Since invasive disease is usually signaled by high levels of hCG that don't go down after the pregnancy has ended, the woman's hCG levels will be checked every two weeks. If the levels don't return to normal by that time, the mole may have become cancerous.

If the hCG level is normal, the woman's hCG will be tested each month for six months, and then every two months for a year.

If the mole has become cancerous, treatment includes removal of the cancerous issue and **chemotherapy.** If the cancer has spread to other parts of the body, radiation will be added. Specific treatment depends on how advanced the cancer is.

Women should make sure not to become pregnant within a year after hCG levels have returned to normal. If a woman were to become pregnant sooner than that, it would be difficult to tell whether the resulting high levels of hCG were caused by the pregnancy or a cancer from the mole.

Prognosis

A woman with a molar pregnancy often goes through the same emotions and sense of loss as does a woman who has a miscarriage. Most of the time, she truly believed she was pregnant and now has suffered a loss of the baby she thought she was carrying. In addition, there is the added worry that the tissue left behind could become cancerous.

In the unlikely case that the mole is cancerous the cure rate is almost 100%. As long as the uterus was not removed, it would still be possible to have a child at a later time.

Resources

BOOKS

Carlson, Karen J., Stephanie A. Eisenstat, and Terra Ziporyn. *The Harvard Guide to Women's Health.* Cambridge, MA: Harvard University Press, 1996.

Ryan, Kenneth J., Ross S. Berkowitz, and Robert L. Barbieri. *Kistner's Gynecology,* 6th ed. St. Louis: Mosby, 1995.

Carol A. Turkington

Hydranencephaly *see* **Congenital brain defects**

Hydrocelectomy

Definition

Hydrocelectomy is a surgical procedure to remove a hydrocele. A hydrocele is collected fluid in the membrane surrounding the testes.

Purpose

Hydrocelectomy is performed to relieve the **pain** or reoccurrence of a hydrocele. Normally, hydroceles are not very painful. They tend to be a soft swelling in the membrane surrounding the testes. As the hydrocele grows, the scrotum gets larger. Hydroceles do not damage the testes. The main symptom is scrotal swelling. There are two types of hydroceles depending on how they form. One type is seen in children, generally shortly after birth. It is caused by a failure of the processus vaginalis to close. Usually, surgery isn't used to treat hydrocele until after two years of age because the processus vaginalis frequently closes by itself if given extra time. In adults, hydroceles develop slowly. Most hydroceles develop because of blocked lymphatic flow. Hydroceles also develop after infection, injury, or local **cancer** tumors. Generally, hydroceles are treated by aspiration of the collected fluid. To do this, a needle is inserted into the scrotum and directed toward the hydrocele. Once there, as much fluid as possible is removed. Hydroceles can reoccur. Rarely, hydroceles grow larger and cause pain. Surgery is used to remove large or painful hydroceles. It is also the recommended procedure to remove hydroceles that reoccur after aspiration. Hydroceles are distinguished from other testicular problems by transillumination and **scrotal ultrasound** examinations.

Precautions

No special precautions are required for hydrocelectomy. It is typically performed on an outpatient basis.

Description

Aspiration of the fluid in a hydrocele is usually successful. However, aspiration may be only a temporary solution because of the potential that the hydrocele will reoccur. Generally, surgical repair of a hydrocele will eliminate the hydrocele. The extent of the surgery depends on whether other factors are present. If the hydrocele is uncomplicated, an incision is made in the scrotum. The hydrocele is cut out, removing the tissues involved in the hydrocele. If there are complications present, such as a **hernia,** an incision is made in the inguinal (groin) area. This approach allows repair of hernias and other complicating factors at the same time.

> ### KEY TERMS
>
> **Aspiration**—The process of removing fluids or gasses from the body by suction.
>
> **Hernia**—The protrusion of an organ or tissue through a wall that normally contains it.
>
> **Hydrocele**—An accumulation of fluid in the membrane surrounding the testes (tunica vaginalis testis).

Patients are placed under general anesthesia for these operations.

Preparation

A physician or nurse will explain the procedure and, in some cases, the need for a temporary drain to be inserted. The drain lessens the chance of infection and prevents fluid build up.

Aftercare

Following surgery, the patient usually only needs a follow-up examination several weeks after the surgery to examine the incision and to check for signs of infection.

Risks

There is a slight risk of infection and internal hemorrhage as well as a chance of excessive bleeding from the surgical incision.

Normal results

There may be swelling of the scrotum for up to a month. The patient is able to resume most activities within 7–10 days, although heavy lifting and sexual activities may be delayed for up to six weeks. The hydrocele does not grow back.

Abnormal results

Swelling that lasts for several months is sometimes a complication of hydrocelectomy. Infection can also occur.

Resources

BOOKS

Hurst, J. W. *Medicine for the Practicing Physician.* Stamford: Appleton and Lange, 1996.

Sabiston, D.C., and H.K. Lyrly *Essentials of Surgery.* Philadelphia: W.B. Saunders Company, 1994.

Way, L.W. *Current Surgical Diagnosis and Treatment.*
Norwalk: Appleton and Lange, 1994.

Hydrocephalus

Definition

Hydrocephalus is an abnormal expansion of cavities (ventricles) within the brain caused by the accumulation of cerebrospinal fluid.

Description

Hydrocephalus is the result of an imbalance between the formation and drainage of cerebrospinal fluid (CSF). Approximately 500 milliliters (about a pint) of CSF is formed within the brain each day, by structures called choroid plexus, with epidermal cells lining chambers called ventricles. Once formed, CSF usually circulates among all the ventricles before it is absorbed and returned to the circulatory system. The normal adult volume of circulating CSF is 150 ml, so that the CSF turn-over rate is more than three times per day. Production is independent of absorption, and reduced absorption causes CSF to accumulate within the ventricles.

Reduced absorption most often occurs when one or more passages connecting the ventricles become blocked, preventing movement of CSF to its drainage sites in the subarachnoid space just inside the skull. This type of hydrocephalus is called "noncommunicating." Reduction in absorption rate can also be caused by damage to the absorptive tissue. This type is called "communicating hydrocephalus."

Both of these types lead to an elevation of the CSF pressure within the brain. This increased pressure squeezes the soft tissues of the brain, distorting and damaging them. In infants whose skull bones have not yet fused, the intracranial pressure is partly relieved by expansion of the skull, so that symptoms may not be as dramatic. Both types of elevated-pressure hydrocephalus may occur from infancy to adulthood.

A third type of hydrocephalus, called "normal pressure hydrocephalus," is marked by ventricle enlargement without an apparent increase in CSF pressure. This type affects mainly the elderly.

Causes & symptoms

Hydrocephalus may be caused by:

• **Congenital brain defects**

• Hemorrhage, either in the ventricles or the subarachnoid space
• Infection of the central nervous system (**syphilis,** herpes, **meningitis, encephalitis,** or **mumps**)
• Tumor.

Symptoms of elevated-pressure hydrocephalus include:

• **Headache**
• **Nausea and vomiting,** especially in the morning

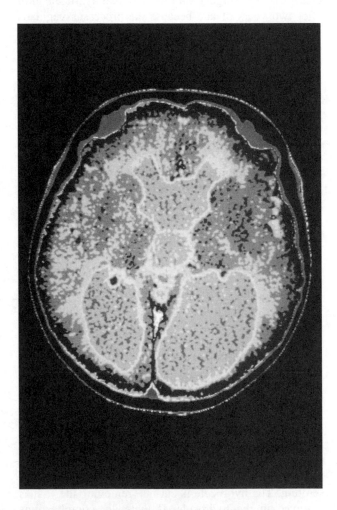

A computed tomography (CT) scan of a brain with hydrocephalus. This scan shows large areas where excessive fluid has collected inside the patient's skull. *(Phototake NYC. Reproduced by permission.)*

- Lethargy

- Gait disturbance

- Double vision

- Subtle difficulties in learning and memory

- Delay in achievement of developmental milestones in children.

Irritability is the most common sign of hydrocephalus in infants and, if untreated, this may lead to lethargy. Bulging of the fontanelle, the soft spot between the skull bones, may also be an early sign. Hydrocephalus in infants prevents fusion of the skull bones, and causes expansion of the skull.

Symptoms of normal pressure hydrocephalus include **dementia,** gait abnormalities, and incontinence (involuntary urination or bowel movements).

Diagnosis

Imaging studies—x ray, **computed tomography scan** (CT scan), ultrasound, and especially **magnetic resonance imaging** (MRI)—are used to assess the presence and location of obstructions, as well as changes in brain tissue that have occurred as a result of the hydrocephalus. Lumbar puncture (spinal tap) may be performed to aid in determining the cause.

Treatment

The primary method of treatment for both elevated- and normal pressure hydrocephalus is surgical installation of a shunt. The shunt is a tube connecting the ventricles to an alternative drainage site, usually the abdomen. The shunt contains a one-way valve to prevent reverse flow. In some cases of non-communicating hydrocephalus, a direct connection can be made between one of the ventricles and the subarachnoid space, allowing drainage without a shunt.

Installation of a shunt requires lifelong monitoring by the patient or family members for signs of recurring hydrocephalus due to obstruction or failure of the shunt.

Some drugs may postpone the need for surgery by inhibiting the production of CSF. These include acetazolamide and furosemide. Other drugs used to delay surgery include glycerol, digoxin, and isosorbide.

Prognosis

Prognosis for elevated-pressure hydrocephalus depends on a wide variety of factors, including the cause, age of onset, and the timing of surgery. Studies indicate that about half of all children who receive appropriate treatment and follow-up will develop IQs greater than 85. Those with hydrocephalus at birth do better than those with later onset due to meningitis. For patients with normal pressure hydrocephalus, shunt installation may lead to improvement in approximately half.

Prevention

Some cases of elevated pressure hydrocephalus may be preventable by preventing or treating the infectious diseases which precede them. Prenatal diagnosis of congenital brain malformation is often possible, offering the option of family planning.

Resources

BOOKS

Bradley, et al. *Neurology in Clinical Practice,* 2nd ed. Butterworth-Heinemann, 1996.

OTHER

The Hydrocephalus Association. 870 Market Street, Suite 955 San Francisco, CA 94102. 415-732-7040. Fax: 415-732-7044.

Hydrochlorothiazide *see* **Diuretics**

Hydrocodone *see* **Opioid analgesics**

Hydrocortisone *see* **Corticosteroids**

Hydrogen peroxide *see* **Antiseptics**

Hydromorphone *see* **Opioid analgesics**

Hydronephrosis

Definition

Hydronephrosis is the swelling of the kidneys when urine flow is obstructed in any of part of the urinary tract. Swelling of the ureter, which always accompanies hydronephrosis, is called hydroureter. Hydronephrosis implies that a ureter and the renal pelvis (the connection of the ureter to the kidney) are overfilled with urine.

Description

The kidneys filter urine out of the blood as a waste product. It collects in the renal pelvis and flows down the ureters into the bladder. The ureters are not simple tubes, but muscular passages that actively propel urine into the bladder. At their lower end is a valve (the ureterovesical junction) that prevents urine from flowing backward into the ureter. The bladder stores urine. The prostate gland

KEY TERMS

Catheter—A tube placed into the body that allows fluids to pass through it.

Contrast agent—Substances that cast shadows on x rays or other imaging methods.

CT and MRI—Two high technology methods of creating images of internal organs. Computerized axial tomography (CT or CAT) uses x rays, while magnetic resonance imaging (MRI) uses magnet fields and radio-frequency signals. Both construct images using a computer.

Cystoscope—A pencil-thin instrument that allows viewing and operating inside the urinary system.

Renal pelvis—The middle section of the kidney where urine first collects after filtration from the blood.

surrounds the bladder outlet in males. Urine then flows through the urethra and out of the body as a waste product.

Because the urinary tract is closed save for the one opening at the bottom, urine cannot escape. Instead, the parts distend. Rupture is rare unless there is violent trauma like an automobile accident.

Obstructed flow anywhere along the drainage route can cause swelling of the upper urinary tract, but if the obstruction is below the bladder, the ureterovesical valve will protect the upper tract to a certain extent. Even then, with no place to go, the urine will back up all the way to its source. Eventually, the back pressure causes kidney function to deteriorate.

Obstruction need not be complete for problems to arise. Intermittent or partial obstruction is far more common than complete blockage, allowing time for the parts to enlarge gradually. Furthermore, if a ureterovesical valve is absent or incompetent, the pressure generated by bladder emptying will force urine backward into the ureter and kidney, causing dilation even without mechanical obstruction.

Causes & symptoms

Causes are numerous. Various congenital deformities of the ureter may sooner or later produce back pressure. **Kidney stones** are a common cause. They form in the renal pelvis and become lodged in the kidney, usually at the ureterovesical junction. In older men, the continued growth of the prostate gland leads commonly to restricted urine flow out of the bladder. **Prostate cancer,** and **cancer** anywhere else along the urine pathways, can

obstruct flow. **Pregnancy** normally causes ureteral obstruction from the pressure of the enlarged uterus (womb) on the ureters.

Symptoms relate to the passage of urine. Sometimes, urine may be difficult to pass, irregular, or uncontrolled. **Pain** from distension of the structures is present. Blood in the urine may be visible, but it is usually microscopic.

In all cases where bodily fluids cannot flow freely, infection is inevitable. Symptoms of urinary infection may include:

- Painful, burning urine.

- Cloudy urine

- Pain in the back, flank, or groin

- **Fever,** sweats, chills, and generalized discomfort.

Patients often mistake a serious urinary infection for the flu.

Diagnosis

If the bladder is significantly distended, it can be felt through the abdomen. An analysis of the urine may reveal blood (if there is a stone), infection, or chemical changes suggesting kidney damage. Blood tests may also detect a decrease in kidney function.

All urinary obstructions will undergo imaging of some sort. Beginning with standard x rays to look for stones, radiologists, physicians specializing in the use of radient energy for diagnostic purposes, will select from a wide array of tests. Ultrasound is simple, inexpensive, and very useful for these conditions. Standard x rays can be enhanced with contrast agents in several ways. If the kidneys are functioning, they will filter an x ray dye out of the blood and concentrate it in the urine, giving excellent pictures and also an assessment of kidney function. For better images of the lower urinary tract, contrast agents can be instilled from below. This is usually done with a cystoscope placed in the bladder. Through the cystoscope, a small tube can be threaded into the ureter through the ureterovesical valve, allowing dye to be injected all the way up to the kidney. CT and MRI scanning provide miraculous detail, more than is often needed for this condition.

Treatment

The obstruction must be relieved, even if it is partial or functional, as in the case of reflux from the bladder. If not, the kidney will ultimately be damaged, infection will appear, or both. The task may be as simple as placing a catheter through a restricting prostate or as complicated as removing a cancerous bladder and rebuilding a new one with a piece of bowel. In some cases, a badly damaged kidney may have to be removed.

Alternative treatment

Catheters or other urinary diversions may be better for weak or ill patients who cannot tolerate more extensive procedures. There is support using botanical medicine that can help the patient using a catheter avoid infections. Consultation with a trained health care practitioner is necessary.

Prognosis

After relief of the obstruction, a kidney may react with a brief flood of urine, but if the obstruction has been of short duration, normal kidney function will return. If one kidney is destroyed, the other will compensate for the lost organ.

Prevention

Kidney stones can be prevented by dietary changes and medication. Prompt evaluation of infections and urinary complaints will usually detect problems early enough to prevent long-term complications.

Resources

BOOKS

Gulmi, Frederick A. "Pathophysiology of urinary tract obstruction." In *Campbell's Urology.* Edited by Patrick C. Walsh, et al. Philadelphia: W. B. Saunders, 1998, pp. 342-380.

Nelson, Waldo E., et al., ed. "Obstruction of the urinary tract." In *Nelson Textbook of Pediatrics.* Philadelphia: W. B. Saunders, 1996, pp. 1534-1542.

Seifter, Julian L. and Barry M. Brenner. "Urinary tract obstruction." In *Harrison's Principles of Internal Medicine.* Edited by Kurt Isselbacher, et al. New York: McGraw-Hill, 1998.

Tierney, Lawrence M., et al., ed. *Current Medical Diagnosis and Treatment.* Stamford, CT: Appleton & Lange, 1996.

Weiss, Robert M. "Physiology and pharmacology of renal pelvis and ureters." In *Campbell's Urology.* Edited by Patrick C. Walsh, et al. Philadelphia: W. B. Saunders, 1998, pp. 855-858.

ORGANIZATIONS

American Association of Kidney Patients. 111 South Parker Street, Suite 405, Tampa, FL 33606. (800)749-2257.

American Kidney Foundation. 6110 Executive Boulevard, #1010, Rockville, MD 20852. (800) 638-8299.

The National Kidney Foundation. 30 East 33rd Street, New York, NY 10016. (800) 622-9010.

J. Ricker Polsdorfer

Hydrotherapy

Definition

Hydrotherapy is a general term for a group of alternative treatments that use water for the relief of various diseases or injuries, or for cleansing the digestive tract. The use of hydrotherapy has a long history as a form of medical treatment. For example, in classical times the Romans and Greeks found sources of water that were considered to have healing properties.

Purpose

Hydrotherapy is used to treat a wide range of conditions, often in conjunction with conventional medical treatment.

Precautions

Some forms of hydrotherapy are not suitable for certain patients. Cold baths should not be given to young children or the elderly. Sauna baths should be avoided by people with heart conditions.

Description

External hydrotherapy

External hydrotherapy involves the immersion of the body in water or the application of water or ice to the body.

TEMPERATURE-BASED TREATMENTS

These treatments are based on the different effects of hot or cold water on the skin and underlying tissues. Hot water (around 100°F/37.8°C) relaxes muscles and causes sweating. It is used to treat arthritis, rheumatism, poor circulation, and sore muscles. Hot water hydrotherapy can be used in combination with **aromatherapy** by adding scented oils to the water. Cold water (60°F/15.6°C) treatments are used to stimulate blood flow in the skin and underlying muscles.

Temperature-based treatments include the application of moist heat or cold to specific parts of the body. The application of moist heat is called fomentation, and is used for chest colds, **influenza**, or arthritis. Cold compresses or ice packs are used in the treatment of sprains, **headaches,** or dental surgery. Body packs, which consist of wet cloth wrapped around the patient, are sometimes used to calm psychiatric patients and for detoxification.

A **sitz bath** is a form of treatment in which the patient sits in a specially constructed tub that allows the lower abdomen to be submerged in water of a different temperature from the water around the feet. Sitz baths are

KEY TERMS

Colonic irrigation—A treatment that uses special equipment to inject water into the rectum and wash out the colon.

Fomentation—The application of warm liquid or moist heat to the surface of the body.

Pack—An application of wet cloth used to treat certain muscular, joint, or psychiatric conditions.

Sauna—A bath that uses dry heat to cause sweating, followed by a swim or shower in cold water.

Sitz bath—A bathtub constructed to allow the hips and feet to be immersed in water of different temperatures.

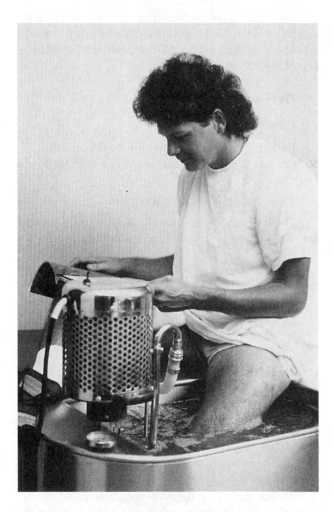

This patient is treating his injured left leg with a whirlpool bath. *(Custom Medical Stock Photo. Reproduced by permission.)*

recommended for **hemorrhoids,** prostate swelling, menstrual cramps, and other genitourinary disorders.

MOTION-BASED TREATMENTS

Motion-based hydrotherapy uses water under pressure in the form of jets, whirlpools, or aerated bubbles to massage the body. It is used to treat joint and muscle injuries as well as **stress** and **anxiety disorders.**

PURIFYING BATHS

Some alternative practitioners recommend bathing in solutions of chlorine bleach, sea salt, lemon juice, turmeric, epsom salts, baking soda, or other substances in order to purify the body of toxins, heavy metal deposits, and radiation.

Internal hydrotherapy

Internal hydrotherapy includes colonic irrigations and **enemas.** Steam baths or inhalation of steam to relieve respiratory congestion are also forms of internal hydrotherapy, as is drinking mineral water to restore the body's electrolyte balance or cleanse the system.

Normal results

Normal results for hydrotherapy are symptomatic relief of the condition for which it was recommended. Additionally, hydrotherapy can strengthen both the individually focused area and the entire body.

Resources

BOOKS

The Holistic Group. ''Some Additional Approaches.'' In *Psychoimmunity & the Healing Process: A Holistic Approach to Immunity & AIDS*, edited by Jason Serinus. Berkeley, CA: Celestial Arts, 1986.

Inglis, Brian, and Ruth West. *The Alternative Health Guide.* New York: Alfred A. Knopf, 1983.

Lowe, Carl, James W. Nechas, and the Editors of *Prevention* Magazine. *Whole Body Healing: Natural Healing with Movement, Exercise, Massage and Other Drug-Free Methods.* Emmaus, PA: Rodale Press, 1983.

Price, Shirley. *Practical Aromatherapy.* London: Thorsons, 1994.

A Visual Encyclopedia of Unconventional Medicine, edited by Ann Hill. New York: Crown Publishers, Inc., 1979.

Rebecca J. Frey

Hydroxzine *see* **Anti-itch drugs**

Hyperactivity *see* **Attention-deficit/ Hyperactivity disorder (ADHD)**

Hyperaldosteronism

Definition

Hyperaldosteronism is a disorder which is defined by the body's overproduction of aldosterone, a hormone that controls sodium and potassium levels in the blood. Its overproduction leads to retention of salt and loss of potassium, which leads to **hypertension** (high blood pressure).

Description

Also known as Conn's syndrome, primary aldosteronism, and secondary aldosteronism, this disorder takes several forms. It often begins with a tumor that produces aldosterone. In fact, approximately 60–70% of the cases of primary aldosteronism result from tumors in the adrenal gland area. Aldosterone is normally produced by the adrenal cortex, or the outer portion of the gland that rests on top of each kidney. Primary aldosteronism is due to adenoma, a typically benign tumor in which the cells form to act as glands or cause the glands on which they rest to overproduce. It can cause a number of problems, most notably hypertension. In secondary aldosteronism, factors outside the adrenal gland may cause overproduction of aldosterone, or overproduction of renin, an enzyme stored in the kidney area that stimulates aldosterone and raises blood pressure. Obstructive renal artery disease may also cause hypertension from elevated renin stimulating aldosterone. **Oral contraceptives** have been known to increase the secretion of aldosterone in some patients. This disorder is more common in women.

Causes & symptoms

Hyperaldosteronism is most often caused by the invasion of adenoma. Other adrenal **cancers** and hyperplasia, or the increase in the bulk of an organ due to increased cell production, may also cause hyperaldosteronism. Those diseases and factors influencing the adrenal and kidney functions may lead to secondary aldosteronism. The primary symptom of hyperaldosteronism is moderate hypertension, or high blood pressure. In addition, a patient may experience **orthostatic hypotension,** or reduced blood pressure when a person stands after lying down. **Constipation,** muscle weakness (sometimes to the point of **periodic paralysis**), excessive urination, excessive thirst, **headache,** and personality changes are also possible symptoms. Some patients will show no obvious symptoms.

Diagnosis

Screening tests can be conducted to pinpoint a diagnosis of hyperaldosteronism. If a patient is taking drugs

to reduce high blood pressure, the physician may order these drugs stopped for a time period before conducting tests, since these drugs will affect results. Blood and urine tests may be conducted to check for levels of aldosterone, potassium levels, or renin activity. A **computed tomography scan** (CT scan) may be ordered to detect tumors as small as five to seven mm. These combined tests approach 95% accuracy for detecting aldosterone-producing adenoma. Laboratory findings recording blood pressure, **edema,** and aldosterone and **plasma renin activity** can help the physician differentiate between primary aldosteronism and secondary aldosteronism.

Treatment

Once the physician has made a diagnosis of hyperaldosteronism, the adrenal glands should be checked for possible adenomas. This can be done through imaging or with a surgical dissection of the gland. Surgical or ablative treatment will vary depending on the number of tumors found. Since more than 60% of hyperaldosteronism cases are caused by these tumors, treatment of the tumors will help eliminate the resulting high blood pressure in many patients. Some patients will receive **antihypertensive drugs,** like **calcium channel blockers,** to control high blood pressure. The use of **diuretics** can help control hypertension by reducing volume. Potassium levels should be considered in the type of diuretic ordered and the levels should be checked throughout treatment. The most widely used drug for treatment of hyperaldosteronism is spironolactone. This drug helps control aldosterone, but should not be prescribed for some patients, especially those with certain kidney diseases. Spironolactone has several possible adverse effects, depending on the dosage. In all cases of hyperaldosteronism, the treatment should be carefully based on the specific type or underlying cause of the disorder.

Alternative treatment

Patients may choose to work with their physician or alternative provider to control hypertension with diet, **stress reduction** (including massage, meditation, **biofeedback,** and **yoga**), and other remedies. Blood pressure elevation needs to be controlled and monitored by frequent blood pressure measurements. There is no alternative treatment known for the underlying adenoma.

Prognosis

Hyperaldosteronism carries with it all the possible complications of high blood pressure, including thickening of arterial walls and a higher risk of **angina,** kidney failure, **stroke,** or **heart attack.** Another possible, and less reversible complication than hypertension, is kidney damage. When primary aldosteronism is caused by a solitary adenoma, the prognosis is good. Once this tumor is removed, blood pressure will drop, and 70% of these patients have full remission. Patients whose hyperaldosteronism results from adrenal hyperplasia will remain hypertensive. However, in up to 70% of patients, blood pressure can be reduced somewhat with drug therapy. Many patients will be faced with the prospect of controlling their hypertension for the remainder of their lives.

Prevention

There is no known prevention for most causes of hyperaldosteronism.

Resources

BOOKS

Tierney, Lawrence M., Stephen J. McPhee, and Maxine A Papadakis. *Current Medical Diagnosis and Treatment.* Stamford, CT: Appleton and Lange, 1998.

ORGANIZATIONS

American Heart Association. 7320 Greenville Ave. Dallas, TX 75231. (214)373-6300. http://www.amhrt.org

American Society of Hypertension. 515 Madison Ave., Suite #1212, New York, NY 10022. (212)644-0650. http://www.ash-us.org

National Heart, Lung and Blood Institute. Building 31, Room 4A21, Bethesda, MD 20892. (301)496-4236. http://www.nhlbi.nih.gov

OTHER

Hypertension Network. http://www.bloodpressure.com

Teresa G. Norris

Hyperbaric oxygenation *see* **Oxygen therapy**

Hyperbilirubinemia *see* **Neonatal jaundice**

Hypercalcemia
Definition

Hypercalcemia is an abnormally high level of calcium in the blood, usually more than 10.5 milligrams per deciliter of blood.

Description

Calcium plays an important role in the development and maintenance of bones in the body. It is also needed in tooth formation and is important in other body functions. Normally, the body maintains a balance between the amount of calcium in food sources and the calcium already available in the body's tissues. The balance can be upset if excess amounts of calcium are eaten or if the body is unable to process the mineral because of disease.

Calcium is one of the most important and most abundant **minerals** in the human body. Dairy products are the major source of calcium. Eggs, green leafy vegetables, broccoli, legumes, nuts, and whole grains provide smaller amounts. Only about 10–30% of the calcium in food is absorbed into the body. Most calcium is found in combination with other dietary components and must be broken down by the digestive system before it can be used. Calcium is absorbed into the body in the small intestine. Its absorption is influenced by such factors as the amount of vitamin D hormone available to aid the process and the levels of calcium already present in the body. As much as 99% of the body's calcium is stored in bone tissue. A healthy person experiences a constant turnover of calcium as bone tissue is built and reshaped. The remaining 1% of the body's calcium circulates in the blood and other body fluids. Circulating calcium plays an important role in the control of many body functions, such as blood clotting, transmission of nerve impulses, muscle contraction, and other metabolic activities. In the

KEY TERMS

Calcium—A silvery-yellow metal that is the basic element of lime and makes up about 3% of the earth's crust. It is the most abundant mineral in the human body. Calcium and phosphorous combine as calcium phosphate, the hard material of bones and teeth.

Hormone—A chemical substance that is carried through the blood to another part of the body, stimulating it to change its function or structure. Many hormones are produced by glands.

Metabolism—All the physical and chemical changes that take place within an organism.

Milk-alkali syndrome—A chronic disorder of the kidneys caused by the ingestion of large amounts of calcium and alkali in the treatment of peptic ulcer. The disorder is reversible in its early stages but can progress to kidney failure.

Mineral—A substance that does not contain carbon (inorganic) and is widely distributed in nature. Minerals play an important role in human metabolism.

Parathyroid hormone (PTH)—A chemical substance produced by the parathyroid glands. This hormone is a major element in regulating calcium in the body.

Vitamin D hormone—Vitamin D is a vitamin that also acts as a hormone. Vitamin D hormone acts with parathyroid hormone to regulate calcium levels in the blood and to supply appropriate amounts of calcium to all cells.

bloodstream, calcium maintains a constant balance with another mineral, phosphate.

Two main control agents are vital in maintaining calcium levels, vitamin D hormone and parathyroid hormone. A hormone is a chemical substance that is formed in one organ or part of the body and carried in the blood to another organ. It can alter the function, and sometimes the structure, of one or more organs.

• Parathyroid hormone (PTH). The four parathyroid glands are endocrine glands located next to the thyroid gland in the neck. A gland is a cell or group of cells that produces a material substance (secretion). When the level of calcium circulating in the blood drops, the parathyroid gland releases its hormone. PTH then acts in three ways to restore the normal blood calcium level. It stimulates the absorption of more calcium in the intestine; it takes more calcium from the bone tissue, and it causes the kidneys to excrete more phosphate.

• Vitamin D hormone. This hormone works with parathyroid hormone to control calcium absorption and affects the deposit of calcium and phosphate in the bone tissue.

The kidneys also help to control calcium levels. Healthy kidneys can increase calcium excretion almost fivefold to maintain normal concentrations in the body. Hypercalcemia can occur when the concentration of calcium overwhelms the ability of the kidneys to maintain balance.

Causes & symptoms

Causes of hypercalcemia

Many different conditions can cause hypercalcemia; the most common are **hyperparathyroidism** and **cancer.**

PRIMARY HYPERPARATHYROIDISM

Primary hyperparathyroidism is the excessive secretion of parathyroid hormone by one or more of the parathyroid glands. It is the most common cause of hypercalcemia in the general population. Women have this condition more frequently than men do, and it is more common in older people. It can appear thirty or more years after radiation treatments to the neck. Ninety percent of the cases of primary hyperparathyroidism are caused by a non-malignant growth on the gland.

Hyperparathyroidism can also occur as part of a rare hereditary disease called **multiple endocrine neoplasia.** In this disease, tumors develop on the parathyroid gland.

CANCER

People with cancer often have hypercalcemia. In fact, it is the most common life-threatening metabolic disorder associated with cancer. Ten to twenty percent of all persons with cancer have hypercalcemia. Cancers of the breast, lung, head and neck, and kidney are frequently associated with hypercalcemia. It also occurs frequently in association with certain cancers of the blood, particularly malignant myeloma. It is seen most often in patients with tumors of the lung (25–35%) and breast (20–40%), according to the National Cancer Institute. Cancer causes hypercalcemia in two ways. When a tumor grows into the bone, it destroys bony tissue (osteolysis). When the bone is not involved, factors secreted by cancer cells can increase calcium levels (humoral hypercalcemia of malignancy). The two mechanisms may operate at the same time.

Because immobility causes an increase in the loss of calcium from bone, cancer patients who are weak and spend most of their time in bed are more prone to hypercalcemia. Cancer patients are often dehydrated because they take in inadequate amounts of food and fluids and often suffer from **nausea and vomiting. Dehydration** reduces the ability of the kidneys to remove excess calcium from the body. Hormones and **diuretics** that increase the amount of fluid released by the body can also trigger hypercalcemia.

OTHER CAUSES

Other conditions can cause hypercalcemia. Excessive intake of vitamin D increases intestinal absorption of calcium. During therapy for peptic **ulcers,** abnormally high amounts of calcium **antacids** are sometimes taken. Over use of antacids can cause milk-alkali syndrome and hypercalcemia. Diseases such as Paget's, in which bone is destroyed or reabsorbed, can also cause hypercalcemia. As in cancer or **paralysis** of the arms and legs, any condition in which the patient is immobilized for long periods of time can lead to hypercalcemia due to bone loss.

Common symptoms

Many patients with mild hypercalcemia have no symptoms and the condition is discovered during routine laboratory screening. Gastrointestinal symptoms include loss of appetite, nausea, vomiting, **constipation,** and abdominal **pain.** There may be a blockage in the bowel. If the kidneys are involved, the individual will have to urinate frequently during both the day and night and will be very thirsty. As the calcium levels rise, the symptoms become more serious. Stones may form in the kidneys and waste products can build up. Blood pressure rises. The heart rhythm may change. Muscles become increasingly weak. The individual may experience mood swings, confusion, **psychosis,** and eventually, **coma** and **death.**

Diagnosis

High levels of calcium in the blood are a good indication of hypercalcemia, but these levels may fluctuate. Calcium levels are influenced by other compounds in the blood that may combine with calcium. Higher calcium and lower phosphate levels may suggest primary hyperparathyroidism. The blood levels of protein (serum albumin) and parathyroid hormone (PTH) are also measured in the diagnosis of hypercalcemia. Too much PTH in the blood may indicate primary hyperparathyroidism. Levels of calcium and phosphate in the urine should also be measured. The medical history and physical condition of the individual must be taken into consideration, especially in the early stages of hypercalcemia when symptoms are mild.

Treatment

The treatment of hypercalcemia depends on how high the calcium level is and what is causing the elevation. Hypercalcemia can be life-threatening and rapid reduction may be necessary. If the patient has normal kidney function, fluids can be given by vein (intravenously) to clear the excess calcium. The amount of fluid taken in and eliminated must be carefully monitored. If the patient's kidneys are not working well, acute hemodyalysis is probably the safest and most effective method to reduce dangerous calcium levels. In this procedure, blood is circulated through tubes made of semipermeable membranes against a special solution that filters out unwanted substances before returning the blood to the body.

Drugs such as furosemide, called loop diuretics, can be given after adequate fluid intake is established. These drugs inhibit calcium reabsorption in the kidneys and promote urine production. Drugs that inhibit bone loss, such as calcitonin, biphosphates, and plicamycin, are helpful in achieving long-term control. Phosphate pills help lower high calcium levels caused by a deficiency in phosphate. Anti-inflammatory agents such as steroids are helpful with some cancers and toxic levels of vitamin D.

Treatment of the underlying cause of the hypercalcemia will also correct the imbalance. Hyperparathyroidism is usually treated by surgical removal of one or more of the parathyroid glands and any tissue, other than the glands themselves, that is producing excessive amounts of the hormone.

The hypercalcemia caused by cancer is difficult to treat without controlling the cancer. Symptoms can be alleviated with fluids and drug therapy as outlined above.

Prognosis

Surgery to remove the parathyroid glands and any misplaced tissue that is producing excessive amounts of hormone succeeds in about 90% of all cases. Outcome is also influenced by whether any damage to the kidneys can be reversed.

Mild hypercalcemia can be controlled through good fluid intake and the use of effective drugs.

Hypercalcemia generally develops as a late complication of cancer and the expected outlook is grim without effective anticancer therapy.

Prevention

People with cancer who are at risk of developing hypercalcemia should be familiar with early symptoms and know when to see a doctor. Good fluid intake (up to four quarts of liquid a day if possible), controlling nausea and vomiting, paying attention to **fevers,** and keeping physically active as much as possible can help prevent problems. Dietary calcium restriction is not necessary because hypercalcemia reduces absorption of calcium in the intestine.

Resources

BOOKS

Shils, Maurice E. et al. *Modern Nutrition in Health and Disease.* Philadelphia: Lea & Febiger, 1994.

Williams, Sue Rodwell. *Essentials of Nutrition and Diet Therapy.* Philadelphia: Mosby, 1997.

OTHER

National Cancer Institute. *Hypercalcemia.* 1998. http://www.graylab.ac.uk/cancernet/304462.html.

Karen Ericson

Hypercoagulation disorders

Definition

Hypercoagulation disorders (or hypercoagulable states or disorders) have the opposite effect of the more common **coagulation disorders.** In hypercoagulation, there is an increased tendency for clotting of the blood, which may put a patient at risk for obstruction of veins and arteries (phlebitis or **pulmonary embolism**).

Description

In normal hemostasis, or the stoppage of bleeding, clots form at the site of the blood vessel's injury. The difference between that sort of clotting and the clotting present in hypercoagulation is that these clots develop in circulating blood.

This disorder can cause clots throughout the body's blood vessels, sometimes creating a condition known as thrombosis. Thrombosis can lead to infarction, or death of tissue, as a result of blocked blood supply to the tissue. However, hypercoagulability does not always lead to thrombosis. In **pregnancy,** and other hypercoagulable states, the incidence of thrombosis is higher than that of the general population, but is still under 10%. However, in association with certain genetic disorders, hypercoagulation disorders may be more likely to lead to thrombosis. Hypercoagulation disorders may also be known as hyperhomocystinemia, antithrombin III deficiency, factor V leyden, and protein C or protein S deficiency.

Causes & symptoms

Hypercoagulation disorders may be acquired or hereditary. Some of the genetic disorders that lead to hypercoagulation are abnormal clotting factor V, variations in fibrinogen, and deficiencies in proteins C and S. Other body system diseases may also lead to these disorders,

KEY TERMS

Antithrombin—Any substance that counters the effect of thrombin, an enzyme that converts fibrinogen into fibrin, leading to blood coagulation.

Congenital—Refers to a condition or disorder present at birth.

Hemostasis—The arrest of bleeding.

Heparin—An anticoagulant, or blood clot "dissolver."

Polycythemia—A condition characterized by an overabundance of red blood cells.

Thalassemia—One of a group of inherited blood disorders characterized by a defect in the metabolism of hemoglobin, or the portion of the red blood cells that transports oxygen throughout the blood stream.

Thrombosis—Formation of a clot in the blood that either blocks, or partially blocks, a blood vessel. The thrombus may lead to infarction, or death of tissue due to a blocked blood supply.

including diabetes, **sickle cell anemia, congenital heart disease,** lupus, **thalassemia,** polycythemia rubra vera, and others. Antithrombin III deficiency is a hereditary hypercoagulation disorder that affects both sexes. Symptoms include obstruction of a blood vessel by a clot (thromboembolic disease), vein inflammation (phlebitis), and ulcers of the lower parts of the legs. The role of proteins C and S is a complex one. In order for coagulation to occur, platelets (small, round fragments in the blood) help contract blood vessels to lessen blood loss and also to help plug damaged blood vessels. However, the conversion of platelets into actual clots is a complicated web involving proteins that are identified clotting factors. The factors are carried in the plasma, or liquid portion of the blood. Proteins C and S are two of the clotting factors that are present in the plasma to help regulate or activate parts of the clotting process. Protein C is considered an anticoagulant. Mutation defects in the proteins may decrease their concentrations in the blood, and may or may not affect their resulting anticoagulant activity. Factor V is an unstable clotting factor also present in plasma. Abnormal factor V resists the changes that normally occur through the influence of protein C, which can also lead to hypercoagulability. Prothrombin, a glycoprotein which converts to thrombin in the early stage of the clotting process, is affected by the presence of these proteins, as well as other clotting factors.

Diagnosis

The diagnosis of hypercoagulation disorders is completed with a combination of **physical examination,** medical history, and blood tests. An accurate medical history is important to determine possible symptoms and causes of hypercoagulation disorders. There are a number of blood tests that can determine the presence or absence of proteins, clotting factors, and **platelet counts** in the blood. Among the tests used to detect hypercoagulation is the Antithrombin III assay. Protein C and Protein S concentrations can be diagnosed with immunoassay or plasma antigen level tests.

Treatment

Coumadin and heparin anticoagulants may be administered to reduce the clotting effects and maintain fluidity in the blood. Heparin is an anticoagulant that prevents thrombus formation and is used primarily for liver and lung clots.

Prognosis

The prognosis for patients with hypercoagulation disorders varies depending on the severity of the clotting and thrombosis. If undetected and untreated, thrombosis could lead to recurrent thrombosis and pulmonary embolism, a potentially fatal problem.

Prevention

Hereditary hypercoagulation disorders may not be prevented. Genetic and blood testing may help determine a person's tendency to develop these disorders.

Resources

BOOKS

Conn, Howard F., Clohecy, Robert J. and Conn, Rex B. *Current Diagnosis.* 9th ed. Philadelphia, PA: W.B. Saunders, 1997.

ORGANIZATIONS

National Heart, Lung and Blood Institute. Building 31, Room 4A21, Bethesda, MD 20892. (301) 496-4236. http://www.nhlbi.nih.gov.

National Hemophilia Foundation. 116 West 32nd St., 11th Floor, New York, NY 10001. 800-42-HANDI. http://wwww.hemophilia.org.

Teresa G. Norris

> **KEY TERMS**
>
> **Ketonuria**—The presence of large amount of ketones in the urine. These byproducts of inadequate breakdown of nutrients indicate that the body is in starvation.

Hyperemesis gravidarum

Definition

Hyperemesis gravidarum means excessive vomiting during **pregnancy.**

Description

In pregnant women, **nausea and vomiting** (morning sickness) are common, affecting up to 80% of pregnancies. Hyperemesis, or extreme nausea and excessive vomiting, occur in about 1% of pregnancies. This condition causes uncontrollable vomiting, severe **dehydration,** and weight loss for the mother. However, hyperemesis gravidarum rarely causes problems for the unborn baby.

Causes & symptoms

The cause of nausea and vomiting during pregnancy is unknown but may be related to the level of certain hormones produced during pregnancy. Hyperemesis is seen more often in first pregnancies and multiple pregnancies (twins, triplets, etc.). The main symptom of hyperemesis is severe vomiting, which causes dehydration and weight loss.

Diagnosis

Although many women with morning sickness feel like they are vomiting everything they eat, they continue to gain weight and are not dehydrated; they do not have hyperemesis gravidarum. Women with this condition will start to show signs of **starvation,** including weight loss. **Physical examination** and laboratory tests of blood and urine samples will be used to help diagnose the condition. One of the most common tests used to help diagnosis and monitor hyperemesis gravidarum is a test for ketones in the urine. Excessive ketones in the urine (ketonuria) indicates that the body is not using carbohydrates from food as fuel and is inadequately trying to break down fat as fuel. Ketonuria is a sign that the body is beginning to operate in starvation mode.

Treatment

Hospitalization is often required. Intravenous fluids with substances that help the body conduct nerve signals (electrolytes) may be given to correct the dehydration and excessive acid in the blood (acidosis). Anti-nausea or sedative medications may be given by injection to stop the vomiting. In some cases, oral medication may be prescribed to control the nausea and vomiting while food is reintroduced. If food cannot be tolerated at all, intravenous nutritional supplements may be necessary. Injections of vitamin B_6, in particular, may help overcome nutritional deficiencies that often occur.

Alternative treatment

The severe vomiting associated with hyperemesis gravidarum requires medical attention. Milder episodes of nausea or vomiting may be reduced with deep breathing and relaxation **exercises.** The use of herbal remedies should be done with extreme caution during pregnancy, especially in the first trimester. Natural remedies to reduce nausea include a teaspoon of cider vinegar in a cup of warm water, or tea made from anise (*Pinpinella anisum*), fennel seed (*Foeniculum vulgare*), red raspberry (*Rubus idaeus*), or ginger (*Zingiber officinale*). Wristbands can be positioned over **acupressure** points on both wrists. **Aromatherapy** with lavender, rose, or chamomile can be soothing, as can smelling ground ginger. Homeopathic remedies—which use extremely diluted solutions as treatments—can be safe and effective for controlling symptoms in some women.

Prognosis

In virtually all cases, the pregnancy can continue to the successful delivery of a healthy baby.

Prevention

Although there is no evidence that hyperemesis gravidarum can be prevented, vomiting during pregnancy sometimes may be lessened. Maintaining a healthy diet, getting adequate sleep, and controlling **stress** may contribute to prevention or improvement of symptoms. Several strategies may help lessen the nausea and vomiting. Eating dry foods and limiting fluid intake may also be helpful. Small meals should be eaten frequently throughout the day, with a protein snack at night. Eating soda crackers before rising from bed in the morning may help prevent early morning nausea. Iron supplements may cause nausea and can be eliminated until the nausea is controlled. Sitting upright for 45 minutes after meals may also help.

Resources

PERIODICALS

Cowan, M.J. "Hyperemesis gravidarum: Implications for home care and infusion therapies." *Journal of Intravenous Nursing* 19 (Jan-Feb 1996): 46-58.

Hallak M., et al. "Hyperemesis gravidarum. Effects on fetal outcome." *Journal of Reproductive Medicine* 41 (Nov 1996): 871-874.

OTHER

Levy, B.T. and P.L. Brown. "Nausea and Vomiting in Pregnancy." In the University of Iowa Family Practice Handbook: Chapter 8: Obstetrics. The Virtual Hospital at http://www.vh.org.

Natural Remedies During Pregnancy: Frequently Asked Questions. http://www.childbirth.org/articles/remedy.html.

Altha Roberts Edgren

Hyperhidrosis

Definition

A disorder marked by excessive sweating. It usually begins at **puberty** and affects the palms, soles, and armpits.

Description

Sweating is the body's way of cooling itself and is a normal response to a hot environment or intense exercise. However, excessive sweating unrelated to these conditions can be a problem for some people. Those with constantly moist hands may feel uncomfortable shaking hands or touching, while others with sweaty armpits and feet may have to contend with the unpleasant odor that results from the bacterial breakdown of sweat and cellular debris (bromhidrosis). People with hyperhidrosis often must change their clothes at least once a day, and their shoes can be ruined by the excess moisture. Hyperhidrosis may also contribute to such skin diseases as athlete's foot (tinea pedis) and contact dermatitis.

Causes & symptoms

Conditions or situations that can trigger hyperhidrosis are varied. They include stressful situations, eating spicy foods, consuming alcohol, the presence of underlying disorders (e.g. tuberculosis, malaria, lymphoma, and diabetes), menopause, hormonal imbalances, and the use of certain drugs. Physicians believe that hyperhidrosis can be linked to a breakdown in communication between the brain and the mechanisms that activate sweating. In addition, a genetic link may also exist: about 40% of people with the condition have a family history of it.

Diagnosis

The condition is diagnosed by patient report and a **physical examination**.

Treatment

Most over-the-counter antiperspirants are not strong enough to effectively prevent hyperhidrosis. To treat the disorder, doctors usually prescribe 20% aluminum chloride hexahydrate solution (Drysol), which the patient applies at night to the affected areas that are then wrapped in a plastic film until morning. Drysol works by blocking the sweat pores. Formaldehyde- and glutaraldehyde-based solutions can also be prescribed; however, formaldehyde may trigger an allergic reaction and glutaraldehyde can stain the skin (for this reason it is primarily applied to the soles). Anticolinergic drugs may also be used. In addition, an electrical device that emits low-voltage current can be held against the skin to reduce sweating. These treatments are usually conducted in a doctor's office on a daily basis for several weeks, followed by weekly visits. Dermatologists also recommend that patients wear clothing made of natural or absorbent fabrics also may help, avoid high-buttoned collars, use talc or cornstarch, and keep underarms shaved.

The only permanent cure for hyperhidrosis of the palms is a surgical procedure. To treat severe excessive sweating, a surgeon can remove a portion of the nerve near the top of the spine that controls palm sweat. However, not very many neurosurgeons in the United States will perform the procedure. Alternatively, it is possible to remove the sweat gland-bearing skin of the armpits, but this is a major procedure that may require skin grafts.

Prognosis

While the condition cannot be cured without radical surgery, it can usually be controlled effectively.

Resources

PERIODICALS

Angerman, Judith E. "Putting a Stop to Sweating." *Good Housekeeping* 221 (July 1, 1995): 162.

ORGANIZATIONS

American Academy of Dermatology. 930 N. Meacham Rd., PO Box 4014 Schaumburg, IL 60168. (708) 330-0230.

Carol A. Turkington

Hyperhomocystinemia *see*
Hypercoagulation disorders

Hyperkalemia

Definition

The normal concentration of potassium in the serum is in the range of 3.5 to 5.0 mM. Hyperkalemia refers to serum or plasma levels of potassium ions above 5.0 mM. The concentration of potassium is often expressed in units of milliequivalents per liter (mEq/L), rather than in units of millimolarity (mM). Both units mean the same thing when applied to concentrations of potassium ions.

Description

A normal adult who weighs about 70 kg contains a total of about 3.6 moles of potassium ions in the body. Most of this potassium (about 98%) occurs inside various cells and organs, where its concentration is about 150 mM. This level is in contrast to the much lower concentration found in the blood serum, where only about 0.4% of the body's potassium resides. Hyperkalemia can be caused by an overall excess of body potassium, or by a shift from inside to outside cells. For example, hyperkalemia can be caused by the sudden release of potassium ions from muscle into the surrounding fluids.

In a normal person, hyperkalemia from too much potassium in the diet is prevented by at least three types of regulatory processes. First, various cells and organs act to prevent hyperkalemia by taking up potassium from the blood. It is also prevented by the action of the kidneys, which excrete potassium into the urine. A third protective mechanism is vomiting. Consumption of a large dose of potassium ions, such as potassium chloride, induces a

KEY TERMS

Acidosis—An abnormally high acid (hydrogen ion) concentration in blood plasma. The unit of acid content is pH, with a lower value indicating more acidic conditions. Blood plasma normally has a pH of 7.35–7.45. Alkaline blood has a pH value greater than pH 7.45. When the blood pH value is less than 7.35, the patient is in acidosis.

vomiting reflex to expel most of the potassium before it can be absorbed.

Causes & symptoms

Hyperkalemia can occur from a variety of causes, including the consumption of too much of a potassium salt; the failure of the kidneys to normally excrete potassium ions into the urine; the leakage of potassium from cells and tissues into the bloodstream; and from acidosis. The most common cause of hyperkalemia is kidney (or renal) disease, which accounts for about three quarters of all cases. Kidney function is measured by the glomerular filtration rate, the rate at which each kidney performs its continual processing and cleansing of blood. The normal glomerular filtration rate is about 100 ml/min. If the kidney is damaged so that the glomerular filtration rate is only 5 ml/min or less, hyperkalemia may result, especially if high-potassium foods are consumed. The elderly are at particular risk, since many regulatory functions of the body do not work well in this population. Elderly patients who are being treated with certain drugs for high blood pressure, such as spironolactone (Aldactone) and triamterene (Dyazide), must especially be monitored for possible hyperkalemia, as these medications promote the retention of potassium by the kidneys.

Hyperkalemia can also be caused by a disease of the adrenal gland called **Addison's disease.** The adrenal gland produces the hormone aldosterone that promotes the excretion of potassium into the urine by the kidney.

Hyperkalemia can also result from injury to muscle or other tissues. Since most of the potassium in the body is contained in muscle, a severe trauma that crushes muscle cells results in an immediate increase in the concentration of potassium in the blood. Hyperkalemia may also result from severe **burns** or infections.

Acidic blood plasma, or acidosis, is an occasional cause of hyperkalemia. Acidosis, which occurs in a number of diseases, is defined as an increase in the concentration of hydrogen ions in the bloodstream. In the body's attempt to correct the situation, hydrogen is taken up by muscle cells out of the blood in an exchange mechanism involving the transfer of potassium ions into the bloodstream. This can abnormally elevate the plasma's concentration of potassium ions. When acidosis is the cause of hyperkalemia, treating the patient for acidosis has two benefits: a reversal of both the acidosis and the hyperkalemia.

Symptoms of hyperkalemia include abnormalities in the behavior of the heart. Heart abnormalities of mild hyperkalemia (5.0 to 6.5 mM potassium) can be detected by an electrocardiogram (ECG or EKG). With severe hyperkalemia (over 8.0 mM potassium), the heart may beat at a dangerously rapid rate (fibrillation) or stop beating entirely (cardiac arrest). Patients with moderate or severe hyperkalemia may also develop nervous symptoms such as tingling of the skin, numbness of the hands or feet, weakness, or a flaccid **paralysis,** which is characteristic of both hyperkalemia and **hypokalemia** (low plasma potassium).

Diagnosis

Hyperkalemia can be measured by acquiring a sample of blood, preparing blood serum, and using a potassium sensitive electrode for measuring the concentration of potassium ions. Alternatively, atomic absorption spectroscopy can be used for measuring potassium. Since high or low potassium levels result in abnormalities in heart function, the electrocardiogram is usually the method of choice for the diagnosis of both hyperkalemia and hypokalemia.

Treatment

Insulin injections are used to treat hyperkalemia in emergency situations. Insulin is a hormone well known for its ability to stimulate the entry of sugar (glucose) into cells. It also provokes the uptake of potassium ions by cells, decreasing potassium ion concentration in the blood. When insulin is used to treat hyperkalemia, glucose is also injected. Serum potassium levels begin to decline within 30 to 60 minutes and remain low for several hours. In non-emergency situations, hyperkalemia can be treated with a low potassium diet. If this does not succeed, the patient can be given a special resin to bind potassium ions. One such resin, sodium polystyrene sulfonate (Kayexalate), remains in the intestines, where it absorbs potassium and forms a complex of resin and potassium. Eventually this complex is excreted in the feces. A typical dose of resin is 15 grams, taken one to four times per day. The correction of hyperkalemia with resin treatment takes at least 24 hours.

Prognosis

The prognosis for specifically correcting hyperkalemia is excellent. However, hyperkalemia is usually caused by kidney failure, an often irreversible and eventually fatal condition.

Prevention

Healthy people are not at risk for hyperkalemia. Patients with renal disease and those on certain diuretic medications must be monitored to prevent its occurrence.

Resources

BOOKS

The American Dietetic Association. *Handbook of Clinical Dietetics.* New Haven, CT: Yale Univ. Press, 1992.

Brody, Tom. *Nutritional Biochemistry.* San Diego, CA: Academic Press, 1998.

Levinsky, N.G. "Fluids and Electrolytes." In *Harrison's Principles of Internal Medicine,* edited by K.J. Isselbacher, et al. Engelwood Cliffs, New Jersey: Prentice-Hall, 1995.

Zeman, F. and D.M. Dey. *Applications in Medical Nutrition Therapy,* 2nd edition. Engelwood Cliffs, New Jersey: Prentice-Hall, 1995.

PERIODICALS

Greenberg, A. "Hyperkalemia: treatment options." *Seminars in Nephrology* 18 (1998): 46-57.

Tom Brody

Hyperkinetic disorder *see* **Attention-deficit/Hyperactivity disorder (ADHD)**

Hyperlipemia *see* **Hyperlipoproteinemia**

Hyperlipidemia *see* **Hyperlipoproteinemia**

Hyperlipoproteinemia

Definition

Hyperlipoproteinemia occurs when there is too much lipid (fat) in the blood. Shorter terms that mean the same thing are hyperlipidemia and hyperlipemia. Dyslipidemia refers to a redistribution of cholesterol from one place to another that increases the risk of vascular disease without increasing the total amount of cholesterol. When more precise terms are needed, hypercholesterolemia and hypertriglycericemia are used.

Description

It is commonly known that oil and water do not mix unless another substance like a detergent is added. Yet

---

KEY TERMS

Atherosclerosis—Hardening of the arteries due to fat (cholesterol) deposits in their walls. Also known as *arteriosclerosis.*

Genetic—Refers to the genes, characteristics inherited from parents.

Inflammation—The body's response to irritation, by releasing chemicals that attack germs and tissues and also repair the damage done.

Lesion—Localized disease or damage.

Pancreatitis—Inflammation of the pancreas.

Serum—The liquid part of blood, from which all the cells have been removed.

---

the body needs to transport both lipids (fats) and water-based blood within a single circulatory system. There must be a way to mix the two, so that essential fatty nutrients can be transported in the blood and so that fatty waste products can be carried away from tissues. The solution is to combine the lipids with protein to form water-soluble packages that can be transported in the blood.

These packages of fats are called lipoproteins. They are a complex mixture of triglycerides, cholesterol, phospholipids and special proteins. Some of these chemicals are fatty nutrients absorbed from the intestines on their way to being made part of the body. Cholesterol is a waste product on its way out of the body through the liver, the bile, and ultimately the bowel for excretion. The proteins and phospholipids make the packages water-soluble.

There are five different sizes of these chemical packages. Each package needs all four chemicals in it to hold everything in solution. They differ in how much of each they contain. If blood serum is spun very rapidly in an ultracentrifuge, these five packages will layer out according to their density. They have, therefore, been named according to their densities—high-density lipoproteins (HDL), low-density lipoproteins (LDL), intermediate-density lipoproteins (IDL), very low density lipoproteins (VLDL), and chylomicrons. Only the HDLs and the LDLs will be discussed in the rest of this article.

If there is not enough detergent in the laundry, the oily stains will remain in the clothes. In the same way, if the balance of chemicals in these packages is not right, cholesterol will stay in tissues rather than being excreted from the body. What is even worse, if the chemical composition of these packages changes, the cholesterol can fall out of the blood and stay where it lands. On the other hand, a different change in the balance can remove cholesterol from tissues where there is too much. This appears to be exactly what is going on in **atherosclerosis**. The lesions contain lots of cholesterol.

The LDLs are overloaded with cholesterol. A minor change in the other chemicals in this package will leave cholesterol behind. The HDLs have a third to a half as much cholesterol. They seem to be able to pick up cholesterol left behind by the LDLs. It seems that atherosclerosis begins with tiny tears at stressed places in the walls of the arteries. Low density lipoproteins from the blood enter these tears, where their chemistry changes enough to leave cholesterol behind. The cholesterol causes irritation; the body responds with inflammation; damage and scarring follow. Eventually the artery gets so diseased blood cannot flow through it. Strokes and **heart attacks** are the result.

But if there are lots of HDLs in the blood, the cholesterol is rapidly picked up and not allowed to cause problems. Women before **menopause** have estrogen (the female hormone), which encourages the formation of HDLs. This is the reason they have so little vascular disease, and why they rapidly catch up to men after menopause, when estrogen levels fall. Replacement of estrogen after menopause sustains the protection through the later years.

Cholesterol is the root of the problem, but like any other root it cannot just be eliminated. Ninety percent of the cholesterol in the body is created there as a waste product of necessary processes. The solution lies in getting it out to the body without clogging the arteries.

Of course the story is much more complex. The body has dozens of chemical processes that make up, break down, and reconfigure all these chemicals. It is these processes that are the targets of intervention in the effort to cure vascular disease.

Diseases

Near the dawn of concern over cholesterol and vascular disease a family of hereditary diseases was identified, all of which produced abnormal quantities of blood fats. These diseases were called dyslipoproteinemias and came in both too much and too little varieties. The hyperlipoproteinemias found their way into five categories, depending on which chemical was in excess.

- Type 1 has a pure elevation of triglycerides in the chylomicron fraction. These people sometimes get **pancreatitis** and abdominal **pains,** but they do not seem to have an increase in vascular disease.

- Type 2 appears in two distinct genetic patterns and a third category, which is by far the most important kind, because everyone is at risk for it. All Type 2s have elevated cholesterol. Some have elevated triglycerides

also. The familial (genetic) versions of Type 2 often develop xanthomas, which are yellow fatty deposits under the skin of the knuckles, elbows, buttocks or heels. They may also have xanthelasmas, smaller yellow patches on the eyelids.

- Type 3 appears in one in 10,000 people and elevates both triglycerides and cholesterol with consequent vascular disease.

- Type 4 elevates only triglycerides and does not increase the risk of vascular disease.

- Type 5 is similar to Type 1.

- Dyslipidemia refers to a normal amount of cholesterol that is mostly in LDLs, where it causes problems.

All but Type 2 are rare and of interest primarily because they give insight into the chemistry of blood fats.

In addition to the above genetic causes of blood fat disorders, a number of acquired conditions can raise lipoprotein levels.

- **Diabetes mellitus,** because it alters the way the body handles its energy needs, also affects the way it handles fats. The result is elevated triglycerides and reduced HDL cholesterol. This effect is amplified by **obesity.**

- **Hypothyroidism** is a common cause of lipid abnormalities. The thyroid hormone affects the rate of many chemical processes in the body, including the clearing of fats from the blood. The consequence is usually an elevation of cholesterol.

- Kidney disease affects the blood's proteins and consequently the composition of the fat packages. It usually raises the LDLs.

- Liver disease, depending on its stage and severity, can raise or lower any of the blood fats.

- Alcohol raises triglycerides. In moderate amounts (if they are very moderate) it raises HDLs and can be beneficial.

- Cigarette smoking lowers HDL cholesterol, as does **malnutrition** and obesity.

Certain medications elevate blood fat levels. Because some of these medications are used to treat heart disease, it has been necessary to reevaluate their usefulness:

- Thiazides, water pills used to treat high blood pressure, can raise both cholesterol and triglycerides.

- Beta-blockers, another class of medication used to treat high blood pressure, cortisone-like drugs, and estrogen can raise triglycerides.

- Progesterone, the **pregnancy** hormone, raises cholesterol.

Not all of these effects are necessarily bad, nor are they necessarily even significant. For instance, estrogen is clearly beneficial. Each effect must be considered in the overall goal of treatment.

Causes & symptoms

A combination of heredity and diet is responsible for the majority of fat disorders. It is not so much the cholesterol in the diet that is the problem, because that accounts for only 10% of the body's store. It is the other fats in the diet that alter the way the body handles its cholesterol. There is a convincing relation between fats in the diet and the incidence of atherosclerosis. The guilty fats are mostly the animal fats, but palm and coconut oil are also harmful. These fats are called saturated fats for the chemical reason that most of their carbon atoms have as many hydrogen atoms attached as they can accommodate. More important than the kind of fat is the amount of fat. For many people, fat is half of their diet. A quarter to a fifth is a much healthier fraction, the rest of the diet being made up of complex carbohydrates and protein.

This disease is silent for decades, until the first episode of heart disease or stroke.

Diagnosis

It would be easier if simple cholesterol and triglyceride tests were all it took to assess the risk of atherosclerosis. But the important information is which package the cholesterol is in—the LDLs or the HDLs. That takes a more elaborate testing process. To complicate matters further, the amount of fats in the blood varies greatly in relation to the last meal—how long ago it was and what kind of food was eaten. A true estimate of the risk comes from several tests several weeks apart all done after at least twelve hours of **fasting.**

Treatment

Diet and lifestyle change are the primary focus for most cholesterol problems. It is a mistake to think that a pill will reverse the effects of a bad diet, obesity, smoking, excess alcohol, stress, and inactivity. Reducing the amount of fat in the diet by at least half is the most important move to make. Much of the food eaten to satisfy a "sweet tooth" is higher in fat than in sugar. A switch away from saturated fats is the next step, but the rush to polyunsaturated fats was ill-conceived. These, and particularly the hydrogenated fats in margarine, have problems of their own. They raise the risk of **cancer** and are considered more dangerous than animal fat by many experts. Theory supports population studies that suggest monounsaturated olive oil may be the healthiest of all.

There is a tremendous push at the end of the 20th century to use lipid-lowering medications. The most pop-ular and most expensive agents, the "statins," hinder the body's production of cholesterol and sometimes damage the liver as a side effect. Their full name is 3-hydroxy-3-methylglutaryl-coemzyme A *(HMG-CoA)* reductase inhibitors. Their generic names are cervistatin, fluvastatin, lovastatin, pravastatin, and simvastatin. Studies show that these do lower cholesterol. Only recently, though, has any evidence appeared that this affects health and longevity. Earlier studies showed, in fact, an increased death rate among users of the first class of lipid-altering agents—the fibric acid derivatives. The chain of events connecting raised HDL and lowered LDL cholesterol to longer, healthier lives is still to be forged.

High-tech methods of rapidly reducing very high blood fat levels are performed for those rare disorders that require it. There are resins that bind cholesterol in the intestines. They taste awful, feel like glue and routinely cause gas, bloating, and **constipation.** For acute cases, there is a filtering system that takes fats directly out of the blood.

Niacin (nicotinic acid) lowers cholesterol very effectively and was the first medication proven to improve overall life expectancy. It can also be liver toxic, and the usual formulation causes a hot flash in many people. This can be overcome by taking a couple of **aspirin**s half-an-hour before the niacin, or by taking a special preparation called "flush free," "inositol-bound" or inositol hexanicotinate. Omega-3 oil is a special kind found mostly in certain kinds of fish. It is beneficial in lowering cholesterol. An herbal alternative called gugulipid, *Commiphora mukul*, an extract of an Indian plant, is supposed to work the same way as the expensive and liver toxic cholesterol-lowering medications.

Alternative treatment

To lower cholesterol, naturopathic medicine, traditional Chinese medicine, and ayurvedic medicine may be considered. Some herbal therapies include gugulipid, alfalfa (*Medicago sativa*), Asian ginseng (*Panax ginseng*), and fenugreek (*Trigonella foenum-graecum*). Garlic (*Allium sativum*) and onions are also reported to have cholesterol-lowering effects. In naturopathic medicine, the liver is considered to be an organ that needs cleansing and rebalancing. The liver is often treated with a botanical formula that will act as a bitter to stimulate bile flow in the liver. Before initiating alternative therapies, medical consultation is strongly advised.

Prognosis

The prognosis is good for Type 1 hyperlipoproteinemia with treatment; without treatment, death may result. For Type 2 the prognosis is poor even with treatment. The prognosis for type 3 is good when the prescribed diet is strictly followed. For types 4 and 5 the prognosis is uncertain, due to the risk of developing premature coronary artery disease and pancreatitis, respectively.

Prevention

Genetic inheritance cannot be changed, but its effects may be modified with proper treatment. Family members of an individual with hyperlipoproteinemia should consider having their blood lipids assessed. The sooner any problems are identified, the better the chances of limiting or preventing the associated health risks. Anyone with a family history of disorders leading to hyperlipoproteinemia also may benefit from genetic testing and counseling to assist them in making reproductive decisions.

Resources

BOOKS

Ginsberg, Henry N. and Ira, J. Goldberg. "Disorders of Lipoprotein Metabolism." In *Harrison's Principles of Internal Medicine,* 14th ed., edited by Anthony S. Fauci, et al. New York: McGraw-Hill, 1998.

Libby, Peter. "Atherosclerosis." In *Harrison's Principles of Internal Medicine,* 14th ed., edited by Anthony S. Fauci, et al. New York: McGraw-Hill, 1998.

Weil, Andrew. *Natural Health, Natural Medicine.* Boston: Houghton Mifflin, 1995.

Witztum, Joseph L. and Daniel Sternberg. "The Hyperlipoproteinemias." In *Cecil Textbook of Medicine,* edited by J. Claude Bennett and and Fred Plum. Philadelphia: W. B. Saunders, 1996.

PERIODICALS

Bays, Harold E. "Drug Therapy for Hyperlipidemia." *Postgraduate Medicine* 91 (1992): 162.

Peters, Wayne L. "Hyperlipidemia: What to Do When Life-Style Changes Aren't Enough." *Postgraduate Medicine* 90 (1991): 213.

ORGANIZATIONS

Inherited High Cholesterol Foundation. 410 Chipeta Way, Room 167, Salt Lake City, UT 84104. (888) 244-2465.

J. Ricker Polsdorfer

Hypermagnesemia *see* **Magnesium imbalance**

Hypermenorrhea *see* **Dysfunctional uterine bleeding**

Hypermetropia *see* **Hyperopia**

Hypernatremia

Definition

The normal concentration of sodium in the blood plasma is 136–145 mM. Hypernatremia is defined as a serum sodium level over 145 mM. Severe hypernatremia, with serum sodium above 152 mM, can result in seizures and **death.**

Description

Sodium is an atom, or ion, that carries a single positive charge. The sodium ion may be abbreviated as Na^+ or as simply Na. Sodium can occur as a salt in a crystalline solid. Sodium chloride (NaCl), sodium phosphate (Na_2HPO_4) and sodium bicarbonate ($NaHCO_3$) are commonly occurring salts. These salts can be dissolved in water or in juices of various foods. Dissolving involves the complete separation of ions, such as sodium and chloride in common table salt (NaCl).

About 40% of the body's sodium is contained in bone. Approximately 2–5% occurs within organs and cells and the remaining 55% is in blood plasma and other extracellular fluids. The amount of sodium in blood plasma is typically 140 mM, a much higher amount than is found in intracellular sodium (about 5 mM). This asymmetric distribution of sodium ions is essential for human life. It makes possible proper nerve conduction, the passage of various nutrients into cells, and the maintenance of blood pressure.

The body continually regulates its handling of sodium. When dietary sodium is too high or low, the intestines and kidneys respond to adjust concentrations to normal. During the course of a day, the intestines absorbs dietary sodium while the kidneys excrete a nearly equal amount of sodium into the urine. If a low sodium diet is consumed, the intestines increase their efficiency of sodium absorption, and the kidneys reduce its release into urine.

The concentration of sodium in the blood plasma depends on two things: the total amount of sodium and water in arteries, veins, and capillaries (the circulatory system). The body uses separate mechanisms to regulate sodium and water, but they work together to correct blood pressure when it is too high or too low. Too high a concentration of sodium, or hypernatremia, can be corrected either by decreasing sodium or by increasing body water. The existence of separate mechanisms that regulate sodium concentration account for the fact that there are numerous diseases that can cause hypernatremia, including diseases of the kidney, pituitary gland, and hypothalamus.

Causes & symptoms

Vasopressin, also called anti-diuretic hormone, is made by the hypothalamus and released by the pituitary gland into the bloodstream. There it travels to the kidney where it reduces the release of water into the urine. With less vasopressin production, the body fails to conserve water, and the result is a trend toward higher plasma sodium concentrations. Hypernatremia may occur in **diabetes insipidus,** a disease that causes excessive urine production. (It is not the same disease as **diabetes mellitus,** a disease resulting from impaired insulin production.) The defect involves either the failure of the hypothalamus to make vasopressin or the failure of the kidney to respond to vasopressin. In either case, the kidney is able to conserve and regulate the body's sodium levels, but is unable to conserve and retain the body's water. Hypernatremia does not occur in diabetes insipidus if the patient is able to drink enough water to keep up with urinary loss, which may be as high as 10 liters per day.

Hypernatremia may occur in unconscious (or comatose) patients due to the inability to drink water. Water is continually lost by evaporation from the lungs and in the urine. If the patient is not given water via infusion, the sodium concentration in the blood may increase and hypernatremia could develop. Hypernatremia can also occur in rare diseases in which the thirst impulse is impaired.

Hypernatremia can also occur accidentally in the hospital when patients are infused with solutions containing sodium, such as sodium bicarbonate for the treatment of acidosis (acidic blood). It can also be accidentally induced with sodium chloride infusions, especially in elderly patients with impaired kidney function.

Hypernatremia can cause neurological damage due to shrinkage of brain cells. Neurological symptoms include confusion, coma, **paralysis** of the lung muscles, and death. The severity of the symptoms is related to how rapidly the hypernatremia developed. Hypernatremia that comes on rapidly does not allow the cells of the brain time to adapt to their new high-sodium environment. Hypernatremia is especially dangerous for children and the elderly.

Diagnosis

Hypernatremia is diagnosed by acquiring a blood sample, preparing plasma, and using a sodium-sensitive electrode for measuring the concentration of sodium ions.

Treatment

Hypernatremia is treated with infusions of a solution of water containing 0.9% sodium chloride (0.9 grams NaCl/100 ml water), which is the normal concentration of sodium chloride in the blood plasma. The infusion is performed over many hours or days to prevent abrupt and dangerous changes in brain cell volume. In emergencies, such as when hypernatremia is causing neurological symptoms, infusions may be conducted with salt solutions containing 0.45% sodium chloride, which is half the normal physiologic level.

Prognosis

The prognosis for treating hypernatremia is excellent, except if neurological symptoms are severe or if overly rapid attempts are made to treat and reverse the condition.

Prevention

Hypernatremia occurs only in unusual circumstances that are not normally under a person's control.

Resources

BOOKS

Levinsky, N.G. "Fluids and electrolytes." In *Harrison's Principles of Internal Medicine,* edited by K.J. Isselbacher, et al. Engelwood Cliffs, New Jersey: Prentice-Hall, 1995.

PERIODICALS

Fried, L.F. and P.M. Palevsky, "Hyponatremia and hypernatremia." *Medical Clinics of North America* 81 (1997): 585-609.

Frizzell, R.T., et al. "Hyponatremia and ultramarathon running." *Journal of the American Medical Association.* 255 (1986): 772-774.

Tom Brody

Hyperopia

Definition

Hyperopia (farsightedness) is the condition of the eye where incoming rays of light reach the retina before they converge into a focused image.

Description

When light goes through transparent but dense material like the materials of the eye's lens system (the lens and cornea), its velocity decreases. If the surface of the dense material is not perpendicular to the incoming light, as is the case with the curved surfaces on lenses and corneas, the direction of the light changes. The greater the curvature of the lens system, the greater the change in the direction of the light.

When parallel light rays from an object go through the lens system of the eye, they are bent so they converge at a point some distance behind the lens. With perfect vision this point of convergence, where the light rays are focused, is on the retina. This happens when the cumulative curvature of the lens plus cornea and the distance from the lens to the retina are just right for each other. The condition where the point of focus of parallel light rays from an object is behind the retina is called hyperopia. This condition exists when the combined curvature of the lens and cornea is insufficient (e.g., flatter than needed for the length of the eyeball). This condition can be equivalently described by saying hyperopia exists when the eyeball is too short for the curvature of its lens system.

There is a connection between the focusing of the lens of the eye (accommodation) and convergence of the eyes (the two eyes turning in to point at a close object.) The best example is during reading. The lens accommodates to make the close-up material clear and the eyes turn in to look at the print and keep it single. Because of this connection between accommodation and convergence, if the lens needs to accommodate to focus for distance (to bring the image back onto the retina) the eyes may appear to turn in even when looking at the distance. This can cause a condition known as accommodative esotropia in children. The eyes turn in and the cause is accommodation because of hyperopia.

Causes & symptoms

Babies are generally born slightly hyperopic. This tends to decrease with age. There is normal variation in eyeball length and curvature of the lens and cornea. Some combinations of these variables give rise to eyes where the cornea is too flat for the distance between the cornea and the retina. If the hyperopia is not too severe the lens

may be able to accommodate and bring the image back onto the retina. This would result in clear distance vision, but the constant focusing might result in **headaches** or eyestrain. If the lens cannot accommodate for the full amount of the hyperopia the distance image would be blurry.

If the eyes are focusing for distance and now the person is looking at a near object, the eyes need to accommodate further. This may result in blurry near objects or headaches during near work.

Depending upon the amount of hyperopia, symptoms can range from none to clear distance vision but blurry near vision, to blurry distance and near vision. Headaches and eyestrain may also occur, particularly when doing near tasks. An eye turned in (esotropia) may be a result of hyperopia, particularly in children. However, because a turned eye may be a result of more serious causes it is very important to have it checked out.

Diagnosis

Because it is possible to have good visual acuity with some degree of hyperopia it is important to relax accommodation before the eye exam. This is done with the use of eyedrops and is called a cycloplegic exam or cycloplegic refraction. The drops relax the accommodation (thus making reading blurry until the drops wear off). Patients will usually be asked to have someone drive them home because of the blurriness. The doctor can then determine the patient's visual status with a hand-held instrument called a retinoscope and/or have the patient read from an eye chart while placing different lenses in front of the patient's eyes. Refractive error is measured in units called diopters (D).

Treatment

The usual treatment for hyperopia is corrective lenses (spectacles or contact lenses).

Different surgical methods to correct hyperopia are under investigation. One approach is to implant corrective contact lenses behind the patient's iris. The first experimental implantable contact lenses were implanted in 1997. Another approach is to surgically increase the curvature of the eye's existing cornea or lens. Although there have been many reports of success using different kinds of lasers to increase corneal curvature, as of 1998 there are still problems with stability and predictability. The introduction of light-activated biologic tissue glue in 1997 holds promise for improvements in those areas.

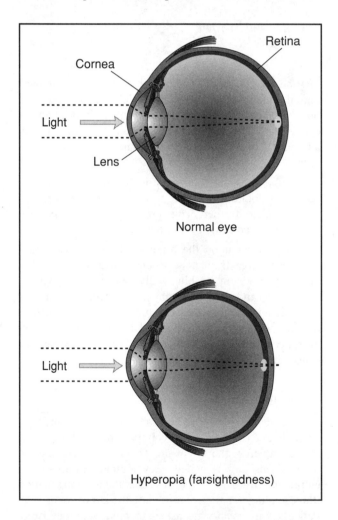

Hyperopia, or farsightedness, is a condition of the eye where incoming rays of light impinge on the retina before converging into a focused image, resulting in difficulty seeing nearby objects clearly. (Illustration by Electronic Illustrators Group.)

Prognosis

The prognosis for fully corrected vision is excellent for patient's with low to moderate amounts of hyperopia. Patient's with very high hyperopia (+ 10.00D or more) may not achieve full correction. Moreover, surgery to correct hyperopia will probably be perfected and approved in the near future.

Hyperopia increases the chances of chronic **glaucoma,** but vision loss from glaucoma is preventable.

Prevention

Hyperopia is usually present at birth, and there is no known way to prevent it.

Resources

BOOKS
Newell, Frank W. *Ophthalmology: Principles and Concepts,* 8th edition. St. Louis: Mosby, 1996.

ORGANIZATIONS
American Academy of Ophthalmology. PO Box 7424, San Francisco, CA 94120-7424. (415) 561-8500. http://www.eyenet.org/.

American Optometric Association. 2420 North Lindburgh Boulevard, St. Louis, MO 63141. (800) 365-2219. http://www.aoanet.org/.

OTHER
Edmiston, D. *Hyperopia* http://eyeinfo.com/hyperopia.html.

Lorraine Lica

Hyperparathyroidism

Definition

Parathyroid glands are four pea-sized glands located just behind the thyroid gland in the front of the neck. The function of parathyroid glands is to produce a hormone called parathyroid hormone (parathormone), which helps regulate calcium and phosphorous in the body. Hyperparathyroidism is the overproduction of this hormone.

Description

Thyroid glands and parathyroid glands, despite their similar name and proximity, are entirely separate, and each produces hormones with different functions. Hyperparathyroidism may be primary or secondary. It most often occurs in those over age 30, and most commonly in patients 50 to 60 years old. It rarely occurs in children or the elderly. Women are affected by the disease up to three times more often than men. It is estimated that 28 of

KEY TERMS

Demineralization—A loss or decrease of minerals in the bones.

Endocrine—Glands and hormone secretions in the body circulation.

Phosphorous—Referring to a chemical element occurring in all living cells.

every 100,000 people in the United States will develop hyperparathyroidism each year.

Normally, parathyroid glands produce the parathormone as calcium levels drop and lower to meet the demands of a growing skeleton, **pregnancy,** or **lactation.** However, when one or more parathyroid glands malfunctions, it can lead to overproduction of the hormone and elevated calcium level in the blood. Therefore, a common result of hyperparathyroidism is **hypercalcemia,** or an abnormally high level of calcium in the blood. Primary hyperparathyroidism occurs as a malfunction of one of the glands, usually as a result of a benign tumor, called adenoma. Secondary hyperparathyroidism occurs as the result of a metabolic abnormality outside the parathyroid glands, which causes a resistance to the function of the parathyroid hormones. Primary hyperparathyroidism is one of the most common endocrine disorders, led only by diabetes and **hyperthyroidism.**

Causes & symptoms

Often, there are no obvious symptoms or suspicion of hyperparathyroidism, and it is first diagnosed when a patient is discovered to be hypercalcemic during a routine blood chemistry profile. Patients may believe they have felt fine, but realize improvements in sleep, irritability, and memory following treatment. When symptoms are present, they may include development of gastric **ulcers** or **pancreatitis** because high calcium levels can cause inflammation and **pain** in the linings of the stomach and pancreas.

Most of the symptoms of hyperparathyroidism are those present as a result of hypercalcemia, such as **kidney stones, osteoporosis,** or bone degradation resulting from the bones giving up calcium. Muscle weakness, central nervous system disturbances such as depression, psychomotor and personality disturbances, and rarely, even **coma** can occur. Patients may also experience **heartburn,** nausea, **constipation,** or abdominal pain. In secondary hyperparathyroidism, patients may show signs of calcium imbalance such as deformities of the long bones. Symptoms of the underlying disease may also be present.

Most commonly, hyperparathyroidism occurs as the result of a single adenoma, or benign tumor, in one of the parathyroid glands. About 90% of all cases of hyperparathyroidism are caused by an adenoma. The tumors are seldom cancerous. They will grow to a much larger size than the parathyroid glands, often to the size of a walnut. Genetic disorders or multiple endocrine tumors can also cause a parathyroid gland to enlarge and oversecrete hormone. In 10% or fewer of patients with primary hyperparathyroidism, there is enlargement of all four parathyroid glands. This condition is called parathyroid hyperplasia.

Diagnosis

Diagnosis of hyperparathyroidism is most often made when a blood test (radioimmunoassay) reveals high levels of parathyroid hormone and calcium. A blood test that specifically measures the amount of parathyroid hormone has made diagnosis simpler. X-ray examinations may be performed to look for areas of diffuse bone demineralization, bone cysts, outer bone absorption and erosion of the long bones of the fingers and toes. Hypercalcemia is mild or intermittent in some patients, but is an excellent indicator of primary hyperparathyroidism. Dual energy x-ray absorptiometry (DEXA or DXA), a tool used to diagnose and measure osteoporosis, is used to show reduction in bone mass for primary hyperparathryroidism patients. Once a diagnosis of hyperparathyroidism is reached, the physician will probably order further tests to evaluate complications. For example, abdominal radiographs might reveal kidney stones.

For secondary hyperparathyroidism, normal or slightly decreased calcium levels in the blood and variable phosphorous levels may be visible. Patient history of familial kidney disease or convulsive disorders may suggest a diagnosis of secondary hyperparathyroidism. Other tests may reveal a disease or disorder, which is causing the secondary hyperparathyroidism.

Treatment

Hyperparathyroidism cases will usually be referred to an endocrinologist, a physician specializing in hormonal problems, or a nephrologist, who specializes in kidney and mineral disorders.

Patients with mild cases of hyperparathyroidism may not need immediate treatment if they have only slight elevations in blood calcium level and normal kidneys and bones. These patients should be regularly checked, probably as often as every six months, by **physical examination** and measurement of kidney function and calcium levels. A bone densitometry measurement should be performed every one or two years. After several years with no worsened symptoms, the length of time between exams may be increased.

Patients with more advanced hyperparathyroidism will usually have all or half of the affected parathyroid gland or glands surgically removed. This surgery is relatively safe and effective. The primary risks are those associated with general anesthesia. There are some instances when the surgery can be performed with the patient under regional, or cervical block, anesthesia. Often studies such as ultrasonography prior to surgery help pinpoint the affected areas.

Alternative treatment

Forcing fluids and reducing intake of calcium-rich foods can help decrease calcium levels prior to surgery or if surgery is not necessary.

Prognosis

Removal of the enlarged parathyroid gland or glands cures the disease 95% of the time and relief of bone pain may occur in as few as three days. In up to 5% of patients undergoing surgery, chronically low calcium levels may result, and these patients will require calcium supplement or vitamin D treatment. Damage to the kidneys as a result of hyperparathyroidism is often irreversible. Prognosis is generally good, however complications of hyperparathyroidism such as osteoporosis, bone **fractures,** kidney stones, peptic ulcers, pancreatitis, and nervous system difficulties may worsen prognosis.

Prevention

Secondary hyperparathyroidism may be prevented by early treatment of the disease causing it. Early recognition and treatment of hyperparathyroidism may prevent hypercalcemia. Since the cause of primary hyperparathyroidism, or the adenoma which causes parathyroid enlargement, is largely unknown, there are not prescribed prevention methods.

Resources

PERIODICALS

Allerheiligen, David A., Joe Schoeber, Robert E. Houston, Virginia K. Mohl, and Karen M. Wildman. "Hyperparathyroidism." *American Family Physician* 58 (April 15, 1998): 1795-1803.

ORGANIZATIONS

Osteoporosis and Related Bone Diseases-National Resource Center. 1150 17th S. NW, Ste. 500, Washington, DC 20036. (800)624-BONE.

The Paget Foundation. 200 Varick Street, Ste. 1004. New York, NY 10014-4810. (800)23-PAGET.

OTHER

Endocrine Web. Endocrine disorder and endocrine surgery. http://www.endocrineweb.com.

Teresa G. Norris

Hyperphosphatemia *see* **Phosphorus imbalance**

Hyperpigmentation

Definition

Hyperpigmentation is the increase in the natural color of the skin.

Description

Melanin, a brown pigment manufactured by certain cells in the skin called melanocytes, is responsible for skin color. Melanin production is stimulated by a pituitary hormone called melanocyte stimulating hormone (MSH). Other pigments appear in the skin much less often.

Causes & symptoms

Darkened spots on the skin come in several varieties. The most ominous is **malignant melanoma,** a very aggressive **cancer** that begins as an innocent mole. The majority of **moles** (nevus), however, are and remain benign (harmless). The average person has several dozen, and certain people with a hereditary excess may have hundreds. Freckles, age spots, and cafe au lait spots, known as ephelides, are always flat and not as dark. Cafe au lait spots are seen mostly in people with another hereditary disorder called neurofibromatosis. "Port wine stains" are congenital dark red blotches on the skin. Other common dark colorations on the skin are called keratosis and consist of locally overgrown layers of skin that are dark primarily because there is more tissue than normal. A few of these turn into skin cancers of a much less dangerous kind than melanoma.

Darkened regions of the skin occur as a result of abnormal tanning when the skin is sensitive to sunlight. Several diseases and many drugs can cause **photosensitivity.** Among the common drugs responsible for this uncommon reaction are birth control pills, **antibiotics** (**sulfonamides** and **tetracyclines**), diuretics, **nonsteroidal anti-inflammatory drugs** (NSAID), **pain** relievers, and a couple psychoactive medications. Some of the same drugs may also cause patches of discolored skin known as localized drug reactions and

KEY TERMS

Addison's disease—A degenerative disease that is characterized by weight loss, low blood pressure, extreme weakness, and dark brown pigmentation of the skin.

Dermatologist—A physician specializing in the study of skin conditions and diseases

Diuretic—A cause of increased urine flow.

Keratosis—A skin disease characterized by an overgrowth of skin, which usually appears discolored.

Lesion—Any localized abnormality.

Melasma—Dark pigmentation of the skin.

Neurofibromatosis—Otherwise known as von Recklinghausen's disease, consists of pigmented skin spots and numerous soft tumors all over the body.

Nevus—Birthmark or mole.

NSAID—Nonsteroidal anti-inflammatory drugs—aspirin, ibuprofen, naproxen, and many others.

Porphyria cutanea tarda—An inherited disease that results in the overproduction of porphyrins.

Syndrome—Common features of a disease or features that appear together often enough to suggest they may represent a single, as yet unknown, disease entity.

representing an allergy to that drug. Sunlight darkens an abnormal chemical in the skin of patients with porphyria cutanea tarda. Several endocrine diseases, some cancers, and several drugs abnormally stimulate melanocytes, usually through an overproduction of MSH. Arsenic poisoning and **Addison's disease** are among these causes. A condition known as acanthosis nigricans is a velvety darkening of skin in folded areas (arm pits, groin, and neck) that can signal a cancer or hormone imbalance.

Of particular note is a condition called melasma (dark pigmentation of the skin), caused by the female hormone estrogen. Normal in **pregnancy,** this brownish discoloration of the face can also happen with birth control pills that contain estrogen.

Overall darkening of the skin may be due to pigmented chemicals in the skin. Silver, gold, and iron each have a characteristic color when visible in the skin. Several drugs and body chemicals, like bilirubin, can end up as deposits in the skin and discolor it.

There are a number of other rare entities that color the skin, each in its own peculiar way. Among these are strange syndromes that seem to be **birth defects** and vitamin and nutritional deficiencies.

Diagnosis

The pattern of discoloration is immediately visible to the trained dermatologist, a physician specializing in skin diseases, and may be all that is required to name and characterize the discoloration. Many of these pigment changes are signs of internal disease that must be identified. Pigmentation changes may also be caused by medication, and the drug responsible for the reaction must be identified and removed.

Treatment

Skin sensitive to sunlight must be protected by shade or **sunscreens** with an SPF of 15 or greater. Skin cancers must be, and unsightly benign lesions may be, surgically removed. **Laser surgery** is an effective removal technique for many localized lesions. Because it spreads so rapidly, melanoma should be immediately removed, as well as some of the surrounding tissue to prevent regrowth.

Prevention

Sunlight is the leading cause of dark spots on the skin, so shade and sunscreens are necessary preventive strategies, especially in people who burn easily.

Resources

BOOKS

Bennett, J. Claude and Fred Plum, ed. *Cecil Textbook of Medicine.* Philadelphia: W. B. Saunders, 1996.

Bolognia, Jean L. and Irwin M. Braverman. ''Skin manifestations of internal disease.'' In *Harrison's Principles of Internal Medicine.* Edited by Kurt Isselbacher, et al. New York: McGraw-Hill, 1998, pp. 318-320.

Mosher, David B. ''Disorders of pigmentation.'' In *Dermatology in General Medicine.* Edited by Thomas B. Fitzpatrick, et al. New York: McGraw-Hill, 1993, pp. 903-995.

PERIODICALS

Bernstein L.J., A.N. Kauvar, M.C. Grossman, and R.G. Geronemus. ''The short- and long-term side effects of carbon dioxide laser resurfacing.'' *Dermatologic Surgery* 23 (July 1997): 519-525.

Fitzpatrick, R.E., M.P. Goldman, N.M. Satur, and W.D. Tope. ''Pulsed carbon dioxide laser resurfacing of photo-aged facial skin.'' *Archives of Dermatology* 132 (April 1996): 395-402.

Rubin, M.G. ''A peeler's thoughts on skin improvement with chemical peels and laser resurfacing.'' *Clinics in Plastic Surgery* 24 (April 1997): 407-409.

Waldorf, H.A., A.N. Kauvar, and R.G. Geronemus. "Skin resurfacing of fine to deep rhytides using a char-free carbon dioxide laser in 47 patients." *Dermatologic Surgery* 21 (November 1995): 940-946.

J. Ricker Polsdorfer

Hyperprolactation *see* **Galactorrhea**

Hypersensitivity pneumonitis

Definition

Hypersensitivity pneumonitis refers to an inflammation of the lungs caused by repeated breathing in of a foreign substance, such an organic dust, a fungus, or a mold. The body's immune system reacts to these substances, called antigens, by forming antibodies, molecules that attack the invading antigen and try to destroy it. The combination of antigen and antibody produces acute inflammation, or pneumonitis (a hypersensitivity reaction), which later can develop into chronic lung disease that impairs the lungs' ability to take oxygen from the air and eliminate carbon dioxide.

Description

Hypersensitivity pneumonitis (HP) is sometimes called "allergic alveolitis." "Allergic" refers to the antigen-antibody reaction, and "alveolitis" means an inflammation of the tiny air sacs in the lungs where oxygen and CO_2 are exchanged, the alveoli. It also is known as "extrinsic" allergic alveolitis, meaning that the antigen that sets up the allergic reaction (also called an allergen) comes from the outside. Most of the antigens that cause this disease come from plant or animal proteins or microorganisms, and many of those affected are exposed either at work or in the course of some hobby or other activity. The first known type of HP, farmer's lung, is caused by antigens from tiny microorganisms living on moldy hay. An example of disease connected with a hobby is pigeon breeder's lung, caused by inhaling protein material from bird droppings or feathers. After a time, very little of the allergenic material is needed to set off a reaction in the lungs.

Roughly one in every 10,000 persons develops some form of HP. A mysterious aspect of this condition is that, even though many persons may be exposed to a particular antigen, only a small number of them will develop the disease. Genetic differences may determine who becomes ill; this remains unclear. Probably between 5% and 15% of all persons who are regularly exposed to organic materials develop HP. Most of those who do get it do *not*

KEY TERMS

Allergen—An outside substance, such as dust or a mold, that, when inhaled, sets off an allregic (hypersensitivity) reaction in the lungs.

Fibrosis—A result of long-standing inflammatory disease in which normal tissue is replaced by scar tissue that is functionally useless.

Granuloma—A collection of inflammatory cells forming a microscopic lesion, many of which are scattered throughout the lung tissue in patients who have had numerous acute episodes of HP.

Hypersensitivity—After the body's immune system attacks an outsider invader (such as organic dust or a fungus) many times, exposure to even a tiny amount of this allergen can provoke a strong inflammatory response the hypersensitivity response.

Pneumonitis—Inflammation of the lung tissues.

Steroid—A natural body substance which may be given orally or by injection, and serves to dampen or even halt inflammation anywhere in the body, including the lungs.

smoke (smoking may create the type of cells that take up antigens and neutralize them). The amount of antigen is an important factor in whether HP will develop and what form it will take. Sudden heavy exposure can produce symptoms in a matter of hours, whereas mild but frequent exposures tend to produce a long-lasting, "smoldering" illness. HP may be more likely to develop in persons exposed to polluted air or industrial fumes.

Typical changes occur in the lungs of persons with HP. In the acute stage, large numbers of inflammatory cells are found throughout the lungs and the air sacs may be filled by a thick fluid mixed with these cells. In the subacute stage, disease extends into the small breathing tubes, or bronchioles, and the inflammatory cells collect into tiny granules called granulomas. Finally, in the chronic stage of HP, the previously inflamed parts of the lungs become scarred and unable to function, as in pulmonary fibrosis.

Causes & symptoms

A number of different types of HP are known, since a wide range of allergens may produce an allergic reaction in the lungs. Many of them produce similar symptoms and abnormal physical findings, but some have their own typical features. Some of the more common forms are:

- Farmer's lung. Can affect any farmer who works with wet hay or other moldy dust. Small farmers who have to directly thresh and handle their hay are most at risk, as are those living in cold and humid areas where damp weather is common.

- Pigeon breeder's lung. Also called "bird fancier's lung," it is second to farmer's lung as the best known type of HP. A substance has been found in pigeon droppings that may cause the allergic reaction, but there may be more than one such substance. Besides pigeons, the disorder may follow exposure to ducks, geese, pheasants, and even canaries. Parakeets produce an especially severe form of disease. Most patients are middle-aged women, who usually care for birds either at home or on bird breeding farms.

- Bagassosis. Caused by bagasse, a substance produced when juice is extracted from sugar cane and is used in making paper and explosives. A fungus is probably responsible. Young and middle-aged men who work in the sugar industry are at risk.

- **Byssinosis.** A similar condition affecting workers who inhale dust from cotton, flax, or hemp.

- Humidifier lung. An acute form of HP caused by inhaling actinomycetes, the same organisms that cause farmer's lung, which grow in contaminated humidifier vents, air conditioners, heating systems, and even saunas.

- Other antigens. HP has been seen in persons working with detergents, silicone, mushrooms, cheese, wood dust, maple bark, coffee, and furs.

In the acute stage, patients with HP begin coughing, develop **fever,** and note tightness in the chest as well as extreme tiredness and aching, four to eight hours after the most recent exposure. Most patients are well aware of the connection between their work (or an activity) and their symptoms. After a time, patients may have trouble breathing. They also may lose their appetite, lose weight, and generally feel ill. Finally, in the chronic stage, the patient will have increasing trouble breathing and may sometimes wheeze. With advanced disease, the skin may appear bluish (because too little oxygen is getting into the blood). When the physician listens to the patient's chest with a stethoscope, there may be crackling sounds or loud **wheezing.** In the late stages, club-shaped fingertips are a sign that the patient has not been getting enough oxygen for an extended period of time.

Diagnosis

No single test can make a definite diagnosis of HP. The key is to relate some specific exposure or activity to episodes of symptoms. The chest x ray may be normal in the acute stage, but later may show a hazy appearance that looks like "ground glass." There may be linear or rounded shadows in the central parts of the lungs. Studies of lung function in the acute stage typically show abnormally small lung volume. The ability to breathe at a fast rate is impaired. Blood from an artery typically has a low level of oxygen. Later, when the lungs have begun to scar, the airways (breathing tubes) are obstructed and the rate of air flow is reduced.

Some experts believe that skin testing can help diagnose HP and show which particular antigen is causing the symptoms. Small amounts of several suspect antigens are injected just beneath the surface of the skin, usually on the arm or back, and the reactions compared to that caused by injecting a harmless salt solution. Another diagnostic test is to place a thin tube into the airways, inject a small amount of fluid, and draw it back up (bronchoalveolar lavage). A very large number of cells called lymphocytes is typical of HP, and mast cells, which are part of the immune system, may also be seen. Rarely, a tissue sample (biopsy) of lung tissue may be taken through a tube placed in the airways and examined under a microscope. Finally, a patient may be "challenged" by actually inhaling a particular antigen in the form of an aerosol and noting whether lung function suddenly becomes worse. This test is usually not necessary.

Treatment

Treatment of HP requires identifying the offending antigen and avoiding further exposure. Although it may sometimes be necessary for a patient to find a totally different type of work, often it is possible to simply perform different duties or switch to a work site where exposure is minimal. In some cases, (like pigeon breeder's lung), wearing a mask can prevent exposure. If acute symptoms are severe, the patient may be treated with a steroid hormone for two to six weeks. This often suppresses the inflammatory response and allows the lungs a chance to recover. In the chronic stage, steroid treatment can delay further damage to the lungs and help preserve their function.

Prognosis

In general, most of the symptoms of HP disappear when the patient is no longer exposed to the causative allergen. The actual chances of complete recovery depend in part on what form of HP is present. Older patients and those exposed repeatedly for long periods after initially developing symptoms tend to have a poorer long-term outlook. The worst outcome is that long repeated episodes of exposure will cause chronic lung inflammation, scar the lungs, and permanently make then unable to properly provide oxygen to the blood. Rarely, a patient will become permanently disabled.

Prevention

It is often not possible to prevent initial episodes of HP, because there is no way of predicting which individuals (such as farmers) will have an allergic reaction to a particular allergen. Once the connection is made between a type of exposure and definite hypersensitivity symptoms, prevention of further episodes is simple as long as further exposure can be avoided.

Exactly how to avoid exposure depends on a person's work or activities and what he or she is reacting to. People with farmer's lung can dry hay thoroughly before storing it. For pigeon breeder's lung (and many other types of HP), a mask can be worn. In many industrial settings, it is possible to take precautions that will limit the amount of allergen that workers will inhale. If it is not possible to avoid exposure altogether, exposure can be timed and strictly minimized.

Resources

BOOKS

Smolley, Lawrence A. and Bryse, Debra F. *Breathe Right Now: A Comprehensive Guide to Understanding and Treating the Most Common Breathing Disorders.* New York: W. W. Norton & Co., 1998.

ORGANIZATIONS

American Lung Association. 432 Park Avenue South, New York, NY 10016. 800-LUNG-USA. http://www.lungusa.org.

Asthma and Allergy Foundation of America. 1125 15th St. NW, Suite 502, Washington, DC 20005. 800-7ASTHMA. http://www.housecall.com/sponsors/nhc/1966vha/aafa.html.

OTHER

University of Wisconsin-Madison Health Sciences Libraries *Healthweb: Pulmonary Medicine.* January 12, 1998. http://www.biostat.wisc.edu/chslib/hw/pulmonar.

David A. Cramer

Hypersomnia *see* **Sleep disorders**

Hypersplenism

Definition

Hypersplenism is a type of disorder which causes the spleen to rapidly and prematurely destroy blood cells.

Description

The spleen is located in the upper left area of the abdomen. One of this organ's major functions is to remove blood cells from the body's bloodstream. In hypersplenism, its normal function accelerates, and it begins to automatically remove cells that may still be normal in function. Sometimes, the spleen will temporarily hold onto up to 90% of the body's platelets and 45% of the red blood cells. Hypersplenism may occur as a primary disease, leading to other complications, or as a secondary disease, resulting from an underlying disease or disorder. Hypersplenism is sometimes referred to as enlarged spleen (splenomegaly). An enlarged spleen is one of the symptoms of hypersplenism. What differentiates hypersplenism is its premature destruction of blood cells.

Causes & symptoms

Hypersplenism may be caused by a variety of disorders. Sometimes, it is brought on by a problem within the spleen itself and is referred to as primary hypersplenism. Secondary hypersplenism results from another disease such as chronic **malaria, rheumatoid arthritis, tuberculosis,** or **polycythemia vera,** a blood disorder. Spleen disorders in general are almost always secondary in nature. Hypersplenism may also be caused by tumors.

Symptoms of hypersplenism include easy bruising, easy contracting of bacterial diseases, **fever,** weakness, heart **palpitations,** and ulcerations of the mouth, legs and feet. Individuals may also bleed unexpectedly and heavily from the nose or other mucous membranes, and from the gastrointestinal or urinary tracts. Most patients will develop an enlarged spleen, anemia, leukopenia, or abnormally low white blood cell counts, or **thrombocytopenia,** a deficiency of circulating platelets in the blood. Other symptoms may be presents that reflect the underlying disease that has caused hypersplenism.

An enlarged spleen can be caused by a variety of diseases, including **hemolytic anemia,** liver **cirrhosis,** leukemia, malignant lymphoma and other infections and inflammatory diseases. Splenomegaly occurs in about 10% of **systemic lupus erythematosus** patients. Sometimes, it is caused by recent viral infection, such as mononucleosis. An enlarged spleen may cause **pain** in the upper left side of the abdomen and a premature feeling of fullness at meals.

Diagnosis

Diagnosis of hypersplenism begins with review of symptoms and patient history, and careful feeling (palpation) of the spleen. Sometimes, a physician can feel an enlarged spleen. X-ray studies, such as ultrasound and **computed tomography scan** (CT scan), may help diagnose an enlarged spleen and possible underlying causes, such as tumors. Blood tests indicate decreases in white blood cells, red blood cells, or platelets. Another test measures red blood cells in the liver and spleen after injection of a radioactive substance, and indicates areas where the spleen is holding on to large numbers of red cells or is destroying them.

Enlarged spleens are diagnosed using a combination of patient history, **physical examination,** including palpation of the spleen, if possible, and diagnostic tests. A history of fever and systemic symptoms may be present because of infection, malaria, or an inflammatory disorder. A complete **blood count** is taken to check counts of young red blood cells. **Liver function tests,** CT scans, and ultrasound exams can also help to detect an enlarged spleen.

Treatment

In secondary hypersplenism, the underlying disease must be treated to prevent further sequestration or destruction of blood cells, and possible spleen enlargement. Those therapies will be tried prior to removal of the spleen (**splenectomy**), which is avoided if possible. In severe cases, the spleen must be removed. Splenectomy will correct the effects of low blood cell concentrations in the blood.

Prognosis

Prognosis depends on the underlying cause and progression of the disease. Left untreated, spleen enlargement can lead to serious complications. Hypersplenism can also lead to complications due to decreased blood cell counts.

Prevention

Some of the underlying causes of hypersplenism or enlarged spleen can be prevented, such as certain forms of anemia and cirrhosis of the liver due to alcohol. In other cases, the hypersplenism may not be preventable, as it is a complication to an underlying disorder.

Resources

BOOKS

Conn, Howard F., Robert J. Clohecy, and Rex B. Conn. *Current Diagnosis.* 9th ed. Philadelphia, PA: WB Saunders Company, 1997.

ORGANIZATIONS

American Liver Foundation. 1425 Pompton Ave., Cedar Grove, NJ 07009. 1-800-GOLIVER (445-4837).

The American Society of Hematology. 1200 19th Street NW, Suite 300, Washington, DC 20036-2422. (202) 857-1118. http://www.hematology.org.

National Heart, Lung and Blood Institute. Building 31, Room 4A21, Bethesda, MD 20892. (301) 496-4236. http://www.nhlbi.nih.gov.

Teresa G. Norris

Hypertension

Definition

Hypertension is high blood pressure. Blood pressure is the force of blood pushing against the walls of arteries as it flows through them. Arteries are the blood vessels that carry oxygenated blood from the heart to the body's tissues.

Description

As blood flows through arteries it pushes against the inside of the artery walls. The more pressure the blood exerts on the artery walls, the higher the blood pressure will be. The size of small arteries also affects the blood pressure. When the muscular walls of arteries are relaxed, or dilated, the pressure of the blood flowing through them is lower than when the artery walls narrow, or constrict.

KEY TERMS

Arteries—Blood vessels that carry blood to organs and other tissues of the body.

Arteriosclerosis—Hardening and thickening of artery walls.

Cushing's syndrome—A disorder in which too much of the adrenal hormone, cortisol, is produced; it may be caused by a pituitary or adrenal gland tumor.

Diastolic blood pressure—Blood pressure when the heart is resting between beats.

Hypertension—High blood pressure.

Renal artery stenosis—Disorder in which the arteries that supply blood to the kidneys constrict.

Sphygmomanometer—An instrument used to measure blood pressure.

Systolic blood pressure—Blood pressure when the heart contracts (beats).

Vasodilator—Any drug that relaxes blood vessel walls.

Ventricle—One of the two lower chambers of the heart.

Blood pressure is highest when the heart beats to push blood out into the arteries. When the heart relaxes to fill with blood again, the pressure is at its lowest point. Blood pressure when the heart beats is called systolic pressure. Blood pressure when the heart is at rest is called diastolic pressure. When blood pressure is measured, the

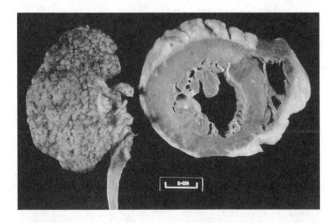

The effects of hypertension on the heart and kidney. Hypertension has caused renal atrophy and scarring, and left ventricular hypertrophy in the sectioned heart (at right). *(Photograph by Dr. E. Walker, Photo Researchers, Inc. Reproduced by permission.)*

systolic pressure is stated first and the diastolic pressure second. Blood pressure is measured in millimeters of mercury (mm Hg). For example, if a person's systolic pressure is 120 and diastolic pressure is 80, it is written as 120/80 mm Hg. The American Heart Association considers blood pressure less than 140 over 90 normal for adults.

Hypertension is a major health problem, especially because it has no symptoms. Many people have hypertension without knowing it. In the United States, about 50 million people age six and older have high blood pressure. Hypertension is more common in men than women and in people over the age of 65 than in younger persons. More than half of all Americans over the age of 65 have hypertension. It is also more common in African-Americans than in white Americans.

Hypertension is serious because people with the condition have a higher risk for heart disease and other medical problems than people with normal blood pressure. Serious complications can be avoided by getting regular blood pressure checks and treating hypertension as soon as it is diagnosed.

If left untreated, hypertension can lead to the following medical conditions:

• Arteriosclerosis, also called **atherosclerosis**

• **Heart attack**

• **Stroke**

• Enlarged heart

• Kidney damage.

Arteriosclerosis is hardening of the arteries. The walls of arteries have a layer of muscle and elastic tissue that makes them flexible and able to dilate and constrict as blood flows through them. High blood pressure can make the artery walls thicken and harden. When artery walls thicken, the inside of the blood vessel narrows. Cholesterol and fats are more likely to build up on the walls of damaged arteries, making them even narrower. Blood clots can also get trapped in narrowed arteries, blocking the flow of blood.

Arteries narrowed by arteriosclerosis may not deliver enough blood to organs and other tissues. Reduced or blocked blood flow to the heart can cause a heart attack. If an artery to the brain is blocked, a stroke can result.

Hypertension makes the heart work harder to pump blood through the body. The extra workload can make the heart muscle thicken and stretch. When the heart becomes too enlarged it cannot pump enough blood. If the hypertension is not treated, the heart may fail.

The kidneys remove the body's wastes from the blood. If hypertension thickens the arteries to the kidneys, less waste can be filtered from the blood. As the condition worsens, the kidneys fail and wastes build up in the blood. Dialysis or a kidney transplant are needed when the kidneys fail. About 25% of people who receive **kidney** dialysis have kidney failure caused by hypertension.

Causes & symptoms

Many different actions or situations can normally raise blood pressure. Physical activity can temporarily raise blood pressure. Stressful situations can make blood pressure go up. When the stress goes away, blood pressure usually returns to normal. These temporary increases in blood pressure are not considered hypertension. A diagnosis of hypertension made only when a person has multiple high blood pressure readings over a period of time.

The cause of hypertension is not known in 90 to 95 percent of the people who have it. Hypertension without a known cause is called primary or essential hypertension.

When a person has hypertension caused by another medical condition, it is called secondary hypertension. Secondary hypertension can be caused by a number of different illnesses. Many people with kidney disorders have secondary hypertension. The kidneys regulate the balance of salt and water in the body. If the kidneys cannot rid the body of excess salt and water, blood pressure goes up. Kidney infections, a narrowing of the arteries that carry blood to the kidneys, called renal artery stenosis, and other kidney disorders can disturb the salt and water balance.

Cushing's syndrome and tumors of the pituitary and adrenal glands often increase levels of the adrenal gland hormones cortisol, adrenalin and aldosterone, which can cause hypertension. Other conditions that can cause hypertension are blood vessel diseases, thyroid gland disorders, some prescribed drugs, **alcoholism** and **pregnancy.**

Even though the cause of most hypertension is not known, some people have risk factors that give them a greater chance of getting hypertension. Many of these risk factors can be changed to lower the chance of developing hypertension or as part of a treatment program to lower blood pressure.

Risk factors for hypertension include:

• Age over 60

• Male sex

• Race

• Heredity

• Salt sensitivity

• **Obesity**

• Inactive lifestyle

• Heavy alcohol consumption

• Use of **oral contraceptives.**

Some risk factors for getting hypertension can be changed, while others cannot. Age, male sex, and race are risk factors that a person can't do anything about. Some people inherit a tendency to get hypertension. People with family members who have hypertension are more likely to develop it than those whose relatives are not hypertensive. A person with these risk factors can avoid or eliminate the other risk factors to lower their chance of developing hypertension.

Diagnosis

Because hypertension doesn't cause symptoms, it is important to have blood pressure checked regularly. Blood pressure is measured with an instrument called a sphygmomanometer. A cloth-covered rubber cuff is wrapped around the upper arm and inflated. When the cuff is inflated, an artery in the arm is squeezed to momentarily stop the flow of blood. Then, the air is let out of the cuff while a stethoscope placed over the artery is used to detect the sound of the blood spurting back through the artery. This first sound is the systolic pressure, the pressure when the heart beats. The last sound heard as the rest of the air is released is the diastolic pressure, the pressure between heart beats. Both sounds are recorded on the mercury gauge on the sphygmomanometer.

Normal blood pressure is defined by a range of values. Blood pressure lower than 140/90 mm Hg is considered normal. A blood pressure around 120/80 mm Hg is considered the best level to avoid heart disease. A number of factors such as **pain,** stress or **anxiety** can cause a temporary increase in blood pressure. For this reason, hypertension is not diagnosed on one high blood pressure reading. If a blood pressure reading is 140/90 or higher for the first time, the physician will have the person return for another blood pressure check. Diagnosis of hypertension usually is made based on two or more readings after the first visit.

Systolic hypertension of the elderly is common and is diagnosed when the diastolic pressure is normal or low, but the systolic is elevated, e.g.170/70 mm Hg. This condition usually co-exists with hardening of the arteries (atherosclerosis).

Blood pressure measurements are classified in stages, according to severity:

• Normal blood pressure: less than 130/85 mm Hg

• High normal: 130–139/85–89 mm Hg

• Mild hypertension: 140–159/90–99 mm Hg

• Moderate hypertension: 160–179/100–109 mm Hg

• Severe hypertension: 180–209/110–119

• Very severe hypertension: 210/120 or higher.

A typical **physical examination** to evaluate hypertension includes:

• Medical and family history

• Physical examination

• Ophthalmoscopy: Examination of the blood vessels in the eye

• **Chest x ray**

• Electrocardiograph (ECG)

• Blood and urine tests.

The medical and family history help the physician determine if the patient has any conditions or disorders that might contribute to or cause the hypertension. A family history of hypertension might suggest a genetic predisposition for hypertension.

The physical exam may include several blood pressure readings at different times and in different positions. The physician uses a stethoscope to listen to sounds made by the heart and blood flowing through the arteries. The pulse, reflexes, and height and weight are checked and recorded. Internal organs are palpated, or felt, to determine if they are enlarged.

Because hypertension can cause damage to the blood vessels in the eyes, the eyes may be checked with a instrument called an ophthalmoscope. The physician will look for thickening, narrowing, or hemorrhages in the blood vessels.

A chest x ray can detect an enlarged heart, other vascular (heart) abnormalities, or lung disease.

An electrocardiogram (ECG) measures the electrical activity of the heart. It can detect if the heart muscle is enlarged and if there is damage to the heart muscle from blocked arteries.

Urine and blood tests may be done to evaluate health and to detect the presence of disorders that might cause hypertension.

Treatment

There is no cure for primary hypertension, but blood pressure can almost always be lowered with the correct treatment. The goal of treatment is to lower blood pressure to levels that will prevent heart disease and other complications of hypertension. In secondary hypertension, the disease that is responsible for the hypertension is treated in addition to the hypertension itself. Successful treatment of the underlying disorder may cure the secondary hypertension.

Treatment to lower blood pressure usually includes changes in diet, getting regular **exercise,** and taking antihypertensive medications. Patients with mild or moderate hypertension who don't have damage to the heart or kidneys may first be treated with lifestyle changes.

Lifestyle changes that may reduce blood pressure by about 5 to 10 mm Hg include:

• Reducing salt intake

• Reducing fat intake

• Losing weight

• Getting regular exercise

• Quitting smoking

• Reducing alcohol consumption

• Managing stress.

Patients whose blood pressure remains higher than 139/90 will most likely be advised to take antihypertensive medication. Numerous drugs have been developed to treat hypertension. The choice of medication will depend on the stage of hypertension, side effects, other medical conditions the patient may have, and other medicines the patient is taking.

Patients with mild or moderate hypertension are initially treated with monotherapy, a single antihypertensive medicine. If treatment with a single medicine fails to lower blood pressure enough, a different medicine may be tried or another medicine may be added to the first. Patients with more severe hypertension may initially be given a combination of medicines to control their hypertension. Combining antihypertensive medicines with different types of action often controls blood pressure with smaller doses of each drug than would be needed for monotherapy.

Antihypertensive medicines fall into several classes of drugs:

• **Diuretics**

• Beta-blockers

• **Calcium channel blockers**

• Angiotensin converting enzyme inhibitors (ACE inhibitors)

• Alpha-blockers

• Alpha-**beta blockers**

• **Vasodilators**

• Peripheral acting adrenergic antagonists

• Centrally acting agonists.

Diuretics help the kidneys eliminate excess salt and water from the body's tissues and the blood. This helps reduce the swelling caused by fluid buildup in the tissues. The reduction of fluid dilates the walls of arteries and lowers blood pressure.

Beta-blockers lower blood pressure by acting on the nervous system to slow the heart rate and reduce the force of the heart's contraction. They are used with caution in patients with **heart failure, asthma,** diabetes, or circulation problems in the hands and feet.

Calcium channel blockers block the entry of calcium into muscle cells in artery walls. Muscle cells need calcium to constrict, so reducing their calcium keeps them more relaxed and lowers blood pressure.

ACE inhibitors block the production of substances that constrict blood vessels. They also help reduce the build-up of water and salt in the tissues. They are often given to patients with heart failure, kidney disease, or diabetes. ACE inhibitors may be used together with diuretics.

Alpha-blockers act on the nervous system to dilate arteries and reduce the force of the heart's contractions.

Alpha-beta blockers combine the actions of alpha and beta blockers.

Vasodilators act directly on arteries to relax their walls so blood can move more easily through them. They lower blood pressure rapidly and are injected in hypertensive emergencies when patients have dangerously high blood pressure.

Peripheral acting adrenergic antagonists act on the nervous system to relax arteries and reduce the force of the heart's contractions. They usually are prescribed together with a diuretic. Peripheral acting adrenergic antagonists can cause slowed mental function and lethargy.

Centrally acting agonists also act on the nervous system to relax arteries and slow the heart rate. They are usually used with other antihypertensive medicines.

Prognosis

There is no cure for hypertension. However, it can be well controlled with the proper treatment. Therapy with a combination of lifestyle changes and antihypertensive medicines usually can keep blood pressure at levels that will not cause damage to the heart or other organs. The key to avoiding serious complications of hypertension is to detect and treat it before damage occurs. Because antihypertensive medicines control blood pressure, but do not cure it, patients must continue taking the medications to maintain reduced blood pressure levels and avoid complications.

Prevention

Prevention of hypertension centers on avoiding or eliminating known risk factors. Even persons at risk because of age, race, or sex or those who have an inherited risk can lower their chance of developing hypertension.

The risk of developing hypertension can be reduced by making the same changes recommended for treating hypertension:

- Reducing salt intake
- Reducing fat intake
- Losing weight
- Getting regular exercise
- Quitting smoking
- Reducing alcohol consumption
- Managing stress.

Resources

BOOKS

Bellenir, Karen and Peter D. Dresser, editors. *Cardiovascular Diseases and Disorders Sourcebook.* Detroit: Omnigraphics, 1995.

Texas Heart Institute. *Heart Owner's Handbook.* New York: John Wiley and Sons, 1996.

ORGANIZATIONS

American Heart Association. 7272 Greenview Avenue, Dallas, TX 75231-4596. (800) AHS-USA1. http://www.amhrt.org/.

National Heart, Lung, and Blood Institute. Information Center. PO Box 30105, Bethesda, MD 20824-0105. (301) 251-1222.

Texas Heart Institute. Heart Information Service, PO Box 20345, Houston, TX 77225-0345. (800) 292-2221.

Toni Rizzo

Hypertensive retinopathy *see* **Retinopathies**

Hyperthermia *see* **Fever**

Hyperthyroidism

Definition

Hyperthyroidism is the overproduction of thyroid hormones by an overactive thyroid.

Description

Located in the front of the neck, the thyroid gland produces the hormones thyroxine (T_4) and triiodothyronine (T_3) that regulate the body's metabolic rate by helping to form protein ribonucleic acid (RNA) and increasing oxygen absorption in every cell. In turn, the production of these hormones are controlled by thyroid-stimulating hormone (TSH) that is produced by the pituitary gland. When production of the thyroid hormones increases despite the level of TSH being produced, hyperthyroidism occurs. The excessive amount of thyroid hormones in the blood increases the body's metabolism, creating both mental and physical symptoms.

The term hyperthyroidism covers any disease which results in overabundance of thyroid hormone. Other names for hyperthyroidism, or specific diseases within the category, include Graves' disease, diffuse toxic **goiter**, Basedow's disease, Parry's disease, and thyrotoxicosis. The disease is 10 times more common in

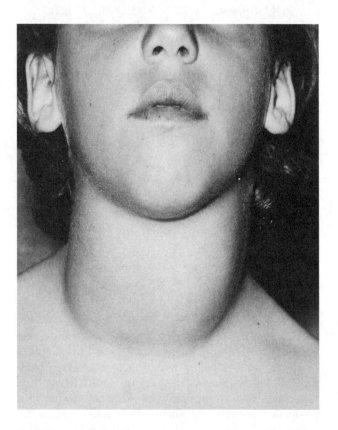

A symptom of hyperthyroidism is the enlargement of the thyroid gland. *(Photograph by Lester V. Bergman, Corbis Images. Reproduced by permission.)*

women than in men, and the annual incidence of hyperthyroidism in the United States is about one per 1,000 women. Although it occurs at all ages, hyperthyroidism is most likely to occur after the age of 15. There is a form of hyperthyroidism called Neonatal Grave's disease, which occurs in infants born of mothers with Graves' disease. Occult hyperthyroidism may occur in patients over 65 and is characterized by a distinct lack of typical symptoms. Diffuse toxic goiter occurs in as many as 80% of patients with hyperthyroidism.

Causes & symptoms

Hyperthyroidism is often associated with the body's production of autoantibodies in the blood which cause the thyroid to grow and secrete excess thyroid hormone. This condition, as well as other forms of hyperthyroidism, may be inherited. Regardless of the cause, hyperthyroidism produces the same symptoms, including weight loss with increased appetite, **shortness of breath** and fatigue, intolerance to heat, heart **palpitations,** increased frequency of bowel movements, weak muscles, **tremors, anxiety,** and difficulty sleeping. Women may also notice decreased menstrual flow and irregular menstrual cycles.

Patients with Graves' disease often have a goiter (visible enlargement of the thyroid gland), although as many as 10% do not. These patients may also have bulging eyes. Thyroid storm, a serious form of hyperthyroidism, may show up as sudden and acute symptoms, some of which mimic typical hyperthyroidism, as well as the addition of **fever,** substantial weakness, extreme restlessness, confusion, emotional swings or **psychosis,** and perhaps even **coma.**

Diagnosis

Physicians will look for physical signs and symptoms indicated by patient history. On inspection, the physician may note symptoms such as a goiter or eye bulging. Other symptoms or family history may be clues to a diagnosis of hyperthyroidism. An elevated body temperature (basal body temperature) above 98.6°F (37°C) may be an indication of a heightened metabolic rate (basal metabolic rate) and hyperthyroidism. A simple blood test can be performed to determine the amount of thyroid hormone in the patient's blood. The diagnosis is usually straightforward with this combination of clinical history, **physical examination,** and routine blood hormone tests. Radioimmunoassay, or a test to show concentrations of **thyroid hormones** with the use of a radioisotope mixed with fluid samples, helps confirm the diagnosis. A thyroid scan is a nuclear medicine procedure involving injection of a radioisotope dye which will tag the thyroid and help produce a clear image of inflammation or involvement of the entire thyroid. Other tests can determine thyroid function and thyroid-stimulating hormone levels. Ultrasonography, **computed tomography scans** (CT scan), and **magnetic resonance imaging** (MRI) may provide visual confirmation of a diagnosis or help to determine the extent of involvement.

Treatment

Treatment will depend on the specific disease and individual circumstances such as age, severity of disease, and other conditions affecting a patient's health.

Antithyroid drugs

Antithyroid drugs are often administered to help the patient's body cease overproduction of thyroid hormones. This medication may work for young adults, pregnant women, and others. Women who are pregnant should be treated with the lowest dose required to maintain thyroid function in order to minimize the risk of **hypothyroidism** in the infant.

Radioactive iodine

Radioactive iodine is often prescribed to damage cells that make thyroid hormone. The cells need iodine to make the hormone, so they will absorb any iodine found in the body. The patient may take an iodine capsule daily for several weeks, resulting in the eventual shrinkage of the thyroid in size, reduced hormone production and a return to normal blood levels. Some patients may receive a single larger oral dose of radioactive iodine to treat the disease more quickly. This should only be done for patients who are not of reproductive age or are not planning to have children, since a large amount can concentrate in the reproductive organs (gonads).

Surgery

Some patients may undergo surgery to treat hyper thyroidism. Most commonly, patients treated with **thyroidectomy,** in the form of partial or total removal of the thyroid, suffer from large goiter and have suffered relapses, even after repeated attempts to address the disease through drug therapy. Some patients may be candidates for surgery because they were not good candidates for iodine therapy, or refused iodine administration. Patients receiving thyroidectomy or iodine therapy must be carefully monitored for years to watch for signs of hypothyroidism, or insufficient production of thyroid hormones, which can occur as a complication of thyroid production suppression.

Alternative treatment

Consumption of foods such as broccoli, brussel sprouts, cabbage, cauliflower, kale, rutabagas, spinach, turnips, peaches, and pears can help naturally suppress thyroid hormone production. Caffeinated drinks and dairy products should be avoided. Under the supervision of a trained physician, high dosages of certain vitamin/mineral combinations can help alleviate hyperthyroidism.

Prognosis

Hyperthyroidism is generally treatable and carries a good prognosis. Most patients lead normal lives with proper treatment. Thyroid storm, however, can be life-threatening and can lead to heart, liver, or kidney failure.

Prevention

There are no known prevention methods for hyperthyroidism, since its causes are either inherited or not completely understood. The best prevention tactic is knowledge of family history and close attention to symptoms and signs of the disease. Careful attention to prescribed therapy can prevent complications of the disease.

Resources

BOOKS

The Burton Goldberg Group. *Alternative Medicine.* Puyallup, WA: Future Medicine Publishing Inc., 1994.

PERIODICALS

Lazarus, John H. ''Hyperthyroidism.'' *The Lancet* 340 (February 1, 1997): 339-342.

ORGANIZATIONS

The Thyroid Foundation of America. 350 Ruth Sleeper Hall - RSL 350, Parkman Street, Boston, MA. 02114. (800)832-8321. http://www.clark.net/pub/tfa.

OTHER

Endocrine Web. Endocrine disorder and endocrine surgery. http://www.endocrineweb.com.

Teresa G. Norris

Hypertrophic cardiomyopathy

Definition

Cardiomyopathy is an ongoing disease process that damages the muscle wall of the lower chambers of the heart. Hypertrophic cardiomyopathy is a form of cardiomyopathy in which the walls of the heart's chambers thicken abnormally. Other names for hypertrophic cardiomyopathy are idiopathic hypertrophic subaortic stenosis and asymmetrical septal hypertrophy.

Description

Hypertrophic cardiomyopathy usually appears in young people, often in athletes. For this reason it is sometimes called athletic heart muscle disease. However, people of any age can develop hypertrophic cardiomyop-

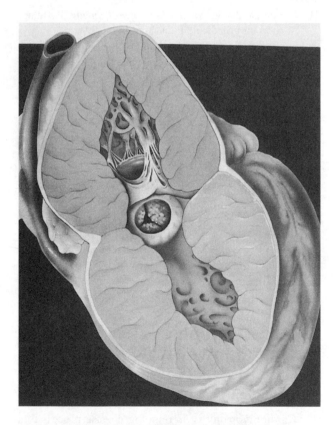

This illustration shows hypertrophic muscle in the heart. The abnormally thick wall of muscle prevents the chambers from stretching to fill up with blood, making the heart less efficient. The extra tissue may also push on the heart valve (center), causing it to leak. *(Illustration by Bryson Biomedical Illustrations, Custom Medical Stock Photo. Reproduced by permission.)*

athy. Often there are no symptoms of hypertrophic cardiomyopathy. Sudden **death** can occur, caused by a heart arrhythmia. The American Heart Association reports that 36% of young athletes who die suddenly have probable or definite hypertrophic cardiomyopathy.

Hypertrophic cardiomyopathy is the result of abnormal growth of the heart muscle cells. The wall between the heart's chambers (the septum) may become so thickened that it blocks the flow of blood through the lower left chamber (left ventricle). The thickened wall may push on the heart valve between the two left heart chambers (mitral valve), making it leaky. The thickened muscle walls also prevent the heart from stretching as much as it should to fill with blood.

Causes & symptoms

The cause of hypertrophic cardiomyopathy is not known. In about one-half of cases, the disease is inherited. An abnormal gene has been identified in these patients. In cases that are not hereditary, a gene that was normal at birth may later become abnormal.

Often people with hypertrophic cardiomyopathy have no symptoms. Unfortunately, the first sign of the condition may be sudden death caused by an abnormal heart rhythm. When symptoms do appear, they include **shortness of breath** on exertion, **dizziness, fainting,** fatigue, and chest **pain.**

Diagnosis

The diagnosis is based on the patient's symptoms (if any), a complete **physical examination,** and tests that detect abnormalities of the heart chambers. Usually, there is an abnormal heart murmur that worsens with the **Valsalva maneuver.** The electrocardiogram (ECG), which provides a record of electrical changes in the heart muscle during the heartbeat, also is typically abnormal.

Sometimes, a routine **chest x ray** may show that the heart is enlarged. **Echocardiography,** a procedure that produces images of the heart's structure, is usually done. These images can show if the heart wall is thickened and if there are any abnormalities of the heart valves.

Treatment

Treatment of hypertrophic cardiomyopathy usually consists of taking medicines and restricting strenuous **exercise.** Drugs called **beta blockers** and **calcium channel blockers** are usually prescribed. Beta blockers reduce the force of the heart's contractions. Calcium channel blockers can help improve the flexibility of the heart muscle walls, allowing them to stretch more. **Antiarrhythmic drugs** may also be given to prevent abnormal heart rhythms.

Patients with hypertrophic cardiomyopathy are also told to avoid strenuous exercise to reduce the risk of passing out or sudden death.

In some cases, if the medications do not help relieve symptoms, surgery may help. In an operation called myotomy-myectomy a piece of the septum is removed to improve blood flow through the heart chamber.

Some patients have **pacemakers** and/or defibrillators implanted to help control the heart rate and rhythm. Pacemakers and defibrillators provide electrical impulses to the heart, which can return the heart beat to a normal rhythm.

If these treatment methods fail and a patient develops **heart failure,** a heart transplant may be necessary.

Prognosis

Some people with hypertrophic cardiomyopathy may not have obstructed blood flow and may never experience symptoms. Others may only experience mild symptoms. With treatment, symptoms may improve. In some patients, the disease may progress to heart failure.

Prevention

While hypertrophic cardiomyopathy cannot be prevented, precautionary measures may prevent sudden deaths. Anyone planning to take part in a program of strenuous competitive exercise should have a check up by a physician first. A physical examination before athletic participation can usually, but not always, detect conditions like hypertrophic cardiomyopathy. Anyone who experiences symptoms of shortness of breath, tiredness, or fainting with exercise should see a physician.

Resources

BOOKS

Bellenir, Karen and Peter D. Dresser, editors. *Cardiovascular Diseases and Disorders Sourcebook.* Detroit: Omnigraphics, 1995.

Texas Heart Institute. *Heart Owner's Handbook.* New York: John Wiley and Sons, 1996.

ORGANIZATIONS

American Heart Association. 7272 Greenview Avenue, Dallas, TX 75231-4596. (800) AHS-USA1. http://www.amhrt.org/.

National Heart, Lung, and Blood Institute. Information Center, PO Box 30105, Bethesda, MD 20824-0105. (301) 251-1222.

Texas Heart Institute. Heart Information Service, PO Box 20345, Houston, TX 77225-0345. (800) 292-2221.

Toni Rizzo

Hypervitaminosis *see* **Vitamin toxicity**

Hypnosis

Definition

Hypnosis is a state described as sleeplike. It is usually induced by another individual for the purpose of tapping into the unconscious mind. As a result of the hypnosis, the subject may experience forgotten or suppressed memories. Hypnosis has also been described as a way to use a person's inherent healing capabilities that usually remain inaccessible to him and outside of his control.

Purpose

Hypnosis can be helpful in relaxation and **pain** reduction by decreasing muscle tension. Hypnosis can also reduce pain by helping the subject visualize and create an alternate reality perceived as being safe and comfortable. Many doctors now use hypnosis to overcome the pain of **headaches,** backaches, **childbirth, cancer,** severe **burns,** and pain and fear resulting from dental procedures. In some cases, surgeons use hypnosis in the operating room, not only to reduce the amount of anesthesia needed by the patient, but also to lessen **anxiety** and postoperative bleeding and swelling. In other instances, hypnosis has been found useful in reducing the severity of **asthma.**

Psychologists use hypnosis in treating patients to overcome negative habits, anxiety, fear and depression. Also, it is commonly used to help patients recall past events, which is useful in psychotherapy. Family physicians have recently begun to use hypnosis to treat psychosomatic illness (physical illnesses or complaints that are largely caused by psychological factors). Professionals in the field of psychotherapy have also found positive results in helping patients control appetite and reduce the levels of drugs necessary in the treatment chronic illness.

Precautions

Because hypnosis can sometimes completely remove or distract people from feeling pain, it is important that a doctor or other appropriate medical specialist assess the underlying medical or psychological condition prior to hypnosis. Another important precaution when dealing with hypnosis is that, despite potential medical benefits of hypnosis, misinterpretation is possible because of the questionable reliability of the memories recalled during hypnosis. Because there is no medical degree required for the practice of hypnotherapy, persons wishing to undergo hypnosis should be sure that the therapist is well trained. It may be helpful to find a therapist who is a licensed professional in a field where hypnotherapy is part of normal practice, such as social workers and psycholo-

KEY TERMS

Anesthesia—The absence of normal sensation, especially sensitivity to pain as induced by an anesthetic substance, or by hypnosis. May be induced for medical or surgical purposes topically, locally, regionally, or generally.

Hypnotherapist—A professional who uses hypnosis as an adjunct to other techniques in psychotherapy

gists. It is important to check credentials and background when choosing a hypnotherapist.

Hypnosis is not to be considered a form of psychotherapy, nor a treatment capable of solving problems immediately or on its own. Problems and habits take time to get implanted in one's life, and it takes considerable amount of time—and often therapy—to remove them.

Description

A hypnotic state results from gradually entering a state of consciousness unlike that of awareness or sleep. During this time, the attention of subjects is withdrawn from their surroundings. Most individuals can easily be hypnotized, but the depth and extent of the hypnotic state varies.

Hypnotherapy is the therapeutic use of hypnosis. In hypnotherapy, hypnosis is used by psychotherapists to modify a patient's behavior. According to the American Association of Professional Hypnotherapists, there is a 75–90% chance of effectively changing behavior with hypnotherapy. Once the patient has seen a hypnotherapist, self-hypnosis can be learned, and is sometimes recommended as part of the treatment plan. Self-hypnosis involves a patient using relaxation techniques and specific signals to clear his mind of extraneous thoughts and sensations.

Preparation

Hypnotherapy requires only that the patient desire to change a certain type of behavior. The hypnotherapist usually prepares for the sessions by asking the subject to stare at an object, suggesting, in a soothing voice, that the eyelids are becoming heavy, that the subject relax, and that he is becoming hypnotized. Then, the hypnotherapist conveys to the subject that it will be effortless to follow the hypnotherapist's suggestions

Aftercare

Coming out of the hypnotic state is as simple as entering it. Waking from the hypnotic state slowly is preferable for optimal results. After hypnosis, subjects report changes in bodily sensations and describe an awareness of having gone into an altered state of mind.

Risks

Because hypnosis can sometimes completely remove or distract people from feeling pain, it is important that a doctor, or other appropriate medical specialist, assess the underlying medical or psychological condition. This assessment is important because, when using hypnosis to reduce pain or other physical symptoms, the pain may be alerting the patient to a problem that needs some other form of medical or psychological treatment. As an example, a **brain tumor** might be causing chronic headaches, and require immediate treatment.

Normal results

Family doctors have begun using hypnosis to treat psychosomatic illness, control appetite, and reduce the need for medication. Because of the utility of using hypnosis to reduce the sensation of pain, it can make it possible for physicians to lower dosages of pain medication in cases of chronic illness. Because hypnosis is actually an intense state of concentration, physicians have now accepted the fact that patients can regulate their own heart rate, circulation, temperature, muscle tension, and other body functions, if necessary.

Abnormal results

Hypnotherapy requires that the patient desire to change a certain type of behavior. Success is greater the more committed the subject is to change. If the patient is reluctant, hypnotherapy may be unsuccessful.

Resources

BOOKS

Sarason, Irwin G., and Barbara R. Sarason. *Abnormal Psychology.* Englewood Cliffs, NJ: Prentice Hall, 1989.

PERIODICALS

Abrams, M. ''Hypnosis & Biofeedback.'' *Good Housekeeping* 218 (March 3, 1994): 104, 106-107.

ORGANIZATIONS

The American Society of Clinical Hypnosis. 2200 East Devon Avenue, Suite 291, Des Plaines, IL 60018-4534. (847) 297-3317.

Jeffrey Peter Larson

Hypnotherapy *see* **Hypnosis**

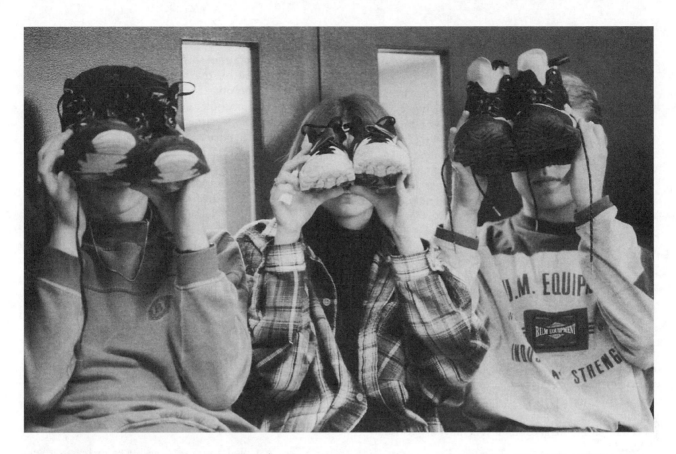

These students peer through their "binoculars" while under hypnosis during a demonstration. They were told they were at the Kentucky Derby and that they were watching the field from the stands. *(Photograph by Gary C. Klein, AP/Wide World Photo. Reproduced by permission.)*

Hypocalcemia

Definition

Hypocalcemia, a low bood calcium level, occurs when the concentration of free calcium ions in the blood falls below 4.0 mg/dL (dL = one tenth of a liter). The normal concentration of free calcium ions in the blood serum is 4.0–6.0 mg/dL.

Description

Calcium is an important mineral for maintaining human helath. It is not only a component of bones and teeth, but is also essential for normal blood clotting and necessary for normal muscle and nerve functions. The calcium ion (Ca^{2+}) has two positive charges. In bone, calcium ions occur as a complex with phosphate to form crystals of calcium phosphate. In the bloodstream, calcium ions also occur in complexes, and here calcium is found combined with proteins and various nutrients. However, in the bloodstream, calcium also occurs in a

free form. Normally, about 47% of the calcium in the blood plasma is free, while 53% occurs in a complexed form. Although all of the calcium in the bloodstream serves a useful purpose, it is only the concentration of free calcium ions which as a direct influence on the functioning of our nerves and muscles. For this reason, the measurement of the concentration of free calcium is more important, in the diagnosis of disease, than measuring the level of total calcium or of complexed calcium. The level of total calcium in the blood serum is normally 8.5–10.5 mg/dL, while the level of free calcium is normally 4–5 mg/dl.

Causes & symptoms

Hypocalcemia can be caused by **hypoparathyroidism,** by failure to produce 1,25-dihydroxyvitamin D, by low levels of plasma magnesium, or by failure to get adequate amounts of calcium or vitamin D in the diet. Hypoparathyroidism involves the failure of the parathyroid gland to make parathyroid hormone. Parathyroid hormone controls and maintains plasma calcium levels. The hormone exerts its effect on the kidneys, where it triggers the synthesis of 1,25-dihydroxyvitamin D. Thus, hypocalcemia can be independently caused by damage to the parathyroid gland or to the kidneys. 1,25-Dihydroxyvitamin D stimulates the uptake of calcium from the diet and the mobilization of calcium from the bone. Bone mobilization means the natural process by which the body dissolves part of the bone in the skeleton in order to maintain or raise the levels of plasma calcium ions.

Low plasma magnesium levels (hypomagnesia) can result in hypocalcemia. Hypomagnesemia can occur with **alcoholism** or with diseases characterized by an inability to properly absorb fat. Magnesium is required for parathyroid hormone to play its part in maintaining plasma calcium levels. For this reason, any disease that results in lowered plasma magnesium levels may also cause hypocalcemia.

Hypocalcimia may also result from the consumption of toxic levels of phosphate. Phosphate is a constituent of certain enema formulas. An enema is a solution that is used to cleanse the intestines via a hose inserted into the rectum. Cases of hypocalcemia have been documented where people swallowed enema formulas, or where an enema has been administered to an infant.

Symptoms of severe hypocalcemia include numbness or tingling around the mouth or in the feet and hands, as well as in muscle spasms in the face, feet, and hands. Hypocalcemia can also result in depression, memory loss, or **hallucinations.** Severe hypocalcemia occurs when serum free calcium is under 3 mg/dL. Chronic and moderate hypocalcemia can result in **cataracts** (damage to the eyes). In this case, the term ''chronic'' means lasting one year or longer.

Diagnosis

Hypocalcemia is diagnosed by acquiring a sample of blood serum and measuring the concentraton of free calcium using a calcium-sensitive electrode. Hypocalcemia has several causes, and hence a full diagnosis requires assessment of health of the parathyroid gland, kidneys, and of plasma magnesium concentration.

Treatment

The method chosen for treatment depends on the exact cause and on the severity of the hypocalcemia. Severe hypocalcemia requires injection of calcium ions, usually in the form of calcium gluconate. Oral calcium supplements are prescribed for long term treatment (nonemergency) of hypocalcemia. The oral supplements may take the form of calcium carbonate, calcium chloride, calcium lactate, or calcium gluconate. Where hypocalcemia results from kidney failure, treatment includes injections of 1,25-dihydroxyvitamin D. Oral vitamin D supplements can increase gastrointestinal absorption of calcium. Where hypocalcemia results from hypoparathyroidism, treatment may include oral calcium, 1,25-dihydroxyvitamin D, or other drugs. Where low serum magnesium levels occur, concurrently with hypocalcemia, the magnesium deficiency must be corrected to effectively treat the hypocalcemia.

Prognosis

The prognosis for correcting hypocalcemia is excellent. However, the eye damage that may result from chronic hypocalcemia cannot be reversed.

Prevention

The first, and most obvious, way to help prevent hypocalcemia is to ensure that adequate amounts of calcium and vitamin D are consumed each day, either in the diet or as supplements. The hypocalcemia that may occur with damage to the parathyroid gland or to the kidneys cannot be prevented. Hypocalcemia resulting from overuse of **enemas** can be prevented by reducing enema usage. Hypocalcemia resulting from magnesium deficiency tends to occur in chronic alcoholics, and this type of hypocalcemia can be prevented by reducing alcohol consumption and increasing the intake of healthful food.

Resources

BOOKS

Brody, Tom. *Nutritional Biochemistry.* San Diego: Academic Press, 1998.

Zeman, F. and D.M. Dey. *Applications in Medical Nutrition Therapy.* 2nd ed. Engelwood Cliffs, NJ: Prentice-Hall, 1995.

PERIODICALS

Sutters, M., C.L. Gaboury, and W.M. Bennett. ''Severe Hyperphosphatemia and Hypocalcemia: A Dilemma in Patient Management.''*Journal of the American Society of Nephrology* 7 (1996): 2056-2061.

Tom Brody

Hypochondriac *see* **Hypochondriasis**

Hypochondriasis

Definition

Hypochondriasis is a mental disorder characterized by excessive fear of or preoccupation with a serious illness, despite medical testing and reassurance to the contrary. It was formerly called hypochondriacal neurosis.

Description

Although hypochondriasis is often considered a disorder that primarily affects adults, it is now increasingly recognized in children and adolescents. In addition, hypochondriasis may develop in elderly people without previous histories of health-related fears. The disorder accounts for about 5% of psychiatric patients and is equally common in men and women.

Causes & symptoms

The causes of hypochondriasis are not precisely known. Children may have physical symptoms that resemble or mimic those of other family members. In adults, hypochondriasis may sometimes reflect a self-centered character structure or a wish to be taken care of by others; it may also have been copied from a parent's behavior. In elderly people, hypochondriasis may be associated with depression or grief. It may also involve biologically based hypersensitivity to internal stimuli.

Most hypochondriacs are worried about being physically sick, although some express fear of insanity. The symptoms reported can range from general descriptions of a specific illness to unusual complaints. In many instances the symptoms reflect intensified awareness of ordinary body functions, such as heartbeat, breathing, or stomach noises. It is important to understand that a hypochondriac's symptoms are not "in the head" in the sense of being delusional. The symptoms are real, but the patient misinterprets bodily functions and attributes them to a serious or even lethal cause.

Diagnosis

The diagnosis is often complicated by the patient's detailed understanding of symptoms and medical terminology from previous contacts with doctors. If a new doctor suspects hypochondriasis, he or she will usually order a complete medical workup in order to rule out physical disease.

Psychological evaluation is also necessary to rule out other disorders that involve feelings of anxiety or complaints of physical illness. These disorders include depression, panic disorder, and schizophrenia with somatic

(physical) delusions. The following features are characteristic of hypochondriasis:

• The patient is not psychotic (out of touch with reality or hallucinating).

• The patient gets upset or blames the doctor when told there is "nothing wrong," or that there is a psychological basis for the problem.

• There is a correlation between episodes of hypochondriacal behavior and stressful periods in the patient's life.

• The behavior has lasted at least six months.

Evaluation of children and adolescents with hypochondriasis should include the possibility of abuse by family members.

Treatment

The goal of therapy is to help the patient (and family) live with the symptoms and to modify thinking and behavior that reinforces hypochondriacal symptoms. This treatment orientation is called supportive, as distinct from insight-oriented, because hypochondriacs usually resist psychological interpretations of their symptoms. Supportive treatment may include medications to relieve **anxiety.** Some clinicians look carefully for "masked" depression and treat with antidepressants.

Follow-up care includes regular physical checkups, because about 30% of patients with hypochondriasis will eventually develop a serious physical illness. The physician also tries to prevent unnecessary medical testing and "doctor shopping" on the patient's part.

Prognosis

From 33–50% of patients with hypochondriasis can expect significant improvement from the current methods of treatment.

Resources

BOOKS

Clark, R. Barkley. "Psychosocial Aspects of Pediatrics & Psychiatric Disorders." In *Current Pediatric Diagnosis & Treatment,* edited by William W. Hay, Jr., et al. Stamford, CT: Appleton & Lange, 1997.

Eisendrath, Stuart J. "Psychiatric Disorders." In *Current Medical Diagnosis & Treatment 1998,* edited by Lawrence M. Tierney, Jr., et al. Stamford, CT: Appleton & Lange, 1997.

Kennedy, Gary J., and Pamela Silverman. "Geriatric Psychiatry." In *Current Diagnosis 9,* edited by Rex B. Conn, et al. Philadelphia: W. B. Saunders Company, 1997.

Nemiah, John C. "Psychoneurotic Disorders." In *The New Harvard Guide to Psychiatry,* edited by Armand M. Nicholi, Jr., Cambridge, MA, and London, UK: The Belknap Press of Harvard University Press, 1988.

"Psychiatric Disorders: The Neuroses." In *The Merck Manual of Diagnosis and Therapy,* vol. I, edited by Robert Berkow, et al. Rahway, NJ: Merck Research Laboratories, 1992.

Stone, Timothy E., and Romaine Hain. "Somatoform Disorders." In *Current Diagnosis 9,* edited by Rex B. Conn, et al. Philadelphia: W. B. Saunders Company, 1997.

Rebecca J. Frey

···

Hypoglycemia

Definition

The condition called hypoglycemia is literally translated as low blood sugar. Hypoglycemia occurs when blood sugar (or blood glucose) concentrations fall below a level necessary to properly support the body's need for energy and stability throughout its cells.

Description

Carbohydrates are the main dietary source of the glucose that is manufactured in the liver and absorbed into the bloodstream to fuel the body's cells and organs. Glucose concentration is controlled by hormones, primarily insulin and glucagon. Glucose concentration is also controlled by epinephrine (adrenalin) and norepinephrine, as well as growth hormone. If these regulators are not working properly, levels of blood sugar can become either excessive (as in hyperglycemia) or inadequate (as in hypoglycemia). If a person has a blood sugar level of 50 mg/dl or less, he or she is considered hypogly-

---

> ## KEY TERMS
> ···
>
> **Adrenal glands**—Two organs that sit atop the kidneys; these glands make and release hormones such as epinephrine.
>
> **Epinephrine**—Also called adrenalin, a secretion of the adrenal glands (along with norepinephrine) that helps the liver release glucose and limits the release of insulin. Norepinephrine is both a hormone and a neurotransmitter, a substance that transmits nerve signals.
>
> **Fructose**—A type of natural sugar found in many fruits, vegetables, and in honey.
>
> **Glucagon**—A hormone produced in the pancreas that raises the level of glucose in the blood. An injectable form of glucagon, which can be bought in a drug store, is sometimes used to treat insulin shock.
>
> **Postprandial**—After eating or after a meal.

cemic, although glucose levels vary widely from one person to another.

Hypoglycemia can occur in several ways.

Drug-induced hypoglycemia

Drug-induced hypoglycemia, a complication of diabetes, is the most commonly seen and most dangerous form of hypoglycemia.

Hypoglycemia occurs most often in diabetics who must inject insulin periodically to lower their blood sugar. While other diabetics are also vulnerable to low blood sugar episodes, they have a lower risk of a serious outcome than do insulin-dependant diabetics. Unless recognized and treated immediately, severe hypoglycemia in the insulin-dependent diabetic can lead to generalized convulsions followed by **amnesia** and unconsciousness. **Death,** though rare, is a possible outcome.

In insulin-dependent diabetics, hypoglycemia known as an insulin reaction or insulin **shock** can be caused by several factors. These include overmedicating with manufactured insulin, missing or delaying a meal, eating too little food for the amount of insulin taken, exercising too strenuously, drinking too much alcohol, or any combination of these factors.

Ideopathic or reactive hypoglycemia

Ideopathic or reactive hypoglycemia (also called postprandial hypoglycemia) occurs when some people eat. A number of reasons for this reaction have been proposed, but no single cause has been identified.

In some cases, this form of hypoglycemia appears to be associated with malfunctions or diseases of the liver, pituitary, adrenals, liver, or pancreas. These conditions are unrelated to diabetes. Children intolerant of a natural sugar (fructose) or who have inherited defects that affect digestion may also experience hypoglycemic attacks. Some children with a negative reaction to **aspirin** also experience reactive hypoglycemia. It sometimes occurs among people with an intolerance to the sugar found in milk (galactose), and it also often begins before diabetes strikes later on.

Fasting hypoglycemia

Fasting hypoglycemia sometimes occurs after long periods without food, but it also happens occasionally following strenuous **exercise,** such as running in a marathon.

Other factors sometimes associated with hypoglycemia include:

• **Pregnancy**

• A weakened immune system

• A poor diet high in simple carbohydrates

• Prolonged use of drugs, including **antibiotics**

• Chronic physical or mental **stress**

• Heartbeat irregularities (**arrhythmias**)

• **Allergies**

• **Breast cancer**

• High blood pressure treated with beta-blocker medications (after strenuous exercise)

• Upper gastrointestinal tract surgery.

Causes & symptoms

When carbohydrates are eaten, they are converted to glucose that goes into the bloodstream and is distributed throughout the body. Simultaneously, a combination of chemicals that regulate how our body's cells absorb that sugar is released from the liver, pancreas, and adrenal glands. These chemical regulators include insulin, glucagon, epinephrin (adrenalin), and norepinephrin. The mixture of these regulators released following digestion of carbohydrates is never the same, since the amount of carbohydrates that are eaten is never the same.

Interactions among the regulators are complicated. Any abnormalities in the effectiveness of any one of the regulators can reduce or increase the body's absorption of glucose. Gastrointestinal enzymes such as amylase and lactase that break down carbohydrates may not be functioning properly. These abnormalities may produce hyperglycemia or hypoglycemia, and can be detected when the level of glucose in the blood is measured.

Cell sensitivity to these regulators can be changed in many ways. Over time, a person's stress level, exercise patterns, advancing age, and dietary habits influence cellular sensitivity. For example, a diet consistently overly rich in carbohydrates increases insulin requirements over time. Eventually, cells can become less receptive to the effects of the regulating chemicals, which can lead to glucose intolerance.

Diet is both a major factor in producing hypoglycemia as well as the primary method for controlling it. **Diets** typical of western cultures contain excess carbohydrates, especially in the form of simple carbohydrates such as sweeteners, which are more easily converted to sugar. In poorer parts of the world, the typical diet contains even higher levels of carbohydrates. Fewer dairy products and meat are eaten, and grains, vegetables, and fruits are consumed. This dietary trend is balanced, however, since people in these cultures eat smaller meals and usually use carbohydrates more efficiently through physical labor.

Early symptoms of severe hypoglycemia, particularly in the drug-induced type of hypoglycemia, resemble an extreme shock reaction. Symptoms include:

• Cold and pale skin

• Numbness around the mouth

• Apprehension

• Heart **palpitations**

• Emotional outbursts

• Hand **tremors**

• Mental cloudiness

• Dilated pupils

• Sweating

• **Fainting.**

Mild attacks, however, are more common in reactive hypoglycemia and are characterized by extreme tiredness. Patients first lose their alertness, then their muscle strength and coordination. Thinking grows fuzzy, and finally the patient becomes so tired that he or she becomes "zombie-like," awake but not functioning. Sometimes the patient will actually fall asleep. Unplanned naps are typical of the chronic hypoglycemic patient, particularly following meals.

Additional symptoms of reactive hypoglycemia include **headaches,** double vision, staggering or inability to walk, a craving for salt and/or sweets, abdominal distress, premenstrual tension, chronic colitis, allergies, ringing in the ears, unusual patterns in the frequency of urination, skin eruptions and inflammations, **pain** in the neck and shoulder muscles, memory problems, and sudden and excessive sweating.

Unfortunately, a number of these symptoms mimic those of other conditions. For example, the depression, **insomnia,** irritability, lack of concentration, crying spells, **phobias,** forgetfulness, confusion, unsocial behavior, and suicidal tendencies commonly seen in nervous system and psychiatric disorders may also be hypoglycemic symptoms. It is very important that anyone with symptoms that may suggest reactive hypoglycemia see a doctor.

Because all of its possible symptoms are not likely to be seen in any one person at a specific time, diagnosing hypoglycemia can be difficult. One or more of its many symptoms may be due to another illness. Symptoms may persist in a variety of forms for long periods of time. Symptoms can also change over time within the same person. Some of the factors that can influence symptoms include physical or mental activities, physical or mental state, the amount of time passed since the last meal, the amount and quality of sleep, and exercise patterns.

Diagnosis

Drug-induced hypoglycemia

Once diabetes is diagnosed, the patient then monitors his or her blood sugar level with a portable machine called a glucometer. The diabetic places a small blood sample on a test strip that the machine can read. If the test reveals that the blood sugar level is too low, the diabetic can make a correction by eating or drinking an additional carbohydrate.

Reactive hypoglycemia

Reactive hypoglycemia can only be diagnosed by a doctor. Symptoms usually improve after the patient has gone on an appropriate diet. Reactive hypoglycemia was diagnosed more frequently 10–20 years ago than today. Studies have shown that most people suffering from its symptoms test normal for blood sugar, leading many doctors to suggest that actual cases of reactive hypoglycemia are quite rare. Some doctors think that people with hypoglycemic symptoms may be particularly sensitive to the body's normal postmeal release of the hormone epinephrine, or are actually suffering from some other physical or mental problem. Others doctors believe reactive hypoglycemia is actually the early onset of diabetes that occurs after a number of years. There continues to be disagreement about the cause of reactive hypoglycemia.

A common test to diagnose hypoglycemia is the extended oral glucose tolerance test. Following an overnight fast, a concentrated solution of glucose is drunk and blood samples are taken hourly for five to six hours. Though this test remains helpful in early identification of diabetes, its use in diagnosing chronic reactive hypoglycemia has lost favor because it can trigger hypoglycemic symptoms in people with otherwise normal glucose readings. Some doctors now recommend that blood sugar be tested at the actual time a person experiences hypoglycemic symptoms.

Treatment

Treatment of the immediate symptoms of hypoglycemia can include eating sugar. For example, a patient can eat a piece of candy, drink milk, or drink fruit juice. Glucose tablets can be used by patients, especially those who are diabetic. Effective treatment of hypoglycemia over time requires the patient to follow a modified diet. Patients are usually encouraged to eat small, but frequent, meals throughout the day, avoiding excess simple sugars (including alcohol), fats, and fruit drinks. Those patients with severe hypoglycemia may require fast-acting glucagon injections that can stabilize their blood sugar within approximately 15 minutes.

Alternative treatment

A holistic approach to reactive hypoglycemia is based on the belief that a number of factors may create the condition. Among them are heredity, the effects of other illnesses, emotional stress, too much or too little exercise, bad lighting, poor diet, and environmental pollution. Therefore, a number of alternative methods have been proposed as useful in treating the condition. Homeopathy, **acupuncture,** and **applied kinesiology,** for example, have been used, as have herbal remedies. One of the herbal remedies commonly suggested for hypoglycemia is a decoction (an extract made by boiling) of gentian (*Gentiana lutea*). It should be drunk warm 15–30 minutes before a meal. Gentian is believed to help stimulate the endocrine (hormone-producing) glands.

In addition to the dietary modifications recommended above, people with hypoglycemia may benefit from supplementing their diet with chromium, which is believed to help improve blood sugar levels. Chromium is found in whole grain breads and cereals, cheese, molasses, lean meats, and brewer's yeast. Hypoglycemics should avoid alcohol, caffeine, and cigarette smoke, since these substances can cause significant swings in blood sugar levels.

Prevention

Drug-induced hypoglycemia

Preventing hypoglycemic insulin reactions in diabetics requires taking glucose readings through frequent blood sampling. Insulin can then be regulated based on those readings. Maintaining proper diet is also a factor. Programmable insulin pumps implanted under the skin have proven useful in reducing the incidence of hypoglycemic episodes for insulin-dependent diabetics. As of late

1997, clinical studies continue to seek additional ways to control diabetes and drug-induced hypoglycemia. Tests of a substance called pramlintide indicate that it may help improve glycemic control in diabetics.

Reactive hypoglycemia

The onset of reactive hypoglycemia can be avoided or at least delayed by following the same kind of diet used to control it. While not as restrictive as the diet diabetics must follow to keep tight control over their disease, it is quite similar.

There are a variety of diet recommendations for the reactive hypoglycemic. Patients should:

• Avoid overeating.

• Never skip breakfast.

• Include protein in all meals and snacks, preferably from sources low in fat, such as the white meat of chicken or turkey, most fish, soy products, or skim milk.

• Restrict intake of fats (particularly saturated fats, such as animal fats), and avoid refined sugars and processed foods.

• Be aware of the differences between some vegetables, such as potatoes and carrots. These vegetables have a higher sugar content than others (like squash and broccoli). Patients should be aware of these differences and note any reactions they have to them.

• Be aware of differences found in grain products. White flour is a carbohydrate that is rapidly absorbed into the bloodstream, while oats take much longer to break down in the body.

• Keep a "food diary." Until the diet is stabilized, a patient should note what and how much he/she eats and drinks at every meal. If symptoms appear following a meal or snack, patients should note them and look for patterns.

• Eat fresh fruits, but restrict the amount they eat at one time. Patients should remember to eat a source of protein whenever they eat high sources of carbohydrate like fruit. Apples make particularly good snacks because, of all fruits, the carbohydrate in apples is digested most slowly.

• Follow a diet that is high in fiber. Fruit is a good source of fiber, as is oatmeal and oat bran, which slows the buildup of sugar in the blood during digestion.

A doctor can recommend a proper diet, and there are many cookbooks available for diabetics. Recipes found in such books are equally effective in helping to control hypoglycemia.

Prognosis

Like diabetes, there is no cure for reactive hypoglycemia, only ways to control it. While some chronic cases will continue through life (rarely is there complete remission of the condition), others will develop into type II (age onset) diabetes. Hypoglycemia appears to have a higher-than-average incidence in families where there has been a history of hypoglycemia or diabetes among their members, but whether hypoglycemia is a controllable warning of oncoming diabetes has not yet been determined by clinical research.

Resources

BOOKS

Eades, Michael R., and Mary Dan. *Protein Power.* New York: Bantam, 1995.

Krimmel, Patricia and Edward Krimmel. *The Low Blood Sugar Handbook.* Bryn Mawr, PA: Franklin Publishers, 1992.

Ruggiero, Roberta. *The Do's and Don'ts of Low Blood Sugar.* Hollywood, FL: Frederick Fell Publishers.

PERIODICALS

Service, F. J. "Hypoglycemic Disorders." *New England Journal of Medicine* (April 27, 1995): pp. 1144-1152.

ORGANIZATIONS

Hypoglycemia Association, Inc. 18008 New Hampshire Ave., PO Box 165, Ashton, MD 20861-0165.

National Hypoglycemia Association, Inc. PO Box 120, Ridgewood, NJ 07451. (201) 670-1189.

Martin Watson Dodge

Hypogonadism

Definition

Hypogonadism is the condition more prevalent in males in which the production of sex hormones and germ cells are inadequate.

Description

Gonads are the organs of sexual differentiation—in the female, they are ovaries; in the male, the testes. Along with producing eggs and sperm, they produce sex hormones that generate all the differences between men and women. If they produce too little sex hormone, then either the growth of the sexual organs or their function is impaired.

The gonads are not independent in their function, however. They are closely controlled by the pituitary

KEY TERMS

Biopsy—Surgical removal of pieces of tissue for examination.

Embryo—Refers to life before birth, specifically the first two months after conception.

Fetus—The unborn person or animal, still in the womb.

Hypothalamus—Part of the brain just above the pituitary that stimulates pituitary gland function.

Ionizing radiation—X rays. Diagnostic x rays are too weak to do damage under normal circumstances, but x rays used to treat cancer must be used with great care.

Undescended testicle—A testicle that is still in the groin and has not made its way into the scrotum.

gland. The pituitary hormones are the same for males and females, but the gonadal hormones are different. Men produce mostly androgens, and women produce mostly estrogens. These two hormones regulate the development of the embryo, determining whether it is a male or a female. They also direct the adolescent maturation of sex organs into their adult form. Further, they sustain those organs and their function throughout the reproductive years. The effects of estrogen reach beyond that to sustain bone strength and protect the cardiovascular system from degenerative disease.

Hormones can be inadequate during or after each stage of development—embryonic and adolescent. During each stage, inadequate hormone stimulation will prevent normal development. After each stage, a decrease in hormone stimulation will result in failed function and perhaps some shrinkage. The organs affected principally by sex hormones are the male and female genitals, both internal and external, and the female breasts. Body hair, fat deposition, bone and muscle growth, and some brain functions are also influenced.

Causes & symptoms

Sex is determined at the moment of conception by sex chromosomes. Females have two X chromosomes, while males have one X and one Y chromosome. If the male sperm with the Y chromosome fertilizes an egg, the baby will be male. This is true throughout the animal kingdom. Genetic defects sometimes result in changes in the chromosomes. If sex chromosomes are involved, there is a change in the development of sexual characteristics.

Female is the default sex of the embryo, so most of the sex organ deficits at birth occur in boys. Some, but not all, are due to inadequate androgen stimulation. The penis may be small, the testicles undescended (cryptorchidism) or various degrees of ''feminization'' of the genitals may be present.

After birth, sexual development does not occur until **puberty.** Hypogonadism most often shows up as an abnormality in boys during puberty. Again, not every defect is due to inadequate hormones. Some are due to too much of the wrong ones. Kallmann's syndrome is a birth defect in the brain that prevents release of hormones and appears as failure of male puberty. Some boys have adequate amounts of androgen in their system but fail to respond to them, a condition known as androgen resistance.

Female problems in puberty are not caused by too little estrogen. Even female reproductive problems are rarely related to a simple lack of hormones, but rather to complex cycling rhythms gone wrong. All the problems with too little hormone happen during **menopause,** which is a normal hypogonadism.

A number of adverse events can damage the gonads and result in decreased hormone levels. The childhood disease **mumps,** if acquired after puberty, can infect and destroy the testicles—a disease called viral orchitis. Ionizing radiation and **chemotherapy,** trauma, several drugs (spironolactone, a diuretic and ketoconazole, an antifungal agent), alcohol, marijuana, heroin, methadone, and environmental toxins can all damage testicles and decrease their hormone production. Severe diseases in the liver or kidneys, certain infections, **sickle cell anemia,** and some cancers also affect gonads. To treat some male cancers, it is necessary to remove the testicles, thereby preventing the androgens from stimulating cancer growth. This procedure, still called castration or *orchiectomy*, removes androgen stimulation from the whole body.

For several reasons the pituitary can fail. It happens rarely after **pregnancy.** It used to be removed to treat advanced breast or **prostate cancer.** Sometimes the pituitary develops a tumor that destroys it. Failure of the pituitary is called **hypopituitarism** and, of course, leaves the gonads with no stimulation to produce hormones.

Besides the tissue changes generated by hormone stimulation, the only other symptoms relate to sexual desire and function. Libido is enhanced by testosterone, and male sexual performance requires androgens. The role of female hormones in female sexual activity is less clear, although hormones strengthen tissues and promote healthy secretions, facilitating sexual activity.

Diagnosis

Presently, there are accurate blood tests for most of the hormones in the body, including those from the pituitary and even some from the hypothalamus. Chromosomes can be analyzed, and gonads can, but rarely are, biopsied.

Treatment

Replacement of missing body chemicals is much easier than suppressing excesses. Estrogen replacement is recommended for nearly all women after menopause for its many beneficial effects. Estrogen can be taken by mouth, injection, or skin patch. It is strongly recommended that the other female hormone, progesterone, be taken as well, because it prevents overgrowth of uterine lining and uterine cancer. Testosterone replacement is available for males who are deficient.

Resources

BOOKS

Carr, Bruce R. and Karen D. Bradshaw. "Disorders of the ovary and female reproductive tract." In *Harrison's Principles of Internal Medicine.* Edited by Kurt Isselbacher, et al. New York: McGraw-Hill, 1998, pp. 2097-2115.

Griffen, James E. and Jean D. Wilson. "Disorders of the testes." In *Harrison's Principles of Internal Medicine.* Edited by Kurt Isselbacher, et al. New York: McGraw-Hill, 1998, pp. 2092-2024.

Matsaumoto, Alvin M. "The Testes." In *Cecil Textbook of Medicine.* Edited by J. Claude Bennett and Fred Plum. Philadelphia: W. B. Saunders, 1996, pp. 1329-1341.

Nelson, Waldo E., et al., ed. "Hypofunction of the ovaries." In *Nelson Textbook of Pediatrics.* Philadelphia: W. B. Saunders, 1996, pp. 1635-1639.

Nelson, Waldo E., et al., ed. "Hypofunction of the testes." In *Nelson Textbook of Pediatrics.* Philadelphia: W. B. Saunders, 1996, pp. 1629-33.

Plymate, Stephen R. "Male hypogonadism." *Principles and Practice of Endocrinology and Metabolism.* Edited by Kenneth L. Becker, et al. Philadelphia: J. B. Lippencott Company, 1995, pp. 1056-1082.

Schimke, R. Neil. "Genetic diseases of endocrinology and metabolism." In *Principles and Practice of Endocrinology and Metabolism.* Edited by Kenneth L. Becker, et al. Philadelphia: J. B. Lippencott Company, 1995, pp. 1551-1553.

PERIODICALS

Rosenberg, M.J., T.D. King, and M.C. Timmons. "Estrogen-androgen for hormone replacement." *Journal of Reproductive Medicine* 42 (July 1997): 394-404.

J. Ricker Polsdorfer

Hypokalemia

Definition

Hypokalemia is a condition of below normal levels of potassium in the blood serum. Potassium, a necessary electrolyte, facilitates nerve impulse conduction and the contraction of skeletal and smooth muscles, including the heart. It also facilitates cell membrane function and proper enzyme activity. Levels must be kept in a proper (homeostatic) balance for the maintenance of health. The normal concentration of potassium in the serum is in the range of 3.5–5.0 mM. Hypokalemia means serum or plasma levels of potassium ions that fall below 3.5 mM. (Potassium concentrations are often expressed in units of milliequivalents per liter [mEq/L], rather than in units of millimolarity [mM], however, both units are identical and mean the same thing when applied to concentrations of potassium ions.)

Hypokalemia can result from two general causes: either from an overall depletion in the body's potassium or from excessive uptake of potassium by muscle from surrounding fluids.

Description

A normal adult weighing about 154 lbs (70 kg) has about 3.6 moles of potassium ions in his body. Most of this potassium (about 98%) occurs inside various cells and organs, where normal concentration are about 150 mM. Blood serum concentrations are much lower—only about 0.4% of the body's potassium is found in blood serum. As noted above, hypokalemia can be caused by the sudden uptake of potassium ions from the bloodstream by muscle or other organs or by an overall depletion of the body's potassium. Hypokalemia due to overall depletion tends to be a chronic phenomenon, while hypokalemia due to a shift in location tends to be a temporary disorder.

Causes & symptoms

Hypokalemia is most commonly caused by the use of **diuretics.** Diuretics are drugs that increase the excretion of water and salts in the urine. Diuretics are used to treat a number of medical conditions, including **hypertension** (high blood pressure), congestive **heart failure,** liver disease, and kidney disease. However, diuretic treatment can have the side effect of producing hypokalemia. In fact, the most common cause of hypokalemia in the elderly is the use of diuretics. The use of furosemide and thiazide, two commonly used diuretic drugs, can lead to hypokalemia. In contrast, spironolactone and triamterene are diuretics that do not provoke hypokalemia.

Other commons causes of hypokalemia are excessive **diarrhea** or vomiting. Diarrhea and vomiting can be produced by infections of the gastrointestinal tract. Due to a variety of organisms, including bacteria, protozoa, and viruses, diarrhea is a major world health problem. It is responsible for about a quarter of the 10 million infant **deaths** that occur each year. Although nearly all of these deaths occur in the poorer parts of Asia and Africa, diarrheal diseases are a leading cause of infant death in the United States. Diarrhea results in various abnormalities, such as **dehydration** (loss in body water), **hyponatremia** (low sodium level in the blood), and hypokalemia.

Because of the need for potassium to control muscle action, hypokalemia can cause the heart to stop beating. Young infants are especially at risk for death from this cause, especially where severe diarrhea continues for two weeks or longer. Diarrhea due to laxative abuse is an occasional cause of hypokalemia in the adolescent or adult. Enema abuse is a related cause of hypokalemia. Laxative abuse is especially difficult to diagnose and treat, because patients usually deny the practice. Up to 20% of persons complaining of chronic diarrhea practice laxative abuse. Laxative abuse is often part of eating disorders, such as **anorexia nervosa** or **bulimia nervosa.** Hypokalemia that occurs with these eating disorders may be life-threatening.

Surprisingly, the potassium loss that accompanies vomiting is only partly due to loss of potassium from the vomit. Vomiting also has the effect of provoking an increase in potassium loss in the urine. Vomiting expels acid from the mouth, and this loss of acid results in alkalization of the blood. (Alkalization of the blood means that the pH of the blood increases slightly.) An increased blood pH has a direct effect on the kidneys. Alkaline blood provokes the kidneys to release excessive amounts of potassium in the urine. So, severe and continual vomiting can cause excessive losses of potassium from the body and hypokalemia.

A third general cause of hypokalemia is prolonged **fasting** and **starvation.** In most people, after three weeks of fasting, blood serum potassium levels will decline to below 3.0 mM and result in severe hypokalemia. However, in some persons, serum potassium may be naturally maintained at about 3.0 mM, even after 100 days of fasting. During fasting, muscle is naturally broken down, and the muscle protein is converted to sugar (glucose) to supply to the brain the glucose which is essential for its functioning. Other organs are able to survive with a mixed supply of fat and glucose. The potassium within the muscle cell is released during the gradual process of muscle breakdown that occurs with starvation, and this can help counteract the trend to hypokalemia during starvation. Eating an unbalanced diet does not cause hypokalemia because most foods, such as fruits (especially bananas, oranges, and melons), vegetables, meat, milk, and cheese, are good sources of potassium. Only foods such as butter, margarine, vegetable oil, soda water, jelly beans, and hard candies are extremely poor in potassium.

Alcoholism occasionally results in hypokalemia. About one half of alcoholics hospitalized for withdrawal symptoms experience hypokalemia. The hypokalemia of alcoholics occurs for a variety of reasons, usually poor nutrition, vomiting, and diarrhea. Hypokalemia can also be caused by **hyperaldosteronism; Cushing's syndrome;** hereditary kidney defects such as Liddle's syndrome, Bartter's syndrom, and Franconi's syndrome; and eating too much licorice.

Symptoms

Mild hypokalemia usually results in no symptoms, while moderate hypokalemia results in confusion, disorientation, weakness, and discomfort of muscles. On occasion, moderate hypokalemia causes cramps during **exercise.** Another symptom of moderate hypokalemia is a discomfort in the legs that is experienced while sitting still. The patient may experience an annoying feeling that can be relieved by shifting the positions of the legs or by stomping the feet on the floor. Severe hypokalemia results in extreme weakness of the body and, on occasion, in **paralysis.** The paralysis that occurs is "flaccid paralysis," or limpness. Paralysis of the muscles of the lungs results in death. Another dangerous result of severe hypokalemia is abnormal heart beat (arrhythmia) that can lead to death from cardiac arrest (cessation of heart beat). Moderate hypokalemia may be defined as serum potassium between 2.5 and 3.0 mM, while severe hypokalemia is defined as serum potassium under 2.5 mM.

Diagnosis

Hypokalemia can be measured by acquiring a sample of blood, preparing blood serum, and using a potassium sensitive electrode for measuring the concentration of potassium ions. Atomic absorption spectroscopy can also be used to measure the potassium ions. Since hypokalemia results in abnormalities in heart behavior, the electrocardiogram is usually used in the diagnosis of hypokalemia. The diagnosis of the cause of hypokalemia can be helped by measuring the potassium content of the urine. Where urinary potassium is under 25 mmoles per day, it means that the patient has experienced excessive losses of potassium due to diarrhea. The urinary potassium test is useful in cases where the patient is denying the practice of laxative or enema abuse. In contrast, where hypokalemia is due to the use of diuretic drugs, the content of potassium in the urine will be high—over 40 mmoles per day.

Treatment

In emergency situations, when severe hypokalemia is suspected, the patient should be put on a cardiac monitor, and respiratory status should be assessed. If laboratory test results show potassium levels below 2.5 mM, intravenous potassium should be given. In less urgent cases, potassium can be given orally in the pill form. Potassium supplements take the form of pills containing potassium chloride (KCl), potassium bicarbonate (KHCO$_3$), and potassium acetate. Oral potassium chloride is the safest and most effective treatment for hypokalemia. Generally, the consumption of 40–80 mmoles of KCl per day is sufficient to correct the hypokalemia that results from diuretic therapy. For many people taking diuretics, potassium supplements are not necessary as long as they eat a balanced diet containing foods rich in potassium.

Prognosis

The prognosis for correcting hypokalemia is excellent. However, in emergency situations, where potassium is administered intravenously, the physician must be careful not to give too much potassium. The administration of potassium at high levels, or at a high rate, can lead to abnormally high levels of serum potassium.

Prevention

Hypokalemia is not a concern for healthy persons, since potassium is present in a great variety of foods. For patients taking diuretics, however, the American Dietetic Association recommends use of a high potassium diet. The American Dietetic Association states that if hypokalemia has already occurred, use of the high potassium diet alone may not reverse hypokalemia. Useful components of a high potassium diet include bananas, tomatoes, cantaloupes, figs, raisins, kidney beans, potatoes, and milk.

Resources

BOOKS

American Dietetic Association. *Handbook of Clinical Dietetics.* New Haven, CT: Yale University Press, 1992.

Brody, Tom. *Nutritional Biochemistry.* San Diego, CA: Academic Press, 1998.

Levinsky, N.G. "Fluids and Electrolytes." In *Harrison's Principles of Internal Medicine*, edited by K.J. Isselbacher, et al. Engelwood Cliffs, NJ: Prentice-Hall, 1995.

Singer, Gary G., and Barry M. Brenner. "Fluid and Electrolyte Disturbances." In *Harrison's Principles of Internal Medicine*, edited by Anthony S. Fauci, et al. New York: McGraw-Hill, 1998.

Zeman, F., and D.M. Dey. *Applications in Medical Nutrition Therapy,* 2nd ed. Engelwood Cliffs, NJ: Prentice-Hall, 1995.

PERIODICALS

Wingo, I.D., and C.S. Wingo. "Hypokalemia— Consequences, Causes, and Correction." *Journal of the American Society of Nephrology* 8 (1997): 1179-1188.

Tom Brody

Hypolipoproteinemia

Definition

Hypolipoproteinemia (or hypolipidemia) is the lack of fat in the blood.

Description

Although quite rare, hypolipoproteinemia is a serious condition. Blood absorbs fat from food in the intestine and transports it as a combined package with proteins and other chemicals like cholesterol. Much of the fat goes straight into the liver for processing. The cholesterol, a waste product, ends up in the bile. The proteins act as vessels, carrying the other chemicals around. These packages of fat, cholesterol, and proteins are called lipoproteins.

Causes & symptoms

Low blood fats can be the result of several diseases, or they can be a primary genetic disease with other associated abnormalities.

• **Malnutrition** is a lack of food, including fats, in the diet.

• Malabsorption is the inability of the bowel to absorb food, causing malnutrition.

- Anemia (too few red blood cells) and **hyperthyroidism** (too much thyroid hormone) also reduce blood fats.

- Rare genetic conditions called hypobetalipoproteinemia and abetalipoproteinemia cause malabsorption plus nerve, eye, and skin problems in early childhood.

- Tangier disease, causes only the cholesterol to be low. It also produces nerve and eye problems in children.

Symptoms are associated more closely with the cause rather than the actual low blood fats.

Diagnosis

Blood studies of the various fat particles help identify both the low and high fat diseases. These tests are often done after an overnight fast to prevent interference from fat just being absorbed from food. Fats and proteins are grouped together and described by density—high-density lipoproteins (HDL), low-density lipoproteins (LDL), and very low-density lipoproteins (VLDL). There are also much bigger particles called chylomicrons. Each contain different proportions of cholesterol, fats, and protein.

Treatment

Supplemental vitamin E helps children with the betalipoprotein deficiencies. There is no known treatment for Tangier disease. Treatment of the causes of the other forms of low blood fats reverses the condition.

Resources

BOOKS

Ginsberg, Henry N. and Ira J. Goldberg. "Disorders Of Lipoprotein Metabolism." In *Harrison's Principles of Internal Medicine.* Edited by Kurt Isselbacher, et al. New York: McGraw-Hill, 1998, p.2144.

J. Ricker Polsdorfer

Hypomagnesemia *see* **Magnesium imbalance**

Hyponatremia

Definition

The normal concentration of sodium in the blood plasma is 136–145 mM. Hyponatremia occurs when sodium falls below 130 mM. Plasma sodium levels of 125 mM or less are dangerous and can result in seizures and **coma.**

Description

Sodium is an atom, or ion, that carries a single positive charge. The sodium ion may be abbreviated as Na^+ or as simply Na. Sodium can occur as a salt in a crystalline solid. Sodium chloride (NaCl), sodium phosphate (Na_2HPO_4) and sodium bicarbonate ($NaHCO_3$) are commonly occurring salts. These salts can be dissolved in water or in juices of various foods. Dissolving involves the complete separation of ions, such as sodium and chloride in common table salt (NaCl).

About 40% of the body's sodium is contained in bone. Approximately 2–5% occurs within organs and cells and the remaining 55% is in blood plasma and other extracellular fluids. The amount of sodium in blood plasma is typically 140 mM, a much higher amount than is found in intracellular sodium (about 5 mM). This asymmetric distribution of sodium ions is essential for human life. It makes possible proper nerve conduction, the passage of various nutrients into cells, and the maintenance of blood pressure.

The body continually regulates its handling of sodium. When dietary sodium is too high or low, the intestines and kidneys respond to adjust concentrations to normal. During the course of a day, the intestines absorbs dietary sodium while the kidneys excrete a nearly equal amount of sodium into the urine. If a low sodium diet is consumed, the intestines increase their efficiency of sodium absorption, and the kidneys reduce its release into urine.

The concentration of sodium in the blood plasma depends on two things: the total amount of sodium and water in arteries, veins, and capillaries (the circulatory system). The body uses separate mechanisms to regulate sodium and water, but they work together to correct blood pressure when it is too high or too low. Too low a concentration of sodium, or hyponatremia, can be corrected either by increasing sodium or by decreasing body water. The existence of separate mechanisms that regulate sodium concentration account for the fact that there are numerous diseases that can cause hyponatremia, including diseases of the kidney, pituitary gland, and hypothalamus.

Causes & symptoms

Hyponatremia can be caused by abnormal consumption or excretion of dietary sodium or water and by diseases that impair the body's ability to regulate them. Maintenance of a low salt diet for many months or excessive sweat loss during a race on a hot day can present a challenge to the body to conserve adequate sodium levels. While these conditions alone are not likely to cause hyponatremia, it can occur under special circumstances. For example, hyponatremia often occurs in patients taking diuretic drugs who maintain a low sodium diet. This is especially of concern in elderly patients, who have a reduced ability to regulate the concentrations of various nutrients in the bloodstream. Diuretic drugs that frequently cause hyponatremia include furosemide (Lasix), bumetanide (Bumex), and most commonly, the thiazides. **Diuretics** enhance the excretion of sodium into the urine, with the goal of correcting high blood pressure. However, too much sodium excretion can result in hyponat!! remi a. Usually only mild hyponatremia occurs in patients taking diuretics, but when combined with a low sodium diet or with the excessive drinking of water, severe hyponatremia can develop.

Severe and prolonged **diarrhea** can also cause hyponatremia. Severe diarrhea, causing the daily output of 8–10 liters of fluid from the large intestines, results in the loss of large amounts of water, sodium, and various nutrients. Some diarrheal diseases release particularly large quantities of sodium and are therefore most likely to cause hyponatremia.

Drinking excess water sometimes causes hyponatremia, because the absorption of water into the bloodstream can dilute the sodium in the blood. This cause of hyponatremia is rare, but has been found in psychotic patients who compulsively drink more than 20 liters of water per day. Excessive drinking of beer, which is mainly water and low in sodium, can also produce hyponatremia when combined with a poor diet.

Marathon running, under certain conditions, leads to hyponatremia. Races of 25–50 miles can result in the loss of great quantities (8 to 10 liters) of sweat, which contains both sodium and water. Studies show that about 30% of marathon runners experience mild hyponatremia during a race. But runners who consume only pure water during a race can develop severe hyponatremia because the drinking water dilutes the sodium in the bloodstream. Such runners may experience neurological disorders as a result of the severe hyponatremia and require emergency treatment.

Hyponatremia also develops from disorders in organs that control the body's regulation of sodium or water. The adrenal gland secretes a hormone called aldosterone that travels to the kidney, where it causes the kidney to retain sodium by not excreting it into the urine. **Addison's disease** causes hyponatremia as a result of low levels of aldosterone due to damage to the adrenal gland. The hypothalamus and pituitary gland are also involved in sodium regulation by making and releasing vasopressin, known as anti-diuretic hormone, into the bloodstream. Like aldosterone, vasopressin acts in the kidney, but it causes it to reduce the amount of water released into urine. With more vasopressin production, the body conserves water, resulting in a lower concentration of plasma sodium. Certain types of **cancer** cells produce vasopressin, leading to hyponatremia.

Symptoms of moderate hyponatremia include tiredness, disorientation, **headache,** muscle cramps, and nausea. Severe hyponatremia can lead to seizures and coma. These neurological symptoms are thought to result from the movement of water into brain cells, causing them to swell and disrupt their functioning.

In most cases of hyponatremia, doctors are primarily concerned with discovering the underlying disease causing the decline in plasma sodium levels. **Death** that occurs during hyponatremia is usually due to other features of the disease rather than to the hyponatremia itself.

Diagnosis

Hyponatremia is diagnosed by acquiring a blood sample, preparing plasma, and using a sodium-sensitive electrode for measuring the concentration of sodium ions. Unless the cause is obvious, a variety of tests are subsequently run to determine if sodium was lost from the urine, diarrhea, or from vomiting. Tests are also used to determine abnormalities in aldosterone or vasopressin levels. The patient's diet and use of diuretics must also be considered.

Treatment

Severe hyponatremia can be treated by infusing a solution of 5% sodium chloride in water into the bloodstream. Moderate hyponatremia due to use of diuretics or an abnormal increase in vasopressin is often treated by instructions to drink less water each day. Hyponatremia due to adrenal gland insufficiency is treated with hormone injections.

Prognosis

Hyponatremia is just one manifestation of a variety of disorders. While hyponatremia can easily be corrected, the prognosis for the underlying condition that causes it varies.

Prevention

Patients who take diuretic medications must be checked regularly for the development of hyponatremia.

Resources

BOOKS

Levinsky, N.G. "Fluids and electrolytes." In *Harrison's Principles of Internal Medicine*, edited by K.J. Isselbacher, et al. Engelwood Cliffs, New Jersey: Prentice-Hall, 1995.

PERIODICALS

Fried, L.F. and P.M. Palevsky, "Hyponatremia and hypernatremia." *Medical Clinics of North America* 81 (1997): 585-609.

Frizzell, R.T. et al., "Hyponatremia and ultramarathon running." *Journal of the American Medical Association* 255 (1986): 772-774.

Tom Brody

Hypoparathyroidism

Definition

Hypoparathyroidism is the result of a decrease in production of parathyroid hormones by the parathyroid glands located behind the thyroid glands in the neck. The result is a low level of calcium in the blood.

Description

Parathyroid glands consist of four pea-shaped glands located on the back and side of the thyroid gland. The gland produces parathyroid hormone which, along with vitamin D and calcitonin, are important for the regulation

---

KEY TERMS

Addison's disease —A disease caused by partial or total failure of adrenocortical (relating to, or derived from the adrenal gland) function, which is characterized by a bronze-like pigmentation of the skin and mucous membranes, anemia, weakness, and low blood pressure.

Autoimmunity —A condition by which the body's defense mechanisms attacks itself.

Calcitonin —A hormone produced by the thyroid gland in human beings, that lowers plasma calcium and phosphate levels without increasing calcium accumulation.

Hashimoto's thyroiditis —The self destruction of the thyroid cells from an autoimmune disorder.

Hormones —A substance produced by one tissue and conveyed by the bloodstream to another to effect physiological activity, such as growth or metabolism.

Pernicious anemia —A severe anemia most often affecting older adults, caused by failure of the stomach to absorb vitamin B12 and characterized by abnormally large red blood cells, gastrointestinal disturbances, and lesions of the spinal cord.

---

of the calcium level in the body. Hypoparathyroidism affects both males and females of all ages.

Causes & symptoms

The accidental removal of the parathyroid glands during neck surgery is the most frequent cause of hypoparathyroidism. Complications of surgery on the parathyroid glands is another common cause of this disorder. There is the possibility of autoimmune genetic disorders causing hypoparathyroidism such as Hashimoto's **thyroiditis, pernicious anemia,** and **Addison's disease.** The destruction of the gland by radiation is a rare cause of hypoparathyroidism. Occasionally, the parathyroids are absent at birth causing low calcium levels and possible convulsions in the newborn. Symptoms in the advanced and continuous stages of hypoparathyroidism include splitting of the nails, inadequate tooth development and **mental retardation** in children, and seizures.

Abnormal low levels of calcium result in irritability of nerves, causing **numbness and tingling** of the hands and feet, with painful-cramp like muscle spasms known as tetany. Laryngeal spasms may also occur causing respiratory obstruction.

Diagnosis

Diagnostic measures begin with the individual's own observation of symptoms. A thorough medical history and physical examination by a physician is always required for an accurate diagnosis. The general practitioner may refer the individual to an endocrinologist, a medical specialist who studies the function of the parathyroid glands as well as other hormone producing glands. Laboratory studies include blood and urine tests to help determine phosphate and calcium levels. X rays are useful to determine any abnormalities in bone density associated with abnormal calcium levels. These autoimmune disorders may accompany hypoparathyroidism, but are not an actual cause of it.

Treatment

In the event of severe muscle spasms, hospitalization may be warranted for calcium injections. Raising carbondioxide levels in the blood, which can decrease muscle spasms, may be achieved in immediate situations by placing a paper bag over the mouth and blowing into it to "reuse" each breath. It is critical to obtain timely periodic laboratory tests to check calcium levels. A high calcium, low-phosphorous diet may be of significance and is directed by the physician or dietitian.

Prognosis

Presently hypoparathyroidism is considered incurable. The disorder requires lifelong replacement therapy to control symptoms. Medical research however, continues to search for a cure.

Prevention

There are no specific preventive measures for hypoparathyroidism. However, careful surgical techniques are critical to reduce the risk of damage to the gland during surgery.

Resources

BOOKS

Chandrasoma, Parakrama and Clive R. Taylor. *Concise Pathology.* East Norwalk, Connecticut: Appleton and Lange, 1991.

ORGANIZATIONS

American Medical Association. Washington office: 1101 Vermont Avenue NW Washington, D.C. 20005. 202-789-7400.

OTHER

1998 thrive@ the healthy living experience HYPOPARA-THYROIDISM. thrive@ the healthy living experience. http://www.thriveonline.com (6/11/98).

Jeffrey Peter Larson

Hypophosphatemia *see* **Phosphorus imbalance**

Hypophysectomy

Definition

Hypophysectomy or hypophysis is the removal of the pituitary gland.

Purpose

The pituitary gland is in the middle of the head. Removing this master gland is a drastic step that was taken in the extreme circumstance of two **cancers** that had escaped all other forms of treatment. Cancers of the female breast and male prostate grow faster in the presence of sex hormones. It used to be that sex hormones could be suppressed only by removing their source, the glands that made them. After the gonads were removed, some cancers continued to grow, so other stimulants to their growth had to removed. At this point, some cancer specialists turned to the pituitary.

With the development of new therapeutic agents and methods, especially new ways to manipulate hormones without removing their source, this type of endocrine surgery has been largely relegated to history. However, tumors develop in the pituitary gland that require removal. Here, the idea is to remove the tumor but partially preserve the gland.

Description

There are several surgical approaches to the pituitary. The surgeon will choose the best one for the specific procedure. The pituitary lies directly behind the nose, and access through the nose or the sinuses is often the best approach. Opening the skull and lifting the frontal lobe of the brain will expose the delicate neck of the pituitary gland. This approach works best if tumors have extended above the pituitary fossa (the cavity in which the gland lies).

Newer surgical methods using technology have made other approaches possible. Stereotaxis is a three-dimensional aiming technique using x rays or scans for guidance. Instruments can be placed in the brain with pinpoint accuracy through tiny holes in the skull. These instruments can then manipulate brain tissue, either to destroy it or remove it. Stereotaxis is also used to direct radiation with similar precision using a gamma knife. Access to some brain lesions can be gained through the blood vessels using tiny tubes and wires guided by x rays.

Preparation

Pituitary surgery is performed by neurosurgeons deep inside the skull. All the patient can do to prepare is keep as healthy as possible and trust that the surgeon will do his usual excellent job. Informed surgical consent is important so that the patient is fully confident of the need for surgery and the expected outcome.

Aftercare

Routine post-operative care is required. In addition, pituitary function will be assessed.

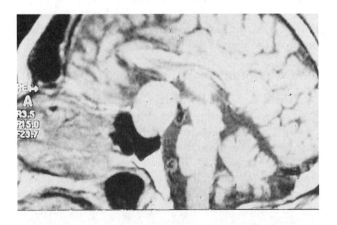

This magnetic resonance imaging (MRI) scan of a human brain indicates a large tumor (left center) on the pituitary gland. *(Custom Medical Stock Photo. Reproduced by permission.)*

Risks

The risks of surgery are multiple. Procedures are painstakingly selected to minimize risk and maximize benefit. Unique to surgery on the pituitary is the risk of destroying the entire gland and leaving the entire endocrine system without guidance. This used to be the whole purpose of hypophysectomy. After the procedure, the endocrinologist, a physician specializing in the study and care of the endocrine system, would provide the patient with all the hormones needed. Patients with no pituitary function did and still do quite well because of the available hormone replacements.

Normal results

Complete removal of the pituitary was the goal for cancer treatment. Today, removal of tumors with preservation of the gland is the goal.

Abnormal results

Tumors may not be completely removed, due to their attachment to vital structures.

Resources

BOOKS

Biller, Beverly M. K. and Gilbert H. Daniels. "Neuroendocrine regulation and diseases of the anterior pituitary and hypothalamus." In *Harrison's Principles of Internal Medicine.* Edited by Kurt Isselbacher, et al. New York: McGraw-Hill, 1998, 1988-1999.

Jameson, J. Larry. "Anterior pituitary." In *Cecil Textbook of Medicine.* Edited by J. Claude Bennett and Fred Plum. Philadelphia: W. B. Saunders, 1996, p.1209.

Youmans, Julian R. "Hypophysectomy." In *Neurological Surgery.* Philadelphia: W. B. Saunders, 1990, pp. 4358-4370.

J. Ricker Polsdorfer

Hypopigmentation *see* **Albinism; Vitiligo**

Hypopituitarism

Definition

Hypopituitarism is loss of function in an endocrine gland due to failure of the pituitary gland to secrete hormones which stimulate that gland's function. The pituitary gland is located at the base of the brain. Patients diagnosed with hypopituitarism may be deficient in one

KEY TERMS

Adenoma—A benign (not threatening or cancerous) tumor that originates in a gland.

Androgen—A hormone that usually stimulates the sex hormones of the male.

Congenital—Present at birth.

Diabetes insipidus—A disorder originating in the pituitary gland which is characterized by excessive thirst and urination.

Endocrine—Refers to the system of internal secretion of substances into the body system from glands.

Hypoglycemia—Abnormal decrease of sugar in the blood.

Hypothyroidism—Deficient activity of the thyroid gland and resulting loss of energy.

single hormone, several hormones, or have complete pituitary failure.

Description

The pituitary is a pea-sized gland located at the base of the brain, and surrounded by bone. The hypothalamus, another endocrine organ in the brain, controls the function of the pituitary gland by providing "hormonal orders." In turn, the pituitary gland regulates the many hormones that control various functions and organs within the body. The posterior pituitary acts as a sort of storage area for the hypothalamus and passes on hormones that control function of the muscles and kidneys. The anterior pituitary produces its own hormones which help to regulate several endocrine functions.

In hypopituitarism, something interferes with the production and release of these hormones, thus affecting the function of the target gland. Commonly affected hormones may include:

Gonadotropin deficiency

Gonadotropin deficiency involves two distinct hormones affecting the reproductive system. Luteinizing hormone (LH) stimulates the testes in men and the ovaries in women. This deficiency can affect fertility in men and women and menstruation in women. Follicle-stimulating hormone (FSH) has similar effects to LH.

Thyroid stimulating hormone deficiency

Thyroid stimulating hormone (TSH) is involved in stimulation of the thyroid gland. A lack of stimulation in the gland leads to **hypothyroidism.**

Adrenocorticotopic hormone deficiency

Also known as corticotropin, adrenocorticotopic hormone (ACTH) stimulates the adrenal gland to produce a hormone similar to cortisone, called cortisol. The loss of this hormone can lead to serious problems.

Growth hormone deficiency

Growth hormone (GH) regulates the body's growth. Patients who lose supply of this hormone before physical maturity will suffer impaired growth. Loss of the hormone can also affect adults.

Other hormone deficiencies

Prolactin stimulates the female breast to produce milk. A hormone produced by the posterior pituitary, antidiuretic hormone (ADH), controls the function of the kidneys. When this hormone is deficient, **diabetes insipidus** can result. However, patients with hypopituitarism rarely suffer ADH deficiency, unless the hypopituitarism is the result of hypothalamus disease.

Multiple hormone deficiencies

Deficiency of a single pituitary hormone occurs less commonly than deficiency of more than one hormone. Sometimes referred to as progressive pituitary hormone deficiency or partial hypopituitarism, there is usually a predictable order of hormone loss. Generally, growth hormone is lost first, then luteinizing hormone deficiency follows. The loss of follicle-stimulating hormone, thyroid stimulating hormone and adrenocorticotopic hormones follow much later. The progressive loss of pituitary hormone secretion is usually a slow process, which can occur over a period of months or years. Hypopituitarism does occasionally start suddenly with rapid onset of symptoms.

Panhypopituitarism

This condition represents the loss 0of all hormones released by the anterior pituitary gland. Panhypopituitarism is also known as complete pituitary failure.

Causes & symptoms

There are three major mechanisms which lead to the development of hypopituitarism. The first involves decreased release of hypothalamic hormones that stimulate pituitary function. The cause of decreased hypothalamic function may be congenital or acquired through interference such as tumors, inflammation, infection, mass lesions or interruption of blood supply. A second category of causes is any event or mass which interrupts the delivery of hormones from the hypothalamus. These may include particular tumors and aneurysms. Damage to the pituitary stalk from injury or surgery can also lead to hypopituitarism.

The third cause of hypopituitarism is damage to the pituitary gland cells. Destroyed cells can not produce the pituitary hormones that would normally be secreted by the gland. Cells may be destroyed by a number of tumors and diseases. Hypopituitarism is often caused by tumors, the most common of which is pituitary adenoma.

Symptoms of hypopituitarism vary with the affected hormones and severity of deficiency. Frequently, patients have had years of symptoms that were nonspecific until a major illness or **stress** occurred. Overall symptoms may include fatigue, sensitivity to cold, weakness, decreased appetite, weight loss and abdominal **pain.** Low blood pressure, **headache** and visual disturbances are other associated symptoms.

Gonadotropin deficiency

Symptoms specific to this hormone deficiency include decreased interest in sex for women and **infertility** in women and men. Women may also have premature cessation of menstruation, hot flashes, vaginal dryness and pain during intercourse. Women who are postmenopausal will not have obvious symptoms such as these and may first present with headache or loss of vision. Men may also suffer **sexual dysfunction** as a result of gonadotropin deficiency. In acquired gonadotropin deficiency, both men and women may notice loss of body hair.

Thyroid stimulating hormone deficiency

Intolerance to cold, fatigue, weight gain, **constipation** and pale, waxy and dry skin indicate thyroid hormone deficiency.

Adrenocorticotopic hormone deficiency

Symptoms of ACTH deficiency include fatigue, weakness, weight loss and low blood pressure. Nausea, pale skin and loss of pubic and armpit hair in women may also indicate deficiency of ACTH.

Growth hormone deficiency

In children, growth hormone deficiency will result in short stature and growth retardation. Symptoms such as **obesity** and skin wrinkling may or may not show in adults and normal release of growth hormone normally declines with age.

Other hormone deficiencies

Prolactin deficiency is rare and is the result of partial or generalized anterior pituitary failure. When present, the symptom is absence of milk production in women. There are no known symptoms for men. ADH deficiency may produce symptoms of diabetes insipidus, such as excessive thirst and frequent urination.

Multiple hormone deficiencies

Patients with multiple hormone deficiencies will show symptoms of one or more specific hormone deficiencies or some of the generalized symptoms listed above.

Panhypopituitarism

The absence of any pituitary function should show symptoms of one or all of the specific hormone deficiencies. In addition to those symptoms, patients may have dry, pale skin that is finely textured. The face may appear finely wrinkled and contain a disinterested expression.

Diagnosis

Once the diagnosis of a single hormone deficiency is made, it is strongly recommended that tests for other hormone deficiencies be conducted.

Gonadotropin deficiency

The detection of low levels of gonadotropin can be accomplished through simple blood tests which measure luteinizing hormone and follicle-stimulating hormone, simultaneously with gonadal steroid levels. The combination of results can indicate to a physician if the cause of decreased hormone levels or function belongs to hypopituitarism or some sort of primary gonadal failure. Diagnosis will vary among men and women.

Thyroid stimulating hormone deficiency

Laboratory tests measuring thyroid function can help determine a diagnosis of TSH deficiency. The commonly used tests are T4 and TSH measurement done simultaneously to determine the reserve, or pool, of thyroid-stimulating hormone.

Adrenocorticotopic hormone deficiency

An insulin tolerance test may be given to determine if cortisol levels rise when **hypoglycemia** is induced. If they do not rise, there is insufficient reserve of cortisol, indicating an ACTH deficiency. If the insulin tolerance test is not safe for a particular patient, a glucagon test offers similar results. A CRH (corticotropin-releasing hormone) test may also be given. It involves injection of CRH to measure, through regularly drawn blood samples, a resulting rise in ACTH and cortisol. Other tests which stimulate ACTH may be ordered.

Growth hormone deficiency

Growth hormone deficiency is measured through the use of insulin-like growth factor I tests, which measure growth factors that are dependent on growth hormones. Sleep and **exercise** studies may also be used to test for growth hormone deficiency, since these activities are known to stimulate growth hormone secretion. Several drugs also induce secretion of growth hormone and may be given to measure hormone response. The standard test for growth hormone deficiency is the insulin-induced hypoglycemia test. This test does carry some risk from the induced hypoglycemia. Other tests include an arginine infusion test, clonidine test and growth-hormone releasing hormone test.

Other hormone deficiencies

If a test calculates normal levels of prolactin, deficiency of the hormone is eliminated as a diagnosis. A TRH (thyrotropin-releasing hormone) simulation test can determine prolactin levels. A number of tests are available to detect ADH levels and to determine diagnosis of diabetes insipidus.

Multiple and general hypopituitarism tests

Physicians should be aware that nonspecific symptoms can indicate deficiency of one or more hormones and should conduct a thorough clinical history. In general, diagnosis of hypopituitarism can be accomplished with a combination of dynamic tests and simple blood tests, as well as imaging exams. Most of these tests can be conducted in an outpatient lab or radiology facility. **Magnetic resonance imaging** (MRI) exams with gadolinium contrast enhancement are preferred imaging exams to study the region of the hypothalamus and pituitary gland. When MRI is not available, a properly conducted **computed tomography scan** (CT scan) exam can take its place. These exams can demonstrate a tumor or other mass, which may be interfering with pituitary function.

Panhypopituitarism

The insulin-induced hypoglycemia, or insulin tolerance test, which is used to determine specific hormone deficiencies, is an excellent test to diagnose panhypopituitarism. This test can reveal levels of growth hormone, ACTH (cortisol) and prolactin deficiency. The presence of insufficient levels of all of these hormones is a good indication of complete pituitary failure. Imaging studies and clinical history are also important.

Treatment

Treatment differs widely, depending on the age and sex of the patient, severity of the deficiency, the number of hormones involved, and even the underlying cause of the hypopituitarism. Immediate hormone replacement is generally administered to replace the specific deficient hormone. Patient education is encouraged to help patients manage the impact of their hormone deficiency on daily life. For instance, certain illnesses, accidents or surgical procedures may have adverse complications due to hypopituitarism.

Gonadotropin deficiency

Replacement of gonadal steroids is common treatment for LH and FSH deficiency. Estrogen for women and testosterone for men will be prescribed in the lowest effective dosage possible, since there can be complications to this therapy. To correct women's loss of libido, small doses of androgens may be prescribed. To restore fertility in men, regular hormone injections may be required. Male and female patients whose hypopituitarism results from hypothalamic disease may be successfully treated with a hypothalamic releasing hormone (GnRH), which can restore gonadal function and fertility.

Thyroid stimulating hormone deficiency

In patients who have hypothyroidism, the function of the adrenal glands will be tested and treated with steroids before administering thyroid hormone replacement.

Adrenocorticotopic hormone deficiency

Hydrocortisone or cortisone in divided doses may be given to replace this hormone deficiency. Most patients require 20 mg or less of hydrocortisone per day.

Growth hormone deficiency

It is essential to treat children suffering from growth hormone deficiency. The effectiveness of growth hormone therapy in adults, particularly elderly adults, is not as well documented. It is thought to help restore normal muscle to fat ratios. Growth hormone is an expensive and cautiously prescribed treatment.

Treatment of multiple deficiencies and panhypopituitarism

The treatment of hypopituitarism is usually very straightforward, but must normally continue for the remainder of the patient's life. Some patients may receive treatment with GnRH, the hypothalamic hormone. In most cases, treatment will be based on the specific deficiency demonstrated. Patients with hypopituitarism should be followed regularly to measure treatment effectiveness and to avoid overtreatment with hormone therapy. If the cause of the disorder is a tumor or lesion, radiation or surgical removal are treatment options. Successful removal may reverse the hypopituitarism. However, even after removal of the mass, **hormone replacement therapy** may still be necessary.

Prognosis

The prognosis for most patients with hypopituitarism is excellent. As long as therapy is continued, many experience normal life spans. However, hypopituitarism is usually a permanent condition and prognosis depends on the primary cause of the disorder. It can be potentially life threatening, particularly when acute hypopituitarism occurs as a result of a large pituitary tumor. Morbidity from the disease has increased, although the cause is not known. It is possible that increased morbidity and **death** are due to overtreatment with hormones. Any time that recovery of pituitary function can occur is preferred to lifelong hormone therapy.

Prevention

There is no known prevention of hypopituitarism, except for prevention of damage to the pituitary/hypothalamic area from injury.

Resources

BOOKS

Conn, R.B., Borer, W.Z., and Snyder, J.W. *Current Diagnosis.* Philadelphia, PA: WB Saunders Company, 1997.

ORGANIZATIONS

Alliance for Genetic Support Groups. 35 Wisconsin Circle, Suite 440. Chevy Chase, MD 20815-7015. http://www.medhelp.org/geneticalliance/.

Human Growth Foundation. 7777 Leesburg Pike, Suite 202-South, Falls Church, VA 22043. 1-800-451-6434. http://www.genetic.org.

OTHER

Health Answers. http://www.healthanswers.com.

Teresa G. Norris

Hypoplastic anemia *see* **Aplastic anemia**

Hypospadias and epispadias

Definition

Misplaced urinary openings are called hypospadias if they are below, and epispadias if they are above, the normal location.

Description

In the male, the opening to the urinary tract is normally at the tip of the penis. In the female, it is between the clitoris and the vagina. Once in about 300 male infants is born with hypospadias, and one in 100,000 is born with epispadias. In females, the incidence of these defects is much less, about one in 500,000. Epispadias is associated with bladder abnormalities, and hypospadias with intersex problems—that is, babies whose sex is not obvious at birth because of related deformities of the sex organs.

In the growing embryo, there is a lot of folding going on. The folds enclose organs and seal their edges to form body cavities. It resembles sewing a pipe into a pillow. Many **birth defects** are caused by failure of the folding process. Incomplete sealing of the edges leaves the organs open to the outside. Small degrees of incompletion leave openings to these organs in the wrong place. Epispadias is a lesser degree of exstrophy of the bladder, wherein the front wall of the bladder does not close. The result is a bladder that is turned inside out and is extruding through the lower abdominal wall. The urethra often remains open in a similar way, all the way down through the front of the pelvis and into the genital area. In this case, the front of the pelvis is widely separated as well.

Hypospadias most often occurs alone, and it can occur at any site along the underside of the penis. If all the possible locations of the opening were present at once, the penis would look like a flute. In the process of sexual differentiation into a male, the urethra is formed by a folding over of tissues that later become the lower side of the penis and scrotum. It is rather like zipping up a jacket. Any defect in the zipping process leaves the opening short of its destination and arrests the completion of the journey. The urethra will not have reached its full length.

In females the urinary opening (the urethral meatus) can be anywhere along the anterior of the vagina, but it is usually well forward and not far from its normal position. Female hypospadias may be associated with abnormalities of the genital tract, since the two are part of the same embryonic process.

Causes & symptoms

All of these urinary tract defects are congenital, which means they appear at birth. They are not hereditary, which means they do not appear more often in blood relatives. Specific causes are not known, although insufficient male hormone influence may be responsible for hypospadias, since it represents incomplete development of the penis.

Diagnosis

Male defects are discovered at birth during the first detailed examination of the newborn. Female urethral defects may not be discovered for some time due to the difficulty in viewing the infant vagina.

Treatment

Reproduction requires that the urethral meatus be close to the tip of the penis. Surgery for these defects is successful 70–80% of the time. Similar or better repair rates can be achieved for females. Males should not be circumcised since the foreskin is often needed for the repair. Hypospadias is more of a nuisance and hindrance to reproduction than a threat to health. If surgery is not an option for some reason, the condition may be allowed to persist. There will be an increased risk of infections in the lower urinary tract.

Resources

BOOKS

Duckett, John W. "Hypospadias." In *Campbell's Urology*. Edited by Patrick C. Walsh, et al. Philadelphia: W. B. Saunders, 1998, pp. 2093-2116.

Gearhart, John P. and Robert D. Jeffs. "Exstrophy-epispadias complex and bladder anomalies." In *Campbell's Urology*. Edited by Patrick C. Walsh, et al. Philadelphia: W. B. Saunders, 1998, pp. 1977-1982.

Nelson, Waldo E., et al., ed. "Anomalies of the penis and urethra." In *Nelson Textbook of Pediatrics*. Philadelphia: W. B. Saunders, 1996, pp. 1546-1548.

Nelson, Waldo E., et al., ed. "Anomalies of the bladder." In *Nelson Textbook of Pediatrics*. Philadelphia: W. B. Saunders, 1996, pp. 1542-1543.

J. Ricker Polsdorfer

Hypotension

Definition

Hypotension is the medical term for low blood pressure.

Description

The pressure of the blood in the arteries rises and falls as the heart and muscles handle demands of daily living, such as **exercise,** sleep and **stress.** Some healthy people have blood pressure well below the average for their age, even though they have a completely normal heart and blood vessels. This is often true of athletes who are in superior shape. The term "hypotension" is usually used only when blood pressure has fallen so far that enough blood can no longer reach the brain, causing **dizziness** and **fainting.**

Causes & symptoms

Postural hypotension is the most common type of low blood pressure. In this condition, symptoms appear after a person sits up or stands quickly. In normal people, the cardiovascular system must make a quick adjustment to raise blood pressure slightly to account for the change in position. For those with postural hypotension, the blood pressure adjustment is not adequate or it doesn't happen. Postural hypotension may occur if someone is taking certain drugs or medicine for high blood pressure. It also happens to diabetics when nerve damage has disrupted the reflexes that control blood pressure.

Many people have a chronic problem with low blood pressure that is not particularly serious. This may include people who require certain medications, who are pregnant, have bad veins, or have arteriosclerosis (hardening of the arteries).

The most serious problem with low blood pressure occurs when there is a sudden drop, which can be life-threatening due to widespread **ischemia** (insufficient supply of blood to an organ due to blockage in an artery). This type of low blood pressure may be due to a wide variety of causes, including:

• Trauma with extensive blood loss

• Serious **burns**

• **Shock** from various causes (e.g. **anaphylaxis**)

• **Heart attack**

• Adrenal failure (Addisonian crisis)

• **Cancer**

• Severe **fever**

• Serious infection (septicemia).

Diagnosis

Blood pressure is a measure of the pressure in the arteries created by the heart contracting. During the day, a normal person's blood pressure changes constantly, depending on activity. Low blood pressure can be diagnosed by taking the blood pressure with a sphygmomanometer. This is a device with a soft rubber cuff that is inflated around the upper arm until it's tight enough to stop blood flow. The cuff is then slowly deflated until the health care worker, listening to the artery in the arm with a stethoscope, can hear the blood first as a beat forcing its way along the artery. This is the systolic pressure. The cuff is then deflated more until the beat disappears and the blood flows steadily through the open artery; this gives the diastolic pressure.

Blood pressure is recorded as systolic (higher) and diastolic (lower) pressures. A healthy young adult has a blood pressure of about 110/75, which typically rises with age to about 140/90 by age 60 (a reading now considered mildly elevated).

Treatment

Treatment of low blood pressure depends on the underlying cause, which can usually be resolved. For those people with postural hypotension, a medication adjustment may help prevent the problem. These individuals may find that rising more slowly, or getting out of bed in slow stages, helps the problem. Low blood pressure with no other symptoms does not need to be treated.

Prognosis

Low blood pressure as a result of injury or other underlying condition can usually be successfully treated if the trauma is not too extensive or is treated in time. Less serious forms of chronic low blood pressure have a good prognosis and do not require treatment.

Resources

BOOKS

Smeltzer, Suzanne C. and Brenda G. Bare. *Brunner and Suddarth's Textbook of Medical and Surgical Nursing,* 8th edition. Philadelphia, PA: Lippincott-Raven Publishers, 1996.

Carol A. Turkington

Hypothermia

Definition

Hypothermia, a potentially fatal condition, occurs when body temperature falls below 95°F (35°C).

Description

Although hypothermia is an obvious danger for people living in cold climates, many cases have occurred when the air temperature is well above the freezing mark. Elderly people, for instance, have succumbed to hypothermia after prolonged exposure to indoor air temperatures of 50–65°F (10–18.3°C). In the United States, hypothermia is primarily an urban phenomenon associated with **alcoholism,** drug **addiction,** mental illness, and cold—water immersion accidents. The victims are often homeless male alcoholics. Officially, 11,817 **deaths** were attributed to hypothermia in the United States from 1979 to 1994, but experts suspect that many fatal cases go unrecognized. Nearly half the victims were 65 or older, with males dominating every age group. Nonwhites were also overrepresented in the statistics. Among males 65 and older, nonwhites outnumbered whites by more than four to one.

Causes & symptoms

Measured orally, a healthy person's body temperature can fluctuate between 97°F (36.1°C) and 100°F (37.8°C). Survival depends on maintaining temperature stability within this range by balancing the heat produced by metabolism with the heat lost to the environment through (for the most part) the skin and lungs. When environmental or other changes cause heat loss to outpace heat production, the brain triggers physiological and behavioral responses to restore the balance. The involuntary muscular activity of shivering, for example, aids heat production by accelerating metabolism. But if the cold stress is too great and the body's defenses are overwhelmed, body temperature begins to fall. Hypothermia is considered to begin once body temperature reaches 95°F (35°C), though even smaller drops in temperature can have an adverse effect.

Hypothermia is divided into two types: primary and secondary. Primary hypothermia occurs when the body's heat-balancing mechanisms are working properly but are subjected to extreme cold, whereas secondary hypothermia affects people whose heat-balancing mechanisms are impaired in some way and cannot respond adequately to moderate or perhaps even mild cold. Primary hypothermia typically involves exposure to cold air or immersion in cold water. The cold air variety usually takes at least several hours to develop, but immersion hypothermia

KEY TERMS

....

Antibiotics—Substances used against microorganisms that cause infection.

Computed tomography—A process that uses x rays to create three-dimensional images of structures inside the body.

Esophagus—A muscular tube through which food and liquids pass on their way to the stomach.

Insulin—A substance that regulates blood glucose levels. Glucose is a sugar.

Magnetic resonance imaging—The use of electromagnetic energy to create images of structures inside the body.

Metabolism—The chemical changes by which the body breaks down food and other substances and builds new substances necessary for life.

Nervous system—The system that transmits information, in the form of electrochemical impulses, throughout the body. It comprises the brain, spinal cord, and nerves.

Rectum—The lower section of the large intestine. The intestines are part of the digestive system.

Stroke—A condition involving loss of blood flow to the brain.

Thyroid—A gland (fluid-secreting structure) in the neck. It plays an important role in metabolism.

will occur within about an hour of entering the water, since water draws heat away from the body much faster than air does. In secondary hypothermia, the body's heat-balancing mechanisms can fail for any number of reasons, including **strokes,** diabetes, **malnutrition,** bacterial infection, thyroid disease, spinal cord injuries (which prevent the brain from receiving crucial temperature-related information from other parts of the body), and the use of medications and other substances that affect the brain or spinal cord. Alcohol is one such substance. In smaller amounts it can put people at risk by interfering with their ability to recognize and avoid cold-weather dangers. In larger amounts it shuts down the body's heat-balancing mechanisms.

Secondary hypothermia is often a threat to the elderly, who may be on medications or suffering from illnesses that affect their ability to conserve heat. Malnutrition and immobility can also put the elderly at risk. Some medical research suggests as well that shivering and blood vessel narrowing—two of the body's defenses against cold—may not be triggered as quickly in older

people. For these and other reasons, the elderly can, over a period of days or even weeks, fall victim to hypothermia in poorly insulated homes or other surroundings that family, friends, and caregivers may not recognize as life threatening. Another risk for the elderly is the fact that hypothermia can easily be misdiagnosed as a stroke or some other common illness of old age.

The signs and symptoms of hypothermia follow a typical course, though the body temperatures at which they occur vary from person to person depending on age, health, and other factors. The impact of hypothermia on the nervous system often becomes apparent quite early. Coordination, for instance, may begin to suffer as soon as body temperature reaches 95°F (35°C). The early signs of hypothermia also include cold and pale skin and intense shivering; the latter stops between 90°F (32.2°C) and 86°F (30°C). As body temperature continues to fall, speech becomes slurred, the muscles go rigid, and the victim becomes disoriented and experiences eyesight problems. Other harmful consequences include **dehydration** as well as liver and kidney failure. Heart rate, respiratory rate, and blood pressure rise during the first stages of hypothermia, but fall once the 90°F (32.2°C) mark is passed. Below 86°F (30°C) most victims are comatose, and below 82°F (27.8°C) the heart's rhythm becomes dangerously disordered. Yet even at very low body temperatures, people can survive for several hours and be successfully revived, though they may appear to be dead.

Diagnosis

Information on the patient's prior health and activities often helps doctors establish a correct diagnosis and treatment plan. Pulse, blood pressure, temperature, and respiration require immediate monitoring. Because the temperature of the mouth is not an accurate guide to the body's core temperature, readings are taken at one or two other sites, usually the ear, rectum, or esophagus. Other diagnostic tools include **electrocardiography,** which is used to evaluate heart rhythm, and blood and urine tests, which provide several kinds of key information; a **chest x ray** is also required. A **computed tomography scan** (CT scan) or **magnetic resonance imaging** (MRI) may be needed to check for head and other injuries.

Treatment

Emergency medical help should be summoned whenever a person appears hypothermic. The danger signs include intense shivering; stiffness and numbness in the arms and legs; stumbling and clumsiness; sleepiness, confusion, disorientation, **amnesia,** and irrational behavior; and difficulty speaking. Until emergency help arrives, a victim of outdoor hypothermia should be brought to shelter and warmed by removing wet clothing and footwear, drying the skin, and wrapping him or her in warm blankets or a sleeping bag. Gentle handling is necessary when moving the victim to avoid disturbing the heart. Rubbing the skin or giving the victim alcohol can be harmful, though warm drinks such as clear soup and tea are recommended for those who can swallow. Anyone who aids a victim of hypothermia should also look for signs of frostbite and be aware that attempting to rewarm a frostbitten area of the body before emergency help arrives can be extremely dangerous. For this reason, frostbitten areas must be kept away from heat sources such as campfires and car heaters.

Rewarming is the essence of hospital treatment for hypothermia. How rewarming proceeds depends on the body temperature. Different approaches are used for patients who are mildly hypothermic (the patient's body temperature is 90–95°F [32.2–35°C]), moderately hypothermic (86–90°F [30–32.2°C]), or severely hypothermic (less than 86°F [30°C]). Other considerations, such as the patient's age or the condition of the heart, can also influence treatment choices.

Mild hypothermia is reversed with passive rewarming. This technique relies on the patient's own metabolism to rewarm the body. Once wet clothing is removed and the skin is dried, the patient is covered with blankets and placed in a warm room. The goal is to raise the patient's temperature by 0.5–2°C an hour.

Moderate hypothermia is often treated first with active external rewarming and then with passive rewarming. Active external rewarming involves applying heat to the skin, for instance by placing the patient in a warm bath or wrapping the patient in electric heating blankets.

Severe hypothermia requires active internal rewarming, which is recommended for some cases of moderate hypothermia as well. There are several types of active internal rewarming. Cardiopulmonary bypass, in which the patient's blood is circulated through a rewarming device and then returned to the body, is considered the best, and can raise body temperature by 1–2°C every 3–5 minutes. However, many hospitals are not equipped to offer this treatment. The alternative is to introduce warm oxygen or fluids into the body.

Hypothermia treatment can also include, among other things, insulin, **antibiotics,** and fluid replacement therapy. When the heart has stopped, both **cardiopulmonary resuscitation** (CPR) and rewarming are necessary. Once a patient's condition has stabilized, he or she may need treatment for an underlying problem such as alcoholism or thyroid disease.

Prognosis

Victims of mild or moderate hypothermia usually enjoy a complete recovery. In regard to severely hypo-

thermic patients, the prognosis for survival varies due to differences in people's physiological responses to cold.

Prevention

People who spend time outdoors in cold weather can reduce heat loss by wearing their clothing loosely and in layers and by keeping their hands, feet, and head well covered (30–50% of body heat is lost through the head). Because water draws heat away from the body so easily, staying dry is important, and wet clothing and footwear should be replaced as quickly as possible. Wind- and water-resistant outer garments are also crucial. Alcohol should be avoided because it promotes heat loss by expanding the blood vessels that carry body heat to the skin.

Preventing hypothermia among the elderly requires vigilance on the part of family, friends, and caregivers. An elderly person's home should be properly insulated and heated, with living areas kept at a temperature of 70°F (21.1°C). Warm clothing and bedding are essential, as are adequate food, rest, and **exercise;** warming the bed and bedroom before going to sleep is also recommended. Older people who live alone should be visited regularly—at least once a day during very cold weather—to ensure that their health remains sound and that they are taking good care of themselves. For help and advice, family members and others can turn to government and social service agencies. Meals on wheels and visiting nurse programs, for instance, may be available, and it may be possible to obtain financial aid for winterizing and heating homes.

Resources

BOOKS

Danzl, Daniel F. "Disturbances Due to Cold." In *Conn's Current Therapy,* edited by Robert E. Rakel. Philadelphia: W.B. Saunders, 1998.

Danzl, Daniel F., Robert S. Pozos, and Murray P. Hamlet. "Accidental Hypothermia." In *Wilderness Medicine: Management of Wilderness and Environmental Emergencies,* edited by Paul S. Auerbach. St. Louis: Mosby, 1995.

Mills, W. J., Jr., and R. S. Pozos. "Low Temperature Effects on Humans." In *Encyclopedia of Human Biology,* edited by Renato Dulbecco. San Diego: Academic Press, 1997.

Petty, Kevin J. "Hypothermia." In *Harrison's Principles of Internal Medicine,* edited by Anthony S. Fauci, et al. New York: McGraw-Hill, 1998.

Howard Baker

Hypothyroidism

Definition

Hypothyroidism, or underactive thyroid, develops when the thyroid gland fails to produce or secrete as much thyroxine (T_4) as the body needs. Because T_4 regulates such essential functions as heart rate, digestion, physical growth, and mental development, an insufficient supply of this hormone can slow life-sustaining processes, damage organs and tissues in every part of the body, and lead to life-threatening complications.

Description

Hypothyroidism is one of the most common chronic diseases in the United States. Symptoms may not appear until years after the thyroid has stopped functioning and they are often mistaken for signs of other illnesses, **menopause,** or aging. Although this condition is believed to affect as many as 11 million adults and children, as many as two of every three people with hypothyroidism may not know they have the disease.

Nicknamed "Gland Central" because it influences almost every organ, tissue, and cell in the body, the thyroid is shaped like a butterfly and located just below the Adam's apple. The thyroid stores iodine the body gets from food and uses this mineral to create T_4. Low T_4 levels can alter weight, appetite, sleep patterns, body temperature, sex drive, and a variety of other physical, mental, and emotional characteristics.

There are three types of hypothyroidism. The most common is primary hypothyroidism, in which the thyroid doesn't produce an adequate amount of T_4. Secondary hypothyroidism develops when the pituitary gland does not release enough of the thyroid-stimulating hormone (TSH) that prompts the thyroid to manufacture T_4. Tertiary hypothyroidism results from a malfunction of the hypothalamus, the part of the brain that controls the endocrine system. Drug-induced hypothyroidism, an adverse reaction to medication, occurs in two of every 10,000 people, but rarely causes severe hypothyroidism.

Hypothyroidism is at least twice as common in women as it is in men. Although hypothyroidism is most common in women who are middle-aged or older, the disease can occur at any age. Newborn infants are tested for congenital thyroid deficiency (cretinism) using a test that measures the levels of thyroxine in the infant's blood. Treatment within the first few months of life can prevent **mental retardation** and physical abnormalities. Older children who develop hypothyroidism suddenly stop growing.

Factors that increase a person's risk of developing hypothyroidism include age, weight, and medical history.

Women are more likely to develop the disease after age 50; men, after age 60. **Obesity** also increases risk. A family history of thyroid problems or a personal history of high cholesterol levels or such autoimmune diseases as lupus, **rheumatoid arthritis,** or diabetes can make an individual more susceptible to hypothyroidism.

Causes & symptoms

Hypothyroidism is most often the result of Hashimoto's disease, also known as chronic thyroiditis (inflammation of the thyroid gland). In this disease, the immune system fails to recognize that the thyroid gland is part of the body's own tissue and attacks it as if it were a foreign body. The attack by the immune system impairs thyroid function and sometimes destroys the gland. Other causes of hypothyroidism include:

• Radiation. Radioactive iodine used to treat **hyperthyroidism** (overactive thyroid) or radiation treatments for head or neck **cancers** can destroy the thyroid gland.

- Surgery. Removal of the thyroid gland because of cancer or other thyroid disorders can result in hypothyroidism.

- Viruses and bacteria. Infections that depress thyroid hormone production usually cause permanent hypothyroidism.

- Medication. Nitroprusside, lithium, or iodides can induce hypothyroidism. Because patients who use these medications are closely monitored by their doctors, this side effect is very rare.

- Pituitary gland malfunction. This is a rare condition in which the pituitary gland fails to produce enough TSH to activate the thyroid's production of T_4.

- Congenital defect. One of every 4,000 babies is born without a properly functioning thyroid gland.

- Diet. Because the thyroid makes T_4 from iodine drawn from food, an iodine-deficient diet can cause hypothyroidism. Adding iodine to table salt and other common foods has eliminated iodine deficiency in the United States. Certain foods (cabbage, rutabagas, peanuts, peaches, soybeans, spinach) can interfere with thyroid hormone production.

- Environmental contaminants. Certain man-made chemicals-such as PCBs-found in the local environment at high levels may also cause hypothyroidism.

Hypothyroidism is sometimes referred to as a ''silent'' disease because early symptoms may be so mild that no one realizes anything is wrong. Untreated symptoms become more noticeable and severe, and can lead to confusion and mental disorders, breathing difficulties, heart problems, fluctuations in body temperature, and **death.**

Someone who has hypothyroidism will probably have more than one of the following symptoms:

- Fatigue
- Decreased heart rate
- Progressive **hearing loss**
- Weight gain
- Problems with memory and concentration
- Depression
- **Goiter** (enlarged thyroid gland)
- Muscle **pain** or weakness
- Loss of interest in sex
- Numb, tingling hands
- Dry skin
- Swollen eyelids
- Dryness, loss, or premature graying of hair
- Extreme sensitivity to cold
- **Constipation**
- Irregular menstrual periods
- Hoarse voice.

Hypothyroidism usually develops gradually. When the disease results from surgery or other treatment for hyperthyroidism, symptoms may appear suddenly and include severe muscle cramps in the arms, legs, neck, shoulders, and back.

It's important to see a doctor if any of these symptoms appear unexpectedly. People whose hypothyroidism remains undiagnosed and untreated may eventually develop myxedema. Symptoms of this rare but potentially deadly complication include enlarged tongue, swollen facial features, hoarseness, and physical and mental sluggishness.

Myxedema **coma** can cause unresponsiveness; irregular, shallow breathing; and a drop in blood pressure and body temperature. The onset of this medical emergency can be sudden in people who are elderly or have been ill, injured, or exposed to very cold temperatures; who have recently had surgery; or who use sedatives or anti-depressants. Without immediate medical attention, myxedema coma can be fatal.

Diagnosis

Diagnosis of hypothyroidism is based on the patient's observations, medical history, **physical examination,** and **thyroid function tests.** Doctors who specialize in treating thyroid disorders (endocrinologists) are most apt to recognize subtle symptoms and physical indications of hypothyroidism. A blood test known as a thyroid-stimulating hormone (TSH) assay, **thyroid nuclear medicine scan,** and **thyroid ultrasound** are used to confirm the diagnosis. A woman being tested for hypothyroidism should let her doctor know if she is pregnant or breastfeeding and all patients should be sure their doctors are aware of any recent procedures involving radioactive materials or contrast media.

The TSH assay is extremely accurate, but some doctors doubt the test's ability to detect mild hypothyroidism. They advise patients to monitor their basal (resting) body temperature for below-normal readings that could indicate the presence of hypothyroidism.

Treatment

Natural or synthetic **thyroid hormones** are used to restore normal (euthyroid) thyroid hormone levels. Synthetic hormones are more effective than natural substances, but it may take several months to determine the correct dosage. Patients start to feel better within 48 hours, but symptoms will return if they stop taking the medication.

Most doctors prescribe levothyroxine sodium tablets, and most people with hypothyroidism will take the medication for the rest of their lives. Aging, other medications, and changes in weight and general health can affect how much replacement hormone a patient needs, and regular TSH tests are used to monitor hormone levels. Patients should not switch from one brand of thyroid hormone to another without a doctor's permission.

Regular **exercise** and a high-fiber diet can help maintain thyroid function and prevent constipation.

Alternative treatment

Alternative treatments are primarily aimed at strengthening the thyroid and will not eliminate the need for thyroid hormone medications. Herbal remedies to improve thyroid function and relieve symptoms of hypothyroidism include bladder wrack (*Fucus vesiculosus*), which can be taken in capsule form or as a tea. Some foods, including cabbage, peaches, radishes, soybeans, peanuts, and spinach, can interfere with the production of thyroid hormones. Anyone with hypothyroidism may want to avoid these foods. The Shoulder Stand **yoga** position (at least once daily for 20 minutes) is believed to improve thyroid function.

Prognosis

Thyroid **hormone replacement therapy** generally maintains normal thyroid hormone levels unless treatment is interrupted or discontinued.

Prevention

Primary hypothyroidism can't be prevented, but routine screening of adults could detect the disease in its early stages and prevent complications.

Resources

BOOKS

The Editors of Time-Life Books. *The Medical Advisor: The Complete Guide to Alternative and Conventional Treatments.* Alexandria, VA: Time-Life Books, 1996.

Langer, Stephen, and James F. Scheer. *Hypothyroidism: The Unsuspected Illness.* Keats Publishing, 1995.

Rosenthal, M. Sara. *The Thyroid Sourcebook: Everything You Need to Know.* Lowell House, 1996.

Wood, Lawrence C., David S. Cooper, and E. Chester Ridgway. *Your Thyroid: A Home Reference.* Ballantine Books, 1996.

PERIODICALS

Dranov, P. "Tired? Wired? It Could Be Your Thyroid." *American Health* (May 1994): 90-93.

Drexler, Madeline. "The Disease Doctors Miss." *McCall's* (October 1996): 112.

"Experts Urge Testing for Sluggish Thyroid." *Tufts University Health & Nutrition Letter* (March 1997): 1.

"Recognizing and Treating Thyroid Problems." *Health After 50* (August 1996): 6.

"Underactive Thyroid" *Mayo Clinic Health Letter* (March 1996): 1-3.

ORGANIZATIONS

American Thyroid Association. Montefiore Medical Center, 111 E. 210th St., Bronx, NY 10467.

Endocrine Society. 4350 East West Highway, Suite 500, Bethesda, MD 20814-4410. (301) 941-0200.

Thyroid Foundation of America, Inc. Ruth Sleeper Hall, RSL 350, Boston, MA 02114-2968. (800) 832-8321 or (617) 726-8500.

Thyroid Society for Education and Research. 7515 S. Main St., Suite 545, Houston, TX 77030. (800) THYROID or (713) 799-9909.

OTHER

"AACE Guidelines for the Evaluation and Treatment of Hyperthyroidism and Hypothyroidism." http://www2.nsysu.edu.tw/hclam/hyperhyp.htm (13 December 1997).

Caroll, Linda. "Routine Screening for Thyroid Disorders Cost-Effective." http://www.pharmacy-web.com/WHP/InfoService/MedTribune/Abstract/M960723c.html (13 December 1997).

"EDRI Federal Project Inventory: Disruption of Thyroid Hormone Action by Environmental Agents - Impact on Brain Development." http://www.epa.gov/endocrine/inventory/NTD-MIL3.html (13 December 1997).

"FAQ on Hashimoto's Thyroiditis." http://www.geocities.com/Athens/3626/hashimoto. html (13 December 1997).

"Hypothyroidism." http://www.cc.nih.gov/drd/test/lung-med/thyrtxt.htm (12 December 1997).

"Hypothyroidism." http://www.intelihealth.com (11 December 1997).

"Hypothyroidism Overview." http://ph.healthpark.com/mds/ov055.htm (14 December 1997).

Mickelson, Alana. "Unmasking Thyroid Disease." Stanford Medicine (Summer 1995). http://www.-med.stanford.edu/center/communications./Stanmed/Summer95/hyroid.html (13 December 1997).

"Thyroid Conditions." http://www.amwa-doc.org/thyroid.html (8 December 1997).

"Thyroid Disorders." http://cpmcnet.columbia.edu/texts/guide/hmg21_0012html (2 December 1997).

Maureen Haggerty

Hypotonic duodenography

Definition

Hypotonic duodenography is an x-ray procedure that produces images of the duodenum. The duodenum is the first part of the small intestine.

Purpose

Hypotonic duodenography may be ordered to detect tumors of the head of the pancreas or the area where the pancreatic and bile ducts meet the small intestine. Lesions causing upper abdominal **pain** may be demonstrated by duodenography, and the procedure can aid in the diagnosis of chronic **pancreatitis.**

Precautions

Some patients with narrowing of the tubes in the upper gastrointestinal tract should not receive duodenography. Patients with certain heart disorders and **glaucoma** are cautioned against receiving an agent called anticholinergic, which is administered during the procedure to lessen intestinal muscle spasms. A hormone called glucagon may also be used to relax the intestines, but its use is not recommended in patients with most forms of diabetes.

Description

Hypotonic duodenography is also referred to as x ray of the duodenum or simply as duodenography. The patient is seated while the radiologist places a catheter in the nose and down into the stomach. Then the patient lies down and the tube is continued to the duodenum. The radiologist is guided in this placement by a fluoroscopic image. (Fluoroscopic equipment shows an immediate x ray. In this case, the x ray shows the location of the catheter as it is moved into the stomach and duodenum.) Next, either the glucagon is administered intravenously or anticholinergic is injected into the patient to relax the muscles of the intestine.

After several minutes, the physician will administer barium through the catheter. Barium is a contrast agent that will help highlight the area on the fluoroscopy screen and x rays. After a few films are taken, some of the barium is withdrawn and air is sent in through the catheter. Additional images are acquired and the catheter is then removed. The procedure takes from 30–60 minutes.

Preparation

Patients are required to fast from midnight before the test until after the test, or about 6–12 hours. Just prior to the exam, patients should remove dentures, glasses, and other objects that may interfere with the procedure. The

patient may be instructed to empty their bladder just prior to duodenography.

Aftercare

The barium should be expelled within two to three days. Extra fluids and/or an agent given by the physician to help encourage bowel movement may aid in barium elimination. Physicians and patients should watch for possible reactions to the anticholinergic or glucagon. If an anticholinergic is used, patients are advised to empty their bladder within a few hours after the exam and to wait two hours for clearing of vision or have someone drive them home. Patients will notice that their stools are chalky white from the barium for one to three days following the procedure.

Risks

Abdominal cramping may occur when the physician instills air into the duodenum, but aside from the discomfort, there are few risks associated with this procedure. Side effects from the contrast, hormones or agents may occur. Those patients with diabetes, heart disease, or glaucoma run the highest risk of reaction and should not receive anticholinergic or glucagon, depending on their specific conditions. Elderly patients or those who are extremely ill, must be closely monitored during the procedure for possible return of fluid, or gastric reflux.

Normal results

The linings of the duodenum and surrounding tissues will look smooth and even. The shape of the head of the pancreas will appear normal and near the duodenal wall.

Abnormal results

Any masses or irregular nodules on the wall of the duodenum may indicate tumors or abnormality of tissue. Tumors of the head of the pancreas or of the opening into the intestine from the pancreatic and bile ducts may be seen. Chronic pancreatitis may be indicated on the x rays. In many instances, follow-up laboratory or imaging studies may be ordered to further study the abnormal findings and confirm a diagnosis.

Resources

BOOKS

Springhouse Corporation. *Illustrated Guide to Diagnostic Tests.* Springhouse, PA: Springhouse Corporation, 1998.

ORGANIZATIONS

American College of Radiology. 1891 Preston White Drive. Reston, VA 22091. (800)ACR-LINE. http://www.acr.org.

Cancer Information Clearinghouse, National Cancer Institute. Building 31, Room 10A24, 9000 Rockville Pike, Bethesda, MD 20892. 800-4-CANCER.

Teresa G. Norris

Hypovolemic shock *see* **Shock**

Hysterectomy

Definition

Hysterectomy is the surgical removal of the uterus. In a total hysterectomy, the uterus and cervix are removed. In some cases, the fallopian tubes and ovaries are removed along with the uterus (called hysterectomy with bilateral **salpingo-oophorectomy**). In a subtotal hysterectomy, only the uterus is removed. In a radical hysterectomy, the uterus, cervix, ovaries, oviducts, lymph nodes, and lymph channels are removed. The type of hysterectomy performed depends on the reason for the procedure. In all cases, menstruation stops and a woman loses the ability to bear children.

Purpose

Hysterectomy is the second most common operation performed in the United States. About 600,000 of these surgeries are done annually. By age 60, approximately one out of every three American women will have had a hysterectomy.

About 10% of hysterectomies are performed to treat **cancer** of the cervix, ovaries, or uterus. Women with cancer in one or more of these organs almost always have the organ(s) removed as one part of their cancer treatment.

The most frequent reason for hysterectomy in the United States is to remove fibroid tumors, accounting for 30% of these surgeries. Fibroid tumors are non-cancerous (benign) growths in the uterus, which can cause pelvic and **low back pain** and heavy or lengthy menstrual periods. They occur in 30–40% of women over age 40, and are three times more likely to be present in African-American women than in Caucasian women. Fibroids do not need to be removed unless they are causing symptoms that interfere with a woman's normal activities.

Treatment of **endometriosis** is the reason for 20% of hysterectomies. The endometrium is the lining of the uterus. Endometriosis is a condition that occurs when the cells from the endometrium begin growing outside the uterus. The outlying endometrial cells respond to the hormones that control the menstrual cycle, bleeding each month the way the lining of the uterus does. This causes irritation of the surrounding tissue, leading to **pain** and scarring.

Another 20% percent of hysterectomies are done because of heavy or abnormal vaginal bleeding that can not be linked to any specific cause and cannot be controlled by other means. The remaining 20% of hysterectomies are performed to treat prolapsed uterus,

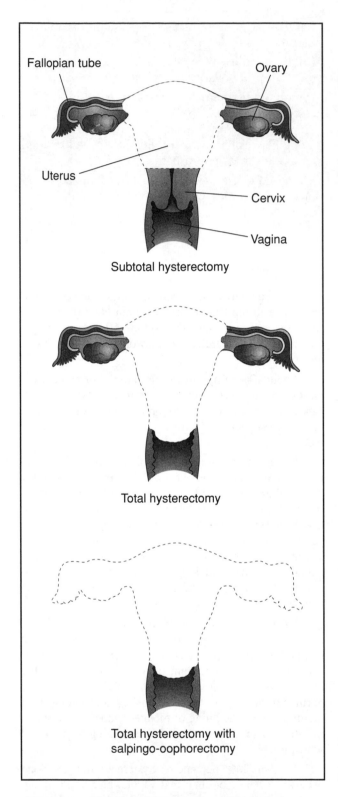

Fallopian tube

Ovary

Uterus

Cervix

Vagina

Subtotal hysterectomy

Total hysterectomy

Total hysterectomy with
salpingo-oophorectomy

**This graphic illustrates three types of hysterectomy and
the organs removed in each type.** *(Illustration by Electronic
Illustrators Group.)*

pelvic inflammatory disease, and endometrial hyperplasia, a potentially precancerous condition.

Total hysterectomy

A total hysterectomy, sometimes called a simple hysterectomy, removes the entire uterus and the cervix. The ovaries are not removed and continue to secrete hormones. Total hysterectomies are always performed in the case of uterine and **cervical cancer.** This is the most common kind of hysterectomy.

Sometimes, in addition to a total hysterectomy a procedure called a bilateral salpingo-oophorectomy is performed. This surgery removes the ovaries and the fallopian tubes. Removal of the ovaries eliminates the main source of the hormone estrogen, so **menopause** occurs immediately. Removal of the ovaries and fallopian tubes is performed in about one-third of hysterectomy operations, often to reduce the risk of ovarian cancer.

Subtotal hysterectomy

If the reason for the hysterectomy is to remove **uterine fibroids,** treat abnormal bleeding, or relieve pelvic pain, it may be possible to remove only the uterus and leave the cervix. This procedure, called a subtotal hysterectomy (or partial hysterectomy), removes the least amount of tissue. The opening to the cervix is left in place. Some women feel that leaving the cervix intact aids in their achieving sexual satisfaction.

Subtotal hysterectomy is easier to perform than a total hysterectomy, but leaves a woman at risk for cervical cancer. She will still need to get yearly pap smears.

Radical hysterectomy

Radical hysterectomies are performed on women with cervical cancer or **endometrial cancer** that has spread to the cervix. A radical hysterectomy removes the uterus, cervix, top part of the vagina, ovaries, fallopian tubes, lymph nodes, lymph channels, and tissue in the pelvic cavity that surrounds the cervix. This type of hysterectomy removes the most tissue and requires the longest hospital stay and longer recovery period.

Precautions

The frequency with which hysterectomies are performed in the United States has been questioned in recent years. It has been suggested that a large number of hysterectomies are performed unnecessarily. The United States has the highest rate of hysterectomies (number of hysterectomies per thousand women) of any country in the world. Also, the frequency of this surgery varies across different regions of the United States. Rates are highest in the South and Midwest.

Women for whom a hysterectomy is recommended should discuss possible alternatives with their doctor and consider getting a second opinion, since this is major surgery with life-changing implications. Alternative treatments exist for many conditions. Whether these alternatives are appropriate for any individual woman is a decision she and her doctor should make together.

As in all major surgery, the health of the patient affects the risk of the operation. Women who have chronic heart or lung diseases, diabetes, or iron-deficiency anemia may not be good candidates for this operation. Heavy smoking, **obesity,** use of steroid drugs, and use of illicit drugs add to the surgical risk.

Description

There are two ways that hysterectomies can be performed. The choice of method depends on the type of hysterectomy, the doctor's experience, and the reason for the hysterectomy.

Abdominal hysterectomy

About 75% of hysterectomies performed in the United States are abdominal hysterectomies. The surgeon makes a four to six inch incision either horizontally across the pubic hair line from hip bone to hip bone or vertically from navel to pubic bone. Horizontal incisions leave a less noticeable scar, but vertical incisions give the surgeon a better view of the abdominal cavity. The blood vessels, fallopian tubes, and ligaments are cut away from the uterus, which is lifted out.

Abdominal hysterectomies take from one to three hours. The hospital stay is three to five days, and it takes four to eight weeks to return to normal activities.

The advantages of an abdominal hysterectomy are that the uterus can be removed even if a woman has internal scarring (adhesions) from previous surgery or her fibroids are large. The surgeon has a good view of the abdominal cavity and more room to work. Also, surgeons have the most experience with this type of hysterectomy. The abdominal incision is more painful than with vaginal hysterectomy and the recovery period is longer.

Vaginal hysterectomy

With a vaginal hysterectomy, the surgeon makes an incision near the top of the vagina. The surgeon then reaches through this incision to cut and tie off the ligaments, blood vessels, and fallopian tubes. Once the uterus is cut free, it is removed through the vagina. The operation takes one to two hours. The hospital stay is usually one to three days, and return to normal activities takes about four weeks.

The advantages of this procedure are that it leaves no visible scar and is less painful. The disadvantage is that it is more difficult for the surgeon to see the uterus and surrounding tissue. This makes complications more common. Large fibroids cannot be removed using this technique. It is

very difficult to remove the ovaries during a vaginal hysterectomy, so this approach may not be possible if the ovaries are involved.

Vaginal hysterectomy can also be performed using a laparoscopic technique. With this surgery, a tube containing a tiny camera is inserted through an incision in the navel. This allows the surgeon to see the uterus on a video monitor. The surgeon then inserts two slender instruments through small incisions in the abdomen and uses them to cut and tie off the blood vessels, fallopian tubes, and ligaments. When the uterus is detached, it is removed though a small incision at the top of the vagina.

This technique, called laparoscopic-assisted vaginal hysterectomy, allows surgeons to perform a vaginal hysterectomy that might be too difficult otherwise. The hospital stay is usually only one day. Recovery time is about two weeks. The disadvantage is that this operation is relatively new and requires great skill by the surgeon.

Any vaginal hysterectomy may have to be converted to an abdominal hysterectomy during surgery if complications develop.

Preparation

Before surgery the doctor will order blood and urine tests. The woman may also meet with the anesthesiologist to evaluate any special conditions that might affect the administration of anesthesia. On the evening before the operation, the woman should eat a light dinner and then avoid eating or drinking anything.

Aftercare

After surgery a woman will feel pain. The degree of discomfort varies, and is generally greatest in abdominal hysterectomies because of the incision. Hospital stays vary from about two days (laparoscopic-assisted vaginal hysterectomy) to five or six days (abdominal hysterectomy with bilateral salpingo-oophorectomy). During the hospital stay, the doctor will probably order more blood tests.

Return to normal activities such as driving and working takes anywhere from two to eight weeks, again depending on the type of surgery. Some women have emotional changes following a hysterectomy. Women who have had their ovaries removed will probably start taking **hormone replacement therapy.**

Risks

Hysterectomy is a relatively safe operation, although like all major surgery it carries risks. These include unanticipated reaction to anesthesia, internal bleeding, blood clots, damage to other organs such as the bladder, and post-surgery infection. The risk of **death** is about 1 in every 1,000 (1/1,000) women having the operation.

Other complications sometimes reported after a hysterectomy include changes in sex drive, weight gain, **constipation,** and pelvic pain. Hot flashes and other symptoms of menopause can occur if the ovaries are removed. Women who have both ovaries removed and who do not take estrogen replacement therapy run an increased risk for heart disease and **osteoporosis** (a condition that causes bones to be brittle). Women with a history of psychological and emotional problems before the hysterectomy are more likely to experience psychological difficulties after the operation.

Normal results

Although there is some concern that hysterectomies may be performed unnecessarily, there are many conditions for which the operation improves a woman's quality of life. In the Maine Woman's Health Study, 71% of women who had hysterectomies to correct moderate or severe painful symptoms reported feeling better mentally, physically, and sexually after the operation.

Resources

BOOKS

Carlson, Karen J., Stephanie A. Eisenstat, and Terra Ziporyn. "Hysterectomy." In *The Harvard Guide to Women's Health,* Cambridge, MA: Harvard University Press, 1996, pp. 308-313.

Griffith, H. Winter. "Hysterectomy." In *The Complete Guide to Symptoms, Illness and Surgery,* 3rd ed. New York: Berkeley Publishing, 1995, pp. 818-825.

ORGANIZATIONS

American Cancer Society. (800) 227-2345. http://www.cancer.org.

National Cancer Institute. (800) 4-CANCER. http://www.nci.nih.gov.

OTHER

Parker, William H. "A Gynecologist's Second Opinion." http://www.gynsecondopinion.com.

Tish Davidson

. . . .

Hysteria

Definition

The term "hysteria" has been in use for over 2000 years and its definition has become broader and more diffuse over time. In modern psychology and psychiatry, hysteria is a feature of hysterical disorders in which a patient experiences physical symptoms that have a psychological, rather than an organic, cause; and histrionic

personality disorder characterized by excessive emotions, dramatics, and attention-seeking behavior.

Description

Hysterical disorders

Patients with hysterical disorders, such as conversion and somatization disorder experience physical symptoms that have no organic cause. Conversion disorder affects motor and sensory functions, while somatization affects the gastrointestinal, nervous, cardiopulmonary, or reproductive systems. These patients are not "faking" their ailments, as the symptoms are very real to them. Disorders with hysteric features typically begin in adolescence or early adulthood.

Histrionic personality disorder

Histrionic personality disorder has a prevalence of approximately 2–3% of the general population. It begins in early adulthood and has been diagnosed more frequently in women than in men. Histrionic personalities are typically self-centered and attention seeking. They operate on emotion, rather than fact or logic, and their conversation is full of generalizations and dramatic appeals. While the patient's enthusiasm, flirtatious behavior, and trusting nature may make them appear charming, their need for immediate gratification, mercurial displays of emotion, and constant demand for attention often alienates them from others.

Causes & symptoms

Hysterical disorders

Hysteria may be a defense mechanism to avoid painful emotions by unconsciously transferring this distress to the body. There may be a symbolic function for this, for example a rape victim may develop paralyzed legs. Symptoms may mimic a number of physical and neurological disorders which must be ruled out before a diagnosis of hysteria is made.

Histrionic personality disorder

According to the *Diagnostic and Statistical Manual of Mental Disorders,* Fourth Edition (*DSM-IV*), individuals with histrionic personality possess at least five of the following symptoms or personality features:

- A need to be the center of attention
- Inappropriate, sexually seductive, or provocative behavior while interacting with others
- Rapidly changing emotions and superficial expression of emotions
- Vague and impressionistic speech (gives opinions without any supporting details)
- Easily influenced by others
- Believes relationships are more intimate than they are.

Diagnosis

Hysterical disorders frequently prove to be actual medical or neurological disorders,which makes it important to rule these disorders out before diagnosing a patient with hysterical disorders. In addition to a patient interview, several clinical inventories may be used to assess the patient for hysterical tendencies, such as the Minnesota Multiphasic Personality Inventory-2 (MMPI-2) or the Millon Clinical Multiaxial Inventory-III (MCMI-III). These tests may be administered in an outpatient or hospital setting by a psychiatrist or psychologist.

Treatment

Hysterical disorders

For people with hysterical disorders, a supportive healthcare environment is critical. Regular appointments with a physician who acknowledges the patient's physical discomfort are important. Psychotherapy may be attempted to help the patient gain insight into the cause of their distress. Use of behavioral therapy can help to avoid reenforcing symptoms.

Histrionic personality disorder

Psychotherapy is generally the treatment of choice for histrionic personality disorder. It focuses on supporting the patient and on helping them develop the skills needed to create meaningful relationships with others.

Prognosis

Hysterical disorders

The outcome for hysterical disorders varies by type. Somatization is typically a lifelong disorder, while conversion disorder may last for months or years. Symptoms of hysterical disorders may suddenly disappear, only to reappear in another form later.

Histrionic personality disorder

Individuals with histrionic personality disorder may be at a higher risk for suicidal gestures, attempts, or threats in an effort to gain attention. Providing a supportive environment for patients with both hysterical disorders and histrionic personality disorder is key to helping these patients.

Resources

BOOKS

American Psychiatric Association. *Diagnostic and Statistical Manual of Mental Disorders,* 4th ed. Washington, DC: American Psychiatric Press, Inc., 1994.

Maxmen, Jerrold S., and Nicholas G. Ward. "Mood Disorders." In *Essential Psychopathology and Its Treatment,* 2nd ed. New York: W.W. Norton, 1995, 206-43.

Shorter, Edward. *From Paralysis to Fatigue: A History of Psychosomatic Illness in the Modern Era.* New York: The Free Press, 1992.

Shorter, Edward. *From the Mind Into the Body: The Cultural Origins of Psychosomatic Symptoms.* New York: The Free Press, 1994.

ORGANIZATIONS

American Psychiatric Association (APA). Office of Public Affairs. 1400 K Street NW, Washington, DC 20005. (202)682-6119. http://www.psych.org/.

American Psychological Association (APA). Office of Public Affairs. 750 First St. NE, Washington, DC 20002-4242. (202)336-5700. http://www.apa.org/.

National Alliance for the Mentally Ill (NAMI). 200 North Glebe Road, Suite 1015, Arlington, VA 22203-3754. (800)950-6264. http://www.nami.org.

Paula Anne Ford-Martin

Hysterosalpingography

Definition

Hysterosalpingography is a procedure where x rays are taken of a woman's reproductive tract after a dye is injected. *Hystero* means uterus and *salpingo* means tubes, so hysterosalpingography literally means to take pictures of the uterus and fallopian tubes. This procedure may also be called hysterography (or HSG).

KEY TERMS

Catheter—A thin tube, usually made of plastic, that is inserted into the body to allow the passage of fluid into or out of a site.

Fallopian tubes—The narrow ducts leading from a woman's ovaries to the uterus. After an egg is released from the ovary during ovulation, fertilization (the union of sperm and egg) normally occurs in the fallopian tubes.

Hysterography—Another term for the x-ray procedure of the uterus and fallopian tubes.

Hysterosalpingogram—The term for the x ray taken during a hysterosalpingography procedure.

Speculum—A plastic or stainless steel instrument that is inserted into the opening of the vagina so the cervix (the opening of the uterus) and interior of the vagina can be examined.

Purpose

Hysterosalpingography is used to determine if the fallopian tubes are open, or if there are any apparent

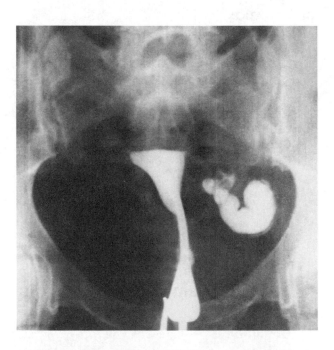

A hysterosalpingogram of the abdomen of a woman whose fallopian tubes are blocked. The fallopian tube (right on image) is blocked near the uterus, the triangular shape at center. The other fallopian tube is obstructed at a point further from the uterus where dilatation has occurred. (Photo Researchers, Inc. Reproduced by permission.)

abnormalities or defects in the uterus. It can be used to detect tumors, scar tissue, or tears in the lining of the uterus. This procedure is often used to help diagnose **infertility** in women. The fallopian tubes are the location where an egg from the ovary joins with sperm to produce a fertilized ovum. If the fallopian tubes are blocked or deformed, the egg may not be able to descend or the sperm may be blocked from moving up to meet the egg. Up to 30% of all cases of infertility are due to damaged or blocked fallopian tubes.

Precautions

This procedure should not be done on women who suspect they might be pregnant or who may have a pelvic infection. Women who have had an allergic reaction to dye used in previous x-ray procedures should inform their doctor.

Description

As with other types of pelvic examinations, the woman will lie on her back on an examination table with her legs sometimes raised in stirrups. The x-ray equipment is placed above the abdomen.

A speculum is inserted into the vagina and a catheter (a thin tube) is inserted into the uterus through the cervix (the opening to the uterus). A small balloon in the catheter is inflated to hold it in place. A liquid water-based or oil-based dye is then injected through the catheter into the uterus. This process can cause cramping, **pain,** and uterine spasms.

As the dye spreads through the reproductive tract, the doctor may watch for blockages or abnormalities on an x-ray monitor. Several x rays will also be taken. The procedure takes approximately 15–30 minutes. The x rays will be developed while the patient waits, but the final reading and interpretation of the x rays by a radiologist (a doctor who specializes in x rays) may not be available for a few days.

Interestingly, sometimes the hysterosalpingography procedure itself can be considered a treatment. The dye used can sometimes open up small blockages in the fallopian tubes. The need for additional test procedures or surgical treatments to deal with infertility should be discussed with the doctor.

Preparation

This procedure is generally done in the x-ray department of a hospital or large clinic. **General anesthesia** is not needed. A pain reliever may be taken prior to the procedure to lessen the severity of cramping.

Aftercare

While no special aftercare is required after a hysterosalpingography, the woman may be observed for some period after the procedure to ensure that she does not have any allergic reactions to the dye. A sanitary napkin may be worn after the procedure to absorb dye that will flow out through the vaginal opening. If a blockage is seen in a tube, the patient may be given an antibiotic. A woman should notify her doctor if she experiences excessive bleeding, extensive pelvic pain, **fever,** or an unpleasant vaginal odor after the procedure. These symptoms may indicate a pelvic infection. Counseling may be necessary to interpret the results of the x rays, and to discuss any additional procedures to treat tubal blockages or uterine abnormalities found.

Risks

Cramps during the procedure are common. Complications associated with hysterosalpingography include abdominal pain, pelvic infection, and allergic reactions. It is also possible that abnormalities of the fallopian tubes and uterus will not be detected by this procedure.

Normal results

A normal hysterosalpingography will show a healthy, normally shaped uterus and unblocked fallopian tubes.

Abnormal results

Blockage of one or both of the fallopian tubes or abnormalities of the uterus may be detected.

Resources

BOOKS

Carlson, Karen J., Stephanie A. Eisenstat, and Terra Ziporyn. ''Infertility: Hysterosalpingogram.'' In *The Harvard Guide to Women's Health.* Cambridge, MA: Harvard University Press, 1996, 326-327.

Faculty Members at The Yale University School of Medicine. ''Hysterosalpingogram.'' In *The Patient's Guide to Medical Tests,* edited by Barry L. Zaret, et al. Boston, MA: Houghton Mifflin Company, 1997, 263-265.

PERIODICALS

Stovall, D. W. ''The Role of Hysterosalpingography in the Evaluation of Infertility.'' *American Family Physician,* 55, 2 (February 1997): 621-628.

ORGANIZATIONS

American Society for Reproductive Medicine. 1209 Montgomery Highway, Birmingham, AL 35216-2809. (205) 978-5000. http://www.asrm.com.

Altha Roberts Edgren

Hysteroscopy

Definition

Hysteroscopy is a procedure that allows a physician to look through the vagina and neck of the uterus (cervix) to inspect the cavity of the uterus. A telescope-like instrument called a hysteroscope is used. Hysteroscopy is used as both a diagnostic and a treatment tool.

Purpose

Diagnostic hysteroscopy may be used to evaluate the cause of **infertility,** to determine the cause of repeated **miscarriages,** or to help locate polyps and fibroids.

The procedure is also used to treat gynecological conditions, often instead of or in addition to **dilatation and curettage** (D&C). A D&C is a procedure for scraping the lining of the uterus. A D&C can be used to take a sample of the lining of the uterus for analysis. Hysteroscopy is an advance over D&C because the doctor can take tissue samples of specific areas or actually see fibroids, polyps, or structural abnormalities.

When used for treatment, the hysteroscope is used with other devices to remove polyps, fibroids, or **IUDs** that have become embedded in the wall of the uterus.

Precautions

The procedure is not performed on women with **cervical cancer, endometrial cancer,** or acute pelvic inflammation.

Description

Diagnostic hysteroscopy is performed in either a doctor's office or hospital. Before inserting the hysteroscope, the doctor injects a local anesthetic around the cervix. Once it has taken effect, the doctor dilates the cervix and then inserts a narrow lighted tube (the hysteroscope) through the cervix to reveal the inside of the uterus. Ordinarily, the walls of the uterus are touching each other. In order to get a better view, the uterus is inflated with carbon dioxide gas or fluid. Hysteroscopy takes about a half hour, and can cost anywhere from $750 to $4,000 depending on the extent of the procedure.

Treatment involving the use of hysteroscopy is usually performed as a day surgical procedure with regional or **general anesthesia.** Tiny surgical instruments are inserted through the hysteroscope, and are used to remove polyps or fibroids. A small sample of tissue lining the uterus is often removed for examination, especially if there is any abnormal bleeding.

Preparation

If the procedure is done in the doctor's office, the patient will be given a mild **pain** reliever before the procedure to ease cramping. The doctor will wash the vagina and cervix with an antiseptic solution.

If the procedure is done in the hospital under general anesthesia, the patient should not eat or drink anything (not even water) after midnight the night before the procedure.

Aftercare

Many women experience light bleeding for several days after surgical hysteroscopy. Mild cramping or pain is common after operative hysteroscopy, but usually

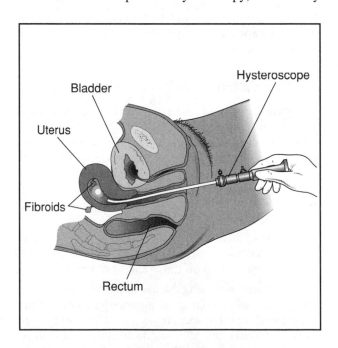

Hysteroscopy is a procedure that allows inspection of the uterus by using a telescope-like instrument called a hysteroscope. *(Illustration by Electronic Illustrators Group.)*

fades away within eight hours. If carbon dioxide gas was used, there may also be some shoulder pain. Nonprescription pain relievers may help ease discomfort. Women may want to take the day off and relax after having hysteroscopy.

Risks

Diagnostic hysteroscopy is a fairly safe procedure that only rarely causes complications. The primary risk is prolonged bleeding or infection, usually following surgical hysteroscopy to remove a growth.

Very rare complications include perforation of the uterus, bowel, or bladder. Surgery under general anesthesia causes the additional risks typically associated with anesthesia.

Patients should alert their health care provider if they develop any of these symptoms:

• Abnormal discharge

• Heavy bleeding

• **Fever** over 101°F (38.3°C)

• Severe lower abdominal pain.

Normal results

A normal, healthy uterus with no fibroids or other growths.

Abnormal results

Using hysteroscopy, the doctor may find **uterine fibroids** or polyps (often the cause of abnormal bleeding) or a septum (extra fold of tissue down the center of the uterus) that can cause infertility. Sometimes, precancerous or malignant growths are discovered.

Resources

BOOKS

Ryan, Kenneth J., Ross S. Berkowitz, and Robert L. Barbieri. *Kistner's Gynecology,* 6th ed. St. Louis: Mosby, 1997.

PERIODICALS

Anon. ''Looking Inside the Uterus.'' *Harvard Women's Health Watch* 4/5 (January 1997): 4-5.

Apgar, B.S., D. Dewitt. ''Diagnostic Hysteroscopy.'' *American Family Physician* 46/5 (November 1992): 19S-24S, 29S-32S, 35S.

Carol A. Turkington

Hysterosonography

Definition

Hysterosonography, which is also called sono-hysterography, is a new noninvasive technique that involves the slow infusion of sterile saline solution into a woman's uterus during ultrasound imaging. Hysterosonography allows the doctor to evaluate abnormal growths inside the uterus; abnormalities of the tissue lining the uterus (the endometrium); or disorders affecting deeper tissue layers. Hysterosonography does not require either radiation or contrast media, or invasive surgical procedures.

Purpose

Hysterosonography is used to evaluate patients in the following groups:

• Peri- or postmenopausal women with unexplained vaginal bleeding.

• Women whose endometrium appears abnormal during baseline ultrasound imaging.

• Women with fertility problems. **Infertility** is sometimes related to polyps, leiomyomas (fibroids), or adhesions inside the uterus. Adhesions are areas of tissue that have grown together to form bands or membranes across the inside of the uterus.

• Women receiving tamoxifen therapy for **breast cancer.**

Hysterosonography is useful as a screening test to minimize the use of more invasive diagnostic procedures, such as tissue biopsies and **dilation and curettage** (D&C). Hysterosonography can also be used as a follow-up after uterine surgery to evaluate its success.

Precautions

Hysterosonography is difficult to perform in patients with certain abnormalities:

• Cervical stenosis. Cervical stenosis means that the lower end of the uterus is narrowed or tightened. It complicates the insertion of a tube (catheter).

• Adhesions or large fibroids. These growths sometimes block the flow of saline fluid into the uterus.

Patients with active **pelvic inflammatory disease** (PID) should not be tested with hysterosonography until the disease is brought under control. Women with chronic PID or heart problems are given **antibiotics** before the procedure.

KEY TERMS

Adhesion—An abnormal union or attachment of two areas of tissue.

Contrast medium—A chemical substance used to make an organ or body part opaque on x ray.

Dilation and curettage (D&C)—A surgical procedure in which the patient's cervix is widened (dilated) and the endometrium is scraped with a scoop-shaped knife (curette).

Endometrium—The tissue that lines the uterus.

Fibroid—Another word for leiomyoma.

Leiomyoma—A benign tumor composed of muscle tissue. Leiomyomas in the uterus are sometimes called fibroids.

Pelvic inflammatory disease (PID)—An inflammation of the fallopian tubes, usually caused by bacterial infection.

Polyp—A growth projecting from the lining of the uterus. Polyps can cause fertility problems or abnormal vaginal bleeding.

Saline solution—A solution of sterile water and salt used in a variety of medical procedures. In hysterosonography, saline solution is used to fill the uterus for diagnostic imaging.

Transvaginal ultrasound (US)—The diagnostic imaging procedure that serves as the baseline for a hysterosonographic examination.

Description

A hysterosonography is preceded by a baseline ultrasound examination performed through the vagina. This allows the doctor to detect an unsuspected **pregnancy** and to assess the thickness and possible abnormalities of the patient's endometrium. The doctor then inserts a catheter into the uterus and injects sterile saline fluid while ultrasound imaging is recorded on film or videotape. The procedure takes about 10 to 15 minutes.

Preparation

Patients do not require special preparation apart from the timing of the procedure. Patients with fertility problems are examined during the first 10 days of the menstrual cycle. Patients who may have polyps are usually examined at a later phase in the cycle. The best time for examining women with fibroids is still under discussion.

Aftercare

Aftercare consists of advising the patient to contact her doctor in case of abnormal bleeding, **fever,** or abdominal **pain.** Some spotting or cramping is common, however, and can usually be treated with **nonsteroidal anti-inflammatory drugs,** such as ibuprofen.

Risks

The chief risks are mild spotting and cramping after the procedure.

Normal results

Normal findings include a symmetrical uterus with a normal endometrium and no visible masses or tumors.

Abnormal results

Abnormal findings include adhesions; polyps; leiomyomas; abnormal thickening of the endometrium; or tissue changes related to tamoxifen (Nolvadex), which is a drug given for breast cancer.

Resources

PERIODICALS

Cullinan, Joanne, et al. ''Sonohysterography: A Technique for Endometrial Evaluation.'' In *RadioGraphics* 15 (May 1995): 501-514.

Huntington, Diane K. ''Invited Commentary.'' In *RadioGraphics* 15 (May 1995): 515-516.

Yoder, Isabel C., and Deborah A. Hall. ''Hysterosalpingography in the 1990s.'' In *American Journal of Roentgenology* 157 (October 1991): 675-683.

Rebecca J. Frey

Ichthyosis

Definition

Derived from the Greek word meaning fish disease, ichthyosis is a congenital dermatological disease that is represented by thick, scaly skin.

Description

Icthyosis is a lifelong defect in skin growth that results in drying and scaling. It can be more or less severe, sometimes accumulating thick scales and cracks that are painful and bleed.

Causes & symptoms

The skin is made up of several layers, supported underneath by a layer of fat that is thicker or thinner depending on location. The lower layers contain blood vessels, the middle layers contain actively growing cells, and the upper layer consists of dead cells that serve as a barrier to the outside world. This barrier is nearly waterproof and highly resistant to infection. Scattered throughout the middle layers are hair follicles, oil and sweat glands, and nerve endings. The upper layer is constantly flaking off and being replaced from beneath by new tissue.

The defect in skin growth and hydration called ichthyosis is inborn. At the least it is unsightly, but it can itch relentlessly, leading to such complications of scratching as **lichen simplex** (**dermatitis** characterized by raw patches of skin). Either the cracking or the scratching can introduce infection, bringing with it many discomforts and complications.

Diagnosis

A dermatologist will make the diagnosis on sight. A search for associated problems will probably lead directly to the many treatments available.

Treatment

Most treatments for ichthyosis are topical, which means they are applied directly to the skin, not taken internally. In its pure form, ichthyosis requires two forms of treatment—a reduction in the amount of scale buildup and moisturizing of the underlying skin. Several agents are available for each purpose. Reduction in the amount of scale is achieved by keratolytics. Among this class of drugs are urea, lactic acid, and salicylic acid. Petrolatum, 60% propylene glycol, and glycerin are successful moisturizing agents, as are the many commercially available products. Increased humidity of the ambient air is also helpful in preventing skin dryness.

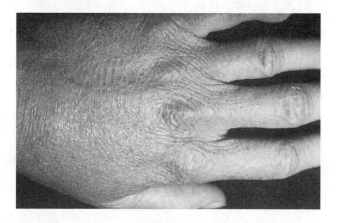

Ichthyosis is characterized by thick, scaly skin, as evident on this person's hand. *(Photograph by Lester V. Bergman, Corbis Images. Reproduced by permission.)*

Because the skin acts as a barrier to the outside environment, medicines have a hard time penetrating, especially through the thick skin of the palms of the hands and the soles of the feet. This resistance is diminished greatly by maceration. Soaking hands in water macerates skin so that it looks like prune skin. Occlusion with rubber gloves or plastic wrap will also macerate skin. Applying medicines and then covering the skin with an occlusive dressing will facilitate entrance of the medicine and greatly magnify its effect.

Secondary treatments are necessary to control pruritus (**itching**) and infection. Commercial products containing camphor, menthol, eucalyptus oil, aloe, and similar substances are very effective as antipruritics. If the skin cracks deeply enough, a pathway for infection is created. **Topical antibiotics** like bacitracin are effective in prevention and in the early stages of these skin infections. Cleansing with hydrogen peroxide inhibits infection as well.

Finally, there are topical and internal derivatives of vitamin A called retinoids, that improve skin growth and are used for bad cases of **acne,** ichthyosis, and other skin conditions.

Prognosis

This condition requires continuous care throughout a lifetime. Properly treated, it is primarily a cosmetic problem.

Resources

BOOKS

Baden, Howard P. "Ichthyosiform Dermatoses." In *Dermatology in General Medicine.* Edited by Thomas B. Fitzpatrick, et al. New York: McGraw-Hill, 1993, pp. 531-544.

Parker, Frank. "Skin Diseases of General Importance." In *Cecil Textbook of Medicine.* Edited by J. Claude Bennett and Fred Plum. Philadelphia: W. B. Saunders, 1996, p. 2204.

J. Ricker Polsdorfer

Icterus *see* **Jaundice**

Idiopathic hypertrophic subaortic stenosis *see* **Hypertrophic cardiomyopathy**

KEY TERMS

Bronchoalveolar lavage—A way of obtaining a sample of fluid from the airways by inserting a flexible tube through the windpipe. Used to diagnose the type of lung disease.

Desquamation—Shedding of the cells lining the insides of the air sacs. A feature of desquamative interstitial pneumonitis.

Idiopathic—A disease whose cause is unknown.

Immune system—A set of body chemicals and specialized cells that attack an invading agent (such as a virus) by forming antibodies that can engulf and destroy it.

Infiltrative—A process whereby inflammatory or other types of disease spread throughout an organ such as the lungs.

Interstitial—Refers to the connective tissue that supports the "working parts" of an organ, in the case of the lungs the air sacs.

Pulmonary fibrosis—A scarring process that is the end result of many forms of long-lasting lung disease.

Idiopathic infiltrative lung diseases

Definition

The term *idiopathic* means "cause unknown." The idiopathic infiltrative lung diseases, also known as interstitial lung diseases, are a group of more than a hundred disorders seen in both adults and (less often) in children, whose cause is unknown but which tend to spread, or "infiltrate" through much or all of the lung tissue. They range from mild conditions that respond well to treatment, to progressive, nonresponsive disease states that severely limit lung function and may cause **death.**

Description

The body produces inflammatory cells in response to a variety of conditions, including a number of different diseases, pollutants, certain infections, exposure to organic dust or toxic fumes and vapors, and various drugs and poisons. When white blood cells and tissue fluid rich in protein collect in the small air sacs of the lungs, or alveoli, the sacs become inflamed (alveolitis). In time, the fluid may solidify and cause scar formation that replaces the normal lung tissue. This process is known as pulmonary fibrosis. In about half of all patients, no specific cause is ever found; they are said to have idiopathic pulmonary fibrosis.

Some patients have special types of interstitial lung disease that may occur in certain types of patients, or feature typical pathological changes when a sample of lung tissue is examined under a microscope. They include:

- Usual interstitial pneumonitis. Disease occurs in a patchy form throughout the lungs. Parts of the lungs can appear normal while others have dense scar tissue and lung cysts, often the end result of pulmonary fibrosis. This disease progresses quite slowly. Both children and adults may be affected.

- Desquamative interstitial pneumonitis. Similar-appearing lesions are present throughout the lungs. Both inflammatory cells and cells that have separated from the air sac linings (''desquamated'') are present. Some researchers believe this is an early form of usual interstitial pneumonitis.

- Lymphocytic interstitial pneumonitis. Most of the cells infiltrating the lungs are the type of white blood cells called lymphocytes. Both the breathing tubes (bronchi) and blood vessels of the lungs become thickened. In children, this condition tends to occur when the immune system is not operating properly as occurs with Acquired immunodeficiency syndrome (**AIDS**).

Causes & symptoms

By definition, the causes of *idiopathic* infiltrative lung diseases are not known. Some forms of pulmonary fibrosis, however, do have specific causes and these may provide a clue as to what may cause idiopathic diseases. Known causes of pulmonary fibrosis include diseases that impair the body's immune function, infection by viruses and the bacterium causing **tuberculosis,** and exposure to mineral dusts such as silica or asbestos, or organic materials such as bird droppings. Other cases of pulmonary fibrosis result from exposure to fumes and vapors, radiation (in industry or medically), and certain drugs used to treat disease.

Patients with interstitial lung disease usually have labored breathing when exerting themselves. Often they **cough** and feel overly tired (''no stamina''). **Wheezing** is uncommon. When the physician listens to the patient's chest with a stethoscope, dry, crackling sounds may be heard. Some patients have vague chest **pain.** When disease progresses, the patient may breathe very rapidly, have mottled blue skin (because of getting too little oxygen), and lose weight. The fingertips may appear thick or club-shaped.

Diagnosis

Both scars in the lung and cysts (air-filled spaces) can be seen on a chest x ray. Up to 10% of patients, however, may have normal x rays even if their symptoms are severe. A special type of x ray, high-resolution **computed tomography scan** (CT scan), often is helpful in adult patients. Tests of lung function will show that the lungs cannot hold enough air with each breath, and there is too little oxygen in the blood, especially after exercising. In a procedure called bronchoalveolar lavage, a tube is placed through the nose and windpipe into the bronchi and a small amount of saline in released and then withdrawn. This fluid then can be analyzed for cells. A tiny piece of lung tissue can be sampled using the same instrument. If necessary, a larger sample (a biopsy) is taken through an incision in the chest wall and examined under a microscope.

Treatment

The first medication given, providing scarring is not too extensive, is usually a steroid drug such as prednisone. An occasional patient will improve dramatically if steroid therapy stops the inflammation. Most patients, however, improve to a limited extent. It may take 6–12 weeks for a patient to begin to respond. Patients must be watched closely for a gain in body weight, high blood pressure, and depression. Steroids can also result in diabetes, ulcer disease, and cataract. Patients treated with steroids are at risk of contracting serious infection. If steroids have not proved effective or have caused serious side-effects, other anti-inflammatory drugs, such as cyclophosphamide (Cytoxan) or azathioprine (Imuran), can be tried. Cytoxan sometimes is combined with a steroid, but it carries its own risks, which include bladder inflammation and suppression of the bone marrow. Some patients will benefit from a bronchodilator drug that relaxes the airways and makes breathing easier.

Some patients with interstitial lung disease, especially children, will need **oxygen therapy.** Usually oxygen is given during sleep or **exercise,** but if the blood oxygen level is very low it may be given constantly. A program of conditioning, training in how to breathe efficiently, energy-saving tips, and a proper diet will help patients achieve the highest possible level of function given the state of their illness. All patients should be vaccinated each year against **influenza.** A last resort for those with very advanced disease who do not respond to medication is **lung transplantation.** This operation is being done more widely, and it is even possible to replace both lungs.

Prognosis

A scoring system based on lung function and x ray appearances has been designed to help monitor a patient's course. In general, idiopathic forms of interstitial lung disease cause a good deal of illness, and a significant numbers of deaths. A majority of patients get worse over time, although survival for many years is certainly possible. An estimated one in five affected children fail to survive. In different series, survival times average between four and ten years. Early diagnosis gives the best chance of a patient recovering, or at least stabilizing. Once the lungs are badly scarred, nothing short of lung transplantation offers hope of restoring lung function. Patients with desquamative interstitial pneumonitis tend to respond well to steroid treatment, and live longer than those with other types of infiltrative lung disease.

Prevention

Since we do not understand what causes idiopathic interstitial lung diseases, there is no way to prevent them. What can be done is to prevent extensive scarring of the lungs by making the diagnosis shortly after the first symptoms develop, and trying steroids or other drugs in hope of suppressing lung inflammation. Every effort should be made to avoid exposure to dusts, gases, chemicals, and even pets. Keeping fit and learning how to breathe efficiently will help maintain lung function as long as possible.

Resources

BOOKS

Berkow, Robert, ed. *Merck Manual of Medical Information: Home Edition.* Whitehouse Station, NJ: Merck Research Laboratories, 1997.

ORGANIZATIONS

American Lung Association. 432 Park Avenue South, New York, NY 10016. 800-LUNG-USA. http://www.lungusa.org.

OTHER

University of Wisconsin-Madison Health Sciences Libraries. *Healthweb: Pulmonary Medicine.* January 12, 1998. http://www.biostat.wisc.edu/chslib/hw/pulmonar.

David A. Cramer

Idiopathic primary renal hematuric/proteinuric syndrome

Definition

This syndrome includes a group of disorders characterized by blood and protein in the urine and by damage to the kidney glomeruli (filtering structures) that may lead to kidney failure.

Description

This syndrome, also known as Berger's disease or IgA nephropathy, arises when internal kidney structure called glomeruli become inflamcd and injured. It can occur at any age, but the great majority of patients are 16–35 when diagnosed. Males seem to be affected more often than females, and whites are more often affected than blacks. Blood in the urine (hematuria), either indicated by a visible change in the color of the urine or detected by laboratory testing, is a hallmark of this syndrome and it may occur continuously or sporadically. The pattern of occurrence is not indicative of the severity of kidney damage.

Causes & symptoms

The glomeruli are the kidney structures that filter the blood and extract waste, which is then excreted as urine. The barrier between the blood and the urine side of the filter mechanism is a membrane only one cell layer thick. Anything that damages the membrane will result in hematuria. Symptoms of idiopathic primary renal hematruic/proteinuric syndrome are caused by inflammation of the glomeruli and deposit of IgA antibodies in kidney tissue. Although a genetic basis for this syndrome is suspected, this has not been proven. Symptoms often appear 24–48 hours after an upper respiratory or gastrointestinal infection. Symptoms of the syndrome include:

- Blood in the urine (hematuria)
- Protein in the urine (proteinuria)
- Pain in the lower back or kidney area
- Elevated blood pressure (20–30% of cases)
- Nephrotic syndrome (less than 10% of cases)
- Swelling (occasionally).

This condition usually does not get worse with time, although renal failure occasionally results. In patients with large amounts of IgA deposits in their glomeruli, the long term prognosis may not be favorable. The syndrome can spontaneously go into remission, although this is more common in children than in adults.

Diagnosis

One of the objectives of diagnosis is to distinguish glomerular from non-glomerular kidney diseases. Idiopathic primary hematuric/proteinuric syndrome involves the glomeruli. The presence of fragmented or distorted red blood cells in the urine is evidence of glomerular disease. A high concentration of protein in the urine is also evidence for glomerular disease. The hematuria associated with this syndrome must be distinguished from that caused by urinary tract diseases, which can also cause a loss of blood into the urine. Biopsy of the patient's kidney shows deposits of IgA antibodies. Detecting IgA-antibody deposits rules out thin membrane disease as the cause of the hematuria and proteinuria. Test values are normal for ASO, complement, rheumatoid factor, antinuclear antibodies, anti-DNase, and cryoglobulins, all of which are associated with different types of kidney disease. A diagnosis of idiopathic primary renal hematuric/proteinuric syndrome is largely made by ruling out other diseases and their causes, leaving this syndrome as the remaining possible diagnosis.

Treatment

Many patients do not need specific treatment, except for those who have symptoms indicating a poor prognosis. Oral doses of corticosteroids are effective in patients with mild proteinuria and good kidney function. Other treatments, such as medications to lower blood pressure, are aimed at slowing or preventing kidney damage. If kidney failure develops, dialysis or kidney transplantation are necessary.

Prognosis

Idiopathic primary renal hematuric/proteinuric syndrome progresses slowly and in many cases does not progress at all. Risk for progression of the disorder is considered higher if there is:

- High blood pressure
- Large amounts of protein in the urine
- Increased levels of urea and creatinine in the blood (indications of kidney function).

About 25–35% of patients may develop kidney failure within about 25 years.

Prevention

Since the underlying causes of this syndrome are so poorly understood, there is no prevention known.

Resources

BOOKS

Brenner, B.M. *The Kidney.* Philadelphia: W.B. Saunders, 1996.

Greenberg, A. *Primer on Kidney Diseases.* San Diego: Academic Press, 1998.

Schrier, R.W., and C.W. Gottschalk. *Diseases of the Kidney.* Boston: Little Brown, 1997.

ORGANIZATIONS

IgA Nephropathy Support Network. 964 Brown Avenue, Huntington Valley, PA 19006. (215) 663–0536.

National Kidney Foundation. 30 E. 33rd Street, Suite 1100, New York, NY 10016. (212) 889–2210.

John Thomas Lohr

Idiopathic thrombocytopenic purpura

Definition

Idiopathic thrombocytopenic purpura, or ITP, is a bleeding disorder caused by an abnormally low level of platelets in the patient's blood. Platelets are small plate-shaped bodies in the blood that combine to form a plug when a blood vessel is injured. The platelet plug then binds certain proteins in the blood to form a clot that stops bleeding. ITP's name describes its cause and two symptoms. Idiopathic means that the disorder has no apparent cause. ITP is now often called immune thrombocytopenic purpura rather than idiopathic because of recent findings that ITP patients have autoimmune antibodies in their blood. **Thrombocytopenia** is another

KEY TERMS

. . . .

Autoimmune disorder—A disorder in which the patient's immune system produces antibodies that destroy some of the body's own products. ITP in adults is thought to be an autoimmune disorder.

Idiopathic—Of unknown cause. Idiopathic refers to a disease that is not preceded or caused by any known dysfunction or disorder in the body.

Petechiae—Small pinpoint hemorrhages in skin or mucous membranes caused by the rupture of capillaries.

Platelet—A blood component that helps to prevent blood from leaking from broken blood vessels. ITP is a bleeding disorder caused by an abnormally low level of platelets in the blood.

Prednisone—A corticosteroid medication that is used to treat ITP. Prednisone works by decreasing the effects of antibody on blood platelets. Long-term treatment with prednisone is thought to decrease antibody production.

Purpura—A skin discoloration of purplish or brownish red spots caused by bleeding from broken capillaries.

Splenectomy—Surgical removal of the spleen.

Thrombocytopenia—An abnormal decline in the number of platelets in the blood.

word for a decreased number of blood platelets. Purpura refers to a purplish or reddish-brown skin rash caused by the leakage of blood from broken capillaries into the skin. Other names for ITP include purpura hemorrhagica and essential thrombocytopenia.

Description

ITP may be either acute or chronic. The acute form is most common in children between the ages of two and six years; the chronic form is most common in adult females between 20 and 40. Between 10% and 20% of children with ITP have the chronic form. ITP does not appear to be related to race, lifestyle, climate, or environmental factors.

ITP is a disorder that affects the overall *number* of blood platelets rather than their function. The normal platelet level in adults is between 150,000 and 450,000/mm3. **Platelet counts** below 50,000 mm3 increase the risk of dangerous bleeding from trauma; counts below 20,000/mm3 increase the risk of spontaneous bleeding.

Causes & Symptoms

In adults, ITP is considered an autoimmune disorder, which means that the body produces antibodies that damage some of its own products—in this case, blood platelets. Some adults with chronic ITP also have other immune system disorders, such as **systemic lupus erythematosus** (SLE). In children, ITP is usually triggered by a virus infection, most often **rubella, chickenpox, measles,** cytomegalovirus, or Epstein-Barr virus. It usually begins about two or three weeks after the infection.

Acute ITP

Acute ITP is characterized by bleeding into the skin or from the nose, mouth, digestive tract, or urinary tract. The onset is usually sudden. Bleeding into the skin takes the form of purpura or petechiae. Purpura is a purplish or reddish-brown rash or discoloration of the skin; petechiae are small round pinpoint hemorrhages. Both are caused by the leakage of blood from tiny capillaries under the skin surface. In addition to purpura and petechiae, the patient may notice that he or she **bruises** more easily than usual. In extreme cases, patients with ITP may bleed into the lungs, brain, or other vital organs.

Chronic ITP

Chronic ITP has a gradual onset and may have minimal or no external symptoms. The low platelet count may be discovered in the course of a routine blood test. Most patients with chronic ITP, however, will consult their primary care doctor because of the purpuric skin rash, **nosebleeds,** or bleeding from the digestive or urinary tract. Women sometimes go to their gynecologist for unusually heavy or lengthy menstrual periods.

The risk factors for the development of chronic ITP include:

• Female sex.

• Age over 10 years at onset of symptoms.

• Slow onset of bruising.

• Presence of other autoantibodies in the blood.

Diagnosis

ITP is usually considered a diagnosis of exclusion, which means that the doctor arrives at the diagnosis by a process of ruling out other possible causes. If the patient belongs to one or more of the risk groups for chronic ITP, the doctor may order a blood test for autoantibodies in the blood early in the diagnostic process.

Physical examination

If the doctor suspects ITP, he or she will examine the patient's skin for bruises, purpuric areas, or petechiae. If the patient has had nosebleeds or bleeding from the mouth or other parts of the body, the doctor will examine these areas for other possible causes of bleeding. Patients with ITP usually look and feel healthy except for the bleeding.

The most important features that the doctor will be looking for during the **physical examination** are the condition of the patient's spleen and the presence of **fever.** Patients with ITP do not have fever whereas patients with lupus and some other types of thrombocytopenia are usually feverish. The doctor will have the patient lie flat on the examining table in order to feel the size of the spleen. If the spleen is noticeably enlarged, ITP is not absolutely ruled out but is a less likely diagnosis.

Laboratory testing

The doctor will order a complete **blood count** (CBC), a test of clotting time, a bone marrow test, and a test for antiplatelet antibodies if it is available in the hospital laboratory. Patients with ITP usually have platelet counts below 20,000/mm3 and prolonged **bleeding time.** The size and appearance of the platelets may be abnormal. The red blood cell count (RBC) and white blood cell count (WBC) are usually normal, although about 10% of patients with ITP are also anemic. The blood marrow test yields normal results. Detection of antiplatelet antibodies in the blood is considered to confirm the diagnosis of ITP.

Treatment

General care and monitoring

There is no specific treatment for ITP. In most cases, the disorder will resolve without medications or surgery within two to six weeks. Nosebleeds can be treated with ice packs when necessary.

General care includes explaining ITP to the patient and advising him or her to watch for bruising, petechiae, or other signs of recurrence. Children should be discouraged from rough contact sports or other activities that increase the risk of trauma. Patients are also advised to avoid using **aspirin** or ibuprofen (Advil, Motrin) as **pain** relievers because these drugs lengthen the clotting time of blood.

Emergency treatment

Patients with acute ITP who are losing large amounts of blood or bleeding into their central nervous system require emergency treatment. This includes **transfusions** of platelets, intravenous immunoglobulins, or prednisone. Prednisone is a steroid medication that decreases the effects of antibody on platelets and eventually lowers antibody production. If the patient has a history of ITP that has not responded to prednisone or immunoglobu-

lins, the surgeon may remove the patient's spleen. This operation is called a **splenectomy.** The reason for removing the spleen when ITP does not respond to other forms of treatment is that the spleen sometimes keeps platelets out of the general blood circulation.

Medications and transfusions

Patients with chronic ITP can be treated with prednisone, immune globulin, or large doses of intravenous gamma globulin. Although 90% of patients respond to immunoglobulin treatment, it is very expensive. About 80% of patients respond to prednisone therapy. Platelet transfusions are not recommended for routine treatment of ITP. If the patient's platelet level does not improve within one to four months, or requires high doses of prednisone, the doctor may recommend splenectomy. All medications for ITP are given either orally or intravenously; intramuscular injection is avoided because of the possibility of causing bleeding into the skin.

Surgery

Between 80% and 85% of adults with ITP have a remission of the disorder after the spleen is removed. Splenectomy is usually avoided in children younger than five years because of the increased risk of a severe infection after the operation. In older children, however, splenectomy is recommended if the child has been treated for 12 months without improvement; if the ITP is very severe or the patient is getting worse; if the patient begins to bleed into the head or brain; and if the patient is an adolescent female with extremely heavy periods.

Prognosis

The prognosis for recovery from acute ITP is good; 80% of patients recover without special treatment. The prognosis for chronic ITP is also good; most patients experience long-term remissions. In rare instances, however, ITP can cause life-threatening hemorrhage or bleeding into the central nervous system.

Resources

BOOKS

"Blood Component Therapy: Platelet Transfusions." In *Internal Medicine On Call,* edited by Steven A. Haist, et al. Stamford, CT: Appleton & Lange, 1991.

Hays, Taru. "Hematologic Disorders." In *Handbook of Pediatrics,* edited by Gerald B. Merenstein, et al. Norwalk, CT: Appleton & Lange, 1994.

"Hematology and Oncology: Immunologic Idiopathic Thrombocytopenic Purpura (ITP)." In *The Merck Manual of Diagnosis and Therapy,,* edited by Robert Berkow, et al. Rahway, NJ: Merck Research Laboratories, 1992.

"Idiopathic Thrombocytopenic Purpura." In *Professional Guide to Diseases,* edited by Stanley Loeb, et al. Springhouse, PA: Springhouse Corporation, 1991.

Linker, Charles A. "Blood." In *Current Medical Diagnosis & Treatment 1998,* edited by Lawrence M. Tierney, Jr., et al. Stamford, CT: Appleton & Lange, 1998.

McMillan, Robert. "Platelet-Mediated Bleeding Disorders." In *Conn's Current Therapy,* edited by Robert E. Rakel, MD. Philadelphia: W. B. Saunders Company, 1998.

"On-Call Problems: Thrombocytopenia." In *Internal Medicine On Call,* edited by Steven A. Haist, et al. Stamford, CT: Appleton & Lange, 1991.

Rebecca J. Frey

IHSS *see* **Hypertrophic cardiomyopathy**

Ileal conduit *see* **Urinary diversion surgery**

Ileocolitis *see* **Crohn's disease**

Ileostomy *see* **Enterostomy**

Ileus

Definition

Ileus is a partial or complete non-mechanical blockage of the small and/or large intestine.

Description

There are two types of **intestinal obstructions,** mechanical and non-mechanical. Mechanical obstructions occur because the bowel is physically blocked and its contents can not pass the point of the obstruction. This happens when the bowel twists on itself (volvulus) or as the result of **hernias,** impacted feces, abnormal tissue growth, or the presence of foreign bodies in the intestines.

Unlike mechanical obstruction, non-mechanical obstruction, called ileus or paralytic ileus, occurs because peristalsis stops. Peristalsis is the rhythmic contraction that moves material through the bowel. Ileus is most often associated with an infection of the peritoneum (the membrane lining the abdomen). It is one of the major causes of bowel obstruction in infants and children.

Another common cause of ileus is a disruption or reduction of the blood supply to the abdomen. Handling the bowel during abdominal surgery can also cause peristalsis to stop, so people who have had abdominal surgery are more likely to experience ileus. When ileus results

---

from abdominal surgery the condition is often temporary and usually lasts only 48-72 hours.

Ileus can also be caused by kidney diseases, especially when potassium levels are decreased. Heart disease and certain **chemotherapy** drugs, such as vinblastine (Velban, Velsar) and vincristine (Oncovin, Vincasar PES, Vincrex), also can cause ileus. Infants with **cystic fibrosis** are more likely to experience meconium ileus (a dark green material in the intestine). Over all, the total rate of bowel obstruction due both to mechanical and non-mechanical causes is one in one thousand people (1/1,000).

Causes & symptoms

When the bowel stops functioning, the following symptoms occur:

- Abdominal cramping
- Abdominal distention
- **Nausea and vomiting**
- Failure to pass gas or stool.

Diagnosis

When a doctor listens with a stethoscope to the abdomen there will be few or no bowel sounds indicating that the intestine has stopped functioning. Ileus can be confirmed by x rays of the abdomen, **computed tomography scans** (CT scans), or ultrasound. It may be necessary to do more invasive tests, such as a **barium enema** or upper GI series, if the obstruction is mechanical. Blood tests also are useful in diagnosing paralytic ileus.

Barium studies are used in cases of mechanical obstruction, but may cause problems by increasing pressure or intestinal contents if used in ileus. Also, in cases of suspected mechanical obstruction involving the gastrointestinal tract (from the small intestine downward) use of barium x rays are contraindicated, since they may contribute to the obstruction. In such cases a barium enema should always be done first.

Treatment

Patients may be treated with supervised bed rest in a hospital and bowel rest—where nothing is taken by mouth and patients are fed intravenously or through the use of a nasogastric tube. A nasogastric tube is a tube inserted through the nose, down the throat, and into the stomach. A similar tube can be inserted in the intestine. The contents are then suctioned out. In some cases, especially where there is a mechanical obstruction, surgery may be necessary.

Drug therapies that promote intestinal motility (ability of the intestine to move spontaneously), such as cisapride and vasopressin (Pitressin), are sometimes prescribed.

Alternative treatment

Alternative practitioners offer few treatment suggestions, but focus on prevention by keeping the bowels healthy through eating a good diet, high in fiber and low in fat. If the case is not a medical emergency, homeopathic treatment and traditional Chinese medicine can recommend therapics that may help to reinstate peristalsis.

Prognosis

The outcome varies depending on the cause of ileus.

Prevention

Most cases of ileus are not preventable. Surgery to remove a tumor or other mechanical obstruction will help prevent a reoccurrence.

Resources

OTHER

Healthanswers. ''Intestinal Obstruction.'' http://www.healthanswers.com/database/ami/converted/000260.html.

Trigan Oncology Associates. ''Bowel Paralysis.'' http://www.trigan.com/ileus.htm.

Tish Davidson

Imipramine *see* **Tricyclic antidepressants**

KEY TERMS

Decubitus ulcers—A pressure sore resulting from ulceration of the skin occurring in persons confined to bed for long periods of time

Ligament—Ligaments are structures that hold bones together and prevent excessive movement of the joint. They are tough, fibrous bands of tissue.

Pneumonia—An acute or chronic disease characterized by inflammation of the lungs and caused by viruses, bacteria, or other microorganisms.

Tendon—Tendons are structures than attach bones to muscles and muscles to other muscles.

Immobilization

Definition

Immobilization refers to the process of holding a joint or bone in place with a splint, cast, or brace. This is done to prevent an injured area from moving while it heals.

Purpose

Splints, casts, and braces support and protect broken bones, dislocated joints, and injured soft tissue, such as tendons and ligaments. Immobilization restricts motion to allow the injured area to heal. It can help reduce **pain**, swelling, and muscle spasm. In some cases, splints and casts are applied after surgical procedures that repair bones, tendons, or ligaments. This allows for protection and proper alignment early in the healing phase.

Precautions

There are no special precautions for immobilization.

Description

When an arm, hand, leg, or foot requires immobilization, the cast, splint, or brace will generally extend from the joint above the injury to the joint below the injury. For example, an injury to the mid calf requires immobilization from the knee to the ankle and foot. Injuries of the hip and upper thigh or shoulder and upper arm require a cast that encircles the body and extends down the injured leg or arm.

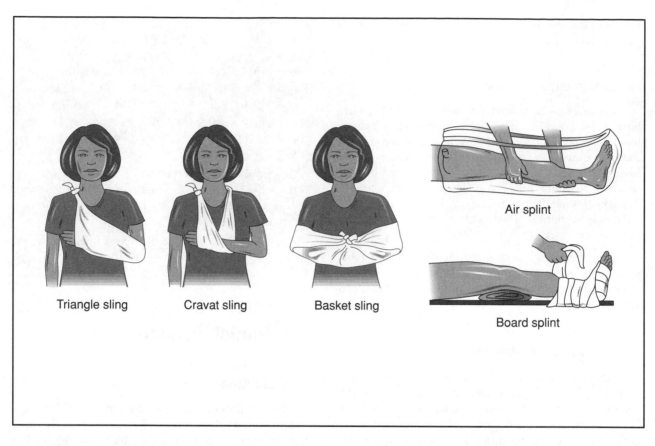

Triangle sling   Cravat sling   Basket sling

Air splint

Board splint

Immobilization refers to the process of immobilizing or fixating the position of a joint, bone, extremity, or torso with a splint, cast, or brace. Immobilization can help reduce pain, swelling, and muscle spasms. The illustrations above feature several types of immobilization techniques. *(Illustration by Electronic Illustrators Group.)*

Casts and splints

Casts are generally used for immobilization of a broken bone. Once the doctor makes sure the two broken ends of the bone are aligned, a cast is put on to keep them in place until they are rejoined through natural healing. Casts are applied by a physician, a nurse, or an assistant. They are custom-made to fit each person, and are usually made of plaster or fiberglass. Fiberglass weighs less than plaster, is more durable, and allows the skin more adequate airflow than plaster. A layer of cotton or synthetic padding is first wrapped around the skin to cover the injured area and protect the skin. The plaster or fiberglass is then applied over this.

Most casts should not be gotten wet. However, some types of fiberglass casts use Gortex padding that is waterproof and allows the person to completely immerse the cast in water when taking a shower or bath. There are some circumstances when this type of cast material can not be used.

A splint is often used to immobilize a dislocated joint while it heals. Splints are also often used for finger injuries, such as **fractures** or baseball finger. Baseball finger is an injury in which the tendon at the end of the finger is separated from the bone as a result of trauma. Splinting also is used to immobilize an injured arm or leg immediately after an injury. Before moving a person who has injured an arm or leg some type of temporary splint should be applied to prevent further injury to the area. Splints may be made of acrylic, polyethylene foam, plaster of paris, or aluminum. In an emergency, a splint can be made from a piece of wood or rolled magazine.

Slings

Slings are often used to support the arm after a fracture or other injury. They are generally used along with a cast or splint, but sometimes are used alone as a means of immobilization. They can be used in an emergency to immobilize the arm until the person can be seen by a doctor. A triangular bandage is placed under the injured arm and then tied around the neck.

Braces

Braces are used to support, align, or hold a body part in the correct position. Braces are sometimes used after a surgical procedure is performed on an arm or leg. They can also be used for an injury. Since some braces can be easily taken off and put back on, they are often used when the person must have physical therapy or **exercise** the limb during the healing process. Many braces can also be adjusted to allow for a certain amount of movement.

Braces can be custom-made or a ready-made brace can be used. The off-the-shelf braces are made in a variety of shapes and sizes. They generally have Velcro straps that make the brace easy to adjust, and to put on and take off. Both braces and splints offer less support and protection than a cast and may not be a treatment option in all circumstances.

Collars

A collar is generally used for neck injuries. A soft collar can relieve pain by restricting movement of the head and neck. They also transfer some of the weight of the head from the neck to the chest. Stiff collars are generally used to support the neck when there has been a fracture in one of the bones of the neck. Cervical collars are widely used by emergency personnel at the scene of injuries when there is a potential neck or **head injury.**

Traction

Immobilization may also be secured by **traction.** Traction involves using a method for applying tension to correct the alignment of two structures (such as two bones) and hold them in the correct position. For example, if the bone in the thigh breaks, the broken ends may have a tendency to overlap. Use of traction will hold them in the correct position for healing to occur. The strongest form of traction involves inserting a stainless steel pin through a bony prominence attached by a horse shoe shaped bow and rope to a pulley and weights suspended over the end of the patient's bed.

Traction must be balanced by counter-traction. This is obtained by tilting the bed and allowing the patient's body to act as a counter-weight. Another technique involves applying weights pulling in the opposite direction.

Traction for neck injuries may be in the form of a leather or cotton cloth halter placed around the chin and lower back of the head. For very severe neck injuries that require maximum traction, tongs that resemble ice tongs are inserted into small holes drilled in the outer skull.

All traction requires careful observation and adjustment by doctors and nurses to maintain proper balance and alignment of the traction with free suspension of the weights.

Immobilzation can also be secured by a form of traction called skin traction. This is a combination of a splint and traction that is applied to the arms or legs by strips of adhesive tape placed over the skin of the arm or leg. Adhesive strips, moleskin, or foam rubber traction strips are applied on the skin. This method is effective only if a moderate amount of traction is required.

Preparation

There are many reasons for immobilization using splints, casts, and braces. Each person should understand his or her diagnosis clearly.

Aftercare

After a cast or splint has been put on, the injured arm or leg should be elevated for 24 to 72 hours. It is recommended that the person lie or sit with the injured arm or leg raised above the level of the heart. Rest combined with elevation will reduce pain and speed the healing process by minimizing swelling.

Fingers or toes can be exercised as much as can be tolerated after casting. This has been found to decrease swelling and prevent stiffness. If excessive swelling is noted, the application of ice to the splint or cast may be helpful.

After the cast, splint, or brace is removed, gradual exercise is usually performed to regain muscle strength and motion. The doctor may also recommend **hydrotherapy, heat treatments,** and other forms of physical therapy.

Risks

For some people, such as those in traction, immobilization will require long periods of bedrest. Lying in one position in bed for an extended period of time can result in sores on the skin (decubitus ulcers) and skin infection. Long periods of bedrest can also cause a build up of fluid in the lungs or an infection in the lungs (**pneumonia**). Urinary infection can also be a result of extended bedrest.

People who have casts, splints, or braces on their arms or legs will generally spend several weeks not using the injured arm or leg. This lack of use can result in decreased muscle tone and shrinkage of the muscle (atrophy). Much of this loss can usually be regained, however, through **rehabilitation** after the injury has healed.

Immobility can also cause psychological **stress.** An individual restricted to a bed with a traction device may become frustrated and bored, and perhaps even depressed, irritable, and withdrawn.

There is the possibility of decreased circulation if the cast, splint, or brace fits too tightly. Excessive pressure over a nerve can cause irritation or possible damage if not corrected. If the cast, splint, or brace breaks or malfunctions, the healing process of the bone or soft tissue can be disrupted and lead to deformity.

Normal results

Normally, the surgical or injured area heals appropriately with the help of immobilization. The form of immobilization can be discontinued, which is followed by an appropriate rehabilitation program under the supervision of a physical therapist to regain range of motion and strength.

Resources

BOOKS

American Red Cross. *Community First Aid and Safety.* St. Louis Mo.: Mosby Year Book Inc., 1993.

PERIODICALS

Gorden, Everett J. "Fractures and Dislocations: An Overview." *Trauma* 37 (Feb.1996): 5-36.

Krock, N. "Immobilizing the Cervical Spine Using a Collar: Complications and Nursing Management." *Nursing Journal* 18 (Mar. 1997):52-55.

OTHER

Casts & Splints the Center for Orthopaedics and Sports Medicine 1211 Johnson Ferry Rd.; Marietta, GA., 30068 770-565-0011 http://www.arthrosc

Griffith, H. "Dislocations or Subluxation" 1998 http://www.thriveonline.com/health/Library/pedillsymp/pedillsymp118.html (3/25/98).

Jeffrey Peter Larson

Immune complex detection *see* **Immune complex test**

Immune complex test

Definition

These tests evaluate the immune system, whose function is to defend the body against invaders such as bacteria and viruses. The immune system also plays a role in the control of **cancer,** and is responsible for the phenomena of allergy, hypersensitivity, and rejection problems when organs or tissue are transplanted.

One of the ways the immune system protects the body is by producing proteins called antibodies. Antibodies are formed in response to another type of protein called an antigen (anything foreign or different from a natural body protein). Immune complex reactions occur when large numbers of antigen-antibody complexes accumulate in the body.

KEY TERMS

Antibody—A (immunogloblin) molecule which interacts with a specific antigen. Antibodies provide protection from microscopic invaders like bacteria.

Antigen—Any substance which is capable under certain circumstances of producing an immune response either from antibodies or T-cells; bacteria are often antigens.

Autoimmune disorder—A disorder caused by a reaction of an individual's immune system against the organs or tissues of the body. Autoimmune processes can have different results: slow destruction of a particular type of cell or tissue, stimulation of an organ into excessive growth, or interference in function.

Biopsy—The removal and examination, usually under a microscope, of tissue from the living body. Used for diagnosis.

Systemic lupus erythematosus—A chronic disease of the connective tissues in the body; characterized by involvement of the skin, joints, kidneys, and serosal membranes (membranes that form the outer covering of organs in the abdomen or chest).

Purpose

The purpose of the immune complex test is to demonstrate circulating immune complexes in the blood, to estimate the severity of immune complex disease, and to monitor response to therapy.

Precautions

Because this test is requested when the physician suspects that a patient's immune system is not functioning properly, special care should be taken during and after blood is drawn. For example, the venipuncture site should be kept clean and dry to avoid any chance of infection.

Description

Immune complexes are normally not detected in the blood. However, when immune complexes are produced faster than they can be cleared by the system, immune complex disease may occur. Examples of such disorders are drug sensitivity, **rheumatoid arthritis,** and a disease called **systemic lupus erythematosus,** or SLE.

The method generally used for detecting immune complexes is examination of tissue obtained by biopsy (removal and examination of tissue sample) and the subsequent use of different staining techniques with specific antibodies. However, since tissue biopsies do not provide information about the level of complexes still in the circulatory system, serum assays obtained from blood samples which indirectly detect circulating immune complexes are useful. However, due to the variability of these complexes, several test methods may be used. Also, as most immune complex assays have not been standardized, more than one test may be required to achieve accurate results.

Preparation

This test requires a blood sample. It is not necessary for the patient to be in a **fasting** (nothing to eat or drink) state before the test.

Risks

Risks for this test are minimal, but may include slight bleeding from the blood-drawing site, **fainting** or feeling lightheaded after venipuncture, or hematoma (blood accumulating under the puncture site).

Normal results

Normally, immune complexes are not detected in the blood.

Abnormal results

The presence of detectable immune complexes in the blood is important in the diagnosis of autoimmune diseases, such as SLE and rheumatoid arthritis. However, for definitive diagnosis, the results of other studies must be considered with the presence of any immune complex. For example, immune complexes are associated with high numbers of a component called antinuclear antibodies in the diagnosis of systemic lupus erythematosus. A different example are the kidneys. Because of their filtering functions, elements in the kidneys called renal glomeruli can be affected by immune complexes. In such cases, renal biopsy is used to provide conclusive evidence for immune complex.

Resources

BOOKS

Cahill, Mathew. *Handbook of Diagnostic Tests*. Springhouse, PA: Springhouse Corporation, 1995.

Jacobs, David S. *Laboratory Test Handbook*. *4th ed*. Cleveland, OH: Lexi-Comp Inc., 1996.

Janis O. Flores

Immunodeficiency

Definition

Immunodeficiency disorders are a group of disorders in which part of the immune system is missing or defective. Therefore, the body's ability to fight infections is impaired. As a result, the person with an immunodeficiency disorder will have frequent infections that are generally more severe and last longer than usual.

Description

The immune system is the body's main system to fight infections. Any defect in the immune system decreases a person's ability to fight infections. A person with an immunodeficiency disorder may get more frequent infections, heal more slowly, and have a higher incidence of some **cancers.**

The normal immune system involves a complex interaction of certain types of cells that can recognize and attack ''foreign'' invaders, such as bacteria, viruses, and fungi. It also plays a role in fighting cancer. The immune system has both innate and adaptive components. Innate immunity is made up of immune protections people are born with. Adaptive immunity develops throughout life. It adapts to fight off specific invading organisms. Adaptive immunity is divided into two components: humoral immunity and cellular immunity.

The innate immune system is made up of the skin (which acts as a barrier to prevent organisms from entering the body), white blood cells called phagocytes, a system of proteins called the complement system, and chemicals called interferon. When phagocytes encounter an invading organism, they surround and engulf it to destroy it. The complement system also attacks bacteria. The elements in the complement system create a hole in the outer layer of the target cell, which leads to the death of the cell.

The adaptive component of the immune system is extremely complex, and is still not entirely understood. Basically, it has the ability to recognize an organism or tumor cell as not being a normal part of the body, and to develop a response to attempt to eliminate it.

The humoral response of adaptive immunity involves a type of cell called B lymphocytes. B lymphocytes manufacture proteins called antibodies (which are also called immunoglobulins). Antibodies attach themselves to the invading foreign substance. This allows the phagocytes to begin engulfing and destroying the organism. The action of antibodies also activates the complement system. The humoral response is particularly useful for attacking bacteria.

The cellular response of adaptive immunity is useful for attacking viruses, some parasites, and possibly cancer cells. The main type of cell in the cellular response is T lymphocytes. There are helper T lymphocytes and killer T lymphocytes. The helper T lymphocytes play a role in recognizing invading organisms, and they also help killer T lymphocytes to multiply. As the name suggests, killer T lymphocytes act to destroy the target organism.

Defects can occur in any component of the immune system or in more than one component (combined immunodeficiency). Different immunodeficiency diseases involve different components of the immune system. The defects can be inherited and/or present at birth (congenital) or acquired.

Congenital immunodeficiency disorders

Congenital immunodeficiency is present at the time of birth, and is the result of genetic defects. Even though more than 70 different types of congenital immunodeficiency disorders have been identified, they rarely occur. Congenital immunodeficiencies may occur as a result of defects in B lymphocytes, T lymphocytes, or both. They can also occur in the innate immune system.

B LYMPHOCYTE DEFICIENCY

If there is an abnormality in either the development or function of B lymphocytes, the ability to make antibodies will be impaired. This allows the body to be susceptible to recurrent infections.

Bruton's agammaglobulinemia, also known as **X-linked agammaglobulinemia,** is one of the most common congenital immunodeficiency disorders. The defect results in a decrease or absence of B lymphocytes, and therefore a decreased ability to make antibodies. People with this disorder are particularly susceptible to infections of the throat, skin, middle ear, and lungs. It is seen only in males because it is caused by a genetic defect on the X chromosome. Since males have only one X chromosome, they always have the defect if the gene is present. Females can have the defective gene, but since they have two X chromosomes, there will be a normal gene on the other X chromosome to counter it. Women may pass the defective gene on to their male children.

Another type of B lymphocyte deficiency involves a group of disorders called selective **immunoglobulin de-ficiency syndomes.** Immunoglobulin is another name for antibody, and there are five different types of immunoglobulins (called IgA, IgG, IgM, IgD, and IgE). The most common type of immunoglobulin deficiency is selective IgA deficiency. The amounts of the other antibody types are normal. Some patients with selective IgA deficiency experience no symptoms, while others have occasional lung infections and **diarrhea.** In another immunoglobulin disorder, IgG and IgA antibodies are deficient and there is increased IgM. People with this disorder tend to get severe bacterial infections.

Common variable immunodeficiency is another type of B lymphocyte deficiency. In this disorder, the production of one or more of the immunoglobulin types is decreased and the antibody response to infections is impaired. It generally develops around the age of 10-20. The symptoms vary among affected people. Most people with this disorder have frequent infections, and some will also experience anemia and **rheumatoid arthritis.** Many people with **common variable immunodeficiency** develop cancer.

T LYMPHOCYTE DEFICIENCIES

Severe defects in the ability of T lymphocytes to mature results in impaired immune responses to infections with viruses, fungi, and certain types of bacteria. These infections are usually severe and can be fatal.

DiGeorge syndrome is a T lymphocyte deficiency that starts during fetal development, but it isn't inherited. Children with **DiGeorge syndrome** either do not have a thymus or have an underdeveloped thymus. Since the thymus is a major organ that directs the production of T-lymphocytes, these patients have very low numbers of T-lymphocytes. They are susceptible to recurrent infections, and usually have physical abnormalities as well. For example, they may have low-set ears, a small receding jawbone, and wide-spaced eyes.

In some cases, no treatment is required for DiGeorge syndrome because T lymphocyte production improves. Either an underdeveloped thymus begins to produce more T lymphocytes or organ sites other than the thymus compensate by producing more T lymphocytes.

COMBINED IMMUNODEFICIENCIES

Some types of immunodeficiency disorders affect both B lymphocytes and T lymphocytes. For example, **severe combined immunodeficiency disease** (SCID) is caused by the defective development or function of these two types of lymphocytes. It results in impaired humoral and cellular immune responses. SCID is usually recognized during the first year of life. It tends to cause a fungal infection of the mouth (thrush), diarrhea, **failure to thrive,** and serious infections. If not treated with a bone marrow transplant, a person with SCID will generally die from infections before age two.

DISORDERS OF INNATE IMMUNITY

Disorders of innate immunity affect phagocytes or the complement system. These disorders also result in recurrent infections.

Acquired immunodeficiency disorders

Acquired immunodeficiency is more common than congenital immunodeficiency. It is the result of an infectious process or other disease. For example, the human immunodeficiency virus (HIV) is the virus that causes acquired immunodeficiency syndrome (**AIDS**). However, this is not the most common cause of acquired immunodeficiency.

Acquired immunodeficiency often occurs as a complication of other conditions and diseases. For example, the most common causes of acquired immunodeficiency are **malnutrition,** some types of cancer, and infections. People who weigh less than 70% of the average weight of persons of the same age and gender are considered to be malnourished. Examples of types of infections that can lead to immunodeficiency are **chickenpox,** cytomegalovirus, German **measles,** measles, tuberculosis, **infectious mononucleosis** (Epstein-Barr virus), chronic hepatitis, lupus, and bacterial and fungal infections.

Sometimes, acquired immunodeficiency is brought on by drugs used to treat another condition. For example, patients who have an organ transplant are given drugs to suppress the immune system so the body will not reject the organ. Also, some **chemotherapy** drugs, which are given to treat cancer, have the side effect of killing cells of the immune system. During the period of time that these drugs are being taken, the risk of infection increases. It usually returns to normal after the person stops taking the drugs.

Causes & symptoms

Congenital immunodeficiency is caused by genetic defects, and they generally occur while the fetus is developing in the womb. These defects affect the development and/or function of one or more of the components of the immune system. Acquired immunodeficiency is the result of a disease process, and it occurs later in life. The causes, as described above, can be diseases, infections, or the side effects of drugs given to treat other conditions.

People with an immunodeficiency disorder tend to become infected by organisms that don't usually cause disease in healthy persons. The major symptoms of most immunodeficiency disorders are repeated infections that heal slowly. These chronic infections cause symptoms that persist for long periods of time. People with chronic infection tend to be pale and thin. They may have skin **rashes.** Their lymph nodes tend to be larger than normal and their liver and spleen may also be enlarged. The lymph nodes are small organs that house antibodies and lymphocytes. Broken blood vessels, especially near the surface of the skin, may be seen. This can result in black-and-blue marks in the skin. The person may loose hair from their head. Sometimes, a red inflammation of the lining of the eye (**conjunctivitis**) is present. They may have crusty appearance in and on the nose from chronic nasal dripping.

Diagnosis

Usually, the first sign that a person might have an immunodeficiency disorder is that they don't improve rapidly when given **antibiotics** to treat an infection. Strong indicators that an immunodeficiency disorder may be present is when rare diseases occur or the patient gets ill from organisms that don't normally cause diseases, especially if the patient gets repeatedly infected. If this happens in very young children it is an indication that a genetic defect may be causing an immunodeficiency disorder. When this situation occurs in older children or young adults, their medical history will be reviewed to determine if childhood diseases may have caused an immunodeficiency disorder. Other possibilities will then be considered, such as recently acquired infections—for example, HIV, hepatitis, tuberculosis, etc.

Laboratory tests are used to determine the exact nature of the immunodeficiency. Most tests are performed on blood samples. Blood contains antibodies, lymphocytes, phagocytes, and complement components; all of the major immune components that might cause immunodeficiency. A blood cell count will determine if the number of phagocytic cells or lymphocytes is below normal. Lower than normal counts of either of these two cell types correlates with immunodeficiencies. The blood cells are also checked for their appearance. Sometimes a person may have normal cell counts, but the cells are structurally defective. If the lymphocyte cell count is low, further testing is usually done to determine whether any particular type of lymphocyte is lower than normal. A lymphocyte proliferation test is done to determine if the lymphocytes can respond to stimuli. The failure to respond to stimulants correlates with immunodeficiency. Antibody levels can be measured by a process called electrophoresis. Complement levels can be determined by immunodiagnostic tests.

Treatment

There is no cure for immunodeficiency disorders. Therapy is aimed at controlling infections and, for some disorders, replacing defective or absent components.

Patients with Bruton's agammaglobulinemia must be given periodic injections of a substance called gamma globulin throughout their lives to make up for their decreased ability to make antibodies. The gamma globulin preparation contains antibodies against common invading bacteria. If left untreated, the disease is usually fatal.

Common variable immunodeficiency also is treated with periodic injections of gamma globulin throughout life. Additionally, antibiotics are given when necessary to treat infections.

Patients with selective IgA deficiency usually do not require any treatment. Antibiotics can be given for frequent infections.

In some cases, no treatment is required for DiGeorge syndrome because T lymphocyte production improves on its own. Either an underdeveloped thymus begins to produce more T lymphocytes or organ sites other than the thymus compensate by producing more T lymphocytes. In some severe cases, a bone marrow transplant or thymus transplant can be done to correct the problem.

For patients with SCID, **bone marrow transplantation** is necessary. In this procedure, healthy bone marrow from a donor who has a similar type of tissue (usually a relative, like a brother or sister) is removed. The bone marrow is a substance that resides in the cavity of bones. It is the factory that produces blood, including some of the white blood cells that make up the immune system. The bone marrow of the person receiving the transplant is destroyed, and is then replaced with marrow from the donor.

Treatment of the HIV infection that causes AIDS consists of drugs called antivirals. These drugs attempt to inhibit the process that the virus goes through to kill T lymphocytes. Several of these drugs used in various combinations with one another can prolong the period of time before the disease becomes apparent. However, this is not a cure. Other treatments for people with AIDS are aimed at the particular infections that arise as a result of the impaired immune system.

In most cases, immunodeficiency caused by malnutrition is reversible. The health of the immune system is directly linked to the nutritional health of the patient. Among the essential nutrients required by the immune system are proteins, **vitamins,** iron, and zinc.

For people being treated for cancer, periodic relief from chemotherapy drugs can restore the function of the immune system.

In general, people with immunodeficiency disorders should maintain a healthy diet. This is because malnutrition can aggravate immunodeficiencies. They should also avoid being near people who have colds or are sick because they can easily acquire new infections. For the same reason, they should practice good personal hygiene, especially dental care. People with immunodeficiency disorders should also avoid eating undercooked food because it might contain bacteria that could cause infection. This food would not cause infection in normal persons, but in someone with an immunodeficiency, food is a potential source of infectious organisms. People with immunodeficiency should be given antibiotics at the first indication of an infection.

Prognosis

The prognosis depends on the type of immunodeficiency disorder. People with Bruton's agammaglobulinemia who are given injections of gamma globulin generally live into their 30s or 40s. They often die from chronic infections, usually of the lung. People with selective IgA deficiency generally live normal lives. They may experience problems if given a blood **transfusion,** and therefore they should wear a Medic Alert bracelet or have some other way of alerting any physician who treats them that they have this disorder.

SCID is the most serious of the immunodeficiency disorders. If a bone marrow transplant is not successfully performed, the child usually will not live beyond two years old.

People with HIV/AIDS are living longer than in the past because of the **antiviral drugs** that became available in the mid 1990s. However, AIDS is still a fatal disease. People with AIDS usually die of opportunistic infections, which are infections that occur because the impaired immune system is unable to fight them.

Prevention

There is no way to prevent a congenital immunodeficiency disorder. However, someone with a congenital immunodeficiency disorder might want to consider getting **genetic counseling** before having children to find out if there is a chance they will pass the defect on to their children.

Some of the infections associated with acquired immunodeficiency can be prevented or treated before they cause problems. For example, there are effective treatments for tuberculosis and most bacterial and fungal infections. HIV infection can be prevented by practicing ''safe sex'' and not using illegal intravenous drugs. These are the primary routes of transmitting the virus. For people who don't know the HIV status of the person with whom they are having sex, safe sex involves using a **condom.**

Malnutrition can be prevented by getting adequate nutrition. Malnutrition tends to be more of a problem in developing countries.

Resources

BOOKS

Abbas, A.K., A. H. Lichtman, and J.S. Pober. *Cellular and Molecular Immunology.* Philadelphia: W.B. Saunders Company, 1997.

Berkow, Robert, Editor in Chief. *Merck Manual of Medical Information.* Whitehouse Station, NJ: Merck Research Laboratories, 1997.

Roitt, Ivan M. *Roitt's Essential Immunology.* Oxford: Blackwell Science Ltd., 1997.

John Thomas Lohr

Immunoelectrophoresis

Definition

Immunoelectrophoresis, also called gamma globulin electrophoresis, or immunoglobulin electrophoresis, is a method of determining the blood levels of three major immunoglobulins: immunoglobulin M (IgM), immunoglobulin G (IgG), and immunoglobulin A (IgA).

Purpose

Immunoelectrophoresis aids in the diagnosis and evaluation of the therapeutic response in many disease states affecting the immune system. It is usually requested when a different type of electrophoresis, called a serum **protein electrophoresis,** has indicated a rise at the immunoglobulin level. Immunoelectrophoresis is also used frequently to diagnose multiple myeloma, a disease affecting the bone marrow.

Precautions

Drugs that may cause increased immunoglobulin levels include therapeutic gamma globulin, hydralazine, isoniazid, phenytoin (Dilantin), procainamide, **oral contraceptives,** methadone, steroids, and **tetanus** toxoid and antitoxin. The laboratory should be notified if the patient has received any **vaccinations** or immunizations in the six months before the test.

It should be noted that, because immunoelectrophoresis is not quantitative, it is being replaced by a procedure called immunofixation, which is more sensitive and easier to interpret.

Description

Immunoelectrophoresis is performed by placing serum on a slide containing a gel designed specifically for the test. An electric current is then passed through the gel, and immunoglobulins, which contain an electric charge, migrate through the gel according to the difference in their individual electric charges. Antiserum is placed alongside the slide to identify the specific type of immunoglobulin present. The results are used to identify different disease entities, and to aid in monitoring the course of

---

KEY TERMS

. . . .

Antibody—A protein manufactured by the white blood cells to neutralize an antigen in the body. In some cases, excessive formation of antibodies leads to illness, allergy, or autoimmune disorders.

Antigen—A substance that can cause an immune response, resulting in production of an antibody, as part of the body's defense against infection and disease. Many antigens are foreign proteins not found naturally in the body, and include germs, toxins, and tissues from another person used in organ transplantation.

Autoimmune disorder—A condition in which antibodies are formed against the body's own tissues, for example, in some forms of arthritis.

---

the disease and the therapeutic response of the patient to such conditions as immune deficiencies, autoimmune disease, chronic infections, chronic viral infections, and intrauterine fetal infections.

There are five classes of antibodies: IgM, IgG, IgA, IgE, and IgD, but immunoelectrophoresis is ordered primarily to test for IgM, IgG, and IgA.

IgM is produced upon initial exposure to an antigen (for example, when a person receives the first tetanus vaccination, antitetanus antibodies of the IgM class are produced 10 to 14 days later). IgM is abundant in the blood but is not normally present in organs or tissues. IgM is primarily responsible for ABO blood grouping and rheumatoid factor, yet is involved in the immunologic reaction to other infections, such as hepatitis. Since IgM does not cross the placenta, an elevation of this immunoglobulin in the newborn indicates intrauterine infection such as **rubella,** cytomegalovirus (CMV) or a sexually transmitted disease (STD).

IgG is the most prevalent type of antibody, comprising approximately 75% of the serum immunoglobulins. IgG is produced upon subsequent exposure to an antigen. As an example, after receiving a second tetanus shot, or booster, a person produces IgG antibodies in five to seven days. IgG is present in both the blood and tissues, and is the only antibody to cross the placenta from the mother to the fetus. Maternal IgG protects the newborn for the first months of life, until the infant's immune system produces its own antibodies.

IgA constitutes approximately 15% of the immunoglobulins within the body. While it is found to some degree in the blood, it is present primarily in the secretions of the respiratory and gastrointestinal tract, in saliva, colostrum (the yellowish fluid produced by the breasts during late **pregnancy** and the first few days after **childbirth),** and in tears. IgA plays an important role in defending the body against invasion of germs through the mucous membrane-lined organs.

IgE is the antibody that causes acute allergic reactions; it is measured to detect allergic conditions. IgD, which constitutes the smallest portion of the immunoglobulins, is rarely evaluated or detected, and its function is not well understood.

Preparation

This test requires a blood sample. The patient should have nothing to eat or drink for 12 hours before the test.

Aftercare

Since this test is ordered when either very low or very high levels of immunoglobulins are suspected, the patient should be alert for any signs of infection after the test, including **fever,** chills, rash, or skin ulcers. Any bone **pain** or tenderness should also be immediately reported to the physician.

Risks

Risks for this test are minimal, but may include slight bleeding from the blood-drawing site, **fainting** or feeling lightheaded after venipuncture, or bruising.

Normal results

Reference ranges vary from laboratory to laboratory and depend upon the method used. For adults, normal values are usually found within the following ranges:

- IgM: 60-290 mg/dL
- IgG: 700-1,800 mg/dL
- IgA: 70-440 mg/dL.

Abnormal results

Increased IgM levels can indicate Waldenstrom's macroglobulinemia, a malignancy caused by secretion of IgM at high levels by malignant lymphoplasma cells. Increased IgM levels can also indicate chromic infections, such as hepatitis or mononucleosis; and autoimmune diseases, like **rheumatoid arthritis.**

Decreased IgM levels can be indicative of AIDS, immunosuppression caused by certain drugs like steroids or dextran, or leukemia.

Increased levels of IgG can indicate chronic liver disease, autoimmune diseases, hyperimmunization reactions, or certain chronic infections, such as **tuberculosis** or **sarcoidosis.**

Decreased levels of IgG can indicate **Wiskott-Aldrich syndrome,** a genetic deficiency caused by inade-

quate synthesis of IgG and other immunoglobulins. Decreased IgG can also be seen with AIDS and leukemia.

Increased levels of IgA can indicate chronic liver disease, chronic infections, or inflammatory bowel disease.

Decreased levels of IgA can be found in ataxia, a condition affecting balance and gait, limb or eye movements and/or speech; and telangiectasia, an increase in the size and number of the small blood vessels in an area of skin, causing redness. Decreased IgA levels are also seen in conditions of low blood protein (hypoproteinemia), and drug immunosuppression.

Resources

BOOKS

Cahill, Mathew. *Handbook of Diagnostic Tests.* Springhouse, PA: Springhouse Corporation, 1995.

Jacobs, David S. *Laboratory Test Handbook,* Fourth Edition. Lexi-Comp Inc., 1996.

Pagana, Kathleen Deska. *Mosby's Manual of Diagnostic and Laboratory Tests.* St. Louis, MO: Mosby, Inc., 1998.

Janis O. Flores

Immunofluorescence test *see* **AIDS tests**

Immunoglobulin *see* **Gammaglobulin**

Immunoglobulin deficiency syndromes

Definition

Immunoglobulin deficiency syndromes are a group of **immunodeficiency** disorders in which the patient has reduced number of or lack of antibodies.

Description

Immunoglobulins (Ig) are antibodies. There are five major classes of antibodies: IgG, IgM, IgA, IgD, and IgE.

- IgG is the most abundant of the classes of immunoglobulins. It is the antibody for viruses, bacteria, and antitoxins. It is found in most tissues and plasma.

- IgM is the first antibody present in an immune response.

- IgA is an early antibody for bacteria and viruses. It is found in saliva, tears, and all other mucous secretions.

- IgD activity is unknown.

KEY TERMS

Antibody—Another term for immunoglobulin. A protein molecule that specifically recognizes and attaches to infectious agents.

T-helper cell—A type of cell that recognizes foreign antigens and activates T- and B-cells in an immune response.

• IgE is present in the respiratory secretions. It is an antibody for parasitic diseases, **Hodgkin's disease,** hay fever, **atopic dermatitis,** and allergic **asthma).**

All antibodies are made by B-lymphocytes (B-cells). Any disease that harms the development or function of B-cells will cause a decrease in the amount of antibodies produced. Since antibodies are essential in fighting infectious diseases, people with immunoglobulin deficiency syndromes become ill more often. However, the cellular immune system is still functional, so these patients are more prone to infection caused by organisms usually controlled by antibodies. Most of these invading germs (microbes) make capsules, a mechanism used to confuse the immune system. In a healthy body, antibodies can bind to the capsule and overcome the bacteria's defenses. The bacteria that make capsules include the streptococci, meningococci, and *Haemophilus influenzae*. These organisms cause such diseases as otitis, **sinusitis, pneumonia, meningitis, osteomyelitis,** septic arthritis, and **sepsis.** Patients with immunoglobulin deficiencies are also prone to some viral infections, including echovirus, enterovirus, and **hepatitis B.** They may also have a bad reaction to the attenuated version of the **polio** virus vaccine.

There are two types of immunodeficiency diseases: primary and secondary. Secondary disorders occur in normally healthy bodies that are suffering from an underlying disease. Once the disease is treated, the immunodeficiency is reversed. Immunoglobulin deficiency syndromes are primary immunodeficiency diseases, occurring because of defective B-cells or antibodies. They account for 50% of all primary immunodeficiencies, and they are, therefore, the most prevalent type of immunodeficiency disorders.

• **X-linked agammaglobulinemia** is an inherited disease. The defect is on the X chromosome and, consequently, this disease is seen more frequently in males than females. The defect results in a failure of B-cells to mature. Mature B-cells are capable of making antibodies and developing "memory," a feature in which the B-cell will rapidly recognize and respond to an infectious agent the next time it is encountered. All classes of antibodies are decreased in agammaglobulinemia.

• Selective IgA deficiency is an inherited disease, resulting from a failure of B-cells to switch from making IgM, the early antibody, to IgA. Although the B-cell numbers are normal, and the B-cells are otherwise normal (they can still make all other classes of antibodies), the amount of IgA produced is limited. This results in more infections of mucosal surfaces, such as the nose, throat, lungs, and intestine.

• Transient hypogammaglobulinemia of infancy is a temporary disease of unknown cause. It is believed to be caused by a defect in the development of T-helper cells (cells that recognize foreign antigens and activate T- and B-cells in an immune response). As the child ages, the number and condition of T-helper cells improves and this situation corrects itself. Hypogammaglobulinemia is characterized by low levels of **gammaglobulin** (antibodies) in the blood. During the disease period, patients have decreased levels of IgG and IgA antibodies. In lab tests, the antibodies that are present do not react well with infectious bacteria.

• **Common variable immunodeficiency** is a defect in both B cells and T-lymphocytes. It results in a near complete lack of antibodies in the blood.

• Ig heavy chain deletions is a genetic disease in which part of the antibody molecule isn't produced. It results in the loss of several antibody classes and subclasses including most IgG antibodies and all IgA and IgE antibodies. The disease occurs because part of the gene for the heavy chain has been lost.

• Selective IgG subclass deficiencies is a group of genetic diseases in which some of the subclasses of IgG are not made. There are four subclasses in the IgG class of antibodies. As the B-cell matures, it can switch from one subclass to another. In these diseases there is a defect in the maturation of the B-cells that results in a lack of switching.

• IgG deficiency with hyper-IgM is a disease that results when the B-cell fails to switch from making IgM to IgG. This produces an increase in the amount of IgM antibodies present and a decrease in the amount of IgGantibodies. This disease is the result of a genetic mutation.

Causes & symptoms

Immunoglobulin deficiencies are the result of congenital defects affecting the development and function of B lymphocytes (B-cells). There are two main points in the development of B-cells when defects can occur. First, B-cells can fail to develop into antibody-producing cells.

X-linked agammablobulinemia is an example of this disease. Secondly, B-cells can fail to make a particular type of antibody or fail to switch classes during maturation. Initially, when B-cells start making antibodies for the first time, they make IgM. As they mature and develop memory, they switch to one of the other four classes of antibodies. Failures in switching or failure to make a subclass of antibody leads to immunoglobulin deficiency diseases. Another mechanism which results in decreased antibody production is a defect in T-helper cells. Generally, defects in T-helper cells are listed as severe combined immunodeficiencies.

Symptoms are persistent and frequent infections, **diarrhea, failure to thrive,** and malabsorption (of nutrients).

Diagnosis

An immunodeficiency disease is suspected when children become ill frequently, especially from the same organisms. The profile of organisms that cause infection in patients with immunoglobulin deficiency syndrome is unique and is preliminary evidence for this disease. Laboratory tests are performed to verify the diagnosis. Antibodies can be found in the blood. Blood is collected and analyzed for the content and types of antibodies present. Depending on the type of immunoglobulin deficiency the laboratory tests will show a decrease or absence of antibodies or specific antibody subclasses.

Treatment

Immunodeficiency diseases can not be cured. Patients are treated with **antibiotics** and immune serum. Immune serum is a source of antibodies. Antibiotics are useful for fighting bacteria infections. There are some drugs that are effective against fungi, but very few drugs that are effective against viral diseases.

Bone marrow transplantation can, in most cases, completely correct the immunodefiency.

Prognosis

Patients with immunoglobulin defiency syndromes must practice impecable health maintenance and care, paying particular attention to optimal dental care, in order to stay in good health.

Resources

BOOKS

Abbas, A.K., A.H. Lichtman, and J.S. Pober. *Cellular and Molecular Immunology.* Philadelphia: W.B. Saunders Company, 1997.

Berkow, Robert, ed. *Merck Manual of Medical Information.* Whitehouse Station, NJ: Merck Research Laboratories, 1997.

Roit, I.M. *Roitt's Essential Immunolgy.* Oxford: Blackwell Science Ltd., 1997.

Jacqueline L. Longe

Immunoglobulin electrophoresis *see*
Immunoelectrophoresis

Immunoglobulins G, A, and M test *see*
Immunoelectrophoresis

Immunologic therapies

Definition

Immunologic therapy is the treatment of disease using medicines that boost the body's natural immune response.

Purpose

Immunologic therapy is used to improve the immune system's natural ability to fight diseases such as **cancer,** hepatitis and **AIDS.** These drugs also may be used to help the body recover from the harmful side effects of treatments such as **chemotherapy** or **radiation therapy.**

Description

Most drugs in this category are artificially-made versions of substances produced naturally in the body. In their natural forms, these substances help defend the body against disease. For example, aldeslcukin (Proleukin) is an artificially-made form of interleukin-2, which helps white blood cells work. Filgrastim (Neupogen) and sargramostim (Leukine) are versions of natural substances called colony stimulating factors, which encourage the bone marrow to make new white blood cells. Another type of drug, epoetin (Epogen, Procrit), stimulates the bone marrow to make new red blood cells. It is an artificially-made version of human erythropoietin, which is made naturally in the body and has the same effect on bone marrow. Thrombopoietin stimulates the production of platelets, disk-shaped bodies in the blood that are important in clotting. Interferons are substances the body produces to fight infections and tumors. Both natural and artificially made interferons are used to treat diseases.

Recommended dosage

The recommended dosage depends on the type of immunologic therapy. For some medicines, the physician

KEY TERMS

AIDS—Acquired immunodeficiency syndrome. A disease caused by infection with the human immunodeficiency virus (HIV). In people with this disease, the immune system breaks down, opening the door to other infections and some types of cancer.

Bone marrow—Soft tissue that fills the hollow centers of bones. Blood cells and platelets (disk-shaped bodies in the blood that are important in clotting) are produced in the bone marrow.

Chemotherapy—Treatment of an illness with chemical agents. The term is usually used to describe the treatment of cancer with drugs.

Clot—A hard mass that forms when blood gels.

Fetus—A developing baby inside the womb.

Hepatitis—Inflammation of the liver caused by a virus, chemical or drug.

Immune response—The body's natural, protective reaction to disease and infection.

Immune system—The system that protects the body against disease and infection through immune responses.

Inflammation—Pain, redness, swelling, and heat that usually develop in response to injury or illness.

Psoriasis—A skin disease in which people have itchy, scaly, red patches on the skin.

Seizure—A sudden attack, spasm, or convulsion.

Shingles—An disease caused by an infection with the Herpes zoster virus, the same virus that causes chickenpox. Symptoms of shingles include pain and blisters along one nerve, usually on the face, chest, stomach, or back.

Sickle cell anemia—An inherited disorder in which red blood cells contain an abnormal form of hemoglobin, a protein that carries oxygen. The abnormal form of hemoglobin causes the red cells to become sickle-shaped. The misshapen cells may clog blood vessels, preventing oxygen from reaching tissues and leading to pain, blood clots and other problems. Sickle cell anemia is most common in people of African descent and in people from Italy, Greece, India, and the Middle East.

will decide the dosage for each patient, taking into account the patient's weight and whether he or she is taking other medicines. Some drugs used in immunologic therapy are given only in a hospital, under a physician's supervision. For those that patients may give themselves, check with the physician who prescribed the medicine or the pharmacist who filled the prescription for the correct dosage.

Most of these drugs come in injectable form. Follow the instructions that come with the medicine for directions on how to prepare and inject it.

Precautions

Aldesleukin

This medicine may temporarily increase the chance of getting infections. It may also lower the number of platelets in the blood, which may interfere with the blood's ability to clot. Taking these precautions may reduce the chance of such problems:

- Avoid people with infections, if possible.

- Be alert to signs of infection, such as **fever,** chills, **sore throat, pain** in the lower back or side, **cough,** hoarseness, or painful or difficult urination. If any of these symptoms occur, get in touch with a physician immediately.

- Be alert to signs of bleeding problems, such as black, tarry stools, tiny red spots on the skin, blood in the urine or stools, or any other unusual bleeding or bruising.

- Take care to avoid cuts or other injuries. Be especially careful when using knives, razors, nail clippers and other sharp objects. Check with a dentist for the best ways to clean the teeth and mouth without injuring the gums. Do not have dental work done without checking with a physician.

- Wash the hands frequently, and avoid touching the eyes or inside of the nose unless the hands have just been washed.

Aldesleukin may make some medical conditions worse, such as **chickenpox, shingles** (herpes zoster), liver disease, lung disease, heart disease, underactive thyroid, **psoriasis,** immune system problems and mental problems. The medicine may increase the chance of seizures (convulsions) in people who are prone to having them. Also, the drug's effects may be greater in people with kidney disease, because their kidneys are slow to clear the medicine from their bodies.

Colony stimulating factors

Certain drugs used in treating cancer reduce the body's ability to fight infections. Although colony stimulating factors help restore the body's natural defenses, the process takes time. Getting prompt treatment for infections is important, even while taking this medicine. Call the physician at the first sign of illness or infection, such as a sore throat, fever or chills.

People with certain medical conditions may have problems if they take colony stimulating factors. In people who have kidney disease, liver disease or conditions caused by inflammation or immune system problems, colony stimulating factors may make these problems worse. People with heart disease may be more likely to have side effects such as water retention and heart rhythm problems when they take these drugs. And people with lung disease may be more likely to have **shortness of breath.** Anyone who has any of these medical conditions should check with his or her physician before using colony stimulating factors.

Epoetin

This medicine may cause seizures (convulsions), especially in people who are prone to having them. Noone who takes these drugs should drive, use machines or do anything else that might be dangerous if he or she has a seizure.

Epoetin helps the body make new red blood cells, but it cannot do its job unless there is plenty of iron in the body. The physician may recommend taking iron supplements or certain **vitamins** that help get iron into the body. Follow the physician's orders to make sure the body has enough iron for this medicine to work. Do not take iron supplements without a physician's consent.

In studies of laboratory animals, epoetin taken during **pregnancy** caused **birth defects,** including damage to the bones and spine. However, the drug has not been reported to cause problems in human babies whose mothers take it. Women who are pregnant or who may become pregnant should check with their physicians for the most up-to-date information on the safety of taking this medicine during pregnancy.

People with certain medical conditions may have problems if they take this medicine. For example, the chance of side effects may be greater in people with high blood pressure, heart or blood vessel disease or a history of blood clots. And epoetin may not work properly in people who have bone problems or **sickle cell anemia.**

Interferons

Interferons may add to the effects of alcohol and other drugs that slow down the central nervous system, such as **antihistamines,** cold medicine, allergy medicine, sleep aids, medicine for seizures, tranquilizers, some pain relievers, and **muscle relaxants.** They may also add to the effects of anesthetics, including those used for dental procedures. Anyone taking interferons should check with his or her physician before taking any of the above.

Some people feel dizzy, unusually tired or less alert than usual while being treated with these drugs. Because

of these possible problems, anyone who takes these drugs should not drive, use machines or do anything else that might be dangerous until they have found out how the drugs affect them.

Interferons often cause flu-like symptoms, including fever and chills. The physician who prescribes this medicine may recommend taking **acetaminophen** (Tylenol) before—and sometimes after—each dose to keep the fever from getting too high. If the physician recommends this, follow his or her instructions carefully.

Like aldesleukin, interferons may temporarily increase the chance of getting infections and may lower the number of platelets in the blood, leading to clotting problems. To help prevent these problems, follow the precautions for reducing the risk of infection and bleeding listed for aldesleukin.

People who have certain medical conditions may have problems if they take interferons. For example, the drugs may worsen some medical conditions, including heart disease, kidney disease, liver disease, lung disease, diabetes, bleeding problems and mental problems. In people who have overactive immune systems, these drugs may make the immune system even more active. People who have shingles or chickenpox or who have recently been exposed to chickenpox may increase their risk of developing severe problems in other parts of the body if they take interferons. And people with a history of seizures or mental problems who take interferons may be at risk of having nervous system problems.

In teenage women, interferons may cause changes in the menstrual cycle. Young women should discuss this possibility with their physicians.

Older people may be more sensitive to the effects of interferons. This may increase the chance of side effects.

These drugs are not known to cause fetal **death,** birth defects or other problems in humans when taken during pregnancy. Women who are pregnant or who may become pregnant should ask their physicians for the latest information on the safety of taking these drugs during pregnancy.

Women who are breastfeeding their babies may need to stop while taking this medicine. Whether interferons pass into breast milk is not known, but because of the chance of serious side effects to the baby, breast-feeding while taking interferon is discouraged. Check with a physician for advice.

General precautions for all types of immunologic therapy

Seeing a physician regularly while being treated with immunologic therapy is important. This gives the physician a chance to make sure the medicine is working and to check for unwanted side effects.

Anyone who has had unusual reactions to drugs used in immunologic therapy should let his or her physician know before taking the drugs again. The physician should also be told about any **allergies** to foods, dyes, preservatives, or other substances.

Side effects

Aldesleukin

In addition to its helpful effects, this medicine may cause serious side effects. Generally, it is given only in a hospital, where medical professionals can watch for early signs of problems. They may also do some medical tests to check for unwanted effects.

Anyone who has breathing problems, fever or chills while being given aldesleukin should check with a physician immediately.

Other side effects should be brought to a physician's attention as soon as possible:

- **Dizziness**
- Drowsiness
- Confusion
- Agitation
- Depression
- **Nausea and vomiting**
- **Diarrhea**
- Sores in the mouth and on the lips
- Tingling of hands or feet
- Decrease in urination
- Weight gain of 5 or more pounds.

Some side effects are usually temporary and do not need medical attention unless they are bothersome. These include dry skin; itchy or burning skin rash or redness followed by peeling; loss of appetite; and a general feeling of illness or discomfort.

Colony stimulating factors

As this medicine starts to work, mild pain may be experienced in the lower back or hips. This is nothing to worry about, and it will usually go away within a few days. If the pain is too uncomfortable, the physician may prescribe a painkiller.

Other possible side effects include **headache,** joint or muscle pain and skin rash or **itching.** These side effects usually go away as the body adjusts to the medicine and do not need medical treatment. If they continue or they interfere with normal activities, check with a physician.

Epoetin

This medicine may cause flu-like symptoms, such as muscle aches, bone pain, fever, chills, shivering, and sweating, within a few hours after it is taken. These symptoms usually go away within 12 hours. If they do not, or if they are troubling, check with a physician. Other possible side effects that do not need medical attention are diarrhea, nausea or vomiting and tiredness or weakness.

Certain side effects should be brought to a physician's attention as soon as possible. These include headache, vision problems, increased blood pressure, fast heartbeat, weight gain and swelling of the face, fingers, lower legs, ankles or feet.

Anyone who has chest pain or seizures after taking epoetin should check with a physician immediately.

Interferons

This medicine may cause temporary hair loss. This may be upsetting, but it is not a sign that something is seriously wrong. The hair should grow back normally after treatment ends.

Many other side effects usually go away during treatment, as the body adjusts to the medicine. These include flu-like symptoms, changes in taste, loss of appetite, nausea and vomiting, skin rash, and unusual tiredness. If these problems do not go away or if they interfere with normal life, check with a physician.

A few more serious side effects should be brought to a physician's attention as soon as possible:

- Confusion
- Difficulty thinking or concentrating
- Nervousness
- Depression
- Sleep problems
- Numbness or tingling in the fingers, toes and face.

General advice on side effects for all types of immunologic therapy

Other side effects are possible with any type of immunologic therapy. Anyone who has unusual symptoms during or after treatment with these drugs should get in touch with his or her physician.

Interactions

Anyone who has immunologic therapy should let the physician know all other medicines he or she is taking. Some combinations of drugs may interact, that can increase or decrease the effects of one or both drugs or may make side effects more likely. Ask the physician whether the possible interactions can interfere with drug therapy or cause harmful effects.

Resources

PERIODICALS

Dale, David C. "Where now for colony-stimulating factors?" *Lancet* 346 (July 15, 1995): 135.

Haynes, Barton F. "New frontiers of immunotherapy for HIV." *Lancet* 347 (December 7, 1996): 1531.

Old, Lloyd J. "Immunotherapy for cancer." (Therapies of the Future) *Scientific American* 275 (September 1996): 136.

Ward, Darrell E. "Taking advantage of the body's healing power." *USA Today Magazine* 123 (May 1995): 68.

Nancy Ross-Flanigan

Immunosuppressant drugs

Definition

Immunosuppressant drugs are medicines that reduce the body's natural defenses against foreign invaders or materials. Used in transplant patients, these drugs help prevent their bodies from rejecting transplanted organs.

Purpose

When an organ, such as a liver, a heart or a kidney, is transplanted from one person (the donor) into another (the recipient), the recipient's immune system has the same response it has to any foreign material. It attacks and tries to destroy the organ. Immunosuppressant drugs help prevent this from happening by subduing the natural immune response. The problem is that the drugs' action also makes the body more vulnerable to infection. For that reason, people who take this medicine need to be especially careful to avoid infections.

In addition to being used to prevent organ rejection, immunosuppressant drugs sometimes are used to treat severe skin disorders such as **psoriasis** and other diseases such as **rheumatoid arthritis, Crohn's disease** (chronic inflammation of the digestive tract) and patchy hair loss (**alopecia** areata).

Description

Immunosuppressant drugs are available only with a physician's prescription and come in tablet, capsule, liquid and injectable forms. Commonly used immunosuppressant drugs include azathioprine (Imuran), cyclosporine (Sandimmune) and tacrolimus (Prograf).

KEY TERMS

Chronic—A word used to describe a long-lasting condition. Chronic conditions often develop gradually and involve slow changes.

Conception—The union of egg and sperm.

Fetus—A developing baby inside the womb.

Immune system—The body's natural defenses against disease and infection.

Inflammation—Pain, redness, swelling, and heat that usually develop in response to injury or illness.

Psoriasis—A skin disease in which people have itchy, scaly, red patches on the skin.

Recommended dosage

The recommended dosage depends on the type and form of immunosuppressant drug and the purpose for which it is being used. Doses may be different for different patients. Check with the physician who prescribed the drug or the pharmacist who filled the prescription for the correct dosage.

Taking this medicine exactly as directed is very important. Never take smaller, larger or more frequent doses, and do not take the drug for longer than directed. The physician will decide exactly how much of the medicine each patient needs. Taking too much may increase the risk of side effects, while taking too little may not do any good. Blood tests often are necessary to make sure that the right amount of the medicine is getting into the body.

Immunosuppressant drugs sometimes are given along with other medicines. Be sure to follow the directions for taking each medicine. If trying to remember when to take each medicine is confusing, ask a health care professional for tips on how to keep them straight.

Do not stop taking an immunosuppressant drug without checking with the physician who prescribed it.

Precautions

Seeing a physician regularly while taking immunosuppressant drugs is important. These regular check-ups will allow the physician to make sure the medicine is working as it should and to watch for unwanted effects. These medicines are very powerful and can cause serious side effects, such as high blood pressure, kidney problems and liver problems. Some side effects may not show up until years after the medicine is used. However, the good these drugs can do may outweigh the possible harm. Anyone who has been advised to take immunosuppressant drugs should thoroughly discuss the risks and benefits with his or her physician

Immunosuppressant drugs lower a person's resistance to infection and can make infections harder to treat. The drugs can also increase the chance of uncontrolled bleeding. Anyone who has a serious infection or injury while taking immunosuppressant drugs should get prompt medical attention and should make sure that the physician in charge knows about the medicine. Check with a physician immediately if signs of infection, such as **fever** or chills, **cough** or hoarseness, **pain** in the lower back or side, or painful or difficult urination, occur. Let the physician know about unusual bruising or bleeding; blood in the urine; bloody or black, tarry stools; or tiny red spots on the skin. Other ways of preventing infection and injury include washing the hands frequently, avoiding sports where injuries may occur, and being careful when using knives, razors, fingernail clippers or other sharp objects. Avoiding contact with people who have infections is also important. In addition, people who are taking or have been taking immunosuppressant drugs should not have immunizations, such as **smallpox vaccinations,** without checking with their physicians. Because of their low resistance to infection, people taking these drugs might get the disease that the vaccine is designed to prevent. People taking immunosuppressant drugs also should avoid contact with anyone who has taken the oral **polio** vaccine, as there is a chance the virus could be passed on to them. Other people living in their home should not take the oral polio va

Immunosuppressant drugs may cause the gums to become tender and swollen or to bleed. If this happens, check with a physician or dentist right away. Regular brushing, flossing, cleaning and gum massage may help prevent this problem. Ask the dentist for advice on how to clean the teeth and mouth without causing injury.

Special conditions

People who have certain medical conditions or who are taking certain other medicines may have problems if they take immunosuppressant drugs. Before taking these drugs, be sure to let the physician know about any of these conditions:

ALLERGIES

Anyone who has had unusual reactions to immunosuppressant drugs in the past should let his or her physician know before taking the drugs again. The physician should also be told about any **allergies** to foods, dyes, preservatives, or other substances.

PREGNANCY

Azathioprine may cause **birth defects** if used during **pregnancy,** or if either the male or female is using it when conception occurs. Anyone taking this medicine should use a barrier method of birth control, such as a diaphragm or **condoms.** Birth control pills should not be used without a physician's approval. Women who become pregnant while taking this medicine should check with their physicians immediately.

The medicine's effects have not been studied in humans during pregnancy. Women who are pregnant or who may become pregnant and who need to take this medicine should check with their physicians.

BREASTFEEDING

Immunosuppressant drugs pass into breast milk and may cause problems in nursing babies whose mothers take it. Breastfeeding is not recommended for women taking this medicine.

OTHER MEDICAL CONDITIONS

People who have certain medical conditions may have problems if they take immunosuppressant drugs. For example:

- People who have **shingles** (herpes zoster) or **chickenpox** or who have recently been exposed to chickenpox may develop severe disease in other parts of their bodies when they take this medicine.

- The medicine's effects may be greater in people with kidney disease or liver disease, because their bodies are slow to get rid of the medicine.

- The effects of oral forms of this medicine may be less in people with intestinal problems, because the medicine cannot be absorbed into the body.

Before using immunosuppressant drugs, people with these or other medical problems should make sure their physicians are aware of their conditions.

USE OF CERTAIN MEDICINES

Taking immunosuppressant drugs with certain other drugs may affect the way the drugs work or may increase the chance of side effects.

Side effects

People who take immunosuppressant drugs may be at higher than normal risk of developing certain kinds of **cancers** later in life. However, the drugs may be necessary to prevent the failure of a life-saving transplant. The possible harm must be carefully weighed against the drugs' benefits. Discussing the medicine's good and bad points with a physician will help a patient decide about whether to take immunosuppressant drugs.

Some side effects of immunosuppressant drugs are minor and usually go away as the body adjusts to the medicine. These include loss of appetite, nausea or vomiting, increased hair growth, and trembling or shaking of the hands. Medical attention is not necessary unless these side effects continue or cause problems.

Check with a physician immediately if any of these side effects occur:

- Unusual tiredness or weakness
- Fever or chills
- Frequent need to urinate.

Interactions

Immunosuppressant drugs may interact with other medicines. When this happens, the effects of one or both drugs may change or the risk of side effects may be greater. For example:

- The effects of azathioprine may be greater in people who take allopurinol, a medicine used to treat **gout.**

- A number of medicines, including female hormones (estrogens), male hormones (androgens), the antifungal drug ketoconazole (Nizoral), the ulcer drug cimetidine (Tagamet) and the **erythromycins** (used to treat infections), may increase the effects of cyclosporine.

- The risk of cancer or infection may be greater when immunosuppressant drugs are combined with certain other drugs which also lower the body's ability to fight disease and infection. These drugs include **corticosteroids** such as prednisone; the **anticancer drugs** chlorambucil (Leukeran), cyclophosphamide (Cytoxan) and mercaptopurine (Purinethol); and the monoclonal antibody muromonab-CD3 (Orthoclone), which also is used to prevent transplanted organ rejection.

Not every drug that may interact with immunosuppressant drugs is listed here. Anyone who takes immunosuppressant drugs should let the physician know all other medicines he or she is taking and should ask whether the possible interactions can interfere with treatment.

Nancy Ross-Flanigan

Impacted tooth

Definition

An impacted tooth is any tooth that is prevented from reaching its normal position in the mouth by tissue, bone, or another tooth.

Description

The teeth that most commonly become impacted are the third molars, also called wisdom teeth. These large teeth are the last to develop, beginning to form when a

person is about nine years old, but not breaking through the gum tissue until the late teens or early twenties. By this time, the jaws have stopped growing and may be too small to accommodate these four additional teeth. As the wisdom teeth continue to move, one or more may become impacted, either by running into the teeth next to them or becoming blocked within the jawbone or gum tissue. An impacted tooth can cause further dental problems, including infection of the gums, displacement of other teeth, or decay. At least one wisdom tooth becomes impacted in nine of every ten people.

Causes & Symptoms

The movement of an erupting wisdom tooth and any subsequent impaction may produce **pain** at the back of

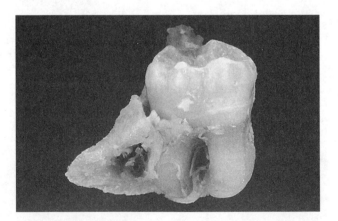

This impacted wisdom tooth, attached to part of the jaw bone, was broken during extraction. *(Photograph by James Stevenson, Photo Researchers, Inc. Reproduced by permission.)*

the jaw. Pain may also be the result of infection, either from decay in any exposed portion of the tooth or from trapped food and plaque in the surrounding gum tissue. Infection typically produces an unpleasant taste when biting down and **bad breath.** Another source of pain may be pericoronitis, a gum condition in which the crown of the incompletely erupted tooth produces inflammation, redness, and tenderness of the gums. Less common symptoms of an impacted tooth are swollen lymph nodes in the neck, difficulty opening the mouth, and prolonged **headache.**

Diagnosis

Upon visual examination, the dentist may find signs of infection or swelling in the area where the tooth is absent or only partially erupted. Dental x rays are necessary to confirm tooth impaction.

Treatment

Because impacted teeth may cause dental problems with few if any symptoms to indicate damage, dentists commonly recommend the removal of all wisdom teeth, preferably while the patient is still a young adult. A dentist may perform an extraction with forceps and local anesthetic if the tooth is exposed and appears to be easily removable in one piece. However, he or she may refer a difficult extraction to an oral surgeon, a specialist who administers either nitrous oxide-oxygen (commonly called ''laughing gas''), an intravenous sedative, or a general anesthetic to alleviate any pain or discomfort during the surgical procedure. Extracting an impacted tooth typically requires cutting through gum tissue to expose the tooth and may require removing portions of bone to free the tooth. The tooth may have to be removed in pieces to minimize destruction to the surrounding structures. The extraction site may or may not require one or more stitches to help the incision heal.

Prognosis

The prognosis is very good when impacted teeth are removed from young healthy adults without complications. Potential complications include postoperative infection, temporary numbness from nerve irritation, jaw fracture, and jaw joint pain. An additional condition which may develop is called dry socket: when a blood clot does not properly form in the empty tooth socket, or is disturbed by an oral vacuum (such as from drinking through a straw or smoking), the bone beneath the socket is painfully exposed to air and food, and the extraction site heals more slowly.

Resources

ORGANIZATIONS

American Association of Oral and Maxillofacial Surgeons. 9700 West Bryn Mawr Avenue, Rosemont, IL 60018-5701. (847) 678-6200. http://www.aaoms.org.

Bethany Thivierge

. . . .

Impedance phlebography

Definition

Impedance phlebography is a non-invasive test that uses electrical monitoring to measure blood flow in veins of the leg. Information from this test helps a doctor to detect **deep vein thrombosis** (blood clots or **thrombophlebitis).**

Purpose

Impedance phlebography may be done in order to:

- Detect blood clots lodged in the deep veins of the leg
- Screen patients who are likely to have blood clots in the leg
- Detect the source of blood clots in the lungs (pulmonary emboli).

Blood clots in the legs can lead to more serious problems. If a clot breaks loose from a leg vein, it may travel to the lungs and lodge in a blood vessel in the lungs. Blood clots are more likely to occur in people who have recently had leg injuries, surgery, **cancer,** or a long period of bed rest.

Precautions

Because this test is not invasive, it can be done on all patients. However, the accuracy of the results will be affected if the patient does not breathe normally or keep the leg muscles relaxed. Compression of the veins because of pelvic tumors or decreased blood flow, due to **shock** or any condition that reduces the amount of blood the heart pumps, may also change the test results.

Description

Impedance phlebography works by measuring the resistance to the transmission of electrical energy (impedance). This resistance changes depending on the volume of blood flowing through the veins. By graphing the impedance, a doctor or technician can tell whether a clot is obstructing blood flow.

Using conductive jelly, the examiner puts electrodes on the patient's calf. These electrodes are connected to an instrument called a plethysmograph which records the changes in electrical resistance which occur during the test.

The patient lies down and raises one leg at a 30° angle, so that the calf is above the level of the heart. The examiner wraps a pressure cuff around the patient's thigh and inflates it to a pressure of 45-60 cm of water for 45 seconds. The plethysmograph records the electrical changes that correspond to changes in the volume of blood in the vein at the time the pressure is exerted and again three seconds after the cuff is deflated. This procedure is repeated several times in both legs.

This test takes 30-45 minutes. Impedance phlebography is also called an impedance test of blood flow or impedance plethysmography.

Preparation

Patients undergoing this test do not need to alter their diet, change their normal activities, or stop taking any medications. They will wear a surgical gown during the test, and be asked to urinate before the test starts. If keeping the legs elevated causes discomfort, mild **pain** medication will be given.

Aftercare

The patient may resume normal or postoperative activities after the test.

Risks

Impedance phlebography is painless and safe. It presents no risk to the patient.

Normal results

Normally, inflating the pressure cuff will cause a sharp rise in the pressure in the veins of the calf because blood flow is blocked. When the cuff is released, the pressure decreases rapidly as the blood flows away.

Abnormal results

If a clot is present, the pressure in the calf veins will already be high. It does not become sharply higher when the pressure cuff is tightened. When the pressure cuff is deflated, the clot blocks the flow of blood out of the calf

vein. The decrease in pressure is not as rapid as when no clot is present and the shape of the resulting graph is different.

Resources

BOOKS

"Impedance Plethysmography." In *Illustrated Guide to Diagnostic Tests.* Springhouse, PA: Springhouse Corp. 1994, pp.923-24.

OTHER

Griffith, H. Winter. *Complete Guide to Medical Tests.* Fisher Books, 1988. http://www.thriveonline.com/health/Library/medtest224.html.

Tish Davidson

Impedance plethysmography *see*
Impedance phlebography

Impedance test of blood flow *see*
Impedance phlebography

. . . .

Impetigo

Definition

Impetigo refers to a very localized bacterial infection of the skin. There are two types, bullous and epidemic.

Description

Impetigo is a skin infection which tends primarily to afflict children. Impetigo caused by the bacteria *Staphylococcus aureus* (also known as staph) affects children of all ages. Impetigo caused by the bacteria called group A streptococci (also know as strep) are most common in children ages two to five.

The bacteria which cause impetigo are very contagious. They can be spread by a child from one part of his or her body to another by scratching, or contact with a towel, clothing, or stuffed animal. These same methods can pass the bacteria on from one person to another.

Impetigo tends to develop in areas of the skin which have already been damaged through some other mechanism (a cut or scrape, burn, insect bite, or pock from **chickenpox**).

Causes & symptoms

The first sign of bullous impetigo is a large bump on the skin, with a clear, fluid-filled top (called a vesicle).

The bump develops a scab-like, honey-colored crust. There is usually no redness or **pain,** although the area may be quite itchy. Ultimately, the skin in this area will become dry, and flake away. Bullous impetigo is usually caused by staph bacteria.

Epidemic impetigo can be caused by staph or strep bacteria, and (as the name implies) is very easily passed between children. Certain factors, such as heat and humidity, crowded conditions, and poor hygiene increase the chance that this type of impetigo will spread rapidly among large groups of children. This type of impetigo involves the formation of a small vesicle surrounded by a circle of reddened skin. The vesicles appear first on the face and legs. When a child has several of these vesicles close together, they may spread to each other. The skin surface may become eaten away (ulcerated), leaving irritated pits. When there are many of these deep, pitting **ulcers,** with pus in the center and brownish-black scabs, the condition is called ecthyma. If left untreated, the type of bacteria causing this type of impetigo has the potential to cause a serious kidney disease, called **glomerulonephritis.** Even when impetigo is initially caused by strep bacteria, the vesicles are frequently secondarily infected with staph bacteria.

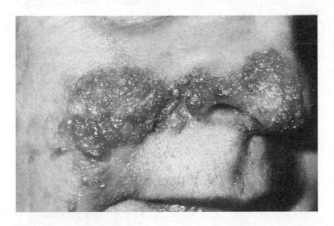

Impetigo is a contagious bacterial skin infection that mostly affects the area around the nose and mouth. Usually caused by staphlococci, this person's impetigo was triggered by herpes simplex. *(Photo Researchers, Inc. Reproduced by permission.)*

Impetigo is usually an uncomplicated skin condition. Left untreated, however, there is a chance of developing a serious disease, including **osteomyelitis** (bone infection), septic arthritis (joint infection), or **pneumonia.** If large quantities of bacteria are present and begin circulating in the bloodstream, the child is in danger of developing an overwhelming systemic infection known as **sepsis.**

Diagnosis

Characteristic appearance of the skin is the usual method of diagnosis, although fluid from the vesicles can be cultured and then examined in an attempt to identify the causative bacteria.

Treatment

Uncomplicated impetigo is usually treated with a topical antibiotic cream called mupirocin. In more serious, widespread cases of impetigo, or when the child has a **fever** or swollen glands, **antibiotics** may be given by mouth or even through a needle placed in a vein (intravenously).

Prognosis

Prognosis for a child with impetigo is excellent. The vast majority of children recover quickly, completely, and uneventfully.

Prevention

Prevention involves good hygiene. Handwashing, never sharing towels, clothing, or stuffed animals, and keeping fingernails well-trimmed are easy precautions to take to avoid spreading the infection from one person to another.

Resources

BOOKS

Darmstad, Gary L., and Al Lane. "The Skin." In *Nelson Textbook of Pediatrics,* edited by Richard Behrman. Philadelphia: W.B. Saunders Co., 1996.

Deresiewicz, Robert L., and Jeffrey Parsonnet. "Staphylococcal Infections." In *Harrison's Principles of Internal Medicine,* edited by Anthony S. Fauci, et al. New York: McGraw-Hill, 1998.

Ryan, Kenneth. "Streptococci." In *Sherris Medical Microbiology: An Introduction to Infectious Diseases,* edited by Kenneth J. Ryan. Norwalk, CT: Appleton and Lange, 1994.

Sherris, John C., and James J. Plorde. In *Sherris Medical Microbiology: An Introduction to Infectious Diseases,* edited by Kenneth J. Ryan. Norwalk, CT: Appleton and Lange, 1994.

Stevens, Dennis L. "Infections of the Skin, Muscle, and Soft Tissues." In *Harrison's Principles of Internal Medicine,* edited by Anthony S. Fauci, et al. New York: McGraw-Hill, 1998.

Stoffman, Phyllis. *The Family Guide to Preventing and Treating 100 Infectious Diseases.* New York: John Wiley and Sons, Inc., 1995.

PERIODICALS

Huerter, Christopher, et al. "Helpful Clues to Common Rashes." *Patient Care* 31, 8 (April 30, 1997): 9+.

Scales. "Bullous Impetigo." *Archives of Pediatrics and Adolescent Medicine* 151, 11 (November 1997): 1168+.

Squires, Sally. "What Your Child Could Catch At School This Year." *Good Housekeeping* 223, 3 (September 1996): 138+.

Rosalyn S. Carson-DeWitt

Implant therapy *see* **Radioactive implants**

Implantable cardioverter-defibrillator

Definition

The implantable cardioverter-defibrillator is an electronic device to treat life-threatening heartbeat irregularities. It is surgically implanted.

Purpose

The implantable cardioverter-defibrillator is used to detect and stop serious ventricular **arrhythmias** and restore a normal heartbeat in people who are at high risk of sudden **death.** The American Heart Association recommends that implantable cardioverter-defibrillators only be considered for patients who have a life-threatening arrhythmia. A recent study by the National Heart, Lung, and Blood Institute demonstrated that implantable cardioverter-defibrillators are the treatment of choice instead of drug therapy for patients who have had a cardiac arrest or **heart attack** and are at risk for developing **ventricular tachycardia,** which is a very rapid heartbeat, or **ventricular fibrillation,** which is an ineffective, irregular heart activity. Other studies suggest that 20% of these high risk patients would die within two years without an implantable cardioverter-defibrillator. With the device, the five-year risk of sudden death drops to five percent.

KEY TERMS

Arrhythmia—A variation of the normal rhythm of the heartbeat.

Cardioverter—A device to apply electric shock to the chest to convert an abnormal heartbeat into a normal heartbeat.

Defibrillation—An electronic process which helps re-establish a normal heart rhythm.

Ventricles—The two large lower chambers of the heart which pump blood to the lungs and the rest of the human body.

Ventricular fibrillation—An arrhythmia in which the heart beats very fast but blood is not pumped out to the body. Ventricular fibrillation can quickly become fatal if not corrected.

Ventricular tachycardia—An arrhythmia in which the heart rate is more than 100 beats per minute.

Precautions

The implantable cardioverter-defibrillator should not be used on patients who faint from causes other than a known life-threatening ventricular arrhythmia, to treat slow heart rates, or during an emergency.

Description

According to the American College of Cardiology, more than 80,000 Americans currently have an implantable cardioverter-defibrillator; 17,000 of these were implanted in 1995 alone. The battery-powered device rescues the patient from a life-threatening arrhythmia by rapid pacing and/or delivering electrical shock(s) to suspend heart activity and then allow it to initiate a normal rhythm. Before the development of the implantable cardioverter-defibrillator, most people who experienced ventricular fibrillation and weren't near a hospital with a well equipped emergency team died within minutes.

The implantable cardioverter-defibrillator is like a mini computer connected to the patient's heart. Newer models weigh less than 10 ounces and can be implanted beneath the skin of the chest in the pectoral region, without major surgery. A lead from the device is then inserted into the heart through a vein. The procedure is performed in an operating room under general anesthesia. Earlier versions of implantable cardioverter-defibrillators were implanted in the abdomen and required open-chest surgery to connect the electrodes to the left and right ventricles.

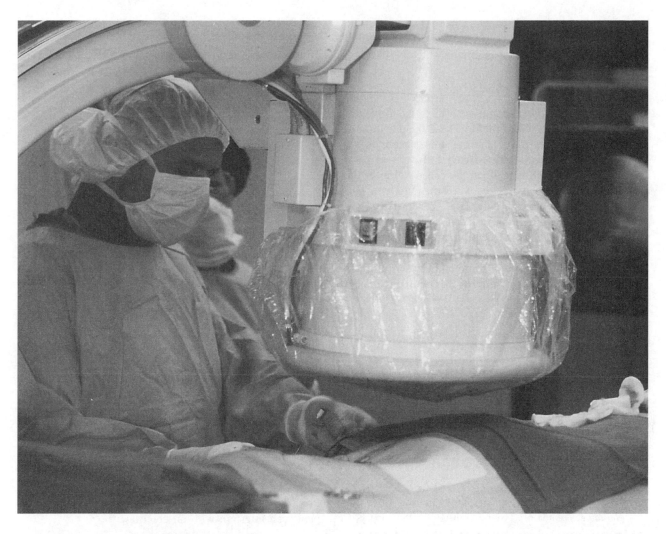

A surgeon implants a defibrillator into a patient. The device is a sophisticated computer that combines a heart pacemaker and defibrillator. *(Photograph by John S. Stewart, AP/Wide World Photo. Reproduced by permission.)*

The implantable cardioverter-defibrillator is set above the patient's **exercise** heart rate. Once the device is in place, many tests will be conducted to ensure that the device is sensing and defibrillating properly. The newer implantable cardioverter-defibrillators last seven or eight years. Technology and procedures continue to evolve.

Preparation

Before the procedure, a complete medical history and physical exam will be done. **Electrocardiography,** special electrophysiologic testing, **chest x ray,** urinalysis, and a blood test are usually also required.

Aftercare

The patient is monitored for arrhythmias and to ensure that the implantable cardioverter-defibrillator is working properly. The physician also watches for signs of infection. Before the patient leaves the hospital, the device is tested again. Anti-arrhythmia drug therapy is necessary in more than half of all patients with implantable cardioverter-defibrillators, but the number of drugs and the dosages are usually reduced. Any time a significant change in anti-arrhythmia medication is made, the device will be tested again.

The patient is taught how the device works, and that the shock it delivers will feel like a punch or kick in the chest. The patient is told to notify his/her physician when the implantable cardioverter-defibrillator delivers a shock, and to go to the emergency room if multiple shocks are sent within a short period of time.

Although most patients with implantable cardioverter-defibrillators are glad that they have the device and feel that it has extended their lives, they do experience fear and **anxiety.** This stems from the sensation of the shock(s), the unpredictable circumstances under which shock(s) occurs, and unknown outcomes.

Risks

There can be serious complications to the implantation of a cardioverter-defibrillator. These include inflammation of the pericardium, the sac that surrounds the heart; heart attack; congestive **heart failure;** and postoperative **stroke.** Serious infections can develop in the area around the device while the patient is initially hospitalized or up to several months later. Death due to the device's failure while being tested during surgery is an uncommon risk. The risk of death from the implantation procedure is about the same as that for a pacemaker, less than one percent. There are also potentially serious risks associated with the device's improper functioning once it is in place.

Resources

BOOKS

DeBakey, M. E., and A.M. Gotto. "Arrhythmias." In *The New Living Heart,* Holbrook, MA: Adams Media Corporation, 1997, pp.133-150.

Texas Heart Institute. "Arrhythmias." In *Texas Heart Institute Heart Owners Handbook.* New York: John Wiley & Sons, 1996, pp. 285-291.

PERIODICALS

"Comparing Implantable Defibrillators and Drug Therapy in Patients with Life-Threatening Arrhythmias." *Modern Medicine* Volume 65, Issue 7 (July 1997):15.

"Computer Software Aids Cardiac Implants." *USA Today* Volume 126, Issue 2633 (February 1998):4.

Daneala Gallagher, et al. "The Impact of the Implantable Cardioverter Defibrillator on Quality of Life." *American Journal of Critical Care* Volume 6, Number 1 (January 1997):16-23.

ORGANIZATIONS

American Heart Association. National Center. 7272 Greenville Avenue, Dallas, TX. 75231-4596. (214) 373-6300. http://www.medsearch.com/pf/profiles/amerh/.

Texas Heart Institute Heart Information Service. P.O. Box 20345, Houston, TX. 77225-0345. 1-800-292-2221. Http://www.tmc.edu/thi/his.html.

OTHER

"Implantable Cardioverter/Defibrillator." *American Heart Association. 1997.* http://207.211.141.25/Heart_and_Stroke_A_Z_guide/.html. (30 March 1998).

"Implantable Defibrillator Can Aid People with Dangerously Irregular Heartbeats." *Cardiovascular Institute of the South.* http://www.cardio.com/articles/defibril.htm (1 April 1998).

"Implantable Defibrillators Prevent Sudden Death. *Reuters.* March 31, 1998.

"Studies Define Role of Defibrillators for Near Future." *North American Society of Pacing and Electrophysiology.* http://www.naspe.org/defib2pr.html (1 April 1998).

Lori De Milto

Impotence

Definition

Impotence, often called erectile dysfunction, is the inability to achieve or maintain an erection long enough to engage in sexual intercourse.

Description

Under normal circumstances, when a man is sexually stimulated, his brain sends a message down the spinal cord and into the nerves of the penis. The nerve endings in the penis release chemical messengers, called neurotransmitters, which signal the corpora cavernosa (the two spongy rods of tissue that span the length of the penis) to relax and fill with blood. As they expand, the corpora cavernosa close off other veins that would normally drain blood from the penis. As the penis becomes engorged with blood, it enlarges and stiffens, causing an erection. Problems with blood vessels, nerves, or tissues of the penis can interfere with an erection.

Causes & symptoms

It is estimated that 10-20 million American men frequently suffer from impotence and that it strikes up to half of all men between the ages of 40 and 70. Doctors used to think that most cases of impotence were psychological in origin, but they now recognize that, at least in older men, physical causes may play a primary role in 60% or more of all cases. In men over the age of 60, the leading cause is **atherosclerosis,** or narrowing of the arteries, which can restrict the flow of blood to the penis. Injury or disease of the connective tissue, such as **Peyronie's disease,** may prevent the corpora cavernosa from completely expanding. Damage to the nerves of the penis, from certain types of surgery or neurological conditions such as **Parkinson's disease** or **multiple sclerosis,** may also cause impotence. Men with diabetes are especially at risk for impotence because of their high risk of both atherosclerosis and a nerve disease called diabetic neuropathy.

Some drugs, including certain types of blood pressure medications, **antihistamines,** tranquilizers (espe-

KEY TERMS

Alprostadil—A smooth muscle relaxant sometimes injected into the penis or applied to the urethral opening to treat impotence.

Atherosclerosis—A disorder in which plaques of cholesterol, lipids, and other debris build up on the inner walls of arteries, narrowing them.

Corpora cavernosa—Rods of spongy tissue found within the penis, which become engorged with blood in order to produce an erection. (The singular form of this term is corpus cavernosum.)

Neurotransmitters—Chemicals that modify or help transmit impulses between nerve synapses.

Papaverine—A smooth muscle relaxant sometimes injected into the penis as a treatment for impotence.

Peyronie's disease—A disease resulting from scarring of the corpus cavernosa, causing painful erections.

Urethra—The small tube that drains urine from the bladder, as well as serving as a conduit for semen during ejaculation in men.

Viagra—An orally administered drug for erectile failure first cleared for marketing in the United States in March 1998.

cially before intercourse), and antidepressants known as **selective serotonin reuptake inhibitors** (SSRIs, including Prozac and Paxil) can interfere with erections. Smoking, excessive alcohol consumption, and illicit drug use may also contribute. In rare cases, low levels of the male hormone testosterone may contribute to erectile failure. Finally, psychological factors, such as **stress,** guilt, or **anxiety,** may also play a role, even when the impotence is primarily due to organic causes.

Diagnosis

When diagnosing the underlying cause of impotence, the doctor begins by asking the man a number of questions about when the problem began, whether it only happens with specific sex partners, and whether he ever wakes up with an erection. (Men whose impotence occurs only with certain partners or who wake up with erections are more likely to have a psychological cause for their impotence.) Sometimes, the man's sex partner is also interviewed. In some cases, marital discord may be a factor.

The doctor also obtains a thorough medical history to find out about past pelvic surgery, diabetes, cardiovascular disease, kidney disease, and any medications the man may be taking. The **physical examination** should include a genital examination, a measurement of blood flow through the penis, hormone tests, and a glucose test for diabetes.

In some cases, nocturnal penile tumescence testing is performed to find out whether the man has erections while asleep. Healthy men usually have about four or five erections throughout the night. The man applies a device to the penis called a Rigiscan before going to bed at night, and the device can determine whether he has had erections. (Again, if a man is able to have normal erections at night, this suggests a psychological cause for his impotence.)

Treatment

Years ago, the standard treatment for impotence was an implantable penile prosthesis or long-term psychotherapy. Although physical causes are now more readily diagnosed and treated, individual or marital counseling is still an effective treatment for impotence when emotional factors play a role. Fortunately, other approaches are now available to treat the physical causes of impotence.

One such approach is vacuum therapy. The man inserts his penis into a clear plastic cylinder and uses a pump to force air out of the cylinder. This forms a partial vacuum around the penis, which helps to draw blood into the corpora cavernosa. The man then places a special ring over the base of the penis to trap the blood inside it. The only side effect with this type of treatment is occasional bruising if the vacuum is left on too long.

Injection therapy involves injecting a substance into the penis to enhance blood flow and cause an erection. The Food and Drug Administration (FDA) approved a drug called alprostadil (Caverject) for this purpose in July of 1995. Alprostadil, which relaxes smooth muscle tissue to enhance blood flow into the penis, must be injected shortly before intercourse. Another, similar drug that is sometimes used is papaverine, which has not yet been approved by the FDA for this use. Either drug may sometimes cause painful erections or **priapism** (uncomfortable, prolonged erections), which must be treated with a shot of epinephrine.

Alprostadil may also be administered into the urethral opening of the penis. In MUSE (medical urethral system for erection), the man inserts a thin tube the width of a vermicelli noodle into his urethral opening and presses down on a plunger to deliver a tiny pellet containing alprostadil into his penis. The drug takes about 10 minutes to work and the erection lasts about an hour. The main side effect is a sensation of pain and burning in the urethra, which can last about 5 to 15 minutes.

In a long-awaited breakthrough, a pill for combating impotence was cleared for marketing by the FDA in March 1998. Called sildenafil citrate (brand name Viagra), the drug boosts levels of a substance called cyclic GMP, which is responsible for widening the blood vessels of the penis. Viagra has been shown to be effective in about 70-80% of men who take it, and it can even work in men with some psychological component to their impotence. Unlike drugs that are injected into the penis, Viagra causes an erection only when the man is sexually aroused. Furthermore, unlike vacuum therapy, injection therapy, and MUSE, taking a pill ahead of time does not interrupt sexual intercourse. In studies, Viagra produced **headaches** in 16% of men who took it, and other side effects included flushing, **indigestion,** and stuffy nose. Nonetheless, only 2.5% of men taking the drug dropped out of the study.

Implantable **penile prostheses** are usually considered a last resort for treating impotence. They are implanted in the corpora cavernosa to make the penis rigid without the need for blood flow. The semirigid type of prosthesis consists of a pair of flexible silicone rods that can be bent up or down. This type of device has a low failure rate but, unfortunately, it causes the penis to always be erect, which can be difficult to conceal under clothing.

The inflatable type of device consists of cylinders that are implanted in the corpora cavernosa, a fluid reservoir implanted in the abdomen, and a pump placed in the scrotum. The man squeezes the pump to move fluid into the cylinders and cause them to become rigid. (He reverses the process by squeezing the pump again.) While these devices allow for intermittent erections, they have a slightly higher malfunction rate than the silicon rods.

Men can return to sexual activity six to eight weeks after implantation surgery. Since implants affect the corpora cavernosa, they permanently take away a man's ability to have a natural erection.

In rare cases, if narrowed or diseased veins are responsible for impotence, surgeons may reroute the blood flow into the corpus cavernosa or remove leaking vessels. However, the success rate with these procedures has been very low, and they are still considered experimental.

Alternative treatment

A number of herbs have been promoted for treating impotence. The most widely touted herbs for this purpose are *Coryanthe yohimbe* (available by prescription as yohimbine, with the trade name Yocon) and gingko (*Gingko biloba*), although neither has been conclusively shown to help the condition in controlled studies. In addition, gingko carries some risk of abnormal blood clotting and should be avoided by men taking blood thinners such as coumadin. Other herbs promoted for treating impotence include true unicorn root (*Aletrius farinosa*), saw palmetto (*Serenoa repens*), ginseng (*Panax ginseng*), and Siberian ginseng (*Eleuthrococcus senticosus*). *Strychnos Nux vomica* has been recommended, especially when impotence is caused by excessive alcohol, cigarettes, or dietary indiscretions, but it can be very toxic if taken improperly, so it should be used only under the strict supervision of a physician trained in its use.

Prognosis

With proper diagnosis, impotence can nearly always be treated or coped with successfully. Unfortunately, fewer than 10% of impotent men seek treatment.

Prevention

There is no specific treatment to prevent impotence. Perhaps the most important measure is to maintain general good health and avoid atherosclerosis—by exercising regularly, controlling weight, controlling **hypertension** and high cholesterol levels, and avoiding smoking. Avoiding excessive alcohol intake may also help.

Resources

BOOKS

The Burton Goldberg Group. *Alternative Medicine: The Definitive Guide.* Fife, WA: Future Medicine Publishing, 1995.

Ryan, George. *Reclaiming Male Sexuality: A Guide to Potency, Vitality, and Prowess.* New York: M. Evans and Company, 1997.

PERIODICALS

"American Urologic Association Issues Treatment Guidelines for Erectile Failure." *American Family Physician* 35 (April 1997): 1967-69.

Burnett, Arthur L. "Erectile Dysfunction: A Practical Approach to Primary Care." *Geriatrics* 53 (February 1998): 36-42.

Church, Paul, and Peta Gilyatt. "Impotence: No Need to Suffer in Secret." *Harvard Health Letter* (May 1996): 4-6.

Leland, John, and Andrew Murr. "A Pill for Impotence?" *Newsweek* (November 17, 1997): 62-67.

Linet, Otto L., and Francis G. Ogring. "Efficacy and Safety of Intracavernosal Alprostadil in Men with Erectile Dysfunction." *New England Journal of Medicine* 334 (April 4, 1996): 873-77.

Lipshultz, Larry I. "Injection Therapy for Erectile Dysfunction." *New England Journal of Medicine* 334 (April 4, 1996): 913-14.

ORGANIZATIONS

American Foundation for Urologic Disease. 1128 North Charles Street, Baltimore, MD 21201. (410) 468-1800.

Impotence Institute of America, Impotents Anonymous. 10400 Little Patuxent Parkway, Suite 485, Columbia, MD 21044-3502. (800) 669-1603.

National Kidney and Urologic Diseases Information Clearinghouse. 3 Information Way, Bethesda, MD 20892-3580. (800) 891-5390.

Robert Scott Dinsmoor

In vitro fertilization

Definition

In vitro fertilization (IVF) is a procedure in which eggs (ova) from a woman's ovary are removed. They are fertilized with sperm in a laboratory procedure, and then the fertilized egg (embryo) is returned to the woman's uterus.

Purpose

IVF is one of several assisted reproductive techniques (ART) used to help infertile couples to conceive a child. If after one year of having sexual intercourse without the use of birth control a woman is unable to get pregnant, **infertility** is suspected. Some of the reasons for infertility are damaged or blocked fallopian tubes, hormonal imbalance, or **endometriosis** in the woman. In the man, low sperm count or poor quality sperm can cause infertility.

IVF is one of several possible methods to increase the chance for an infertile couple to become pregnant. Its use depends on the reason for infertility. IVF may be an option if there is a blockage in the fallopian tube or endometriosis in the woman or low sperm count or poor quality sperm in the man. There are other possible treatments for these conditions, such as surgery for blocked tubes or endometriosis, which may be tried before IVF.

IVF will not work for a woman who is not capable of ovulating or a man who is not able to produce at least a few healthy sperm.

Precautions

The screening procedures and treatments for infertility can become a long, expensive, and sometimes, disappointing process. Each IVF attempt takes at least an entire menstrual cycle and can cost $5000-$10,000, which may or may not be covered by health insurance. The **anxiety** of dealing with infertility can challenge both

---

KEY TERMS

Fallopian tubes—In a woman's reproductive system, a pair of narrow tubes that carry the egg from the ovary to the uterus.

GIFT—Stands for gamete intrafallopian tube transfer. This is a process where eggs are taken from a woman's ovaries, mixed with sperm, and then deposited into the woman's fallopian tube.

ICSI—Stands for intracytoplasmic sperm injection. This process is used to inject a single sperm into each egg before the fertilized eggs are put back into the woman's body. The procedure may be used if the male has a low sperm count.

ZIFT—Stands for zygote intrafallopian tube transfer. In this process of in vitro fertilization, the eggs are fertilized in a laboratory dish and then placed in the woman's fallopian tube.

---

individuals and their relationship. The added **stress** and expense of multiple clinic visits, testing, treatments, and surgical procedures can become overwhelming. Couples may want to receive counseling and support through the process.

Description

In vitro fertilization is a procedure where the joining of egg and sperm takes place outside of the woman's body. A woman may be given fertility drugs before this procedure so that several eggs mature in the ovaries at the same time. Eggs (ova) are removed from a woman's ovaries using a long, thin needle. The physician gets access to the ovaries using one of two possible procedures. One procedure involves inserting the needle through the vagina (transvaginally). The physician guides the needle to the location of the ovaries with the help of an ultrasound machine. In the other procedure, called **laparoscopy,** a small thin tube with a viewing lens is inserted through an incision in the navel. This allows the physician to see inside the patient, and locate the ovaries, on a video monitor.

Once the eggs are removed, they are mixed with sperm in a laboratory dish or test tube. (This is where the term *test tube baby* comes from.) The eggs are monitored for several days. Once there is evidence that fertilization has occurred and the cells begin to divide, they are then returned to the woman's uterus.

In the procedure to remove eggs, enough may be gathered to be frozen and saved (either fertilized or unfertilized) for additional IVF attempts.

IVF has been used successfully since 1978, when the first child to be conceived by this method was born in England. Over the past 20 years, thousands of couples have used this method of ART or similar procedures to conceive.

Other types of assisted reproductive technologies might be used to achieve **pregnancy.** A procedure called intracytoplasmic sperm injection (ICSI) uses a manipulation technique that must be performed using a microscope to inject a single sperm into each egg. The fertilized eggs can then be returned to the uterus, as in IVF. In gamete intrafallopian tube transfer (GIFT) the eggs and sperm are mixed in a narrow tube and then deposited in the fallopian tube, where fertilization normally takes place. Another variation on IVF is zygote intrafallopian tube transfer (ZIFT). As in IVF, the fertilization of the eggs occurs in a laboratory dish. And, similar to GIFT, the embryos are placed in the fallopian tube (rather than the uterus as with IVF).

Preparation

Once a woman is determined to be a good candidate for in vitro fertilization, she will generally be given "fertility drugs" to stimulate ovulation and the development of multiple eggs. These drugs may include gonadotropin releasing hormone agonists (GnRHa), Pergonal, Clomid, or human chorionic gonadotropin (hcg). The maturation of the eggs is then monitored with ultrasound tests and frequent blood tests. If enough eggs mature, the physician will perform the procedure to remove them. The woman may be given a sedative prior to the procedure. A local anesthetic agent may also be used to reduce discomfort during the procedure.

Aftercare

After the IVF procedure is performed the woman can resume normal activities. A pregnancy test can be done approximately 12-14 days later to determine if the procedure was successful.

Risks

The risks associated with in vitro fertilization include the possibility of **multiple pregnancy** (since several embryos may be implanted) and **ectopic pregnancy** (an embryo that implants in the fallopian tube or in the abdominal cavity outside the uterus). There is a slight risk of ovarian rupture, bleeding, infections, and complications of anesthesia. If the procedure is successful and pregnancy is achieved, the pregnancy would carry the same risks as any pregnancy achieved without assisted technology.

Normal results

Success rates vary widely between clinics and between physicians performing the procedure. A couple has about a 10% chance of becoming pregnant each time the procedure is performed. Therefore, the procedure may have to be repeated more than once to achieve pregnancy.

Abnormal results

An ectopic or multiple pregnancy may abort spontaneously or may require termination if the health of the mother is at risk.

Resources

BOOKS
"Assisted Reproductive Technologies." In *The Merck Manual,* 16th ed., edited by Robert Berkow. Rahway, NJ: Merck & Co., Inc., 1992, pp. 1772-1773.

Carlson, Karen J., Stephanie A. Eisenstat, and Terra Ziporyn. *The Harvard Guide to Women's Health.* Cambridge, Massachusetts: Harvard University Press, 1996.

Sher, G. V.M. Davis, and J. Stoess. *In Vitro Fertilization: The A.R.T. of Making Babies.* 1st ed. New York: Facts On File, Inc., 1995.

PERIODICALS
Blackwell, R. E. "Clinical Treatment of Infertility: A Practicable Algorithm." *Drug Benefit Trends* 8, no. 1 (1996): 17, 21-22, 38.

ORGANIZATIONS
American Society for Reproductive Medicine. 1209 Montgomery Highway, Birmingham, AL 35216-2809. (205) 978-5000. asrm@asrm.com. http://www.asrm.com.

Center for Fertility and In Vitro Fertilization Loma Linda University. 11370 Anderson Street, Loma Linda, CA 92354. (909) 796-4851. http://www.llu.edu/llumc/fertility.

Resolve (Education, support and advocacy for those struggling with infertility). 1310 Broadway, Somerville, MA 02144. (617) 623-0744. resolveinc@aol.com. http://www.resolve.org.

OTHER
In vitro Fertilization: A Teacher's Guide from Newton's Apple. http://www.pbs.org/ktca/newtons/11/invitro.html.

Infertility at http://www.healthy.net/library/books/hoffman/reproductive/infertility.htm.

Altha Roberts Edgren

Incentive spirometry *see* **Inhalation therapies**

Inclusion blennorrhea *see* **Inclusion conjunctivitis**

Inclusion conjunctivitis

Definition

Inclusion conjunctivitis is an inflammation of the conjunctiva (the membrane that lines the eyelids and covers the white part, or sclera, of the eyeball) by *Chlamydia trachomatis*. Chlamydia is a sexually transmitted organism.

Description

Inclusion conjunctivitis, known as neonatal inclusion conjunctivitis in the newborn and adult inclusion conjunctivitis in the adult, is also called inclusion blennorrhea, chlamydial **conjunctivitis,** or swimming pool conjunctivitis. This disease affects four of 1,000 (0.4%) live births. Approximately half of the infants born to untreated infected mothers will develop the disease.

Causes & symptoms

Inclusion conjunctivitis in the newborn results from passage through an infected birth canal and develops 5-14 days after birth. Both eyelids and conjunctivae are swollen. There may be a discharge of pus from the eyes.

Most instances of adult inclusion conjunctivitis result from exposure to infected genital secretions. It is transmitted to the eye by fingers and occasionally by the water in swimming pools, poorly chlorinated hot tubs, or by sharing makeup. In adult inclusion conjunctivitis, one eye is usually involved, with a stringy discharge of mucus and pus. There may be little bumps called follicles inside the lower eyelid and the eye is red. Occasionally, the condition damages the cornea, causing cloudy areas and a growth of new blood vessels (neovascularization).

Diagnosis

Inclusion conjunctivitis is usually considered when the patient has a follicular conjunctivitis that will not go away, even after using **topical antibiotics.** Diagnosis depends upon tests performed on the discharge from the eye. Gram stains determine the type of microorganism, while culture and sensitivity tests determine which antibiotic will kill the harmful microorganism. Conjunctival scraping determines whether chlamydia is present in cells taken from the conjunctiva.

Treatment

Treatment in the newborn consists of administration of tetracycline ointment to the conjunctiva and erythromycin orally or through intravenous therapy for fourteen days. The mother should be treated for cervicitis and the father for **urethritis,** even if they do not have symptoms of these diseases.

In adults, tetracycline ointment or drops should be applied to the conjunctiva and oral tetracycline, amoxacillin, or erythromycin should be taken for three weeks, or doxycycline for one week.

Patients should have weekly checkups so the doctor can monitor the healing.

Oral tetracycline should not be administered to children whose permanent teeth have not erupted. It should also not be given to nursing or pregnant women.

Prognosis

Untreated inclusion conjunctivitis in the newborn persists for 3-12 months and usually heals; however, there may be scarring or neovascularization. In the adult, if left untreated, the disease may continue for months and cause corneal neovascularization. Even if treated, **antibiotics** usually do not reverse damage that may have occurred, but they may help prevent it if given early enough.

Prevention

The neonatal infection may be prevented by instilling erythromycin ointment in the conjunctival cul-de-sac at birth. It is not prevented by silver nitrate.

Chlamydia is a contagious, sexually transmitted disease. Some systemic symptoms include a history of vaginitis, **pelvic inflammatory disease,** or urethritis. Patients with symptoms of these diseases should be treated by a physician.

Resources

BOOKS

Newell, Frank W. *Ophthalmology: Principles and Concepts.* Boston, MA: Mosby, 1996.

ORGANIZATIONS

American Academy of Ophthalmology. P.O. Box 7424, San Francisco CA 94120-7424. (415) 561-8500. http://www.eyenet.org.

American Optometric Association. 243 North Lindbergh Blvd., St. Louis, MO 63141. (314) 991-4100. http://www.aoanet.org.

Lorraine T. Steefel

Incompetent cervix

Definition

A cervix (the structure at the bottom of the uterus) that is incompetent is abnormally weak, and therefore it can gradually widen during **pregnancy.** Left untreated, this can result in repeated pregnancy losses or premature delivery.

Description

Incompetent cervix is the result of an anatomical abnormality. Normally, the cervix remains closed throughout pregnancy until labor begins. An incompetent cervix gradually opens due to the pressure from the developing fetus after about the 13th week of pregnancy. The cervix begins to thin out and widen without any contractions or labor. The membranes surrounding the fetus bulge down into the opening of the cervix until they break, resulting in the loss of the baby or a very premature delivery.

Causes & symptoms

Some factors that can contribute to the chance of a woman having an incompetent cervix include trauma to the cervix, physical abnormality of the cervix, or having been exposed to the drug diethylstilbestrol (DES) in the mother's womb. Some women have cervical incompetence for no obvious reason.

Diagnosis

Incompetent cervix is suspected when a woman has three consecutive spontaneous pregnancy losses during the second trimester (the fourth, fifth and sixth months of the pregnancy). The likelihood of this happening by random chance is less than 1%. Spontaneous losses due to incompetent cervix account for 20-25% of all second trimester losses. A spontaneous second trimester pregnancy loss is different from a **miscarriage,** which usually happens during the first three months of pregnancy.

KEY TERMS

Diethylstilbestrol (DES)—DES is a drug given to women a generation ago to prevent miscarriage. At that time it was not known that female children born of women who had been given DES would show a higher rate for cervical and other reproductive abnormalities, as well as a rare form of vaginal cancer, when they reached reproductive age.

Effacement—The thinning out of the cervix that normally occurs along with dilation shortly before delivery.

Preterm labor—Labor before the thirty-seventh week of pregnancy.

The physician can check for abnormalities in the cervix by performing a manual examination or by an ultrasound test. The physician can also check to see if the cervix is prematurely widened (dilated). Because incompetent cervix is only one of several potential causes for this, the patient's past history of pregnancy losses must also be considered when making the diagnosis.

Treatment

Treatment for incompetent cervix is a surgical procedure called cervical cerclage. A stitch (suture) is used to tie the cervix shut to give it more support. It is most effective if it is performed somewhere between 14-16 weeks into the pregnancy. The stitch is removed near the end of pregnancy to allow for a normal birth.

Cervical cerclage can be performed under spinal, epidural, or general anesthesia. The patient will need to stay in the hospital for one or more days. The procedure to remove the suture is done without the need for anesthesia. The vagina is held open with an instrument called a speculum and the stitch is cut and removed. This may be slightly uncomfortable, but should not be painful.

Some possible risks of cerclage are premature rupture of the amniotic membranes, infection of the amniotic sac, and preterm labor. The risk of infection of the amniotic sac increases as the pregnancy progresses. For a cervix that is dilated 3 centimeters (cm), the risk is 30%.

After cerclage, a woman will be monitored for any preterm labor. The woman needs to consult her obstetrician immediately if there are any signs of contractions.

Cervical cerclage can not be performed if a woman is more than 4 cm dilated, if the fetus has already died in her uterus, or if her amniotic membranes are torn and her water has broken.

Prognosis

The success rate for cerclage correction of incompetent cervix is good. About 80-90% of the time women deliver healthy infants. The success rate is higher for cerclage done early in pregnancy.

Resources

BOOKS

Barber, Hugh R. K., David H. Fields, and Sherwin A. Kaufman. "Infertility." In *Quick Reference to OB-GYN Procedures*. Philadelphia: Lippincott, 1990, pp. 33-34; 119-120.

OTHER

Weiss, Robin. "Incompetent Cervix." In *The Mining Co. Guide to Pregnancy/Childbirth*. http://www.pregnancy.miningco.com/library/weekly/aa011298.htm. 8 (March 1998).

Tish Davidson

Indapamide *see* **Diuretics**

Indigestion

Definition

Indigestion, which is sometimes called **dyspepsia,** is a general term covering a group of nonspecific symptoms in the digestive tract. It is often described as a feeling of fullness, bloating, nausea, **heartburn,** or gassy discomfort in the chest or abdomen. The symptoms develop during meals or shortly afterward. In most cases, indigestion is a minor problem that often clears up without professional treatment.

Description

Indigestion or dyspepsia is a widespread condition, estimated to occur in 25% of the adult population of the United States. Most people with indigestion do not feel sick enough to see a doctor; nonetheless, it is a common reason for office visits. About 3% of visits to primary care doctors are for indigestion.

Causes & symptoms

Physical causes

The symptoms associated with indigestion have a variety of possible physical causes, ranging from commonplace food items to serious systemic disorders:

KEY TERMS

Dyspepsia—Another name for indigestion.

Endoscope—A slender tubular instrument used to examine the inside of the stomach.

Gastroesophageal reflux disease (GERD)—A disorder of the lower end of the esophagus, caused by stomach acid flowing backward into the esophagus and irritating the tissues.

H_2 antagonist—A type of drug that relieves indigestion by reducing the production of stomach acid.

Heartburn—A popular term for an uncomfortable burning sensation in the stomach and lower esophagus, sometimes caused by the reflux of small amounts of stomach acid.

Helicobacter pylori—A gram- negative rod-shaped bacterium that lives in the tissues of the stomach and causes inflammation of the stomach lining.

Motility—The movement or capacity for movement of an organism or body organ. Indigestion is sometimes caused by abnormal patterns in the motility of the stomach.

Peptic ulcer disease (PUD)—A stomach disorder marked by corrosion of the stomach lining due to the acid in the digestive juices.

Prokinetic—A drug that works to speed up the emptying of the stomach and the motility of the intestines.

Reflux—The backward flow of a body fluid or secretion. Indigestion is sometimes caused by the reflux of stomach acid into the esophagus.

• Diet. Milk, milk products, alcoholic beverages, tea, and coffee cause indigestion in some people because they stimulate the stomach's production of acid.

• Medications. Certain prescription drugs as well as over-the- counter medications can irritate the stomach lining. These medications include **aspirin,** NSAIDs, some **antibiotics,** digoxin, theophylline, **corticosteroids,** iron (ferrous sulfate), **oral contraceptives,** and **tricyclic antidepressants.**

• Disorders of the pancreas and gallbladder. These include inflammation of the gallbladder or pancreas, **cancer** of the pancreas, and **gallstones.**

- Intestinal parasites. Parasitic infections that cause indigestion include **amebiasis,** fluke and tapeworm infections, **giardiasis,** and strongyloidiasis.

- Systemic disorders, including diabetes, thyroid disease, collagen vascular disease.

- Cancers of the digestive tract.

- Conditions associated with women's reproductive organs. These conditions include menstrual cramps, **pregnancy,** and **pelvic inflammatory disease.**

Psychologic and emotional causes

Indigestion often accompanies an emotional upset, because the part of the nervous system involved in the so-called "fight-or-flight" response also affects the digestive tract. People diagnosed with **anxiety** or **somatoform disorders** frequently have problems with indigestion. Many people in the general population, however, will also experience heartburn, "butterflies in the stomach," or stomach cramps when they are in upsetting situations—such as school examinations, arguments with family members, crises in their workplace, and so on. Some people's digestive systems appear to react more intensely to emotional **stress** due to hypersensitive nerve endings in their intestinal tract.

Specific gastrointestinal disorders

In some cases, the patient's description of the symptoms suggests a specific digestive disorder as the cause of the indigestion. Some doctors classify these cases into three groups:

ESOPHAGITIS TYPE

Esophagitis is an inflammation of the tube that carries food from the throat to the stomach (the esophagus). The tissues of the esophagus can become irritated by the flow (reflux) of stomach acid backward into the lower part of the esophagus. If the patient describes the indigestion in terms of frequent or intense heartburn, the doctor will consider gastroesophageal reflux disease (GERD) as a possible cause. GERD is a common disorder in the general population, affecting about 30% of adults.

PEPTIC ULCER TYPE

Patients who smoke and are over 45 are more likely to have indigestion of the peptic ulcer type. This group also includes people who find that their indigestion is relieved by taking **antacids** or eating a small amount of food. Patients in this category are often found to have *Helicobacter pylori* infections. *H. pylori* is a rod-shaped bacterium that lives in the tissues of the stomach and causes irritation of the mucous lining of the stomach walls. Most people with *H. pylori* infections do not develop chronic indigestion, but the organism appears to cause peptic ulcer disease (PUD) in a vulnerable segment of the population.

NONULCER TYPE

Most cases of chronic indigestion—as many as 65%—fall into this third category. Nonulcer dyspepsia is sometimes called functional dyspepsia because it appears to be related to abnormalities in the way that the stomach empties its contents into the intestine. In some people, the stomach empties either too slowly or too rapidly. In others, the stomach's muscular contractions are irregular and uncoordinated. These disorders of stomach movement (motility) may be caused by hypersensitive nerve endings in the stomach tissues. Patients in this group are likely to be younger than 45 and have a history of taking medications for anxiety or depression.

Diagnosis

Patient history

Because indigestion is a nonspecific set of symptoms, patients who feel sick enough to seek medical attention are likely to go to their primary care doctor. The history does not always point to an obvious diagnosis. The doctor can, however, use the process of history-taking to evaluate the patient's mood or emotional state in order to assess the possibility of a psychiatric disturbance. In addition, asking about the location, intensity, timing, and recurrence of the indigestion can help the doctor weigh the different diagnostic possibilities.

An important part of the history-taking is asking about symptoms that may indicate a serious illness. These warning symptoms include:

- Weight loss

- Persistent vomiting

- Difficulty or **pain** in swallowing

- Vomiting blood or passing blood in the stools

- Anemia.

Imaging studies

If the doctor thinks that the indigestion should be investigated further, he or she will order an endoscopic examination of the stomach. An endoscope is a slender tube-shaped instrument that allows the doctor to look at the lining of the patient's stomach. If the patient has indigestion of the esophagitis type or nonulcer type, the stomach lining will appear normal. If the patient has PUD, the doctor will be able to see breaks or ulcerated areas in the tissue. He or she may also order ultrasound imaging of the abdomen, or a radionuclide scan to evaluate the motility of the stomach.

Laboratory tests

BLOOD TESTS

If the patient is over 45, the doctor will have the patient's blood analyzed for a complete blood cell count, measurements of liver enzyme levels, electrolyte and serum calcium levels, and thyroid function.

TESTS FOR *HELICOBACTER PYLORI*

Doctors can now test patients for the presence of *H. pylori* without having to take a tissue sample from the stomach. One of these noninvasive tests is a blood test and the other is a breath test.

Treatment

Since most cases of indigestion are not caused by serious disorders, many doctors prefer to try medications and other treatment measures before ordering an endoscopy.

Diet and stress management

Many patients benefit from the doctor's reassurance that they do not have a serious or fatal disorder. Cutting out alcoholic beverages and drinks containing **caffeine** often helps. The patient may also be asked to keep a record of food intake, daily schedule, and symptom severity. Food diaries sometimes reveal psychologic or dietary factors that influence indigestion.

Medications

Patients with the esophagitis type of indigestion are often treated with H_2 antagonists. H_2 antagonists are drugs that block the secretion of stomach acid. They include ranitidine (Zantac) and famotidine (Pepcid).

Patients with motility disorders may be given prokinetic drugs. Prokinetic medications speed up the emptying of the stomach and increase intestinal motility. They include metoclopramide (Reglan) and cisapride (Propulsid). These drugs relieve symptoms in 60-80% of patients.

Removal of H. pylori

It is not clear that patients with *H. pylori* infections who have *not* developed gastric **ulcers** need to have the bacterium removed. Some studies indicate, however, that these patients may benefit from antibiotic therapy.

Alternative treatment

Herbal medicine

Practitioners of **Chinese traditional herbal medicine** might recommend medicines derived from peony (*Paeonia lactiflora*), hibiscus (*Hibiscus sabdariffa*), or hare's ear (*Bupleurum chinense*) to treat indigestion.

Western herbalists are likely to prescribe fennel (*Foeniculum vulgare*), lemon balm (*Melissa officinalis*), or peppermint (*Mentha piperita*) to relieve stomach cramps and heartburn.

Homeopathy

Homeopaths tailor their remedies to the patient's overall personality profile as well as the specific symptoms. Depending on the patient's reaction to the indigestion and some of its likely causes, the homeopath might choose *Gelsemium* (*Gelsemium sempervirens*), *Carbo vegetalis*, *Nux vomica*, or *Pulsatilla* (*Pulsatilla nigricans*).

Other treatments

Some alternative treatments are aimed at lowering the patient's stress level or changing attitudes and beliefs that contribute to indigestion. These therapies and practices include **Reiki, reflexology, hydrotherapy,** therapeutic **massage, yoga,** and **meditation.**

Prognosis

Most cases of mild indigestion do not need medical treatment. For patients who consult a doctor and are given an endoscopic examination, 5-15% are diagnosed with GERD and 15-25% with PUD. About 1% of patients who are endoscoped have **stomach cancer.** Most patients with functional dyspepsia do well on either H_2 antagonists or prokinetic drugs, depending on the cause of their indigestion.

Prevention

Indigestion can often be prevented by attention to one's diet, general stress level, and ways of managing stress. Specific preventive measures include:

• Stop smoking.

• Cutting down on or eliminating alcohol, tea, or coffee.

• Avoiding foods that are highly spiced or loaded with fat.

• Eating slowly and keeping mealtimes relaxed.

• Practicing yoga or meditation.

• Not taking aspirin or other medications on an empty stomach.

• Keeping one's weight within normal limits.

Resources

OTHER

Indigestion. http://www.thriveonline.com/health/Library/illsymp/illness299.html (6 April 1998).

Rebecca J. Frey

Indinavir *see* **Protease inhibitors**

Indirect Coombs' test *see* **Coombs' tests**

Indium scan of the body

Definition

A scanning procedure in which a patient's white blood cells are first labeled with the radioactive substance indium, and then the patient's body is scanned as a way of tracking the white blood cells at the site of possible infection.

Purpose

The procedure is used to detect inflammatory processes in the body such as infections. By labelling the leukocytes (white blood cells), radiologists or nuclear medicine specialists can then watch their migration toward an **abscess** or other infection.

Description

A nuclear medicine technologist withdraws about 50 ml. of blood. White blood cells are collected, exposed to indium, and reinjected by IV back into the patient.

The scan is scheduled for between 18 and 24 hours after the white blood cells have been labelled with indium. (In some cases, more scanning may be scheduled 48 hours after labelling).

For the scan, the patient lies on a special scanning table, as either a single camera passing underneath the table or two cameras (one above the table and one underneath) are placed as close as possible to the body, slowly scanning the person's body.

The radiologist may need extra pictures, but these take only a few minutes each.

While the patient must remain perfectly still during the scan, there should be no discomfort.

Aftercare

After the scan, the patient should be able to continue with normal daily activities with no problems.

Risks

The only risk during this scanning procedure could be to a patient who is pregnant, as with any type of injectable radioactive substance. If the woman is pregnant, the radiologist must be notified; if the scan is cleared, the radiologist may use a lower dosage of indium.

Normal results

The scan should reveal no infection or pathology.

Abnormal results

The scan will reveal details, such as location, about an infection in the patient's body.

Carol A. Turkington

Induction of labor

Definition

Induction of labor involves using artificial means to assist the mother in delivering her baby.

Purpose

Labor is brought on, or induced, when the **pregnancy** has extended significantly beyond the expected delivery date and the mother shows no signs of going into labor. Generally, if the unborn baby is more than two weeks past due, labor will be induced. In most cases, a mother delivers her baby between 38-42 weeks of pregnancy. This usually means that labor is induced if the pregnancy has lasted more than 42 weeks. Labor is also induced if the mother is suffering from diseases (preeclampsia, chronic **hypertension**), if there is an Rh blood incompatibility between the baby and the mother, or if the mother or baby has a medical problem that requires delivery of the baby (like a premature rupture of the membranes).

Description

The uterus is the hollow female organ that supports the development and nourishment of the unborn baby

KEY TERMS

Cesarean section—Delivery of a baby through an incision in the mother's abdomen instead of through the vagina; also called a C-section.

Preeclampsia—Hypertension (high blood pressure) experienced during pregnancy.

Rh blood incompatibility—A blood type problem between mother (who is Rh negative) and baby (who is Rh positive), making the immune system of the mother attack her unborn baby. During delivery of the first pregnancy, the mother's immune system becomes sensitive to the Rh positive blood of the baby. The mother's system may then attack later pregnancies and cause severe illness or death to those babies.

Vasoconstriction—Constriction of a blood vessel.

during pregnancy. Sometimes labor is induced by the rupturing the amniotic membrane to release amniotic fluid. This is an attempt to mimic the normal process of "breaking water" that occurs early in the normal birth process. This method is sometimes enough stimulation to induce contractions in the mother's uterus. If labor fails to start, drugs are used.

Most labor is induced by using the drug Pitocin, a synthetic form of oxytocin. Oxytocin is a natural hormone produced in the body by the pituitary gland. During normal labor, oxytocin causes contractions. When labor does not occur naturally, the doctor may give the mother Pitocin to start the contractions. Pitocin makes the uterus contract with strength and force almost immediately. This drug is given through a vein in a steady flow that allows the doctor to control the amount the mother is given.

Sometimes vaginal gels are used to induce labor. Normally, the baby will pass through the opening of the uterus (the cervix) into the birth canal during delivery. Because of this, the cervix softens and begins to enlarge (dilate) during the early part of labor to make room for the baby to pass through. The cervix will continue to dilate, and the contractions will eventually push the baby out of the mother's body. When labor needs to be induced, the cervix is often small, hard, and not ready for the process. The doctor may need to prepare or "ripened" the cervix to induce labor. The hormone prostaglandin in a gel form may be applied high in the vagina to soften and dilate the cervix, making the area ready for labor. This may be enough to stimulate contractions on its own. More often, prostaglandin gel is used in conjunction with Pitrocin.

If all attempts to induce labor fail, a **cesarean section** is performed.

Risks

Once labor has been induced, the unborn baby is monitored to guard against a reduction in its oxygen supply, or hypoxia. The drugs used to induce labor cause vasoconstriction, which can decrease blood supply to the unborn baby. Throughout the process, the baby's heart rate is monitored by an electronic device placed on top of the mother's abdomen. The heart rate is one sign that the unborn baby is getting enough oxygen and remains healthy. Once the membranes are broken, prolonged labor may result in infection to either the newborn or the mother.

Normal results

Once labor is induced and the cervix has dilated, labor usually proceeds normally. When performed properly, induced labor is a safe procedure for both mother and baby.

Resources

BOOKS

Berkow, Robert, et al. *The Merck Manual of Medical Information,* Home ed. Whitehouse Station, NJ: Merck Research Laboratories, 1997.

"Induction of Labor." In *The American Medical Association Encyclopedia of Medicine.* New York: Random House, 1989.

"Induction of Labor." In *Columbia University College of Physicians and Surgeons Complete Home Medical Guide.* New York: Random House, 1985.

John T. Lohr

Infant respiratory distress syndrome *see* **Respiratory distress syndrome**

Infantile paralysis *see* **Polio**

Infarct avid imaging *see* **Technetium heart scan**

Infarction *see* **Stroke**

. . . .

Infection control

Definition

Infection control refers to policies and procedures
used to minimize the risk of spreading infections, especially in hospitals and health care facilities.

Purpose

The purpose of infection control is to reduce the
occurrence of infectious diseases. These diseases are
usually caused by bacteria or viruses and can be spread
by human to human contact, animal to human contact,
human contact with an infected surface, airborne transmission through tiny droplets of infectious agents suspended in the air, and, finally, by a common vehicle such
as food or water.

Infection control in hospitals

Infections obtained in hospitals are also called nosocomial infections. They occur in approximately 5% of all
hospital patients. This results in increased time spent in
the hospital and, in some cases, **death.** There are many
reasons nosocomial infections are common, one of which
is that many hospital patients have a weakened immune
system which makes them more susceptible to infections.
This weakened immune system can be caused either by
the patient's diseases or by treatments given to the patient. Second, many medical procedures can increase the
risk of infection by introducing infectious agents into the
patient. Thirdly, many patients are admitted to hospitals
because of infectious disease. These infectious agents can
then be transferred from patient to patient by hospital
workers or visitors.

Infection control has become a formal discipline in
the United States since the 1950s, due to the spread of
staphylococcal infections in hospitals. Because there is
both the risk of health care providers acquiring infections
themselves, and of them passing infections on to patients,
the Centers for Disease Control and Prevention have
established guidelines for infection control procedures. In
addition to hospitals, infection control is important in
nursing homes, clinics, child care centers, and restau-
rants, as well as in the home.

Threat of emerging infectious diseases

Due to constant changes in our lifestyles and envi-
ronments, there are constantly new diseases that people
are susceptible to, making protection from the threat of
infectious disease urgent. Many new contagious diseases
have been identified in the past 30 years, such as **AIDS,**
Ebola, and hantavirus. Increased travel between conti-
nents makes the worldwide spread of disease a bigger
concern than it once was. Additionally, many common
infectious diseases have become resistant to known treatments.

Problems of antibiotic resistance

Because of the overuse of **antibiotics,** many bacteria
have developed a resistance to common antibiotics. This
means that newer antibiotics must continually be developed in order to treat an infection. However, further
resistance seems to come about almost simultaneously.
This indicates to many scientists that it might become
more and more difficult to treat infectious diseases. The
use of antibiotics outside of medicine also contributes to
increased antibiotic resistance. One example of this is the
use of antibiotics in animal husbandry. These negative

SELECTED INFECTIOUS DISEASES AND CORRESPONDING TREATMENT

Disease	Symptoms	Transmittal	Treatment
Chicken pox	Rash, low-grade fever	Person to person	None
Common cold/ Influenza	Runny nose, sore throat, cough, fever, headache, muscle aches	Person to person	None
Hepatitis	Jaundice, flu-like symptoms	Sexual contact with an infected person, contaminated blood, food, or water	None
Legionnaire's Disease	Flu symptoms, pneumonia, diarrhea, vomiting, kidney failure, respiratory failure	Air conditioning or water systems	Antibiotics
Measles	Skin rash, runny nose and eyes, fever, cough	Person to person	None
Meningitis	Neck pain, headache, pain caused by exposure to light, fever, nausea, drowsiness	Person to person	Antibiotics for bacterial meningitis, hospital care for viral meningitis
Mumps	Swelling of salivary glands	Person to person	Anti-inflammatory drugs
Ringworm	Skin rash	Contact with infected animal or person	Antifungal drugs applied topically
Tetanus	Lockjaw, other spasms	Soil infection of wounds	Antibiotics, antitoxins, muscle relaxers

trends can only be reversed by establishing a more rational use of antibiotics through treatment guidelines.

Description

The goals of infection control programs are: immunizing against preventable diseases, defining precautions that can prevent exposure to infectious agents, and restricting the exposure of health care workers to an infectious agent. An infection control practitioner is a specially trained professional, oftentimes a nurse, who oversees infection control programs.

Commonly recommended precautions to avoid and control the spread of infections include:

• Vaccinate against diseases for which a vaccine is available.

• Wash hands often.

• Cook food thoroughly.

• Use antibiotics only as directed.

• See a doctor for infections that do not heal.

• Avoid areas with a lot of insects.

• Be cautious around unfamiliar animals.

• Do not engage in unprotected sex or in intravenous drug use.

• Inquire about infectious diseases when you travel.

Because of the higher risk of spreading infectious disease in a hospital setting, higher levels of precautions are taken there. Typically, health care workers wear gloves with all patients, since it is difficult to know whether a transmittable disease is present or not. Patients who have a known transmittable infectious disease are isolated to decrease the risk of transmitting the infectious agent to another person. Hospital workers who come in contact with infected patients must wear gloves and gowns to decrease the risk of carrying the infectious agent to other patients. All articles of equipment that are used in an **isolation** room are decontaminated before reuse. Patients who are immunocompromised may be put in protective isolation to decrease the risk of infectious agents being brought into their room. Any hospital worker with infections, including colds, are restricted from that room.

Hospital infections can also be transmitted through the air. Thus care must be taken when handling infected materials so as to decrease the numbers of infectious agents that become airborne. Special care should also taken with hospital ventilation systems to prevent recirculation of contaminated air.

Resources

BOOKS

Edmond, Michael B., and Richard P. Wenzel. ''Infection Control.'' In *Principles and Practice of Infectious Diseases,* edited by G.L. Mandell, J. E. Bennett, and R. Dolin. New York: Churchill Livingston, 1995.

PERIODICALS

''Plagued by Cures.'' *Economist* 344 (Nov. 22, 1997): 95-97.

Williams, Rosamund J., and David L. Heymann. ''Containment of Antibiotic Resistance.'' *Science* 279 (Feb. 20, 1998): 1153-1154.

Winik, Lyric W. ''Before The Next Epidemic Strikes.'' *Parade Magazine* (Feb. 8, 1998): 6-7.

ORGANIZATIONS

National Center for Infectious Disease, Centers for Disease Control and Prevention. 1600 Clifton Rd. NE, Atlanta, GA 30333. http://www.cdc.gov and http://www.cdc.gov/ncidod/ncid.htm.

Cindy L. Jones

Infectious arthritis

Definition

Infectious arthritis, which is sometimes called septic arthritis or pyogenic arthritis, is a serious infection of the joints characterized by pain, fever, occasional chills, inflammation and swelling in one or more joints, and loss of function in the affected joints. It is considered a medical emergency.

KEY TERMS

Arthrocentesis—A procedure in which the doctor inserts a needle into the patient's joint to withdraw fluid for diagnostic testing or to drain infected fluid from the joint.

Pyogenic arthritis—Another name for infectious arthritis. Pyogenic means that pus is formed during the disease process.

Sepsis—Invasion of the body by disease organisms or their toxins. Generalized sepsis can lead to shock and eventual death.

Septic arthritis—Another name for infectious arthritis.

Synovial fluid (SF)—A fluid secreted by tissues surrounding the joints that lubricates the joints.

Description

Infectious arthritis can occur in any age group, including newborns and children. In adults, it usually affects the wrists or one of the patient's weight-bearing joints—most often the knee—although about 20% of adult patients have symptoms in more than one joint. Multiple joint infection is common in children and typically involves the shoulders, knees, and hips.

Some groups of patients are at greater risk for developing infectious arthritis. These high-risk groups include:

- Patients with chronic **rheumatoid arthritis.**
- Patients with certain systemic infections, including **gonorrhea** and HIV infection. Women and male homosexuals are at greater risk for gonorrheal arthritis than are male heterosexuals.
- Patients with certain types of **cancer.**
- IV drug abusers and alcoholics.
- Patients with artificial (prosthetic) joints.
- Patients with diabetes, **sickle cell anemia,** or **systemic lupus erythematosus** (SLE).
- Patients with recent joint injuries or surgery, or patients receiving medications injected directly into a joint.

Causes & symptoms

In general, infectious arthritis is caused by the spread of a bacterial, viral, or fungal infection through the bloodstream to the joint. The disease agents may enter the joint directly from the outside as a result of an injury or a surgical procedure, or they may be carried to the joint by the blood from infections elsewhere in the body. The specific organisms vary somewhat according to age group. Newborns are most likely to acquire gonococcal infections of the joints from a mother with gonorrhea. Children may also acquire infectious arthritis from a hospital environment, often as a result of catheter placement. The organisms involved are usually either *Haemophilus influenzae* (in children under two years of age) or *Staphylococcus aureus*. In older children or adults, the infectious organisms include *Streptococcus pyogenes* and *Streptococcus viridans* as well as *Staphylococcus aureus*. *Staphylococcus epidermidis* is usually involved in joint infections related to surgery. Sexually active teenagers and adults frequently develop infectious arthritis from *Neisseria gonorrhoeae* infections. Older adults are often vulnerable to joint infections caused by gram-negative bacilli, including *Salmonella* and *Pseudomonas.*

Infectious arthritis often has a sudden onset, but symptoms sometimes develop over a period of three to 14 days. The symptoms include swelling in the infected joint and pain when the joint is moved. Infectious arthritis in the hip may be experienced as pain in the groin area that becomes much worse if the patient tries to walk. In 90% of cases, there is some leakage of tissue fluid into the affected joint. The joint is sore to the touch; it may or may not be warm to the touch, depending on how deep the infection lies within the joint. In most cases the patient will have fever and chills, although the fever may be only low-grade. Children sometimes develop **nausea and vomiting.**

Septic arthritis is considered a medical emergency because of the damage it causes to bone as well as cartilage, and its potential for creating **septic shock,** which is a potentially fatal condition. *Staphylococcus aureus* is capable of destroying cartilage in one or two days. Destruction of cartilage and bone in turn leads to dislocations of the joints and bones. If the infection is caused by bacteria, it can spread to the blood and surrounding tissues, causing **abscesses** or even blood poisoning. The most common complication of infectious arthritis is **osteoarthritis.**

Diagnosis

The diagnosis of infectious arthritis depends on a combination of laboratory testing with careful history-taking and **physical examination** of the affected joint. It is important to keep in mind that infectious arthritis can coexist with other forms of arthritis, **gout, rheumatic fever, Lyme disease,** or other disorders that can cause a combination of joint pain and fever. In some cases, the doctor may consult a specialist in orthopedics or rheumatology to avoid misdiagnosis.

Patient history

The patient's history will tell the doctor whether he or she belongs to a high-risk group for infectious arthritis. Sudden onset of joint pain is also important information.

Physical examination

The doctor will examine the affected joint for swelling, soreness, warmth, and other signs of infection. Location is sometimes a clue to diagnosis; infection of an unusual joint, such as the joints between the breastbone and collarbone, or the pelvic joints, often occurs in drug abusers.

Laboratory tests

Laboratory testing is necessary to confirm the diagnosis of infectious arthritis. The doctor will perform an arthrocentesis, which is a procedure that involves withdrawing a sample of synovial fluid (SF) from the joint with a needle and syringe. SF is a lubricating fluid secreted by tissues surrounding the joints. Patients should be warned that arthrocentesis is a painful procedure. The fluid sample is sent for culture in the sealed syringe. SF from infected joints is usually streaked with pus or looks cloudy and watery. Cell counts usually indicate a high level of white cells; a level higher than 100,000 cells/mm3 or a neutrophil proportion greater than 90% suggests septic arthritis. A Gram's stain of the culture obtained from the SF is usually positive for the specific disease organism.

Doctors sometimes order a biopsy of the synovial tissue near the joint if the fluid sample is negative. Cultures of other body fluids, such as urine, blood, or cervical mucus, may be taken in addition to the SF culture.

Diagnostic imaging

Diagnostic imaging is not helpful in the early stages of infectious arthritis. Destruction of bone or cartilage does not appear on x rays until 10-14 days after the onset of symptoms. Imaging studies are sometimes useful if the infection is in a deep-seated joint.

Treatment

Infectious arthritis requires usually requires several days of treatment in a hospital, with follow-up medication and physical therapy lasting several weeks or months.

Medications

Because of the possibility of serious damage to the joint or other complications if treatment is delayed, the patient will be started on intravenous **antibiotics** before the specific organism is identified. After the disease organism has been identified, the doctor may give the patient a drug that targets the specific bacterium or virus. Nonsteroidal anti-inflammatory drugs are usually given for viral infections.

Intravenous antibiotics are given for about two weeks, or until the inflammation has disappeared. The patient may then be given a two- to four-week course of oral antibiotics.

Surgery

In some cases, surgery is necessary to drain fluid from the infected joint. Patients who need surgical drainage include those who have not responded to antibiotic treatment, those with infections of the hip or other joints that are difficult to reach with arthrocentesis, and those with joint infections related to gunshot or other penetrating **wounds.**

Patients with severe damage to bone or cartilage may need **reconstructive surgery,** but it cannot be performed until the infection is completely gone.

Monitoring and supportive treatment

Infectious arthritis requires careful monitoring while the patient is in the hospital. The doctor will drain the joint on a daily basis and remove a small sample of fluid for culture to check the patient's response to the antibiotic.

Infectious arthritis often causes intense pain. Patients are given medications to relieve pain, together with hot compresses or ice packs on the affected joint. In some cases the patient's arm or leg is put in a splint to protect the sore joint from accidental movement. Recovery can be speeded up, however, if the patient practices range-of-motion exercises to the extent that the pain allows.

Prognosis

The prognosis depends on prompt treatment with antibiotics and drainage of the infected joint. About 70% of patients will recover without permanent joint damage. However, many patients will develop osteoarthritis or deformed joints. Children with infected hip joints sometimes suffer damage to the growth plate. If treatment is delayed, infectious arthritis has a mortality rate between 5% and 30% due to septic shock and **respiratory failure.**

Prevention

Some cases of infectious arthritis are preventable by lifestyle choices. These include avoidance of self-injected drugs; sexual abstinence or monogamous relationships; and prompt testing and treatment for suspected cases of gonorrhea. Patients receiving corticosteroid injections into the joints for osteoarthritis may want to

weigh this treatment method against the increased risk of infectious arthritis.

Resources

BOOKS

"Bedside Procedures: Joint Aspiration (Arthrocentesis)." In *Surgery On Call,* edited by Leonard G. Gomella, and Alan T. Lefor. Stamford, CT: Appleton & Lange, 1996.

Bradford, David S., et al. "Orthopedics." In *Current Surgical Diagnosis & Treatment,* edited by Lawrence W. Way. Stamford, CT: Appleton & Lange, 1994.

Eilert, Robert E. "Bones & Joints." In *Handbook of Pediatrics,* edited by Gerald B. Merenstein, et al. Norwalk, CT: Appleton & Lange, 1994.

Gilliland, Bruce C., and Robert G. Petersdorf. "Infectious Arthritis." In *Harrison's Principles of Internal Medicine,* edited by Eugene Braunwald, et al. New York: McGraw-Hill Book Company, 1987.

Hellman, David B., "Arthritis & Musculoskeletal Disorders." In *Current Medical Diagnosis & Treatment 1998,* edited by Lawrence M. Tierney, Jr., et al. Stamford, CT: Appleton & Lange, 1998.

"Musculoskeletal and Connective Tissue Disorders: Infectious Arthritis." In *The Merck Manual of Diagnosis and Therapy*, edited by Robert Berkow, et al. Rahway, NJ: Merck Research Laboratories, 1992.

Nanagara, Ratanavadee, et al. "Septic Arthritis." In *Current Diagnosis 9,* edited by Rex B. Conn, et al. Philadelphia: W. B. Saunders Company, 1997.

"On-Call Problems: Joint Swelling." In *Internal Medicine On Call,* edited by Steven A. Haist, et al. Stamford, CT: Appleton & Lange, 1991.

"Septic Arthritis." In *Professional Guide to Diseases,* edited by Stanley Loeb, et al. Springhouse, PA: Springhouse Corporation, 1991.

Theodosakis, Jason, et al. *The Arthritis Cure.* New York: St. Martin's Paperbacks, 1997.

Rebecca J. Frey

Infectious hepatitis *see* **Hepatitis A**

. . . .

Infectious mononucleosis

Definition

Infectious mononucleosis is a contagious illness caused by the Epstein-Barr virus that can affect the liver, lymph nodes, and oral cavity. While mononucleosis is not usually a serious disease, its primary symptoms of fatigue and lack of energy can linger for several months.

KEY TERMS

Antibody—A specific protein produced by the immune system in response to a specific foreign protein or particle called an antigen.

Herpes viruses—A group of viruses that can cause cold sores, shingles, chicken pox, and congenital abnormalities. The Epstein-Barr virus which causes mononucleosis belongs to this group of viruses.

Reye's syndrome—A very serious, rare disease, most common in children, which involves an upper respiratory tract infection followed by brain and liver damage.

Description

Infectious mononucleosis, frequently called "mono" or the "kissing disease," is caused by the Epstein-Barr virus (EBV) found in saliva and mucus. The virus affects a type of white blood cell called the B lymphocyte producing characteristic atypical lymphocytes that may be useful in the diagnosis of the disease.

While anyone, even young children, can develop mononucleosis, it occurs most often in young adults between the ages of 15 and 35 and is especially common in teenagers. The mononucleosis infection rate among college students who have not previously been exposed to EBV has been estimated to be about 15%. In younger children, the illness may not be recognized.

The disease typically runs its course in four to six weeks in people with normally functioning immune systems. People with weakened or suppressed immune systems, such as **AIDS** patients or those who have had organ transplants, are particularly vulnerable to the potentially serious complications of infectious mononucleosis.

Causes and symptoms

The EBV that causes mononucleosis is related to a group of herpes viruses, including those that cause **cold sores**, chicken pox, and **shingles.** Most people are exposed to EBV at some point during their lives. Mononucleosis is most commonly spread by contact with virus-infected saliva through coughing, sneezing, kissing, or sharing drinking glasses or eating utensils.

In addition to general weakness and fatigue, symptoms of mononucleosis may include any or all of the following:

- **Sore throat** and/or swollen tonsils
- **Fever** and chills
- **Nausea and vomiting,** or decreased appetite

- Swollen lymph nodes in the neck and armpits
- **Headaches** or joint **pain**
- Enlarged spleen
- **Jaundice**
- Skin rash.

Complications that can occur with mononucleosis include a temporarily enlarged spleen or inflamed liver. In rare instances, the spleen may rupture, producing sharp pain on the left side of the abdomen, a symptom that warrants immediate medical attention. Additional symptoms of a ruptured spleen include light headedness, rapidly beating heart, and difficulty breathing. Other rare, but potentially life-threatening, complications may involve the heart or brain. The infection may also cause significant destruction of the body's red blood cells or platelets.

Symptoms do not usually appear until four to seven weeks after exposure to EBV. An infected person can be contagious during this incubation time period and for as many as five months after the disappearance of symptoms. Also, the virus will be excreted in the saliva intermittently for the rest of their lives, although the individual will experience no symptoms. Contrary to popular belief, the EBV is not highly contagious. As a result, individuals living in a household or college dormitory with someone who has mononucleosis have a very small risk of being infected unless they have direct contact with the person's saliva.

Diagnosis

If symptoms associated with a cold persist longer than two weeks, mononucleosis is a possibility; however, a variety of other conditions can produce similar symptoms. If mononucleosis is suspected, a physician will typically conduct a **physical examination,** including a "Monospot" antibody blood test that can indicate the presence of proteins or antibodies produced in response to infection with the EBV. These antibodies may not be detectable, however, until the second or third weeks of the illness. Occasionally, when this test is inconclusive, other blood tests may be conducted.

Treatment

The most effective treatment for infectious mononucleosis is rest and a gradual return to regular activities. Individuals with mild cases may not require bed rest but should limit their activities. Any strenuous activity, athletic endeavors, or heavy lifting should be avoided until the symptoms completely subside, since excessive activity may cause the spleen to rupture.

The sore throat and **dehydration** that usually accompany mononucleosis may be relieved by drinking water and fruit juices. Gargling salt water or taking throat lozenges may also relieve discomfort. In addition, taking over-the-counter medications, such as **acetaminophen** or ibuprofen, may relieve symptoms, but **aspirin** should be avoided because mononucleosis has been associated with **Reye's syndrome,** a serious illness aggravated by aspirin.

While **antibiotics** do not affect EBV, the sore throat accompanying mononucleosis can be complicated by a streptococcal infection, which can be treated with antibiotics. Cortisone anti-inflammatory medications are also occasionally prescribed for the treatment of severely swollen tonsils or throat tissues.

Prognosis

While the severity and length of illness varies, most people diagnosed with mononucleosis will be able to return to their normal daily routines within two to three weeks, particularly if they rest during this time period. It may take two to three months before a person's usual energy levels return. One of the most common problems in treating mononucleosis, particularly in teenagers, is that people return to their usual activities too quickly and then experience a relapse of symptoms. Once the disease has completely run its course, the person cannot be re-infected.

Prevention

Although there is no way to avoid becoming infected with EBV, paying general attention to good hygiene and avoiding sharing beverage glasses or having close contact with people who have mononucleosis or cold symptoms can help prevent infection.

Resources

BOOKS

The Merck Manual, 16th edition. Whitehouse Station, NJ: Merck & Co., 1992.

PERIODICALS

Baily, Eugene R. "Diagnosis and Treatment of Infectious Mononucleosis." *American Family Physician* (March 1994): 879-887.

ORGANIZATIONS

National Institute of Allergy and Infectious Diseases, National Institutes of Health Bethesda, MD 20892.

OTHER

Mayo Health Oasis. "Mononucleosis: A Tiresome Disease." http://www.mayo.ivi.com/mayo/9701/htm/mono.htm.

New York State Department of Health, Communicable Disease Fact Sheet. http://www.nyhealth@health.state.ny.us. Revised December 1996.

Susan J. Montgomery

. . . .

Infertility

Definition

Infertility is the failure of a couple to conceive a **pregnancy** after trying to do so for at least one full year. In primary infertility, pregnancy has never occurred. In secondary infertility, one or both members of the couple have previously conceived, but are unable to conceive again after a full year of trying.

Description

Currently, in the United States, about 20% of couples struggle with infertility at any given time. Infertility has increased as a problem over the last 30 years. Some studies pin the blame for this increase on social phenomena, including the tendency for marriage to occur at a later age, which means that couples are trying to start families at a later age. It is well known that fertility in women decreases with increasing age, as illustrated by the following statistics:

- Infertility in married women ages 16-20 = 4.5%

- Infertility in married women ages 35-40 = 31.8%

- Infertility in married women over the age of 40 = 70%.

Nowadays, individuals often have multiple sexual partners before they marry and try to have children. This increase in numbers of sexual partners has led to an increase in **sexually transmitted diseases.** Scarring from these infections, especially from **pelvic inflammatory disease** (a serious infection of the female reproductive organs, most commonly caused by **gonorrhea**) seems to be in part responsible for the increase in infertility noted. Furthermore, use of some forms of the contraceptive called the intrauterine device (**IUD**) contributed to an increased rate of pelvic inflammatory disease, with subsequent scarring. However, newer IUDs do not lead to this increased rate of infection.

To understand issues of infertility, it is first necessary to understand the basics of human reproduction. Fertilization occurs when a sperm from the male merges with an egg (ovum) from the female, creating a zygote that contains genetic material (DNA) from both the father and the mother. If pregnancy is then established, the

KEY TERMS

Blastocyst—A cluster of cells representing multiple cell divisions that have occurred in the fallopian tube after successful fertilization of an ovum by a sperm. This is the developmental form which must leave the fallopian tube, enter the uterus, and implant itself in the uterus to achieve actual pregnancy.

Cervix—The opening from the vagina, which leads into the uterus.

Embryo—The stage of development of a baby between the second and eighth weeks after conception.

Endometrium—The lining of the uterus.

Fallopian tube—The tube leading from the ovary into the uterus. Just as there are two ovaries, there are two Fallopian tubes.

Fetus—A baby developing in the uterus from the third month to birth.

Ovary—The female organ in which eggs (ova) are stored and mature.

Ovum (plural: ova)—The reproductive cell of the female, which contains genetic information and participates in the act of fertilization. Also popularly called the egg.

Semen—The fluid that contains sperm, which is ejaculated by the male.

Sperm—The reproductive cell of the male, which contains genetic information and participates in the act of fertilization of an ovum.

Spermatogenesis—The process by which sperm develop to become mature sperm, capable of fertilizing an ovum.

Zygote—The result of the sperm successfully fertilizing the ovum. The zygote is a single cell that contains the genetic material of both the mother and the father.

zygote will develop into an embryo, then a fetus, and ultimately a baby will be born.

The male contribution to fertilization and the establishment of pregnancy is the sperm. Sperm are small cells which carry the father's genetic material. This genetic material is contained within the oval head of the sperm. The sperm are mixed into a fluid called semen, which is discharged from the penis during sexual intercourse. The whip-like tail of the sperm allows the sperm to swim up the female reproductive tract, in search of the egg it will try to fertilize.

The female makes many contributions to fertilization and the establishment of pregnancy. The ovum is the cell that carries the mother's genetic material. These ova develop within the ovaries. Once a month, a single mature ovum is produced, and leaves the ovary in a process called ovulation. This ovum enters a tube leading to the uterus (the fallopian tube). The ovum needs to meet up with the sperm in the fallopian tube if fertilization is to occur.

When fertilization occurs, the resulting cell (which now contains genetic material from both the mother and the father) is called the zygote. This single cell will divide into multiple other cells within the fallopian tube, and the resulting cluster of cells (called a blastocyst) will then move into the womb (uterus). The uterine lining (endometrium) has been preparing itself to receive a pregnancy by growing thicker. If the blastocyst successfully reaches the inside of the uterus and attaches itself to the wall of the uterus, then implantation and pregnancy have been achieved.

Causes & symptoms

Unlike most medical problems, infertility is an issue requiring the careful evaluation of two separate individuals, as well as an evaluation of their interactions with each other. In about 3-4% of couples, no cause for their infertility will be discovered. About 40% of the time, the root of the couple's infertility is due to a problem with the male partner; about 40% of the time, the root of the infertility is due to the female partner; and about 20% of the time, there are fertility problems with both the man and the woman.

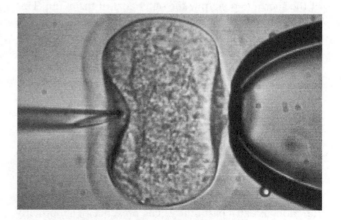

A microscopic image of a needle (left) injecting sperm cells directly into a human egg (center). The broad object at right is a pipette used to hold the ovum steady. (Phototake NYC. Reproduced by permission.)

The main factors involved in causing infertility, listing from the most to the least common, include:

• Male problems: 35%

• Ovulation problems: 20%

• Tubal problems: 20%

• Endometriosis: 10%

• Cervical factors: 5%.

Male factors

Male infertility can be caused by a number of different characteristics of the sperm. To check for these characteristics, a sample of semen is obtained and examined under the microscope (**semen analysis**). Four basic characteristics are usually evaluated:

• Sperm count refers to the number of sperm present in a semen sample. The normal number of sperm present in just one milliliter (ml) of semen is over 20 million. An individual with only 5-20 million sperm per ml of semen is considered subfertile, an individual with less than 5 million sperm per ml of semen is considered infertile.

• Sperm are also examined to see how well they swim (sperm motility) and to be sure that most have normal structure.

• Not all sperm within a specimen of semen will be perfectly normal. Some may be immature, and some may have abnormalities of the head or tail. A normal semen sample will contain no more than 25% abnormal forms of sperm.

• Volume of the semen sample is important. An abnormal amount of semen could affect the ability of the sperm to successfully fertilize an ovum.

Another test can be performed to evaluate the ability of the sperm to penetrate the outer coat of the ovum. This is done by observing whether sperm in a semen sample can penetrate the outer coat of a guinea pig ovum; fertilization cannot occur, of course, but this test is useful in predicting the ability of the individual's sperm to penetrate a human ovum.

Any number of conditions result in abnormal findings in the semen analysis. Men can be born with testicles that have not descended properly from the abdominal cavity (where testicles develop originally) into the scrotal sac, or may be born with only one instead of the normal two testicles. Testicle size can be smaller than normal. Past infection (including **mumps**) can affect testicular function, as can a past injury. The presence of abnormally large veins (varicocele) in the testicles can increase testicular temperature, which decreases sperm count. History of having been exposed to various toxins, drug use, excess alcohol use, use of anabolic steroids, certain medi-

cations, diabetes, thyroid problems, or other endocrine disturbances can have direct effects on the formation of sperm (spermatogenesis). Problems with the male anatomy can cause sperm to be ejaculated not out of the penis, but into the bladder, and scarring from past infections can interfere with ejaculation.

Treatment of male infertility includes addressing known reversible factors first; for example, discontinuing any medication known to have an effect on spermatogenesis or ejaculation, as well as decreasing alcohol intake, and treating thyroid or other endocrine disease. Varicoceles can be treated surgically. Testosterone in low doses can improve sperm motility.

Other treatments of male infertility include collecting semen samples from multiple ejaculations, after which the semen is put through a process that allows the most motile sperm to be sorted out. These motile sperm are pooled together to create a concentrate that can deposited into the female partner's uterus at a time that coincides with ovulation. In cases where the male partner's sperm is proven to be absolutely unable to cause pregnancy in the female partner, and with the consent of both partners, donor sperm may be used for this process. Depositing the male partner's sperm or donor sperm by mechanical means into the female partner are both forms of artificial insemination.

Ovulatory problems

The first step in diagnosing ovulatory problems is to make sure that an ovum is being produced each month. A woman's morning body temperature is slightly higher around the time of ovulation. A woman can measure and record her temperatures daily and a chart can be drawn to show whether or not ovulation has occurred. Luteinizing hormone (LH) is released just before ovulation. A simple urine test can be done to check if LH has been released around the time that ovulation is expected.

Treatment of ovulatory problems depends on the cause. If a thyroid or pituitary problem is responsible, simply treating that problem can restore fertility. (The thyroid and pituitary glands release hormones that also are involved in regulating a woman's menstrual cycle.) Medication can also be used to stimulate fertility. The most commonly used of these are called Clomid and Pergonal. These drugs increase the risk of multiple births (twins, triplets, etc.).

Pelvic adhesions & endometriosis

Pelvic adhesions and endometriosis can cause infertility by preventing the sperm from reaching the egg or interfering with fertilization.

Pelvic adhesions are fibrous scars. These scars can be the result of past infections, such as pelvic inflammatory disease, or infections following abortions or prior births. Previous surgeries can also leave behind scarring.

Endometriosis may lead to pelvic adhesions. Endometriosis is the abnormal location of uterine tissue outside of the uterus. When uterine tissue is planted elsewhere in the pelvis, it still bleeds on a monthly basis with the start of the normal menstrual period. This leads to irritation within the pelvis around the site of this abnormal tissue and bleeding, and may cause scarring.

Pelvic adhesions cause infertility by blocking the fallopian tubes. The ovum may be prevented from traveling down the fallopian tube from the ovary or the sperm may be prevented from traveling up the fallopian tube from the uterus.

A hysterosalpingogram (HSG) can show if the fallopian tubes are blocked. This is an x-ray exam that tests whether dye material can travel through the patient's fallopian tubes. A few women become pregnant following this x-ray exam. It is thought that the dye material in some way helps flush out the tubes, decreasing any existing obstruction. Scarring also can be diagnosed by examining the pelvic area through the use of a scope that can be inserted into the abdomen through a tiny incision made near the naval. This scoping technique is called **laparoscopy.**

Pelvic adhesions can be treated during laparoscopy. The adhesions are cut using special instruments. Endometriosis can be treated with certain medications, but may also require surgery to repair any obstruction caused by adhesions.

Cervical factors

The cervix is the opening from the vagina into the uterus through which the sperm must pass. Mucus produced by the cervix helps to transport the sperm into the uterus. Injury to the cervix or scarring of the cervix after surgery or infection can result in a smaller than normal cervical opening, making it difficult for the sperm to enter. Injury or infection can also decrease the number of glands in the cervix, leading to a smaller amount of cervical mucus. In other situations, the mucus produced is the wrong consistency (perhaps too thick) to allow sperm to travel through. In addition, some women produce antibodies (immune cells) that are specifically directed to identify sperm as foreign invaders and to kill them.

Cervical mucus can be examined under a microscope to diagnose whether cervical factors are contributing to infertility. The interaction of a live sperm sample from the male partner and a sample of cervical mucus from the female partner can also be examined. This procedure is called a post-coital test.

Treatment of cervical factors includes **antibiotics** in the case of an infection, steroids to decrease production of anti-sperm antibodies, and artificial insemination techniques to completely bypass the cervical mucus.

Treatment

Assisted reproductive techniques include **in vitro fertilization** (IVF), gamete intrafallopian transfer (GIFT), and zygote intrafallopian tube transfer (ZIFT). These are usually used after other techniques to treat infertility have failed.

In vitro fertilization involves the use of a drug to induce the simultaneous release of many eggs from the female's ovaries, which are retrieved surgically. Meanwhile, several semen samples are obtained from the male partner, and a sperm concentrate is prepared. The ova and sperm are then combined in a laboratory, where several of the ova may be fertilized. Cell division is allowed to take place up to the embryo stage. While this takes place, the female may be given drugs to ensure that her uterus is ready to receive an embryo. Three or four of the embryos are transferred to the female's uterus, and the wait begins to see if any or all of them implant and result in an actual pregnancy.

Success rates of IVF are still rather low. Most centers report pregnancy rates between 10-20%. Since most IVF procedures put more than one embryo into the uterus, the chance for a multiple birth (twins or more) is greatly increased in couples undergoing IVF.

GIFT involves retrieval of both multiple ova and semen, and the mechanical placement of both within the female partner's fallopian tubes, where one hopes that fertilization will occur. ZIFT involves the same retrieval of ova and semen, and fertilization and growth in the laboratory up to the zygote stage, at which point the zygotes are placed in the fallopian tubes. Both GIFT and ZIFT seem to have higher success rates than IVF.

Prognosis

It is very hard to obtain statistics regarding the prognosis of infertility because many different problems may exist within and individual or couple trying to conceive. In general, it is believed that of all couples who undergo a complete evaluation of infertility followed by treatment, about half will ultimately have a successful pregnancy. Of those couples who do not choose to undergo evaluation or treatment, about 5% will go on to conceive after a year or more of infertility.

Resources

BOOKS

Hornstein, Mark D., and Daniel Schust. ''Infertility.'' In *Novak's Gynecology,* edited by Jonathan S. Berek. Baltimore: Williams and Wilkins, 1996.

Martin, Mary C. "Infertility" In *Current Obstetric and Gynecologic Diagnosis and Treatment,* edited by Alan H. Cecherney and Martin L. Pernoll. Norwalk, CT: 1994.

PERIODICALS

Intrator, Nancy. "What To Do If You Can't Get Pregnant." *Cosmopolitan* (December 1995): 154+.

Mastroianni, Luigi, et al. "Helping Infertile Patients." *Patient Care* (October 15, 1997): 103+.

Rosenbaum, Joshua. "Beat the Clock: Treatments for Infertility." *American Health* (December 1995): 70+.

Trantham, Patricia. "The Infertile Couple." *American Family Physician* (September 1, 1996): 1001+.

ORGANIZATIONS

American Society for Reproductive Medicine. 1209 Montgomery Highway, Birmingham, AL 35216-2809. (205)978-5000. http://www.asrm.com.

International Center for Infertility Information Dissemination. http://www.inciid.org.

Rosalyn S. Carson-DeWitt

Infertility drugs

Definition

Infertility drugs are medicines that help bring about **pregnancy.**

Purpose

Infertility is the inability of a man and woman to achieve pregnancy after at least a year of having regular sexual intercourse without any type of birth control. There are many possible reasons for infertility, and finding the most effective treatment for a couple may involve many tests to find the problem. For pregnancy to occur, the woman's reproductive system must release eggs regularly—a process called ovulation. The man must produce healthy sperm that are able to reach and unite with an egg. And once an egg is fertilized, it must travel to the woman's uterus (womb), become implanted and remain there to be nourished.

If a couple is infertile because the woman is not ovulating, infertility drugs may be prescribed to stimulate ovulation. The first step usually is to try a drug such as clomiphene. If that doesn't work, human chorionic gonadotropin (HCG) may be tried, usually in combination with other infertility drugs.

Clompiphene and HCG may also be used to treat other conditions in both males and females.

Description

Clomiphene (Clomid, Serophene) comes in tablet form and is available only with a physician's prescription. Human chorionic gonadotropin is given as an injection, only under a physician's supervision.

Recommended dosage

The dosage may be different for different patients. Check with the physician who prescribed the drug or the pharmacist who filled the prescription for the correct dosage.

Clomiphene must be taken at certain times during the menstrual cycle. Be sure to follow directions exactly.

Precautions

Seeing a physician regularly while taking infertility drugs is important.

Treatment with infertility drugs increases the chance of multiple births. Although this may seem like a good thing to couples who want children very badly, multiple fetuses can cause problems during pregnancy and delivery and can even threaten the babies' survival.

Having intercourse at the proper time in the woman's menstrual cycle helps increase the chance of pregnancy. The physician may recommend using an ovulation prediction test kit to help determine the best times for intercourse.

Some people feel dizzy or lightheaded, or less alert when using clomiphene. The medicine may also cause blurred vision and other vision changes. Anyone who takes clomiphene should not drive, use machines or do anything else that might be dangerous until they have found out how the drugs affect them.

Questions remain about the safety of long-term treatment with clomiphene. Women should not have more than 6 courses of treatment with this drug and should ask their physicians for the most up-to-date information about its use.

Special conditions

People who have certain medical conditions or who are taking certain other medicines may have problems if they take infertility drugs. Before taking these drugs, be sure to let the physician know about any of these conditions:

ALLERGIES

Anyone who has had unusual reactions to infertility drugs in the past should let his or her physician know before taking the drugs again. The physician should also be told about any **allergies** to foods, dyes, preservatives, or other substances.

PREGNANCY

Clomiphene may cause **birth defects** if taken during pregnancy. Women who think they have become pregnant while taking clomiphene should stop taking the medicine immediately and check with their physicians.

OTHER MEDICAL CONDITIONS

Infertility drugs may make some medical conditions worse. Before using infertility drugs, people with any of these medical problems should make sure their physicians are aware of their conditions:

• Endometriosis

• Fibroid tumors of the uterus

• Unusual vaginal bleeding

• Ovarian cyst

• Enlarged ovaries

• Inflamed veins caused by blood clots

• Liver disease, now or in the past

• Depression.

USE OF CERTAIN MEDICINES

Taking infertility drugs with certain other medicines may affect the way the drugs work or may increase the chance of side effects.

Side effects

When used in low doses for a short time, clomiphene and HCG rarely cause side effects. However, anyone who has stomach or pelvic **pain** or bloating while taking either medicine should check with a physician immediately. Infertility drugs may also cause less serious symptoms such as hot flashes, breast tenderness or swelling, heavy menstrual periods, bleeding between menstrual periods, nausea or vomiting, **dizziness,** lightheadedness, irritability, nervousness, restlessness, **headache,** tiredness, sleep problems, or depression. These problems usually go away as the body adjusts to the drug and do not require medical treatment unless they continue or they interfere with normal activities.

Other side effects are possible. Anyone who has unusual symptoms after taking infertility drugs should get in touch with a physician.

Interactions

Infertility drugs may interact with other medicines. When this happens, the effects of one or both of the drugs may change or the risk of side effects may be greater. Anyone who takes infertility drugs should let the physician know all other medicines she is taking.

Resources

PERIODICALS

Randal, Judith. "Trying to outsmart infertility." *FDA Consumer* 25 (May 1991): 22.

Nancy Ross-Flanigan

. . . .

Infertility therapies

Definition

Infertility is the inability of a man and a woman to conceive a child through sexual intercourse. There are many possible reasons for the problem, which can involve the man, the woman, or both partners. Various treatments are available that enable a woman to become pregnant; the correct one will depend on the specific cause of the infertility.

Purpose

Infertility treatment is aimed at enabling a woman to have a baby by treating the man, the woman, or both partners. During normal conception of a child, the man's sperm will travel to the woman's fallopian tubes, where, if conditions are right, it will encounter an egg that has been released from the ovary. The sperm will fertilize the egg, which will enter the uterus where it implants and begins to divide, forming what's called an embryo. The embryo will develop during **pregnancy** into a baby.

Infertility treatment attempts to correct or compensate for any abnormalities in this process that prevent the fertilization of an egg or development of an embryo.

Precautions

It's important for a couple contemplating infertility treatment to examine their own ideas and feelings about the process and consider ethical objections before the woman becomes pregnant from such treatment.

Description

About 90% of women who are trying to get pregnant and use no birth control will do so within one year. If, after one year of having frequent sexual intercourse with no **contraception** a couple has not conceived, they should seek the advice of a physician. Tests can be performed to look for possible infertility problems.

Treating an underlying infection or illness is the first step in infertility treatment. The physician may also suggest improving general health, dietary changes, reducing **stress,** and counseling.

Treatments

Low sperm count treatments

The most common cause of male infertility is failure to produce enough healthy sperm. For fertilization to happen, the number of sperm cells in the man's semen (the fluid ejected during sexual intercourse) must be sufficient, and the sperm cells must have the right shape, appearance, and activity (motility).

Defects in the sperm can be caused by an infection resulting from a **sexually transmitted disease,** a blockage caused by a **varicose vein** in the scrotum (varicocele), an endocrine imbalance, or problems with other male reproductive organs (such as the testicles, prostate gland, or seminal vesicles).

If a low sperm count is the problem, it's possible to restore fertility by:

• Treating underlying infections.

• Timing sex to coincide with the time the woman is ovulating, which means that the egg is released from the ovary and is beginning to travel down the fallopian tube (the site of fertilization).

• Having sex less often to build up the number of sperm in the semen.

• Treating any endocrine imbalance with drugs.

• Having a surgical procedure to remove a varicocele (varicocelectomy).

Fertility drugs

If infertility is due to a woman's failure to release eggs from the ovary (ovulate), fertility drugs can help bring hormone levels into balance, stimulating the ovaries and triggering egg production.

Surgical repair

In some women, infertility is due to blocked fallopian tubes. The egg is released from the ovary, but the sperm is prevented from reaching it because of a physical obstruction in the fallopian tube. If this is the case, surgery may help repair the damage. Microsurgery can sometimes repair the damage to scarred fallopian tubes if it is not too severe. Not all tube damage can be repaired, however, and most tubal problems are more successfully treated with **in vitro fertilization.**

Fibroid tumors in the uterus also may cause infertility, and they can be surgically treated. **Endometriosis,** a condition in which parts of the lining of the uterus become imbedded on other internal organs (such as the ovaries or fallopian tubes) may contribute to infertility. It may be necessary to surgically remove the endometrial tissue to improve fertility.

Artificial insemination

Artificial insemination may be tried if sperm count is low, the man is impotent, or the woman's vagina creates a hostile environment for the sperm. The procedure is not always successful. In this procedure, the semen is collected and placed into the woman's cervix with a small syringe at the time of ovulation. From the cervix, it can travel to the fallopian tube where fertilization takes place. If the partner's sperm count is low, it can be mixed with donor sperm before being transferred into the uterus.

If there is no sperm in the male partner's semen, then artificial insemination can be performed using a donor's sperm obtained from a sperm bank.

Assisted reproductive technologies

Some fertility treatments require removal of the eggs and/or sperm and manipulation of them in certain ways in a laboratory to assist fertilization. These techniques are called assisted reproductive technologies.

IN VITRO FERTILIZATION (IVF)

When infertility can't be treated by other means or when the cause is not known, it's still possible to become pregnant through in vitro fertilization (IVF), a costly, complex procedure that achieves pregnancy 20% of the time.

In this procedure, a woman's eggs are removed by withdrawing them with a special needle. Attempts are then made to fertilize the eggs with sperm from her partner or a donor. This fertilization takes place in a petri dish in a laboratory. The fertilized egg (embryo) is then returned to the woman's uterus.

Often, three to six fertilized eggs are returned at the same time into the uterus. Usually one or two of the embryos survive and grow into fetuses, but sometimes three or more fetuses result.

A child born in this method is popularly known as a "test tube baby," but in fact the child actually develops inside the mother. Only the fertilization of the egg takes place in the laboratory.

INTRACYTOPLASMIC SPERM INJECTION (ICSI)

In a variation of IVF called intracytoplasmic sperm injection (ICSI), single sperm cells are injected directly into each egg. This may be helpful for men with severe infertility.

GAMETE INTERFALLOPIAN TRANSFER (GIFT)

In this technique, sperm and eggs are placed directly into the woman's fallopian tubes to encourage fertilization to occur naturally. This procedure is done with the help of **laparoscopy.** In laparoscopy, a small tube with a viewing lens at one end is inserted into the abdomen through a small incision. The lens allows the physician to see inside the patient on a video monitor.

ZYGOTE INTRAFALLOPIAN TRANSFER (ZIFT)

If infertility is caused by a low sperm count, zygote intrafallopian transfer (ZIFT) can be tried. This technique combines GIFT and IVF. This procedure is also called a "tubal embryo transfer."

In this technique, in-vitro fertilization is first performed, so that the actual fertilization takes place and is confirmed in the laboratory. Two days later, instead of placing the embryo in the uterus, the physician performs laparoscopy to place the embryos in the fallopian tube, much like the GIFT procedure.

A woman must have at least one functioning fallopian tube in order to participate in ZIFT.

Preparation

Couples who are having fertility problems may want to limit or avoid:

- Tobacco
- Alcohol
- **Caffeine**

- Stress
- Tight-fitting undershorts (men)
- Hot tubs, saunas and steam rooms (high temperatures can kill sperm).

Risks

Women who take fertility drugs have a higher likelihood of getting pregnant with more than one child at once. There are also rare but serious side effects to fertility drugs.

Normal results

Typically, at least half of all couples who are infertile will respond to treatment with a successful pregnancy. For those who cannot become pregnant with treatment or insemination, surrogate parenting or adopting may be a workable option.

Resources

BOOKS

Berger, Gary S., et al. *The Couple's Guide to Infertility.* New York: Doubleday, 1994.

Carlson, Karen J., Stephanie A. Eisenstat, and Terra Ziporyn. *The Harvard Guide to Women's Health.* Cambridge, MA: Harvard University Press, 1996.

Cunningham, F. Gary, Paul C. Macdonald, et al. *Williams Obstetrics.* 20th ed. Stamford, CT: Appleton & Lange, 1997.

Ryan, Kenneth J., Ross S. Berkowitz, and Robert L. Barbieri. *Kistner's Gynecology.* 6th ed. St. Louis: Mosby, 1995.

ORGANIZATIONS

American Society for Reproductive Medicine. 1209 Montgomery Highway, Birmingham, AL 35216. (205) 978-5000.

RESOLVE, Inc. 1310 Broadway, Somerville, MA 02144. (617) 623-0744.

Carol A. Turkington

Influenza

Definition

Usually referred to as the flu or grippe, influenza is a highly infectious respiratory disease. The disease is caused by certain strains of the influenza virus. When the virus is inhaled, it attacks cells in the upper respiratory tract, causing typical flu symptoms such as fatigue, **fever** and chills, a hacking **cough,** and body aches. Influenza victims are also susceptible to potentially life-threatening secondary infections. Although the stomach or intestinal "flu" is commonly blamed for stomach upsets and **diarrhea,** the influenza virus rarely causes gastrointestinal symptoms. Such symptoms are most likely due to other organisms such as rotavirus, *Salmonella*, *Shigella*, or *Escherichia coli*.

Description

The flu is considerably more debilitating than the **common cold.** Influenza outbreaks occur suddenly, and infection spreads rapidly. The annual **death** toll attributable to influenza and its complications averages 20,000 in

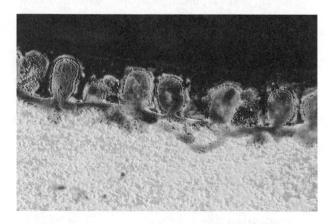

A transmission electron microscopy (TEM) image of influenza viruses budding from the surface of an infected cell. *(Photo Researchers, Inc. Reproduced by permission.)*

the United States alone. In the 1918-1919 Spanish flu pandemic, the death toll reached a staggering 20-40 million worldwide. Approximately 500,000 of these fatalities occurred in America.

Influenza outbreaks occur on a regular basis. The most serious outbreaks are pandemics, which affect millions of people worldwide and last for several months. The 1918-1919 influenza outbreak serves as the primary example of an influenza pandemic. Pandemics also occurred in 1957 and 1968 with the Asian flu and Hong Kong flu, respectively. The Asian flu was responsible for 70,000 deaths in the United States, while the Hong Kong flu killed 34,000.

Epidemics are widespread regional outbreaks that occur every two to three years and affect 5-10% of the population. The Russian flu in the winter of 1977 is an example of an epidemic. A regional epidemic is shorter lived than a pandemic, lasting only several weeks. Finally, there are smaller outbreaks each winter that are confined to specific locales.

The earliest existing descriptions of influenza were written nearly 2,500 years ago by the ancient Greek physician, Hippocrates. Historically, influenza was ascribed to a number of different agents, including "bad air" and several different bacteria. It was not until 1933 that the causative agent was identified as a virus.

There are three types of influenza viruses, identified as A, B, and C. Influenza A can infect a range of species, including humans, pigs, horses, and birds, but only humans are infected by types B and C. Influenza A is responsible for most flu cases, while infection with types B and C virus are less common and cause a milder illness.

Causes & symptoms

Approximately one to four days after infection with the influenza virus, the victim is hit with an array of symptoms. "Hit" is an appropriate term, because symptoms are sudden, harsh, and unmistakable. Typical influenza symptoms include the abrupt onset of a **headache,** dry cough, and chills, rapidly followed by overall achiness and a fever that may run as high as 104°F (40°C). As the fever subsides, nasal congestion and a **sore throat** become noticeable. Flu victims feel extremely tired and weak and may not return to their normal energy levels for several days or even a couple of weeks.

Influenza complications usually arise from bacterial infections of the lower respiratory tract. Signs of a secondary respiratory infection often appear just as the victim seems to be recovering. These signs include high fever, intense chills, chest **pains** associated with breathing, and a productive cough with thick yellowish green sputum. If these symptoms appear, medical treatment is necessary. Other secondary infections, such as sinus or ear infections, may also require medical intervention. Heart and lung problems, and other chronic diseases, can be aggravated by influenza, which is a particular concern with elderly patients.

With children and teenagers, it is advisable to be alert for symptoms of **Reye's syndrome,** a rare, but serious complication. Symptoms of Reye's syndrome are **nausea and vomiting,** and more seriously, neurological problems such as confusion or **delirium.** The syndrome has been associated with the use of **aspirin** to relieve flu symptoms.

Diagnosis

Although there are specific tests to identify the flu virus strain from respiratory samples, doctors typically rely on a set of symptoms and the presence of influenza in the community for diagnosis. Specific tests are useful to determine the type of flu in the community, but they do little for individual treatment. Doctors may administer tests, such as **throat cultures,** to identify secondary infections.

Treatment

Essentially, a bout of influenza must be allowed to run its course. Symptoms can be relieved with bed rest and by keeping well hydrated. A steam vaporizer may make breathing easier, and pain relievers will take care of the aches and pain. Food may not seem very appetizing, but an effort should be made to consume nourishing food. Recovery should not be pushed too rapidly. Returning to normal activities too quickly invites a possible relapse or complications.

Drugs

Since influenza is a viral infection, **antibiotics** are useless in treating it. However, antibiotics are frequently used to treat secondary infections.

Over-the-counter medications are used to treat flu symptoms, but it is not necessary to purchase a medication marketed specifically for flu symptoms. Any medication that is designed to relieve symptoms, such as pain and coughing, will provide some relief. Medications containing alcohol, however, should be avoided because of the dehydrating effects of alcohol. The best medicine for symptoms is simply an analgesic, such as aspirin, **acetaminophen,** or naproxen. Without a doctor's approval, aspirin is generally not recommended for people under 18 owing to its association with Reye's syndrome, a rare aspirin-associated complication seen in children recovering from the flu. To be on the safe side, children should receive acetaminophen or ibuprofen to treat their symptoms.

There are two **antiviral drugs** marketed for use in the United States. These may be useful in treating individuals who have weakened immune systems or who are at-risk for developing serious complications of influenza but may be allergic to the flu vaccine. The first is amantadine hydrochloride, which is marketed under the names Symmetrel (syrup), Symadine (capsule) and Amantadine-hydrochloride (capsule and syrup). The second antiviral is rimantadine hydrochloride, trade name Flumandine (tablet and syrup). These two drugs are chemically related and are only effective against type A influenza viruses. Both drugs can cause side effects such as nervousness, **anxiety,** lightheadedness, and nausea, with side effects more likely to occur with amantadine. Severe side effects include seizures, delirium, and hallucination, but are rare and are nearly always limited to people who have kidney problems, **seizure disorders,** or psychiatric disorders.

Alternative treatment

There are several alternative treatments that may help in fighting off the virus and recovering from the flu, in addition to easing flu symptoms.

- Acupuncture and acupressure. Both are said to stimulate natural resistance, relieve nasal congestion and headaches, fight fever, and calm coughs, depending on the acupuncture and acupressure points used.

- Aromatherapy. Aromatherapists recommend gargling daily with one drop each of the essential oils of tea tree (*Melaleuca* spp.) and lemon mixed in a glass of warm water. If already suffering from the flu, two drops of tea tree oil in a hot bath may help ease the symptoms. Essential oils of eucalyptus (*Eucalyptus globulus*) or peppermint (*Mentha piperita*) added to a steam vaporizer may help clear chest and nasal congestion.

- Herbal remedies. Herbal remedies can be used stimulate the immune system (echinacea), as antivirals (*Hydrastis canadensis*) goldenseal and garlic (*Allium sativum*), or directed at whatever symptoms arise as a result of the flu. For example, an infusion of boneset (*Eupatroium perfoliatum*) may counteract aches and fever, and yarrow (*Achillea millefolium*) or elderflower tinctures may combat chills.

- Homeopathy. To prevent flu, a homeopathic remedy called *Oscillococcinum* may be taken at the first sign of flu symptoms and repeated for a day or two. Other homeopathic remedies recommended vary according to the specific flu symptoms present. *Gelsemium* (*Gelsemium sempervirens*) is recommended to combat weakness accompanied by chills, a headache, and nasal congestion. *Bryonia* (*Bryonia alba*) may be used to treat muscle aches, headaches, and a dry cough. For restlessness, chills, hoarseness, and achy joints, poison ivy (*Rhus toxicodendron*) is recommended. Finally, for achiness and a dry cough or chills, *Eupatorium perfoliatum* is suggested.

- Hydrotherapy. A bath to induce a fever will speed recovery from the flu by creating an environment in the body where the flu virus cannot survive. The patient should take a bath as hot as he/she can tolerate and remain in the bath for 20–30 minutes. While in the bath, the patient drinks a cup of yarrow or elderflower tea to induce sweating. During the bath, a cold cloth is held on the forehead or at the nape of the neck to keep the temperature down in the brain. The patient is assisted when getting out of the bath (he/she may feel weak or dizzy) and then gets into bed and covers up with layers of blankets to indue more sweating.

- Vitamins. For adults, 2–3 grams of vitamin C daily may help prevent the flu. Increasing the dose to 5–7 grams per day during the flu can felp fight the infection. (The dose should be reduced if diarrhea develops.)

Prognosis

Following proper treatment guidelines, healthy people under the age of 65 usually suffer no long-term consequences associated with flu infection. The elderly and the chronically ill are at greater risk for secondary infection and other complications, but they can also enjoy a complete recovery.

Most people recover fully from an influenza infection, but it should not be viewed complacently. Influenza is a serious disease, and approximately 1 in 1,000 cases proves fatal.

Prevention

The Centers for Disease Control and Prevention recommend that people get an influenza vaccine injection each year before flu season starts. In the United States, flu season typically runs from late December to early March. Vaccines should be received two to six weeks prior to the onset of flu season to allow the body enough time to establish immunity. Adults only need one dose of the yearly vaccine, but children under nine years of age who have not previously been immunized should receive two doses with a month between each dose.

Each season's flu vaccine contains three virus strains that are the most likely to be encountered in the coming flu season. When there is a good match between the anticipated flu strains and the strains used in the vaccine, the vaccine is 70-90% effective in people under 65. Because immune response diminishes somewhat with age, people over 65 may not receive the same level of protection from the vaccine, but even if they do contract the flu, the vaccine diminishes the severity and helps prevent complications.

The virus strains used to make the vaccine are inactivated and will not cause the flu. In the past, flu symptoms were associated with vaccine preparations that were not as highly purified as modern vaccines, not to the virus itself. In 1976, there was a slightly increased risk of developing **Guillain-Barré syndrome,** a very rare disorder, associated with the swine flu vaccine. This association occurred only with the 1976 swine flu vaccine preparation and has never recurred.

Serious side effects with modern vaccines are extremely unusual. Some people experience a slight soreness at the point of injection, which resolves within a day or two. People who have never been exposed to influenza, particularly children, may experience one to two days of a slight fever, tiredness, and muscle aches. These symptoms start within 6-12 hours after the **vaccination.**

It should be noted that certain people should not receive an influenza vaccine. Infants six months and younger have immature immune systems and will not benefit from the vaccine. Since the vaccines are prepared using hen eggs, people who have severe **allergies** to eggs or other vaccine components should not receive the influenza vaccine. As an alternative, they may receive a course of amantadine or rimantadine, which are also used as a protective measure against influenza. Other people who might receive these drugs are those that have been immunized after the flu season has started or who are immunocompromised, such as people with advanced HIV disease. Amantadine and rimantadine are 70-90% effective in preventing influenza.

Certain groups are strongly advised to be vaccinated because they are at-risk for influenza-related complications:

- All people 65 years and older

- Residents of nursing homes and chronic-care facilities, regardless of age

- Adults and children who have chronic heart or lung problems, such as **asthma**

- Adults and children who have chronic metabolic diseases, such as diabetes and renal dysfunction, as well as severe anemia or inherited hemoglobin disorders

- Children and teenagers who are on long-term aspirin therapy

- Women who will be in their second or third trimester during flu season or women who are nursing

- Anyone who is immunocompromised, including HIV-infected persons, **cancer** patients, organ transplant recipients, and patients receiving steroids, **chemotherapy,** or **radiation therapy**

- Anyone in contact with the above groups, such as teachers, care givers, health-care personnel, and family members

- Travelers to foreign countries.

An individual need not be in one of the at-risk categories listed above, however, to receive a flu vaccination. Anyone who wants to forego the discomfort and inconvenience of an influenza attack may receive the vaccine.

Resources

BOOKS

Levine, Arthur J. "The Influenza A Virus." In *Viruses.* New York: Scientific American Library, 1992.

PERIODICALS

Centers for Disease Control and Prevention. "Prevention and Control of Influenza: Recommendations of the Advisory Committee on Immunization Practices (ACIP)." *Morbidity and Mortality Weekly Report,* 46 (15) (April 25, 1997).

Novitt-Moren, Anne. "Holidays' Biggest Spoilers: Colds and Flu." *Current Health 2,* 4 (24) (December 1997): 6.

Saul, Helen. "Flu Vaccines Wanted: Dead or Alive." *New Scientist,* (February 18, 1995): 26.

Zimmerman, Richard K., Frederick L. Ruben, and Ellen R. Ahwesh. "Influenza, Influenza Vaccine, and Amantadine/Rimantadine." *Journal of Family Practice,* 45 (2) (August 1997): 107.

ORGANIZATIONS

Centers for Disease Control and Prevention. 1600 Clifton Road, NE, Atlanta, Georgia 30333. (888) CDC-FACTS (888-232-3228). http://www.cdc.gov/.

Julia Barrett

Infrequent menstruation *see* **Oligomenorrhea**

Inguinal hernia *see* **Hernia**

Inhalation therapies

Definition

Inhalation therapies are a group of respiratory, or breathing, treatments designed to help restore or improve breathing function in patients with a variety of diseases, conditions, or injuries. The treatments range from at-home **oxygen therapy** for patients with chronic obstructive pulmonary disease to mechanical ventilation for

---

patients with acute **respiratory failure.** Inhalation therapies usually include the following categories:

- Oxygen therapy

- Incentive spirometry

- Continuous positive airway pressure (CPAP)

- Oxygen chamber therapy

- Mechanical ventilation

- Newborn life support.

Purpose

Inhalation therapies are ordered for various stages of diseases which are causing progressive or sudden respiratory failure. Although physicians generally follow guidelines to assign specific therapy according the type and stage of a disease, the ultimate decision is based on a number of tests indicating pulmonary function and the presence or absence of oxygen in body organs and tissues.

Oxygen therapy

Oxygen therapy is most commonly ordered to support patients with **emphysema** and other chronic obstructive pulmonary disease (COPD). The oxygen therapy is usually ordered once decreased oxygen saturation in the blood or tissues is demonstrated. Oxygen therapy may also be used in the hospital setting to help return a patient's breathing and oxygen levels to normal.

Incentive spirometry

Spirometry is a diagnostic method for measuring gases and respiratory function. Incentive spirometry may be ordered to help patients practice and improve controlled breathing. It may be ordered after surgery to the abdomen, lungs, neck, or head.

Continuous positive airway pressure (CPAP)

Common uses of continuous positive airway pressure include **sleep apnea, respiratory distress syndrome** in infants, and **adult respiratory distress syndrome.** Signs of **atelectasis** (absence of gas from the lungs) or abnormalities of the lower airways may also indicate CPAP.

Oxygen chamber therapy

Oxygen chamber therapy is ordered for various causes that indicate immediate need for oxygen saturation in the blood. Divers with decompression illness, climbers in high altitude, patients suffering from severe carbon dioxide poisoning, and children or adults in acute respiratory distress may require oxygen chamber therapy. In recent years, physicians have also used the forced pressure of oxygen chambers to help heal **burns** and other **wounds,** since the pressure under which the oxygen is delivered can reach areas that are blocked off or suffering from poor circulation.

Mechanical ventilation

Mechanical ventilation is ordered for patients in acute respiratory distress, and is often used in an intensive care situation. In some cases, mechanical ventilation is a final attempt to continue the breathing function in a patient and may be considered "life-sustaining."

Newborn life support

Newborn babies, particularly those who were premature, may require inhalation therapies immediately upon birth, since the lungs are among the last organs to fully develop. Some newborns suffer from serious respiratory problems or birth complications, such as respiratory distress syndrome, neonatal wet lung syndrome, apnea of **prematurity** or persistent fetal circulation, which may require inhalation therapies.

Precautions

There are numerous indications for not prescribing various inhalation therapies.

Oxygen therapy

Patients and family members who smoke should not have oxygen prescribed or should avoid smoking in the area to prevent combustion. Sedatives should be avoided for patients on oxygen therapy.

Incentive spirometry

Patients who are unable or unwilling to properly and consistently practice incentive spirometry as prescribed should not receive this form of treatment.

Continuous positive airway pressure (CPAP)

Patients unable or unwilling to comply with the physician's instructions for use of CPAP are not likely to have it prescribed. Extremely obese patients may have less success with this form of therapy for the treatment of sleep apnea.

Oxygen chamber therapy

Complications may arise from this form of treatment and during transport to or from the oxygen chamber. Therefore, some patients may not receive enough benefit to outweigh possible complications. All patients, particularly children, must be carefully monitored.

Mechanical ventilation

Use of mechanical ventilation will be carefully weighed against benefit and possible risks. Some patients will require sedation to prevent fighting of the ventilator, which can increase the risk of complications.

Newborn life support

Not all infants with breathing problems will require measures as severe as mechanical ventilation. The physician will make the determination based on weight and condition of the infant. Newborns with patent ductus arteriosis, a handicap affecting the pulmonary artery, are more likely to suffer pulmonary hemorrhage from mechanical ventilation.

Description

Oxygen therapy

Once a patient shows hypoxemia, or decreased oxygen in arterial blood, supplemental oxygen may be ordered. The main purpose of the oxygen is to prevent damage to vital organs resulting from inadequate oxygen supply. The lowest possible saturation will be given to keep the patient's measurements at a minimum acceptable level. The oxygen is administered through a mask or nasal tube, or sometimes directly into the trachea. The amount of oxygen prescribed is measured in liters of flow per minute. Patients with chronic hypoxemia, most likely in late stages of COPD, will often receive long-term oxygen therapy.

Most patients will receive their long-term oxygen therapy through home oxygen use. A physician must prescribe home oxygen and levels will be monitored to ensure that the correct amount of oxygen is administered. Some patients will receive oxygen therapy only at night or when exercising.

The choice of type of home oxygen systems will vary depending on availability, cost considerations, and the mobility of the patient. Those patients who are ambulatory, especially those who work, will need a system with a small portable tank. Depending on the system chosen, frequent deliveries of oxygen and filling of portable tanks will be necessary.

In the case of respiratory distress in newborns or adults, oxygen therapy may be attempted before mechanical ventilation since it is a noninvasive and less expensive choice. Oxygen has been found effective in treating patients with other diseases such as **cystic fibrosis,** chronic congestive **heart failure,** or other lung diseases.

Incentive spirometry

Incentive spirometry is also referred to as sustained maximal inspiration. It is designed to mimic natural sighs and yawns. A device provides positive feedback when a patient inhales at a predetermined rate and sustains the breath for a specific period of time. This helps teach the patient to take long, slow, and deep breaths. A spirometer, or equipment that measures pulmonary function, is provided to the patient and a respiratory therapist will work with the patient to demonstrate and explain the technique. Once patients show mastery of the technique, they are instructed to practice the exercises frequently on their own.

Continuous positive airway pressure (CPAP)

Patients with sleep apnea will receive continuous positive airway pressure to prevent upper airway collapse. It is usually administered through a tight-fitting mask as humidified oxygen. The pressure of flow is constant during both exhaling and inhaling and the level of pressure is determined based on each individual. Most patients undergoing CPAP in a hospital setting will receive continuous monitoring of some vital signs and periodic sampling of blood gas values.

Oxygen chamber therapy

Also known as hyperbaric oxygen chamber or hyperbaric oxygen therapy (HBO), this treatment delivers pure oxygen under pressure equal to that of 2-3 times normal atmospheric pressure. For years, this treatment has been especially effective on scuba divers who suffer from the ''bends,'' or decompression illness. The patient enters the chamber, a plastic cylinder-shaped structure that is normally transparent. In most cases, just one patient will enter by being rolled into the chamber on a type of stretcher. Once inside, the oxygen will be delivered under forced pressure and the patient is free to read, nap, or listen to the radio. The therapy usually lasts one hour, although it can take up to five hours in serious decompression cases. Before exiting the chamber, the pressure will eventually be lowered to normal atmospheric level.

Mechanical ventilation

In general, mechanical ventilation replaces or supports the normal ventilatory lung function of a patient. Although normally delivered in a hospital, often to treat serious illness, mechanical ventilation may be performed at home under the order and supervision of a physician and home health agency. The patient will usually be intubated and the ventilator machine ''takes over'' the breathing function.

There are several modes and methods of mechanical ventilation, each offering different advantages and disadvantages. In assist/control ventilation, the oldest mode of ventilation, the physician predetermines settings and the ventilator delivers a breath each time the patient makes an effort to inhale. In synchronized intermittent mandatory ventilation, the machine senses a patient's effort to inhale and delivers the preset amount. The amount cannot be increased by the patient's effort. Pressure-control ventilation involves the physician's selection of a peak pressure and this method is most useful for patients suffering from obstructive airways disease. In cases of severe hypoventilation, an endotracheal tube must be inserted. If a patient will be on mechanical ventilation for more than two weeks, a tracheostomy, or surgical incision, will be performed for placement of the breathing tubes.

There are other modes of ventilation that may be used, including high-frequency ventilation, a newer technique that delivers 100 to 200 breaths per minute to the patient. The breaths are delivered through a humidified, high-pressure gas jet. High-frequency ventilation may be ordered when a patient does not respond to conventional mechanical ventilation or for certain conditions and circumstances.

Newborn life support

Premature infants, especially those born before the 28th week of gestation, have underdeveloped breathing muscles and immature structures within the lungs. These infants will require breathing support, often in the form of mechanical ventilation. The support delivers warm, humidified, oxygen-enriched gases either by oxygen hood or through mechanical ventilation. In serious cases, the infant may require mechanical ventilation with CPAP or positive-end expiratory pressure (PEEP) through a tightly fitting face mask or even by endotracheal intubation.

Need for continued resuscitation for newborns depends not only on gestational age, but on signs indicating ineffective breathing, including color, heart rate, and respiratory effort. CPAP will be delivered through nasal or endotracheal tubes with a continuous-flow ventilator specifically designed for infants. An alarm system alerts the neonatal staff to problems and monitoring of breathing and other vital functions will accompany the therapy. As respiratory distress syndrome begins to resolve, usually in four or five days, the type of support will be reduced accordingly and the infant may be weaned from the ventilator and moved to only CPAP or an oxygen hood.

Preparation

Preparation for any of these treatments is normally not necessary, and in fact, these therapies may be administered as a result of an emergency situation. Some of the methods, particularly incentive spirometry, or at-home oxygen or ventilation, will require education and cooperation with a home health agency or respiratory therapist. Pretreatment testing of various indicators of respiratory function and oxygen saturation will be performed to determine exact needs of individual patients.

Aftercare

Pulmonary function tests and other tests will be performed to verify that treatments have been successful or to monitor and adjust treatments. Mechanical ventilation will require weaning from the equipment and may also require care for the area surrounding the intubation.

Risks

Inhalation therapies may carry risks, complications or side effects including:

Oxygen therapy

At-home oxygen therapy carries risk if improper care is taken to follow instructions when handling the oxygen. Patients are cautioned not to smoke near the oxygen supply and to keep the supply away from other sources that may cause electrical spark, flames, or intense heat. Patients on home oxygen therapy should avoid use of sedatives.

Incentive spirometry

The major risk associated with incentive spirometry relates to improper use. Patients must be carefully instructed in the technique and monitored periodically for compliance and improvement. Barotrauma, injury to the middle ear or sinuses caused by imbalance between the affected cavity and the outside, or ambient pressure, can result form incentive spirometry. A patient may also suffer discomfort or fatigue.

Continuous positive airway pressure (CPAP)

The effectiveness of CPAP may be limited if patients do not cooperate. Possible side effects of CPAP include skin abrasions from the mask, leakage from the tube or mask, nasal congestion, nasal or oral dryness, or discomfort from the pressure of delivery.

Oxygen chamber therapy

Hyperbaric oxygen therapy is painless. The only risk would be associated with improper administration of the pressure levels, which should not occur, since respiratory staff and the supervising physician should be thoroughly trained in performance of this therapy. The drawback to hyperbaric oxygen treatment is the limited availability of chambers. Many cities do not have readily available chambers.

Mechanical ventilation

The biggest risk of mechanical ventilation is sometimes considered to be a patient's dependence on the machine and the difficulty of weaning the patient. The physician will carefully select and monitor the mode of ventilation, the machine's settings, and the patient's progress to prevent this complication. A patient may therefore be left on a ventilator after sufficient progress is made to gradually wean breathing dependence.

Intubation and mechanical ventilation are frightening and uncomfortable for many patients and they may fight the ventilator. If this occurs, the physician may order a sedative to ensure cooperation and effectiveness of the therapy. Intubation often results in irritation to the trachea and larynx. Tracheostomy is associated with risk of bleeding, **pneumothorax,** local infection, and increased incidence of aspiration.

Newborn life support

Infants are continuously monitored to determine even small changes in breathing function. Mechanical ventilation can result in increases in respiratory distress or other complications. It is possible for the ventilator to be accidentally disconnected and staff is trained to watch for signs or alarms indicating disconnection. Mechanical ventilation increases risk of infection in premature babies. Complications of PEEP or CPAP may include pneumothorax or decreased cardiac output.

Normal results

Oxygen therapy

In the case of COPD, oxygen therapy does not treat the disease but can prolong life, quality of life, and onset of more serious symptoms. Effective oxygen therapy for any patient should lead to improved or sustained levels of oxygen in arterial blood.

Incentive spirometry

With proper use of incentive spirometry, the physician should observe improved pulse rate, decreased respiratory rate, improved respiratory muscle performance, and other indicators of improved function. Lung function following lung resection should show marked improvement following incentive spirometry.

Continuous positive airway pressure

Successful CPAP will result in reduction in apnea for those suffering from sleep apnea. A study reported on in 1998 demonstrated that CPAP was effective in the majority of patients with sleep apnea, with the exception of significantly obese patients with blood gas values that were worse during waking hours at rest and at exercise. Hospitalized patients on CPAP therapy should show improvement in blood gas and other pulmonary measurements as expected by the treating physician.

Oxygen chamber therapy

Divers undergoing emergency treatment in a hyperbaric chamber should show immediate improvement in oxygen levels throughout the body, regardless of blood flow restrictions, after one or two treatments. Those patients receiving oxygen chamber therapy for difficult wounds may continue to receive treatments daily for several weeks before satisfactory results are reached. Patients with carbon dioxide poisoning should show improvement in or recovery of neurologic function. Results of hyperbaric chamber therapy depend largely on how quickly the patient was brought to the chamber, as well as the severity of the initial condition.

Mechanical ventilation

Successful mechanical ventilation will result in gradual decrease in dependence on the ventilator and weaning from the machine. Reduction of therapy to another form, such as CPAP or oxygen therapy, indicates that ventilation has worked as expected. In the case of COPD, exacerbation may be successfully treated with mechanical ventilation and the patient may return to home oxygen therapy. Pediatric patients will demonstrate normal growth and development as a normal result of long-term mechanical ventilation at home. Some patients, particularly those in a hospital intensive care unit, will not be able to breathe again without the ventilator and families and physicians will face tough choices about continued life support.

Newborn life support

Neonates will be constantly monitored to measure lung function. Those measurements will help caregivers determine if and when mechanical ventilation can be reduced and CPAP or oxygen mask begun. CPAP is considered successful when the infant's respiratory rate is reduced by 30-40%, a chest radiograph shows improved lung volume and appearance, stabilization of oxygen levels is documented and caregivers observe improvement in the infant's comfort. Evidence that there is no infection from ventilation is also considered normal. In some cases, inhalation therapy, including mechanical ventilation, will not work and the infant's parents and physicians will face tough decisions about invasive procedures with associated high risks or cessation of life support.

Resources

ORGANIZATIONS

American Association for Respiratory Care. 11030 Ables Lane, Dallas, TX 75229. (972) 243-2272, Fax (972) 484-2720.

American Lung Association. 1-800-LUNG-USA. (1-800-586-4872). http://www.lungusa.org.

National Heart, Lung and Blood Institute. Building 31, Room 4A21, Bethesda, MD 20892. (301)496-4236. http://www.nhlbi.nih.gov.

OTHER

Hyperbaric Research and Treatment Center. http://www.hyperbaricrx.com.

Teresa G. Norris

Inner ear infection *see* **Labyrinthitis**

Insomnia

Definition

Insomnia is the inability to obtain an adequate amount or quality of sleep. The difficulty can be in falling asleep, remaining asleep, or both. People with insomnia do not feel refreshed when they wake up. Insomnia is a common symptom affecting millions of people that may be caused by many conditions, diseases, or circumstances.

Description

Sleep is essential for mental and physical restoration. It is a cycle with two separate states: rapid eye movement (REM), the stage in which most dreaming occurs; and non-REM (NREM). Four stages of sleep take place during NREM: stage I, when the person passes from relaxed wakefulness; stage II, an early stage of light sleep; stages III and IV, which are increasing degrees of deep sleep. Most stage IV sleep (also called delta sleep), occurs in the first several hours of sleep. A period of REM sleep normally follows a period of NREM sleep.

Insomnia is more common in women and older adults. People who are divorced, widowed, or separated are more likely to have the problem than those who are married, and it is more frequently reported by those with lower socioeconomic status. Short-term, or transient, insomnia is a common occurrence and usually lasts only a few days. Long-term, or chronic insomnia lasts more than three weeks and increases the risk for injuries in the home, at the workplace, and while driving because of daytime sleepiness and decreased concentration. Chronic insomnia can also lead to **mood disorders** like depression.

Causes & symptoms

Transient insomnia is often caused by a temporary situation in a person's life, such as an argument with a loved one, a brief medical illness, or **jet lag.** When the situation is resolved or the precipitating factor disappears, the condition goes away, usually without medical treatment.

Chronic insomnia usually has different causes, and there may be more than one. These include:

- A medical condition or its treatment, including **sleep apnea**
- Use of substances such as **caffeine,** alcohol, and nicotine
- Psychiatric conditions such as mood or **anxiety disorders**
- **Stress,** such as sadness caused by the loss of a loved one or a job
- Disturbed sleep cycles caused by a change in work shift
- Sleep-disordered breathing, such as snoring
- Periodic jerky leg movements (*nocturnal myoclonus*), which happen just as the individual is falling asleep
- Repeated nightmares or panic attacks during sleep.

Another cause is excessive worrying about whether or not a person will be able to go to sleep, which creates so much **anxiety** that the individual's bedtime rituals and behavior actually trigger insomnia. The more one worries about falling asleep, the harder it becomes. This is called psychophysiological insomnia.

Symptoms of insomnia

People who have insomnia do not start the day refreshed from a good night's sleep. They are tired. They may have difficulty falling asleep, and commonly lie in bed tossing and turning for hours. Or the individual may go to sleep without a problem but wakes in the early hours of the morning and is either unable to go back to sleep, or drifts into a restless unsatisfying sleep. This is a common symptom in the elderly and in those suffering from depression. Sometimes sleep patterns are reversed and the individual has difficulty staying awake during the day and takes frequent naps. The sleep at night is fitful and frequently interrupted.

Diagnosis

The diagnosis of insomnia is made by a physician based on the patient's reported signs and symptoms. It can be useful for the patient to keep a daily record for two weeks of sleep patterns, food intake, use of alcohol, medications, **exercise,** and any other information recommended by the physician. If the patient has a bed partner, information can be obtained about whether the patient snores or is restless during sleep. This, together with a medical history and **physical examination,** can help confirm the doctor's assessment.

A wide variety of healthcare professionals can recognize and treat insomnia, but when a patient with chronic insomnia does not respond to treatment, or the condition is not adequately explained by the patient's physical, emotional, or mental circumstances, then more extensive testing by a specialist in **sleep disorders** may be warranted.

Treatment

Treatment of insomnia includes alleviating any physical and emotional problems that are contributing to the condition and exploring changes in lifestyle that will improve the situation.

Changes in behavior

Patients can make changes in their daily routine that are simple and effective in treating their insomnia. They should go to bed only when sleepy and use the bedroom only for sleep. Other activities like reading, watching television, or snacking should take place somewhere else. If they are unable to go to sleep, they should go into another room and do something that is relaxing, like reading. Watching television should be avoided because it has an arousing effect. The person should return to bed only when they feel sleepy. Patients should set the alarm and get up every morning at the same time, no matter how much they have slept, to establish a regular sleep-wake pattern. Naps during the day should be avoided, but if absolutely necessary, than a 30 minute nap early in the afternoon may not interfere with sleep at night.

Another successful technique is called sleep-restriction therapy, which restricts the amount of time spent in bed to the actual time spent sleeping. This approach allows a slight sleep debt to build up, which increases the individual's ability to fall asleep and stay asleep. If a patient is sleeping five hours a night, the time in bed is limited to 5-5 1/2 hours. The time in bed is gradually increased in small segments, with the individual rising at the same time each morning; at least 85% of the time in bed must be spent sleeping.

Drug therapy

Medications given for insomnia include sedatives, tranquilizers, and **antianxiety drugs.** All require a doctor's prescription and may become habit-forming. They can lose effectiveness over time and can reduce alertness during the day. The medications should be taken two to four times daily for approximately three to four weeks, though this will vary with the physician and patient. If the insomnia is related to depression, then an antidepressant medication may be helpful. Over-the-counter drugs such as **antihistamines** are not very effective in bringing about sleep and can affect the quality of sleep.

Other measures

Relaxing before going to bed will help a person fall asleep faster. Learning to substitute pleasant thoughts for unpleasant ones (imagery training) is a technique that can be very helpful in reducing worry. Another effective measure is the use of audiotapes which combine the sounds of nature with soft relaxing music. These, alone or in combination with other relaxation techniques, can safely promote sleepiness.

Changes in diet and exercise routines can also have a have a beneficial effect. Dietary items to be avoided include drinks that contain caffeine such as coffee, tea and colas, chocolate (which contains a stimulant), and alcohol, which initially makes a person sleepy but a few hours later can have the opposite effect. Maintaining a comfortable bedroom temperature, reducing noise and eliminating light are also helpful. Regularly scheduled morning or afternoon exercise can relax the body. This should be done 3-4 times a week and be sufficient to produce a light sweat.

Alternative treatments

Many alternative treatments are effective in treating both the symptom of insomnia and its underlying causes. Incorporating relaxation techniques into bedtime rituals will help a person go to sleep faster, as well as improve the quality of sleep. These methods include **meditation, massage,** breathing exercises, and a warm bath, scented with rose, lavender (*Lavendula officinalis*), marjoram, or chamomile (*Matricaria recutita*). Eating a healthy diet rich in calcium, magnesium, and the B **vitamins** is also beneficial. A high protein snack like yogurt before going to bed is recommended, or a cup of herb tea made with chamomile, hops (*Humulus lupulus*), passionflower (*Passiflora incarnata*), or St-John's-Wort (*Hypericum perforatum*) to encourage relaxation. **Acupuncture** and **biofeedback** have also proven useful.

Prevention

Prevention of insomnia centers around promotion of a healthy lifestyle. A balance of rest, recreation and exercise in combination with stress management, regular physical examinations, and a healthy diet can do much to reduce the risk.

Resources

BOOKS

Boyd, Mary Ann, and Mary Ann Nihart. *Psychiatric Nursing: Contemporary Practice.* Philadelphia, PA: Lippincott, 1998.

The Burton Goldberg Group. *Alternative Medicine: The Definitive Guide.* Fife, WA: Future Medicine Publishing, 1995.

Frisch, Noreen Cavan, and Lawrence E. Frisch. *Psychiatric Mental Health Nursing.* Albany, NY: Delmar, 1988.

ORGANIZATIONS

American Sleep Disorders Association. 6301 Bandel Road, Suite 101, Rochester, MN 55901. http://www.asda.org/.

OTHER

American Family Physician. Volume 49, Number 6, May 1, 1994. *Patient Information: Insomnia and What You Can Do to Sleep Better.* http://srvr.third-wave.com/tricounty/insomnia.html (1998.)

Children's Hospital of Iowa. *What to Do When You Can't Sleep.* 1995. http://www.vh.org/Patients/IHB/Fam . . . tice/AFP/January1995/Insomnia.html (1998.)

Donald Gardner Barstow

Insulin *see* **Antidiabetic drugs**

Insulin tolerance test *see* **Growth hormone tests**

Intelligence tests *see* **Stanford-Binet intelligence scales; Wechsler intelligence test**

Intention tremor *see* **Tremors**

Interferon *see* **Antiviral drugs; Immunologic therapies**

Interleukin-2 *see* **Immunologic therapies**

Internal fetal monitoring *see* **Electronic fetal monitoring**

Internuclear ophthalmoplegia *see* **Ophthalmoplegia**

Interpositional reconstruction *see* **Arthroplasty**

Intersex states

Definition

Intersex states are conditions where a newborn's sex organs (genitals) look unusual, making it impossible to identify the sex of the baby from its outward appearance.

Description

All developing babies start out with external sex organs that look female. If the baby is male, the internal sex organs mature and begin to produce the male hormone testosterone. If the hormones reach the tissues correctly, the external genitals that looked female change into the scrotum and penis. Sometimes, the genetic sex (as indicated by chromosomes) may not match the appearance of the external sex organs. About 1 in every 2,000 births results in a baby whose sex organs look unusual.

Patients with intersex states can be classified as a true hermaphrodite, a female pseudohermaphrodite, or a male pseudohermaphrodite. This is determined by examining the internal and external structures of the child.

A true hermaphrodite is born with both ovaries and testicles. They also have mixed male and female external genitals. This condition is extremely rare.

A female pseudohermaphrodite is a genetic female. However, the external sex organs have been masculinized and look like a penis. This may occur if the mother takes the hormone progesterone to prevent a

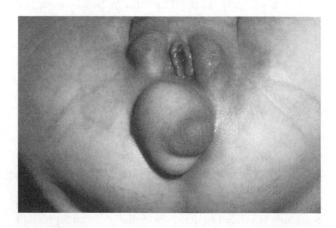

This infant was born with female and male genitalia.
(Photography by Mike Peres, Custom Medical Stock Photo. Reproduced by permission.)

miscarriage, but more often it is caused by an overproduction of certain hormones.

A male pseudohermaphrodite is a genetic male. However, the external sex organs fail to develop normally. Intersex males may have testes and a female-like vulva, or a very small penis.

Causes & symptoms

Any abnormality in chromosomes or sex hormones, or in the unborn baby's response to the hormones, can lead to an intersex state in a newborn.

Intersex states may also be caused by a condition called **congenital adrenal hyperplasia,** which occurs in about 1 out of every 5,000 newborns. This disease blocks the baby's metabolism and can cause a range of symptoms, including abnormal genitals.

Diagnosis

When doctors are uncertain about a newborn's sex, a specialist in infant hormonal problems is consulted as soon as possible. Ultrasound can locate a uterus behind the bladder and can determine if there is a cervix or uterine canal. Blood tests can check the levels of sex hormones in the baby's blood, and chromosome analysis (called karyotyping) can determine sex. Explorative surgery or a biopsy of reproductive tissue may be necessary. Only after thorough testing can a correct diagnosis and determination of sex be made.

Treatment

Treatment of intersex states is controversial. Traditional treatment assigns sex according to test results, the potential for the child to identify with a sex, and the ease of genital surgery to make the organs look more normal. Treatment may then include **reconstructive surgery** followed by hormone therapy. Babies born with congenital adrenal hyperplasia can be treated with cortisone-type drugs and sometimes surgery.

Counseling should be given to the entire family of an intersex newborn. Families should explore all available medical and surgical options. Counseling should also be provided to the child when he or she is old enough.

Prognosis

Since the mid-1950s, doctors have typically assigned a sex to an intersex infant based on how easy reconstructive surgery would be. The American Academy of Pediatrics states that children with these types of genitals can be raised successfully as members of either sex, and recommends surgery within the first 15 months of life.

Some people are critical of this approach, including intersex adults who were operated on as children. The remolded genitals do not function sexually and can be the source of lifelong **pain.** They suggest that surgery be delayed until the patient can make informed choices about surgery and intervention.

Resources

BOOKS

Carlson, Karen J., Stephanie A. Eisenstat, and Terra Ziporyn. "Hermaphroditism." In *The Harvard Guide to Women's Health.* Cambridge, MA: Harvard University Press, 1996, 289-290.

Cunningham, F. Gary, et al. *Williams Obstetrics,* 20th ed. Stamford, CT: Appleton & Lange, 1997.

Johnson, Robert V., ed. *Mayo Clinic Complete Book of Pregnancy and Baby's First Year.* New York: William Morrow and Company, Inc., 1994, 387-388.

Ryan, Kenneth J., Ross S. Berkowitz, and Robert L. Barbieri. "Medical Genetics." In *Kistner's Gynecology,* 6th Edition. St. Louis, MO: Mosby, 1997.

PERIODICALS

Johnson, Kate. "Doctors Asked to Delay Sex-Assignment Surgery." *Ob-Gyn News,* (March 1, 1997): 30.

ORGANIZATIONS

Ambiguous Genitalia Support Network. PO Box 313, Clements, CA 95227. (209) 727-0313.

Intersex Society. PO Box 31791, San Francisco, CA 94131.

Carol A. Turkington

Interstitial therapy *see* **Radioactive implants**

Intestinal culture *see* **Stool culture**

Intestinal obstructions

Definition

Intestinal obstruction is the partial or complete mechanical or nonmechanical blockage of the small or large intestine.

Description

There are two types of intestinal obstructions—mechanical and nonmechanical. Mechanical obstructions occur because the bowel is physically blocked and its contents cannot get past the obstruction. Mechanical obstructions can occur for several reasons. Sometimes the

KEY TERMS

Electrolytes—Salts and minerals that ionize in body fluids. Electrolytes control the body's fluid balance as well as performing other important functions.

Gangrene—The death of soft tissue in any part of the body when the blood supply is obstructed.

Ileus—Obstruction of the intestines caused by the absence of peristalsis.

Intussusception—The slipping or telescoping of one part of the intestine into the section next to it.

Meconium—A greenish fecal material that forms the first bowel movement of an infant.

Peristalsis—The waves of muscular contraction in the intestines that push the food along during the process of digestion.

Strangulated obstruction—An obstruction in which a loop of the intestine has its blood supply cut off.

Volvulus—A twisting of the intestine that causes an obstruction.

bowel twists on itself (volvulus) or telescopes into itself (intussusception). Mechanical obstruction can also result from **hernias**, impacted feces, abnormal tissue growth, the presence of foreign bodies in the intestines, or inflammatory bowel disease (**Crohn's disease**). Nonmechanical obstruction, called **ileus**, occurs because the wavelike muscular contractions of the intestine (peristalsis) that ordinarily move food through the digestive tract stop.

Mechanical obstruction in infants

Infants under one year of age are most likely to have intestinal obstruction caused by meconium ileus, volvulus, and intussusception. Meconium ileus, which is the inability to pass the first fecal excretion after birth (meconium), is a disorder of newborns. It is an early clue that the infant has **cystic fibrosis.** In meconium ileus, the material that is blocking the intestine is thick and stringy, rather than the collection of mucus and bile that is passed by normal infants. The abnormal meconium must be removed with an enema or through surgery.

Volvulus is the twisting of either the small or large bowel. The twisting may cut off the blood supply to the bowel, leading to tissue death (**gangrene**). This development is called a strangulating obstruction.

In intussusception, the bowel telescopes into itself like a radio antenna folding up. Intussusception is most common in children between the ages of three and nine months, although it also occurs in older children. Almost twice as many boys suffer intussusception as girls. It is, however, difficult for doctors to predict which infants will suffer from intestinal obstruction.

Mechanical obstruction in adults

Obstructions in adults are usually caused by tumors, trauma, volvulus, the presence of foreign bodies such as **gallstones,** or hernias. Volvulus occurs most often in elderly adults and psychiatrically disturbed patients. Intussusception in adults is usually associated with tumors in the bowel, whether benign or malignant.

Causes & symptoms

One of the earliest signs of mechanical intestinal obstruction is abdominal **pain** or cramps that come and go in waves. Infants typically pull up their legs and cry in pain, then stop crying suddenly. They will then behave normally for as long as 15-30 minutes, only to start crying again when the next cramp begins. The cramping results from the inability of the muscular contractions of the bowel to push the digested food past the obstruction.

Vomiting is another symptom of intestinal obstruction. The speed of its onset is a clue to the location of the obstruction. Vomiting follows shortly after the pain if the obstruction is in the small intestine but is delayed if it is in the large intestine. The vomited material may be fecal in character. When the patient has a mechanical obstruction, the doctor will first hear active, high-pitched gurgling and splashing bowel sounds while listening with a stethoscope. Later these sounds decrease, then stop. If the blockage is complete, the patient will not pass any gas or feces. If the blockage is only partial, however, the patient may have **diarrhea.** Initially there is little or no **fever.**

When the material in the bowel cannot move past the obstruction, the body reabsorbs large amounts of fluid and the abdomen becomes sore to the touch and swollen. The balance of certain important chemicals (electrolytes) in the blood is upset. Persistent vomiting can cause the patient to become dehydrated. Without treatment, the patient can suffer **shock** and kidney failure.

Strangulation occurs when a loop of the intestine is cut off from its blood supply. Strangulation occurs in about 25% of cases of small bowel obstruction. It is a serious condition that can progress to gangrene within six hours.

Diagnosis

Imaging studies

If the doctor suspects intestinal obstruction based on the **physical examination** and patient history, he or she will order x rays, a **computed tomography scan** (CT scan), or an ultrasound evaluation of the abdomen. In many cases the patient is given a **barium enema.** Barium sulfate, which is a white powder, is inserted through the rectum and the intestinal area is photographed. Barium acts as a contrast material and allows the location of the obstruction to be pinpointed on film.

Laboratory tests

The first blood test of a patient with an intestinal obstruction usually gives normal results, but later tests indicate electrolyte imbalances. There is no way to determine if an obstruction is simple or strangulated except surgery.

Treatment

Initial assessment

All patients with suspected intestinal obstruction are hospitalized. Treatment must be rapid, because strangulating obstructions can be fatal. The first step in treatment is inserting a nasogastric tube to suction out the contents of the stomach and intestines. The patient is then given intravenous fluids to prevent **dehydration** and correct electrolyte imbalances.

Nonsurgical approaches

Surgery can be avoided for some patients. In some cases of volvulus, guiding a rectal tube into the intestines will straighten the twisted bowels. In infants, a barium enema may reverse intussusception in 50-90%. An air enema is sometimes used instead of a barium enema. This treatment successfully relieves the obstruction in many infants. The children are usually hospitalized for observation for two to three days after these procedures. In patients with only partial obstruction, a barium enema may dissolve the blockage.

Surgical treatment

If these efforts fail, surgery is necessary. Strangulated obstructions require emergency surgery. The obstructed area is removed and part of the bowel is cut away. If the obstruction is caused by tumors, polyps, or scar tissue, they are removed. Hernias, if present, are repaired. **Antibiotics** are given to reduce the possibility of infection.

Alternative treatment

Alternative practitioners offer few suggestions for treatment. They focus on preventive strategies, particularly the use of high-fiber **diets** to keep the bowels healthy through regular elimination.

Prognosis

Mortality

Untreated intestinal obstructions can be fatal. The bowel either strangulates or perforates, causing massive infection. With prompt treatment, however, most patients recover without complications.

Recurrence

As many as 80% of patients whose volvulus is treated without surgery have recurrences. Recurrences in infants with intussusception are most likely to happen during the first 36 hours after the blockage has been cleared. The mortality rate for unsuccessfully treated infants is 1-2%.

Prevention

Most cases of intestinal obstruction are not preventable. Surgery to remove tumors, polyps, or gallstones helps prevent recurrences.

Resources

BOOKS

''Intestinal Obstruction.'' In *The Merck Manual of Diagnosis and Therapy,*, edited by Robert Berkow, et al. Rahway, NJ: Merck Research Laboratories, 1992.

OTHER

Healthanswers. ''Intestinal Obstruction.'' www.healthanswers.com/database/ami/converted/ 000260.html.

University of New Brunswick Nursing Faculty. ''Intussusception: A Case Study for Nurses.'' http:// www.unb.ca/courses/nur4284/intu.htm.

Tish Davidson

Intestinal polyps

Definition

The word polyp refers to any overgrowth of tissue from the surface of mucous membranes. Intestinal polyps grow out of the lining of the small and large bowels.

KEY TERMS

Autosomal dominance—A pattern of heredity in which a trait is inherited without respect to sex and from either parent. The hereditary diseases associated with intestinal polyps are all autosomal dominant.

Colectomy—Surgical removal of the large bowel.

Intussusception—The slipping of one section of the intestine inside an adjoining section. Intussusception can be caused by small intestinal polyps.

Mucosal—Refers to tissues that produce mucus, such as the digestive, genital and urinary tracts.

Neoplasm—A new growth of abnormal tissue.

Peristalsis—The rhythmic contractions of muscular tubes like the intestines that carry the contents along the tube.

Sigmoid—The S-shaped curve of the large intestine where the colon joins the rectum.

Polyps come in a variety of shapes—round, droplet, and irregular being the most common.

Description

Polyps are one of many forms of tissue overproduction that can occur in the body. Cells in many body tissues sometimes keep growing beyond their usual limits. Medical scientists call this process *neoplasia*, which means simply "new growth." An individual overgrowth is called a neoplasm. In most cases these growths are limited, and the result is a benign swelling or mass of cells called a tumor. If the new growth occurs on the surface of the tissue instead of inside an organ it is often called a polyp. **Cancer** is another type of neoplasm marked by unlimited tissue growth. The essential feature that distinguishes cancer from nonmalignant neoplasms is that it does not stop growing.

Intestinal polyps are a common form of neoplasm. All intestinal polyps arise from the inner lining of the intestinal wall. This layer of mucosal tissue does the work of digestion. About 30% of the general population will develop intestinal polyps at some point in life, with the likelihood increasing with age. Most of these polyps are never noticed during a person's lifetime because they cause no problems. They are often discovered accidentally at **autopsy**. The primary importance of intestinal polyps is that 1% of them become cancerous. Because the polyps that eventually turn malignant cannot be identified in advance, they are all suspect.

Location of intestinal polyps

The chances of a polyp's becoming cancerous depend to some extent on its location within the digestive tract.

COLON

Ninety-five percent of all intestinal polyps develop inside the large bowel. There are several hereditary diseases that produce large numbers of intestinal polyps. These disorders include:

- **Familial polyposis** of the colon.
- Gardner's syndrome.
- Lynch's syndrome.
- Turcot's syndrome.
- Peutz-Jeghers syndrome.
- Juvenile polyposis.

All of these disorders are inherited in what is called an autosomal dominant pattern. This pattern means that the disorders are not sex-linked and that a child can inherit the disorder from either parent. In all of these hereditary disorders, the intestinal polyps appear during or after **puberty.** The first four diseases on the list have such a high rate of cancer of the large bowel (colon)—virtually 100% by the age of 40—that persons diagnosed with any of them should have the colon removed surgically in early adulthood.

STOMACH

The stomach's lining is host to polyps of a similar appearance, but there is no agreement as to their potential for becoming **stomach cancer.**

SMALL INTESTINE

Polyps in the small bowel do not seem to have malignant potential. Instead they can produce obstruction in either of two ways. A large polyp can obstruct the bowel by its sheer size. Smaller polyps can be picked up by the rhythmic contractions (peristalsis) of the intestines and pull the part of the bowel to which they are attached into the adjoining section. The result is a telescoping of one section of bowel into another, called intussusception.

Causes & symptoms

Population studies of colon cancer suggest that diet plays an important role in the disease, and by implication in the formation of colon polyps. The most consistent interpretation of these data is that animal fats—though not vegetable fats—are the single most important dietary factor. Lack of fiber in the diet may also contribute to polyp formation. Other types of polyps are too rare to produce enough data for evaluation.

Most polyps cause no symptoms. Large ones eventually cause intestinal obstruction, which produces cramping abdominal **pain** with **nausea and vomiting.** As colon polyps evolve into cancers, they begin to produce symptoms that include bleeding and altered bowel habits.

Diagnosis

Routine screening for bowel cancer is recommended for everyone over the age of 40. Screening may be as simple as testing the stool for blood or as elaborate as **colonoscopy.** Colonoscopy is a procedure in which the doctor threads an instrument called a colonoscope up through the entire large bowel. Most polyps are in the lower segment of the colon, called the sigmoid colon. These polyps can be seen with a shorter scope called a sigmoidoscope. X ray imaging can also used to look for polyps. For x rays, the colon is first filled with barium, which is a white substance that shows up as a shadowed area on the film. The colon can also be filled with barium and air, which is called a double contrast study.

Because polyps take about five years to turn into cancers, routine examinations are recommended every three years.

Treatment

All polyps should be removed as preventive care. Most of them can be taken out through a colonoscope. Complications like obstruction and intussusception are surgical emergencies.

Prevention

Patients with hereditary disorders associated with polyps must undergo total colectomy early in adult life. All children of parents with these disorders should be screened early in adulthood, because half of them will have the same disease. For the bulk of the population, increased dietary fiber and decreased animal fat are the best preventives known at present. For the occasional intestinal polyp that arises in spite of good dietary habits, routine screening should prevent it from becoming cancerous.

Resources

BOOKS

Levin, Bernard. "Neoplasms of the Large and Small Intestines." In *Cecil Textbook of Medicine,* edited by J. Claude Bennett, and Fred Plum. Philadelphia: W. B. Saunders, 1996.

Mayer, Robert J. "Gastrointestinal Tract Cancer." In *Harrison's Principles of Internal Medicine,* edited by Anthony S. Fauci, et al. New York: McGraw-Hill, 1998.

Silverstein, Fred E. "Gastrointestinal Endoscopy." In *Harrison's Principles of Internal Medicine,* edited by Anthony S. Fauci, et al. New York: McGraw-Hill, 1998.

J. Ricker Polsdorfer

Intestinal strangulation *see* **Intestinal obstructions**

Intoxication confusional state *see* **Delirium**

Intracavity therapy *see* **Radioactive implants**

Intracranial abscess *see* **Brain abscess**

Intrauterine device *see* **IUD**

Intrauterine growth retardation

Definition

Intrauterine growth retardation (IUGR) occurs when the unborn baby is at or below the 10th weight percentile for his or her age (in weeks).

Description

There are standards or averages in weight for unborn babies according their age in weeks. When the baby's weight is at or below the 10th percentile for his or her age, it is called intrauterine growth retardation or fetal growth restriction. These babies are smaller than they should be for their age. How much a baby weighs at birth depends not only on how many weeks old it is, but the rate at which it has grown. This growth process is complex and delicate. There are three phases associated with the development of the baby. During the first phase, cells multiply in the baby's organs. This occurs from the beginning of development through the early part of the fourth month. During the second phase, cells continue to multiply and the organs grow. In the third phase (after 32 weeks of development), growth occurs quickly and the baby may gain as much as 7 ounces per week. If the delicate process of development and weight gain is disturbed or interrupted, the baby can suffer from restricted growth.

IUGR is usually classified as symmetrical or asymmetrical. In symmetrical IUGR, the baby's head and body are proportionately small. In asymmetrical IUGR, the baby's brain is abnormally large when compared to the liver. In a normal infant, the brain weighs about three times more than the liver. In asymmetrical IUGR, the brain can weigh five or six times more than the liver.

Causes & symptoms

Doctors think that the two types of IUGR may be linked to the time during development that the problem occurs. Symmetrical IUGR may occur when the unborn baby experiences a problem during early development. Asymmetrical IUGR may occur when the unborn baby experiences a problem during later development. While not true for all asymmetrical cases, doctors think that sometimes the placenta may allow the brain to get more oxygen and nutrition while the liver gets less.

There are many IUGR risk factors involving the mother and the baby. A mother is at risk for having a growth restricted infant if she:

• Has had a previous baby who suffered from IUGR

• Is small in size

• Has poor weight gain and nutrition during **pregnancy**

• Is socially deprived

• Uses substances (like tobacco, narcotics, alcohol) that can cause abnormal development or **birth defects**

• Has a vascular disease (like preeclampsia)

• Has chronic kidney disease

• Has a low total blood volume during early pregnancy

• Is pregnant with more than one baby

• Has an antibody problem that can make successful pregnancy difficult (antiphospholipid antibody syndrome).

Additionally, an unborn baby may suffer from IUGR if it has:

• Exposure to an infection, including German **measles** (**rubella**), cytomegalovirus, **tuberculosis, syphilis,** or **toxoplasmosis**

• A birth defect (like a severe cardiovascular defect)

• A chromosome defect, especially trisomy 18 (**Edwards' syndrome**)

• A primary disorder of bone or cartilage

• A chronic lack of oxygen during development (hypoxia)

• Placenta or umbilical cord defects

• Developed outside of the uterus.

Diagnosis

IUGR can be difficult to diagnose and in many cases doctors are not able to make an exact diagnosis until the baby is born. A mother who has had a growth restricted baby is at risk of having another during a later pregnancy. Such mothers are closely monitored during pregnancy. The length in weeks of the pregnancy must be carefully determined so that the doctor will know if development and weight gain are appropriate. Checking the mother's weight and abdomen measurements can help diagnose cases when there are no other risk factors present. Measuring the girth of the abdomen is often used as a tool for diagnosing IUGR. During pregnancy, the healthcare provider will use a tape measure to record the height of the upper portion of the uterus (the uterine fundal height). As the pregnancy continues and the baby grows, the uterus stretches upward in the direction of the mother's head. Between 18 and 30 weeks of gestation, the uterine fundal height (in cm.) equals the weeks of gestation. If the uterine fundal height is more than 2-3 cm below normal, then IUGR is suspected. Ultrasound is used to evaluate the growth of the baby. Usually, IUGR is diagnosed after week 32 of pregnancy. This is during the phase of rapid growth when the baby should be gaining more weight. IUGR caused by genetic factors or infection may sometimes be detected earlier.

Treatment

There is no treatment that improves fetal growth, but IUGR babies who are at or near term have the best outcome if delivered promptly. If IUGR is caused by a problem with the placenta and the baby is otherwise healthy, early diagnosis and treatment of the problem may reduce the chance of a serious outcome.

Prognosis

Babies who suffer from IUGR are at an increased risk for **death,** low blood sugar (**hypoglycemia**), low body temperature (**hypothermia**), and abnormal development of the nervous system. These risks increase with the severity of the growth restriction. The growth that occurs after birth cannot be predicted with certainty based on the size of the baby when it is born. Infants with asymmetrical IUGR are more likely to catch up in growth after birth than are infants who suffer from prolonged symmetrical IUGR. However, as of 1998, doctors cannot reliably predict an infant's future progress. Each case is unique. Some infants who have IUGR will develop normally, while others will have complications of the nervous system or intellectual problems like **learning**

disorders. If IUGR is related to a disease or a genetic defect, the future of the infant is related to the severity and the nature of that disorder.

Resources

BOOKS

Cunningham, F. Gary, et al. *Williams Obstetrics,* 20th ed. Stamford, CT: Appleton & Lange, 1997.

Linda Jones

Intravenous nutrition *see* **Nutrition through an intravenous line**

Intravenous pyelography *see* **Intravenous urography**

Intravenous rehydration

Definition

Sterile water solutions containing small amounts of salt or sugar, are injected into the body through a tube attached to a needle which is inserted into a vein.

Purpose

Fever, vomiting, and **diarrhea** can cause a person to become dehydrated fairly quickly. Infants and children are especially vulnerable to **dehydration.** Patients can become dehydrated due to an illness, surgery, or accident. Athletes who have overexerted themselves may also require rehydration with IV fluids. An IV for rehydration can be used for several hours to several days, and is generally used if a patient cannot drink fluids.

Precautions

Patients receiving IV therapy need to be monitored to ensure that the IV solutions are providing the correct amounts of fluids and **minerals** needed. People with kidney and heart disease are at increased risk for overhydration, so they must be carefully monitored when receiving IV therapy.

Description

Basic IV solutions are sterile water with small amounts of sodium (salt) or dextrose (sugar) supplied in bottles or thick plastic bags that can hang on a stand mounted next to the patient's bed. Additional minerals like potassium and calcium, **vitamins,** or drugs can be

---

KEY TERMS

Intravenous—Into a vein; a needle is inserted into a vein in the back of the hand, inside the elbow, or some other location on the body. Fluids, nutrients, and drugs can be injected.

---

added to the IV solution by injecting them into the bottle or bag with a needle.

Preparation

A doctor orders the IV solution and any additional nutrients or drugs to be added to it. The doctor also specifies the rate at which the IV will be infused. The IV solutions are prepared under the supervision of a doctor, pharmacist, or nurse, using sanitary techniques that prevent bacterial contamination. Just like a prescription, the IV is clearly labeled to show its contents and the amounts of any additives. The skin around the area where the needle is inserted is cleaned and disinfected. Once the needle is in place, it will be taped to the skin to prevent it from dislodging.

Aftercare

Patients need to take fluids by mouth before an IV solution is discontinued. After the IV needle is removed, the site should be inspected for any signs of bleeding or infection.

Risks

There is a small risk of infection at the injection site. It is possible that the IV solution may not provide all of the nutrients needed, leading to a deficiency or an imbalance. If the needle becomes dislodged, it is possible that the solution may flow into tissues around the injection site rather than into the vein.

Resources

BOOKS

Josephson, Dianne. *Intravenous Therapy for Nurses.* Albany, NY: Delmar Publishers, 1998.

"Water, Electrolyte, Mineral, and Acid-Base Metabolism." In *The Merck Manual.* 16th ed. Rahway, NJ: Merck, 1992.

PERIODICALS

Castellani, J.W., et al. "Intravenous vs. Oral Rehydration: Effects on Subsequent Exercise-Heat Stress." *Journal of Applied Physiology* 82(March 1997): 799–806.

OTHER

Martinez-Bianchi, Viviana, Michelle Rejman-Peterson, and Mark A. Graber. ''Pediatrics: Vomiting, Diarrhea, and Dehydration.'' In *University of Iowa Family Practice Handbook*. 3rd ed. http://www.vh.org/Providers/ClinRef/FPHandbook/Chapter10/17-10.html.

Toth, Peter P. ''Gastoenterology: Acute Diarrhea.'' In *University of Iowa Family Practice Handbook*. 3rd ed. http://www.vh.org/Providers/ClinRef/FPHandbook/Chapter04/01-4.html.

Altha Roberts Edgren

Intravenous urography

Definition

Intravenous urography is a test which x rays the urinary system using intravenous dye for diagnostic purposes.

Of the many ways to obtain images of the urinary system, the intravenous injection of a contrast agent has been traditionally considered the best. The kidneys excrete the dye into the urine. X rays can then create pictures of every structure through which the urine passes.

The procedure has several variations and many names.

- Intravenous pyelography (IVP).

- Urography.

- Pyelography.

- Antegrade pyelography differentiates this procedure from ''retrograde pyelography,'' which injects dye into the lower end of the system, therefore flowing backward or ''retrograde.'' Retrograde pyelography is better able to define problems in the lower parts of the system and is the only way to get x rays if the kidneys are not working well.

- Nephrotomography is somewhat different in that the x rays are taken by a moving x ray source onto a film moving in the opposite direction. By accurately coordinating the movement, all but a single plane of tissue is blurred, and that plane is seen without overlying shadows.

Every method available gives good pictures of this system, and the question becomes one of choosing among many excellent alternatives. Each condition has special requirements, while each technique has distinctive benefits and drawbacks.

- Nuclear scans rely on the radiation given off by certain atoms. Chemicals containing such atoms are injected into the bloodstream. They reach the kidneys, where images are constructed by measuring the radiation emitted. The radiation is no more dangerous than standard x rays. The images require considerable training to interpret, but unique information is often available using this technology. Different chemicals can concentrate the radiation in different types of tissue. This technique may require several days for the chemical to concentrate at its destination. It also requires a special detector to create the image.

- Ultrasound is a quick, safe, simple, and inexpensive way to obtain views of internal organs. Although less detailed than other methods, it may be sufficient.

- Retrograde pyelography is better able to define problems in the lower parts of the system and is the only way to get x rays if the kidneys are not working well. Dye is usually injected through an instrument (cystoscope) passed into the bladder through the urethra.

- **Computed tomography scans** (CT or CAT scanning) uses the same kind of radiation used in x rays, but it collects information by computer in such a way that three dimensional images can be constructed, eliminating interference from nearby structures. CT scanning requires a special apparatus.

- **Magnetic resonance imaging** (MRI) uses magnetic fields and radio frequency signals, instead of ionizing radiation, to create computerized images. This form of energy is entirely safe as long as the patient has no metal on board. The technique is far more versatile than CT scanning. MRI requires special apparatus and, because of the powerful magnets needed, even a special building all by itself. It is quite expensive.

Purpose

Most diseases of the kidneys, ureters, and bladder will yield information to this procedure, which actually has two phases. First, it requires a functioning kidney to filter the dye out of the blood into the urine. The time required for the dye to appear on x rays correlates accurately with kidney function. The second phase gives detailed anatomical images of the urinary tract. Within the first few minutes the dye "lights up" the kidneys, a phase called the nephrogram. Subsequent pictures follow the dye down the ureters and into the bladder. A final film taken after urinating reveals how well the bladder empties.

IVPs are most often done to assess structural abnormalities or obstruction to urine flow. If kidney function is at issue, more films are taken sooner to catch the earliest phase of the process.

- Stones, tumors and congenital malformations account for many of the findings.

- Kidney cysts and **cancers** can be seen.

- Displacement of a kidney or ureter suggests a space-occupying lesion like a cancer pushing it out of the way.

- Bad valves where the ureters enter the bladder will often show up.

- **Bladder cancers** and other abnormalities are often outlined by the dye in the bladder.

- An **enlarged prostate** gland will show up as incomplete bladder emptying and a bump at the bottom of the bladder.

Precautions

The only serious complication of an IVP is allergy to the iodine-containing dye that is used. Such an allergy is rare, but it can be dramatic and even lethal. Emergency measures taken immediately are usually effective.

Description

IVPs are usually done in the morning. In the x ray suite, the patient will undress and lie down. There are two methods of injecting the dye. An intravenous line can be established, through which the dye will be consistently fed through the body during the procedure. The other method is to give the dye all at once through a needle that is immediately withdrawn. X rays are taken until the dye has reached the bladder, an interval of half an hour or less. The patient will be asked to empty the bladder before one last x ray.

Preparation

Emptying the bowel with **laxatives** or **enemas** prevents bowel shadows from obscuring the details of the urinary system. An empty stomach prevents the complications of vomiting, a rare effect of the contrast agent. Therefore, the night before the IVP the patient will be asked to evacuate the bowels and to drink sparingly.

Risks

Allergy to the contrast agent is the only risk. Anyone with a possible iodine allergy or a previous reaction to x ray dye must be particularly careful to inform the x ray personnel.

Resources

BOOKS

Merrill, Vinta. *Atlas of roentgenographic positions and standard radiologic procedures.* Saint Louis, MO: The C.V. Mosby Company, 1975.

J. Ricker Polsdorfer

Intussusception *see* **Intestinal obstructions**

Iodine *see* **Antiseptics**

Iodine deficiency *see* **Mineral deficiency**

Iodine excess: Copper excess *see* **Mineral toxicity**

Iodine uptake test *see* **Thyroid nuclear medicine scan**

Ipratropium *see* **Bronchodilators**

I.Q. tests *see* **Stanford-Binet intelligence scales; Wechsler intelligence test**

Iridocyclitis *see* **Uveitis**

Iritis *see* **Uveitis**

Iron deficiency anemia

Definition

Anemia can be caused by iron deficiency, folate deficiency, vitamin B_{12} deficiency, and other causes. The term iron deficiency anemia means anemia that is due to iron deficiency. Iron deficiency anemia is characterized by the production of small red blood cells. When examined under a microscope, the red blood cells also appear pale or light colored. For this reason, the anemia that occurs with iron deficiency is also called hypochronic microcytic anemia.

KEY TERMS

Hematocrit—The proportion of whole blood in the body, by volume, that is composed of red blood cells.

Hemoglobin—Hemoglobin is an iron-containing protein that resides within red blood cells. Hemoglobin accounts for about 95% of the protein in the red blood cell.

Protoporphyrin IX—Protoporphyrin IX is a protein. The measurement of this protein is useful for the assessment of iron status. Hemoglobin consists of a complex of a protein plus heme. Heme consists of iron plus protoporphyrin IX. Normally, during the course of red blood cell formation, protoporphyrin IX acquires iron, to generate heme, and the heme becomes incorporated into hemoglobin. However, in iron deficiency, protophoryrin IX builds up.

Recommended Dietary Allowance (RDA)—The Recommended Dietary Allowances (RDAs) are quantities of nutrients of the diet that are required to maintain human health. RDAs are established by the Food and Nutrition Board of the National Academy of Sciences and may be revised every few years.

Description

Iron deficiency anemia is the most common type of anemia throughout the world. In the United States, iron deficiency anemia occurs to a lesser extent than in developing countries because of the higher consumption of red meat and the practice of food fortification (addition of iron to foods by the manufacturer). Anemia in the United States is caused by a variety of sources, including excessive losses of iron in menstrual fluids and excessive bleeding in the gastrointestinal tract. In developing countries located in tropical climates, the most common cause of iron deficiency anemia is infestation with hookworm.

Causes & symptoms

Infancy is a period of increased risk for iron deficiency. The human infant is born with a built-in supply of iron, which can be tapped during periods of drinking low-iron milk or formula. Both human milk and cow milk contain rather low levels of iron (0.5-1.0 mg iron/liter). However, the iron in human milk is about 50% absorbed by the infant, while the iron of cow milk is only 10% absorbed. During the first six months of life, growth of the infant is made possible by the milk in the diet and by the infant's built-in supply. However, premature infants have a lower supply of iron and, for this reason, it is recommended that pre-term infants (beginning at 2 months of age) be given oral supplements of 7 mg iron/day, as ferrous sulfate. Iron deficiency can be provoked where infants are fed formulas that are based on unfortified cow milk. For example, unfortified cow milk is given free of charge to mothers in Chile. This practice has the fortunate result of preventing general **malnutrition,** but the unfortunate result of allowing the development of mild iron deficiency.

The normal rate of blood loss in the feces is 0.5-1.0 ml per day. These losses can increase with **colorectal cancer.** About 60% of colorectal cancers result in further blood losses, where the extent of blood loss is 2-10 ml/day. **Cancer** of the colon and rectum can provoke losses of blood, resulting in iron deficiency anemia. The fecal blood test is widely used to screen for the presence of cancer of the colon or rectum. In the absence of testing, colorectal cancer may be first detected because of the resulting iron deficiency anemia.

Infection with hookworm can provoke iron deficiency and iron deficiency anemia. The hookworm is a parasitic worm. It thrives in warm climates, including in the southern United States. The hookworm enters the body through the skin, as through bare feet. The hookworm then migrates to the small intestines where it attaches itself to the villi (small sausage-shaped structures in the intestines that are used for the absorption of all nutrients). The hookworm provokes damage to the villi, resulting in blood loss, and they produce anti-coagulants which promote continued bleeding. Each worm can provoke the loss of up to 0.25 ml of blood per day.

Bleeding and blood losses through gastrointestinal tract can be provoked by colorectal cancer and hookworms, as mentioned above, but also by **hemorrhoids,** anal fissures, **irritable bowel syndrome,** aspirin-induced bleeding, blood clotting disorders, and diverticulosis (a condition caused by an abnormal opening from the intestine or bladder). Several genetic diseases exist which lead to bleeding diorders, and these include **hemophilia** A, hemophilia B, and **von Willebrand's disease.** Of these, only von Willebrand's disease leads to gastrointestinal bleeding.

The symptoms of iron deficiency anemia include weakness and fatigue. These symptoms result because of the lack of function of the red blood cells, and the reduced ability of the red blood cells to carry iron to exercising muscles. Iron deficiency can also affect other tissues, including the tongue and fingernails. Prolonged iron deficiency can result in changes of the tongue, and it may become smooth, shiny, and reddened. This condition is called glossitis. The fingernails may grow abnormally, and acquire a spoon-shaped appearance.

Decreased iron intake is a contributing factor in iron deficiency and iron deficiency anemia. The iron content of cabbage, for example, is about 1.6 mg/kg food, while that of spinach (33 mg/kg), lima beans (15 mg/kg), potato (14 mg/kg), tomato (3 mg/kg), apples (1.5 mg/kg), raisins (20 mg/kg), whole wheat bread (43 mg/kg), eggs (20 mg/kg), canned tuna (13 mg/kg), chicken (11 mg/kg), beef (28 mg/kg), corn oil (0.6 mg/kg), and peanut butter (6.0 mg/kg), are indicated. One can see that apples, tomatoes, and vegetable oil are relatively low in iron, while whole wheat bread and beef are relatively high in iron. The assessment of whether a food is low or high in iron can also be made by comparing the amount of that food eaten per day with the recommended dietary allowance (RDA) for iron. The RDA for iron for the adult male is 10 mg/day, while that for the adult woman is 15 mg/day. The RDA during **pregnancy** is 30 mg/day. The RDA for infants of 0-0.5 years of age is 6 mg/day, while that for infants of 0.5-1.0 years of age is 10 mg/day. The RDA values are based on the assumption that the consumer eats a mixture of plant and animal foods.

The above list of iron values alone may be deceptive, since the availability of iron in fruits, vegetables, and grains is very low, while that the availability from meat is much higher. The availability of iron in plants ranges from only 1-10%, while that in meat, fish, chicken, and liver is 20-30%. The term availability means the percent of dietary iron that is absorbed via the gastrointestinal tract to the bloodstream. Non-absorbed iron is lost in the feces.

Interactions between various foods can influence the absorption of dietary iron. Vitamin C can increase the absorption of dietary iron. Orange juice is a rich source of vitamin C. Thus, if a plant food, such as rice, is consumed with orange juice, then the orange juice can enhance the absorption of the iron of the rice. Vitamin C is also added to infant formulas, and the increased use of formulas fortified with both iron and vitamin C have led to a marked decline in anemia in infants and young children in the United States (Dallman, 1989). In contrast, if rice is consumed with tea, certain chemicals in the tea (tannins) can reduce the absorption of the iron. Phytic acid is a chemical that naturally occurs in legumes, cereals, and nuts. Phytic acid, which can account for 1-5% of the weight of these foods, is a potent inhibitor of iron absorption. The increased availability of the iron in meat products is partly due to the fact that heme-iron is absorbed to a greater extent than free iron salts, and to a greater extent than iron in the phytic acid/iron complex. Nearly all of the iron in plants is nonheme-iron. Much of the iron in meat is nonheme-iron as well. The nonheme-iron in meat, fish, chicken and liver may be about 20% available. The heme-iron of meat may be close to 30% available. The most available source of iron is human milk (50% availability).

Diagnosis

Iron deficiency anemia in infants is defined as a hemoglobin level below 109 mg/ml of whole blood, and a **hematocrit** of under 33%. Anemia in adult males is defined as a hemoglobin under 130 mg/ml and a hematocrit of under 38%. Anemia in adult females is defined as hemoglobin under 120 mg/ml and a hematocrit of under 32%. Anemia in pregnant women is defined as hemoglobin of under 110 mg/ml and hematocrit of under 31%.

When an abnormally high presence of blood is found in the feces during a fecal occult blood test, the physician needs to examine the gastrointestinal tract to determine the cause of bleeding. Here, the diagnosis for iron deficiency anemia includes the examination using a sigmoidoscope. The sigmoidoscope is an instrument that consists of a flexible tube that permits examination of the colon to a distance of 60 cm. A **barium enema,** with an x ray, may also be used to detect abnormalities that can cause bleeding.

The diagnosis of iron deficiency anemia should include a test for oral iron absorption, where evidence suggests that oral iron supplements fail in treating anemia. The oral iron absorption test is conducted by eating 64 mg iron (325 mg ferrous sulfate) in a single dose. Blood samples are then taken after 2 hours and 4 hours. The iron content of the blood serum is then measured. The concentration of iron should rise by an increment of about 22 micromolar, where iron absorption is normal. Lesser increases in concentration mean that iron absorption is abnormal, and that therapy should involve injections or infusions of iron.

Treatment

Oral iron supplements (pills) may contain various iron salts. These iron salts include ferrous sulfate, ferrous gluconate, or ferrous fumarate. Injections and infusions of iron can be carried out with a preparation called iron dextran. In patients with poor iron absorption (by the gut), therapy with injection or infusion is preferable over oral supplements. Treatment of iron deficiency anemia sometimes requires more than therapy with iron. Where iron deficiency was provoked by hemorrhoids, surgery may prove essential to prevent recurrent iron deficiency anemia. Where iron deficiency is provoked by bleeding due to aspirin treatment, aspirin should be discontinued. Where iron deficiency is provoked by hookworm infections, therapy for this parasite should be used, along with protection of the feet by wearing shoes whenever walking in hookworm-infested soil.

Prognosis

The prognosis for treating and curing iron deficiency anemia is excellent. Perhaps the main problem is failure to take iron supplements. In cases of pregnant women, the health care worker may recommend taking 100-200 mg iron/day. This dose is rather high, and can lead to nausea, **diarrhea,** or abdominal **pain** in 10-20 % of women taking this dose. The reason for using this high dose is to effect a rapid cure for anemia, where the anemia is detected at a mid-point during the pregnancy. The above problems of sideeffects and noncompliance can be avoided by taking iron doses (100-200 mg) only once a week, where supplements are initiated some time prior to conception, or continuously throughout the fertile period of life. The problem of compliance is not an issue where infusions are used, however a fraction of patients treated with iron infusions experience sideeffects, such as flushing, **headache,** nausea, **anaphylaxis,** or seizures. A number of studies have shown that iron deficiency anemia in infancy can result in reduced intelligence, where intelligence was measured in early childhood. It is not certain if iron supplementation of children with reduced intelligence, due to iron-deficiency anemia in infancy, has any influence in allowing a "catch-up" in intellectual development.

Prevention

In the healthy population, all of the mineral deficiencies can be prevented by the consumption of inorganic nutrients at levels defined by the RDA. Iron deficiency anemia in infants and young children can be prevented by the use of fortified foods. Liquid cow milk-based infant formulas are generally supplemented with iron (12 mg/L). The iron in liquid formulas is added as ferrous sulfate or ferrous gluconate. Commercial infant cereals are also fortified with iron, and here small particles of elemental iron are added. The levels used are about 0.5 gram iron/kg dry cereal. This amount of iron is about 10-fold greater than that of the iron naturally present in the cereal.

Resources

BOOKS

Brody, Tom. *Nutritional Biochemistry.* San Diego, CA: Academic Press, 1998.

"Food and Nutrition Board." *Recommended Dietary Allowances.* Washington, D.C.: National Academy Press, 1989.

PERIODICALS

Pennington, J., S. Schoen, G. Salmon, B. Young, R. Johnson, and R. Marts."Composition of core foods of the U.S. food supply, 1982-1991."*Journal of Food Composition and Analysis* 8 (1995): 129-169.

Swain, R., B. Kaplan, and E. Montgomery. "Iron deficiency anemia."*Postgraduate Medicine* 100 (1996): 181-193.

Walter, T., P. Pino, F. Pizarro, and B. Lozoff. "Prevention of iron-deficiency anemia: comparison of high- and low-iron formulas in term healthy infants after six months of life."*Journal of Pediatrics* 132 (1998): 635-640.

Tom Brody

Iron overload *see* **Hemochromatosis**

Iron tests

Definition

Iron tests are a group of blood tests that are done to evaluate the iron level in blood serum, the body's capacity to absorb iron, and the amount of iron actually stored in the body. Iron is an essential trace element; it is necessary for the formation of red blood cells and certain enzymes. At the other extreme, high levels of iron can be poisonous.

Purpose

There are four different types of tests that measure the body's iron levels and storage. They are called iron level tests, total iron-binding capacity (TIBC) tests, ferritin tests, and transferrin tests. These tests are given for several reasons:

• To help in the differential diagnosis of different types of anemia.

• To assess the severity of anemia and monitor the treatment of patients with chronic anemia.

• To evaluate protein depletion and other forms of **malnutrition.**

• To check for certain liver disorders.

• To evaluate the possibility of chronic gastrointestinal bleeding. Blood loss from the digestive tract is a common cause of **iron deficiency anemia.**

• To help diagnose certain unusual disorders, including iron poisoning, **thalassemia,** hemosiderosis, and **hemochromatosis.**

A serum iron test can be used without the others to evaluate cases of iron poisoning.

Precautions

Patients should not have their blood tested for iron within four days of a blood **transfusion** or tests and treatments that use radioactive materials. Recent high

KEY TERMS

Anemia—A disorder marked by low hemoglobin levels in red blood cells, which leads to a deficiency of oxygen in the blood.

Ferritin—A protein found in the liver, spleen, and bone marrow that stores iron.

Hemochromatosis—A disorder of iron absorption characterized by bronze-colored skin. It can cause painful joints, diabetes, and liver damage if the iron concentration is not lowered.

Hemosiderosis—An overload of iron in the body resulting from repeated blood transfusions. Hemosiderosis occurs most often in patients with thalassemia.

Iron poisoning—A potentially fatal condition caused by swallowing large amounts of iron dietary supplements. Most cases occur in children who have taken adult- strength iron formulas. The symptoms of iron poisoning include vomiting, bloody diarrhea, convulsions, low blood pressure, and turning blue.

Plasma—The liquid part of blood.

Siderophilin—Another name for transferrin.

Thalassemia—A hereditary form of anemia that occurs most frequently in people of Mediterranean origin.

Transferrin—A protein in blood plasma that carries iron derived from food intake to the liver, spleen, and bone marrow.

stress levels or sleep deprivation are additional reasons for postponing iron tests.

Blood samples for iron tests should be taken early in the morning because serum iron levels vary during the day. This precaution is especially important in evaluating the results of iron replacement therapy.

Description

Iron tests are performed on samples of the patient's blood, withdrawn from a vein into a vacuum tube. The amount of blood taken is between 6 mL and 10 mL (1/3 of a fluid ounce). The procedure, which is called a venipuncture, takes about five minutes.

Iron level test

The iron level test measures the amount of iron in the blood serum that is being carried by a protein (transferrin) in the blood plasma.

Medications and substances that can cause *increased* iron levels include chloramphenicol, estrogen preparations, dietary iron supplements, alcoholic beverages, methyldopa, and birth control pills.

Medications that can cause *decreased* iron levels include ACTH, colchicine, deferoxamine, methicillin, and testosterone.

Total iron-binding capacity (TIBC) test

The TIBC test measures the amount of iron that the blood would carry if the transferrin were fully saturated. Since transferrin is produced by the liver, the TIBC can be used to monitor liver function and nutrition.

Medications that can cause *increased* TIBC levels include fluorides and birth control pills.

Medications that can cause *decreased* TIBC levels include chloramphenicol and ACTH.

Transferrin test

The transferrin test is a direct measurement of transferrin—which is also called siderophilin—levels in the blood. Some laboratories prefer this measurement to the TIBC. The saturation level of the transferrin can be calculated by dividing the serum iron level by the TIBC.

Ferritin test

The ferritin test measures the level of a protein in the blood that stores iron for later use by the body.

Medications that can cause *increased* ferritin levels include dietary iron supplements. In addition, some diseases that do not directly affect the body's iron storage can cause artificially high ferritin levels. These disorders include infections, late stage **cancers**, lymphomas, and severe inflammations. Alcoholics often have high ferritin levels.

Preparation

Patient history

Before patients are tested for iron, they should be checked for any of the following factors:

• Prescription medications that affect iron levels, absorption, or storage

• Blood transfusion or radioactive medications within the last four days

• Recent extreme stress or sleep deprivation

• Recent eating habits. Test results can be affected by eating large amounts of iron-rich foods shortly before the blood test.

Fasting

Patients scheduled for an iron level, TIBC, or transferrin test should fast for 12 hours before the blood is drawn. They are allowed to drink water. Patients scheduled for a ferritin test do not need to fast but they should not have any alcoholic beverages before the test.

Aftercare

Aftercare consists of routine care of the area around the venipuncture.

Risks

The primary risk is the possibility of a bruise or swelling in the area of the venipuncture. The patient can apply moist warm compresses if there is any discomfort.

Normal results

Iron level test

Normal serum iron values are as follows:

- Adult males: 75-175 micrograms/dL
- Adult females: 65-165 micrograms/dL
- Children: 50-120 micrograms/dL
- Newborns: 100-250 micrograms/dL.

TIBC test

Normal TIBC values are as follows:

- Adult males: 300-400 micrograms/dL
- Adult females: 300-450 micrograms/dL.

Transferrin test

Normal transferrin values are as follows:

- Adult males: 200-400 mg/dL
- Adult females: 200-400 mg/dL
- Children: 203-360 mg/dL
- Newborns: 130-275 mg/dL.

Normal transferrin saturation values are between 30-40%.

Ferritin test

Normal ferritin values are as follows:

- Adult males: 20-300 ng/mL
- Adult females: 20-120 ng/mL
- Children (one month): 200-600 ng/mL
- Children (two to five months): 50-200 ng/mL
- Children (six months to 15 years): 7-140 ng/mL
- Newborns: 25-200 ng/mL.

Abnormal results

Iron level test

Serum iron level is *increased* in thalassemia, hemochromatosis, severe hepatitis, liver disease, **lead poisoning,** acute leukemia, and kidney disease. It is also increased by multiple blood transfusions and intramuscular iron injections.

Iron levels above 350-500 micrograms/dL are considered toxic; levels over 1000 micrograms/dL indicate severe iron poisoning.

Serum iron level is *decreased* in iron deficiency anemia, chronic blood loss, chronic diseases (lupus, **rheumatoid arthritis**), late **pregnancy,** chronically heavy menstrual periods, and thyroid deficiency.

TIBC test

The TIBC is *increased* in iron deficiency anemia, **polycythemia** vera, pregnancy, blood loss, severe hepatitis, and the use of birth control pills.

The TIBC is *decreased* in malnutrition, severe **burns,** hemochromatosis, anemia caused by infections and chronic diseases, **cirrhosis** of the liver, and kidney disease.

Transferrin test

Transferrin is *increased* in iron deficiency anemia, pregnancy, **hormone replacement therapy** (HRT), and the use of birth control pills.

Transferrin is *decreased* in protein deficiency, liver damage, malnutrition, severe burns, kidney disease, chronic infections, and certain genetic disorders.

Ferritin test

Ferritin is *increased* in liver disease, iron overload from hemochromatosis, certain types of anemia, acute leukemia, **Hodgkin's disease, breast cancer,** thalassemia, infections, inflammatory diseases, and hemosiderosis. Ferritin levels may be normal or slightly above normal in patients with kidney disease.

Ferritin is *decreased* in chronic iron deficiency and severe protein depletion.

Resources

BOOKS

Fischbach, Frances Talaska. *A Manual of Laboratory and Diagnostic Tests.* Philadelphia and New York: Lippincott, 1996.

Mosby's Diagnostic and Laboratory Test Reference, edited by Kathleen Deska Pagana, and Timothy James Pagana. St. Louis: Mosby-Year Book, Inc., 1997.

Springhouse Corporation. *Everything You Need to Know About Medical Tests,* edited by Michael Shaw et al. Springhouse, PA: Springhouse Corporation, 1996.

Rebecca J. Frey

Iron-binding capacity test *see* **Iron tests**

Iron-utilization anemias *see* **Sideroblastic anemias**

Irregular bite *see* **Malocclusion**

Irritable bowel syndrome

Definition

Irritable bowel syndrome (IBS) is a common intestinal condition characterized by abdominal **pain** and cramps; changes in bowel movements (**diarrhea, constipation,** or both); gassiness; bloating; nausea; and other symptoms. There is no cure for IBS. Much about the condition remains unknown or poorly understood; however, dietary changes, drugs, and psychological treatment are often able to eliminate or substantially reduce its symptoms.

Description

IBS is the name people use today for a condition that was once called—among other things—colitis, mucous colitis, spastic colon, nervous colon, spastic bowel, and functional bowel disorder. Some of these names reflected the now outdated belief that IBS is a purely psychological disorder, a product of the patient's imagination. Although modern medicine recognizes that **stress** can trigger IBS attacks, medical specialists agree that IBS is a genuine physical disorder—or group of disorders—with specific identifiable characteristics.

No one knows for sure how many Americans suffer from IBS. Surveys indicate a range of 10-20%, with perhaps as many as 30% of Americans experiencing IBS at some point in their lives. IBS normally makes its first appearance during young adulthood, and in half of all cases symptoms begin before age 35. Women with IBS outnumber men by two to one, for reasons that are not yet understood. IBS is responsible for more time lost from work and school than any medical problem other than the **common cold.** It accounts for a substantial proportion of the patients seen by specialists in diseases of the digestive system (gastroenterologists). Yet only half—possibly as few as 15%—of IBS sufferers ever consult a doctor.

KEY TERMS

Anus—The opening at the lower end of the rectum.

Crohn's disease—A disease characterized by inflammation of the intestines. Its early symptoms may resemble those of IBS.

Defecation—Passage of feces through the anus.

Feces—Undigested food and other waste that is eliminated through the anus. Feces are also called fecal matter or stools.

Lactose—A sugar found in milk and milk products. Some people are lactose intolerant, meaning they have trouble digesting lactose. Lactose intolerance can produce symptoms resembling those of IBS.

Peristalsis—The periodic waves of muscular contractions that move food through the intestines during the process of digestion.

Ulcerative colitis—A disease that inflames and causes breaks (ulcers) in the colon and rectum, which are parts of the large intestine.

Causes & symptoms

Symptoms

The symptoms of IBS tend to rise and fall in intensity rather than growing steadily worse over time. They always include abdominal pain, which may be relieved by defecation; diarrhea or constipation; or diarrhea alternating with constipation. Other symptoms—which vary from person to person—include cramps; gassiness; bloating; nausea; a powerful and uncontrollable urge to defecate (urgency); passage of a sticky fluid (mucus) during bowel movements; or the feeling after finishing a bowel movement that the bowels are still not completely empty. The accepted diagnostic criteria—known as the Rome criteria—require at least three months of continuous or recurrent symptoms before IBS can be confirmed. According to Christine B. Dalton and Douglas A. Drossman in the *American Family Physician,* an estimated 70% of IBS cases can be described as "mild;" 25% as "moderate;" and 5% as "severe." In mild cases the symptoms are slight. As a general rule, they are not present all the time and do not interfere with work and other normal activities. Moderate IBS occasionally disrupts normal activities and may cause some psychological problems. People with severe IBS often find living a normal life impossible and experience crippling psychological problems as a result. For some the physical pain is constant and intense.

Causes

Researchers remain unsure about the cause or causes of IBS. It is called a functional disorder because it is thought to result from changes in the activity of the major part of the large intestine (the colon). After food is digested by the stomach and small intestine, the undigested material passes in liquid form into the colon, which absorbs water and salts. This process may take several days. In a healthy person the colon is quiet during most of that period except after meals, when its muscles contract in a series of wavelike movements called peristalsis. Peristalsis helps absorption by bringing the undigested material into contact with the colon wall. It also pushes undigested material that has been converted into solid or semisolid feces toward the rectum, where it remains until defecation. In IBS, however, the normal rhythm and intensity of peristalsis is disrupted. Sometimes there is too little peristalsis, which can slow the passage of undigested material through the colon and cause constipation. Sometimes there is too much, which has the opposite effect and causes diarrhea. A Johns Hopkins University study found that healthy volunteers experienced 6–8 contractions of the colon each day, compared with up to 25 contractions a day for volunteers suffering from IBS with diarrhea, and an almost complete absence of contractions among constipated IBS volunteers. In addition to differences in the number of contractions, many of the IBS volunteers experienced powerful spasmodic contractions affecting a larger-than-normal area of the colon—''like having a Charlie horse in the gut,'' according to one of the investigators.

DIET

Some kinds of food and drink appear to play a key role in triggering IBS attacks. Food and drink that healthy people can ingest without any trouble may disrupt peristalsis in IBS patients, which probably explains why IBS attacks often occur shortly after meals. Chocolate, milk products, **caffeine** (in coffee, tea, colas, and other drinks), and large quantities of alcohol are some of the chief culprits. Other kinds of food have also been identified as problems, however, and the pattern of what can and cannot be tolerated is different for each person. Characteristically, IBS symptoms rarely occur at night and disrupt the patient's sleep.

STRESS

Stress is an important factor in IBS because of the close nervous system connections between the brain and the intestines. Although researchers do not yet understand all of the links between changes in the nervous system and IBS, they point out the similarities between mild digestive upsets and IBS. Just as healthy people can feel nauseated or have an upset stomach when under stress, people with IBS react the same way, but to a greater degree. Finally, IBS symptoms sometimes intensify during menstruation, which suggests that female reproductive hormones are another trigger.

Diagnosis

Diagnosing IBS is a fairly complex task because the disorder does not produce changes that can be identified during a **physical examination** or by laboratory tests. When IBS is suspected, the doctor (who can be either a family doctor or a specialist) needs to determine whether the patient's symptoms satisfy the Rome criteria. The doctor must rule out other conditions that resemble IBS, such as **Crohn's disease** and **ulcerative colitis.** These disorders are ruled out by questioning the patient about his or her physical and mental health (the medical history), performing a physical examination, and ordering laboratory tests. Normally the patient is asked to provide a stool sample that can be tested for blood and intestinal parasites. In some cases x rays or an internal examination of the colon using a flexible instrument inserted through the anus (a sigmoidoscope or colonoscope) is necessary. The doctor also may ask the patient to try a lactose-free diet for two or three weeks to see whether lactose intolerance is causing the symptoms.

Treatment

Dietary changes, sometimes supplemented by drugs or psychotherapy, are considered the key to successful treatment. The following approach, offered by Dalton and Drossman, is typical of the advice found in the medical literature on IBS. The authors tie their approach to the severity of the patient's symptoms:

Mild symptoms

Dalton and Drossman recommend a low-fat, high-fiber diet. Problem-causing substances such as lactose, caffeine, beans, cabbage, cucumbers, broccoli, fatty foods, alcohol, and medications should be identified and avoided. Bran or 15-25 grams a day of an over-the-counter psyllium laxative (Metamucil or Fiberall) may also help both constipation and diarrhea. The patient can still have milk or milk products if lactose intolerance is not a problem. People with irregular bowel habits—particularly constipated patients—may be helped by establishing set times for meals and bathroom visits.

Moderate symptoms

The advice given by Dalton and Drossman in mild cases applies here as well. They also suggest that patients keep a diary of symptoms for two or three weeks, covering daily activities including meals, and emotional responses to events. The doctor can then review the diary with the patient to identify possible problem areas.

Although a high-fiber diet remains the standard treatment for constipated patients, such **laxatives** as lactulose (Chronulac) or sorbitol may be prescribed. Loperamide (Imodium) and cholestyramine (Questran) are suggested for diarrhea. Abdominal pain after meals can be reduced by taking **antispasmodic drugs** such as hyoscyamine (Anaspaz, Cystospaz, or Levsin) or dicyclomine (Bemote, Bentyl, or Di-Spaz) before eating.

Dalton and Drossman also suggest psychological counseling or behavioral therapy for some patients to reduce **anxiety** and to learn to cope with the pain and other symptoms of IBS. Relaxation therapy, **hypnosis, biofeedback,** and **cognitive-behavioral therapy** are examples of behavioral therapy.

Severe symptoms

When IBS produces constant pain that interferes with everyday life, **antidepressant drugs** can help by blocking pain transmission from the nervous system. Dalton and Drossman also underscore the importance of an ongoing and supportive doctor-patient relationship.

Alternative treatment

Alternative and mainstream approaches to IBS treatment overlap to a certain extent. Like mainstream doctors, alternative practitioners advise a high-fiber diet to reduce digestive system irritation. They also suggest avoiding alcohol, caffeine, and fatty, gassy, or spicy foods. Recommended stress management techniques include **yoga, meditation,** hypnosis, biofeedback, and **reflexology.** Reflexology is a technique of foot massage that is thought to relieve diarrhea, constipation, and other IBS symptoms.

Alternative medicine also emphasizes such herbal remedies as ginger (*Zingiber officinale*), buckthorn (*Rhamnus purshiana*), and enteric-coated peppermint oil. Enteric coating prevents digestion until the peppermint oil reaches the small intestine, thus avoiding irritation of the upper part of the digestive tract. Chamomile (*Matricaria recutita*), valerian (*Valeriana officinalis*), rosemary (*Rosemarinus officinalis*), lemon balm (*Melissa officinalis*), and other herbs are recommended for their antispasmodic properties. The list of alternative treatments for IBS is in fact quite long. It includes **aromatherapy,** homeopathy, **hydrotherapy,** juice therapy, **acupuncture, chiropractic, osteopathy, naturopathic medicine,** and **Chinese traditional herbal medicine.**

Prognosis

IBS is not a life-threatening condition. It does not cause intestinal bleeding or inflammation, nor does it cause other bowel diseases or **cancer.** Although IBS can last a lifetime, in up to 30% of cases the symptoms eventually disappear. Even if the symptoms cannot be eliminated, with appropriate treatment they can usually be brought under control to the point where IBS becomes merely an occasional inconvenience. Treatment requires a long-term commitment, however; six months or more may be needed before the patient notices substantial improvement.

Resources

BOOKS

The Burton Goldberg Group. *Alternative Medicine: The Definitive Guide.* Puyallup, WA: Future Medicine Publishing, 1993.

Lynn, Richard B., and Lawrence S. Friedman. "Irritable Bowel Syndrome." In *Harrison's Principles of Internal Medicine,* edited by Anthony S. Fauci, et al. New York: McGraw-Hill, 1998.

PERIODICALS

Dalton, Christine B., and Douglas A. Drossman. "Diagnosis and Treatment of Irritable Bowel Syndrome." *American Family Physician* (February 1997): 875 + .

Hendricks, Melissa. "Bowels in an Uproar." *Johns Hopkins Magazine* (April 1997). http://www.jhu.edu/~jhumag/ 0497web/gastro1.html (1 May 1998).

"Irritable Bowel Syndrome: Treating the Mind to Treat the Body." *Tufts University Health & Nutrition Letter* (September 1997): 4 + .

Maxwell, P. R., M. A. Mendall, and D. Kumar. "Irritable Bowel Syndrome." *The Lancet* 350(1997): 1691 + .

ORGANIZATIONS

International Foundation for Functional Gastrointestinal Disorders. PO Box 17864, Milwaukee, WI 53217. (888) 964-2001. http://www.execpc.com/iffgd.

National Digestive Diseases Information Clearinghouse. 2 Information Way, Bethesda, MD 20892-3570. http:// www.niddk.nih.gov/health/digest/nddic.htm.

Howard Baker

Ischemia

Definition

Ischemia is an insufficient supply of blood to an organ, usually due to a blocked artery.

Description

Myocardial ischemia is an intermediate condition in **coronary artery disease** during which the heart tissue is slowly or suddenly starved of oxygen and other nutrients.

KEY TERMS

Atherosclerosis—A process in which the walls of the arteries thicken due to the accumulation of plaque in the blood vessels. Atherosclerosis is the cause of most coronary artery disease.

Coronary artery disease—A narrowing or blockage, due to atherosclerosis, of the arteries that provide oxygen and nutrients to the heart. When blood flow is cut-off, the result is a heart attack.

Plaque—A deposit of fatty and other substances that accumulate in the lining of the artery wall.

Stroke—A sudden decrease or loss of consciousness caused by rupture or blockage of a blood vessel by a blood clot or hemorrhage in the brain. Ischemic strokes are caused by blood clots in a cerebral artery.

Eventually, the affected heart tissue will die. When blood flow is completely blocked to the heart, ischemia can lead to a **heart attack.** Ischemia can be silent or symptomatic. According to the American Heart Association, up to four million Americans may have silent ischemia and be at high risk of having a heart attack with no warning.

Symptomatic ischemia is characterized by chest **pain** called **angina** pectoris. The American Heart Association estimates that nearly seven million Americans have angina pectoris, usually called angina. Angina occurs more frequently in women than in men, and in blacks and Hispanics more than in whites. It also occurs more frequently as people age—25% of women over the age of 85 and 27% of men who are 80-84 years old have angina.

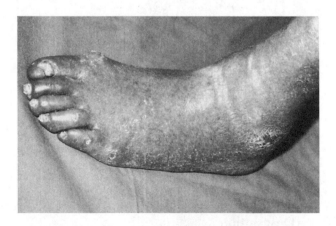

This patient's foot is affected with ischemia. Ischemia occurs when there is an insufficient supply of blood to a specific organ or tissue. *(Photograph by Dr. P. Marazzi, Photo Researchers, Inc. Reproduced by permission.)*

People with angina are at risk of having a heart attack. Stable angina occurs during exertion, can be quickly relieved by resting or taking nitroglycerine, and lasts from three to twenty minutes. Unstable angina, which increases the risk of a heart attack, occurs more frequently, lasts longer, is more severe, and may cause discomfort during rest or light exertion.

Ischemia can also occur in the arteries of the brain, where blockages can lead to a **stroke.** About 80-85% of all strokes are ischemic. Most blockages in the cerebral arteries are due to a blood clot, often in an artery narrowed by plaque. Sometimes, a blood clot in the heart or aorta travels to a cerebral artery. A **transient ischemic attack** (TIA) is a "mini-stroke" caused by a temporary deficiency of blood supply to the brain. It occurs suddenly, lasts a few minutes to a few hours, and is a strong warning sign of an impending stroke. Ischemia can also effect intestines, legs, feet and kidneys. Pain, malfunctions, and damage in those areas may result.

Causes & symptoms

Ischemia is almost always caused by blockage of an artery, usually due to atherosclerotic plaque. Myocardial ischemia is also caused by blood clots (which tend to form on plaque), artery spasms or contractions, or any of these factors combined. Silent ischemia is usually caused by emotional or mental **stress** or by exertion, but there are no symptoms. Angina is usually caused by increased oxygen demand when the heart is working harder than usual, for example, during **exercise,** or during mental or physical stress. According to researchers at Harvard University, physical stress is harder on the heart than mental stress. A TIA is caused by a blood clot briefly blocking a cerebral artery.

Risk factors

The risk factors for myocardial ischemia are the same as those for coronary artery disease. For TIA, coronary artery disease is also a risk factor.

• Heredity. People whose parents have coronary artery disease are more likely to develop it. African-Americans are also at higher risk.

• Sex. Men are more likely to have heart attacks than women, and to have them at a younger age.

• Age. Men who are 45 years of age and older and women who are 55 years of age and older are considered to be at risk.

• Smoking. Smoking increases both the chance of developing coronary artery disease and the chance of dying from it. Second hand smoke may also increase risk.

• High cholesterol. Risk of developing coronary artery disease increases as blood cholesterol levels increase.

When combined with other factors, the risk is even greater.

- High blood pressure. High blood pressure makes the heart work harder, and with time, weakens it. When combined with **obesity,** smoking, high cholesterol, or diabetes, the risk of heart attack or stroke increases several times.

- Lack of physical activity. Lack of exercise increases the risk of coronary artery disease.

- **Diabetes mellitus.** The risk of developing coronary artery disease is seriously increased for diabetics.

- Obesity. Excess weight increases the strain on the heart and increases the risk of developing coronary artery disease, even if no other risk factors are present. Obesity increases blood pressure and blood cholesterol, and can lead to diabetes.

- Stress and anger. Some scientists believe that stress and anger can contribute to the development of coronary artery disease. Stress increases the heart rate and blood pressure and can injure the lining of the arteries. Angina attacks often occur after anger, as do many heart attacks and strokes.

Angina symptoms include:

- A tight, squeezing, heavy, burning, or **choking** pain that is usually beneath the breastbone—the pain may spread to the throat, jaw, or one arm

- A feeling of heaviness or tightness that isn't painful

- A feeling similar to gas or **indigestion**

- Attacks brought on by exertion and relieved by rest.

If the pain or discomfort continues or intensifies, immediate medical help should be sought, ideally within 30 minutes.

TIA symptoms include:

- Sudden weakness, tingling, or numbness, usually in one arm or leg or both the arm and leg on the same side of the body, as well as sometimes in the face

- Sudden loss of coordination

- Loss of vision or double vision

- Difficulty speaking

- Vertigo and loss of balance.

Diagnosis

Diagnostic tests for myocardial ischemia include: resting, exercise, or ambulatory electrocardiograms; scintigraphic studies (radioactive heart scans); echocardiography; coronary **angiography;** and, rarely, positron emission tomography. Diagnostic tests for TIA include physician review of symptoms, **computed to-** mography scans (CT scans), carotid artery ultrasound (**Doppler ultrasonography**), and **magnetic resonance imaging.** Angiography is the best test for ischemia of any organ.

An electrocardiogram (ECG) shows the heart's activity and may reveal a lack of oxygen. Electrodes covered with conducting jelly are placed on the patient's chest, arms, and legs. Impulses of the heart's activity are recorded on paper. The test takes about 10 minutes and is performed in a physician's office. About 25% of patients with angina have normal electrocardiograms. Another type of electrocardiogram, the exercise **stress test,** measures response to exertion when the patient is exercising on a treadmill or a stationary bike. It is performed in a physician's office or an exercise laboratory and takes 15 to 30 minutes. This test is more accurate than a resting ECG in diagnosing ischemia. Sometimes an ambulatory ECG is ordered. For this test, the patient wears a portable ECG machine called a Holter monitor for 12, 24, or 48 hours.

Myocardial perfusion scintigraphy and radionuclide angiography are nuclear studies involving the injection of a radioactive material (e.g., thallium) which is absorbed by healthy tissue. A gamma scintillation camera displays and records a series of images of the radioactive material's movement through the heart. Both tests are usually performed in a hospital's nuclear medicine department and take about 30 minutes to an hour. A perfusion scan is sometimes performed at the end of a stress test.

An echocardiogram uses sound waves to create an image of the heart's chambers and valves. The technician applies gel to a hand-held transducer then presses it against the patient's chest. The heart's sound waves are converted into an image on a monitor. Performed in a cardiology outpatient diagnostic laboratory, the test takes 30 minutes to an hour. It can reveal abnormalities in the heart wall that indicate ischemia, but it doesn't evaluate the coronary arteries directly.

Coronary angiography is the most accurate diagnostic technique, but it is also the most invasive. It shows the heart's chambers, great vessels, and coronary arteries by using a contrast solution and x ray technology. A moving picture is recorded of the blood flow through the coronary arteries. The patient is awake, but sedated, and connected to ECG electrodes and an intravenous line. A local anesthetic is injected. The cardiologist then inserts a catheter into a blood vessel and guides it into the heart. Coronary angiography is performed in a **cardiac catheterization** laboratory and takes from half an hour to two hours.

Positron emission tomography (PET) is a noninvasive nuclear test used to evaluate the heart tissue. A PET scanner traces high-energy gamma rays released from radioactive particles to provide three-dimensional images of the heart tissue. Performed at a hospital, it usually takes from one hour to one hour and 45 minutes. PET is very expensive and not widely available.

Computed tomography scans (CT scans) and magnetic resonance imaging (MRI) are computerized scanning methods. CT scanning uses a thin x-ray beam to show three-dimensional views of soft tissues. It is performed at a hospital or clinic and takes less than a minute. MRI uses a magnetic field to produce clear, cross-sectional images of soft tissues. The patient lies on a table which slides into a tunnel-like scanner. It is usually performed at a hospital and takes about 30 minutes.

Treatment

Angina is treated with drug therapy and surgery. Drugs such as nitrates, beta-blockers, and **calcium channel blockers** relieve chest pain, but they cannot clear blocked arteries. **Aspirin** helps prevent blood clots. Surgical procedures include percutaneous transluminal coronary **angioplasty** and coronary artery bypass graft surgery.

Nitroglycerin is the classic treatment for angina. It quickly relieves pain and discomfort by opening the coronary arteries and allowing more blood to flow to the heart. **Beta blockers** reduce the amount of oxygen required by the heart during stress. Calcium channel blockers help keep the arteries open and reduce blood pressure. Aspirin helps prevent blood clots from forming on plaques.

Percutaneous transluminal coronary angioplasty and coronary artery bypass graft surgery are invasive procedures which improve blood flow in the coronary arteries. Percutaneous transluminal coronary angioplasty is a nonsurgical procedure in which a catheter tipped with a balloon is threaded from a blood vessel in the thigh into the blocked artery. The balloon is inflated, compressing the plaque to enlarge the blood vessel and open the blocked artery. The balloon is deflated and the catheter is removed. The procedure is performed by a cardiologist in a hospital and generally requires a two-day stay. Sometimes a metal stent is placed in the artery to prevent closing of the artery.

In coronary artery bypass graft, called bypass surgery, a detour is built around the coronary artery blockage with a healthy leg vein or chest wall artery. The healthy vein or artery then supplies oxygen-rich blood to the heart. Bypass surgery is major surgery appropriate for patients with blockages in two or three major coronary arteries or severely narrowed left main coronary arteries, as well as those who have not responded to other treatments. It is performed in a hospital under general anesthesia using a heart-lung machine to support the patient while the healthy vein or artery is attached to the coronary artery.

There are several experimental surgical procedures: **atherectomy,** where the surgeon shaves off and removes strips of plaque from the blocked artery; laser angioplasty, where a catheter with a laser tip is inserted to burn or break down the plaque; and insertion of a metal coil, called a stent, that can be implanted permanently to keep a blocked artery open. This stenting procedure is becoming more common. Another experimental procedure uses a laser to drill channels in the heart muscle to increase blood supply.

TIAs are treated by drugs that control high blood pressure and reduce the likelihood of blood clots and surgery. Aspirin is commonly used and anticoagulants are sometimes used to prevent blood clots. In some cases, carotid **endarterectomy** surgery is performed to help prevent further TIAs. The procedure involves removing arterial plaque from inside blood vessels.

The use of **chelation therapy,** a long-term injection by a physician of a cocktail of synthetic amino acid, ethylenediaminetetracetric acid, and anticoagulant drugs and nutrients, is controversial.

Alternative treatment

Ischemia can be life-threatening. Although there are alternative treatments for angina, traditional medical care may be necessary. Prevention of the cause of ischemia, primarily atherosclerosis, is primary. This becomes even more important for people with a family history of heart disease. Dietary modifications, especially the reduction or elimination of saturated fats (primarily found in meat), are essential. Increased fiber (found in fresh fruits and vegetables, grains, and beans) can help the body eliminate excessive cholesterol through the stools. Exercise, particularly aerobic exercise, is essential for circulation health. Not smoking will prevent damage from smoke and the harmful substances it contains.

Abana, a mixture of herbs and **minerals** used in **ayurvedic medicine,** can reduce the frequency and severity of angina attacks. Western herbal medicine recommends hawthorn (*Crataegus laevigata* or *C. oxyacantha*) to relieve long-term angina, since it strengthens the contractility of the heart muscles. Nutritional supplements and botanical medicines that act as antioxidants, for example, vitamins C and E, selenium, gingko (*Gingko biloba*), bilberry (*Vaccinium myrtillus*), and hawthorn, can help prevent initial arterial injury that can lead to the formation of plaque deposits. Cactus (*Cactus grandiflorus*) is a homeopathic remedy used for pain relief during an attack. Mind/body relaxation techniques such as **yoga** and **biofeedback** can help control strong emotions and stress.

Prognosis

In many cases, ischemia can be successfully treated, but the underlying disease process of **atherosclerosis** is usually not "cured." New diagnostic techniques enable doctors to identify ischemia earlier. New technologies and surgical procedures can prevent angina from leading to a heart attack or TIA from resulting in a stroke. The outcome for patients with silent ischemia has not been well established.

Prevention

A healthy lifestyle, including eating right, getting regular exercise, maintaining a healthy weight, not smoking, drinking in moderation, not using illegal drugs, controlling **hypertension,** and managing stress are practices that can reduce the risk of ischemia progressing to a heart attack or stroke.

A healthy diet includes a variety of foods that are low in fat, especially saturated fat; low in cholesterol; and high in fiber. Plenty of fruits and vegetables should be eaten and sodium should be limited. Fat should comprise no more than 30% of total daily calories. Cholesterol should be limited to about 300 mg and sodium to about 2,400 mg per day.

Moderate aerobic exercise lasting about 30 minutes four or more times per week is recommended for maximum heart health, according to the Centers for Disease Control and Prevention and the American College of Sports Medicine. Three 10-minute exercise periods are also beneficial. If any risk factors are present, a physician's clearance should be obtained before starting exercise.

Maintaining a desirable body weight is also important. People who are 20% or more over their ideal body weight have an increased risk of developing coronary artery disease or stroke.

Smoking has many adverse effects on the heart and arteries, so should be avoided. Heart damage caused by smoking can be improved by quitting. Several studies have shown that ex-smokers face the same risk of heart disease as non-smokers within five to ten years of quitting.

Excessive drinking can increase risk factors for heart disease. Modest consumption of alcohol, however, can actually protect against coronary artery disease. The American Heart Association defines moderate consumption as one ounce of alcohol per day—roughly one cocktail, one 8-ounce glass of wine, or two 12-ounce glasses of beer.

Commonly used illegal drugs can seriously harm the heart and should never be used. Even stimulants like ephedra and **decongestants** like pseudoephedrine can be harmful to patients with hypertension or heart disease.

Treatment should be sought for hypertension. High blood pressure can be completely controlled through lifestyle changes and medication. Stress, which can increase the risk of a heart attack or stroke, should also be managed. While it cannot always be avoided, it can be controlled.

Resources

BOOKS

American Heart Association. *Heart Attack Treatment, Prevention, Recovery.* New York: Time Books, 1996.

"Angina." In *The Alternative Advisor: The Complete Guide to Natural Therapies & Alternative Treatments.* Alexandria, VA: Time-Life Books, 1997.

DeBakey, Michael E. and Antonio M. Gotto Jr. "Coronary Artery Disease," and "Stroke." In *The New Living Heart.* Holbrook, MA: Adams Media Corporation, 1997.

Iskandrian, A.S. and Mario S. Verani. "Scintigraphic Techniques in Acute Ischemic Syndromes." In *Nuclear Cardiac Imaging: Principles and Applications,* 2nd ed. Philadelphia: F.A. Davis, 1996.

Tierney, Lawrence M. Jr, Stephen J. McPhee, and Maxine A. Papadakis. "Coronary Heart Disease (Arteriosclerotic Coronary Artery Disease; Ischemic Heart Disease)." In *Current Medical Diagnosis & Treatment,* 36th ed. Stamford, CT: Appleton & Lange, 1997.

PERIODICALS

Geraci, Ron and Duane Swierczynski. "Short Strokes." *Men's Health* (September 1997): 56.

"How Mental Stress Taxes the Heart." *Harvard Health Letter* (March 1997):2.

ORGANIZATIONS

American Heart Association. National Center. 7272 Greenville Avenue, Dallas, TX 75231-4596. (214) 373-6300. http://www.medsearch.com/pf/profiles/amerh/.

National Heart, Lung, and Blood Institute Information Center. P.O. Box 30105, Bethesda, MD 20824-0105. http://www.nhlbi.gov/nhlbi/nhbli.htm.

Texas Heart Institute Heart Information Service. P.O. Box 20345, Houston, TX 77225-0345. 1-800-292-2221. http://www.tmc.edu/thi/his.html.

OTHER

"Transient Ischemic Attack." *American Academy of Neurology.* 1997. http://www.aan.com/public/tran.html (25 March 1998).

Lori De Milto

Isocarboxazid *see* **Monoamine oxidase inhibitors**

Isokinetic exercises *see* **Exercise**

Isolation

Definition

Isolation refers to the precautions that are taken in the hospital to prevent the spread of an infectious agent from an infected or colonized patient to susceptible persons.

Purpose

Isolation practices are designed to minimize the transmission of infection in the hospital, using current understanding of the way infections can transmit. Isolation should be done in a user friendly, well-accepted, inexpensive way that interferes as little as possible with patient care, minimizes patient discomfort, and avoids unnecessary use.

Precautions

The type of precautions used should be viewed as a flexible scale that may range from the least to the most demanding methods of prevention. These methods should always take into account that differences exist in the way that diseases are spread. Recognition and understanding of these differences will avoid use of insufficient or unnecessary interventions.

Description

Isolation practices can include placement in a private room or with a select roommate, the use of protective barriers such as masks, gowns and gloves, a special emphasis on handwashing (which is always very important), and special handling of contaminated articles. Because of the differences among infectious diseases, more than one of these precautions may be necessary to prevent spread of some diseases but may not be necessary for others.

The Centers for Disease Control and Prevention (CDC) and the Hospital Infection Control Practice Advisory Committee (HICPAC) have led the way in defining the guidelines for hospital-based infection precautions. The most current system recommended for use in hospitals consists of two levels of precautions. The first level is Standard Precautions which apply to all patients at all times because signs and symptoms of infection are not always obvious and therefore may unknowingly pose a risk for a susceptible person. The second level is known as Transmission-Based Precautions which are intended for individuals who have a known or suspected infection with certain organisms.

Frequently, patients are admitted to the hospital without a definite diagnosis, but with clues to suggest an

---

infection. These patients should be isolated with the appropriate precautions until a definite diagnosis is made.

Standard Precautions

Standard Precautions define all the steps that should be taken to prevent spread of infection from person to person when there is an anticipated contact with:

- Blood
- Body fluids
- Secretions, such as phlegm
- Excretions, such as urine and feces (not including sweat) whether or not they contain visible blood
- Nonintact skin, such as an open wound
- Mucous membranes, such as the mouth cavity.

Standard Precautions includes the use of one or combinations of the following practices. The level of use will always depend on the anticipated contact with the patient:

- Handwashing, the most important infection control method
- Use of latex or other protective gloves
- Masks, eye protection and/or face shield
- Gowns
- Proper handling of soiled patient care equipment
- Proper environmental cleaning
- Minimal handling of soiled linen
- Proper disposal of needles and other sharp equipment such as scalpels
- Placement in a private room for patients who cannot maintain appropriate cleanliness or contain body fluids.

Transmission Based Precautions

Transmission Based Precautions may be needed in addition to Standard Precautions for selected patients who are known or suspected to harbor certain infections. These precautions are divided into three categories that reflect the differences in the way infections are transmitted. Some diseases may require more than one isolation category.

AIRBORNE PRECAUTIONS

Airborne Precautions prevent diseases that are transmitted by minute particles called droplet nuclei or contaminated dust particles. These particles, because of their size, can remain suspended in the air for long periods of time; even after the infected person has left the room. Some examples of diseases requiring these precautions are **tuberculosis, measles,** and **chickenpox.**

A patient needing Airborne Precautions should be assigned to a private room with special ventilation requirements. The door to this room must be closed at all possible times. If a patient must move from the isolation room to another area of the hospital, the patient should be wearing a mask during the transport. Anyone entering the isolation room to provide care to the patient must wear a special mask called a respirator.

DROPLET PRECAUTIONS

Droplet Precautions prevent the spread of organisms that travel on particles much larger than the droplet nuclei. These particles do not spend much time suspended in the air, and usually do not travel beyond a several foot range from the patient. These particles are produced when a patient **coughs,** talks, or sneezes. Examples of disease requiring droplet precautions are meningococcal **meningitis** (a serious bacterial infection of the lining of the brain), **influenza, mumps,** and German measles **(rubella).**

Patients who require Droplet Precautions should be placed in a private room or with a roommate who is infected with the same organism. The door to the room may remain open. Health care workers will need to wear masks within 3 ft of the patient. Patients moving about the hospital away from the isolation room should wear a mask.

CONTACT PRECAUTIONS

Contact Precautions prevent spread of organisms from an infected patient through direct (touching the patient) or indirect (touching surfaces or objects that that been in contact with the patient) contact. Examples of patients who might be placed in Contact Precautions are those infected with:

• Antibiotic-resistant bacteria

• Hepatitis A

• Scabies

• Impetigo

• Lice.

This type of precaution requires the patient to be placed in a private room or with a roommate who has the same infection. Health care workers should wear gloves when entering the room. They should change their gloves if they touch material that contains large volumes of organisms such as soiled dressings. Prior to leaving the room, health care workers should remove the gloves and wash their hands with medicated soap. In addition, they may need to wear protective gowns if there is a chance of contact with potentially infective materials such as **diarrhea** or wound drainage that cannot be contained or if there is likely to be extensive contact with the patient or environment.

Patient care items, such as a stethoscope, that are used for a patient in Contact Precautions should not be shared with other patients unless they are properly cleaned and disinfected before reuse. Patients should leave the isolation room infrequently.

Resources

BOOKS

Edmond, M. "Isolation." In *A Practical Handbook for Hospital Epidemiologists,* edited by L.A. Herwaldt and M.D. Decker. Thorofare, NJ: Slack Inc., 1998.

Garner, J.S. "Universal Precautions and Isolation Systems." In *Hospital Infections,* edited by J.V. Bennett and P.S. Brachman. Boston: Little, Brown, 1992.

PERIODICALS

U.S. Department of Health and Human Services. Centers for Disease Control and Prevention. "Draft Guideline for Isolation Precautions in Hospitals." *Federal Register* 59(1994): 55552-55570.

Suzanne M. Lutwick

Isometric exercises *see* **Exercise**

Isoniazid *see* **Antituberculosis drugs**

Isosorbide dinitrate *see* **Antiangina drugs**

Isotonic exercises *see* **Exercise**

Isotretinoin *see* **Antiacne drugs**

Isradipine *see* **Calcium channel blockers**

Itching

Definition

Itching is an intense, distracting irritation or tickling sensation that may be felt all over the skin's surface, or confined to just one area. The medical term for itching is "pruritus."

Description

Itching instinctively leads most people to scratch the affected area. Different people can tolerate different amounts of itching, and anyone's threshold of tolerance can be changed due to **stress,** emotions, and other factors. In general, itching is more severe if the skin is warm, and if there are few distractions. This is why people tend to notice itching more at night.

Causes & symptoms

The reason for the sensation of itching is not well understood. While itching is the most noticeable symptom in many skin diseases, but it doesn't necessary mean that a person who feels itchy has a disease.

Stress and emotional upset can make itching worse, no matter what the underlying cause. If emotional problems are the primary reason for the itch, the condition is known as psychogenic itching. Some people become convinced that their itch is caused by a parasite; this conviction is often linked to burning sensations in the tongue, and may be caused by a major psychiatric disorder.

Generalized itching

Itching that occurs all over the body may indicate a medical condition such as **diabetes mellitus,** liver disease, kidney failure, **jaundice,** thyroid disorders (and rarely, **cancer).** Blood disorders such as leukemia, and lymphatic conditions such as **Hodgkin's disease** may sometimes cause itching as well.

Some people may develop an itch without a rash when they take certain drugs (such as **aspirin,** codeine, cocaine); others may develop an itchy red "drug rash" or **hives** because of an allergy to a specific drug.

Itching also may be caused when any of the family of hookworm larvae penetrate the skin. This includes swimmer's itch and creeping eruption caused by cat or dog hookworm, and ground itch caused by the "true" hookworm.

Many skin conditions cause an itchy rash. These include:

- **Atopic dermatitis**
- **Chickenpox**

KEY TERMS

Atopic dermatitis—An intensely itchy inflammation often found on the face of people prone to allergies. In infants and early childhood, it's called infantile eczema.

Creeping eruption—Itchy irregular, wandering red lines on the foot made by burrowing larvae of the hookworm family and some roundworms.

Dermatitis herpetiformis—A chronic very itchy skin disease with groups of red lesions that leave spots behind when they heal. It is sometimes associated with cancer of an internal organ.

Eczema—A superficial type of inflammation of the skin that may be very itchy and weeping in the early stages; later, the affected skin becomes crusted, scaly, and thick. There is no known cause.

Hodgkin's disease—A type of cancer characterized by a slowly-enlarging lymph tissue; symptoms include generalized itching.

Lichen planus—A noncancerous, chronic itchy skin disease that causes small, flat purple plaques on wrists, forearm, ankles.

Neurodermatitis—An itchy skin disease (also called lichen simplex chronicus) found in nervous, anxious people.

Psoriasis—A common, chronic skin disorder that causes red patches anywhere on the body. Occasionally, the lesions may itch.

Scabies—A contagious parasitic skin disease characterized by intense itching.

Swimmer's itch—An allergic skin inflammation caused by a sensitivity to flatworms that die under the skin, causing an itchy rash.

- **Contact dermatitis**
- **Dermatitis** herpetiformis (occasionally)
- Eczema
- Fungus infections (such as **athlete's foot**)
- Hives (urticaria)
- Insect bites
- Lice
- **Lichen planus**
- Neurodermatitis (**lichen simplex** chronicus)
- **Psoriasis** (occasionally)
- **Scabies.**

On the other hand, itching all over the body can be caused by something as simple as bathing too often, which removes the skins natural oils and may make the skin too dry and scaly.

Localized itching

Specific itchy areas may occur if a person comes in contact with soap, detergents, and wool or other rough-textured, scratchy material. Adults who have **hemorrhoids,** anal fissure, or persistent **diarrhea** may notice itching around the anus (called ''pruritus ani''). In children, itching in this area is most likely due to worms.

Intense itching in the external genitalia in women (''pruritus vulvae'') may be due to **candidiasis,** hormonal changes, or the use of certain spermicides or vaginal suppositories, ointments, or deodorants.

It's also common for older people to suffer from dry, itchy skin (especially on the back) for no obvious reason. Younger people also may notice dry, itchy skin in cold weather. Itching is also a common complaint during **pregnancy.**

Diagnosis

Itching is a symptom that is quite obvious to its victim. Someone who itches all over should seek medical care. Because itching can be caused by such a wide variety of triggers, a complete physical exam and medical history will help diagnose the underlying problem. A variety of blood and stool tests may help determine the underlying cause.

Treatment

Antihistamines such as diphenhydramine (Benadryl) can help relieve itching caused by hives, but won't affect itching from other causes. Most antihistamines also make people sleepy, which can help patients sleep who would otherwise be awake from the itch.

Specific treatment of itching depends on the underlying condition that causes it. In general, itchy skin should be treated very gently. While scratching may temporarily ease the itch, in the long run scratching just makes it worse. In addition, scratching can lead to an endless cycle of itch—scratch—more itching.

To avoid the urge to scratch, a person can apply a cooling or soothing lotion or cold compress when the urge to scratch occurs. Soaps are often irritating to the skin, and can make an itch worse; they should be avoided, or used only when necessary.

Creams or ointments containing cortisone may help control the itch from insect bites, contact dermatitis or eczema. Cortisone cream should not be applied to the face unless a doctor prescribes it.

Probably the most common cause of itching is dry skin. There are a number of simple things a person can do to ease the annoying itch:

- Don't wear tight clothes
- Avoid synthetic fabrics
- Don't take long baths
- Wash the area in lukewarm water with a little baking soda
- For generalized itching, take a lukewarm shower
- Try a lukewarm oatmeal (or Aveeno) bath for generalized itching
- Apply bath oil or lotion (without added colors or scents) right after bathing.

People who itch as a result of mental problems or stress should seek help from a mental health expert.

Prognosis

Most cases of itching go away when the underlying cause is treated successfully.

Prevention

There are certain things people can do to avoid itchy skin. Patients who tend toward itchy skin should:

- Avoid a daily bath
- Use only lukewarm water when bathing
- Use only gentle soap
- Pat dry, not rub dry, after bathing, leaving a bit of water on the skin
- Apply a moisture-holding ointment or cream after the bath
- Use a humidifier in the home.

Patients who are allergic to certain substances, medications, and so on can avoid the resulting itch if they avoid contact with the allergen. Avoiding insect bites, bee stings, poison ivy and so on can prevent the resulting itch. Treating sensitive skin carefully, avoiding over-drying of the skin, and protecting against diseases that cause itchy **rashes** are all good ways to avoid itching.

Resources

BOOKS

Donahue, Peggy Jo. *Relief from Chronic Skin Problems.* New York: Dell Publishing, 1992.

Olbricht, Suzanne, Michael Bigby, and Kenneth Arndt. *Manual of Clinical Problems in Dermatology.* Boston: Little, Brown, 1992.

Turkington, Carol A., and Jeffrey S. Dover. *Skin Deep: An A to Z of Skin Disorders, Treatments and Health.* New York: Facts on File, 1998.

PERIODICALS
Bogin, Rob. "Don't Scratch That Itch." *Rocky Mountain News* (Oct. 5, 1997): 6F.

Carol A. Turkington

Itraconazole *see* **Systemic antifungal drugs**

IUD

Definition

An IUD is an intrauterine device made of plastic and/or copper that is inserted into the womb (uterus) by way of the vaginal canal. One type releases a hormone (progesterone), and is replaced each year. The second type is made of copper and can be left in place for five years. The most common shape in current use is a plastic "T" which is wrapped with copper wire.

Purpose

IUDs are used to prevent **pregnancy** and are considered to be 95-98% effective. It should be noted that IUDs offer no protection against the acquired immunodeficiency syndrome (**AIDS**) virus or other **sexually transmitted diseases** (STDs).

Precautions

IUDs are placed in the uterus by physicians. Prior to placement the doctor will take a medical history, do a **physical examination,** and take a **Pap test.** Women who have had tubal pregnancies, an abnormal Pap smear, or abnormal vaginal bleeding are generally disqualified from using this form of **contraception.** Also, women who have STDs, an allergy to copper, severe **pain** with periods (menstruation), sex with multiple partners, or who are currently pregnant are not eligible for an IUD. There are no age restrictions.

Description

There is continuing controversy over exactly how IUDs prevent pregnancy. Some researchers think pregnancy is controlled by preventing conception (fertilization), while others believe that the devices prevent embryo attachment to the uterine wall (implantation).

IUDs which release a hormone may prevent pregnancy in several ways. Since one hormonal response is a thickening of the mucous at the entrance to the uterus, it is more difficult for the sperm to gain entry. This prevents the sperm from reaching an ovum. At the same time, the

lining of the uterus becomes thinner, making it more difficult for a fertilized egg to implant itself in the uterus. The copper device slowly releases copper which is believed to weaken and perhaps kill sperm. An alternate explanation is that these objects "sweep" the uterus, dislodging any fertilized egg that attempts to implant itself. In addition, both devices tend to cause a mild inflammatory reaction in the lining of the uterus which also has an adverse impact on implantation.

Preparation

After the physician approves the use of an IUD, the woman's genital area is washed thoroughly with soap and water in preparation of IUD insertion. The opening into the uterus (cervix) will also be cleaned with an antiseptic such as an iodine solution. Actual IUD insertion takes about five minutes, during which a local anesthesia is used to reduce any discomfort associated with the procedure. A plastic string connected to the IUD will hang out of the uterus into the vagina. The string is used to periodically check the position of the IUD.

Aftercare

The woman will be taught to watch for the signs and symptoms of potential complications and how to check the string, which should be done at least once a week. To check the string, the woman should first wash her hands with soap and water. From a squatting position, or with one foot elevated (such as on a chair), she should gently insert her finger into the vagina until she the cervix. If she cannot feel the string, if the string feel longer than it should, or if she can feel part of the IUD she should notify her physician immediately. Additional information that needs to be reported includes painful intercourse and unusual discharge from the vagina.

Risks

Serious risks are rare, but include heavy bleeding, pain, infection, cramps, **pelvic inflammatory disease,** perforation of the uterus, and **ectopic pregnancy.**

Resources

BOOKS

Dickason, Elizabeth Jean, Bonnie Lang Silverman, and Judith A. Kaplan. *Maternal-Infant Nursing Care.* St. Louis, MO: Mosby-Year Book Inc., 1998.

Gorrie, Trula Meyers, Emily Slone McKinney, and Sharon Smith Murray. *Foundations of Maternal-Newborn Nursing.* Philadelphia, PA: W.B. Saunders Company, 1998.

Nichols, Francine H. and Elaine Zwelling. *Maternal-Newborn Nursing: Theory and Practice.* Philadelphia, PA: W. B. Saunders Company, 1997.

Olds, Sally B., Marcia L. London, and Patricia Wieland Ladewig. *Maternal-Newborn Nursing: A Family Centered Approach.* Menlo Park, CA: Addison-Wesley, 1996.

ORGANIZATIONS

Planned Parenthood Federation of America Inc. 810 Seventh Avenue, New York, NY 10019. 800-669-0156. http://www.plannedparenthood.org/.

OTHER

"The Copper IUD: Typical Questions." *Network* 16 (Winter 1996). http://reservoir.fhi.org/fp/fppubs/network/v16-2/nt16210.html (February 11, 1998).

Intrauterine Device (IUD). Planned Parenthood League of Massachusetts. http://www.pplm.org/iud.html (February 11, 1998).

The IUD (Intrauterine Device): Answers to Your Questions. AVSC International. http://www.avsc.org/iud.html (February 4, 1998).

Keller, Sarah. "IUDs Block Fertilization." *Network* 16 (Winter 1996). http://reservoir.fhi.org/fp/fppubs/network/v16-2/nt1623.html.

Keller, Sarah. "Contraceptive Update: LNg IUD Offers Less Bleeding." *Network* 16 (Winter 1996). http://reservoir.fhi.org/fp/fppubs/network/v16-2/nt1629.html (February 11, 1998).

Donald Gardner Barstow

Ivory bones *see* **Osteopetroses**

IVP *see* **Intravenous urography**

Ivy method *see* **Bleeding time**

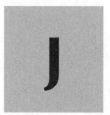

J

Japanese encephalitis

Definition

Japanese encephalitis is an infection of the brain caused by a virus. The virus is transmitted to humans by mosquitoes.

Description

The virus that causes Japanese encephalitis is called an arbovirus, which is an arthropod-borne virus. Mosquitoes are a type of arthropod. Mosquitoes in a number of regions carry this virus and are responsible for passing it along to humans. Many of these areas are in Asia, including Japan, Korea, China, India, Thailand, Indonesia, Malaysia, Vietnam, Taiwan, and the Philippines. Areas where the disease-causing arbovirus is always present are referred to as being endemic for the disease. In such areas, blood tests will reveal that more than 70% of all adults have been infected at some point with the arbovirus.

Because the virus that causes Japanese encephalitis is carried by mosquitoes, the number of people infected increases during those seasons when mosquitoes are abundant. This tends to be in the warmest, rainiest months. In addition to humans, other animals like wild birds, pigs, and horses are susceptible to infection with this arbovirus. Because the specific type of mosquito carrying the Japanese encephalitis arbovirus frequently breeds in rice paddies, the disease is considered to be primarily a rural problem.

Causes & symptoms

The virus is transferred to a human when an infected mosquito sucks that person's blood. Once in the body, the virus travels to various glands where it multiplies. The virus can then enter the bloodstream. Ultimately, the virus settles in the brain, where it causes serious problems.

KEY TERMS

Antibody—A type of cell made by the immune system that has the ability to recognize markers (antigens) on the surface of invading organisms, like bacteria and viruses.

Encephalitis—A swelling of the brain, potentially causing serious brain damage.

Endemic—Naturally and consistently present in a certain geographical region.

Japanese encephalitis begins with **fever,** severe **headache,** nausea, and vomiting. As the tissue covering the brain and spinal cord (the meninges) becomes infected and swollen, the patient will develop a stiff and painful neck. By day two or three, the patient begins to suffer the effects of swelling in the brain. These effects include:

- Problems with balance and coordination

- **Paralysis** of some muscle groups

- **Tremors**

- Seizures

- Lapses in consciousness

- A stiff, mask-like appearance of the face.

The patient becomes dehydrated and loses weight. If the patient survives the illness, the fever will decrease by about day seven and the symptoms will begin to improve by about day 14. Other patients will continue to have extremely high fevers and their symptoms will get worse. In these cases, **coma** and then **death** occur in 7-14 days. Many patients who recover have permanent disabilities due to brain damage.

Diagnosis

Most diagnostic techniques for Japanese encephalitis do not yield results very quickly. The diagnosis is made primarily on the basis of the patient's symptoms and the knowledge of the kinds of illnesses endemic to a particular geographic region.

Immunofluorescence tests, where special viral markers react with human antibodies that have been tagged with a fluorescent chemical, are used to verify the disease. However, these results tend to be unavailable until week two of the infection. Other tests involve comparing the presence and quantity of particular antibodies in the blood or spinal fluid during week one with those present during week two of the illness.

Treatment

There are no treatments available to stop or slow the progression of Japanese encephalitis. Only the symptoms of each patient can be treated. Fluids are given to decrease **dehydration** and medications are given to decrease fever and pain. Medications are available to attempt to decrease brain swelling. Patients in a coma may require mechanical assistance with breathing.

Prognosis

While the majority of people infected with arbovirus never become sick, those who develop Japanese encephalitis become very ill. Some outbreaks have a 50% death rate. A variety of long-term problems may haunt those who recover from the illness. These problems include:

- Movement difficulties where the arms, legs, or body jerks or writhes involuntarily

- Shaking

- Paralysis

- Inability to control emotions

- Loss of mental abilities

- Mental disturbances, including **schizophrenia** (which may affect as many as 75% of Japanese encephalitis survivors).

Young children are most likely to have serious, long-term problems after an infection.

Prevention

A three-dose vaccine is available for Japanese encephalitis and is commonly given to young children in areas where the disease is endemic. Travelers to these regions can also receive the vaccine.

Controlling the mosquito population with insecticides is another preventive measure. Visitors to regions with high rates of Japanese encephalitis should take precautions (like using mosquito repellents and sleeping under a bed net) to avoid contact with mosquitoes.

Resources

BOOKS

Douglas, R. Gordon. "Other Arthropod-Borne Viruses." In *Cecil Textbook of Medicine,* edited by J. Claude Bennett and Fred Plum. Philadelphia: W. B. Saunders, 1996.

Ray, C. George. "Arthropod-Borne and Other Zoonotic Viruses." In *Sherris Medical Microbiology: An Introduction to Infectious Diseases,* edited by Kenneth J. Ryan. Norwalk, CT: Appleton & Lange, 1994.

ORGANIZATIONS

Centers for Disease Control and Prevention. (404) 332-4559. http://www.cdc.gov/travel/travel.html.

Rosalyn S. Carson-DeWitt

Jaundice

Definition

Jaundice is a condition in which a person's skin and the whites of the eyes are discolored yellow due to an increased level of bile pigments in the blood resulting from liver disease. Jaundice is sometimes called icterus, from a Greek word for the condition.

Description

In order to understand jaundice, it is useful to know about the role of the liver in producing bile. The most important function of the liver is the processing of chemical waste products like cholesterol and excreting them into the intestines as bile. The liver is the premier chemical factory in the body—most incoming and outgoing chemicals pass through it. It is the first stop for all nutrients, toxins, and drugs absorbed by the digestive tract. The liver also collects chemicals from the blood for processing. Many of these outward-bound chemicals are excreted into the bile. One particular substance, bilirubin, is yellow. Bilirubin is a product of the breakdown of hemoglobin, which is the protein inside red blood cells. If bilirubin cannot leave the body, it accumulates and discolors other tissues. The normal total level of bilirubin in blood serum is between 0.2 mg/dL and 1.2 mg/dL. When it rises to 3 mg/dL or higher, the person's skin and the whites of the eyes become noticeably yellow.

Bile is formed in the liver. It then passes into the network of hepatic bile ducts, which join to form a single tube. A branch of this tube carries bile to the gallbladder,

KEY TERMS

Ampulla of Vater—The widened portion of the duct through which the bile and pancreatic juices enter the intestine. Ampulla is a Latin word for a bottle with a narrow neck that opens into a wide body.

Anemia—A condition in which the blood does not contain enough hemoglobin.

Biliary system/Bile ducts—The gall bladder and the system of tubes that carries bile from the liver into the intestines.

Bilirubin—A reddish pigment excreted by the liver into the bile as a breakdown product of hemoglobin.

Crigler-Najjar syndrome—A moderate to severe form of hereditary jaundice.

Erythroblastosis fetalis—A disorder of newborn infants marked by a high level of immature red blood cells (erythroblasts) in the infant's blood.

Gilbert's syndrome—A mild hereditary form of jaundice.

Glucose-6-phosphate dehydrogenase (G6PD) deficiency—A hereditary disorder that can lead to episodes of hemolytic anemia in combination with certain medications.

Hemoglobin—The red chemical in blood cells that carries oxygen.

Hemolysis—The destruction or breakdown of red blood cells.

Hepatic—Refers to the liver.

Icterus—Another name for jaundice.

Microangiopathic—Pertaining to disorders of the small blood vessels.

Pancreas—The organ beneath the stomach that produces digestive juices, insulin, and other hormones.

Sickle cell disease—A hereditary defect in hemoglobin synthesis that changes the shape of red cells and makes them more fragile.

Splenectomy—Surgical removal of the spleen.

where it is stored, concentrated, and released on a signal from the stomach. Food entering the stomach is the signal that stimulates the gallbladder to release the bile. The tube, which is now called the common bile duct, continues to the intestines. Before the common bile duct reaches the intestines, it is joined by another duct from the pancreas. The bile and the pancreatic juice enter the intestine through a valve called the ampulla of Vater. After entering the intestine, the bile and pancreatic secretions together help in the process of digestion.

Causes & symptoms

There are many different causes for jaundice, but they can be divided into three categories based on where they start—before, in, or after the liver (pre-hepatic, hepatic and post-hepatic). When bilirubin begins its life cycle, it cannot be dissolved in water. The liver changes it so that it is soluble in water. These two types of bilirubin are called unconjugated (insoluble) and conjugated (soluble). Blood tests can easily distinguish between these two types of bilirubin.

Hemoglobin and bilirubin formation

Bilirubin begins as hemoglobin in the blood-forming organs, primarily the bone marrow. If the production of

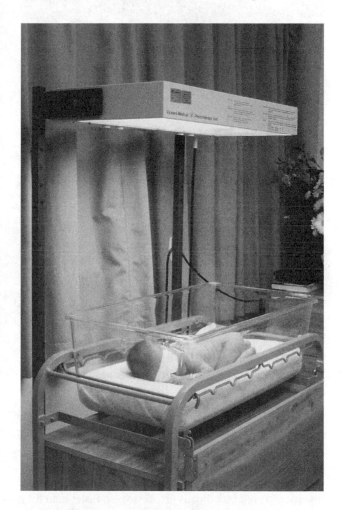

A newborn baby undergoes phototherapy with visible blue light to treat his jaundice. (Photograph by Ron Sutherland, Photo Researchers, Inc. Reproduced by permission.)

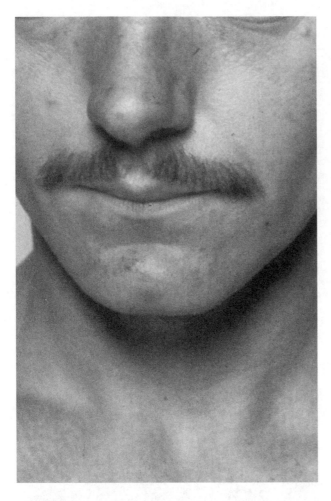

This patient suffers from obstructive jaundice, which is often caused by gallstones. *(Custom Medical Stock Photo. Reproduced by permission.)*

red blood cells (RBCs) falls below normal, the extra hemoglobin finds its way into the bilirubin cycle and adds to the pool.

Once hemoglobin is in the red cells of the blood, it circulates for the life span of those cells. The hemoglobin that is released when the cells die is turned into bilirubin. If for any reason the RBCs die at a faster rate than usual, bilirubin can accumulate in the blood and cause jaundice.

Hemolytic disorders

Many disorders speed up the death of red blood cells. The process of red blood cell destruction is called hemolysis, and the diseases that cause it are called hemolytic disorders. If red blood cells are destroyed faster than they can be produced, the patient develops anemia. Hemolysis can occur in a number of diseases, disorders, conditions, and medical procedures:

- **Malaria.** The malaria parasite develops inside red blood cells. When it is mature it breaks the cell apart and swims off in the blood. This process happens to most of the parasites simultaneously, causing the intermittent symptoms of the disease. When enough cells burst at once, jaundice may result from the large amount of bilirubin formed from the hemoglobin in the dead cells. The pigment may reach the urine in sufficient quantities to cause "blackwater fever," an often lethal form of malaria.

- Side effects of certain drugs. Some common drugs can cause hemolysis as a rare but sudden side effect. These medications include some antibiotic and anti-**tuberculosis** medicines; drugs that regulate the heartbeat; and levodopa, a drug used to treat **Parkinson's disease.**

- Certain drugs in combination with a hereditary enzyme deficiency known as glucose-6-phosphate dehydrogenase (G6PD). G6PD is a deficiency that affects over 200 million people in the world. Some of the drugs listed above are more likely to cause hemolysis in people with G6PD. Other drugs cause hemolysis only in people with this disorder. Most important among these drugs are anti-malarial medications such as quinine, and **vitamins** C and K.

- Poisons. Snake and spider venom, certain bacterial toxins, copper, and some organic industrial chemicals directly attack the membranes of red blood cells.

- Artificial heart valves. The inflexible moving parts of heart valves damage RBCs as they flutter back and forth. This damage is one reason to recommend pig valves and valves made of other organic materials.

- Hereditary RBC disorders. There are a number of hereditary defects that affect the blood cells. There are many genetic mutations that affect the hemoglobin itself, the best-known of which is sickle cell disease. Such hereditary disorders as spherocytosis weaken the outer membrane of the red cell. There are also inherited defects that involve the internal chemistry of RBCs.

- Enlargement of the spleen. The spleen is an organ that is located near the upper end of the stomach and filters the blood. It is supposed to filter out and destroy only worn-out RBCs. If it has become enlarged, it filters out normal cells as well. Malaria, other infections, **cancers** and leukemias, some of the hereditary **anemias** mentioned above, obstruction of blood flow from the spleen—all these and many more diseases can enlarge the spleen to the point where it removes too many red blood cells.

- Diseases of the small blood vessels. Hemolysis that occurs in diseased small blood vessels is called microangiopathic hemolysis. It results from damage caused by rough surfaces on the inside of the capillaries. The RBCs squeeze through capillaries one at a time and can easily be damaged by scraping against the vessel walls.

- **Immune reactions to RBCs.** Several types of cancer and immune system diseases produce antibodies that react with RBCs and destroy them. In 75% of cases, this reaction occurs all by itself, with no underlying disease to account for it.

- **Transfusions.** If a patient is given an incompatible blood type, hemolysis results.

- Kidney failure and other serious diseases. Several diseases are characterized by defective blood coagulation that can destroy red blood cells.

- **Erythroblastosis fetalis.** Erythroblastosis fetalis is a disease of newborns marked by the presence of too many immature red blood cells (erythroblasts) in the baby's blood. When a baby's mother has a different blood type, antibodies from the mother may leak into the baby's circulation and destroy blood cells. This reaction can produce severe hemolysis and jaundice in the newborn. Rh factor incompatibility is the most common cause.

- High bilirubin levels in newborns. Even in the absence of blood type incompatibility, the newborn's bilirubin level may reach threatening levels.

Normal jaundice in newborns

Normal newborn jaundice is the result of two conditions occurring at the same time—a pre-hepatic and a hepatic source of excess bilirubin. First of all, the baby at birth immediately begins converting hemoglobin from a fetal type to an adult type. The fetal type of hemoglobin was able to extract oxygen from the lower levels of oxygen in the mother's blood. At birth the infant can extract oxygen directly from his or her own lungs and does not need the fetal hemoglobin any more. So fetal hemoglobin is removed from the system and replaced with adult hemoglobin. The resulting bilirubin loads the system and places demands on the liver to clear it. But the liver is not quite ready for the task, so there is a period of a week or so when the liver has to catch up. During that time the baby is jaundiced.

Hepatic jaundice

Liver diseases of all kinds threaten the organ's ability to keep up with bilirubin processing. **Starvation,** circulating infections, certain medications, hepatitis, and **cirrhosis** can all cause hepatic jaundice, as can certain hereditary defects of liver chemistry, including Gilbert's syndrome and Crigler-Najjar syndrome.

Post-hepatic jaundice

Post-hepatic forms of jaundice include the jaundices caused by failure of soluble bilirubin to reach the intestines after it has left the liver. These disorders are called obstructive jaundices. The most common cause of obstructive jaundice is the presence of **gallstones** in the ducts of the biliary system. Other causes have to do with **birth defects** and infections that damage the bile ducts; drugs; infections; cancers; and physical injury. Some drugs—and **pregnancy** on rare occasions—simply cause the bile in the ducts to stop flowing.

Symptoms and complications associated with jaundice

Certain chemicals in bile may cause **itching** when too much of them ends up in the skin. In newborns, insoluble bilirubin may get into the brain and do permanent damage. Long-standing jaundice may upset the balance of chemicals in the bile and cause stones to form. Apart from these potential complications and the discoloration of skin and eyes, jaundice by itself is inoffensive. Other symptoms are determined by the disease producing the jaundice.

Diagnosis

Physical examination

In many cases the diagnosis of jaundice is suggested by the appearance of the patient's eyes and complexion. The doctor will ask the patient to lie flat on the examining table in order to feel (palpate) the liver and spleen for enlargement and to evaluate any abdominal **pain.** The location and severity of abdominal pain and the presence or absence of fever help the doctor to distinguish between hepatic and obstructive jaundice.

Laboratory tests

Disorders of blood formation can be diagnosed by more thorough examination of the blood or the bone marrow, where blood is made. Occasionally a bone marrow biopsy is required, but usually the blood itself will reveal the diagnosis. The spleen can be evaluated by an ultrasound examination or a nuclear scan if the **physical examination** has not yielded enough information.

Liver disease is usually assessed from blood studies alone, but again a biopsy may be necessary to clarify less obvious conditions. A **liver biopsy** is performed at the bedside. The doctor uses a thin needle to take a tiny core of tissue from the liver. The tissue sample is sent to the laboratory for examination under a microscope.

Assessment of jaundice in newborns

Newborns are more likely to have problems with jaundice if:

• They are premature.

• They are Asian or Native Americans.

• They have been bruised during the birth process.

• They have lost too much weight during the first few days.

• They are born at high altitude.

• The mother has diabetes.

• Labor had to be induced.

Imaging studies

Disease in the biliary system can be identified by imaging techniques, of which there are many. X rays are taken a day after swallowing a contrast agent that is secreted into the bile. This study gives functional as well as anatomical information. There are several ways of injecting x ray dye directly into the bile ducts. It can be done through a thin needle pushed straight into the liver or through a scope passed through the stomach that can inject dye into the Ampulla of Vater. CT and MRI scans are very useful for imaging certain conditions like cancers in and around the liver or gall stones in the common bile duct.

Treatment

Jaundice in newborns

Newborns are the only major category of patients in whom the jaundice itself requires attention. Because the insoluble bilirubin can get into the brain, the amount in the blood must not go over certain levels. If there is reason to suspect increased hemolysis in the newborn, the bilirubin level must be measured repeatedly during the first few days of life. If the level of bilirubin shortly after birth threatens to go too high, treatment must begin immediately. Exchanging most of the baby's blood was the only way to reduce the amount of bilirubin until a few decades ago. Then it was discovered that bright blue light will render the bilirubin harmless. Now jaundiced babies are fitted with eye protection and placed under bright fluorescent lights. The light chemically alters the bilirubin in the blood as it passes through the baby's skin.

Hemolytic disorders

Hemolytic diseases are treated, if at all, with medications and blood transfusions, except in the case of a large spleen. Surgical removal of the spleen (**splenectomy**) can sometimes cure **hemolytic anemia.** Drugs that cause hemolysis or arrest the flow of bile must be stopped immediately.

Hepatic jaundice

Most liver diseases have no specific cure, but the liver is so robust that it can heal from severe damage and regenerate itself from a small remnant of its original tissue.

Post-hepatic jaundice

Obstructive jaundice frequently requires a surgical cure. If the original passageways cannot be restored, surgeons have several ways to create alternate routes. A popular technique is to sew an open piece of intestine over a bare patch of liver. Tiny bile ducts in that part of the liver will begin to discharge their bile into the intestine, and pressure from the obstructed ducts elsewhere will find release in that direction. As the flow increases, the ducts grow to accommodate it. Soon all the bile is redirected through the open pathways.

Prevention

Erythroblastosis fetalis can be prevented by giving an Rh negative mother a gamma globulin solution called RhoGAM whenever there is a possibility that she is developing antibodies to her baby's blood. G6PD hemolysis can be prevented by testing patients before giving them drugs that can cause it. Medication side effects can be minimized by early detection and immediate cessation of the drug. Malaria can often be prevented by certain precautions when traveling in tropical or subtropical countries. These precautions include staying in after dark; using prophylactic drugs such as mefloquine; and protecting sleeping quarters with mosquito nets treated with insecticides and mosquito repellents.

Resources

BOOKS

Balistreri, William F. "Manifestations of Liver Disease." In *Nelson Textbook of Pediatrics,* edited by Waldo E. Nelson, et al. Philadelphia: W. B. Saunders, 1996.

"Jaundice." In *Sleisenger & Fordtran's Gastrointestinal and Liver Disease,* edited by Mark Feldman, et al. Philadelphia: W. B. Saunders, 1998.

Kaplan, Lee M., and Kurt J. Isselbacher. "Jaundice." In *Harrison's Principles of Internal Medicine,* edited by Kurt Isselbacher et al. New York: McGraw-Hill, 1998.

McQuaid, Kenneth R. "Alimentary Tract." In *Current Medical Diagnosis and Treatment,* edited by Lawrence M. Tierney, Jr., et al. Stamford, CT: Appleton & Lange, 1996.

Scharschmidt, Bruce F. "Bilirubin Metabolism, Hyperbilirubinemia, and Approach to the Jaundiced Patient." In *Cecil Textbook of Medicine*, edited by J. Claude Bennett, and Fred Plum. Philadelphia: W. B. Saunders, 1996.

ORGANIZATIONS

American Liver Foundation. 1425 Pompton Avenue, Cedar Grove, New Jersey 07009. 800 223-0179.

J. Ricker Polsdorfer

Jaw wiring

Definition

Jaw wiring, also known as maxillomandibular fixation, is a surgical procedure where metal pins and wires are anchored into the jaw bones and surrounding tissues to keep the jaw from moving.

Purpose

Sports injuries, automobile accidents, falls, or fistfights are a few of the situations where the jaw might be fractured or broken. In these cases, jaw wiring may be necessary to keep the bones aligned and stable while the jaw heals. The presence of **cancer** or other diseased tissues may make removal and reconstruction of the jaw necessary. Wiring the jaws shut has been used in the past as a weight loss aid in cases of extreme **obesity** where other treatments had failed, although this procedure is rarely used for that purpose today.

Precautions

Traumatic injuries to the face can cause damage to facial nerves and salivary glands and ducts. These injuries can also leave scars that may require additional surgery to correct.

Description

Jaw wiring surgery can be performed by an oral or maxillofacial surgeon (a specially trained dentist), or by an otolaryngologist (a doctor specializing in surgeries of the head and neck). The procedure may be done in a medical or dental office if the office is staffed and equipped to handle this type of surgery. More often, this surgery is performed in a hospital or medical center surgical area. If jaw wiring is required due to an injury, the surgeon may set the fracture immediately before swelling sets in. It is also possible to wait (up to several weeks) until the swelling goes down and some of the soft tissue injuries have healed, prior to wiring the jaw fracture.

The surgeon realigns the fractured bones. Every effort is made to restore the shape and appearance of the original jaw line. If any teeth were damaged, repair or replacement may be done at the same time. Small incisions may be made through the skin and surrounding tissue so the pins and wires can be set into the jawbone to hold the fracture together. To prevent the lower jaw from moving during healing, pins and wires may be inserted into the top jaw, as well. The upper and lower jaws are then wired together in order to stabilize the fracture.

As with other types of bone **fractures,** the jaw may take several weeks to heal. Another type of jaw **immobilization** that has been developed more recently, rigid fixation uses small metal plates and screws rather than pins and wires to secure the jaw bones. The main benefit of this technique is that the jaws do not have to be wired shut, allowing the patient to return to a more normal lifestyle sooner.

Preparation

X rays of the fractured area may be taken prior to surgery. Depending on the extent of the facial injury or condition to be corrected, the patient may receive a sedative for relaxation, a local anesthetic drug to numb the area, and/or an anesthetic agent to induce unconsciousness prior to the surgery.

Aftercare

A patient whose jaw has been wired will not be able to eat solid foods for several weeks. In order for the bone and surrounding tissues to heal, it is important to maintain adequate nutrition. A liquid diet that can be consumed through a straw, will be required. Soft, precooked foods can be liquefied in a blender, however, it may be difficult for the patient to consume adequate calories, protein, **vitamins,** and **minerals** with this type of diet. Liquid diet formulas may be a good alternative. The patient will also have to be taught how to care for the mouth, teeth, and injured area while the wires are in place.

Risks

It is possible that scarring may occur due to the need to make small incisions in the skin in order to insert the wires. With any surgical procedure, there are risks associated with the anesthetic drugs used and the possibility of infection. If there is a risk that the patient may vomit, the jaw wiring may pose a **choking** hazard. It may be recommended that wire cutters be kept available in case the wires need to be cut in an emergency situation.

Resources

BOOKS

''Jaw Wiring.'' In *Nutrition and Diet Therapy Reference Dictionary,* 4th ed., New York, NY:Chapman & Hall, 1996.

ORGANIZATIONS

American Association of Oral & Maxillofacial Surgeons. 9700 West Bryn Mawr Avenue; Rosemont, IL 60018-5701; (847) 678-6200.

American Dental Association. 211 E. Chicago Avenue; Chicago, IL 60611; (312) 440-2500.

OTHER

''Know the Score on Facial Sports Injuries'' Iowa Health Book: Otolaryngology; Virtual Hospital Website: http://www.vh.org/Patients/IHB/Oto/AAO/SportsInjuries.html.

''Topic: Maxillofacial Trauma'' Connecticut Maxillofacial Surgeons Website: http://www.cmsllc.com/toptrm.html.

Altha Roberts Edgren

JC virus infection *see* **Progressive multifocal leukoencephalopathy**

Jejunostomy *see* **Enterostomy**

Jet lag

Definition

Jet lag is a condition marked by fatigue and irritability that is caused from air travel through changing time zones.

Description

Living organisms are accustomed to periods of night and day alternating at set intervals. Most of the body's regulating hormones follow this cycle, known as circa-

dian rhythm. In Latin, *circa* means almost and *dies* means day. These cycles are not by themselves exactly 24 hours long, hence the ''circa.'' Each chemical has its own cycle of highs and lows, interacting with and influencing the other cycles. Body temperature, sleepiness, thyroid function, growth hormone, metabolic processes, and the newly discovered sleep hormone melatonin all cycle with daylight. There is a direct connection between the retina (where light hits the back of the eye) and the part of the brain that controls all these hormones. Artificial light has some effect, but sunlight has much more.

When people are without clocks in a compartment that is completely closed to sunlight, most of them fall into a circadian cycle of about 25 hours. Normally, all the regulating chemicals follow one another in order like threads in a weaving pattern. Every morning the sunlight resets the cycle, stimulating the leading chemicals and thus compensating for the difference between the 24 hour day and the 25 hour innate rhythm.

This was fine for centuries. It even accommodated those early navigators like Magellan who sailed slowly around the world. Each day the sun reset the clock and all the cycles fell into place. Today, technology has surpassed adaptability, at least momentarily. In a single day, we can completely reverse the night-day rhythm by flying to the other side of the earth. The chemicals are thrown into confusion like an armada without a compass or flagship. Most people reset their rhythms within a few days, demonstrating the adaptability of the human species. Some people, however, have upset rhythms that last indefinitely.

Causes & symptoms

Traveling through a few time zones at a time is not as disruptive to circadian rhythms as traveling around the world can be. Because the intrinsic day is longer than the earthly day, it is also easier to travel West than East. Beyond the normal limits, jet lag will occur. The foremost symptom is altered sleep pattern—sleepiness during the day, **insomnia** during the night. Jet lag may also include **indigestion** and trouble concentrating. Sometimes the cycle continues to run at 25 or more hours because it is not reset by daylight. Individuals afflicted by jet lag will alternate in and out of a normal day-night cycle.

Treatment

Exposure to bright morning sunlight cures jet lag after a few days in most people. A few will have prolonged sleep phase difficulties. For these, there is one curious treatment that has achieved success. By forcing one's self into a 27 hour day, complete with the appropriate stimulation from bright light, all the errant chemical cycles will be able to catch up during one week of recycling.

Alternative treatment

Drinking a lot of water to prevent **dehydration** can limit or prevent jet lag. As much movement as possible during a flight helps keep circulation moving nutrients and waste through the body and aids in elimination. All antioxidants help to decrease the effects of jet lag. Extra doses of **vitamins** A, C, and E, as well as zinc and selenium, two days before and two days after a flight help to alleviate jet lag. Homeopathic remedies can assist in the transition of time and space. For individuals who are biochemically deficient in melatonin, increased intake of this hormone is believed to help combat jet lag.

Prognosis

Jet lag usually lasts from 24-48 hours after travel has taken place. In that short time period, the body adjust to the time changes, and with enough rest, it returns to normal circadian rhythm.

Prevention

Eating a high protein diet that is low in calories before intended travel may help reduce the effects of jet lag.

Resources

BOOKS

Czeisler, Charles A., and Gary S. Richardson. "Disorders of Sleep and Circadian Rhythms." In *Harrison's Principles of Internal Medicine,* edited by Anthony S. Fauci, et al. New York: McGraw-Hill, 1998.

Molitch, Mark E. "The Neuroendocrine System." In *Cecil Textbook of Medicine,* edited by J. Claude Bennett and Fred Plum. Philadelphia: W. B. Saunders, 1996.

PERIODICALS

Delagrange, P., and B. Guardiola-Lemaitre. "Melatonin, Its Receptors, and Relationships with Biological Rhythm Disorders." *Clinical Neuropharmacology* 20(December 1997): 482-510.

Dijk, D.J., et al. "Light Treatment for Sleep Disorders: Consensus Report. II. Basic Properties of Circadian Physiology and Sleep Regulation." *Journal of Biological Rhythms* 10(June 1995): 113-125.

Garfinkel D. and N. Zisapel. "The Use of Melatonin for Sleep." *Nutrition* 14(January 1998): 53-55.

Hastings, M.H. "Central Clocking." *Trends in Neurosciences* 20(October 1997): 459-464.

Hastings, M.H. "Circadian Clocks." *Current Biology* 7(November 1, 1997): R670-672.

Hinton, S.C., and W.H. Meck. "The 'Internal Clocks' of Circadian and Interval Timing." *Endeavour* 21(1997): 82-87.

Kraft, M., and R.J. Martin. "Chronobiology and Chronotherapy in Medicine." *Disease-A-Month* 41(August 1995): 501-575.

Paulson, E. "Travel Statement on Jet Lag." *CMAJ* 155(July 1, 1996): 61-66.

Sack, R.L., and A.J. Lewy. "Melatonin as a Chronobiotic: Treatment of Circadian Desynchrony in Night Workers and the Blind." *Journal of Biological Rhythms* 12(December 1997): 595-603.

Samel, A., and H.M. Wegmann. "Bright Light: a Countermeasure for Jet Lag?" *Chronobiology International* 14(March 1997): 173-183.

Wagner, D.R. "Disorders of the Circadian Sleep-Wake Cycle." *Neurologic Clinics* 14(August 1996): 651-670.

Waterhouse, J., D. Minors, and P. Redfern. "Some Comments on the Measurement of Circadian Rhythms After Time-Zone Transitions and During Night Work." *Chronobiology International* 14(March 1997): 125-132.

Zhdanova, I.V., and R.J. Wurtman. "Efficacy of Melatonin as a Sleep-Promoting Agent." *Journal of Biological Rhythms* 12(December 1997): 644-650.

J. Ricker Polsdorfer

Jock itch *see* **Ringworm**

Joint aspiration *see* **Joint fluid analysis**

Joint biopsy

Definition

A joint or synovial membrane biopsy refers to a procedure where a sample of the joint lining or synovial membrane is taken.

Purpose

A joint biopsy is performed to determine why a joint is painful or swollen. It is usually reserved for more difficult cases where the diagnosis is not clear. The test can be used to diagnose bacterial or fungal infections, an abnormal buildup of iron, **cancer,** or other diseases.

Precautions

The procedure must be done under very sterile conditions to reduce the risk of infection.

Description

The test is performed either in the doctor's office, clinic, or hospital by a surgeon. There are many different ways to perform this biopsy: through an incision in the joint; with a scope inserted in the joint; or, more typically, by the insertion of a sharp instrument through the skin. The procedure can be taken from any joint, but the most common joint requiring biopsy is the knee. A sharp instrument (trocar) is pushed into the joint space. A needle with an attached syringe is inserted into the joint to withdraw fluid for laboratory analysis. The surgeon may instill numbing medicine into the joint and along the needle track before the needle is withdrawn. The trocar and then the biopsy needle is inserted and specimens taken. After the specimen is taken, both the trocar and the biopsy needle are removed, a bandage is placed over the joint, and the samples are sent to pathology for analysis.

Preparation

Blood tests will be done to check that blood clots properly. A mild sedative may be given before the procedure. With the patient lying down, the skin over the joint is disinfected and a local anesthetic is injected into the skin and tissue just below the skin.

Aftercare

The joint will need rest for at least one day. Normal activity can resume if there is no increased pain or swelling.

Risks

There is a chance of joint swelling or tenderness. Rarely, bleeding and infection can occur in the joint, or the biopsy needle could break off or strike a nerve or blood vessel. The risk of infection is higher if the patient has an immune deficiency.

Resources

BOOKS

"Arthrocentesis, Synovial Fluid Analysis and Synovial Biopsy." In *Primer on Rheumatic Diseases,* edited by H. Ralph Schumacher. Atlanta, GA: Arthritis Foundation, 1993.

Schumacher, H. Ralph Jr. "Synovial Fluid Analysis and Synovial Biopsy." In *Textbook of Rheumatology,* edited by William N. Kelley et al. Philadelphia: WB Saunders Company, 1997.

PERIODICALS

Beaule, V. et al. "Synovial Membrane: Percutaneous Biopsy." *Radiology* 177(1990):581-585

Jeanine Barone

Joint endoscopy *see* **Arthroscopy**

Joint fluid analysis

Definition

Joint fluid analysis, also called synovial fluid analysis, or arthrocentesis, is a procedure used to assess joint-related abnormalities, such as in the knee or elbow.

Purpose

The purpose of a joint fluid analysis is to identify the cause of swelling in the joints, to relieve **pain** and distention from fluid accumulation in the joint, and to diagnose certain types of arthritis and inflammatory joint diseases. The test is also a method to determine whether an infection, either bacterial or fungal, exists within the joint.

Precautions

Joint fluid analysis should not be performed on any patient who is uncooperative, especially if the patient cannot or will not keep the joint immobile throughout the procedure. Patients with certain infections should be excluded from the procedure, particularly those who have a local infection along the proposed needle track. The joint space should be accessible. Therefore, a poorly accessible joint space, such as in hip aspiration in an obese patient, should not be subject to this procedure.

KEY TERMS

Aspirate—The removal by suction of a fluid from a body cavity using a needle.

Bursae—A closed sac lined with a synovial membrane and filled with fluid, usually found in areas subject to friction, such as where a tendon passes over a bone.

Hematoma—A localized mass of blood that is confined within an organ or tissue.

Synovial fluid—A transparent lubricating fluid secreted in a sac to protect an area where a tendon passes over a bone.

Description

The test is also called arthrocentesis, joint tap, and closed joint aspiration. Normal synovial fluid is a clear or pale-yellow fluid found in small amounts in joints, bursae (fluid-filled sac found on points of friction, like joints), and tendon sheaths. The procedure is done by passing a needle into a joint space and sucking out (aspirating) synovial fluid for diagnostic analysis. When the sample is sent to the laboratory, the fluid is analyzed for color, clarity, quantity, and chemical composition. It is also examined microscopically to check for the presence of bacteria and other cells.

The procedure takes about 10 minutes. Prior to the procedure, any risks that are involved should be explained to the patient. No intravenous pain medications or sedatives are required, although the patient will be given a local anesthetic.

The patient is asked to lie on their back and remain relaxed. The local anesthetic, typically an injection of lidocaine, is then administered. The clinician is usually seated next to the patient. Then the clinician marks exactly where the needle is to enter. As the needle enters the joint, a "pop" may be felt or heard. This is normal. Correct placement of the needle in the joint space is normally painless. At this point, the clinician slowly drains some of the fluid into the syringe. The needle is then withdrawn and adhesive tape is placed over the needle site.

Preparation

Glucose, or sugar, in the joint can be a signal of arthritis. If the clinician will be doing a glucose test, the patient will be asked to fast for 6-12 hours preceding the procedure. If not, there is no special preparation required for a joint fluid analysis.

Aftercare

Some post-procedural pain may be experienced. For this reason, the patient should arrange to be driven home by someone else. Aftercare of the joints will depend on the results of the analysis.

Risks

While joint fluid analysis is generally a safe procedure, especially when performed on a large, easily accessible joint, such as the knee, some risks are possible. Some of the complications to the procedure, although rare, include infection at the site of the needle stick, an accumulation of blood (hematoma) formation, local pain, injury to cartilage, tendon rupture, and nerve damage.

Normal results

The results of a normal joint fluid analysis include fluid of a clear or pale-yellow color and the absence of bacteria, fungus, and other cells, such as white blood cells.

Abnormal results

The results of an abnormal joint fluid analysis include fluid that is turbid, or cloudy. Also, white blood cells and other blood cells may be found, from which the clinician can make a diagnosis and arrive at a treatment for the joint problem. An abnormal result can indicate an infection caused by a bacteria, or **tuberculosis.** Or, there might be inflammation that is caused by **gout, rheumatoid arthritis,** or **osteoarthritis.**

Resources

BOOKS

Arnold, William J., and Robert W. Ike. "Specialized Procedures in the Management of Patients with Rheumatic Diseases." In *Cecil Textbook of Medicine,* edited by James B. Wyngaarden, et al. Philadelphia: W.B. Saunders Company, 1992.

Ron Gasbarro

Joint infection *see* **Infectious arthritis**

Joint radiography *see* **Arthrography**

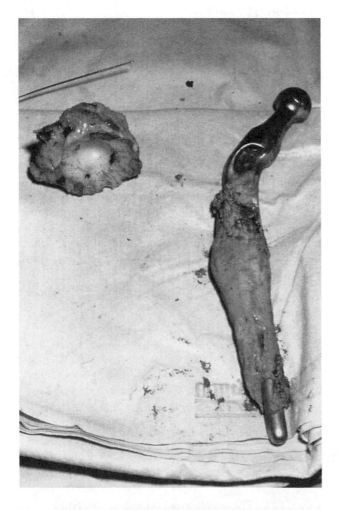

The components of a prosthetic hip joint, removed due to loosening. On the right is the metal shaft encased in the cement which fixed it to the inside of the femur. On the left is the plastic socket. *(Custom Medical Stock Photo. Reproduced by permission.)*

Joint replacement

Definition

Joint replacement is the surgical replacement of a joint with an artificial prosthesis.

Purpose

Great advances have been made in joint replacement since the first hip replacement was performed in the United States in 1969. Improvements have been made in the endurance and compatibility of materials used and the surgical techniques to install artificial joints. Custom joints can be made using a mold of the original joint that duplicate the original with a very high degree of accuracy.

The most common joints to be replaced are hips and knees. There is ongoing work on elbow and shoulder replacement, but some joint problems are still treated with joint resection (the surgical removal of the joint in question) or interpositional reconstruction (the reassembly of the joint from constituent parts).

Seventy percent of joint replacements are performed because arthritis has caused the joint to stiffen and become painful to the point where normal daily activities are no longer possible. If the joint does not respond to conservative treatment such medication, weight loss, activity restriction, and use of walking aids such as a cane, joint replacement is considered appropriate.

Patients with **rheumatoid arthritis** or other connective tissue diseases may also be candidates for joint replacement, but the results are usually less satisfactory in those patients. Elderly people who fall and break their hip often undergo hip replacement when the probability of successful bone healing is low.

More than 170,000 hip replacements are performed in the United States each year. Since the lifetime of the artificial joint is limited, the best candidates for joint replacement are over age 60.

Precautions

Joint replacements are performed successfully on an older- than-average group of patients. People with diseases that interfere with blood clotting are not good candidates for joint replacement. Joint replacement surgery should not be done on patients with infection, or any heart, kidney or lung problems that would make it risky to undergo **general anesthesia.**

Description

Joint replacements are performed under general or regional anesthesia in a hospital by an orthopedic sur-

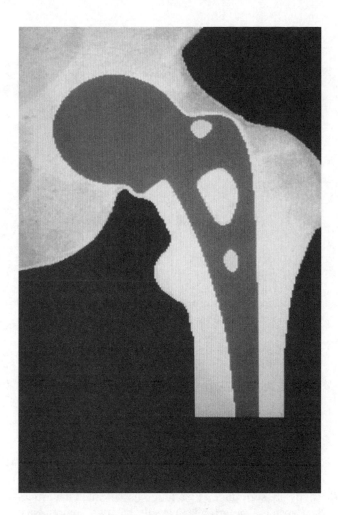

A false color x-ray image of the human pelvis showing a prosthetic hip joint. *(Custom Medical Stock Photo. Reproduced by permission.)*

geon. Some medical centers specialize in joint replacement, and these centers generally have a higher success rate than less specialized facilities. The specific techniques of joint replacement vary depending on the joint involved.

Hip Replacement

The surgeon makes an incision along the top of the thigh bone (femur) and pulls the thigh bone away from the socket of the hip bone (the acetabulum). An artificial socket made of metal coated with polyethylene (plastic) to reduce friction is inserted in the hip. The top of the thigh bone is cut, and a piece of artificial thigh made of metal is fitted into the lower thigh bone on one end and the new socket on the other.

The artificial hip can either be held in place by a synthetic cement or by natural bone in-growth. The cement is an acrylic polymer. It assures good locking of the prosthesis to the remaining bone. However, bubbles left

in the cement after it cures may act as weak spots, causing the development of cracks. This promotes loosening of the prosthesis later in life. If additional surgery is needed, all the cement must be removed before surgery can be performed.

An artificial hip fixed by natural bone in-growth requires more precise surgical techniques to assure maximum contact between the remaining natural bone and the prosthesis. The prosthesis is made so that it contains small pores that encourage the natural bone to grow into it. Growth begins 6 to 12 weeks after surgery. The short term outcome with non-cemented hips is less satisfactory, with patients reporting more thigh pain, but the long term outlook is better, with fewer cases of hip loosening in non-cemented hips. The trend is to use the non-cemented technique. Hospital stays last from four to eight days.

Knee Replacement

The doctor puts a tourniquet above the knee, than makes a cut to expose the knee joint. The ligaments surrounding the knee are loosened, then the shin bone and thigh bone are cut and the knee removed. The artificial knee is then cemented into place on the remaining stubs of those bones. The excess cement is removed, and the knee is closed. Hospital stays range from three to six days.

In both types of surgery, preventing infection is very important. **Antibiotics** are given intravenously and continued in pill form after the surgery. Fluid and blood loss can be great, and sometimes blood **transfusions** are needed.

Preparation

Many patients choose to donate their own blood for transfusion during the surgery. This prevents any blood incompatibility problems or the transmission of bloodbourne diseases.

Prior to surgery, all the standard preoperative blood and urine tests are performed, and the patient meets with the anesthesiologist to discuss any special conditions that affect the administration of anesthesia. Patients receiving general anesthesia should not eat or drink for ten hours prior to the operation.

Aftercare

Immediately after the operation the patient will be catheterized so that he or she will not have to get out of bed to urinate. The patient will be monitored for infection. Antibiotics are continued and pain medication is prescribed. Physical therapy begins (first passive **exercises,** then active ones) as soon as possible using a walker, cane, or crutches for additional support. Long term care of the artificial joint involves refraining from heavy activity and heavy lifting, and learning how to sit, walk, how to get out of beds, chairs, and cars so as not to dislocate the joint.

Risks

The immediate risks during and after surgery include the development of blood clots that may come loose and block the arteries, excessive loss of blood, and infection. Blood thinning medication is usually given to reduce the risk of clots forming. Some elderly people experience short term confusion and disorientation from the anesthesia.

Although joint replacement surgery is highly successful, there is an increased risk of nerve injury. Dislocation or fracture of the hip joint is also a possibility. Infection caused by the operation can occur as long as a year later and can be difficult to treat. Some doctors add antibiotics directly to the cement used to fix the replacement joint in place. Loosening of the joint is the most common cause of failure in hip joints that are not infected. This may require another joint replacement surgery in about 12% of patients within a 15-year period following the first procedure.

Normal results

Over 90% of patients receiving hip replacements achieve complete relief from pain and significant improvement in joint function. The success rate is slightly lower in knee replacements, and drops still more for other joint replacement operations.

Resources

PERIODICALS

Siopack, Jorge, and Harry Jergensen. ''Total Hip Arthroplasty.'' In *Western Journal of Medicine* (March, 1995): 43-50.

Tish Davidson

Joint resection *see* **Arthroplasty**

Joint x rays *see* **Arthrography**

Juvenile arthritis

Definition

Juvenile arthritis (JA) refers to a number of different conditions, all of which strike children, and all of which have joint inflammation as their major manifestation.

Description

The skeletal system of the body is made up of different types of the strong, fibrous tissue known as connective tissue. Bone, cartilage, ligaments, and tendons are all forms of connective tissue which have different compositions, and thus different characteristics.

The joints are structures which hold two or more bones together. Some joints (synovial joints) allow for movement between the bones being joined (called articulating bones). The simplest model of a synovial joint involves two bones, separated by a slight gap called the joint cavity. The ends of each articular bone are covered by a layer of cartilage. Both articular bones and the joint cavity are surrounded by a tough tissue called the articular capsule. The articular capsule has two components: the fibrous membrane on the outside, and the synovial membrane (or synovium) on the inside. The fibrous membrane may include tough bands of fibrous tissue called ligaments, which are responsible for providing support to the joints. The synovial membrane has special cells and many capillaries (tiny blood vessels). This membrane produces a supply of synovial fluid which fills the joint cavity, lubricates it, and helps the articular bones move smoothly about the joint.

In JA, the synovial membrane becomes intensely inflamed. Usually thin and delicate, the synovium becomes thick and stiff, with numerous infoldings on its surface. The membrane becomes invaded by white blood cells, which produce a variety of destructive chemicals. The cartilage along the articular surfaces of the bones may be attacked and destroyed, and the bone, articular capsule, and ligaments may begin to be worn away (eroded). These processes severely interfere with movement in the joint.

JA specifically refers to chronic arthritic conditions which affect a child under the age of 16 years, and which last for a minimum of three to six months. JA is often characterized by a waxing and waning course, with flares separated by periods of time during which no symptoms are noted (remission). Some literature refers to JA as juvenile **rheumatoid arthritis,** although most types of JA differ significantly from the adult disease called rheumatoid arthritis, in terms of symptoms, progression, and prognosis.

Causes & symptoms

A number of different causes have been sought to explain the onset of JA. There seems to be some genetic link, based on the fact that the tendency to develop JA sometimes runs in a particular family, and based on the fact that certain genetic markers are more frequently found in patients with JA and other related diseases. Many researchers have looked for some infectious cause for JA, but no clear connection to a particular organism has ever been made. JA is considered by some to be an autoimmune disorder. **Autoimmune disorders** occur when the body's immune system mistakenly identifies the body's own tissue as foreign, and goes about attacking those tissues, as if trying to rid the body of an invader (such as a bacteria, virus, or fungi). While an autoimmune mechanism is strongly suspected, certain markers of such a mechanism (such as rheumatoid factor, often present in adults with such disorders) are rarely present in children with JA.

Joint symptoms of arthritis may include stiffness, **pain,** redness and warmth of the joint, and swelling. Bone in the area of an affected joint may grow too quickly, or too slowly, resulting in limbs which are of different lengths. When the child tries to avoid moving a painful joint, the muscle may begin to shorten from disuse. This is called a contracture.

Symptoms of JA depend on the particular subtype. JA is classified by the symptoms which appear within the first six months of the disorder:

• Pauciarticular JA: This is the most common and the least severe type of JA, affecting about 40-60% of all JA patients. This type of JA affects fewer than four joints, usually the knee, ankle, wrist, and/or elbow. Other more general (systemic) symptoms are usually absent, and the child's growth usually remains normal. Very few children (less than 15%) with pauciarticular JA end up with deformed joints. Some children with this form of JA experience painless swelling of the joint. Some children with JA have a serious inflammation of structures within the eye, which if left undiagnosed and untreated could even lead to blindness. While many children have cycles of flares and remissions, in some children the disease completely and permanently resolves within a few years of diagnosis.

• Polyarticular JA: About 40% of all cases of JA are of this type. More girls than boys are diagnosed with this form of JA. This type of JA is most common in children up to age three, or after the age of 10. Polyarticular JA affects five or more joints simultaneously. This type of JA usually affects the small joints of both hands and both feet, although other large joints may be affected as well. Some patients with arthritis in their knees will experience a different rate of growth in each leg. Ultimately, one leg will grow longer than the other. About half of all patients with polyarticular JA have arthritis of the spine and/or hip. Some patients with polyarticular JA will have other symptoms of a systemic illness, including **anemia** (low red blood cell count), decreased growth rate, low appetite, low-grade **fever,** and a slight rash. The disease is most severe in those children who are diagnosed in early adolescence. Some of these children will test positive for a marker present in other autoimmune disorders, called rheumatoid factor (RF). RF is found in adults who have rheumatoid arthritis. Children who are positive for RF tend to have a more severe course, with a disabling form of arthritis which destroys and deforms the joints. This type of arthritis is thought to be the adult form of rheumatoid arthritis occurring at a very early age.

• Systemic onset JA: Sometimes called Still disease (after a physician who originally described it), this type of JA occurs in about 10-20% off all patients with JA. Boys and girls are equally affected, and diagnosis is usually made between the ages of 5-10 years. The initial symptoms are not usually related to the joints. Instead, these children have high fevers; a rash; decreased appetite and weight loss; severe joint and muscle pain; swollen lymph nodes, spleen, and liver; and serious anemia. Some children experience other complications, including inflammation of the sac containing the heart (**pericarditis**); inflammation of the tissue lining the chest cavity and lungs (pleuritis); and inflammation of the heart muscle (**myocarditis**). The eye inflammation often seen in pauciarticular JA is uncommon in systemic onset JA. Symptoms of actual arthritis begin later in the course of systemic onset JA, and they often involve the wrists and ankles. Many of these children continue to have periodic flares of fever and systemic symptoms throughout childhood. Some children will go on to develop a polyarticular type of JA.

• Spondyloarthropathy: This type of JA most commonly affects boys older than eight years of age. The arthritis occurs in the knees and ankles, moving over time to include the hips and lower spine. Inflammation of the eye may occur occasionally, but usually resolves without permanent damage.

• Psoriatic JA: This type of arthritis usually shows up in fewer than four joints, but goes on to include multiple joints (appearing similar to polyarticular JA). Hips, back, fingers, and toes are frequently affected. A skin condition called **psoriasis** accompanies this type of arthritis. Children with this type of JA often have pits or ridges in their fingernails. The arthritis usually progresses to become a serious, disabling problem.

Diagnosis

Diagnosis of JA is often made on the basis of the child's collection of symptoms. Laboratory tests often show normal results. Some nonspecific indicators of inflammation may be elevated, including white blood cell count, **erythrocyte sedimentation rate,** and a marker called C-reactive protein. As with any chronic disease, anemia may be noted. Children with an extraordinarily early onset of the adult type of rheumatoid arthritis will have a positive test for rheumatoid factor.

Treatment

Treating JA involves efforts to decrease the amount of inflammation, in order to preserve movement. Medications which can be used for this include nonsteroidal anti-inflammatory agents (such as ibuprofen and naproxen). Oral (by mouth) steroid medications are effective, but have many serious side effects with long-term use. Injections of steroids into an affected joint can be helpful. Steroid eye drops are used to treat eye inflammation. Other drugs which have been used to treat JA include methotrexate, sulfasalazine, penicillamine, and hydroxychloroquine. Physical therapy and **exercises** are often recommended in order to improve joint mobility and to strengthen supporting muscles. Occasionally, splints are used to rest painful joints and to try to prevent or improve deformities.

Alternative treatment

Alternative treatments that have been suggested for arthritis include juice therapy, which can work to detoxify the body, helping to reduce JA symptoms. Some recommended fruits and vegetables to include in the juice are carrots, celery, cabbage, potatoes, cherries, lemons, beets, cucumbers, radishes, and garlic. Tomatoes and other vegetables in the nightshade (potatoes, eggplant, red and green peppers) are discouraged. As an adjunct therapy, **aromatherapy** preparations utilize cypress, fennel, and lemon. **Massage** oils include rosemary, benzoin, chamomile, camphor, juniper, and lavender. Other types of therapy which have been used include **acupuncture, acupressure,** and body work. Nutritional supplements that may be beneficial include large amounts of antioxi-dants (**vitamins** C, A, E, zinc, selenium, and flavenoids), as well as B vitamins and a full complement of minerals (including boron, copper, manganese). Other nutrients that assist in detoxifying the body, including methionine, cysteine, and other amino acids, may also be helpful. A number of autoimmune disorders, including JA, seem to have a relationship to food allergies. Identification and elimination of reactive foods may result in a decrease in JA symptoms. Constitutional homeopathy can also work to quiet the symptoms of JA and bring about balance to the whole person.

Prognosis

The prognosis for pauciarticular JA is quite good, as is the prognosis for spondyloarthropathy. Polyarticular JA carries a slightly worse prognosis. RF-positive polyarticular JA carries a difficult prognosis, often with progressive, destructive arthritis and joint deformities. Systemic onset JA has a variable prognosis, depending on the organ systems affected, and the progression to polyarticular JA. About 1-5% of all JA patients die of such complications as infection, inflammation of the heart, or kidney disease.

Prevention

Because so little is known about what causes JA, there are no recommendations available for how to avoid developing it.

Resources

BOOKS

Kredich, Deborah Welt. "Juvenile Rheumatoid Arthritis." In *Rudolph's Pediatrics,* edited by Abraham M. Rudolph. Stamford, CT: Appleton & Lange, 1996.

Olson, Judyann C. "Rheumatic Diseases of Childhood." In *Principles and Practice of Pediatrics,* edited by Frank A. Oski, et al. Philadelphia: J.B. Lippincott Company, 1994.

Schaller, Jane Green. "Juvenile Rheumatoid Arthritis." In *Nelson Textbook of Pediatrics,* edited by Richard Behrman. Philadelphia: W.B. Saunders Co., 1996.

ORGANIZATIONS

American College of Rheumatology. 60 Executive Park South, Suite 150, Atlanta, GA 30329. (404) 633-1870. http://www.rheumatology.org.

Arthritis Foundation, 1330 West Peachtree St., Atlanta, GA 30309. (404) 872-7100. http://www.arthritis.org.

Rosalyn S. Carson-DeWitt

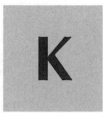

Kaposi's sarcoma

Definition

Kaposi's sarcoma produces pink, purple, or brown tumors on the skin, mucous membranes, or internal organs. It was a very rare form of **cancer,** primarily affecting elderly men of Mediterranean and eastern European background, until the 1980s, when it began to appear among **AIDS** patients. Milder forms of the disease can be managed successfully with topical agents and therapies; widespread disease requires **chemotherapy.**

Description

Investigators recognize four distinct forms of Kaposi's sarcoma (KS). The first form, called classic KS, was described by the Austrian dermatologist Moricz Kaposi more than a century ago. Classic KS usually affects older men of Mediterranean or eastern European backgrounds by producing tumors on the lower legs. Though at times painful and disfiguring, they are not generally life-threatening. The second form of the disease, African endemic KS, primarily affects boys and men. It can appear as classic KS, or in a more deadly form that quickly spreads to tissues below the skin, the bones and lymph system, leading to **death** within a few years of diagnosis. Another form of KS, iatrogenic KS, is observed in kidney and liver transplant patients who take immunosuppressive drugs to prevent rejection of their organ transplant. Iatrogenic KS usually reverses after the immunosuppressive drug is stopped. The fourth form of KS, AIDS-related KS, emerged as one of the first illnesses observed among those with AIDS. Unlike classic KS, AIDS-related KS tumors generally appear on the upper body, including the head, neck, and back. The tumors also can appear on the soft palate and gum areas of the mouth, and in more advanced cases, they can be found in the stomach and intestines, the lymph nodes, and the lungs.

Causes & symptoms

A variety of factors appear to contribute to the development of KS:

• Genetic predisposition. People with classic KS, and those who develop the tumors after transplantation, are more likely than others to possess a genetically determined immune factor called HLA-DR. Cases of KS that run in families, however, are rare.

• Sex hormones. The fact that the disease is more likely to afflict men than women suggests sex hormones, such as testosterone in men, may stimulate the growth of KS tumors, and that estrogen in women may retard their growth.

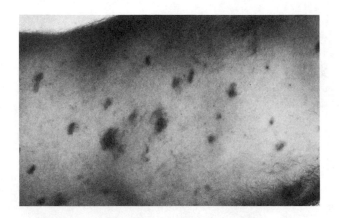

Kaposi's sarcoma usually appears on the lower extremities, as evidenced on this patient's hip. *(Custom Medical Stock Photo. Reproduced by permission.)*

• Immune suppression. Liver, kidney, and bone marrow patients who take immunosuppressive drugs to prevent transplant rejection frequently develop KS lesions. Similarly, KS has been observed in patients receiving systemic treatment with high-dose **corticosteroids,** which also suppresses the immune system. Immune suppression is the hallmark of AIDS.

• Infectious, sexually transmitted agent. AIDS-related KS is ten times more likely to appear in homosexual or bisexual men with AIDS than it is to appear in IV drug users, hemophiliacs, or women. In addition, the propor-

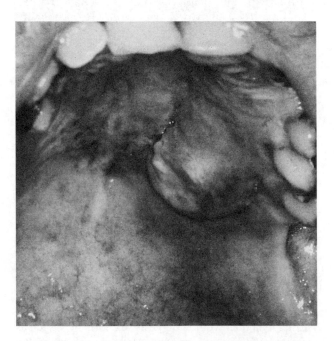

This HIV-positive patient is afflicted with Kaposi's sarcoma inside the mouth. *(Custom Medical Stock Photo. Reproduced by permission.)*

tion of AIDS patients who develop KS has decreased markedly as safer-sex practices have become more widespread. A number of viruses have been proposed as possible causes. They include cytomegalovirus and human papilloma virus, fragments of which have been found in KS tumor specimens. A more likely candidate, however, is a new herpes virus that has been called human herpes virus 8 (HHV-8) or KS-associated herpes virus (KSHV). Since fragments of the virus were first disclosed in KS samples in 1994, they have since been found in KS samples taken from patients with classic KS, African endemic KS, and KS in transplant patients. Fragments of HHV-8, however, have also been found in patients who have other skin diseases but who do not have KS.

Diagnosis

Many physicians will diagnose KS based on the appearance of the skin tumors and the patient's medical history. Unexplained **cough** or chest pain, as well as unexplained stomach or intestinal pain or bleeding, could suggest that the disease has moved beyond the skin. The most certain diagnosis can be achieved by taking a biopsy sample of a suspected KS lesion and examining it under high-power magnification. For suspected involvement of internal organs, physicians will use a bronchoscope to examine the lungs or an endoscope to view the stomach and intestinal tract.

Treatment

There is no single best treatment for KS. Treatments range from topical agents for mild disease with few tumors to more aggressive systemic chemotherapy for more serious KS that has spread to large areas of skin or the internal organs. Physicians will frequently combine topical, radiation, and various systemic chemotherapy drugs, depending on the sites of the body affected, the speed at which it is progressing, and the patient's overall health, among other considerations.

Local therapy

When the number of KS tumors is small and the disease appears to be progressing slowly, physicians will consider destroying the lesions with **cryotherapy** (using a liquid nitrogen spray or probe to freeze the tumor); injections directly into the tumor of vinblastine (a drug also used for systemic chemotherapy); or **radiation therapy** targeted at the tumor sites.

Systemic chemotherapy

With widespread KS lesions over the body surface, or evidence of spread to other parts of the body, physicians will consider systemic chemotherapy drugs, either alone or in a variety of combinations. Combination therapy generally produces a better response, with fewer toxic side effects associated with large doses of any single drug. Among the chemotherapy agents that physicians will consider using are vinblastine, bleomycin, and doxorubicin. A new class of chemotherapy drugs, called liposomally encapsulated drugs, appears to produce good results with fewer toxic side effects than do more conventional chemotherapy drugs.

Antiviral therapy

Evidence suggests that for some individuals, the class of AIDS drugs called **protease inhibitors,** in combination with other anti-HIV drugs, can reduce the levels of detectable HIV in the blood to nearly zero, and in some patients stabilize or reverse KS tumors. More research is needed in this area. Since the discovery of HHV-8, interest in an antiviral approach to KS has increased. There is no evidence, however, that two **antiviral drugs** commonly prescribed for herpes, acyclovir and ganciclovir, have any effect on the disease. One study of 20,000 patients with HIV and AIDS found that those who took foscarnet, another antiviral medication that works in a different way than acyclovir and ganciclovir, were less likely to develop KS tumors.

A number of other treatments for KS are under investigation, including:

• Interferon-alpha. Interferon-alpha is made by the body and has powerful effects on the immune system. Investigators have tried injecting it directly into lesions, and also in combination with other anti-HIV drugs such as zidovudine, with some success.

• Retinoids. These derivatives of vitamin A have long been used to treat **acne** and other skin diseases. Investigators are evaluating both topical preparations of these drugs as well as systemic versions.

• Laser therapy. In patients with small tumors, some investigators report success using lasers to destroy KS lesions. The reappearance of new tumors, may be high, however.

Alternative treatment

The Bastyr University AIDS Research Study has been investigating and collecting data on treatment for KS and other opportunistic conditions that are AIDS-related. Among the treatments under investigation are nutritional and herbal therapies (both internal and external). Bastyr University is located in Seattle, Washington.

Prognosis

The prognosis for patients with classic KS is good. Tumors can frequently be controlled and patients fre-

quently die of other causes before any serious spread. African endemic KS can progress rapidly and lead to premature death, despite treatment. In AIDS-related KS, milder cases can frequently be controlled; the prognosis for more advanced and rapidly progressing cases is less certain and dependent on the patient's overall medical condition. There are indications that KS can be stabilized or reversed in patients whose level of HIV in the blood is reduced to undetectable levels via antiretroviral therapy.

Prevention

Safer sex practices may help to prevent AIDS-related KS by decreasing the risk of transmission of HHV-8. Treatment with antiretrovirals and protease inhibitors may help to preserve the function of the immune system in HIV patients and delay the appearance and progression of KS lesions.

Resources

BOOKS

Fitzpatrick, Thomas B., et al. *Color Atlas and Synopsis of Clinical Dermatology.* New York: McGraw-Hill, 1997.

Sams, W. Mitchell Jr., et al. *Principles and Practice of Dermatology.* New York: Churchill Livingstone, 1996.

PERIODICALS

Krown, Susan E. "Acquired Immunodeficiency Syndrome-Associated Kaposi's Sarcoma." *Medical Clinics of North America* 81(March 1997): 471-494.

Myskowski, Patricia L., and Rosaline Ahkami. "Advances in Kaposi's Sarcoma." *Dermatologic Clinics* 15(January 1997): 177-188.

Sung, Jennifer C.Y., et al. "Kaposi's Sarcoma: Advances in Tumor Biology and Pharmacotherapy." *Pharmacotherapy* 17(1997): 670-683.

ORGANIZATIONS

American Academy of Dermatology. 930 N. Meacham Road, PO Box 4014, Schaumburg, IL 60168-4014. (847) 330-0230. http://www.aad.org.

Gay Men's Health Crisis. 119 West 24th Street, New York, NY 10011. (212) 807-6664. http://www.gmhc.org.

Richard H. Camer

Kawasaki syndrome

Definition

Kawasaki syndrome is a potentially fatal inflammatory disease that affects several organ systems in the body, including the heart, circulatory system, mucous

KEY TERMS

Aneurysm—Dilation of an artery caused by thinning and weakening of the vessel wall.

Arrythmia—Abnormal heart rhythm.

Arteritis—Inflammation of an artery.

Cardiomegaly—An enlarged heart.

Conjunctivae—The mucous membranes that cover the exposed area of the eyeball and line the inner surface of the eyelids.

Exanthem—A skin eruption associated with a disease, usually one accompanied by fever as in Kawasaki syndrome.

Gangrene—The death of soft tissue in a part of the body, usually caused by obstructed circulation.

Hepatitis—Inflammation of the liver.

Meningitis—Inflammation of the membranes, called the meninges, covering the brain and spinal cord.

Mucocutaneous lymph node syndrome (MLNS)—Mucocutaneous lymph node syndrome, another name for Kawasaki syndrome. The name comes from the key symptoms of the disease, which involve the mucous membranes of the mouth and throat, the skin, and the lymph nodes.

Myocarditis—Inflammation of the heart muscle.

Stevens-Johnson syndrome—A severe inflammatory skin eruption that occurs as a result of an allergic reaction or respiratory infection.

T cell—A type of white blood cell that develops in the thymus gland and helps to regulate the immune system's response to infections or malignancy.

membranes, skin, and immune system. It occurs primarily in infants and children but has also been identified in adults as old as 34 years. Its cause is unknown.

Description

Kawasaki syndrome, also called mucocutaneous lymph node syndrome (MLNS), is an inflammatory disorder with potentially fatal complications affecting the heart and its larger arteries. Nearly twice as many males are affected as females. Although persons of Asian descent are affected more frequently than either black or white individuals, there does not appear to be a distinctive geographic pattern of occurrence. Eighty percent of cases involve children under the age of four. Although the disease usually appears in individuals, it sometimes affects several members of the same family and occasionally occurs in small epidemics.

Causes & symptoms

The specific cause of Kawasaki syndrome is unknown, although the disease resembles infectious illnesses in many ways. It has been suggested that Kawasaki syndrome represents an allergic reaction or other unusual response to certain types of infections. Some researchers think that the syndrome may be caused by the interaction of an immune cell, called the T cell, with certain poisons (toxins) secreted by bacteria.

Kawasaki syndrome has an abrupt onset, with **fever** as high as 104°F (40°C) and a rash that spreads over the patient's chest and genital area. The fever is followed by a characteristic peeling of the skin beginning at the fingertips and toenails. In addition to the body rash, the patient's lips become very red, with the tongue developing a ''strawberry'' appearance. The palms, soles, and mucous membranes that line the eyelids and cover the exposed portion of the eyeball (conjuntivae) become purplish-red and swollen. The lymph nodes in the patient's neck may also become swollen. These symptoms may last from two weeks to three months, with relapses in some patients.

In addition to the major symptoms, about 30% of patients develop joint **pains** or arthritis, usually in the large joints of the body. Others develop **pneumonia, diarrhea,** dry or cracked lips, **jaundice,** or an inflammation of the membranes covering the brain and spinal cord (**meningitis**). A few patients develop symptoms of inflammation in the liver (hepatitis), gallbladder, lungs, or tonsils.

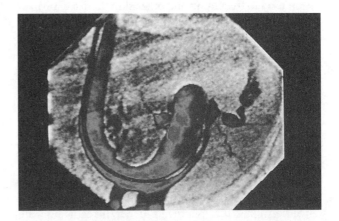

An angiogram showing abnormal coronary arteries in a child suffering from Kawasaki's disease. The coronary arteries are abnormal and weakened in that they bulge into balloon shapes, or aneurysms, along their lengths. This illness occurs in children between the ages of 1-2 years. (*Photograph by Mehau Kulyk, Photo Researchers, Inc. Reproduced by permission.*)

About 20% of patients with Kawasaki syndrome develop complications of the cardiovascular system. These complications include inflammation of the heart tissue (**myocarditis**), disturbances in heartbeat rhythm (**arrhythmias**), and areas of blood vessel dilation (aneurysms) in the coronary arteries. Other patients may develop inflammation of an artery (arteritis) in their arms or legs. Complications of the heart or arteries begin to develop around the tenth day after the illness begins, when the fever and rash begin to subside. A few patients may develop **gangrene,** or the death of soft tissue, in their hands and feet. The specific causes of these complications are not yet known.

Diagnosis

Because Kawasaki syndrome is primarily a disease of infants and young children, the disease is most likely to be diagnosed by a pediatrician. The physician will first consider the possible involvement of other diseases that cause fever and skin **rashes,** including **scarlet fever, measles, Rocky Mountain spotted fever, toxoplasmosis** (a disease carried by cats), juvenile **rheumatoid arthritis,** and a blistering and inflammation of the skin caused by reactions to certain medications (Stevens-Johnson syndrome).

Once other diseases have been ruled out, the patient's symptoms will be compared with a set of diagnostic criteria. The patient must have a fever lasting five days or longer that does not respond to antibiotics, together with four of the following five symptoms:

- Inflammation of the conjunctivae of both eyes with no discharge

- At least one of the following changes in the mucous membranes of the mouth and throat: ''strawberry'' tongue; cracked lips; or swollen throat tissues

- At least one of the following changes in the hands or feet: swelling caused by excess fluid in the tissues; peeling of the skin; or abnormal redness of the skin

- A skin eruption or rash associated with fever (exanthem) on the patient's trunk

- Swelling of the lymph nodes in the neck to a size greater than 1.5 cm.

Since the cause of Kawasaki syndrome is unknown, there are no laboratory tests that can confirm the diagnosis. The following test results, however, are associated with the disease:

- Blood tests show a high white blood cell count, high **platelet count,** a high level of protein in the blood serum, and mild anemia.

- **Chest x ray** may show enlargement of the heart (cardiomegaly).

- Urine may show the presence of pus or an abnormally high level of protein.

- An electrocardiogram may show changes in the heartbeat rhythm.

In addition to these tests, it is important to take a series of echocardiograms during the course of the illness because 20% of Kawasaki patients will develop coronary aneurysms or arteritis that will not appear during the first examination.

Treatment

Kawasaki syndrome is usually treated with a combination of **aspirin,** to control the patient's fever and skin inflammation, and high doses of intravenous immune globulin to reduce the possibility of coronary artery complications. Some patients with heart complications may be treated with drugs that reduce blood clotting or may receive corrective surgery.

Follow-up care includes two to three months of monitoring with chest x rays, **electrocardiography,** and **echocardiography.** Treatment with aspirin is often continued for several months.

Prognosis

Most patients with Kawasaki syndrome will recover completely, but about 1-2% will die as a result of blood clots forming in the coronary arteries or as a result of a **heart attack.** Deaths are sudden and unpredictable. Almost 95% of fatalities occur within six months of infection, but some have been reported as long as 10 years afterward. Long-term follow-up of patients with aneurysms indicates that about half show some healing of the aneurysm. The remaining half has a high risk of heart complications in later life.

Resources

BOOKS

Abzug, Mark J. ''Infectious Diseases: Bacterial, Spirochetal, Protozoal, Metazoal, & Mycotic.'' In *Handbook of Pediatrics,* edited by Gerald B. Merenstein, et al. Norwalk, CT: Appleton & Lange, 1994.

''Childhood Infections: Kawasaki Syndrome.'' In *The Merck Manual of Diagnosis and Therapy,* Vol. II, edited by Robert Berkow, et al. Rahway, NJ: Merck Research Laboratories, 1992.

Shaffer, Elizabeth M., et al. ''Heart.'' In *Handbook of Pediatrics,* edited by Gerald B. Merenstein, et al. Norwalk, CT: Appleton & Lange, 1994.

Shandera, Wayne X., and Maria E. Carlini. ''Infectious Diseases: Viral & Rickettsial.'' In *Current Medical Diagnosis & Treatment 1998,* edited by Lawrence M. Tierney Jr., et al. Stamford, CT: Appleton & Lange, 1997.

Wolfe, Robert R., et al. "Cardiovascular Diseases." In *Current Pediatric Diagnosis & Treatment,* edited by William W. Hay Jr., et al. Stamford, CT: Appleton & Lange, 1997.

Rebecca J. Frey

Keloid *see* **Skin lesions**

Keneda device *see* **Spinal instrumentation**

Keratitis

Definition

Keratitis is an inflammation of the cornea, the transparent membrane that covers the colored part of the eye (iris) and pupil of the eye.

Description

There are many types and causes of keratitis. Keratitis occurs in both children and adults. Organisms cannot generally invade an intact, healthy cornea. However, certain conditions can allow an infection to occur. For example, a scratch can leave the cornea open to infection. A very dry eye can also decrease the cornea's protective mechanisms.

Risk factors that increase the likelihood of developing this condition include:

- Poor contact lens care; overuse of contact lenses

- Illnesses or other factors that reduces the body's ability to overcome infection

- **Cold sores, genital herpes,** and other viral infections

- Crowded, dirty living conditions; poor hygiene

- Poor nutrition (especially a deficiency of Vitamin A, which is essential for normal vision).

Some common types of keratitis are listed below, however there are many other forms.

Herpes simplex keratitis

A major cause of adult eye disease, herpes simplex keratitis may lead to:

- Chronic inflammation of the cornea

- Development of tiny blood vessels in the eye

- Scarring

- Loss of vision

- Glaucoma.

This infection generally begins with inflammation of the membrane lining the eyelid (conjunctiva) and the portion of the eyeball that comes into contact with it. It usually occurs in one eye. Subsequent infections are characterized by a pattern of lesions that resemble the veins of a leaf. These infections are called dendritic keratitis and aid in the diagnosis.

Recurrences may be brought on by **stress,** fatigue, or ultraviolet light (UV) exposure (e.g., skiing or boating increase the exposure of the eye to sunlight; the sunlight reflects off of the surfaces). Repeated episodes of dendritic keratitis can cause sores, permanent scarring, and numbness of the cornea.

Recurrent dendritic keratitis is often followed by disciform keratitis. This condition is characterized by clouding and deep, disc-shaped swelling of the cornea and by inflammation of the iris.

It is very important not to use topical **corticosteroids** with herpes simplex keratitis as it can make it much worse, possibly leading to blindness.

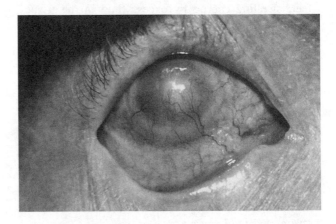

Close-up of a damaged cornea due to complications following cataract surgery. *(Custom Medical Stock Photo. Reproduced by permission.)*

Bacterial keratitis

People who have bacterial keratitis wake up with their eyelids stuck together. There can be **pain,** sensitivity to light, redness, tearing, and a decrease in vision. This condition, which is usually aggressive, can be caused by wearing soft contact lenses overnight. One study found that overnight wear can increase risk by 10-15 times more than if wearing daily wear contact lenses. Improper lens care is also a factor. Contaminated makeup can also contain bacteria.

Bacterial keratitis makes the cornea cloudy. It may also cause **abscesses** to develop in the stroma, which is located beneath the outer layer of the cornea.

Fungal keratitis

Usually a consequence of injuring the cornea in a farm-like setting or in a place where plant material is present, fungal keratitis often develops slowly. This condition:

- Usually affects people with weakened immune systems
- Often results in infection within the eyeball
- May cause stromal abscesses.

Peripheral ulcerative keratitis

Peripheral ulcerative keratitis is also called marginal keratolysis or peripheral rheumatoid ulceration. This condition is often associated with active or chronic:

- **Rheumatoid arthritis**
- **Relapsing polychondritis** (connective-tissue inflammation)
- **Wegener's granulomatosis,** a rare condition characterized by kidney disease and development of nodules in the respiratory tract.

Superficial punctate keratitis

Often associated with the type of viruses that cause upper respiratory infection (adenoviruses), superficial punctate keratitis is characterized by destruction of pinpoint areas in the outer layer of the cornea (epithelium). One or both eyes may be affected.

Acanthamoeba keratitis

This pus-producing condition is very painful. It is a common source of infection in people who wear soft or rigid contact lenses. It can be found in tap water, soil, and swimming pools.

Photokeratitis

Photokeratitis or snowblindness is caused by excess exposure to UV light. This can occur with sunlight, suntanning lamps, or a welding arc. It is called snowblindness because the sunlight is reflected off of the snow. It therefore can occur in water sports as well, because of the reflection of light off of the water. It is very painful and may occur several hours after exposure. It may last one to two days.

Interstitial keratitis

Also called parenchymatous keratitis, interstitial keratitis is a chronic inflammation of tissue deep within the cornea. Interstitial keratitis is rare in the United States. Interstitial keratitis affects both eyes and usually occurs as a complication of congenital or acquired **syphilis.** In congenital syphilis it can occur between age two and **puberty.** It may also occur in people with **tuberculosis, leprosy,** or other diseases.

Causes & symptoms

In summary, keratitis can be caused by:

- Bacterial, viral, or fungal infections
- Dry eyes resulting from disorders of the eyelid or diminished ability to form tears
- Exposure to very bright light
- **Foreign objects** that injure or become lodged in the eye
- Sensitivity or allergic reactions to eye makeup, dust, pollen, pollution, or other irritants
- **Vitamin A deficiency,** which people with normal diets rarely develop.

Symptoms of keratitis include, but are not limited to:

- Tearing
- Pain
- Sensitivity to light
- Inflammation of the eyelid
- Decrease in vision
- Redness.

Diagnosis

A case history will be taken and the vision will be tested. Examination with a slit lamp, an instrument that's a microscope and focuses a beam of light on the eye is important for diagnosis. The cornea can be examined with fluorescein, a yellow dye which will highlight defects in the cornea. Deeper layers of the cornea can also be examined with the slit lamp. Infiltrates, hazy looking areas in the cornea, can be seen by the doctor and will aid in the diagnosis. Samples of infectious matter removed from the eye will be sent for laboratory analysis.

Treatment

Antibiotics, antifungals, and antiviral medication will be used to treat the appropriate organism. Broad spectrum antibiotics will be used immediately, but once the lab analysis determines the offending organism the medication may be changed. Sometimes more than one medication is necessary. It depends upon the infection, but the patient should be clear on how often and how to use the medications.

A sterile, cotton-tipped applicator may be used to gently remove infected tissue and allow the eye to heal more rapidly. **Laser surgery** is sometimes performed to destroy unhealthy cells, and some severe infections require corneal transplants.

Antifungal, antibiotic, or antiviral eyedrops or ointments are usually prescribed to cure keratitis, but they should be used only by patients under a doctor's care. Inappropriate prescriptions or over-the-counter preparations can make symptoms more severe and cause tissue deterioration. Topical corticosteroids can cause great harm to the cornea in patient's with herpes simplex keratitis.

A patient with keratitis may wear a patch to protect the healing eye from bright light, foreign objects, the lid rubbing against the cornea, and other irritants. Sometimes a patch can make it worse, so again, the patient must discuss with the doctor whether or not a patch is necessary. The patient will probably return every day to the eye doctor to check on the progress.

Although early detection and treatment can cure most forms of keratitis, the infection can cause:

• Glaucoma

• Permanent scarring

• Ulceration of the cornea

• Blindness.

Prevention

Children and adults who wear contact lenses should always use sterile lens-cleaning and disinfecting solutions. Tap water is not sterile and should not be used to clean contact lenses. It is important to go for follow-up checkups because small defects in the cornea can occur without the patient being aware of it. Do not overwear contact lenses. Remove them if the eyes become red or irritated. Replace contact lenses when scheduled to do so. Proteins and other things can deposit on the contacts, leading to an increased risk of infection. Rinse contact lens cases in hot water every night, if possible, and let them air dry. Replace contact lens cases every three months. Organisms have been cultured from contact lens cases.

Eating a well-balanced diet and wearing protective glasses when working or playing in potentially dangerous situations can reduce anyone's risk of developing keratitis. Protective goggles can even be worn mowing the lawn so that if twigs are tossed up they can't hurt the eye. Goggles or sunglasses with UV coatings can help protect against damage from UV light.

Resources

BOOKS

Current Medical Diagnosis and Treatment 1998, edited by Tierney, Lawrence M., Jr., et al. Stamford, CT: Appleton & Lange, 1998.

ORGANIZATIONS

American Academy of Ophthalmology. P.O. Box 7424, San Francisco CA. 94120-7424. (415) 561-8500. http://www.eyenet.org.

American Optometric Association. 243 North Lindbergh Blvd., St. Louis, MO 63141. (314) 991-4100. http://www.aoanet.org.

National Eye Institute. 9000 Rockville Pike, Bethesda, MD 20892-0001 (301) 496-3123. http://www.nei.nih.gov/nei/pubpat.htm.

Prevent Blindness America. 500 East Remington Road, Schaumburg, IL 60173. (800) 331-2020. http://www.prevent-blindness.org.

OTHER

Infection-causing Organism Dictates Microbial Keratitis Treatment. http://www.slackinc.com/eye/pcon/199603/kera.html (21 May 1998).

Keratitis. http://www.thriveonline.com/health/Library/illsymp/illness308.html (20 May 1998).

The Merck Manual: Opthalmologic disorders. http://www.merck.com/ (21 May 1998).

To Avoid Infection, Make RGP Patients Aware of Tap Water Risk. http://www.slackinc.com/eye/pcon/199603/taph20.htm (21 May 1998).

Maureen Haggerty

Keratomalacia *see* **Vitamin A deficiency**

Ketoconazole *see* **Antifungal drugs, systemic**

Ketorolac *see* **Nonsteroidal anti-inflammatory drugs**

Kidney angiogram *see* **Angiography**

Kidney biopsy

Definition

Kidney biopsy is a medical procedure in which a small piece of tissue is removed from the kidney for microscopic examination.

Purpose

The test is usually done to diagnose kidney disease and to evaluate the extent of damage to the kidney. A biopsy is also frequently ordered to detect the reason for acute renal failure when normal office procedures and tests fail to establish the cause. In addition, information regarding the progression of the disease and how it is responding to medical treatment can be obtained from a biopsy. Occasionally a biopsy may be done to confirm a diagnosis of **kidney cancer,** to determine its aggressiveness, and decide on the mode of treatment.

Precautions

The biopsy is not recommended for patients who have any uncontrollable bleeding disorders. Platelets are blood cells that play an important role in the blood clotting process. If the bleeding disorder is caused by a low **platelet count** (less than 50,000 per cubic millimeter of blood), then a platelet **transfusion** can be done just before performing the biopsy.

Description

The kidneys, a pair of organs that are shaped like beans, lie on either side of the backbone, just above the waist. The periphery (parenchyma) of the kidney is made up of tiny tubes. These tubes filter and clean the blood by taking out the waste products and making urine. The urine is collected in the central portion of the kidney. Tubes called ureters drain the urine from the kidney into the bladder, where it is held until it is voided from the body.

A kidney specialist (nephrologist) performs the biopsy. It can be done either in the doctor's office or in a local hospital. The patient may be given a calming drug before the procedure to help him relax. The skin and muscles on the back overlying the site that is to be biopsied may be numbed with **local anesthesia.**

The patient will be asked to lie face down and a pad or a rolled towel may be placed under the stomach. Either the left or the right kidney may be biopsied depending on the results of the imaging tests: x rays, **computed tomography scans** (CT scans), **magnetic resonance imaging** (MRI), and ultrasound. The area that will be biopsied is cleaned with an antiseptic solution and sterile drapes are placed on it. The skin is numbed with local

---

KEY TERMS

Biopsy—The surgical removal and microscopic examination of living tissue for diagnostic purposes.

Computed tomography (CT) scan—A medical procedure in which a series of x rays are taken and put together by a computer in order to form detailed pictures of areas inside the body.

Magnetic resonance imaging (MRI)—A medical procedure used for diagnostic purposes in which pictures of areas inside the body can be created using a magnet linked to a computer.

Nephrologist—A doctor who specializes in the diseases and disorders of the kidneys.

Renal ultrasound—A painless and non-invasive procedure in which sound waves are bounced off the kidneys. These sound waves produce a pattern of echoes that are then used by the computer to create pictures of areas inside the kidney (sonograms).

---

anesthesia. A small incision is made on the skin with a scalpel blade. Using a long needle, the physician injects local anesthesia into the incision so that it infiltrates down to the kidney. The biopsy needle is then advanced slowly through the incision. The patient is asked to hold his or her breath each time the needle is pushed forward. Once the wall (capsule) of the kidney has been penetrated, the patient can breathe normally. The tissue is collected for examination and the needle is withdrawn. The needle may be re-inserted into another part of the kidney so that tissue is collected from at least three different areas. The tissue samples are sent to the laboratory for examination. The entire procedure may last about an hour.

Preparation

Before performing the biopsy, the doctor should be made aware of all the medications that the patient is taking. The doctor should also be told whether the patient is allergic to any medications. The procedure and the risks of the procedure are explained to the patient and the necessary consent forms are obtained. The patient should be told that a kidney biopsy requires a 24-hour stay in the hospital after the biopsy.

Some doctors order blood tests to check for clotting problems before performing the biopsy. The patient's blood type may also be determined in case a transfusion becomes necessary.

Aftercare

Immediately after the biopsy, pulse, respiration, and temperature (vital signs) are measured. If they are stable, the patient is instructed to lie flat in bed for at least 12 hours. The pulse and blood pressure are checked at regular intervals by the nursing staff. All urine voided by the patient in the first 12-24 hours is examined in the laboratory for blood cells.

If bleeding is severe, iron levels in the blood drop significantly, or the patient complains of severe **pain** at the biopsy site, the physician should be contacted immediately. After the patient goes home, he should avoid heavy lifting, vigorous **exercise,** and contact sports for at least one or two weeks.

Risks

The risks of a kidney biopsy are very small. Severe bleeding may occur after the procedure. There is also a slight chance that an infection or a lump of blood under the skin that looks black and blue (hematoma) may develop. In most cases, the hematoma disappears by itself and does not cause any pain. However, severe pain or a drop in blood pressure and iron levels in the blood indicates that the hematoma is expanding. This condition could lead to complications and should be reported immediately to the doctor.

Very rarely, the patient may develop high blood pressure (**hypertension**), and the bleeding may be severe enough to require a transfusion. In extremely rare circumstances, the kidney may rupture, or the surrounding organs (pancreas, bowel, spleen, and liver) may be punctured. **Death** occurs in about one in 3000 cases.

Normal results

The results are normal if no abnormalities can be seen in the tissue samples with the naked eye, with an electron microscope or through staining with a fluorescent dye (immunofluorescence).

Abnormal results

Any abnormalities in the size, color, and consistency of the sample will be reported as an abnormal result. In addition, any change in the structure of the renal tubules, the presence of red blood cells, or abnormalities in the cells are considered an abnormal result. If cancerous changes are detected in the kidney cells, they are further characterized in order to determine the stage of the tumor and decide on the appropriate mode of treatment.

Resources

BOOKS

Berkow, Robert, ed. *The Merck Manual of Diagnosis and Therapy.* 16th ed. Rahway, NJ: Merck Research Laboratories, 1992.

Segen, Joseph C., and Joseph Stauffer. *The Patient's Guide to Medical Tests. Everything You Need to Know about the Tests Your Doctor Prescribes.* New York: Facts On File, 1998.

Sobel, David S., and T. Ferguson. *The People's Book of Medical Tests.* New York: Summit Books, 1985.

ORGANIZATIONS

National Kidney Cancer Association. 1234 Sherman Avenue, Suite 203, Evanston, IL 60202-1375. (800) 850-9132.

National Kidney Foundation. 30 East 33rd Street, New York, NY 10016. (800) 622-9010. http://www.kidney.org.

Lata Cherath

· ·

Kidney cancer

Definition

Kidney cancer is a disease in which the cells in certain tissues of the kidney start to grow uncontrollably and form tumors. Renal cell carcinoma, which occurs in the cells lining the kidneys (epithelial cells), is the most common type of kidney cancer. Eighty-five percent of all kidney tumors are renal cell carcinomas. **Wilms' tumor** is a rapidly developing **cancer** of the kidney most often found in children under four years of age.

Description

The kidneys are a pair of organs shaped like kidney beans that lie on either side of the spine just above the waist. Inside each kidney are tiny tubes (tubules) that filter and clean the blood, taking out the waste products and making urine. The urine that is made by the kidney passes through a tube called the ureter into the bladder. Urine is held in the bladder until it is discharged from the body. Renal cell carcinoma generally develops in the lining of the tubules that filter and clean the blood. Cancer that develops in the central portion of the kidney (where the urine is collected and drained into the ureters) is known as transitional cell cancer of the renal pelvis. Transitional cell cancer is similar to **bladder cancer.**

Kidney cancer accounts for 3% of all cancers. According to the American Cancer Society, approximately 30,000 new cases of kidney cancer will be found in 1998. Kidney cancer occurs most often in men over the age of

KEY TERMS

Biopsy—The surgical removal and microscopic examination of living tissue for diagnostic purposes.

Bone scan—An x-ray study in which patients are given an intravenous injection of a small amount of a radioactive material that travels in the blood. When it reaches the bones, it can be detected by x ray to make a picture of their internal structure.

Chemotherapy—Treatment with anticancer drugs.

Computed tomography (CT) scan—A medical procedure in which a series of x-ray images are made and put together by a computer to form detailed pictures of areas inside the body.

Hematuria—Blood in the urine.

Immunotherapy—Treatment of cancer by stimulating the body's immune defense system.

Intravenous pyelogram (IVP)—A procedure in which a dye is injected into a vein in the arm. The dye travels through the body and concentrates in the urine to be discharged. It outlines the kidneys, ureters, and the urinary bladder. An x-ray image is then made and any abnormalities of the urinary tract are revealed.

Magnetic resonance imaging (MRI)—A medical procedure used for diagnostic purposes in which pictures of areas inside the body can be created using a magnet linked to a computer.

Nephrectomy—A medical procedure in which the kidney is surgically removed.

Radiation therapy—Treatment with high-energy radiation from x-ray machines, cobalt, radium, or other sources.

Renal ultrasound—A painless and non-invasive procedure in which sound waves are bounced off the kidneys. These sound waves produce a pattern of echoes that are then used by the computer to create pictures of areas inside the kidney (sonograms).

40. Men are twice as likely as women are to have cancer of the kidney.

Causes & symptoms

The causes of kidney cancer are unknown, but men seem to have twice the risk of contracting the disease. There is a strong association between cigarette smoking and kidney cancer. Cigarette smokers are twice as likely as non-smokers are to develop kidney cancer. Working around coke ovens has been shown to increase people's risk of developing this cancer. Certain types of painkillers that contain the chemical phenacetin are associated with kidney cancer. The United States government discontinued use of **analgesics** containing phenacetin about 20 years ago. **Obesity** may be yet another risk factor for kidney cancer. Some studies show a loose association between exposure to cadmium and asbestos and kidney cancer.

The most common symptom of kidney cancer is blood in the urine (hematuria). Other symptoms include painful urination, pain in the lower back or on the sides, abdominal pain, a lump or hard mass that can be felt in the kidney area, unexplained weight loss, **fever,** weakness, fatigue, and high blood pressure.

Diagnosis

A diagnostic examination for kidney cancer includes taking a thorough medical history and making a complete **physical examination** in which the doctor will probe (palpate) the abdomen for lumps. Blood tests will be ordered to check for changes in blood chemistry caused by substances released by the tumor. Laboratory tests may show abnormal levels of iron in the blood. Either a low red blood cell count (anemia) or a high red blood cell count (erythrocytosis) may accompany kidney cancer. Occasionally, patients will have high calcium levels.

If the doctor suspects kidney cancer, an intravenous pyelogram (IVP) may be ordered. An IVP is an x-ray test in which a dye in injected into a vein in the arm. The dye travels through the body, and when it is concentrated in the urine to be discharged, it outlines the kidneys, ureters, and the urinary bladder. On an x-ray image, the dye will reveal any abnormalities of the urinary tract. The IVP may miss small kidney cancers.

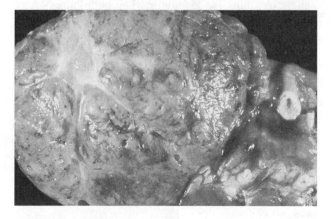

An extracted cancerous kidney. (Custom Medical Stock Photo. Reproduced by permission.)

Renal ultrasound is a diagnostic test in which sound waves are used to form an image of the kidneys. Ultrasound is a painless and non-invasive procedure that can be used to detect even very small kidney tumors. Imaging tests such as **computed tomography scans** (CT scans) and **magnetic resonance imaging** (MRI) can be used to evaluate the kidneys and the surrounding organs. These tests are used to check whether the tumor has spread outside the kidney to other organs in the abdomen. If the patient complains of bone pain, a special x ray called a bone scan may be ordered to rule out spread to the bones. A **chest x ray** may be taken to rule out spread to the lungs.

A **kidney biopsy** is used to positively confirm the diagnosis of kidney cancer. During this procedure, a small piece of tissue is removed from the tumor and examined under a microscope. The biopsy will give information about the type of tumor, the cells that are involved, and the aggressiveness of the tumor (tumor stage).

Treatment

Each person's treatment is different and depends on several factors. The location, size, and extent of the tumor have to be considered in addition to the patient's age, general health, and medical history.

The primary treatment for kidney cancer that has not spread to other parts of the body is surgical removal of the diseased kidney (**nephrectomy**). Because most cancers affect only one kidney, the patient can function well on the one remaining. Two types of surgical procedure are used. Radical nephrectomy removes the entire kidney and the surrounding tissue. Sometimes, the lymph nodes surrounding the kidney are also removed. Partial nephrectomy removes only part of the kidney along with the tumor. This procedure is used either when the tumor is very small or when it is not practical to remove the entire kidney. It is not practical to remove a kidney when the patient has only one kidney or when both kidneys have tumors. There is a small (5%) chance of missing some of the cancer.

Radiation therapy, which consists of exposing the cancer cells to high-energy gamma rays from an external source, generally destroys cancer cells with minimal damage to the normal tissue. Side effects are nausea, tiredness, and stomach upsets. These symptoms disappear when the treatment is over. In kidney cancer, radiation therapy has been shown to alleviate pain and bleeding, especially when the cancer is inoperable. However, it has not proven to be of much use in destroying the kidney cancer cells. Therefore radiation therapy is not used very often.

Treatment of kidney cancer with anti-cancer drugs (**chemotherapy**) has not produced good results. However, new drugs and new combinations of drugs continue to be tested in clinical trials.

Immunotherapy, a form of treatment in which the body's immune system is harnessed to help fight the cancer, is a new mode of therapy that is being tested for kidney cancer. Clinical trials with substances produced by the immune cells (interleukin-2 and interferon) have shown some promise in destroying kidney cancer cells. These substances have been approved for use but they can be very toxic and produce severe side effects. The benefits derived from the treatment have to be weighed very carefully against the side effects in each case.

Prognosis

Because kidney cancer is often caught early and sometimes progresses slowly, the chances of a surgical cure are good. It is also one of the few cancers for which there are well-documented cases of spontaneous remission without therapy.

Prevention

The exact cause of kidney cancer is not known, so it is not possible to prevent all cases. However, because a strong association between kidney cancer and tobacco has been shown, avoiding tobacco is the best way to lower one's risk of developing this cancer. Using care when working with cancer-causing agents such as asbestos and cadmium and eating a well-balanced diet may also help prevent kidney cancer.

Resources

BOOKS

Berkow, Robert, ed. *The Merck Manual of Diagnosis and Therapy.* 16th ed. Rahway, NJ: Merck Research Laboratories, 1992.

Dollinger, Malin, Ernest H. Rosenbaum, and Greg Cable. *Everyone's Guide to Cancer Therapy. How Cancer Is Diagnosed, Treated, and Managed Day to Day.* Toronto: Somerville House Books Limited, 1994.

Morra, Marion, and Eve Potts *Choices.* New York: Avon Books, 1994.

Murphy, Gerald P., Lois B. Morris, and Dianne Lange. *Informed Decisions: The Complete Book of Cancer Diagnosis, Treatment and Recovery.* New York: Viking, 1997.

ORGANIZATIONS

American Cancer Society (National Headquarters). 1599 Clifton Road, N.E., Atlanta, GA 30329. (800) 227-2345. http://www.cancer.org.

Cancer Research Institute (National Headquarters). 681 Fifth Avenue, New York, NY 10022. (800) 992-2623. http://www.cancerresearch.org.

National Cancer Institute. 9000 Rockville Pike, Building 31, Room 10A16, Bethesda, MD 20892. (800) 422-6237. http://www.nci.nih.gov.

National Kidney Cancer Association. 1234 Sherman Avenue, Suite 203, Evanston, IL 60202-1375. (800) 850-9132.

National Kidney Foundation. 30 East 33rd Street, New York, NY 10016. (800) 622-9010. http://www.kidney.org.

Lata Cherath

Kidney dialysis *see* **Dialysis, kidney**

Kidney failure *see* **Acute kidney failure; Chronic kidney failure**

Kidney function tests

Definition

Kidney function tests is a collective term for a variety of individual tests and procedures that can be done to evaluate how well the kidneys are functioning.

Purpose

The kidneys, the body's natural filtration system, perform many vital functions, including removing metabolic waste products from the bloodstream, regulating the body's water balance, and maintaining the pH (acidity/ alkalinity) of the body's fluids. Approximately one and a half quarts of blood per minute are circulated through the kidneys, where waste chemicals are filtered out and eliminated from the body (along with excess water) in the form of urine. Kidney function tests help to determine if the kidneys are performing their tasks adequately.

Precautions

A complete history should be taken prior to kidney function tests to assess the patient's food and drug intake. A wide variety of prescription and over-the-counter medications can affect blood and urine kidney function test results, as can some food and beverages.

Description

Many conditions can affect the ability of the kidneys to carry-out their vital functions. Some lead to a rapid (acute) decline in kidney function; others lead to a gradual (chronic) decline in function. Both result in a build-up of toxic waste substances in the blood. A number of clinical laboratory tests that measure the levels of substances normally regulated by the kidneys can help deter-

---

KEY TERMS

Blood urea nitrogen (BUN)—The nitrogen portion of urea in the bloodstream. Urea is a waste product of protein metabolism in the body.

Creatinine—The metabolized by-product of creatine, an organic acid that assists the body in producing muscle contractions. Creatinine is found in the bloodstream and in muscle tissue. It is removed from the blood by the kidneys and excreted in the urine.

Osmolality—A measurement of urine concentration that depends on the number of particles dissolved in it. Values are expressed as milliosmols per kilogram (mOsm/kg) of water.

Urea—A by-product of protein metabolism that is formed in the liver. Because urea contains ammonia, which is toxic to the body, it must be quickly filtered from the blood by the kidneys and excreted in the urine.

---

mine the cause and extent of kidney dysfunction. These tests are done on urine samples, as well as on blood samples.

Urine tests

There are a variety of urine tests that assess kidney function. A simple, inexpensive screening test, called a routine **urinalysis,** is often the first test administered if kidney problems are suspected. A small, randomly collected urine sample is examined physically for things like color, odor, appearance, and concentration (specific gravity); chemically for substances such a protein, glucose, and pH (acidity/ alkalinity); and microscopically for the presence of cellular elements (red blood cells, white blood cells, and epithelial cells), bacteria, crystals, and casts (structures formed by the deposit of protein, cells, and other substances in the kidneys' tubules). If results indicate a possibility of disease or impaired kidney function, one or more of the following additional tests is usually performed to more specifically diagnose the cause and the level of decline in kidney function.

• Creatinine clearance test. This test evaluates how efficiently the kidneys clear a substance called creatinine from the blood. Creatinine, a waste product of muscle energy metabolism, is produced at a constant rate that is proportional to the muscle mass of the individual. Because the body does not recycle it, all of the creatinine filtered by the kidneys in a given amount of time is excreted in the urine, making creatinine clearance a very specific measurement of kidney function. The test is performed on a timed urine specimen—a cumulative sample collected over a two to twenty-four hour period. Determination of the blood creatinine level is also required to calculate the urine clearance.

• Urea clearance test. Urea is a waste product that is created by protein metabolism and excreted in the urine. The urea clearance test requires a blood sample to measure the amount of urea in the bloodstream and two urine specimens, collected one hour apart, to determine the amount of urea that is filtered, or cleared, by the kidneys into the urine.

• Urine osmolality test. Urine osmolality is a measurement of the number of dissolved particles in urine. It is a more precise measurement than specific gravity for evaluating the ability of the kidneys to concentrate or dilute the urine. Kidneys that are functioning normally will excrete more water into the urine as fluid intake is increased, diluting the urine. If fluid intake is decreased, the kidneys excrete less water and the urine becomes more concentrated. The test may be done on a urine sample collected first thing in the morning, on multiple timed samples, or on a cumulative sample collected over a twenty-four hour period. The patient will typically be prescribed a high-protein diet for several days before the test and asked to drink no fluids the night before the test.

• Urine protein test. Healthy kidneys filter all proteins from the bloodstream and then reabsorb them, allowing no protein, or only slight amounts of protein, into the urine. The persistent presence of significant amounts of protein in the urine, then, is an important indicator of kidney disease. A positive screening test for protein (included in a routine urinalysis) on a random urine sample is usually followed-up with a test on a 24-hour urine sample that more precisely measures the quantity of protein.

Blood tests

There are also several blood tests that can aid in evaluating kidney function. These include:

• **Blood urea nitrogen test** (BUN). Urea is a by-product of protein metabolism. This waste product is formed in the liver, then filtered from the blood and excreted in the urine by the kidneys. The BUN test measures the amount of nitrogen contained in the urea. High BUN levels can indicate kidney dysfunction, but because blood urea nitrogen is also affected by protein intake and liver function, the test is usually done in conjunction with a blood creatinine, a more specific indicator of kidney function.

• **Creatinine test.** This test measures blood levels of creatinine, a by-product of muscle energy metabolism that, like urea, is filtered from the blood by the kidneys and excreted into the urine. Production of creatinine depends on an individual's muscle mass, which usually fluctuates very little. With normal kidney function, then, the amount of creatinine in the blood remains relatively constant and normal. For this reason, and because creatinine is affected very little by liver function, an elevated blood creatinine is a more sensitive indication of impaired kidney function than the BUN.

• Other blood tests. Measurement of the blood levels of other elements regulated in part by the kidneys can also be useful in evaluating kidney function. These include sodium, potassium, chloride, bicarbonate, calcium, magnesium, phosphorus, protein, uric acid, and glucose.

Preparation

Patients will be given specific instructions for collection of urine samples, depending on the test to be performed. Some timed urine tests require an extended collection period of up to 24 hours, during which time the patient collects all urine voided and transfers it to a specimen container. Refrigeration and/or preservatives are typically required to maintain the integrity of such urine specimens. Certain dietary and/or medication restrictions may be imposed for some of the blood and urine tests. The patient may also be instructed to avoid **exercise** for a period of time before a test.

Aftercare

If medication was discontinued prior to a urine kidney function test, it may be resumed once the test is completed.

Risks

Risks for these tests are minimal, but may include slight bleeding from a blood-drawing site, hematoma (accumulation of blood under a puncture site), or **fainting** or feeling light-headed after venipuncture. In addition, suspension of medication or dietary changes imposed in preparation for some blood or urine tests may trigger side-effects in some individuals.

Normal results

Normal values for many tests are determined by the patient's age and sex. Reference values can also vary by laboratory, but are generally within the ranges that follow.

Urine tests

- Creatinine clearance. For a 24-hour urine collection, normal results are 90-139 ml/min for adult males less than 40 years old, and 80-125 ml/min for adult females less than 40 years old. For people over 40, values decrease by 6.5 ml/min for each decade of life.

- Urea clearance. With maximum clearance, normal is 64-99 ml/min.

- Urine osmolality. With restricted fluid intake (concentration testing), osmolality should be greater than 800 mOsm/kg of water. With increased fluid intake (dilution testing), osmolality should be less than 100 mOSm/kg in at least one of the specimens collected.

- Urine protein. A 24-hour urine collection should contain no more than 150 mg of protein.

Blood tests

- Blood urea nitrogen (BUN). 8-20 mg/dl.

- Creatinine. 0.8-1.2 mg/dl for males, and 0.6-0.9 mg/dl for females.

Abnormal results

Low clearance values for creatinine and urea indicate diminished ability of the kidneys to filter these waste products from the blood and excrete them in the urine. As clearance levels decrease, blood levels of creatinine and urea nitrogen increase. Since it can be affected by other factors, an elevated BUN, by itself, is suggestive, but not diagnostic, for kidney dysfunction. An abnormally elevated blood creatinine, a more specific and sensitive indicator of kidney disease than the BUN, is diagnostic of impaired kidney function.

Inability of the kidneys to concentrate the urine in response to restricted fluid intake, or to dilute the urine in response to increased fluid intake during osmolality testing may indicate decreased kidney function. Because the kidneys normally excrete almost no protein in the urine, its persistent presence, in amounts that exceed the normal 24-hour urine value, usually indicates some type of kidney disease as well.

Resources

BOOKS

Bock, G.H., E.J. Ruley, and M.P. Moore. *A Parent's Guide to Kidney Disorders.* Minneapolis, MN: Univ. of Minnesota Press, 1993.

Brenner, Barry M., and Floyd C. Rector, Jr., eds. *The Kidney.* Philadelphia, PA: W.B. Saunders Company, 1991.

Cameron, J.S. *Kidney Failure: The Facts.* New York, NY: Oxford Univ. Press, 1996.

Fischbach, Frances Talaska. *A Manual of Laboratory & Diagnostic Tests,* 5th ed. Philadelphia, PA: J.B. Lippincott Company, 1996.

Pagana, Kathleen Deska, and Timothy James Pagana. *Mosby's Diagnostic and Laboratory Desk Reference,* 3rd ed. St. Louis, MO: Mosby-Year Book, Inc., 1997.

ORGANIZATIONS

National Kidney Foundation (NKF). 30 East 33rd Street, New York, NY 10016. (800)622-9020. http://www.kidney.org.

Paula Anne Ford-Martin

Kidney nuclear medicine scan

Definition

A kidney nuclear medicine scan, or study, is a simple outpatient test that involves administering small amounts of radioactive substances, called tracers, into the body and then imaging the kidneys and bladder with a special camera. The images obtained can help in the diagnosis and treatment of certain kidney diseases.

Purpose

While many tests, such as x rays, ultrasound exams, or **computed tomography scans** (CT scans), can reveal the structure of the kidneys (its anatomy), the kidney nuclear medicine scan is unique in that it reveals how the kidneys are functioning. This is valuable information in helping a doctor make a diagnosis. Therefore, the kidney nuclear medicine scan is performed primarily to see how well the kidneys are working and, at the same time, they can identify some of the various structures that make up the kidney.

Precautions

If a patient is pregnant, it is generally recommended that she not have a kidney nuclear medicine scan. The unborn baby is more sensitive to radiation than an adult. If a woman thinks she might be pregnant, she should inform her doctor of this too.

Women who are breastfeeding should also inform their doctor. The doctor may recommend the woman stop breastfeeding for a day or two after a kidney nuclear medicine scan, depending on the particular tracer that was used since the tracer can accumulate in breast milk.

Description

Nuclear medicine is a branch of radiology that uses radioactive materials to diagnose or treat various diseases. These radioactive materials (tracers) may also be called radiopharmaceuticals, and they accumulate (collect) in specific organs in the body. Radiopharmaceuticals are able to yield valuable information about the particular organ being studied.

Whether outside the body or inside the body, tracers emit radioactive signals, called gamma rays, which can be collected and counted by a special device, called a gamma camera. The images of the kidney that the camera produces are called renal scans.

The kidney nuclear medicine scan can be performed on an outpatient basis, usually by a nuclear medicine technologist. The technologist helps prepare the patient for the exam by positioning him or her on an exam table or cart in the imaging area. The patient's position is usually flat on the back. The patient must lie still during imaging to prevent blurring of the images that will be taken. The technologist positions the camera as close to the kidney (or kidneys) as possible to obtain the best images.

In the next step of the procedure, the technologist injects the radiopharmaceutical into the patient. This may be done with one single injection or through an intravenous (IV) line. Immediately after the tracer is injected, imaging begins. It is important to obtain images right away because the tracer's radioactivity begins to diminish (decay). The time required for one-half of the tracer's activity to decay is called the tracer's half-life (T 1/2). The half-life is unique to each radiopharmaceutical. Also, it is important to see the kidney in its immediate state.

Serial pictures are taken with the gamma camera and may be seen on a computer or TV-like screen. The camera doesn't emit radiation, it only records it. The images then are stored on film.

A kidney nuclear medicine scan ranges from 45 minutes to three hours in length, depending on the goals of the test. But the test typically takes about an hour to an hour-and-a-half.

Once the images and curves are obtained, the nuclear medicine physician or radiologist analyzes, or reads, them. Various information can be provided to the doctor through these, depending on the test that was performed. A variety of kidney nuclear medicine studies are available for a doctor to help in making diagnoses. It is important to understand that kidney nuclear medicine scans are good at identifying when there is an abnormality, but they do not always identify the specific problem. They are very useful in providing information about how the various parts of the kidneys function, which, in turn, can assist in making a diagnosis.

Studies may be performed to determine the rate at which the kidney's are filtering a patient's blood. These studies use a radiopharmaceutical, called Technetium DTPA (Tc 99m DTPA). This radiopharmaceutical also can identify obstruction (blockage) in the collecting system. To study how well the tubules and ducts of the kidney are functioning, the radiopharmaceutical Technetium MAG3 is used. Studying tubular function is a good indicator of overall renal function. In many renal diseases, one of the first things that disappears or diminishes is the tubular function.

Candidates for a kidney nuclear medicine scan are patients who have:

- Renal failure or chronic renal failure
- Obstruction in their urine collection systems
- Renal artery stenosis
- A kidney transplant.

Preparation

No preparation is necessary for a kidney nuclear medicine scan. The doctor may ask the patient to refrain from certain medications, however, before the scan if the medications might interfere with the test. For example, if a scan is being performed to study renal artery stenosis, the patient may have to refrain from taking medications for **hypertension.**

Aftercare

Patients can resume their normal daily activities immediately after the test. Most tracers are passed naturally from the body, though drinking fluids after a kidney nuclear medicine scan can help flush the tracer into the urine and out of the body more quickly.

Risks

Nuclear medicine procedures are very safe. Unlike some of the dyes that may be used in x-ray studies, radioactive tracers rarely cause side effects. There are no long-lasting effects of the tracers themselves, because they have no functional effects on the body's tissues.

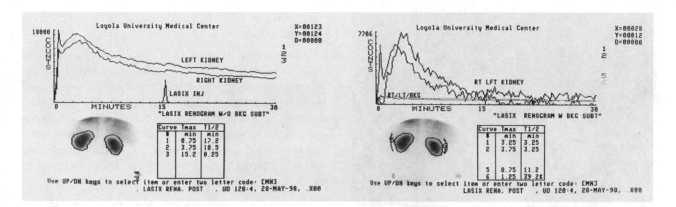

A computer-generated time activity curve generated from a renal scan. This time activity curve looks at the radiation count over a period of time. *(Photograph by Collette L. Placek. Reproduced by permission.)*

Normal results

The test reveals normal kidney function for age and medical situation.

Abnormal results

The test reveals a change in function that may be attributable to a disease process, such as obstruction or a malfunctioning kidney. If the test is abnormal, the patient may be recalled another day for a repeat study, performed differently, to narrow the list of causes.

Resources

BOOKS

Henkin, Robert, et al. *Nuclear Medicine.* St. Louis, MO: Mosby, 1996.

Maisey, Michael. *Clinical Nuclear Medicine,* 2nd ed. New York, NY: Chapman and Hall, 1991.

PERIODICALS

McBiles, Mike. "Correlative Imaging of the Kidney." *Seminars in Nuclear Medicine* 24 (3)(July 1994): 219-233.

Taylor Jr., Andrew, and Joseph V. Nally. "Clinical Applications of Renal Scintigraphy." *American Journal of Radiology,* 164(January 1995): 31-41.

ORGANIZATIONS

Society of Nuclear Medicine. 1850 Samuel Morse Drive, Reston, VA 20190-5316. (800) 633-2665.

OTHER

Interview with Robert H. Wagner, MD., Assistant Professor of Radiology, Section of Nuclear Medicine, Loyola University Medical Center. May 28, 1998 & June 5, 1998.

Collette L. Placek

Kidney removal *see* **Nephrectomy**

Kidney stones

Definition

Kidney stones are solid accumulations of material that form in the tubal system of the kidney. Kidney stones cause problems when they block the flow of urine through or out of the kidney. When the stones move along the ureter, they cause severe **pain.**

Description

Urine is formed by the kidneys. Blood flows into the kidneys, and specialized tubes (nephrons) within the kidneys allow a certain amount of fluid from the blood, and certain substances dissolved in that fluid, to flow out of the body as urine. Sometimes, a problem causes the dissolved substances to become solid again. Tiny crystals may form in the urine, meet, and cling together to create a larger solid mass called a kidney stone.

Many people do not ever find out that they have stones in their kidneys. These stones are small enough to allow the kidney to continue functioning normally, never causing any pain. These are called "silent stones." Kidney stones cause problems when they interfere with the normal flow of urine. They can block (obstruct) the flow down the tube (the ureter) that carries urine from the kidney to the bladder. The kidney is not accustomed to experiencing any pressure. When pressure builds from backed-up urine, the kidney may swell (**hydronephrosis**). If the kidney is subjected to this pressure for

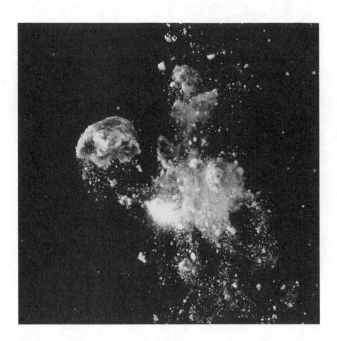

This kidney stone is being fragmented by sound waves.
(FPG International. Reproduced by permission.)

some time, it may cause damage to the delicate kidney structures. When the kidney stone is lodged further down the ureter, the backed-up urine may also cause the ureter to swell (hydroureter). Because the ureters are muscular tubes, the presence of a stone will make these muscular tubes spasm, causing severe pain.

About 10% of all people will have a kidney stone in his or her lifetime. Kidney stones are most common among:

- Caucasians
- Males
- People over the age of 30
- People who have had kidney stones previously
- Relatives of kidney stone patients.

Causes & symptoms

Kidney stones can be composed of a variety of substances. The most common types of kidney stones include:

- Calcium stones. About 80% of all kidney stones fall into this category. These stones are composed of either calcium and phosphate, or calcium and oxalate. People with calcium stones may have other diseases that cause them to have increased blood levels of calcium. These diseases include primary parathyroidism, **sarcoidosis, hyperthyroidism, renal tubular acidosis, multiple myeloma,** hyperoxaluria, and some types of **cancer.** A

diet heavy in meat, fish, and poultry can cause calcium oxalate stones.

- Struvite stones. About 10% of all kidney stones fall into this category. This type of stone is composed of magnesium ammonium phosphate. These stones occur most often when patients have had repeated urinary tract infections with certain types of bacteria. These bacteria produce a substance called urease, which increases the urine pH and makes the urine more alkaline and less acidic. This chemical environment allows struvite to settle out of the urine, forming stones.

- Uric acid stones. About 5% of all kidney stones fall into this category. Uric acid stones occur when increased amounts of uric acid circulate in the bloodstream. When the uric acid content becomes very high, it can no longer remain dissolved and solid bits of uric acid settle out of the urine. A kidney stone is formed when these bits of uric acid begin to cling to each other within the kidney, slowly growing into a solid mass. About half of all patients with this type of stone also have deposits of uric acid elsewhere in their body, commonly in the joint of the big toe. This painful disorder is called **gout.** Other causes of uric acid stones include **chemotherapy** for cancer, certain bone marrow disorders where blood cells are over-produced, and an inherited disorder called **Lesch-Nyhan syndrome.**

- Cystine stones. About 2% of all kidney stones fall into this category. Cystine is a type of amino acid, and people with this type of kidney stone have an abnormality in the way their bodies process amino acids in the diet.

Patients who have kidney stones usually do not have symptoms until the stones pass into the ureter. Prior to this, some people may notice blood in their urine. Once the stone is in the ureter, however, most people will experience bouts of very severe pain. The pain is crampy and spasmodic, and is referred to as ''**colic**''. The pain usually begins in the flank region, the area between the lower ribs and the hip bone. As the stone moves closer to the bladder, a patient will often feel the pain radiating along the inner thigh. In women, the pain may be felt in the vulva. In men, the pain may be felt in the testicles. Nausea, vomiting, extremely frequent and painful urination, and obvious blood in the urine are common. **Fever** and chills usually means that the ureter has become obstructed, allowing bacteria to become trapped in the kidney causing a kidney infection (**pyelonephritis**).

Diagnosis

Diagnosing kidney stones is based on the patient's history of the very severe, distinctive pain associated with the stones. Diagnosis includes laboratory examination of a urine sample and an x-ray examination. During the passage of a stone, examination of the urine almost always reveals blood. A number of x-ray tests are used to diagnose kidney stones. A plain x ray of the kidneys, ureters, and bladder may or may not reveal the stone. A series of x rays taken after injecting iodine dye into a vein is usually a more reliable way of seeing a stone. This procedure is called an intravenous pyelogram (IVP). The dye "lights up" the urinary system as it travels. In the case of an obstruction, the dye will be stopped by the stone or will only be able to get past the stone at a slow trickle.

When a patient is passing a kidney stone, it is important that all of his or her urine is strained through a special sieve. This is to make sure that the stone is caught. The stone can then be sent to a special laboratory for analysis so that the chemical composition of the stone can be determined. After the kidney stone has been passed, other tests will be required in order to understand the underlying condition that may have caused the stone to form. Collecting urine for 24 hours, followed by careful analysis of its chemical makeup, can often determine a number of reasons for stone formation.

Treatment

A patient with a kidney stone will say that the most important aspect of treatment is adequate pain relief. Because the pain of passing a kidney stone is so severe, narcotic pain medications (like morphine) are usually required. It is believed that stones may pass more quickly if the patient is encouraged to drink large amounts of water (2-3 quarts per day). If the patient is vomiting or unable to drink because of the pain, it may be necessary to provide fluids through a vein. If symptoms and urine tests indicate the presence of infection, **antibiotics** will be required.

Although most kidney stones will pass on their own, some will not. Surgical removal of a stone may become necessary when a stone appears too large to pass. Surgery may also be required if the stone is causing serious obstructions, pain that cannot be treated, heavy bleeding, or infection. Several alternatives exist for removing stones. One method involves inserting a tube into the bladder and up into the ureter. A tiny basket is then passed through the tube, and an attempt is made to snare the stone and pull it out. Open surgery to remove an obstructing kidney stone was relatively common in the past, but current methods allow the stone to be crushed with shock waves (called **lithotripsy**). These shock waves may be aimed at the stone from outside of the body by passing the necessary equipment through the bladder and into the ureter. The shock waves may be aimed at the stone from inside the body by placing the instrument through a tiny incision located near the stone. The stone fragments may then pass on their own or may be removed through the incision. All of these methods reduce the patient's recovery time considerably when compared to the traditional open operation.

Alternative treatment

Alternative treatments for kidney stones include the use of herbal medicine, homeopathy, **acupuncture, acupressure, hypnosis,** or **guided imagery** to relieve pain. Starfruit (*Averrhoa carambola*) is recommended to increase the amount of urine a patient passes and to relieve pain. Dietary changes can be made to reduce the risk of future stone formation and to facilitate the resorption of existing stones. Supplementation with magnesium, a smooth muscle relaxant, can help reduce pain and facilitate stone passing. Homeopathy and herbal medicine, both western and Chinese, recommend a number of remedies that may help prevent kidney stones.

Prognosis

A patient's prognosis depends on the underlying disorder causing the development of kidney stones. In most cases, patients with uncomplicated calcium stones will recover very well. About 60% of these patients, however, will have other kidney stones. Struvite stones are particularly dangerous because they may grow extremely large, filling the tubes within the kidney. These are called staghorn stones and will not pass out in the urine. They will require surgical removal. Uric acid stones may also become staghorn stones.

Prevention

Prevention of kidney stones depends on the type of stone and the presence of an underlying disease. In almost all cases, increasing fluid intake so that a person consistently drinks several quarts of water a day is an important preventative measure. Patients with calcium stones may benefit from taking a medication called a diuretic, which has the effect of decreasing the amount of calcium passed in the urine. Eating less meat, fish, and chicken may be helpful for patients with calcium oxalate stones. Other items in the diet that may encourage calcium oxalate stone formation include beer, black pepper, berries, broccoli, chocolate, spinach, and tea. Uric acid stones may require treatment with a medication called allopurinol. Struvite stones will require removal and the patient should receive an antibiotic. When a disease is identified as the cause of stone formation, treatment specific to that disease may lessen the likelihood of repeated stones.

Resources

BOOKS

Asplin, John R., et al. "Nephrolithiasis." In *Harrison's Principles of Internal Medicine,* edited by Anthony S. Fauci, et al. New York: McGraw-Hill, 1998.

Fishman, Mark C., et al. *Medicine.* Philadelphia: J. B. Lippincott Co., 1996.

PERIODICALS

Goshorn, Janet. "Kidney Stones: Strategies for Managing This Common, Excruciating Condition." *American Journal of Nursing,* 96 (9)(September 1996): 40+.

"New Advice Regarding the Treatment of Kidney Stones." *HealthFacts,* 22 (11)(November 1997): 2.

Squires, Sally. "New Guidelines Issued for Kidney Stones." *The Washington Post,* 120 (280)(October 7, 1997): WH7.

Trivedi, Bhairvi K. "Nephrolithiasis: How It Happens and What To Do About It." *Postgraduate Medicine,* 100 (6)(December 1996): 63+.

ORGANIZATIONS

American Foundation for Urologic Disease. 300 West Pratt St., Baltimore, MD 21201-2463. (800) 242-2383.

National Kidney Foundation. 30 East 33rd St., New York, NY 10016. (800) 622-9010.

Rosalyn S. Carson-DeWitt

Kidney transplantation

Definition

Kidney transplantation is a surgical procedure to remove a healthy, functioning kidney from a living or brain-dead donor and implant it into a patient with non-functioning kidneys.

Purpose

Kidney transplantation is performed on patients with **chronic kidney failure,** or end-stage renal disease (ESRD). ESRD occurs when a disease or disorder damages the kidneys so that they are no longer capable of adequately removing fluids and wastes from the body or of maintaining the proper level of certain kidney-regulated chemicals in the bloodstream. Without long-term dialysis or a kidney transplant, ESRD is fatal.

Precautions

Patients with a history of heart disease, lung disease, **cancer,** or hepatitis may not be suitable candidates for receiving a kidney transplant.

Description

Kidney transplantation involves surgically attaching a functioning kidney, or graft, from a brain-dead organ donor (a cadaver transplant) or from a living donor, to a patient with ESRD. Living donors may be related or unrelated to the patient, but a related donor has a better chance of having a kidney that is a stronger biological "match" for the patient.

The surgical procedure to remove a kidney from a living donor is called a *nephrectomy*. The kidney donor is administered **general anesthesia** and an incision is made on the side or front of the abdomen. The blood vessels connecting the kidney to the donor are cut and clamped, and the ureter is also cut between the bladder and kidney and clamped. The kidney and an attached section of ureter is removed from the donor. The vessels and ureter in the donor are then tied off and the incision is sutured together again. A similar procedure is used to harvest cadaver kidneys, although both kidneys are typically removed at once, and blood and cell samples for **tissue typing** are also taken.

Laparoscopic **nephrectomy** is a form of minimally-invasive surgery using instruments on long, narrow rods to view, cut, and remove the donor kidney. The surgeon views the kidney and surrounding tissue with a flexible videoscope. The videoscope and surgical instruments are maneuvered through four small incisions in the abdomen.

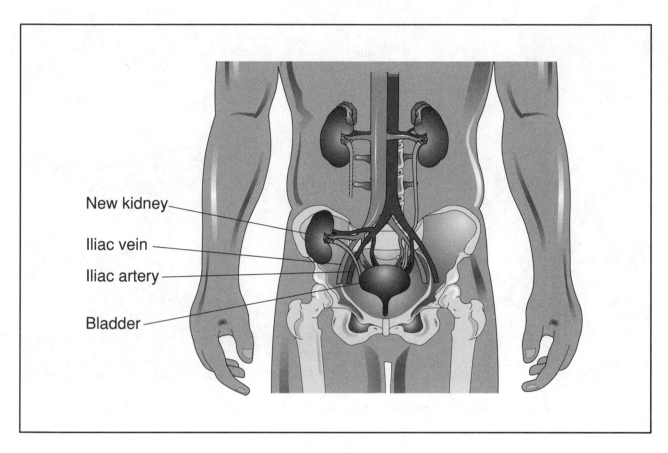

New kidney

Iliac vein

Iliac artery

Bladder

Kidney transplantation involves the surgical attachment of a functioning kidney, or graft, from a donor to a patient with end-stage renal disease (ESRD). During the procedure, the surgeon makes an incision in the patient's flank and implants the new kidney above the pelvic bone and below the non-functioning kidney by suturing the kidney artery and vein to the patient's iliac artery and vein. The ureter of the new kidney is then attached directly to the bladder of the patient. *(Illustration by Electronic Illustrators Group.)*

Once the kidney is freed, it is secured in a bag and pulled through a fifth incision, approximately 3 in (7.6 cm) wide, in the front of the abdominal wall below the navel. Although this surgical technique takes slightly longer than a traditional nephrectomy, preliminary studies have shown that it promotes a faster recovery time, shorter hospital stays, and less post-operative **pain** for kidney donors.

Once removed, kidneys from live donors and cadavers are placed on ice and flushed with a cold preservative solution. The kidney can be preserved in this solution for 24-48 hours until the transplant takes place. The sooner the transplant takes place after harvesting the kidney, the better the chances are for proper functioning.

During the transplant operation, the kidney recipient patient is typically under general anesthesia and administered **antibiotics** to prevent possible infection. A catheter

is placed in the bladder before surgery begins. An incision is made in the flank of the patient and the surgeon implants the kidney above the pelvic bone and below the existing, non-functioning kidney by suturing the kidney artery and vein to the patient's iliac artery and vein. The ureter of the new kidney is attached directly to the bladder of the kidney recipient. Once the new kidney is attached, the patient's existing, diseased kidneys may or may not be removed, depending on the circumstances surrounding the kidney failure.

Since 1973, Medicare has picked up 80% of ESRD treatment costs, including the costs of transplantation for both the kidney donor and recipient. Medicare also covers 80% of immunosuppressive medication costs for up to three years, although federal legislation was under consideration in early 1998 that may remove the time limit on these benefits. To qualify for Medicare ESRD

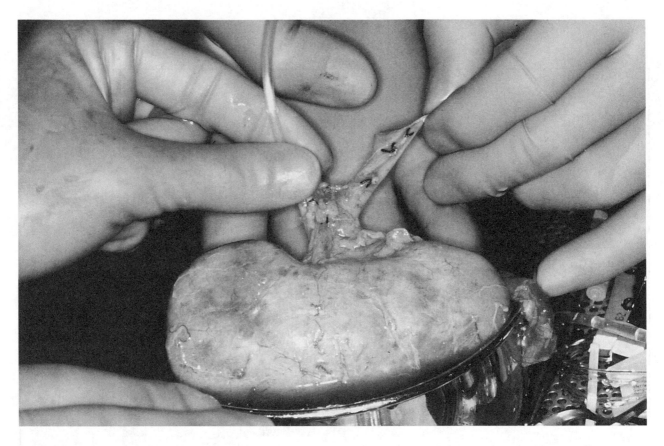

A human kidney is being prepped by medical personnel prior to transplantation. *(Photograph by Brad Nelson, Custom Medical Stock Photo. Reproduced by permission.)*

benefits, a patient must be insured or eligible for benefits under Social Security, or be a spouse or child of an eligible American. Private insurance and state Medicaid programs often cover the remaining 20% of treatment costs.

Preparation

Patients with chronic renal disease who need a transplant and do not have a living donor register with United Network for Organ Sharing (UNOS) will be placed on a waiting list for a cadaver kidney transplant. UNOS is a non-profit organization that is under contract with the federal government to administer the Organ Procurement and Transplant Network (OPTN) and the national Scientific Registry of Transplant Recipients (SR). Kidney availability is based on the patient's health status. The most important factor is that the kidney be compatible to the patient's body. A human kidney has a set of six antigens, substances that stimulate the production of antibodies. (Antibodies then attach to cells they recognize as foreign and attack them.) Donors are tissue-matched for 0 to 6 of the antigens, and compatibility is determined by the number and strength of those matched pairs. Patients with a living donor who is a close relative have the best chance of a close match.

Potential kidney donors undergo a complete medical history and **physical examination** to evaluate their suitability for donation. Extensive blood tests are performed on both donor and recipient. The blood samples are used to tissue type for antigen matches, and confirm that blood types are compatible. A panel of reactive antibody (PRA) is performed by mixing white blood cells from the donor and serum from the recipient to ensure that the recipient antibodies will not have a negative reaction to the donor antigens. A urine test is performed on the donor to evaluate his kidney function. In some cases, a special dye that shows up on x rays is injected into an artery, and x rays are taken to show the blood supply of the donor kidney (a procedure called an arteriogram).

Once compatibility is confirmed and the physical preparations for kidney transplantation are complete, both donor and recipient may undergo a psychological or psychiatric evaluation to ensure that they are emotionally prepared for the transplant procedure and aftercare regimen.

Aftercare

Kidney donors and recipients will experience some discomfort in the area of the incision. Pain relievers are administered following the transplant operation. Patients may also experience numbness, caused by severed nerves, near or on the incision.

A regimen of immunosuppressive, or anti-rejection, medication is prescribed to prevent the body's immune system from rejecting the new kidney. Common immunosuppressants include cyclosporine, prednisone, and azathioprine. The kidney recipient will be required to take immunosuppressants for the life span of the new kidney. Intravenous antibodies may also be administered after transplant surgery. Daclizumab, a monoclonal antibody, is a promising new therapy that can be used in conjunction with standard immunosuppressive medications to reduce the incidence of organ rejection.

Transplant recipients may need to adjust their dietary habits. Certain immunosuppressive medications cause increased appetite or sodium and protein retention, and the patient may have to adjust his or her intake of calories, salt, and protein to compensate.

Risks

As with any surgical procedure, the kidney transplantation procedure carries some risk for both a living donor and a graft recipient. Possible complications include infection and bleeding (hemorrhage). The most common complication for kidney recipients is a urine leak. In approximately 5% of kidney transplants, the ureter suffers some damage, which results in the leak. This problem is usually correctable with follow-up surgery.

The biggest risk to the recovering transplant recipient is not from the operation or the kidney itself, but from the immunosuppressive medication he or she must take. Because these drugs suppress the immune system, the patient is susceptible to infections such as cytomegalovirus (CMV) and varicella (**chickenpox**). The immunosuppressants can also cause a host of possible side effects, from high blood pressure to **osteoporosis.** Prescription and dosage adjustments can lessen side effects for some patients.

Normal results

The new kidney may start functioning immediately, or may take several weeks to begin producing urine. Living donor kidneys are more likely to begin functioning earlier than cadaver kidneys, which frequently suffer some reversible damage during the kidney transplant and storage procedure. Patients may have to undergo dialysis for several weeks while their new kidney establishes an acceptable level of functioning.

The success of a kidney transplant graft depends on the strength of the match between donor and recipient and the source of the kidney. Cadaver kidneys have a four-year survival rate of 66%, compared to an 80.9% survival rate for living donor kidneys. However, there have been cases of cadaver and living, related donor kidneys functioning well for over 25 years.

Studies have shown that after they recover from surgery, kidney donors typically have no long-term complications from the loss of one kidney, and their remaining kidney will increase its functioning to compensate for the loss of the other.

Abnormal results

A transplanted kidney may be rejected by the patient. Rejection occurs when the patient's immune system recognizes the new kidney as a foreign body and attacks the kidney. It may occur soon after transplantation, or several months or years after the procedure has taken place. Rejection episodes are not uncommon in the first weeks after transplantation surgery, and are treated with high-dose injections of **immunosuppressant drugs.** If a rejection episode cannot be reversed and kidney failure continues, the patient will typically go back on dialysis. Another transplant procedure can be attempted at a later date if another kidney becomes available.

Resources

BOOKS

Brenner, Barry M., and Floyd C. Rector Jr., eds. *The Kidney.* Philadelphia: W.B. Saunders Company, 1991.

Cameron, J.S. *Kidney Failure: The Facts* New York: Oxford University Press, 1996.

Ross, Linda M. ed. *Kidney and Urinary Tract Diseases and Disorders Sourcebook.* Vol. 21. Health Reference Series. Detroit: Omnigraphics, Inc., 1997.

U.S. Renal Data System. *USRDS 1997 Annual Data Report.* Bethesda, MD: The National Institutes of Health, National Institute of Diabetes and Digestive and Kidney Diseases, 1996.

PERIODICALS

Okie, Susan. "New Surgery Makes Kidney Donation Easier." *Washington Post* 120, no. 154(June 3, 1997):WH5.

ORGANIZATIONS

American Association of Kidney Patients (AAKP), 100 S. Ashley Drive, Suite 280, Tampa, FL 33602. (800)749-2257. http://www.aakp.org/.

American Kidney Fund (AKF). Suite 1010, 6110 Executive Boulevard, Rockville, MD 20852. (800)638-8299. http://www.arbon.com/kidney/.

National Kidney Foundation (NKF). 30 East 33rd Street, New York, NY 10016. (800)622-9020. http://www.kidney.org/.

United Network for Organ Sharing (UNOS). (888)894-6361. Richmond, VA. http://www.unos.org/.

United States Renal Data System (USRDS). USRDS Coordinating Center, 315 W. Huron, Suite 240, Ann Arbor, MI 48103. (313)998-6611. http://www.med.umich.edu/usrds/.

OTHER

Transweb. http://www.transweb.org/.

Paula Anne Ford-Martin

Kidney ultrasound *see* **Abdominal ultrasound**

Kidney, ureter, and bladder x-ray study

Definition

A kidney, ureter, and bladder (KUB) x-ray study is an abdominal x ray. Despite its name, KUB does not show the ureters and only sometimes shows the kidneys and bladder and, even then, with uncertainty.

Purpose

The KUB study is a diagnostic test used to detect **kidney stones** and to diagnose some gastrointestinal disorders. The KUB is also used as a follow-up procedure after the placement of devices such as ureteral stents and nasogastric or nasointestinal tubes (feeding tubes) to verify proper positioning.

Precautions

Because of the risks of radiation exposure to the fetus, pregnant women are advised to avoid this x-ray procedure.

A KUB study is a preliminary screening test for kidney stones, and should be followed by a more sophisticated series of diagnostic tests [such as an **abdominal ultrasound, intravenous urography,** or **computed tomography scan** (CT scan)] if kidney stones are suspected.

Description

A KUB is typically a single x-ray procedure. The patient lies flat on his back on an x-ray table. An x-ray

plate is placed underneath him near the small of the back, and the x-ray camera is aimed at his abdomen. The patient is asked to hold his breath and lie still while the x ray is taken. Sometimes a second KUB will be ordered, with the patient standing, or if unable to do so, lying on his side.

Preparation

A KUB study requires no special diet, fluid restrictions, medications, or other preparation. The patient is

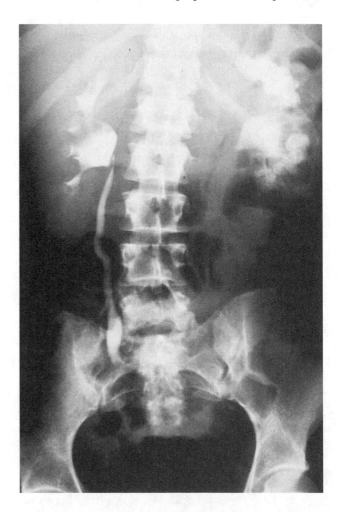

An x-ray image of a human torso and abdomen showing a blocked ureter. *(Custom Medical Stock Photo. Reproduced by permission.)*

typically required to wear a hospital gown or similar attire and to remove all jewelry so the x-ray camera has an unobstructed view of the abdomen. A lead apron may be placed over the abdominal areas of the body not being x rayed to shield the patient from unnecessary radiation.

Aftercare

No special aftercare treatment or regimen is required for a KUB study.

Risks

Because the KUB study is an x-ray procedure, it does involve minor exposure to radiation.

Normal results

Normal KUB x-ray films show two kidneys of a similar size and shape. A normal amount of intestinal gas is seen.

Abnormal results

Abnormal KUB films may show calculi (**kidney stones**). If both kidneys are visible, it may be possible to diagnose renal size discrepancies. The films may also show too much bowel gas indicating possible obstruction or soft tissue masses.

Resources

BOOKS

Kevles, Bettyann. *Naked to the Bone: Medical Imaging in the Twentieth Century.* New Brunswick, NJ: Rutgers University Press, 1997.

Pagana, Kathleen Deska, and Timothy James Pagana. *Mosby's Diagnostic and Laboratory Test Reference,* 3rd edition. St. Louis, MO: Mosby 1997.

Paula Anne Ford-Martin

Kinesiology, applied

Definition

Kinesiology is a series of tests that locate weaknesses in specific muscles reflecting imbalances throughout the body. Then specific **massages** or **acupressure** techniques are used in an attempt to rebalance what has been revealed by the kinesiology tests. Thus, kinesiology is used as both an assessment tool and as a limited therapeutic modality.

KEY TERMS

Acupressure—A form of acupuncture in which certain points of the body are pressed with the fingers and hands to release energy blocks.

Alleviate—To make something easier to be endured.

Complementary—Something that serves to fill out or complete something else.

Deficiency—A shortage of something necessary for health.

Diagnostic—The art or act of identifying a disease from its signs and symptoms.

Flaccid—Flabby, limp, weak.

Meridian—In traditional Chinese medicine, the channels which run beneath the skin through which the body's energy flows.

Spasm—An involuntary, sudden, violent contraction of a muscle or a group of muscles.

Purpose

Kinesiology claims to be a healing system that detects and corrects imbalances in the body before they develop into a disease, and which restores overall system balance and harmony. It is used to alleviate muscle, bone, and joint problems, treat all manner of aches and **pains,** and correct many areas of imbalance and discomfort.

Precautions

Since interpretation of the muscle tests is both complex and subjective, it should only be performed by a licensed health professional trained to look for "subclinical" symptoms (those which have not yet become a major problem). Kinesiology, itself, is more of a diagnostic technique and should not be thought of as a cure for any particular problem.

Description

Traditionally, the word "kinesiology" refers simply to the study of muscles and body movement. In 1964, however, American chiropractor George J. Goodheart founded what has become known as **applied kinesiology** when he linked oriental ideas about energy flow in the body with western techniques of muscle testing. First, Goodheart noted that all muscles are related to other muscles. He observed that for each movement a muscle makes, there is another muscle or group of muscles involved with that movement; one muscle contracts while another one relaxes. So when he was presented with a painful, overly-tight muscle, he would observe and treat the opposite, and necessarily weak, muscle to restore balance. This was then a very new technique.

Further, Goodheart argued that there is a definite and real connection between muscles, glands, and organs, and that by testing the strength of certain muscles he could learn about the health or condition of the gland or organ to which it was related.

Applied kinesiology is based on the idea that the body is an interacting unit made of different parts that interconnect and affect each other. Everything we do affects the body as a whole; therefore, a problem in one area can cause trouble in another area. According to kinesiology, the muscles eventually register and reflect anything that is wrong with any part of the body, whether physical or mental. Thus, a particular digestive problem might show up in the related and corresponding muscles of the legs. By testing the strength of certain muscles, the kinesiologist claims to be able to gain access to the body's communication system, and, thus, to read the health status of each of the body's major components.

The manual testing of muscles or muscle strength is not new, and was used in the late 1940s to evaluate muscle function and strength and to assess the extent of an injury. Applied kinesiology measures whether a muscle is stuck in the "on" position, acting like a tense muscle spasm, or is stuck "off," appearing weak or flaccid. It is called manual testing because it is done without instruments, using only the kinesiologist's fingertip pressure. During the first and longest appointment which lasts about an hour, the kinesiologist conducts a complete consultation, asking about the patient's history and background. During the **physical examination,** patients sit or lie down, then the kinesiologist holds the patient's leg or arm to isolate a particular muscle. The practitioner then touches a point on the body which he believes is related to that muscle, and, with quick, gentle, and painless pressure, pushes down on the limb. Patients are asked to resist this pressure, and, if they cannot, an imbalance is suspected in the related organ, gland, or body part. This diagnostic technique uses muscles to find the cause of a problem, and is based on traditional Chinese medicine and its idea that the body has common energy meridians, or channels, for both organs and muscles. Kinesiologists also claim that they are able to locate muscle weaknesses that stem from a variety of causes such as **allergies,** mineral and vitamin deficiencies, as well as from problems with the lymph system. Once the exact cause is determined, the kinesiologist uses his fingertips to work the appropriate corresponding acupressure points in order to rebalance the flow of energy and restore health. Often he will recommend a complementary program of nutrition therapy.

Risks

There are no major risks associated with this gentle, noninvasive therapy. It is generally safe for people of all ages and has no side effects.

Normal results

If applied kinesiology does what it claims, patients should expect muscle testing to discover the cause of their physical complaint and to be told how to correct it.

Resources

BOOKS

Burton Goldberg Group. *Alternative Medicine: The Definitive Guide.* Puyallup, WA: Future Medicine Publishing, Inc., 1993.

Holdway, Ann. *Kinesiology: Muscle Testing and Energy Balancing for Health and Well-Being.* Rockport, MA: Element Books Ltd., 1995.

Kastner, Mark, and Hugh Burroughs. *Alternative Healing.* New York: Henry Holt and Company, 1996.

Levy, Susan L., and Carol R. Lehr. *Your Body Can Talk.* Prescott, AZ: Hohm Press, 1996.

PERIODICALS

Gelb, Harold, and Paula M. Siegel. "Applied Kinesiology: Relieving Internal Stresses and Pain." *Science Digest* (August 1980): 28-33.

ORGANIZATIONS

International College of Applied Kinesiology. P.O. Box 905. Lawrence, KS 66044-9005 (913) 542-1801.

Leonard C. Bruno

Kleine-Levin syndrome *see* **Sleep disorders**

Klinefelter syndrome

Definition

Klinfelter syndrome is a genetic disorder affecting males. People with this syndrome are born with at least one extra X chromosome.

Description

Chromosomes are found in every cell in the body. Chromosomes contain genes, structures that direct the growth and functioning of all the cells and systems in the body. In other words, chromosomes are responsible for passing on hereditary traits from parents to child, like eye color, height, nose shape, etc. Chromosomes also determine whether the child will be male or female. Normally,

KEY TERMS

Chromosomes—Spaghetti-like structures located within the nucleus (or central portion) of each cell. Chromosomes contain the genetic information necessary to direct the development and functioning of all cells and systems in the body.

a person has a total of 46 chromosomes in each cell, two of which are responsible for determining that individual's sex. These two sex chromosomes are called X and Y. The combination of these two types of chromosomes determines the sex of a child. Females have two X chromosomes (the XX combination); males have one X and one Y chromosome (the XY combination).

In Klinefelter syndrome, a problem very early in development results in an abnormal number and arrangement of chromosomes. Most commonly, a male with Klinefelter syndrome will be born with 47 chromosomes in each cell, rather than the normal number of 46. The extra chromosome is an X chromosome. This means that rather than having the normal XY combination, the male has an XXY combination. Some Klinefelter patients have more complex chromosomal errors, including the presence of 48, 49, or even 50 chromosomes. All of the extra chromosomes are Xs.

Klinefelter syndrome is one of the most common chromosomal abnormalities. About 1 in every 1,000 infant boy is born with some variation of this disorder.

Causes & symptoms

The cause of Klinefelter syndrome is unknown, although it has been noted that the disorder is seen more frequently among the children of older mothers.

The presence of more than one X chromosome in a male results in a delay in **puberty.** The testicles and the penis tend to be smaller than normal, and **infertility** is common. The testicles may remain up in the abdomen, instead of descending into the scrotum as is normal. Body hair decreases and breast size increases. Sexual drive is often below normal. Boys with Klinefelter syndrome tend to be tall and thin.

While it was once believed that all boys with Klinefelter syndrome were mentally retarded, doctors now know that the disorder can exist without retardation. However, children with Klinefelter syndrome frequently have difficulty with language, including learning to speak, read, and write. Some children have difficulty with social skills and tend to be more shy, anxious, or immature than their peers. Overly aggressive behavior has also been noted.

The greater the number of X chromosomes present, the greater the disability. Boys with several extra X chromosomes have distinctive facial features, more severe retardation, deformities of bony structures, and even more disordered development of male features.

Diagnosis

Diagnosis of Klinefelter syndrome is made by examining chromosomes for evidence of more than one X chromosome present in a male. Other abnormalities of sex hormones are common, including a low level of the male hormone testosterone.

Treatment

There is no treatment available to change chromosomal makeup. However, delayed puberty and decreased sexual drive can both be treated with injections of a testosterone preparation about every three weeks.

Prognosis

While many men with Klinefelter syndrome go on to live normal lives, nearly 100% of these men will be sterile (unable to produce a child). Because men with Klinefelter syndrome have enlarged breasts, they have nearly the same chance of developing **breast cancer** as do women. Lung disease and certain rare tumors are also increased in patients with Klinefelter syndrome.

Resources

BOOKS

DiGeorge, Angelo M. "Klinefelter Syndrome." In *Harrison's Principles of Internal Medicine,* edited by Anthony S. Fauci, et al. New York: McGraw-Hill, 1998.

PERIODICALS

Sotos, Juan F. "Genetic Disorders Associated with Overgrowth." *Clinical Pediatrics,* 36 (1)(January 1997): 39+.

Rosalyn S. Carson-DeWitt

Knee replacement *see* **Joint replacement**

Kneecap removal

Definition

Kneecap removal, or patellectomy, is the surgical removal of the patella, commonly called the kneecap.

Purpose

Kneecap removal is done under three circumstances:

• When the kneecap is fractured or shattered

• When the kneecap dislocates easily and repeatedly

• When degenerative arthritis of the kneecap causes extreme **pain.**

A person of any age can break a kneecap in an accident. When the bone is shattered beyond repair, the kneecap is removed. No prosthesis or artificial replacement part is put in its place.

Dislocation of the kneecap is most common in young girls between the ages of 10-14. Initially, the kneecap will pop back into place of its own accord, but pain may continue. If dislocation occurs too often, or the kneecap doesn't go back into place correctly, the patella may rub the other bones in the knee, causing an arthritis-like condition. Some people are born with **birth defects** that cause the kneecap to dislocate frequently.

Degenerative arthritis of the kneecap, also called patellar arthritis or *chondromalacia patellae*, can cause enough pain that it is necessary to remove the kneecap. As techniques of **joint replacement** have improved, arthritis in the knee is more frequently treated with total knee replacement.

Precautions

People who have had their kneecap removed for degenerative arthritis and then later have to have a total knee replacement are more likely to have problems with the stability of their artificial knee than those who only have total knee replacement. This is because the realigned muscles and tendons provide less support once the kneecap is removed.

Description

Kneecap removal is performed under either general or local anesthesia at a hospital or freestanding surgical center, by an orthopedic surgeon. The surgeon makes an incision around the kneecap. Then, the muscles and tendons attached to the kneecap are cut and the kneecap is removed. Next, the muscles are sewed back together, and the skin is closed with sutures or clips that stay in place about one week. Any hospital stay is generally brief.

Preparation

Prior to surgery, x rays and other diagnostic tests are done on the knee to determine if removing the kneecap is the appropriate treatment. Pre-operative blood and urine tests are also done.

Aftercare

Pain relievers may be prescribed for a few days. The patient will initially need to use a cane, or crutches, to walk. Physical therapy **exercises** to strengthen the knee should be begun immediately. Driving should be avoided for several weeks. Full recovery can take months.

Risks

Risks involved with kneecap removal are similar to those that occur in any surgical procedure, mainly allergic reaction to anesthesia, excessive bleeding, and infection.

Normal results

People who have kneecap removal because of a broken bone or repeated dislocations have the best chance for complete recovery. Those who have this operation because of arthritis may have less successful results, and later need a total knee replacement.

Resources

BOOKS

Griffith, H. Winter. ''Kneecap Removal.'' In *The Complete Guide to Symptoms, Illness and Surgery,* 3rd ed. New York: Berkeley Publishing, 1995, 834-35.

Tish Davidson

KOH test

Definition

The KOH test takes its name from the chemical formula for potassium hydroxide (KOH), which is the substance used in the test. The test, which is also called a potassium hydroxide preparation, is done to rapidly diagnose fungal infections of the hair, skin, or nails. A sample of the infected area is analyzed under a microscope following the addition of a few drops of potassium hydroxide.

KEY TERMS

Dermatophyte—A type of fungus that causes diseases of the skin, including tinea or ringworm.

KOH—The chemical formula for potassium hydroxide, which is used to perform the KOH test. The tests is also called a potassium hydroxide preparation.

Thrush—A disease of the mouth, caused by *Candida albicans* and characterized by a whitish growth and ulcers. It can be diagnosed with the KOH test.

Tinea—A superficial infection of the skin, hair, or nails, caused by a fungus and commonly known as ringworm.

Purpose

The primary purpose of the KOH test is the differential diagnosis of infections produced by dermatophytes and *Candida albicans* from other skin disorders. Dermatophytes are a type of fungus that invade the top layer of the skin, hair, or nails, and produce an infection commonly known as **ringworm,** technically known as tinea. It can appear as "jock itch" in the groin or inner thighs (tinea cruris); on the feet (tinea pedis); on the scalp and hair (tinea capitis); and on the nails (tinea unguium). Tinea versicolor appears anywhere on the skin and produces characteristic unpigmented patches. Tinea unguium affects the nails.

Similar symptoms of redness, scaling, and **itching** can be caused by other conditions, such as eczema and **psoriasis.** The KOH test is a quick, inexpensive test—often done in a physician's office—to see if these symptoms are caused by a dermatophyte. If a dermatophyte is found, treatment is started immediately; further tests are seldom necessary.

A yeast (candidal) infection of the skin or a mucous membrane, such as the mouth, often produces a white cheesy material at the infection site. This type of infection, known as thrush, is also identified with the KOH test.

Description

The KOH test involves the preparation of a slide for viewing under the laboratory microscope. KOH mixed with a blue-black dye is added to a sample from the infected tissues. This mixture makes it easier to see the dermatophytes or yeast under the microscope. The KOH dissolves skin cells, hair, and debris; the dye adds color.

The slide is gently heated to speed up the action of the KOH. Finally the slide is examined under a microscope.

Dermatophytes are easily recognized under the microscope by their long branch-like structures. Yeast cells look round or oval. The dermatophyte that causes tinea versicolor has a characteristic spaghetti-and-meatballs appearance.

If the KOH test is done in the doctor's office, the results are usually available while the person waits. If the test is sent to a laboratory, the results will be ready the same or following day. The KOH test is covered by insurance when medically necessary.

Preparation

The physician selects an infected area from which to collect the sample. Scales and cells from the area are scraped using a scalpel. If the test is to be analyzed immediately, the scrapings are placed directly onto a microscope slide. If the test will be sent to a laboratory, the scrapings are placed in a sterile covered container.

Normal results

A normal, or negative, KOH test shows no fungi (no dermatophytes or yeast).

Abnormal results

Dermatophytes or yeast seen on a KOH test indicate the person has a fungal infection. Follow-up tests are usually unnecessary.

Resources

PERIODICALS

Crissey, John Thorne. "Common Dermatophyte Infections. A Simple Diagnostic Test and Current Management." *Postgraduate Medicine* (February, 1998): 191-192, 197-198, 200, 205.

Nancy J. Nordenson

Köhler's disease *see* **Osteochondroses**

Korean hemorrhagic fever *see* **Hantavirus infections**

Korsakoff's psychosis *see* **Korsakoff's syndrome**

Korsakoff's syndrome

Definition

Korsakoff's syndrome is a memory disorder which is caused by a deficiency of vitamin B$_1$, also called thiamine.

Description

In the United States, the most common cause of thiamine deficiency is **alcoholism.** Other conditions which cause thiamine deficiency occur quite rarely, but can be seen in patients undergoing dialysis (a procedure used primarily for patients suffering from kidney failure, during which the patient's blood circulates outside of the body, is mechanically cleansed, and then is circulated back into the body), pregnant women with a condition called **hyperemesis gravidarum** (a condition of extreme morning sickness, during which the woman vomits up nearly all fluid and food intake), and patients after surgery who are given vitamin-free fluids for a prolonged period of time. Thiamine deficiency is an important cause of disability in developing countries where the main source of food is polished rice (rice with the more nutritious outer husk removed).

An associated disorder, Wernicke's syndrome, often precedes Korsakoff's syndrome. In fact, they so often occur together that the spectrum of symptoms produced during the course of the two diseases is frequently referred to as Wernicke-Korsakoff syndrome. The main symptoms of Wernicke's syndrome include ataxia (difficulty in walking and maintaining balance), **paralysis** of some of the muscles responsible for movement of the eyes, and confusion. Untreated Wernicke's will lead to **coma** and then **death.**

Causes

One of the main reasons that alcoholism leads to thiamine deficiency has to do with the high-calorie nature of alcohol. A person with a large alcohol intake often, in essence, substitutes alcohol for other, more nutritive calorie sources. Food intake drops off considerably, and multiple vitamin deficiencies develop. Furthermore, it is believed that alcohol increases the body's requirements for B **vitamins,** at the same time interfering with the absorption of thiamine from the intestine and impairing the body's ability to store and use thiamine. Direct neurotoxic (poisonous damage to the nerves) effects of alcohol may also play some role.

Thiamine is involved in a variety of reactions which provide energy to the neurons (nerve cells) of the brain. When thiamine is unavailable, these reactions cannot be carried out, and the important end-products of the reactions are not produced. Furthermore, certain other substances begin to accumulate, and are thought to cause damage to the vulnerable neurons. The area of the brain believed to be responsible for the symptoms of Korsakoff's syndrome is called the diencephalon, specifically the structures called the mamillary bodies and the thalamus.

Symptoms

An individual with Korsakoff's syndrome displays much difficulty with memory. The main area of memory affected is the ability to learn new information. Usually, intelligence and memory for past events is relatively unaffected, so that an individual may remember what occurred 20 years previously, but is unable to remember what occurred 20 minutes ago. This memory defect is referred to as anterograde **amnesia,** and leads to a peculiar symptom called "confabulation," in which a person suffering from Korsakoff's fills in the gaps in his or her memory with fabricated or imagined information. For instance, a person may insist that a doctor to whom he or she has just been introduced is actually an old high school classmate, and may have a lengthy story to back this up. When asked, as part of a memory test, to remember the name of three objects which the examiner listed ten minutes earlier, a person with Korsakoff's may list three entirely different objects and be completely convincing in his or her certainty. In fact, one of the hallmarks of Korsakoff's is the person's complete unawareness of the memory defect, and complete lack of worry or concern when it is pointed out.

Diagnosis

Whenever someone has a possible diagnosis of alcoholism, and then has the sudden onset of memory difficulties, it is important to seriously consider the diagnosis of Korsakoff's syndrome. While there is no specific laboratory test to diagnose Korsakoff's syndrome in a patient, a careful exam of the individual's mental state should be rather revealing. Although the patient's ability to confabulate answers may be convincing, checking the patient's retention of factual information (asking, for example, for the name of the current president of the United States), along with the patient's ability to learn new information (repeating a series of numbers, or recalling the names of three objects ten minutes after having been asked to memorize them) should point to the diagnosis. Certainly a patient known to have just begun recovery from Wernicke's syndrome, who then begins displaying memory difficulties, would be very likely to have developed Korsakoff's syndrome. A **physical examination** may also show signs of Wernicke's syndrome, such as **peripheral neuropathy.**

Treatment

Treatment of both Korsakoff's and Wernicke's syndromes involves the immediate administration of thiamine. In fact, any individual who is hospitalized for any reason and who is suspected of being an alcoholic, should receive thiamine. The combined Wernicke-Korsakoff syndrome has actually been precipitated in alcoholic patients hospitalized for other medical illnesses, due to the administration of thiamine-free intravenous fluids (intravenous fluids are those fluids containing vital sugars and salts which are given to the patient through a needle inserted in a vein). Also, the vitamin therapy may be impaired by the feeding of carbohydrates prior to the giving of thiamine; since carbohydrates cannot be metabolized with thiamine.

Prognosis

Fifteen to twenty percent of all patients hospitalized for Wernicke's syndrome will die of the disorder. Although the degree of ataxia nearly always improves with treatment, half of those who survive will continue to have some permanent difficulty walking. The paralysis of the eye muscles almost always resolves completely with thiamine treatment. Recovery from Wernicke's begins to occur rapidly after thiamine is given. Improvement in the symptoms of Korsakoff's syndrome, however, can take months and months of thiamine replacement. Furthermore, patients who develop Korsakoff's syndrome are almost universally memory-impaired for the rest of their lives. Even with thiamine treatment, the memory deficits tend to be irreversible, with less than 20% of patients

even approaching recovery. The development of Korsakoff's syndrome often results in an individual requiring a supervised living situation.

Prevention

Prevention depends on either maintaining a diet with a sufficient intake of thiamine, or supplementing an inadequate diet with vitamin preparations. Certainly, one of the most important forms of prevention involves treating the underlying alcohol **addiction.**

Resources

BOOKS

Messing, Robert. "Nutritional Disorders of the Nervous System." In *Cecil Textbook of Medicine,* edited by J. Claude Bennett and Fred Plum. Philadelphia: W.B. Saunders, 1996.

Rossor, Martin. "Disorders of Higher Cerebral Cortical Function and Behavioral Neurology." In *Brain's Diseases of the Nervous System,* edited by John Walton. New York: Oxford Medical Publications, 1993.

Schuckit, Marc Alan. *Educating Yourself About Drugs and Alcohol.* New York: Plenum Press, 1995.

PERIODICALS

Langlais, Philip J. "Alcohol-Related Thiamine Deficiency." *Alcohol Health and Research World* (Spring 1995): p. 113.

ORGANIZATIONS

National Institute on Alcoholism Abuse and Alcoholism. 6000 Executive Boulevard - Willco Building, Bethesda, Maryland 20892-7003. http://www.niaaa.nih.gov.

Rosalyn S. Carson-DeWitt

Krabbe's disease *see* **Lipidoses**

KUB *see* **Kidney, ureter, and bladder x ray study**

Kwashiorkor *see* **Protein-energy malnutrition**

Kyphosis

Definition

Kyphosis is the extreme curvature of the upper back also known as a hunchback.

KEY TERMS

Congenital—Present at birth.

Dwarfism—A congenital disease of bone growth that results in short stature and weak bones.

Orthopedic—Refers to surgery on the supporting structures of the body—bones, joints, ligaments, muscles.

Osteoporosis—A weakening of bones due to calcium loss that affects post-menopausal women.

Scheuermann's disease—Juvenile kyphosis due to damaged bone in the spinal vertebrae.

Description

The upper back bone (thoracic region), is normally curved forward. If the curve exceeds 50° it is considered abnormal (kyphotic).

Causes & symptoms

Kyphosis can be divided into three ages of acquisition—birth, old age, and the time in between.

- Spinal **birth defects** can result in a fixed, exaggerated curve. Vertebrae can be fused together, shaped wrong, extraneous, or partially missing. Congenital and hereditary defects in bone growth weaken bone and result in exaggerated curves wherever gravity or muscles pull on them. Dwarfism is such a defect.

- During life, several events can distort the spine. Because the natural tendency of the thoracic spine is to curve forward, any weakness of the supporting structures will tend in that direction. A diseased thoracic vertebra (a spine bone) will ordinarily crumble its forward edge first, increasing the kyphotic curve. Conditions that can do this include **cancer, tuberculosis,** Scheuermann's disease, and certain kinds of arthritis. Healthy vertebra will fracture forward with rapid deceleration injuries, such as in car crashes when the victim is not wearing a seat belt.

- Later in life, kyphosis is caused from **osteoporosis,** bone weakness, and crumbling forward.

The **stress** caused by kyphosis produces such symptoms as an increase in musculoskeletal **pains, tension headaches,** back aches, and joint pains.

Diagnosis

A quick look at the back will usually identify kyphosis. X rays of the spine will confirm the diagnosis and identify its cause.

Treatment

Congenital defects have to be repaired surgically. The procedures are delicate, complicated, and lengthy. Often orthopedic hardware must be placed to stabilize the back bone. At other times, a device called a Milwaukee brace can hold the back in place from the outside. Fitting Milwaukee braces comfortably is difficult because they tend to rub and cause sores.

Kyphosis acquired during the younger years requires treatment directed at the cause, such as medications for tuberculosis. Surgical reconstruction or bracing may also be necessary.

Kyphosis induced by osteoporosis is generally not treated except to prevent further bone softening.

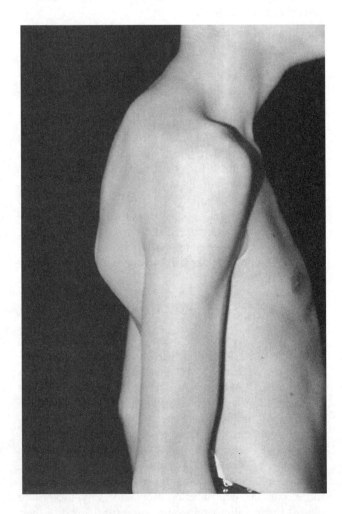

This patient's spine shows excessive backward curvature at the level of the upper chest. *(Custom Medical Stock Photo. Reproduced by permission.)*

Prognosis

Congenital kyphosis may be alleviated to some extent by surgery and bracing. Kyphosis occurring later in life may worsen over time.

Prevention

Preventing osteoporosis is within the grasp of modern medicine. Menopausal women must start early with estrogen replacement, calcium supplementation, and appropriate **exercise.** The treatment must continue through the remainder of life. Evidence suggests that a high calcium intake even during younger years delays the onset of symptomatic osteoporosis. Dairy products are the major dietary sources of calcium.

Resources

BOOKS

Canale, S. Terry, ed. "Kyphosis." In *Campbell's Operative Orthopedics.* St. Louis, MO: Mosby, 1998, pp.2941-2961.

Finkelstein, Joel S. "Osteoporosis." In *Cecil Textbook of Medicine,* edited by J. Claude Bennett and Fred Plum. Philadelphia: W. B. Saunders, 1996, pp.1379-1384.

Krane, Stephen M., and Alan L. Schiller. " Hyperostosis, fibrous dysplasia and other dysplasias of bone and cartilage." In *Harrison's Principles of Internal Medicine,* edited by Kurt Isselbacher, et al. New York: McGraw-Hill, 1998, pp.2369-2375.

Krane, Stephen M., and Michael F. Holick. "Metabolic bone disease." In *Harrison's Principles of Internal Medicine,* edited by Kurt Isselbacher. et al. New York: McGraw-Hill, 1998, pp. 2247-2259.

PERIODICALS

Boachie-Adjei, O., and B. Lonner. "Spinal Deformity." *Pediatric Clinics of North America* 43 (August 1996): 883-897.

Boachie-Adjei, O., and R.G. Squillante. "Tuberculosis of the Spine." *Orthopedic Clinics of North America* 27 (January 1996): 95-103.

Hawker, G.A. "The Epidemiology of Osteoporosis." *Journal of Rheumatology* 45 (August 1996): 2-5.

Winter R.B., J.E. Lonstein, and O. Boachie-Adjei. "Congenital Spinal Deformity." *Instructional Course Lectures. Minnesota Spine Center, Minneapolis, USA* 45 (1996): 117-127.

ORGANIZATIONS

Arthritis Foundation. 1330 W. Peachtree St. PO Box 7669, Atlanta, GA 30357-0669. (800) 283-7800. http://www.arthritis.org.

National Osteoporosis Foundation. 1150 17th Street, Suite 500 NW, Washington, DC 20036-4603. (800) 223-9994 (202) 223-2226. http://www.nof.org.

Osteoporosis and Related Bone Diseases-National Resource Center. 1150 17th Street, NW, Suite 500, Washington, DC 20036-4603. (800) 624-bone. http://www.osteo.org.

J. Ricker Polsdorfer

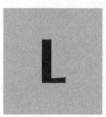

Labor and delivery *see* **Childbirth**

Labor induction *see* **Induction of labor**

Labyrinthitis

Definition

Labyrinthitis is an inflammation of the inner ear that is often a complication of **otitis media.** It is caused by the spread of bacterial or viral infections from the head or respiratory tract into the inner ear.

Description

Labyrinthitis is characterized by **dizziness** or feelings of **motion sickness** caused by disturbance of the sense of balance.

Causes & symptoms

Causes

The disease agents that cause labyrinthitis may reach the inner ear by one of three routes:

- Bacteria may be carried from the middle ear or the membranes that cover the brain.

- The viruses that cause **mumps, measles, influenza,** and colds may reach the inner ear following an upper respiratory infection.

- The **rubella** virus can cause labyrinthitis in infants prior to birth.

  Labyrinthitis can also be caused by toxic drugs.

Symptoms

The primary symptoms of labyrinthitis are vertigo (dizziness), accompanied by **hearing loss** and a sensation of ringing in the ears called tinnitus. Vertigo occurs be-

cause the inner ear controls the sense of balance as well as hearing. Some patients also experience **nausea and vomiting** and spontaneous eye movements in the direction of the unaffected ear. Bacterial labyrinthitis may produce a discharge from the infected ear.

Diagnosis

The diagnosis of labyrinthitis is based on a combination of the patient's symptoms and history—especially a history of a recent upper respiratory infection. The doctor will test the patient's hearing, and order a laboratory culture to identify the organism if the patient has a discharge.

If there is no history of a recent infection, the doctor will order extra tests in order to exclude injuries to the brain or **Meniere's disease.**

Treatment

Medication

Patients with labyrinthitis are given **antibiotics,** either by mouth or intravenously to clear up the infection. They may also be given meclizine (Antivert, Bonine) for vertigo and nausea.

Surgery

Some patients require surgery to drain the inner and middle ear.

Supportive care

Patients with labyrinthitis should rest in bed for three to five days until the acute dizziness subsides. Patients who are dehydrated by repeated vomiting may need intravenous fluid replacement. In addition, patients are advised to avoid driving or similar activities for four to six weeks after the acute symptoms subside, because they may have occasional dizzy spells during that period.

Prognosis

Most patients with labyrinthitis recover completely, although it often takes five to six weeks for the vertigo to disappear completely and the patient's hearing to return to normal. In a few cases the hearing loss is permanent.

Prevention

The most effective preventive strategy includes prompt treatment of middle ear infections, as well as monitoring of patients with mumps, measles, influenza, or colds for signs of dizziness or hearing problems.

Resources

BOOKS

Baloh, Robert W.. "Episodic Vertigo." In *Conn's Current Therapy,* edited by Robert E. Rakel. Philadelphia: W. B. Saunders Company, 1998.

Borer, William Z., and Duane W. Taebel. "Nausea, Vomiting, and Dyspepsia." In *Current Diagnosis 9,* edited by Rex B. Conn, et al. Philadelphia: W. B. Saunders Company, 1997.

Jackler, Robert K., and Michael J. Kaplan. "Ear, Nose, & Throat." In *Current Medical Diagnosis & Treatment 1998,* edited by Lawrence M. Tierney, Jr., et al. Stamford, CT: Appleton & Lange, 1997.

"Labyrinthitis." In *Professional Guide to Diseases,* edited by Stanley Loeb, et al. Springhouse, PA: Springhouse Corporation, 1991.

"Otolaryngology: Purulent Labyrinthitis." In *The Merck Manual of Diagnosis and Therapy,* vol. II, edited by Robert Berkow, et al. Rahway, NJ: Merck Research Laboratories, 1992.

Rowe, Lee D. "Otolaryngology— Head & Neck Surgery." In *Current Surgical Diagnosis & Treatment,* edited by Lawrence W. Way. Stamford, CT: Appleton & Lange, 1994.

Rebecca J. Frey

Laceration repair

Definition

A laceration is a wound caused by a sharp object producing edges that may be jagged, dirty, or bleeding. Lacerations most often affect the skin, but any tissue may be lacerated, including subcutaneous fat, tendon, muscle, or bone.

Purpose

A laceration should be repaired if it:

* Continues to bleed after application of pressure for ten to fifteen minutes
* Is more than one-eighth to one-fourth inch deep
* Exposes fat, muscle, tendon, or bone
* Causes a change in function surrounding the area of the laceration
* Is dirty or has visible debris in it
* Is located in an area where an unsightly scar is undesirable.

Precautions

Lacerations are less likely to become infected if they are repaired soon after they occur. Many physicians will not repair a laceration that is more than eight hours old because the risk of infection is too great.

Description

Laceration repair mends a tear in the skin or other tissue. The procedure is similar to repairing a tear in clothing. Primary care physicians, emergency room physicians, and surgeons usually repair lacerations. The four goals of laceration repair are to stop bleeding, prevent infection, preserve function, and restore appearance. Insurance companies do pay for the procedure. Cost depends upon the severity and size of the laceration.

Before repairing the laceration, the physician thoroughly examines the wound and the underlying tendons or nerves. If nerves or tendons have been injured, a surgeon may be needed to complete the repair. The laceration is cleaned by removing any foreign material or debris. Removing **foreign objects** from penetrating **wounds** can sometimes cause bleeding, so this type of wound must be cleaned very carefully. The wound is then irrigated with saline solution and a disinfectant. The disinfecting agent may be mild soap or a commercial preparation. An antibacterial agent may be applied.

Once the wound has been cleansed, the physician anesthetizes the area of the repair by injecting a local

KEY TERMS

Debridement—The act of removing any foreign material and damaged or contaminated tissue from a wound to expose surrounding healthy tissue.

anesthetic. The physician may trim edges that are jagged or extremely uneven. Tissue that is too damaged to heal must be removed (**debridement**) to prevent infection. If the laceration is deep, several absorbable stitches (sutures) are placed in the tissue under the skin to help bring the tissue layers together. Suturing also helps eliminate any pockets where tissue fluid or blood can accumulate.

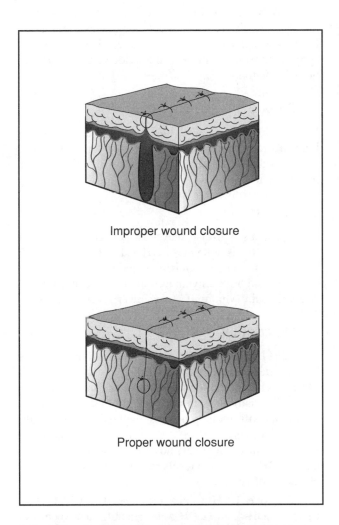

Improper wound closure

Proper wound closure

A laceration is a traumatic break in the skin caused by a sharp object producing edges that may be jagged, dirty, or bleeding. The underlying tissue may also be severed. In such instances, the physician may place absorbable sutures in the tissue to help bring the edges together before the skin is sutured close. (Illustration by Electronic Illustrators Group.)

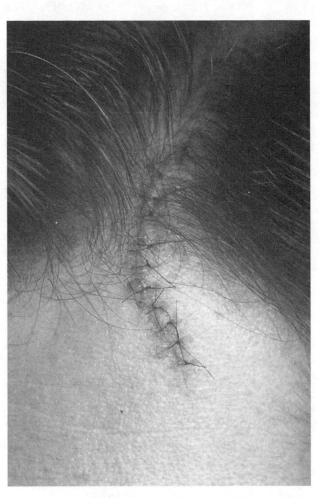

Eleven sutures are necessary to close up the laceration on this person's forehead. (Custom Medical Stock Photo. Reproduced by permission.)

The skin wound is closed with sutures. Suture material used on the surface of a wound is usually non-absorbable and will have to be removed later. A light dressing or an adhesive bandage is applied for 24-48 hours. In areas where a dressing is not feasible, an antibiotic ointment can be applied. If the laceration is the result of a human or animal bite, if it is very dirty, or if the patient has a medical condition that alters wound healing, oral **antibiotics** may be prescribed.

Aftercare

The laceration is kept clean and dry for at least 24 hours after the repair. Light bathing is generally permitted after 24 hours if the wound is not soaked. The physician will provide directions for any special wound care. Sutures are removed 3-14 days after the repair is completed. Timing of suture removal depends on the location of the laceration and physician preference.

The repair should be observed frequently for signs of infection, which include redness, swelling, tenderness, drainage from the wound, red streaks in the skin surrounding the repair, chills, or **fever.** If any of these occur, the physician should be contacted immediately.

Risks

The most common complication of any laceration repair is infection. Risk of infection can be minimized by cleansing the wound thoroughly. Wounds from bites or dirty objects or wounds that have a large amount of dirt in them are most likely to become infected.

All lacerations will heal with a scar. Wounds that are repaired with sutures are less likely to develop scars that are unsightly, but no one can predict how wounds will heal and who will develop unsightly scars. Plastic surgery can improve the appearance of many scars.

Resources

BOOKS

Snell, George. "Laceration Repair." In *Procedures for Primary Care Physicians,* edited by John L. Pfenninger and Grant C. Fowler. St. Louis: Mosby, 1994.

OTHER

Caring for cuts and scrapes at home. Mayo Health Oasis. Mayo Clinic. http://www.mayohealth.org/mayo/9611/htm/cuts_sb.htm.

Cuts and Scrapes. Mayo Health Oasis. Mayo Clinic. http://www.mayohealth.org/mayo/9611/htm/cuts.htm.

Laceration Repair. Thriveonline.com. http://www.thriveonline.com/health/Library/surgery/surgery164.html.

Mary Jeanne Krob

Lacerations *see* **Wounds**

Lacrimal sac infection *see* **Dacryocystitis**

Lactate dehydrogenase isoenzymes test

Definition

The enzyme lactate dehydrogenase (also known as lactic dehydrogenase, or LDH) is found in the cells of almost all body tissues. The enzyme is especially concentrated in the heart, liver, red blood cells, kidneys, muscles, brain, and lungs. The total LDH can be further separated into five components or fractions labeled by number: LDH-1, LDH-2, LDH-3, LDH-4, and LDH-5.

Each of these fractions, called isoenzymes, is used mainly by a different set of cells or tissues in the body. For this reason, the relative amounts of a particular isoenzyme of LDH in the blood can provide valuable diagnostic information.

Purpose

The LDH isoenzymes test assists in differentiating **heart attack, anemia,** lung injury, or liver disease from other conditions that may cause the same symptoms (differential diagnosis).

Precautions

Strenuous **exercise** may raise levels of total LDH, specifically the isoenzymes LDH-1, LDH-2, and LDH-5. Alcohol, anesthetics, **aspirin,** narcotics, procainamide, fluorides, and mithramycin may also raise levels of LDH. Ascorbic acid (vitamin C) can lower levels of LDH.

Description

LDH is found in the cells of almost all body tissues. When certain conditions injure cells in tissues containing LDH, it is released into the bloodstream. Because LDH is so widely distributed throughout the body, analysis of total LDH will not help make a diagnosis of a particular disease. Because this enzyme is actually composed of five different isoenzymes, however, analysis of the different LDH isoenzyme levels in the blood can help in the diagnosis of some diseases.

The five LDH isoenzymes are: LDH-1, LDH-2, LDH-3, LDH-4, and LDH-5. In general, each isoenzyme is used mostly by the cells in a specific tissue. LDH-1 is found mainly in the heart. LDH-2 is primarily associated with the system in the body that defends against infection (reticuloendothelial system). LDH-3 is found in the lungs and other tissues, LDH-4 in the kidney, placenta, and pancreas, and LDH-5 in liver and striated (skeletal) muscle. Normally, levels of LDH-2 are higher than those of the other isoenzymes.

Certain diseases have classic patterns of elevated LDH isoenzyme levels. For example, an LDH-1 level higher than that of LDH-2 is indicative of a heart attack or injury; elevations of LDH-2 and LDH-3 indicate lung injury or disease; elevations of LDH-4 and LDH-5 indicate liver or muscle disease or both. A rise of all LDH isoenzymes at the same time is diagnostic of injury to multiple organs. For example, a heart attack with congestive **heart failure** may cause symptoms of lung and liver congestion. Advanced **cancer** and autoimmune diseases such as lupus can also cause this pattern.

One of the most important diagnostic uses for the LDH isoenzymes test is in the differential diagnosis of myocardial infarction or heart attack. The total LDH level rises within 24-48 hours after a heart attack, peaks in two to three days, and returns to normal in approximately five to ten days. This pattern is a useful tool for a delayed diagnosis of heart attack. The LDH-1 isoenzyme level, however, is more sensitive and specific than the total LDH. Normally, the level of LDH-2 is higher than the level of LDH-1. An LDH-1 level higher than that of LDH-2, a phenomenon known as "flipped LDH," is strongly indicative of a heart attack. The flipped LDH usually appears within 12-24 hours after a heart attack. In about 80% of cases, flipped LDH is present within 48 hours of the incident. A normal LDH-1/LDH-2 ratio is considered reliable evidence that a heart attack has not occurred.

It should be noted that two conditions might cause elevated LDH isoenzymes at the same time and that one may confuse the other. For example, a patient with **pneumonia** may also be having an acute heart attack. In this instance, the LDH-1 level would rise with the LDH-2 and LDH-3. Because of this complication, some laboratories measure only the LDH-1 and consider an elevated LDH level with LDH-1 higher than 40% to be diagnostic of heart damage. LDH isoenzymes test is not used much anymore for diagnosis of heart attack. Tests for the protein troponin, which is found in myocardial cells, have been found to be more accurate.

Preparation

This test requires a blood sample. The patient need not fast (nothing to eat or drink) before the test unless requested to do so by the physician.

Risks

Risks for this test are minimal. The patient may experience slight bleeding from the blood-drawing site, **fainting** or feeling lightheaded after the vein is punctured (venipuncture), or an accumulation of blood under the puncture site (hematoma).

Normal results

Reference values for normal levels of LDH isoenzymes vary from laboratory to laboratory but can generally be found within the following ranges:

- LDH-1: 17-27%
- LDH-2: 27-37%
- LDH-3: 18-25%
- LDH-4: 8-16%
- LDH-5: 6-16%.

Abnormal results

Increased levels of LDH-1 are seen in myocardial infarction, red blood cell diseases like **hemolytic anemia,** kidney disease including **kidney transplantation** rejection, and testicular tumors. Increased levels of LDH-2 are found in lung diseases such as pneumonia and congestive heart failure, as well as in lymphomas and other tumors. Elevations of LDH-3 are significant in lung disease and certain tumors. Elevations of LDH-4 are greatly increased in **pancreatitis.** High levels of LDH-5 are found in liver disease, intestinal problems, and skeletal muscle disease and injury, such as **muscular dystrophy** and recent muscular trauma.

Diffuse disease or injury (for example, collagen disease, **shock,** low blood pressure) and advanced solid-tumor cancers cause significant elevations of all LDH isoenzymes at the same time.

Resources

BOOKS

Cahill, Mathew. *Handbook of Diagnostic Tests.* Springhouse, Pennsylvania: Springhouse Corporation, 1995.

Jacobs, David S., ed. *Laboratory Test Handbook.* 4th ed. Hudson, Ohio: Lexi Comp Inc., 1996.

Pagana, Kathleen Deska, and Timothy James Pagana. *Mosby's Manual of Diagnostic and Laboratory Tests.* St. Louis: Mosby, Inc., 1998.

Janis O. Flores

Lactate dehydrogenase test

Definition

Lactate dehydrogenase, also called lactic dehydrogenase, or LDH, is an enzyme found in the cells of many body tissues, including the heart, liver, kidneys, skeletal muscle, brain, red blood cells, and lungs. It is responsible for converting muscle lactic acid into pyruvic acid, an essential step in producing cellular energy.

Purpose

Lactic dehydrogenase is present in almost all body tissues, so the LDH test is used to detect tissue alterations and as an aid in the diagnosis of **heart attack,** anemia, and liver disease. Newer injury markers are becoming more useful than LDH for heart attack diagnosis.

Precautions

Because the LDH enzyme is so widely distributed throughout the body, cellular damage causes an elevation of the total serum LDH. As a result, the diagnostic usefulness of this enzyme by itself is not as valuable as determination of the five fractions that comprise the LDH. These fractions are called isoenzymes and are better indicators of disease than is the total LDH. The fractions are LDH-1, LDH-2, LDH-3, LDH-4, and LDH-5. A normal total LDH level does not mean that individual isoenzyme levels should not be measured. Individual isoenzyme ranges can help differentiate a diagnosis.

Description

When disease or injury affects tissues containing LDH, the cells release LDH into the bloodstream, where it is identified in higher than normal levels. For example, when a person has a heart attack, the LDH level begins to rise about 12 hours after the attack and usually returns to normal within 5-10 days. The LDH is also elevated in diseases of the liver, in certain types of **anemia,** and in cases of excessive destruction of cells, as in **fractures,** trauma, muscle damage, and **shock.**

Cancers can also elevate LDH level. Additionally, some patients have chronically elevated LDH with no identifiable cause and no apparent consequence.

Preparation

This test requires a blood sample. It is not necessary for the patient to fast (nothing to eat or drink) before the test unless the physician requests it.

Risks

Risks for this test are minimal, but may include slight bleeding from the blood-drawing site, **fainting** or feeling lightheaded after venipuncture, or hematoma (blood accumulating under the puncture site).

Normal results

Reference ranges for total LDH vary from laboratory to laboratory. Normal values are also higher in childhood. For adults, in most laboratories, the range can be up to approximately 200 units/L, but is usually found within 45-90 U/L.

Abnormal results

Due to the fact that many common disease processes cause elevations in the total LDH level, a breakdown of the five different isoenzymes that make up the total LDH is often helpful for diagnosis. In certain disorders, the total LDH may be within normal limits, but individual isoenzyme elevations can indicate specific organ or tissue damage. For example, the LDH-2 fraction is normally greater than LDH-1 in the blood. After an acute heart attack, however, the LDH-1 rises over the LDH-2 in what is known as a "flipped LDH."

Certain diagnoses can be assisted by determination of the total LDH. One example is **infectious mononucleosis,** in which the LDH is usually more elevated than a liver enzyme called AST. Conversely, in cases of viral hepatitis, the liver enzymes AST and ALT are greatly increased over the LDH.

Resources

BOOKS

Cahill, Mathew. *Handbook of Diagnostic Tests.* Springhouse, PA: Springhouse Corporation, 1995.

Jacobs, David S. *Laboratory Test Handbook,* Fourth Edition. Hudson, OH: Lexi-Comp Inc., 1996.

Pagana, Kathleen Deska. *Mosby's Manual of Diagnostic and Laboratory Tests.* St. Louis: Mosby, Inc., 1998.

Janis O. Flores

· ·

Lactation

Definition

Lactation is the medical term for breastfeeding, a natural method of feeding an infant from birth to the time he or she can eat solid food. Human milk contains the ideal amount of nutrients for the infant, and provides

KEY TERMS

Bromocriptine—A drug used to treat Parkinson's disease that can decrease a woman's milk supply.

Ergotamine—A drug used to prevent or treat migraine headaches. This can cause vomiting, diarrhea, and convulsions in infants.

Lithium—A drug used to treat manic depression (bipolar disorder) that can be transmitted in breast milk.

Methotrexate—An anticancer drug also used to treat arthritis that can suppress an infant's immune system when taken by a nursing mother.

important protection from diseases through the mother's natural defenses.

Description

Early in a woman's **pregnancy** her milk-producing glands begin to prepare for her baby's arrival, and by the sixth month of pregnancy the breasts are ready to produce milk. Immediately after the baby is born, the placenta is delivered. This causes a hormone in the woman's body (prolactin) to activate the milk-producing glands. By the third to fifth day, the woman's breasts fill with milk.

Then, as the baby continues to suck each day, nursing triggers the continuing production of milk. The baby's sucking stimulates nerve endings in the nipple, which signal the mother's pituitary gland to release oxytocin, a hormone that causes the mammary glands to release milk to the nursing baby. This is called the "let-down reflex." While the baby's sucking is the primary stimulus for this reflex, a baby's cry, thoughts of the baby, or the sound of running water also may trigger the response. Frequent nursing will lead to increased milk production.

Breast milk cannot be duplicated by commercial baby food formulas, although both contain protein, fat, and carbohydrates. In particular, breast milk changes to meet the specific needs of a baby. The composition of breast milk changes as the baby grows, to meet the baby's changing needs. Most important, breast milk contains substances called antibodies from the mother that can protect the child against illness and **allergies.** Antibodies are part of the body's natural defense system against infections and other agents that can cause disease. Breast milk also helps a baby's own immune system mature faster. As a result, breast-fed babies have fewer ear infections, **diarrhea, rashes,** allergies, and other medical problems than bottle-fed babies.

There are many other benefits to breast milk. Because it is easily digested, babies do not get constipated. Breast-fed babies have fewer speech impediments, and they have good cheekbone development and jaw alignment.

Breastfeeding is also good for the mother. The act of breastfeeding releases hormones that stimulate the uterus to contract, helping it to return to normal size after delivery and reducing the risk of bleeding. The act of producing milk burns calories, which helps the mother to lose excess weight gained during pregnancy. Breastfeeding also may be related to a lower risk of **breast cancer, ovarian cancer,** or **cervical cancer.** This benefit is stronger the younger a woman is when she breastfeeds; women who breastfeed before age 20 and nurse for at least six months have a 50% drop in the risk for **breast cancer.**

In addition, breastfeeding does not involve any formulas, bottles and nipples, or sterilizing equipment. Breast milk is free, and saves money by eliminating the need to buy formula, bottles, and nipples. Because breast-fed babies are healthier, health care costs for breast-fed infants are lower.

Procedure

Breastfeeding should begin as soon as possible after birth, and should continue every two to three hours. However, all babies are different; some need to nurse almost constantly at first, while others can go much longer between feedings. A baby should be fed at least 8-12 times in 24 hours. Because breast milk is easily digested, a baby may be hungry again as soon as one and one-half hours after the last meal.

Mothers should wear comfortable, loose, front-opening clothes and a good nursing bra. Mothers should find a comfortable chair with lots of pillows, supporting the arm and back. Feet should rest on a low footstool, with knees raised slightly. The baby should be level with the breast. The new mother may have to experiment with different ways of holding the baby before finding one that is comfortable for both the mother and baby.

Some babies have no trouble breastfeeding, while others may need some assistance. Once the baby begins to suck, the mother should make sure that the entire dark area around the nipple is in the baby's mouth. This will help stimulate milk flow, allowing the baby to get enough milk. It will also prevent nipple soreness.

Breastfeeding mothers will usually offer the baby both breasts at each feeding. Breastfeeding takes about 15-20 minutes on each side. After stopping the feeding on one side, the mother should burp the baby before beginning the feeding on the other breast. If the baby falls asleep at the breast, the next feeding should begin with the breast that was not nursed.

Mothers can tell if the baby is getting enough milk by checking diapers; a baby who is wetting between four to six disposable diapers (six to eight cloth) and who has three or four bowel movements in 24 hours is getting enough milk.

Nursing problems

New mothers may experience nursing problems, including:

* Engorged breasts. Breasts that are too full can prevent the baby from sucking. Expressing milk manually or with a breast pump can help.

* Sore nipples. In the early weeks nipples may become sore; a nipple shield can ease discomfort.

* Infection. Soreness and inflammation on the breast surface or a **fever** in the mother, may be an indication of breast infection. **Antibiotics** and continued nursing on the affected side may solve the problem.

Prognosis

There are no rules about when to stop breastfeeding. A baby needs breast milk for at least the first year of life; as long as a baby eats age-appropriate solid food, the mother may nurse for several years.

Prevention

Most common illnesses can not be transmitted via breast milk. However, some viruses, including HIV (the virus that causes **AIDS**) can be passed in breast milk; for this reason, women who are HIV-positive should not breastfeed.

Many medications have not been tested in nursing women, so it is not known if these drugs can affect a breast-fed child. A nursing woman should always check with her doctor before taking any medications, including over-the-counter drugs.

These drugs are not safe to take while nursing:

* Radioactive drugs for some diagnostic tests

* **Chemotherapy** drugs for **cancer**

* Bromocriptine

* Ergotamine

* Lithium

* Methotrexate

* Street drugs (including marijuana, heroin, amphetamines)

* Tobacco.

Resources

BOOKS

Cunningham, F. Gary, et al. *Williams Obstetrics.* 20th ed. Stamford, Ct: Appleton & Lange, 1997.

Franck, Irene, and David Brownstone. *The Parents' Desk Reference.* New York: Prentice Hall, 1991.

Johnson, Robert V. *Mayo Clinic Complete Book of Pregnancy and Baby's First Year.* New York: William Morrow and Co., 1994.

PERIODICALS

Newman, Jack. "How Breast Milk Protects Newborns." *Scientific American* 273(December 1995):676.

ORGANIZATIONS

International Lactation Consultants Assoc. 201 Brown Ave., Evanston, IL 60202. (708) 260-8874.

La Leche League International. 1400 North Meacham Rd., Schaumburg, IL 60173. (800) LA-LECHE.

National Alliance for Breastfeeding Advocacy. 254 Conant Rd., Weston, MA 02193. (617) 893-3553.

Carol A. Turkington

Lactic acid test

Definition

Lactic acid is a weak acid produced by cells during chemical processes in the body that do not require oxygen (anaerobic metabolism). Anaerobic metabolism occurs only when too little oxygen is present for the more usual aerobic metabolism. Lactic acid is a contributing factor in muscle cramps. It is also produced in tissues when conditions such as **heart attack** or **shock** reduce the blood supply responsible for carrying oxygen. Normally, lactic acid is removed from the blood by the liver. When an excess of lactic acid accumulates for any reason, the result is a condition called lactic acidosis.

Purpose

The lactic acid test is used as an indirect assessment of the oxygen level in tissues and to determine the cause and course of lactic acidosis.

Precautions

During blood collection, the patient should be instructed to relax the hand. Clenching and unclenching the fist will cause a build-up of potassium and lactic acid from the hand muscles that will falsely elevate the levels.

KEY TERMS

Acidosis—A disturbance of the balance of acid to base in the body causing an accumulation of acid or loss of alkali (base). There are two types of acidosis: metabolic and respiratory. One of the most common causes of metabolic acidosis is an overdose of aspirin. Respiratory acidosis is caused by impaired breathing caused by conditions such as severe chronic bronchitis, bronchial asthma, or airway obstruction.

Description

The degree of acidity is an important chemical property of blood and other body fluids. Acidity is expressed on a pH scale where 7.0 is neutral, above 7.0 is basic (alkaline), and below 7.0 is acidic. A strong acid has a very low pH (near 1.0). A strong base has a very high pH (near 14.0). Blood is normally slightly alkaline or basic. It has a pH range of 7.35-7.45. The balance of acid to base in blood is precisely controlled. Even a minor deviation from the normal range can severely affect many organs.

Lactic acid (present in the blood as lactate ion) is a product of the breakdown of glucose to generate energy. It is found primarily in muscle cells and red blood cells. The lactate concentration in the blood depends on the rates of energy production and metabolism. Levels may increase significantly during **exercise.**

Together, lactate and another substance called pyruvate form a reversible reaction regulated by the oxygen supply to the blood and tissues. When oxygen levels are deficient, pyruvate converts to lactate; when they are adequate, lactate converts to pyruvate. When the liver fails to metabolize lactose sufficiently or when too much pyruvate converts to lactate, lactic acidosis occurs. Measurement of blood lactate levels is recommended for all patients with symptoms of lactic acidosis. Testing is generally indicated if the blood pH level falls below 7.25-7.35.

Because of the close relationship between pyruvate and lactate, comparison of blood levels of the two substances can provide reliable information about tissue oxidation. However, pyruvate measurement is technically difficult and seldom performed. Lactic acid is measured more often, in either venous or arterial blood samples.

Preparation

This test requires a blood sample. The patient should have nothing to eat or drink (**fasting**) from midnight the night before the test. Because lactic acid is produced by exertion, the patient should rest for at least one hour before the test.

Risks

Risks for this test are minimal. The patient may experience slight bleeding from the blood-drawing site, **fainting** or feeling lightheaded after puncture of the vein (venipuncture), or an accumulation of blood under the puncture site (hematoma).

Normal results

Reference values vary from laboratory to laboratory but can be found within the following ranges:

* Venous blood: 4.5-19.8 mg/dL
* Arterial blood: 4.5-14.4 mg/dL.

Abnormal results

High blood lactate levels, together with decreased oxygen in tissues, may be caused by strenuous muscle exercise, shock, hemorrhage, severe infection in the blood stream, heart attack, or cardiac arrest. When tissue oxygenation is low for no apparent reason, increased lactate levels may be caused by systemic disorders like diabetes, leukemia, liver disease, or kidney failure. Defects in enzymes may also be responsible, as in glycogen storage disease (von Gierke's disease). Lactate is also increased in certain instances of intestinal obstruction.

Lactic acidosis can be caused by taking large doses of **acetaminophen** and alcohol and by intravenous infusion of epinephrine, glucagon, fructose, or sorbitol. Antifreeze **poisoning** can also cause lactic acidosis. In rare instances, a diabetic medication, metformin (Glucophage), causes lactic acidosis. People with weak kidneys should not take metformin.

Resources

BOOKS

Cahill, Mathew. *Handbook of Diagnostic Tests.* Springhouse, Pennsylvania: Springhouse Corporation, 1995.

Jacobs, David S., ed. *Laboratory Test Handbook.* 4th ed. Hudson, Ohio: Lexi-Comp Inc., 1996.

Pagana, Kathleen Deska, and Timothy James Pagana. *Mosby's Manual of Diagnostic and Laboratory Tests.* St. Louis: Mosby, Inc., 1998.

Janis O. Flores

Lactogen test *see* **Prolactin test**

Lactogenic hormone test *see* **Prolactin test**

Lactose intolerance *see* **Carbohydrate intolerance**

Lambliasis *see* **Giardiasis**

Laminectomy *see* **Disk removal**

Lamivudine *see* **Antiretroviral drugs**

Langerhans-cell histiocytosis *see* **Histiocytosis X**

Language disturbance *see* **Aphasia**

Laparoscopic cholecystectomy *see* **Cholecystectomy**

Laparoscopy

Definition

Laparoscopy is a type of surgical procedure in which a small incision is made, usually in the navel, through which a viewing tube (laparoscope) is inserted. The viewing tube has a small camera on the eyepiece. This allows the doctor to examine the abdominal and pelvic organs on a video monitor connected to the tube. Other small incisions can be made to insert instruments to perform procedures. Laparoscopy can be done to diagnose conditions or to perform certain types of operations. It is less invasive than regular open abdominal surgery (laparotomy).

Purpose

Laparoscopy was first used by gynecologists to diagnose and treat conditions relating to the female reproductive organs: uterus, fallopian tubes, and ovaries. It is now used for a wider range of procedures, including operations that in the past required open surgery, such as removal of the appendix (**appendectomy**) and gallbladder removal (**cholecystectomy**).

Diagnostic procedure

As a diagnostic procedure, laparoscopy is done to determine the cause of pelvic **pain** or gynecological symptoms that cannot be confirmed by a physical exam or ultrasound. For example, a laparoscopic examination can identify **ovarian cysts, endometriosis, ectopic pregnancy,** or blocked fallopian tubes. It is an important tool when trying to determine the cause of **infertility.**

Laparoscopy can also be used to examine the appendix, gallbladder, or liver.

Operative procedure

As an operative procedure, laparoscopy is used for female sterilization (**tubal ligation**), some vaginal hysterectomies, treating an ectopic pregnancy, treating endometriosis, and to collect eggs for **in vitro fertilization.** It also is a useful technique for taking a biopsy, aspirating a cyst, or locating and removing an intrauterine device (**IUD**) that has perforated the uterus. Laparoscopy can be used as an alternative to open surgery for some nongynecologic operations, such as removal of the appendix, gallstones, or gallbladder.

While many of these procedures can be done using regular open surgery, laparoscopy usually involves less pain, less risk, less scarring, and faster recovery. Because

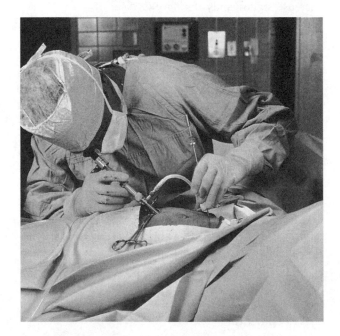

This surgeon is performing a laparoscopic procedure on a patient. *(Photo Researchers, Inc. Reproduced by permission.)*

laparoscopy is so much less invasive than traditional abdominal surgery, patients can leave the hospital sooner.

Description

Laparoscopy is a surgical procedure that is usually done in the hospital under general anesthesia, although it also can be done under local anesthesia. Before starting the procedure, a catheter is inserted through the urethra to empty the bladder, and the skin of the abdomen is cleaned.

After the patient is anesthetized, a hollow needle is inserted into the abdomen in or near the navel, and carbon dioxide gas is pumped through the needle to expand the abdomen. This allows the surgeon a better view of the internal organs. The laparoscope is then inserted through this incision to look at the internal organs. The image from the camera attached to the end of laparoscope is seen on a video monitor.

Sometimes, other small incisions are made to insert other instruments which are used to lift the tubes and ovaries for examination or to perform surgical procedures.

Some common reasons for having a diagnostic laparoscopy are:

• Infertility. A laparoscopy can determine if there are anatomical abnormalities, endometriosis, blocked fallopian tubes, or some other reason for infertility. A dye may be injected through the cervical canal to see if the fallopian tubes are open. If the tubes are open, the dye will be seen spilling out the ends.

• Pelvic pain. There are many possible causes of pelvic pain that can be diagnosed with laparoscopy. These include endometriosis, ovarian cysts, ectopic pregnancy, **pelvic inflammatory disease** (PID), and uterine abnormalities.

Some common laparoscopic operative procedures are:

• Tubal ligation. In this procedure, the fallopian tubes are sealed or cut to prevent subsequent pregnancies.

• Ectopic pregnancy. If a fertilized egg becomes embedded outside the uterus, usually in the fallopian tube, an operation must be performed to remove the developing embryo. This often can be done with laparoscopy.

• Endometriosis. This is a condition in which tissue from inside the uterus is found outside the uterus in other parts of (or on organs within) the pelvic cavity. This can cause cysts to form. Endometriosis is diagnosed with laparoscopy, and in some cases the cysts and other tissue can be removed during laparoscopy.

• **Hysterectomy.** This procedure to remove the uterus can, in some cases, be performed using laparoscopy.

The uterus is cut away with the aid of the laparoscopic instruments and then the uterus is removed through the vagina.

• Ovarian masses. Tumors or cysts in the ovaries can be removed using laparoscopy.

• Appendectomy. This surgery to remove an inflamed appendix required open surgery in the past. It is now routinely performed with laparoscopy.

• Cholecystectomy. Like appendectomy, this procedure to remove the gall bladder used to require open surgery. Now it can be performed with laparoscopy, in some cases.

Preparation

Patients should not eat or drink after midnight on the night before the procedure.

Aftercare

Nurses will check the patient's vital signs of patients who had general anesthesia after the operation. If there are no complications, the patient may leave the hospital within four to eight hours. (Traditional abdominal surgery requires a hospital stay of four days).

There may be some slight pain or throbbing at the incision sites in the first day or so after the procedure. The gas that is used to expand the abdomen may cause discomfort under the ribs or in the shoulder for a few days.

Depending on the reason for the laparoscopy in gynecological procedures, some women may experience some vaginal bleeding.

Many patients can return to work within a week of surgery and most are back to work within two weeks.

Risks

Laparoscopy is a relatively safe procedure, especially if the physician is experienced in the technique. The risk of complications is less than 0.5%.

The procedure carries a slight risk of puncturing an organ, which could cause blood to seep into the abdominal cavity. Puncturing the intestines could allow intestinal contents to seep into the cavity. These are serious complications and major surgery may be required to correct the problem. For operative procedures, there is the possibility that it may become apparent that open surgery is required.

In rare cases, one of the following complications may occur:

• Hemorrhage

• Inflammation of the abdominal cavity lining

• **Abscess**

• Problems related to general anesthesia.

Normal results

In diagnostic procedures, normal results would indicate no abnormalities or disease of the organs that were examined.

Abnormal results

A diagnostic laparoscopy may reveal abnormalities or diseases, such as ovarian tumors or cysts, tumors, pelvic inflammatory disease, **cirrhosis,** endometriosis, fibroid tumors, or an accumulation of fluid in the cavity.

Resources

BOOKS

Carlson, Karen J., Stephanie A. Eisenstat, and Terra Ziporyn. *The Harvard Guide to Women's Health.* Cambridge, MA: Harvard University Press, 1996.

Cunningham, F. Gary, Paul C. MacDonald, et al. *Williams Obstetrics,* 20th ed. Stamford, Ct: Appleton & Lange, 1997.

Ryan, Kenneth J., Ross S. Berkowitz, and Robert L. Barbieri. *Kistner's Gynecology,* 6th ed. St. Louis: Mosby, 1997.

Carol A. Turkington

Laryngeal cancer *see* **Head and neck cancer**

Laryngectomy

Definition

A laryngectomy is a surgical procedure involving the removal of the voicebox and other surrounding structures as a treatment for **cancer** of the larynx. Whether the procedure involves a partial or complete laryngectomy is dependent upon the precise location and involvement of the tumor.

Purpose

Surgery or surgery combined with radiation may be recommended for newly diagnosed patients, or for those in which the tumor has not responded to radiation.

Description

During this operation, the surgeon performs a tracheostomy, an opening in the front of the neck through to the

trachea (air passage to the lungs). A tube, called a trach, keeps this new airway open. A partial laryngectomy involves removal of only part of the voice box, and after recovery from the surgery, the trach tube is removed. The patient's ability to speak is preserved; the voice however, may be hoarse or weak. In a total laryngectomy, the whole voice box is removed, and the patient, referred to as a laryngectomee, breathes through the opening in his neck, called a stoma.

Preparation

As with any surgical procedure, the patient will be required to sign a consent form after the procedure is thoroughly explained. Blood and urine studies, along with chest x ray and EKG may be ordered as the doctor deems necessary. If a complete laryngectomy is planned, it may be helpful to meet with the speech-language pathologist and/or an established larygectomee for discussion of post-operative expectations and moral support.

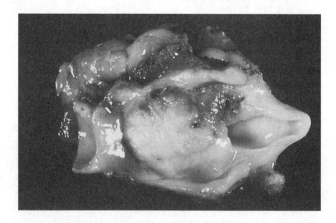

A pathology photograph of an extracted tumor found on the larynx. *(Custom Medical Stock Photo. Reproduced by permission.)*

Aftercare

As with any major surgery, the blood pressure, pulse and respirations will be monitored. The patient will be encouraged to turn, **cough** and deep breathe, to help mobilize secretions in the lungs. Humidification of air to the stoma and suctioning of the secretions may be also ordered by the physician to prevent obstruction of airflow. Initially the trach tube in the stoma will be cleaned and changed at regular intervals; once the tube is removed, a thin covering (laryngectomy bib or scarf) should be worn to prevent dust or other foreign matter from entering the tracheostomy.

An alternate method of communication should be used, such as writing, gesturing or pointing. A partial laryngectomy patient usually can speak within a week or two after surgery. A speech pathologist will work with a complete laryngectomee to explore various new ways of communicating. One method is espheageal speech, in which the laryngectomee learns how to "swallow" air down into the esophagus and creates sounds by releasing the air. Most patients can resume activities before surgery. Special precautions are indicated during showering or shaving; special instruction and equipment is also required for those who wish to swim or water ski, as it would be very dangerous for water to enter the windpipe and lungs through the stoma.

Regular follow-up visits are very important following treatment for cancer of the larynx. There is a higher than average risk for developing a new cancer in the mouth, throat, or other areas of the head or neck. There are many self-help and support groups available to help patients meet others who face similar problems.

Resources

BOOKS

Dollinger, Malin. *Everyone's Guide to Cancer Therapy* Toronto: Somerville House Books Limited, 1994.

Monahan, Frances. *Medical-Surgical Nursing* Philadelphia: W. B. Saunders Company, 1998.

Suddarth, Doris. *The Lippincott Manual of Nursing Practice* Philadelphia: J. B. Lippincott, 1991.

ORGANIZATIONS

American Cancer Society. National Headquarters, 1599 Clifton Road NE, Atlanta, GA 30329. 800(ACS)-2345).

American Speech-Language-Hearing Association(ASHA). Consumer Division, 10801 Rockville Pike, Rockville, MD 20852. 800-638-TALK.

Cancer Information Service. National Cancer Institute, Building 31, Room 10A19, 9000 Rockville Pike, Bethesda, MD 20892. (800)4-CANCER.

International Association of Laryngectomees(IAL). 1559 Clifton Road NE, Atlanta, GA 30329, 800-ACS-2345.

OTHER

Cancer of the Larynx:information and assistance http://members.aol.com/fantamtwo/cancer1.htm.(25May1998).

Cancer of the Larynx http://www.medicinenet.com/mainmenu/encyclop/ARTICLE/Art.L/larynC.htm. (25May1998).

Kathleen Dredge Wright

Laryngitis

Definition

Laryngitis is caused by inflammation of the larynx, resulting in hoarseness of the voice.

Description

When air is breathed in (inspired), it passes through the nose and the nasopharynx or through the mouth and the oropharynx. These are both connected to the larynx, a tube made of cartilage. The vocal cords, responsible for setting up the vibrations necessary for speech, are located within the larynx. The air continues down the larynx to the trachea. The trachea then splits into two branches, the left and right bronchi (bronchial tubes). These bronchi branch into smaller air tubes which run within the lungs, leading to the small air sacs of the lungs (alveoli).

Either food, liquid, or air may be taken in through the mouth. While air goes into the larynx and the respiratory system, food and liquid are directed into the tube leading to the stomach, the esophagus. Because food or liquid in the bronchial tubes or lungs could cause a blockage or lead to an infection, the airway must be protected. The epiglottis is a leaf-like piece of cartilage extending upwards from the larynx. The epiglottis can close down over the larynx when someone is eating or drinking, preventing these substances from entering the airway.

In laryngitis, the tissues below the level of the epiglottis are swollen and inflamed. This causes swelling around the area of the vocal cords, so that they cannot vibrate normally. A hoarse sound to the voice is very characteristic of laryngitis. Laryngitis is a very common problem, and often occurs during the course of an upper respiratory tract infection (cold).

Causes & symptoms

Laryngitis is caused almost 100% of the time by a virus. The same viruses which cause the majority of simple upper respiratory infections (colds, etc.) are responsible for laryngitis. These include parainfluenzae vi-

KEY TERMS

Epiglottis—A leaf-like piece of cartilage extending upwards from the larynx, which can close like a lid over the trachea to prevent the airway from receiving any food or liquid being swallowed.

Larynx—The part of the airway lying between the pharynx and the trachea.

Nasopharynx—The part of the airway into which the nose leads.

Oropharynx—The part of the airway into which the mouth leads.

Trachea—The part of the airway which leads into the bronchial tubes.

rus, **influenza** virus, respiratory syncytial virus, rhinovirus, coronavirus, and echovirus. Extremely rarely, bacteria such as Group A streptococcus, M. catarrhalis, or that which causes **tuberculosis** may cause laryngitis. In people with faulty immune systems (particular due to acquired immunodeficiency syndrome, or **AIDS**), infections with fungi may be responsible for laryngitis.

Symptoms usually begin along with, or following, symptoms of a cold. A sore, scratchy throat, **fever,** runny nose, achiness, and fatigue may all occur. Difficulty swallowing sometimes occurs with **streptococcal infections.** The patient may **cough** and wheeze. Most characteristically, the patient's voice will sound strained, hoarse, and raspy.

In extremely rare cases, the swelling of the larynx may cause symptoms of airway obstruction. This is more common in infants, because the diameter of their airways is so small. In that case, the baby may have a greatly

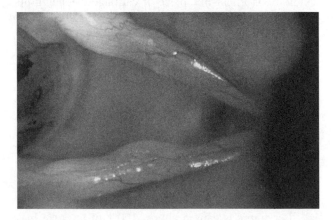

An endoscopic view of a patient's vocal cords with laryngitis. (*Custom Medical Stock Photo. Reproduced by permission.*)

increased respiratory rate, and exhibit loud high-pitched sounds with breathing (called **stridor**).

Diagnosis

Diagnosis is usually made by learning the history of a cold followed by hoarseness. The throat usually appears red and somewhat swollen. Listening to the chest and back with a stethoscope may reveal some harsh **wheezing** sounds with inspiration (breathing in).

In long-standing (chronic laryngitis), tuberculosis may be suspected. Using a scope called a laryngoscope, examination of the airway will show redness, swelling, small bumps of tissue called nodules, and irritated pits in the tissue called ulcerations. Special skin testing (TB testing) will reveal that the individual has been exposed to the bacteria causing TB.

Treatment

Treatment of a simple, viral laryngitis simply addresses the symptoms. Gargling with warm salt water, **pain** relievers such as **acetaminophen,** the use of vaporizers to create moist air, and rest will help the illness resolve within a week.

In an infant who is clearly struggling for air, it may be necessary to put in an artificial airway for a short period of time. This is very rarely needed.

An individual with tubercular laryngitis is treated with a combination of medications used to treat classic TB. In people with fungal laryngitis, a variety of antifungal medications are available.

Alternative treatment

Alternative treatments include **aromatherapy** inhalations made with benzoin, lavender, frankincense, thyme, and sandalwood. Decoctions (extracts made by boiling an herb in water) or infusions (extracts made by steeping an herb in boiling water) can be made with red sage (*Salvia officinalis* var. *rubra*) and yarrow (*Achillea millefolium*) or with licorice (*Glycyrrhiza glabra*). These are used for gargling, and are said to reduce pain. Echinacea (*Echinacea* spp.) tincture taken in water every hour for 48 hours is recommended to boost the immune system. Antiviral herbs, including usnea (*Usnea* spp.), lomatium (*Lomatium dissectum*), and ligusticum (*Ligusticum porteri*), may help hasten recovery from laryngitis. Homeopathic remedies are recommended based on the patient's symptoms. Some people may get relief from placing cold compresses on the throat.

Prognosis

Prognosis for laryngitis is excellent. Recovery is complete, and usually occurs within a week's time.

Prevention

Prevention of laryngitis is the same as for any upper respiratory infections. The only way to even attempt to prevent such illnesses is by good handwashing, and by avoiding situations where one might come in contact with people who might be sick. However, even with relatively good hygiene practices, most people will get about five to six colds per year. It is unpredictable which of these may lead to laryngitis.

Resources

BOOKS

Durand, Marlene, et al. "Laryngitis, Croup, and Epiglottitis." In *Harrison's Principles of Internal Medicine,* edited by Anthony S. Fauci, et al. New York: McGraw-Hill, 1998.

Orenstein, David. "Acute Inflammatory Upper Airway Obstruction." In *Nelson Textbook of Pediatrics,* edited by Richard Behrman. Philadelphia: W.B. Saunders Co., 1996.

Ray, C. George, and Kenneth J. Ryan. "Middle and Lower Respiratory Tract Infections." In *Sherris Medical Microbiology: An Introduction to Infectious Diseases,* edited by Kenneth J. Ryan. Norwalk, CT: Appleton and Lange, 1994.

Stoffman, Phyllis. *The Family Guide to Preventing and Treating 100 Infectious Diseases.* New York: John Wiley and Sons, Inc., 1995.

ORGANIZATIONS

American Academy of Otolaryngology-Head and Neck Surgery, Inc. One Prince Street, Alexandria VA 22314-3357. (703) 836-4444.

Rosalyn S. Carson-DeWitt

Laryngoscopy

Definition

Laryngoscopy refers to a procedure used to view the inside of the larynx (the voice box).

Description

The purpose and advantage of seeing inside the larynx is to detect tumors, foreign bodies, nerve or structural injury, or other abnormalities. Two methods allow the larynx to be seen directly during the examination. In one, a flexible tube with a fiber-optic device is threaded through the nasal passage and down into the throat. The other method uses a rigid viewing tube passed directly from the mouth, through the throat, into the larynx. A

KEY TERMS

Endoscopic tube—a tube that is inserted into a hollow organ permitting a physician to see the inside it.

---

light and lens affixed to the endoscope are used in both methods. The endoscopic tube may also be equipped to suction debris or remove material for biopsy. **Bronchoscopy** is a similar, but more extensive procedure in which the tube is continued through the larynx, down into the trachea and bronchi.

Preparation

Laryngoscopy is done in the hospital with a local anesthetic spray to minimize discomfort and suppress the gag reflex. Patients are requested not to eat for several hours before the examination.

Aftercare

If the throat is sore, soothing liquids or lozenges will probably relieve any temporary discomfort.

Risks

This procedure carries no serious risks, although the patient may experience soreness of the throat or **cough** up small amounts of blood until the irritation subsides.

Normal results

A normal result would be the absence of signs of disease or damage.

Abnormal results

An abnormal finding, such as a tumor or an object lodged in the tissue, would either be removed or described for further medical attention.

Jill S. Lasker

Larynx removal *see* **Laryngectomy**

Laser-assisted in-situ keratomileusis *see* **Photorefractive keratectomy and laser-assisted in-situ keratomileusis**

Laser surgery

Definition

Laser (light amplification by stimulated emission of radiation) surgery uses an intensely hot, precisely focused beam of light to remove or vaporize tissue and control bleeding in a wide variety of non-invasive and minimally invasive procedures.

Purpose

Laser surgery is used to:

- Cut or destroy tissue that is abnormal or diseased without harming healthy, normal tissue

- Shrink or destroy tumors and lesions

- Cauterize (seal) blood vessels to prevent excessive bleeding.

Precautions

Anyone who is thinking about having laser surgery should ask his doctor to:

- Explain why laser surgery is likely to be more beneficial than traditional surgery

- Describe his experience in performing the laser procedure the patient is considering.

Because some lasers can temporarily or permanently discolor the skin of Blacks, Asians, and Hispanics, a dark-skinned patient should make sure that his surgeon has successfully performed laser procedures on people of color.

Some types of laser surgery should not be performed on pregnant women or on patients with severe cardiopulmonary disease or other serious health problems.

Description

The first working laser was introduced in 1960. The device was initially used to treat diseases and disorders of the eye, whose transparent tissues gave ophthalmic surgeons a clear view of how the narrow, concentrated beam was being directed. Dermatologic surgeons also helped pioneer laser surgery, and developed and improved upon many early techniques and more refined surgical procedures.

Types of lasers

The three types of lasers most often used in medical treatment are the:

- Carbon dioxide (CO_2) laser. Primarily a surgical tool, this device converts light energy to heat strong enough to minimize bleeding while it cuts through or vaporizes tissue.

- Neodymium:yttrium-aluminum-garnet (Nd:YAG) laser. Capable of penetrating tissue more deeply than other lasers, the Nd:YAG makes blood clot quickly and can enable surgeons to see and work on parts of the body that could otherwise be reached only through open (invasive) surgery.

- Argon laser. This laser provides the limited penetration needed for eye surgery and superficial skin disorders. In a special procedure known as photodynamic therapy (PDT), this laser uses light-sensitive dyes to shrink or dissolve tumors.

Laser applications

Sometimes described as ''scalpels of light,'' lasers are used alone or with conventional surgical instruments in a diverse array of procedures that:

- Improve appearance

- Relieve **pain**

- Restore function

- Save lives.

Laser surgery is often standard operating procedure for specialists in:

- Cardiology

- Dentistry

- Dermatology

- Gastroenterology (treatment of disorders of the stomach and intestines)

- Gynecology

- Neurosurgery

- Oncology (**cancer** treatment)

- Ophthalmology (treatment of disorders of the eye)

- Orthopedics (treatment of disorders of bones, joints, muscles, ligaments, and tendons)

- Otolaryngology (treatment of disorders of the ears, nose, and throat)

- Pulmonary care (treatment of disorders of the respiratory system

- Urology (treatment of disorders of the urinary tract and of the male reproductive system).

Routine uses of lasers include erasing **birthmarks,** skin discoloration, and skin changes due to aging, and removing benign, precancerous, or cancerous tissues or tumors. Lasers are used to stop snoring, remove tonsils, remove or transplant hair, and relieve pain and restore

KEY TERMS

Argon—A colorless, odorless gas.

Astigmatism—A condition in which one or both eyes cannot filter light properly and images appear blurred and indistinct.

Canker sore—A blister-like sore on the inside of the mouth that can be painful but is not serious.

Carbon dioxide—A heavy, colorless gas that dissolves in water.

Cardiopulmonary resuscitation—An emergency procedure used to restore circulation and prevent brain death to a person who has collapsed, is unconscious, is not breathing, and has no pulse.

Cauterize—To use heat or chemicals to stop bleeding, prevent the spread of infection, or destroy tissue.

Cornea—The outer, transparent lens that covers the pupil of the eye and admits light.

Endometriosis—An often painful gynecologic condition in which endometrial tissue migrates from the inside of the uterus to other organs inside and beyond the abdominal cavity.

Glaucoma—A disease of the eye in which increased pressure within the eyeball can cause gradual loss of vision.

Invasive surgery—A form of surgery that involves making an incision in the patient's body and inserting instruments or other medical devices into it.

Nearsightedness—A condition in which one or both eyes cannot focus normally, causing objects at a distance to appear blurred and indistinct. Also called myopia.

Ovarian cyst—A benign or malignant growth on an ovary. An ovarian cyst can disappear without treatment or become extremely painful and have to be surgically removed.

Vaporize—To dissolve solid material or convert it into smoke or gas.

Varicose veins—Swollen, twisted veins, usually occurring in the legs, that occur more often in women than in men.

function in patients who are too weak to undergo major surgery. Lasers are also used to treat:

- **Angina** (chest pain)

- Cancerous or non-cancerous tumors that cannot be removed or destroyed

- Cold and **canker sores,** gum disease, and tooth sensitivity or decay

- **Ectopic pregnancy** (development of a fertilized egg outside the uterus)

- **Endometriosis**

- Fibroid tumors

- Gallstones

- **Glaucoma,** mild-to-moderate nearsightedness and **astigmatism,** and other conditions that impair sight

- **Migraine headaches**

- Non-cancerous enlargement of the prostate gland

- **Nosebleeds**

- **Ovarian cysts**

- Ulcers

- **Varicose veins**

- Warts

- And numerous other conditions, diseases, and disorders.

Advantages of laser surgery

Often referred to as "bloodless surgery," laser procedures usually involve less bleeding than conventional surgery. The heat generated by the laser keeps the surgical site free of germs and reduces the risk of infection. Because a smaller incision is required, laser procedures often take less time (and cost less money) than traditional surgery. Sealing off blood vessels and nerves reduces bleeding, swelling, scarring, pain, and the length of the recovery period.

Disadvantages of laser surgery

Although many laser surgeries can be performed in a doctor's office rather than in a hospital, the person guiding the laser must be at least as thoroughly trained and highly skilled as someone performing the same procedure in a hospital setting. The American Society for Laser Medicine and Surgery, Inc. urges that:

- All operative areas be equipped with oxygen and other drugs and equipment required for **cardiopulmonary resuscitation (CPR)**

- Non-physicians performing laser procedures be properly trained, licensed, and insured

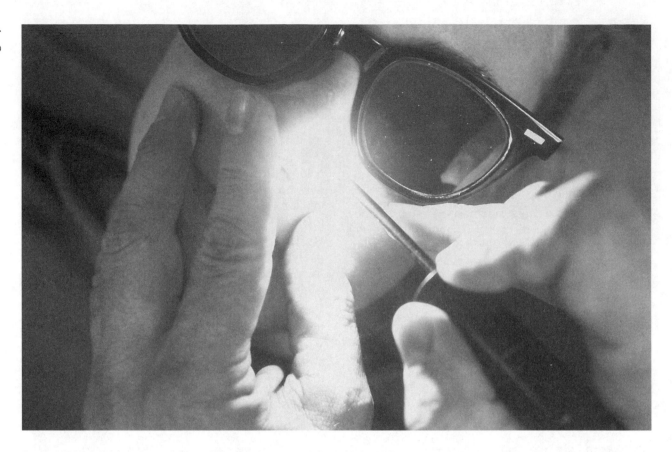

Cosmetic laser surgery in progress. The wavelengths of the laser's light can be matched to a specific target, enabling the physician to destroy the capillaries near the skin's surface without damaging the surrounding tissue. *(Photograph by Will & Deni McIntyre, Photo Researchers, Inc. Reproduced by permission.)*

• A qualified and experienced supervising physician be able to respond to and manage unanticipated events or other emergencies within five minutes of the time they occur

• Emergency transportation to a hospital or other acute-care facility be available whenever laser surgery is performed in a non-hospital setting.

Imprecisely aimed lasers can burn or destroy healthy tissue.

Preparation

Because laser surgery is used to treat so many dissimilar conditions, the patient should ask his physician for detailed instructions about how to prepare for a specific procedure. Diet, activities, and medications may not have to be limited prior to surgery, but some procedures require a **physical examination** and a medical history that:

• Determines the patient's general health and current medical status

• Describes how the patient has responded to other illnesses, hospital stays, and diagnostic or therapeutic procedures

• Clarifies what the patient expects the outcome of the procedure to be.

Aftercare

Most laser surgeries can be performed on an outpatient basis, and patients are usually permitted to leave the hospital or medical office when their vital signs have stabilized. A patient who has been sedated should not be discharged:

• Until he has recovered from the anesthesia and knows who and where he is

• Unless he is accompanied by a responsible adult.

The doctor may prescribe analgesic (pain-relieving) medication, and should provide easy-to-understand written instructions that describe how the patient's recovery should progress and what to do in case complications or emergency arise.

Risks

Like traditional surgery, laser surgery can be complicated by:

• Hemorrhage

• Infection

• Perforation (piercing) of an organ or tissue.

Laser surgery can also involve risks that are not associated with traditional surgical procedures. Being careless or not practicing safe surgical techniques can severely burn the patient's lungs or even cause them to explode. Patients must wear protective eye shields while undergoing laser surgery on any part of the face near the eyes or eyelids, and the United States Food and Drug Administration (FDA) has said that both doctors and patients must use special protective eyewear whenever a CO_2 laser is used.

Laser beams can burn or destroy healthy tissue, cause injuries that are painful and sometimes permanent, and actually compound problems they are supposed to solve. Errors or inaccuracies in laser surgery can worsen a patient's vision, for example, and lasers can scar and even change the skin color of some patients.

Normal results

The nature and severity of the problem, the skill of the surgeon performing the procedure, and the patient's general health and realistic expectations are among the factors that influence the outcome of laser surgery. Successful procedures can enable patients to:

• Feel better

• Look younger

• Enjoy longer, fuller, more active lives.

A patient who is considering any kind of laser surgery should ask his doctor to provide detailed information about what the outcome of the surgery is expected to be, what the recovery process will involve, and how long it will probably be before he regains a normal appearance and can resume his normal activities.

Abnormal results

A person who is considering any type of laser surgery should ask his doctor to provide specific and detailed information about what could go wrong during the procedure and what the negative impact on the patient's health or appearance might be.

Lighter or darker skin may appear, for example, when a laser is used to remove sun damage or age spots from an olive-skinned or dark-skinned individual. This abnormal pigmentation may or may not disappear in time.

Scarring or rupturing of the cornea is uncommon, but laser surgery on one or both eyes can:

• Increase sensitivity to light or glare

• Reduce night vision

• Permanently cloud vision, or cause sharpness of vision to decline throughout the day.

Signs of infection following laser surgery include:

• Burning

• Crusting of the skin

• **Itching**

• Pain

• Scarring

• Severe redness

• Swelling.

Resources

BOOKS

Carlson, Karen J., et al. *The Harvard Guide to Women's Health.* Cambridge, Massachusetts: Harvard University Press, 1996.

PERIODICALS

"Laser Procedures for Nearsightedness." *FDA Consumer* (January-February 1996): 2.

"Laser Resurfacing Slows the Hands of Time." *Harvard Health Letter* (August 1996): 4-5.

"Lasers." *Mayo Clinic Health Letter* (July 1994): 1-3.

"Lasers: Bright Lights of the Medical World." *Cosmopolitan* (May 1995): 262-265.

"Lasers for Skin Surgery." *Harvard Women's Health Watch* (March 1997): 2-3.

"Lasers — Hope or Hype?" *American Health* (June 1994): 68-72, 103.

"The Light Fantastic." *Helix* (Winter 1989): 3-9.

"New Cancer Therapies That Ease Pain, Extend Life." *Cancer Smart* (June 1997): 8-10.

"New Laser Surgery for Angina." *HealthNews* (May 6, 1997): 3-4.

"Saving Face." *Essence* (August 1997): 24, 26, 28.

"Under the Gun." *Mirabella* (January/February 1996): 108-110.

"What a Laser Can and Cannot Do." *San Jose Mercury News* (February 1994): 22, 24.

ORGANIZATIONS

American Society for Dermatologic Surgery. 930 North Meacham Road, Schaumburg, IL 60173-6016. (847) 330-9830. http://www.asds-net.org.

American Society for Laser Medicine and Surgery, Inc. 2404 Stewart Square, Wausau, WI 54401 (715) 845-9283 http://www.as/ms.org/index.html.

Cancer Information Service. (800) 422-6237.

National Cancer Institute. http://www.rex.nci.nih.gov.

OTHER

ASLMS Guidelines for Office-Based Laser Procedures. http://www.as/ms.org/offbased.html (19 March 1998).

Facts About Laser Surgery. http://www.glaucoma.org/fs-laser-sur.html (12 March 1998).

Refractive Eye Surgery. http://www.mayohealth.org/mayo/9707/htm/refract.htm (15 March 1998).

What is Laser? http://www.asds_.net.org/laser.html (19 March 1998).

Maureen Haggerty

LASIK *see* **Photorefractive keratectomy and laser-assisted in-situ keratomileusis**

Lassa fever *see* **Hemorrhagic fevers**

Laxatives

Definition

Laxatives are products that promote bowel movements.

Purpose

Laxatives are used to treat **constipation** — the passage of small amounts of hard, dry stools, usually fewer than three times a week. People who are constipated may find it difficult and even painful to have bowel movements. They may also feel bloated, sluggish, and generally uncomfortable and may have other symptoms such as a dull **headache** and **low back pain.** But these symptoms do not always mean that laxatives are necessary. A great deal of misunderstanding exists about their use. Many people believe that they are constipated and should take a laxative if they do not have a bowel movement every day or if their stools are sometimes hard. However, a wide range in normal bowel habits exists, depending on the individual and his or her diet. Some people have bowel movements as often as three times a day, some only three times a week. Anything within this range is considered normal. In addition, some people's stools are naturally firmer than others.

Occasional constipation can often be treated without laxatives. Increasing the amount of fiber in the diet, drinking enough water and other liquids, such as fruit and vegetable juices, exercising regularly, and setting aside time every day to have a bowel movement are the first steps. These measures will also help prevent constipation from occurring again. If these methods do not relieve the problem, a physician may suggest using a laxative for a

---

> **KEY TERMS**
>
> **Aspartame**—A low-calorie, artificial sweetener.
>
> **Carbohydrates**—Compounds, such as cellulose, sugar, and starch, that contain only carbon, hydrogen, and oxygen, and are a major part of the diets of people and other animals.
>
> **Colon**—The large intestine.
>
> **Fiber**—Carbohydrate material in food that cannot be digested.
>
> **Phenylketonuria**—(PKU) A genetic disorder in which the body lacks an important enzyme. If untreated, the disorder can lead to brain damage and mental retardation.
>
> **Stool**—The solid waste that is left after food is digested. Stool forms in the intestines and passes out of the body through the anus.

limited time. A physician should always be the one to decide when a laxative is needed and which type of laxative should be used.

Description

Laxatives come in various forms — liquids, tablets, suppositories, powders, granules, capsules, chewing gum, chocolate-flavored wafers, and caramels. The basic types of laxatives are bulk-forming laxatives, lubricant laxatives, stool softeners (also called emollient laxatives), and stimulant laxatives.

Bulk-forming laxatives

Bulk-forming laxatives contain materials, such as cellulose and psyllium, that pass through the digestive tract without being digested. In the intestines, these materials absorb liquid and swell, making the stool soft, bulky, and easier to pass. The bulky stool then stimulates the bowel to move. Laxatives in this group include such brands as FiberCon, Fiberall, and Metamucil.

Lubricant laxatives

Mineral oil is the mostly widely used lubricant laxative. Taken by mouth, the oil coats the stool. This keeps the stool moist and soft and makes it easier to pass. Lubricant laxatives are often used for patients who need to avoid straining — after abdominal surgery, for example.

Stool softeners (emollient laxatives)

As their name suggests, stool softeners make stools softer and easier to pass by increasing their moisture content. This type of laxative does not really stimulate bowel movements, but it makes it possible to have bowel movements without straining. Stool softeners are best used to prevent constipation in people who need to avoid straining — because of recent surgery, for example. However, they are not very effective at treating existing constipation. Docusate (Colace, Sof-Lax) is an example of a stool softener.

Stimulant laxatives

Ingredients in these laxatives stimulate muscles and nerves in the intestines. This helps move the stool along. Although these laxatives are popular and effective, they should be used with care, as they are more likely than other types to cause side effects. They may also work more quickly and powerfully than other laxatives. Examples of stimulant laxatives are bisacodyl (Correctol) and senna (Senokot).

Precautions

Laxatives are among the most widely misused over-the-counter medicines. The overuse of laxatives can lead the body to depend on them. When used regularly over a long time, laxatives can damage nerve cells in the colon, and the colon can lose its natural ability to contract. This makes constipation worse. Overuse of certain laxatives can weaken the bones and cause other serious problems. Because of these possible problems, do not use laxatives unless told to do so by a physician. If a physician has recommended a laxative, use it only as directed. Do not take it more often or for a longer period than recommended.

Occasional, temporary constipation usually results from an improper diet, too little **exercise,** changes in daily routines, or the use of certain medicines, such as pain relievers, **antidepressant drugs, diuretics** (water pills), and some **antacids.** However, constipation can also be caused by a number of diseases. See a physician for any of the following symptoms:

• Persistent constipation in a person who has always had regular bowel movements

• Constipation that does not get better with the proper use of laxatives

• Rectal bleeding or blood in the stool

• Pain when having a bowel movement

• Loss of appetite or unexplained weight loss

• Bloating that continues or gets worse

• Nausea

• Vomiting

• Continuing abdominal pain or cramps

• Sores or irritation in the anal area.

Do not use stool softeners, such as docusate (Colace) and lubricant laxatives, such as mineral oil, at the same time. This may cause unwanted side effects, such as watery **diarrhea.**

People whose gag reflexes do not work properly (such as people who have had **strokes**) should not use mineral oil laxatives. They may inhale small amounts of mineral oil, which could lead to inflammation of the lungs and possible **pneumonia.**

Some types of laxatives contain large amounts of sugar. People who have diabetes or who must limit their intake of sugar or other carbohydrates should read package labels carefully or check with a pharmacist before using laxatives.

People with **phenylketonuria** should be aware that sugar-free laxatives may contain aspartame.

When using a stimulant laxative, such as bisacodyl (Correctol), take the smallest recommended amount. Do not use this type of laxative on a daily basis.

Some stimulant laxatives can turn stools or urine pinkish or red. This is a harmless, temporary effect that should go away when the person stops taking the medicine.

Bulk-forming laxatives must be taken with at least 8 oz. of water or other liquid. If the laxative is taken without enough fluid, it may form a mass that can block the throat, esophagus, or bowel.

Anyone who develops a skin rash while taking a laxative should stop taking it immediately and call a physician.

Older people

Older people are especially likely to have constipation. People in this age group should be careful not to overuse laxatives and should instead manage their constipation with proper diet and exercise when possible. When laxatives are necessary, the bulk-forming types (such as FiberCon and Metamucil) are best for older people. Stimulants and lubricants should be avoided.

Children

Bowel habits vary in children, as they do in adults. In general, children should not be given laxatives unless a physician has directed it.

Special conditions

People with certain medical conditions or who are taking certain other medicines can have problems if they take laxatives. Before using a laxative, be sure to let the physician know about any of these conditions:

ALLERGIES

People who are sensitive to psyllium or who have respiratory disorders may have severe reactions if they inhale dry particles of psyllium (found in some bulk-forming laxatives, such as Metamucil). The risk of this problem can be reduced by using a spoon to add the powder to liquid in a glass, rather than pouring the powder directly from the container. Anyone who has had unusual reactions to laxatives in the past should let his or her physician know before taking the drugs again. The physician should also be told about any **allergies** to foods, dyes, preservatives, or other substances.

PREGNANCY

Bulk-forming laxatives (such as Metamucil and FiberCon) and stool softeners (such as Colace) are the only kinds recommended for pregnant women. Stimulants and lubricants should be avoided.

BREASTFEEDING

Some kinds of laxatives may pass into breast milk. Women who are breastfeeding should check with their physicians before using laxatives.

OTHER MEDICAL CONDITIONS

Before using laxatives, people with any of these medical problems should make sure their physicians are aware of their conditions:

- Kidney disease
- Past or present disease affecting the gastrointestinal tract
- Past surgery on the gastrointestinal tract
- **Hypercalcemia** (abnormally high amount of calcium in the blood)
- Throat problems
- Swallowing problems
- Partial bowel obstruction.

USE OF CERTAIN MEDICINES

Taking laxatives with certain other drugs may affect the way the drugs work or may increase the chance of side effects.

Recommended dosage

Recommended dosage depends on the type of laxative. Always take laxatives exactly as the physician directs. If using non-prescription (over-the-counter) types, follow the directions on the package label. Never take larger or more frequent doses, and do not take the drug for longer than directed.

Side effects

Serious side effects are not common, but may occur. If any of the following side effects occur, check with the physician who prescribed the medicine as soon as possible:

For bulk-forming laxatives

- Breathing problems
- Swallowing problems
- Skin rash or **itching**
- Intestinal blockage.

For stool softeners (emollient laxatives)

- Skin rash.

For stimulant laxatives

- Confusion
- Unusual tiredness or weakness
- Skin rash
- Irregular heartbeat
- Muscle cramps.

Less common side effects, such as cramping, diarrhea, nausea, belching, throat irritation, or skin irritation around the rectal area also may occur and do not need medical attention unless they do not go away or they interfere with normal activities.

Other rare side effects are possible. Anyone who has unusual symptoms after taking laxatives should get in touch with his or her physician.

Interactions

Some laxatives may make it more difficult for the body to absorb other medicines taken by mouth. For example, bulk-forming laxatives may interfere with the absorption of **aspirin,** the blood-thinning **anticoagulant drug** warfarin (Coumadin), **digitalis drugs,** and other drugs. Other types of laxatives, such as docusate (Colace), increase the absorption of other drugs taken by mouth. Anyone who is taking any other medicines should check with a physician or pharmacist before using a laxative.

The stimulant laxative bisacodyl (Correctol) should not be taken with drugs that reduce stomach acid, such as cimetidine (Tagamet), ranitidine (Zantac), and omeprazole (Prilosec). This drug also should not be taken within 1 hour of drinking milk.

Resources

PERIODICALS

"Constipation, Laxatives and Dietary Fiber." *HealthTips* (April 1993): 9.

"Overuse Hazardous: Laxatives Rarely Needed." (Includes related article on types of laxatives.) *FDA Consumer* (April 1991): 33.

ORGANIZATIONS

National Digestive Diseases Information Clearinghouse. 2 Information Way, Bethesda, MD 20892-3570. nddic@aerie.com. http://www.niddk.nih.gov/Brochures/NDDIC.htm.

Nancy Ross-Flanigan

Lazy eye *see* **Amblyopia**

LCM *see* **Lymphocytic choriomeningitis**

LDH isoenzymes test *see* **Lactate dehydrogenase isoenzymes test**

LDH test *see* **Lactate dehydrogenase test**

Lead poisoning

Definition

Lead poisoning occurs when a person swallows or inhales lead in any form. The result can be damage to the brain, nerves, and many other parts of the body. Acute lead poisoning, which is relatively rare, occurs when a large amount of lead is taken into the body over a short period of time. Chronic lead poisoning, which is a common problem in children, occurs when small amounts of lead are taken in over a longer period.

Description

Lead can damage almost every system in the human body, and it can also cause high blood pressure (**hypertension**). It is particularly harmful to the developing brain of fetuses and young children. The higher the level of lead in a child's blood, and the longer this elevated level lasts, the greater the chance of ill effects. Over the long term, lead poisoning in a child can lead to learning disabilities, behavior problems, and even **mental retardation.** At very high levels, lead poisoning can cause seizures, **coma,** and even **death.**

About one out of every six children in the United States has a high level of lead in the blood, according to

---

> ## KEY TERMS
>
> **Chelation therapy**—Treatment with chemicals that bind to a poisonous metal and help the body pass it in urine at a faster rate.
>
> **Dimercaprol (BAL)**—A chemical agent used to remove excess lead from the body.
>
> **Edetate calcium disodium (EDTA calcium)**—A chemical agent used to remove excess lead from the body.
>
> **Penicillamine (Cuprimine, Depen)**—A drug used to treat medical problems (such as excess copper in the body and rheumatoid arthritis) and to prevent kidney stones. It is also sometimes prescribed to remove excess lead from the body.
>
> **Succimer (Chemet)**—A drug used to remove excess lead from the body.

the Agency for Toxic Substances and Disease Registry. Many of these children are exposed to lead through peeling paint in older homes. Others are exposed through dust or soil that has been contaminated by old paint or past emissions of leaded gasoline. Since children between the ages of 12-36 months are apt to put things in their mouths, they are more likely than older children to take in lead. Pregnant women who come into contact with lead can pass it along to the fetus.

Over 80% of American homes built before 1978 have lead-based paint in them, according to the Centers for Disease Control and Prevention (CDC). The older the home, the more likely it is to contain lead paint, and the higher the concentration of lead in the paint is apt to be. Some homes also have lead in the water pipes or plumbing. People may have lead in the paint, dust, or soil around their homes or in their drinking water without knowing it, since lead can't be seen, smelled, or tasted. Because lead doesn't break down naturally, it can continue to cause problems until it is removed.

Causes & symptoms

Before scientists knew how harmful it could be, lead was widely used in paint, gasoline, water pipes, and many other products. Today house paint is almost lead-free, gasoline is unleaded, and household plumbing is no longer made with lead materials. Still, remnants of the old hazards remain. Following are some sources of lead exposure:

- Lead-based paint. This is the most common source of exposure to large amounts of lead among preschoolers. Children may eat paint chips from older homes that

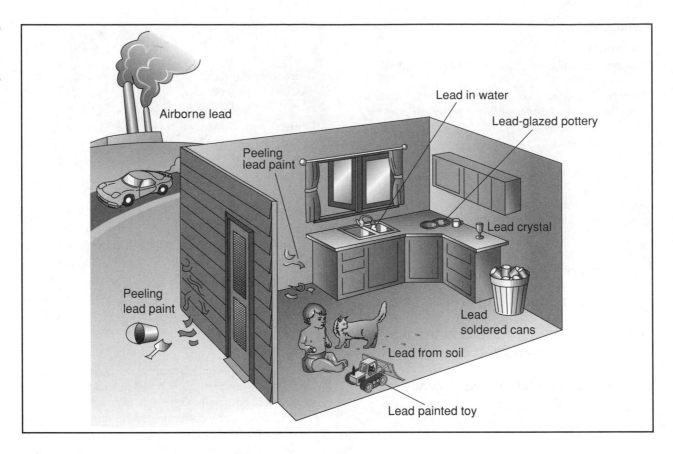

Continuous exposure to lead can damage nearly every system in the human body and is particularly harmful to the developing brain of fetuses and young children. Common sources of lead exposure include lead-based paint; dust and soil; drinking water; food from cans; and eating utensils, such as plates and drinking glasses, that are lead-based. *(Illustration by Electronic Illustrators Group.)*

have fallen into disrepair. They may also chew on painted surfaces such as windowsills. In addition, paint may be disturbed during remodeling.

- Dust and soil. These can be contaminated with lead from old paint or past emissions of leaded gasoline. In addition, pollution from operating or abandoned industrial sites and smelters can find its way into the soil, resulting in soil contamination.

- Drinking water. Exposure may come from lead water pipes, found in many homes built before 1930. Even newer copper pipes may have lead solder. Also, some new homes have brass faucets and fittings that can leach lead.

- Jobs and hobbies. A number of activities can expose participants to lead. These include making pottery or stained glass, refinishing furniture, doing home repairs, and using indoor firing ranges. When adults take part in such activities, they may inadvertently expose children

to lead residue that is on their clothing or on scrap materials.

- Food. Imported food cans often have lead solder. Also, lead is found in leaded crystal glassware and some imported or old ceramic dishes. In addition, food may be contaminated by lead in the water or soil.

- Folk medicines. Certain folk medicines (for example, alarcon, alkohl, azarcon, bali goli, coral, ghasard, greta, liga, pay-loo-ah, and rueda) and traditional cosmetics (kohl, for example) contain large amounts of lead.

Chronic lead poisoning

New evidence suggests that lead may be harmful to children even at low levels that were once thought to be safe, and the risk of damage rises as blood levels of lead increase. The symptoms of chronic lead poisoning take time to develop, however. Children can appear healthy despite having high levels of lead in their blood. Over time, though, problems such as the following may arise:

- Learning disabilities
- Hyperactivity
- Mental retardation
- Slowed growth
- **Hearing loss**
- **Headaches.**

Lead poisoning is also harmful to adults, in whom it can cause high blood pressure, digestive problems, nerve disorders, memory loss, and muscle and joint pain. In addition, it can lead to difficulties during **pregnancy,** as well as cause reproductive problems in both men and women.

Acute lead poisoning

Acute lead poisoning, while less common, shows up more quickly and can be fatal. Symptoms such as the following may occur:

- Severe abdominal pain
- **Diarrhea**
- **Nausea and vomiting**
- Weakness of the limbs
- Seizures
- Coma.

Diagnosis

A high level of lead in the blood can be detected with a simple blood test. In fact, testing is the only way to know for sure if children without symptoms have been exposed to lead, since they can appear healthy even as long-term damage occurs. The CDC recommends testing all children at 12 months of age and, if possible, again at 24 months. Testing should start at six months for children at risk for lead poisoning. Based on these test results and a child's risk factors, the doctor will then decide whether further testing is needed and how often. In some states, more frequent testing is required by law.

Children at risk

Children with an increased risk of lead poisoning include those who:

- Live in or regularly visit a house built before 1978 in which chipped or peeling paint is present.
- Live in or regularly visit a house that was built before 1978 where remodeling is planned or underway.
- Have a brother or sister, housemate, or playmate who has been diagnosed with lead poisoning.

- Live with an adult whose job or hobby involves exposure to lead.
- Live near an active lead smelter, battery-recycling plant, or other industry that can create lead pollution.

Adults at risk

Testing is also important for adults whose job or hobby puts them at risk for lead poisoning. This includes people who take part in the following activities:

- Glazed pottery or stained glass making
- Furniture refinishing
- Home renovation
- Target shooting at indoor firing ranges
- Battery reclamation
- Precious metal refining
- Radiator repair
- Art restoration.

Treatment

The first step in treating lead poisoning is to avoid further contact with lead. For adults, this usually means making changes at work or in hobbies. For children, it means finding and removing sources of lead in the home. In most states, the public health department can help assess the home and identify lead sources.

If the problem is lead paint, a professional with special training should remove it. This is not a do-it-yourself project. Scraping or sanding lead paint creates large amounts of dust that can poison people in the home. This dust can stay around long after the work is completed. In addition, heating lead paint can release lead into the air. For these reasons, lead paint should only be removed by someone who knows how to do the job safely and has the equipment to clean up thoroughly. Occupants, especially children and pregnant women, should leave the home until the cleanup is finished.

Chelation therapy

If blood levels of lead are high enough, the doctor may also prescribe **chelation therapy.** This refers to treatment with chemicals that bind to the lead and help the body pass it in urine at a faster rate. There are four chemical agents that may be used for this purpose, either alone or in combination. Edetate calcium disodium (EDTA calcium) and dimercaprol (BAL) are given through an intravenous line or in shots, while succimer (Chemet) and penicillamine (Cuprimine, Depen) are taken by mouth. (Although many doctors prescribe penicillamine for lead poisoning, this use of the drug has not been approved by the Food and Drug Administration.)

Alternative treatment

Changes in diet are no substitute for medical treatment. However, getting enough calcium, zinc, and protein may help reduce the amount of lead the body absorbs. Iron is also important, since people who are deficient in this nutrient absorb more lead. Garlic and thiamine, a B-complex vitamin, have been used to treat lead poisoning in animals. However, their usefulness in humans for this purpose has not been proved. Nutritional, botanical, and **homeopathic medicines** can be administered once the source is removed, to help correct any imbalances brought on by lead toxicity.

Prognosis

If acute lead poisoning reaches the stage of seizures and coma, there is a high risk of death. Even if the person survives, there is a good chance of permanent brain damage. The long-term effects of lower levels of lead can also be permanent and severe. However, if chronic lead poisoning is caught early, these negative effects can be limited by reducing future exposure to lead and getting proper medical treatment.

Prevention

Many cases of lead poisoning can be prevented. These steps can help:

- Keep the areas where children play as clean and dust-free as possible.

- Wash pacifiers and bottles when they fall to the floor, and wash stuffed animals and toys often.

- Make sure children wash their hands before meals and at bedtime.

- Mop floors and wipe windowsills and other chewable surfaces, such as cribs, twice a week with a solution of powdered dishwasher detergent in warm water.

- Plant bushes next to an older home with painted exterior walls to keep children at a distance.

- Plant grass or another ground cover in soil that is likely to be contaminated, such as soil around a home built before 1960 or located near a major highway.

- Have household tap water tested to find out if it contains lead.

- Use only water from the cold-water tap for drinking, cooking, and making baby formula, since hot water is likely to contain higher levels of lead.

- If the cold water hasn't been used for six hours or more, run it for several seconds, until it becomes as cold as it will get, before using it for drinking or cooking. The more time water has been sitting in the pipes, the more lead it may contain.

- If you work with lead in your job or hobby, change your clothes before you go home.

- Do not store food in open cans, especially imported cans.

- Do not store or serve food in pottery meant for decorative use.

Resources

BOOKS

Centers for Disease Control and Prevention. *Screening Young Children for Lead Poisoning: Guidance for State and Local Public Health Officials.* Atlanta, GA: CDC, 1997.

Upton, Arthur C., and Eden Graber, eds. *Staying Healthy in a Risky Environment: The New York University Medical Center Family Guide.* New York: Simon & Schuster, 1993.

PERIODICALS

Centers for Disease Control and Prevention. ''Adult Blood Lead Epidemiology and Surveillance—United States, Second Quarter, 1995.'' *Morbidity and Mortality Weekly Report* 44(October 27, 1995): 801-803.

Committee on Drugs, American Academy of Pediatrics. ''Treatment Guidelines for Lead Exposure in Children.'' *Pediatrics* 96(July 1995): 155-160.

Krucoff, Carol. ''Lead Alert.'' *Child* (August 1996): 64-65, 67.

Trachtenbarg, David E. ''Getting the Lead Out.'' *Postgraduate Medicine* 99(March 1996): 201-202, 207-208, 211-214, 216, 218.

ORGANIZATIONS

National Center for Environmental Health, Centers for Disease Control and Prevention. Mail Stop F-29, 4770 Buford Highway N.E., Atlanta, GA 30341-3724. (888) 232-6789. http://www.cdc.gov/nceh/ncehhome.htm.

National Lead Information Center, National Safety Council. 1025 Connecticut Ave. N.W., Suite 1200, Washington, DC 20036. (800) LEAD-FYI (general information), (800) 424-LEAD (detailed information or questions). http://www.nsc.org/ehc/lead.htm.

Office of Water Resources Center, Environmental Protection Agency. Mail Code (4100), Room 2615 East Tower Basement, 401 M St. S.W., Washington, DC 20460. (800) 426-4791. http://www.epa.gov/ow/.

Linda Wasmer Smith

Learning disorders

Definition

Learning disorders are academic difficulties experienced by children and adults of average to above-average intelligence. People with learning disorders have difficulty with reading, writing, mathematics, or a combination of the three. These difficulties significantly interfere with academic achievement or daily living.

Description

Learning disorders, or disabilities, affect approximately 2 million children between the ages of 6-17 (5% of public school children). These children have specific impairments in acquiring, retaining, and processing information. Standardized tests place them well below their IQ range in their area of difficulty. The three main types of learning disorders are reading disorders, mathematics disorders, and disorders of written expression.

Reading disorders

Reading disorders are the most common type of learning disorder. Children with reading disorders have difficulty recognizing and interpreting letters and words (dyslexia). They aren't able to recognize and decode the sounds and syllables (phonetic structure) behind written words and language in general. This condition lowers accuracy and comprehension in reading.

Mathematics disorders

Children with mathematics disorders (dyscalculia) have problems recognizing and counting numbers correctly. They have difficulty using numbers in everyday settings. Mathematics disorders are typically diagnosed in the first few years of elementary school when formal teaching of numbers and basic math concepts begins. Children with mathematics disorders usually have a co-existing reading disorder, a disorder of written expression, or both.

Disorders of written expression

Disorders of written expression typically occur in combination with reading disorders or mathematics disorders or both. The condition is characterized by difficulty with written compositions (dysgraphia). Children with this type of learning disorder have problems with spelling, punctuation, grammar, and organizing their thoughts in writing.

Causes & symptoms

Learning disorders are thought to be caused by neurological abnormalities that trigger impairments in the

regions of the brain that control visual and language processing and attention and planning. These traits may be genetically linked. Children from families with a history of learning disorders are more likely to develop disorders themselves. Learning difficulties may also be caused by medical conditions such as a traumatic brain injury or brain infections such as **encephalitis** or **meningitis.**

The defining symptom of a learning disorder is academic performance that is markedly below a child's age and grade capabilities and measured IQ. Children with a reading disorder may confuse or transpose words or letters and omit or add syllables to words. The written homework of children with disorders of written expression is filled with grammatical, spelling, punctuation, and organizational errors. The child's handwriting is often extremely poor. Children with mathematical disorders are often unable to count in the correct sequence, to name numbers, and to understand numerical concepts.

Diagnosis

Problems with vision or hearing, mental disorders (depression, **attention-deficit/hyperactivity disorder**), **mental retardation,** cultural and language differences, and inadequate teaching may be mistaken for learning disorders or complicate a diagnosis. A comprehensive medical, psychological, and educational assessment is critical to making a clear and correct diagnosis.

A child thought to have a learning disorder should undergo a complete medical examination to rule out an organic cause. If none is found, a psychoeducational assessment should be performed by a psychologist, psychiatrist, neurologist, neuropsychologist, or learning specialist. A complete medical, family, social, and educational history is compiled from existing medical and school records and from interviews with the child and the child's parents and teachers. A series of written and verbal tests are then given to the child to evaluate his or her cognitive and intellectual functioning. Commonly used tests include the Wechsler Intelligence Scale for Children (WISC-III), the Woodcock-Johnson Psychoeducational Battery, the Peabody Individual Achievement

Test-Revised (PIAT-R) and the California Verbal Learning Test (CVLT). Federal legislation mandates that this testing is free of charge within the public school system.

Treatment

Once a learning disorder has been diagnosed, an individual education plan (IEP) is developed for the child in question. IEPs are based on psychoeducational test findings. They provide for annual retesting to measure a child's progress. Learning-disordered students may receive special instruction within a regular general education class or they may be taught in a special education or learning center for a portion of the day.

Common strategies for the treatment of reading disorders focus first on improving a child's recognition of the sounds of letters and language through phonics training. Later strategies focus on comprehension, retention, and study skills. Students with disorders of written expression are often encouraged to keep journals and to write with a computer keyboard instead of a pencil. Instruction for students with mathematical disorders emphasizes real-world uses of math, such as balancing a checkbook or comparing prices.

Prognosis

The high school dropout rate for children with learning disabilities is almost 40%. Children with learning disabilities that go undiagnosed or are improperly treated may never achieve functional literacy. They often develop serious behavior problems as a result of their frustration with school. The key to helping these students reach their fullest potential is early detection and the implementation of an appropriate individualized education plan. The prognosis is good for a large percentage of children with reading disorders that are identified and treated early. Learning disorders continue into adulthood, but with proper educational and vocational training, an individual can complete college and pursue a challenging career.

Resources

BOOKS

American Psychiatric Association. *Diagnostic and Statistical Manual of Mental Disorders*. 4th ed. Washington, DC: American Psychiatric Press, Inc., 1994.

Church, Robin P., M.E.B. Lewis, and Mark L. Batshaw. "Learning Disabilities." In *Children with Disabilities*, edited by Mark L. Batshaw. 4th ed. Baltimore: Paul H. Brookes, 1997.

Hallowell, Edward. *When You Worry About the Child You Love*. New York: Simon & Schuster, 1996.

Osman, Betty B. *Learning Disabilities and ADHD: A Family Guide to Living and Learning Together*. New York: John Wiley & Sons, 1997.

PERIODICALS

Baringa, Marcia. "Learning Defect Identified in Brain." *Science*. 273(August 1996): 867-868.

Stage, Frances K. and Nancy V. Milne. "Invisible Scholars: Students With Learning Disabilities." *Journal of Higher Education* 67(July-August 1996): 426-45.

ORGANIZATIONS

National Center for Learning Disabilities (NCLD). 381 Park Avenue South, Suite 1401, New York, NY 10016. (410) 296-0232. http://www.ncld.org/.

The Learning Disabilities Association of America (LDA). 4156 Library Road, Pittsburgh, PA 15234-1349. (412) 341-1515. http://www.ldanatl.org/.

The National Adult Literacy and Learning Disabilities Center (National ALLD Center). 1875 Connecticut Avenue, NW, Washington, DC 20009-1202. (800) 953-2553. http://www.nifl.gov/nalldtop.htm/.

OTHER

The Interactive Guide to Learning Disabilities for Parents, Teachers, and Children. http://www.ldonline.org/.

Paula Anne Ford-Martin

Leeches

Definition

Leeches are bloodsucking worms with segmented bodies. They belong to the same large classification of worms as earthworms and certain oceanic worms.

Leeches can primarily be found in freshwater lakes, ponds, or rivers. They range in size from 0.2 in (5 mm) to nearly 18 in (45 cm) and have two characteristic suckers located at either end of their bodies. Leeches consume the blood of a wide variety of animal hosts, ranging from fish to humans. To feed, a leech first attaches itself to the host using the suckers. One of these suckers surrounds the leech's mouth, which contains three sets of jaws that bite into the host's flesh, making a Y-shaped incision. As the leech begins to feed, its saliva releases chemicals that dilate blood vessels, thin the blood, and deaden the pain of the bite. Because of the saliva's effects, a person bitten by a leech may not even be aware of it until afterwards, when he or she sees the incision and the trickle of blood that is difficult to stop.

For centuries, leeches were a common tool of doctors, who believed that many diseases were the result of "imbalances" in the body that could be stabilized by releasing blood. For example, leeches were sometimes attached to veins in the temples to treat headaches. Advances in medical knowledge led doctors to abandon bloodletting and the use of leeches in the mid-nineteenth century. In recent years, however, doctors have found a new purpose for leeches—helping to restore blood circulation to grafted or severely injured tissue.

Purpose

There are many occasions in medicine, mostly in surgery and trauma care, when blood accumulates and causes trouble. Leeches can be used to reduce the swelling of any tissue that is holding too much blood. This problem is most likely to occur in two situations:

- Trauma. Large blood clots resulting from trauma can threaten tissue survival by their size and pressure. Blood clots can also obstruct the patient's airway.

- Surgical procedures involving reattachment of severed body parts or tissue reconstruction following **burns.** In these situations it is difficult for the surgeon to make a route for blood to leave the affected part and return to the circulation. The hardest part of reattaching severed extremities like fingers, toes and ears is to reconnect the tiny veins. If the veins are not reconnected, blood will accumulate in the injured area. A similar situation occurs when plastic surgeons move large flaps of skin to replace skin lost to burns, trauma or radical surgery. The

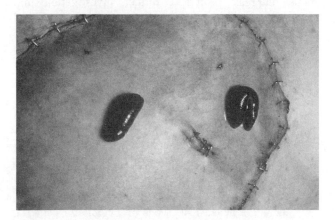

These leeches are being used to reduce venous congestion, or excessive amounts of blood in the blood vessels. *(Photograph by Michael English, M.D., Custom Medical Stock Photo. Reproduced by permission.)*

skin flaps often drain blood poorly, get congested, and begin to die. Leeches have come to the rescue in both situations.

Precautions

It is important to use only leeches that have been raised in the laboratory under sterile conditions in order to protect patients from infection. Therapeutic leeches belong to one of two species—*Hirudo michaelseni* or *Hirudo medicinalis.*

Description

One or more leeches are applied to the swollen area, depending on the size of the graft or injury, and left on for several hours. The benefits of the treatment lie not in the amount of blood that the leeches ingest, but in the anti-bloodclotting (**anticoagulant**) enzymes in the saliva that allow blood to flow from the bite for up to six hours after the animal is detached, effectively draining away blood that could otherwise accumulate and cause tissue death. Leech saliva has been described as a better anticoagulant than many currently available to treat **strokes** and **heart attacks.** Active investigation of the chemicals in leech saliva is currently under way, and one anticoagulant drug, hirudin, is derived from the tissues of *Hirudo medicinalis.*

Aftercare

The leeches are removed by pulling them off or by loosening their grip with cocaine, heat, or acid. The used leeches are then killed by placing them in an alcohol solution and disposed of as a biohazard. Proper care of the patient's sore is important, as is monitoring the rate at which it bleeds after the leech is removed. Any clots that form at the wound site during treatment should be removed to ensure effective blood flow.

Risks

Infection is a constant possibility until the sore heals. It is also necessary to monitor the amount of blood that the leeches have removed from the patient, since a drop in red blood cell counts could occur in rare cases of prolonged bleeding.

Resources

PERIODICALS

Adams, J. F., and L. F. Lassen. ''Leech Therapy for Venous Congestion Following Myocutaneous Pectoralis Flap Reconstruction.'' *ORL - Head & Neck Nursing* 13(1) (Winter 1995): 12-14.

Daane, S., et al. "Clinical Use of Leeches in Reconstructive Surgery." *American Journal of Orthopedics* 26(8) (August 1997): 528-532.

de Chalain, T., et al. "Successful Use of Leeches in the Treatment of Purpura Fulminans." *Annals of Plastic Surgery* 35(3) (September 1995): 300-306.

de Chalain, T. M. "Exploring the Use of the Medicinal Leech: A Clinical Risk-Benefit Analysis." *Source Journal of Reconstructive Microsurgery* 12(3) (April 1996): 165-172.

de Chalain, T., and G. Jones. "Replantation of the Avulsed Pinna: 100 Percent Survival with a Single Arterial Anastomosis and Substitution of Leeches for a Venous Anastomosis." *Plastic & Reconstructive Surgery* 95(7) (June 1995): 1275-1279.

Godfrey, K. "Uses of Leeches and Leech Saliva in Clinical Practice." *Nursing Times* 93(9) (Feb 26-Mar 4, 1997): 62-63.

Goessl, C., et al. "Leech Therapy for Massive Scrotal Mematoma Following Percutaneous Transluminal Angioplasty." *Journal of Urology* 158(2) (August 1997): 545.

Haycox, C. L., et al. "Indications and Complications of Medicinal Leech Therapy." *Journal of the American Academy of Dermatology* 33(6) (December 1995): 1053-1055.

Iafolla, A. K. "Medicinal Leeches in the Postoperative Care of Bladder Exstrophy." *Journal of Perinatology* 15(2) (March-April 1995): 135-138.

Lee, N. J., and N. S. Peckitt. "Treatment of a Sublingual Hematoma with Medicinal Leeches: Report of Case." *Journal of Oral & Maxillofacial Surgery* 54(1) (January 1996): 101-103.

Pantuck, A. J., et al. "Penile Replantation Using the Leech *Hirudo medicinalis*." *Urology* 48(6) (December 1996): 953-956.

Piascik, P. "Medicinal Leeches: Ancient Therapy Is a Source of Biotech Drugs." *Journal of the American Pharmaceutical Association* NS37(3) (1997): 285-286.

Smeets, I. M., and I. Engelberts. "The Use of Leeches in a Case of Post-Operative Life-Threatening Macroglossia." *Journal of Laryngology & Otology* 109(5) (May 1995): 442-444.

Van Wingerden, J. J., and J. H. Oosthuizen. "Use of the Local Leech *Hirudo michaelseni* in Reconstructive Plastic and Hand Surgery." *South African Journal of Surgery* 35(1) (February 1997): 29-31.

Wallis, R. B. "Hirudins: From Leeches to Man." *Seminars in Thrombosis & Hemostasis* 22(2) (1996): 185-196.

J. Ricker Polsdorfer

Left ventricular failure *see* **Heart failure**

Leg veins x ray *see* **Venography**

Legg-Calvé-Perthes disease *see* **Osteochondroses**

Legionella micdadei infection *see* **Legionnaires' disease**

Legionella pneumophila infection *see* **Legionnaires' disease**

Legionellosis *see* **Legionnaires' disease**

Legionnaires' disease

Definition

Legionnaires' disease is a type of **pneumonia** caused by *Legionella* bacteria. The bacterial species responsible for Legionnaires' disease is *L. pneumophila*. Major symptoms include **fever,** chills, muscle aches, and a **cough** that is initially nonproductive. Definitive diagnosis relies on specific laboratory tests for the bacteria, bacterial antigens, or antibodies produced by the body's immune system. As with other types of pneumonia, Legionnaires' disease poses the greatest threat to people who are elderly, ill, or immunocompromised.

Description

Legionella bacteria were first identified as a cause of pneumonia in 1976, following an outbreak of pneumonia among people who had attended an American Legion convention in Philadelphia, Pennsylvania. This eponymous outbreak prompted further investigation into *Legionella* and it was discovered that earlier unexplained pneumonia outbreaks were linked to the bacteria. The earliest cases of Legionnaires' disease were shown to have occurred in 1965, but samples of the bacteria exist from 1947.

Exposure to the *Legionella* bacteria doesn't necessarily lead to infection. According to some studies, an estimated 5-10% of the American population show serologic evidence of exposure, the majority of whom do not develop symptoms of an infection. *Legionella* bacteria account for 2-15% of the total number of pneumonia cases requiring hospitalization in the United States.

There are at least 40 types of *Legionella* bacteria, half of which are capable of producing disease in humans. A disease that arises from infection by *Legionella* bacteria is referred to as legionellosis. The *L. pneumophila bacterium*, the root cause of Legionnaires' disease,

KEY TERMS

Antibody—A molecule created by the immune system in response to the presence of an antigen. It serves to recognize the invader and help defend the body from infection.

Antigen—A molecule, such as a protein, which is associated with a particular infectious agent. The immune system uses this molecule as the identifying characteristic of the infectious invader.

Culture—A laboratory system for growing bacteria for further study.

DNA probe—An agent that binds directly to a predefined sequence of nucleic acids.

Immunocompromised—Refers to conditions in which the immune system is not functioning properly and cannot adequately protect the body from infection.

Immunoglobulin—The protein molecule that serves as the primary building block of antibodies.

Immunosuppressive therapy—Medical treatment in which the immune system is purposefully thwarted. Such treatment is necessary, for example, to prevent organ rejection in transplant cases.

Legionellosis—A disease caused by infection with a Legionella bacterium.

Media—Substance which contains all the nutrients necessary for bacteria to grow in a culture.

Phagocytosis—The "ingestion" of a piece of matter by a cell.

causes 90% of legionellosis cases. The second most common cause of legionellosis is the *L. micdadei* bacterium, which produces the Philadelphia pneumonia-causing agent.

Approximately 10,000-40,000 people in the United States develop Legionnaires' disease annually. The people who are the most likely to become ill are over age 50. The risk is greater for people who suffer from health conditions such as malignancy, diabetes, lung disease, or kidney disease. Other risk factors include immunosuppressive therapy and cigarette smoking. Legionnaires' disease has occurred in children, but typically it has been confined to newborns receiving respiratory therapy, children who have had recent operations, and children who are immunosuppressed. People with HIV infection and **AIDS** do not seem to contract Legionnaires' disease with any greater frequency than the rest of the population,

however, if contracted, the disease is likely to be more severe compared to other cases.

Cases of Legionnaires' disease that occur in conjunction with an outbreak, or epidemic, are more likely to be diagnosed quickly. Early diagnosis aids effective and successful treatment. During epidemic outbreaks, fatalities have ranged from 5% for previously healthy individuals to 24% for individuals with underlying illnesses. Sporadic cases (that is, cases unrelated to a wider outbreak) are harder to detect and treatment may be delayed pending an accurate diagnosis. The overall fatality rate for sporadic cases ranges from 10-19%. The outlook is bleaker in severe cases that require respiratory support or dialysis. In such cases, fatality may reach 67%.

Causes & symptoms

Legionnaires' disease is caused by inhaling *Legionella* bacteria from the environment. Typically, the bacteria are dispersed in aerosols of contaminated water. These aerosols are produced by devices in which warm water can stagnate, such as air-conditioning cooling towers, humidifiers, shower heads, and faucets. There have also been cases linked to whirlpool spa baths and water misters in grocery store produce departments. Aspiration of contaminated water is also a potential source of infection, particularly in hospital-acquired cases of Legionnaires' disease. There is no evidence of person-to-person transmission of Legionnaires' disease.

Once the bacteria are in the lungs, cellular representatives of the body's immune system (alveolar macrophages) congregate to destroy the invaders. The typical macrophage defense is to phagocytose the invader and demolish it in a process analogous to swallowing and digesting it. However, the *Legionella* bacteria survive being phagocytosed. Instead of being destroyed within the macrophage, they grow and replicate, eventually kill-

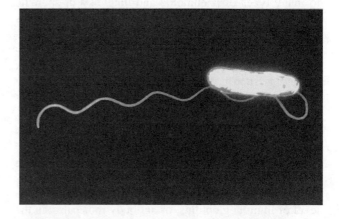

A transmission electron microscopy (TEM) image of *Legionella pneumophila*, **the bacteria which causes Legionnaires' disease.** *(Custom Medical Stock Photo. Reproduced by permission.)*

ing the macrophage. When the macrophage dies, many new *Legionella* bacteria are released into the lungs and worsen the infection.

Legionnaires' disease develops 2-10 days after exposure to the bacteria. Early symptoms include lethargy, **headaches,** fever, chills, muscle aches, and a lack of appetite. Respiratory symptoms such as coughing or congestion are usually absent. As the disease progresses, a dry, hacking cough develops and may become productive after a few days. In about a third of Legionnaires' disease cases, blood is present in the sputum. Half of the people who develop Legionnaires' disease suffer **shortness of breath** and a third complain of breathing-related chest **pain.** The fever can become quite high, reaching 104°F (40°C) in many cases, and may be accompanied by a decreased heart rate.

Although the pneumonia affects the lungs, Legionnaires' disease is accompanied by symptoms that affect other areas of the body. About half the victims experience **diarrhea** and a quarter have **nausea and vomiting** and abdominal pain. In about 10% of cases, acute renal failure and scanty urine production accompany the disease. Changes in mental status, such as disorientation, confusion, and **hallucinations,** also occur in about a quarter of cases.

In addition to Legionnaires' disease, *L. pneumophila* legionellosis also includes a milder disease, Pontiac fever. Unlike Legionnaires' disease, Pontiac fever does not involve the lower respiratory tract. The symptoms usually appear within 36 hours of exposure and include fever, headache, muscle aches, and lethargy. Symptoms last only a few days and medical intervention is not necessary.

Diagnosis

The symptoms of Legionnaires' disease are common to many types of pneumonia and diagnosis of sporadic cases can be difficult. The symptoms and **chest x rays** that confirm a case of pneumonia are not useful in differentiating between Legionnaires' disease and other pneumonias. If a pneumonia case involves multisystem symptoms, such as diarrhea and vomiting, and an initially dry cough, laboratory tests are done to definitively identify *L. pneumophila* as the cause of the infection.

If Legionnaires' disease is suspected, several tests are available to reveal or indicate the presence of *L. pneumophila* bacteria in the body. Since the immune system creates antibodies against infectious agents, examining the blood for these indicators is a key test. The level of immunoglobulins, or antibody molecules, in the blood reveals the presence of infection. In microscopic examination of the patient's sputum, a fluorescent stain linked to antibodies against *L. pneumophila* can uncover the presence of the bacteria. Other means of revealing the bacteria's presence from patient sputum samples include isolation of the organism on culture media or detection of the bacteria by DNA probe. Another test detects *L. pneumophila* antigens in the urine.

Treatment

Most cases of *Legionella* pneumonia show improvement within 12-48 hours of starting antibiotic therapy. The antibiotic of choice has been erythromycin, sometimes paired with a second antibiotic, rifampin. Tetracycline, alone or with rifampin, is also used to treat Legionnaires' disease, but has had more mixed success in comparison to erythromycin. Other **antibiotics** that have been used successfully to combat *Legionella* include doxycycline, clarithromycin, fluorinated quinolones, and trimethoprim/sulfamethoxazole.

The type of antibiotic prescribed by the doctor depends on several factors including the severity of infection, potential **allergies,** and interaction with previously prescribed drugs. For example, erythromycin interacts with warfarin, a blood thinner. Several drugs, such as **penicillins** and **cephalosporins,** are ineffective against the infection. Although they may be deadly to the bacteria in laboratory tests, their chemical structure prevents them from being absorbed into the areas of the lung where the bacteria are present.

In severe cases with complications, antibiotic therapy may be joined by respiratory support. If renal failure occurs, dialysis is required until renal function is recovered.

Prognosis

Appropriate medical treatment has a major impact on recovery from Legionnaires' disease. Outcome is also linked to the victim's general health and absence of complications. If the patient survives the infection, recovery from Legionnaires' disease is complete. Similar to other types of pneumonia, severe cases of Legionnaires' disease may cause scarring in the lung tissue as a result of the infection. Renal failure, if it occurs, is reversible and renal function returns as the patient's health improves. Occasionally, fatigue and weakness may linger for several months after the infection has been successfully treated.

Prevention

Since the bacteria thrive in warm stagnant water, regularly disinfecting ductwork, pipes, and other areas that may serve as breeding areas is the best method for preventing outbreaks of Legionnaires' disease. Most outbreaks of Legionnaires' disease can be traced to specific points of exposure, such as hospitals, hotels, and other places where people gather. Sporadic cases are harder to determine and there is insufficient evidence to point to exposure in individual homes.

Resources

BOOKS

Edelstein, Paul H. and Richard D. Meyer. "Legionella Pneumonias." In *Respiratory Infections: Diagnosis and Management,* 3rd Edition, James E. Pennington, editor. New York: Raven Press, Ltd., 1994.

Johnson, Caroline C. and Sydney M. Finegold. "Pyogenic Bacterial Pneumonia, Lung Abscess, and Empyema." In *Volume 1: Textbook of Respiratory Medicine,* 2nd Edition, John F. Murray and Jay A. Nadel, editors. Philadelphia: W.B. Saunders Company, 1994.

PERIODICALS

Shuman, H.A., M. Purcell, G. Segal, L. Hales, and L.A. Wiater. "Intracellular Multiplication of *Legionella pneumophila*: Human Pathogen of Accidental Tourist?" *Current Topics in Microbiology and Immunology* 225 (1998): 99.

Stout, Janet E. and Victor L. Yu. "Legionellosis," *The New England Journal of Medicine* 337 (September 4, 1997): 682.

Julia Barrett

Leiomyomas *see* **Uterine fibroids**

Leishmaniasis

Definition

Leishmaniasis refers to several different illnesses caused by infection with an organism called a protozoan.

Description

Protozoa are considered to be the most simple organisms in the animal kingdom. They are all single-celled. The types of protozoa which cause leishmaniasis are carried by the blood-sucking sandfly. The sandfly is referred to as the disease vector, simply meaning that the infectious agent (the protozoan) is carried by the sandfly and passed on to other animals or humans in whom the protozoan will set up residence and cause disease. The animal or human in which the protozoan then resides is referred to as the host.

Once the protozoan is within the human host, the human's immune system is activated to try to combat the invader. Specialized immune cells called macrophages work to swallow up the protozoa. Usually, this technique kills a foreign invader, but these protozoa can survive and

---

KEY TERMS

Host—The organism (such as a monkey or human) in which another organism (such as a virus or bacteria) is living.

Larynx—The part of the airway lying between the pharynx and the trachea.

Leishman-Donovan body—A body of a (trypanosomatid) protozoa at a particular and characteristic stage in its life cycle; the infectious (trypanosomatid) protozoa can cause leishmaniasis, and is relatively easy to identify at that stage.

Lesion—A disruption of the normal structure and function of a tissue by some disease process.

Macrophage—A cell of the immune system which engulfs and digests foreign invaders such as bacteria and viruses in an attempt to stop them from causing disease within the body.

Protozoa—A group of organisms which are the smallest members of the animal kingdom, consisting of a single cell.

Ulceration—An area of pitting and irritation.

Vector—A carrier organism (such as a fly or mosquito) which serves to deliver a virus (or other agent of infection) to a host.

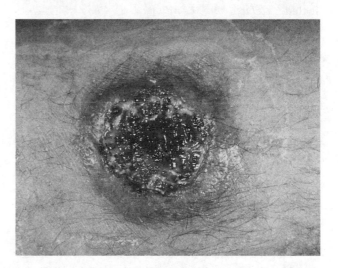

This condition, also called an oriental sore, is caused by the protozoan *L. tropica*. *(Photograph by Lester V. Bergman, Corbis Images. Reproduced by permission.)*

flourish within macrophages. The protozoa multiply within the macrophages, ultimately causing the macrophage to burst open. The protozoa are released, and take up residence within other neighboring cells.

At this point, the course of the disease caused by the protozoa is dependent on the specific type of protozoa, and on the type of reaction the protozoa elicits from the immune system. There are several types of protozoa which cause leishmaniasis, and they cause different patterns of disease progression.

At any one time, about 20 million people throughout the world are infected with leishmaniasis. While leishmaniasis exists as a disease in 88 countries around the globe, some countries are hit harder than others. These include Bangladesh, India, Nepal, Sudan, Afghanistan, Brazil, Iran, Peru, Saudi Arabia, and Syria. Other areas which harbor the causative protozoa include China, many countries throughout Africa, Mexico, Central and South America, Turkey, and Greece. Although less frequent, cases have occurred in the United States, in Texas.

In some areas of southern Europe, leishmaniasis is becoming an important disease which infects people with weakened immune systems. In particular, individuals with acquired immunodeficiency syndrome (**AIDS**) are at great risk of this infection.

Causes & symptoms

There are a number of types of protozoa which can cause leishmaniasis. Each type exists in specific locations, and there are different patterns to the kind of disease each causes. The overall species name is Leishmania (commonly abbreviated L.). The specific types include: *L. Donovani, L. Infantum, L. Chagasi, L. Mexicana, I.. Amazonensis, L. Tropica, L. Major, L. Aethiopica, L. Brasiliensis, L. Guyaensis, L. Panamensis, L. Peruviana.* Some of the names are reflective of the locale in which the specific protozoa is most commonly found, or in which it was first discovered.

Localized cutaneous leishmaniasis

This type of disease occurs most commonly in China, India, Asia Minor, Africa, the Mediterranean Basin, and Central America. It has occurred in an area ranging from northern Argentina all the way up to southern Texas. It is called different names in different locations, including chiclero ulcer, bush **yaws,** uta, oriental sore, Aleppo boil, and Baghdad sore.

This is perhaps the least drastic type of disease caused by any of the Leishmania. Several weeks or months after being bitten by an infected sandfly, the host may notice an itchy bump (lesion) on an arm, leg, or face. Lymph nodes in the area of this bump may be swollen. Within several months, the bump develops a crater (ulceration) in the center, with a raised, reddened ridge around it. There may be several of these lesions near each other, and they may spread into each other to form one large lesion. Although localized cutaneous leishmaniasis usually heals on its own, it may take as long as year. A depressed, light-colored scar usually remains behind. Some lesions never heal, and may invade and destroy the tissue below. For example, lesions on the ears may slowly, but surely, invade and destroy the cartilage which supports the outer ear.

Diffuse cutaneous leishmaniasis

This type of disease occurs most often in Ethiopia, Brazil, Dominican Republic, and Venezuela.

The lesions of diffuse cutaneous leishmaniasis are very similar to those of localized cutaneous leishmaniasis, except they are spread all over the body. The body's immune system apparently fails to battle the protozoa, which are free to spread throughout. The characteristic lesions resemble those of the dread biblical disease, **leprosy.**

Mucocutaneous leishmaniasis

This form of leishmaniasis occurs primarily in the tropics of South America. The disease begins with the same sores noted in localized cutaneous leishmaniasis. Sometimes these primary lesions heal, other times they spread and become larger. Some years after the first lesion is noted (and sometimes several years after that lesion has totally healed), new lesions appear in the mouth and nose, and occasionally in the area between the genitalia and the anus (the perineum). These new lesions are particularly destructive and painful. They erode underlying tissue and cartilage, frequently eating through the septum (the cartilage which separates the two nostrils). If the lesions spread to the roof of the mouth and the larynx (the part of the wind pipe which contains the vocal cords), they may prevent speech. Other symptoms include **fever,** weight loss, anemia (low red blood cell count). There is always a large danger of bacteria infecting the already open sores.

Visceral leishmaniasis

This type of leishmaniasis occurs India, China, the southern region of Russia, and throughout Africa, the Mediterranean, and South and Central America. It is frequently called Kala-Azar or Dumdum fever.

In this disease, the protozoa uses the bloodstream to travel to the liver, spleen, lymph nodes, and bone marrow. Fever may last for as long as eight weeks, disappear, and then reappear again. The lymph nodes, spleen, and liver are often quite enlarged. Weakness, fatigue, loss of appetite, **diarrhea,** and weight loss are common. Kala-azar translates to mean "black fever." The name kala-azar comes from a characteristic of this form of leishmaniasis. Individual with light-colored skin take on a darker, grayish skin tone, particularly of their face and hands. A variety of lesions appear on the skin.

Diagnosis

Diagnosis for each of these types of leishmaniasis involves taking a scraping from a lesion, preparing it in a laboratory, and examining it under a microscope to demonstrate the causative protozoan. Other methods that have been used include culturing a sample piece of tissue in a laboratory to allow the protozoa to multiply for easier microscopic identification; injecting a mouse or hamster with a solution made of scrapings from a patient's lesion to see if the animal develops a leishmaniasis-like disease; and demonstrating the presence in macrophages of the characteristic-appearing protozoan, called Leishman-Donovan bodies.

In some forms of leishmaniasis, a skin test (similar to that given for TB) may be used. In this test, a solution containing a small bit of the protozoan antigen (cell markers which cause the human immune system to react) is injected or scratched into a patient's skin. In a positive reaction, cells from the immune system will race to this spot, causing a characteristic skin lesion. Not all forms of leishmaniasis cause a positive skin test, however.

Treatment

The treatment of choice for all forms of leishmaniasis is a type of drug containing the element antimony. These include sodium sitogluconate, and meglumin antimonate. When these types of drugs do not work, other medications with anti-protozoal activity are utilized, including amphotericin B, pentamidine, flagyl, and allopurinol.

Prognosis

The prognosis for leishmaniasis is quite variable, and depends on the specific strain of infecting protozoan, as well as the individual patient's immune system response to infection. Localized cutaneous leishmaniasis may require no treatment. Although it may take many months, these lesions usually heal themselves completely. Only rarely do these lesions fail to heal and become more destructive.

Disseminated cutaneous leishmaniasis may smolder on for years without treatment, ultimately causing **death** when the large, open lesions become infected with bacteria.

Mucocutaneous leishmaniasis is often relatively resistant to treatment. Untreated visceral leishmaniasis has a 90% death rate, but only a 10% death rate with treatment.

Prevention

Prevention involves protecting against sandfly bites. Insect repellents used around homes, on clothing, on skin, and on bednets (to protect people while sleeping) are effective measures.

Reducing the population of sandflies is also an important preventive measure. In areas where leishmaniasis is very common, recommendations include clearing the land of trees and brush for at least 984 ft (300 m) around all villages, and regularly spraying the area with insecticides. Because rodents often carry the protozoan which causes leishmaniasis, careful rodent control should be practiced. Dogs, which also carry the protozoan, can be given a simple blood test and then either treated or put to sleep.

Resources

BOOKS

Herwaldt, Barbara. "Leishmaniasis." In *Harrison's Principles of Internal Medicine,* edited by Anthony S. Fauci, et al. New York: McGraw-Hill, 1998.

Plorde, James J. "Flagellate Infections." In *Sherris Medical Microbiology: An Introduction to Infectious Diseases,* edited by Kenneth J. Ryan. Norwalk, CT: Appleton and Lange, 1994.

Plorde, James J. "Introduction to Pathogenic Parasites." In *Sherris Medical Microbiology: An Introduction to Infectious Diseases,* edited by Kenneth J. Ryan. Norwalk, CT: Appleton and Lange, 1994.

PERIODICALS

Ablon, Glynis R., and Ted Rosen. "Protozoan Skin Infections: The World Traveler and the Unwanted Companion." *Consultant* 35 (April 1995): 461 +.

Farley, Dixie. "Treating Tropical Diseases." *FDA Consumer* 31 (January/February 1997): 26 +.

Farley, Dixie. "Tropical Diseases: Travelers Take Note." *Consumer Research Magazine* 80 (May 1997): 27 +.

Gradoni, L., et al. "Treatment of Mediterranean Visceral Leishmaniasis." *World Health Organization* 73 (March/April 1995): 191 +.

Hashim, Faisal A. "Neurologic Changes in Visceral Leishmaniasis." *The Journal of the American Medical Association*" 274 (5 July 1995): 6E.

ORGANIZATIONS

Centers for Disease Control and Prevention. (404) 332-4559. http://www.cdc.gov/travel/travel.html

Rosalyn S. Carson-Dewitt

Leprosy

Definition

Leprosy is a slowly progressing bacterial infection that affects the skin, peripheral nerves in the hands and feet, and mucous membranes of the nose, throat, and eyes. Destruction of the nerve endings causes the the affected areas to lose sensation. Occasionally, because of the loss of feeling, the fingers and toes become mutilated and fall off, causing the deformities that are typically associated with the disease.

Description

Leprosy is also known as Hansen's disease after G. A. Hansen who in 1878 identified the bacillus *Mycobacterium leprae* that caused the disease.

The infection is characterized by abnormal changes of the skin. These changes, called lesions, are at first flat and red. Upon enlarging, they have irregular shapes and a characteristic appearance. The lesions are typically darker in color around the edges with discolored pale centers. Because the organism grows best at lower temperatures the leprosy bacillus has a preference for the skin, the mucous membranes and the nerves. Infection in and destruction of the nerves leads to sensory loss. The loss of sensation in the fingers and toes increases the risk of injury. Inadequate care causes infection of open **wounds. Gangrene** may also follow, causing body tissue to die and become deformed.

Because of the disabling deformities associated with it, leprosy has been considered one of the most dreaded diseases since biblical times, though much of what was called leprosy in the Old Testament most likely was not the same disease. Its victims were often shunned by the community, kept at arm's length, or sent to a leper colony. Many people still have misconceptions about the disease. Contrary to popular belief, it is not highly communicable and is extremely slow to develop. Household contacts of most cases and the medical personnel caring for Hansen's disease patients are not at particular risk. It is very curable, although the treatment is long-term, requiring multiple medications.

The World Health Organization (WHO) puts the number of identified leprosy cases in the world, at the beginning of 1997, at about 890,000. Seventy percent of all cases are found in just three countries: India, Indonesia, and Myanamar (Burma). The infection can be acquired, however, in the Western Hemisphere as well.

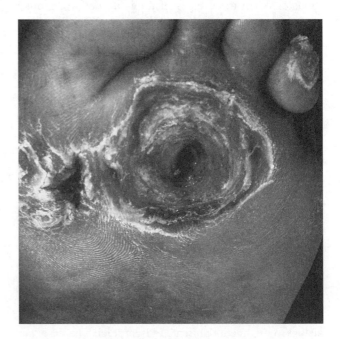

Lesions such as these are characteristic of leprosy.
(Phototake NYC. Reproduced by permission.)

Cases also occur in some areas of the Caribbean and even in southern Texas and Louisiana.

Causes & symptoms

The organism that causes leprosy is a rod-shaped bacterium called *Mycobacterium leprae*. This bacterium is related to *Mycobacterium tuberculosis*, the causative agent of **tuberculosis**. Because special staining techniques involving acids are required to view these bacteria under the microscope, they are referred to as acid-fast bacilli (AFB).

When *Mycobacterium leprae* invades the body, one of two reactions can take place. In tuberculoid leprosy (TT), the milder form of the disease, the body's immune cells attempt to seal off the infection from the rest of the body by surrounding the offending pathogen. Because this response by the immune system occurs in the deeper layers of the skin, the hair follicles, sweat glands, and nerves can be destroyed. As a result, the skin becomes dry and discolored and loses its sensitivity. Involvement of nerves on the face, arms, or legs can cause them to enlarge and become easily felt by the doctor. This finding is highly suggestive of TT. The scarcity of bacteria in this type of leprosy leads to it being referred to as paucibacillary (PB) leprosy. Seventy to eighty percent of all leprosy cases are of the tuberculoid type.

In lepromatous (LL) leprosy, which is the second and more contagious form of the disease, the body's immune system is unable to mount a strong response to the invading organism. Hence, the organism multiplies freely in the skin. This type of leprosy is also called the multibacillary (MB) leprosy, because of the presence of large numbers of bacteria. The characteristic feature of this disease is the appearance of large nodules or lesions all over the body and face. Occasionally, the mucous membranes of the eyes, nose, and throat may be involved. Facial involvement can produce a lion-like appearance (leonine facies). This type of leprosy can lead to blindness, drastic change in voice, or mutilation of the nose. Leprosy can strike anyone; however, children seem to be more susceptible than adults.

Well-defined **skin lesions** that are numb are the first symptoms of tuberculoid leprosy. Lepromatous leprosy is characterized by a chronic stuffy nose due to invasion of the mucous membranes, and the presence of nodules and lesions all over the body and face.

The incubation period varies anywhere from six months to ten years. On an average, it takes four years for the symptoms of tuberculoid leprosy to develop. Probably because of the slow growth of the bacillus, lepromatous leprosy develops even more slowly, taking an average of eight years for the initial lesions to appear.

It is not very clear how the leprosy bacillus is transmitted from person to person. Inhaling bacteria that are present in dust is thought to be one of the modes of transmission. However, even among people who live in the same household as the patient and are in close contact, only 5% get leprosy. It is obviously not a highly communicable disease. The incidence of leprosy is highest in the poverty belt of the globe. Therefore, environmental factors such as unhygienic living conditions, overpopulation, and **malnutrition** may also be contributing factors favoring the infection. The nine-banded armadillo is susceptible to this disease but it is still unclear if human infection is related to exposure to this animal.

Diagnosis

One of the hallmarks of leprosy is the presence of AFB in smears taken from the skin lesions, nasal scrapings, or tissue secretions. In patients with LL leprosy, the bacilli are easily detected; however, in TT leprosy the bacteria are very few and almost impossible to find. In such cases, a diagnosis is made based on the clinical signs and symptoms, the type and distribution of skin lesions, and history of having lived in an endemic area.

The signs and symptoms characteristic of leprosy can be easily identified by a health worker after a short training period. There is no need for a laboratory investigation to confirm a leprosy diagnosis, except in very rare circumstances.

In an endemic area, if smears from an individual show the presence of AFB, or if he has typical skin lesions, he should definitely be regarded as having leprosy. Usually, there is slight discoloration of the skin and loss of skin sensitivity. Thickened nerves accompanied by weakness of muscles supplied by the affected nerve are very typical of the disease. One characteristic occurrence is a foot drop where the foot cannot be flexed upwards, affecting the ability to walk.

Treatment

The most widely used drug for leprosy is dapsone. However, emergence of dapsone-resistant strains prompted the introduction of multi-drug therapy. The multi-drug therapy includes dapsone, refampin (also known as rifampicin), and clofazimine, all of which are powerful antibacterial drugs. Patients with MB leprosy are usually treated with all three drugs, while patients with PB leprosy are only given refampin and dapsone. Usually three months after starting treatment, a patient ceases being infectious, though not everyone with this disease is necessarily infectious before treatment. Depending on the type of leprosy, the time required for treatment may vary from six months to two years or more.

Each of the drugs have minor side effects. Dapsone can cause nausea, **dizziness, palpitations, jaundice** and rash. A doctor should be contacted immediately if a rash develops. Dapsone also interacts with the second drug, refampin. Refampin increases the metabolizing of dapsone in the body, requiring an adjustment of the dapsone dosage. Refampin may also cause muscle cramps, or nausea. If jaundice, flu-like symptoms or a rash appear, a doctor should be contacted immediately. The third drug, clofazimine may cause severe abdominal **pain** and **diarrhea,** as well as discoloration of the skin. Red to brownish black discoloration of the skin and bodily fluids, including sweat, may persist for months to years after use.

Thalidomide, the most famous agent of **birth defects** in the 20th century, is now being used to treat complications of leprosy and similar diseases. Thalidomide regulates the immune response by suppressing a protein, tumor necrosis factor-alpha.

Leprosy patients should be aware that treatment itself can cause a potentially serious immune system response called a lepra reaction. When antibiotics kill *M. leprae,* antigens (the proteins on the surface of the organism that initiate the body's immune system response) are released from the dying bacteria. In some people, when the antigens combine with the antibodies to *M. Leprae* in the bloodstream, a reaction called erythema nodosum leprosum may occur, resulting in new lesions and peripheral nerve damage. Cortisone-type medications and, increasingly, thalidomide are used to minimize the effects of lepra reactions.

Prognosis

Leprosy is curable; however, the deformities and nerve damage associated with leprosy are often irreversible. Preventions or rehabilitation of these defects is an integral part of management of the disease. **Reconstructive surgery,** aimed at preventing and correcting deformities, offers the greatest hope for disabled patients. Sometimes, the deformities are such that the patients will not benefit from this type of surgery.

Comprehensive care involves teaching patients to care for themselves. If the patients have significant nerve damage or are at high risk of developing deformities, they must be taught to take care of their insensitive limbs, similar to diabetics with lower leg nerve damage. Lacking the sensation of pain, the patients should constantly check themselves to identify cuts and **bruises.** If adequate care is not taken, these wounds become festering sores and a source of dangerous infection. Physiotherapy **exercises** are taught to the patients to maintain a range of movement in finger joints and prevent the deformities from worsening. Prefabricated standardized splints are available and are extremely effective in correcting and preventing certain common deformities in leprosy. Special kinds of footwear have been designed for patients with insensitive feet in order to prevent or minimize the progression of foot ulcers.

Prevention

By early diagnosis and appropriate treatment of infected individuals, even a disease as ancient as leprosy can be controlled. People who are in immediate contact with the leprosy patient should be tested for leprosy. Annual examinations should also be conducted on these people for a period of five years following their last contact with an infectious patient. Some physicians have advocated dapsone treatment for people in close household contact with leprosy patients.

The WHO Action Program for the Elimination of Leprosy has adopted a resolution calling for the reduction of leprosy's prevalence to less than one case per 10,000 people by the year 2000. In order to make this possible, educating people about the disease and raising their awareness is of utmost importance. The tuberculosis BCG vaccine, used in many areas of the world, may have an effect in decreasing the incidence of leprosy.

Resources

BOOKS

"Bacterial and Mycotic Infections: Leprosy." In *Microbiology,* 3rd ed., edited by B. D. Davis, et al. New York: Harper & Row Publishers, 1980.

Krane, Stephen M., and Michael F. Holick. "Mycobacterial Diseases: Leprosy." In *Harrison's Principles of Internal Medicine,* edited by R.G. Petersdorf, et al. New York: McGraw-Hill, 1994.

Zinsser, Hans. *Zinsser Microbiology,* 19th ed., edited by Wolfgang K. Joklik, et al. Norfolk, CT: Appleton and Lange, 1988.

PERIODICALS

Binford, Chapman et al. "Leprosy." *Journal of the American Medical Association* 247 (April 23-30, 1982): 2283-2292.

ORGANIZATIONS

American Leprosy Missions. 1 ALM Way, Greenville, SC 29601. (1-800-LEPROSY).

British Leprosy Relief Association, LEPRA. Fairfax House, Causton Road, Colchester, Essex CO1 1PU, UK.

INFOLEP, Leprosy Information Services. Postbus 95005,1090 HA, Amsterdam, Netherlands. Infolep@antenna.nl.

WHO/LEP, Action Programme for the Elimination of Leprosy. 20 Avenue Appia CH-1211, Geneva 27, Suisse. (http://www.who.ch/programmes/lep/lep_home.htm).

OTHER

National Institutes of Health. Leprosy. http://www.search.info.nih.gov.

U.S. government. Leprosy. http://www.healthfinder.nih.gov.

Lata Cherath

Leptospirosis

Definition

Leptospirosis is a febrile disease (**fever**) caused by infection with the bacteria *Leptospira interrogans*. The disease can range from very mild and symptomless to a more serious, even life threatening form, that may be associated with kidney (renal) failure.

Description

An infection by the bacterium *Leptospira interrogans* goes by different names in different regions. Alternate names for leptospirosis include mud fever, swamp fever, sugar cane fever, and Fort Bragg fever. More severe cases of leptospirosis are called Weil's syndrome or icterohemorrhagic fever. This disease is commonly found in tropical and subtropical climates but occurs worldwide.

As of the mid 1980s, there were 35-60 cases of leptospirosis reported in the United States each year. Most cases occur in Hawaii, followed by the south Atlantic, Gulf, and Pacific coastal states. However, because of the nonspecific symptoms of leptospirosis, it is believed that the occurrence in the United States is actually much higher. Leptospirosis occurs year-round in the United States, but about half of the cases occur between July and October.

Leptospirosis is a disease of animals and can be a very serious problem in the livestock industry. *Leptospira* bacteria have been found in dogs, rats, livestock, mice, voles, rabbits, hedgehogs, skunks, possums, frogs, fish, snakes, and certain birds and insects. Infected animals will pass the bacteria in their urine for months, or even years. In the United States, rats and dogs are more commonly linked with human leptospirosis than other animals.

Humans are considered "accidental hosts" and become infected with *Leptospira interrogans* by coming into contact with urine from infected animals. This is either through direct contact with urine, or through contact with soil, water, or plants that have been contaminated by animal urine. *Leptospira interrogans* can survive for as long as six months outdoors under favorable conditions. Leptospira bacteria can enter the body through cuts or other skin damage or through mucous membranes (such as the inside of the mouth and nose). It is believed that the bacteria may be able to pass through intact skin, but this is not known.

Once past the skin barrier, the bacteria enter the blood stream and rapidly spread throughout the body. The infection causes damage to the inner lining of blood

KEY TERMS

Hemodialysis—The removal of waste products from the blood stream in patients with kidney failure. Blood is removed from a vein, passed through a dialysis machine, and then put back into a vein.

Jarisch-Herxheimer reaction—A rare reaction to the dead bacteria in the blood stream following antibiotic treatment.

Meningitis—Inflammation of tissues in the brain and spinal cord. Aseptic meningitis refers to meningitis with no bacteria present in the cerebral spinal fluid.

vessels. The liver, kidneys, heart, lungs, central nervous system, and eyes may be affected.

There are two stages in the disease process. The first stage is during the active Leptospira infection and is called the "bacteremic," or "septicemic," phase. The bacteremic phase lasts from three to seven days and presents as typical flu-like symptoms. During this phase, bacteria can be found in the patient's blood and cerebrospinal fluid. The second stage, or "immune phase," occurs either immediately after the bacteremic stage or after a 1-3 day symptom-free period. The immune phase can last up to one month. During the immune phase, symptoms are milder but **meningitis** (inflammation of spinal cord and brain tissues) is common. Bacteria can be isolated only from the urine during this second phase.

Causes & symptoms

Leptospirosis is caused by an infection with the bacterium *Leptospira interrogans*. The bacteria are spread through contact with urine from infected animals. Persons at an increased risk for leptospirosis include farmers, miners, animal health care workers, fish farmers and processors, sewage and canal workers, cane harvesters, and soldiers. High risk activities include care of pets, hunting, trail biking, freshwater swimming, rafting, canoeing, kayaking, and participating in sports in muddy fields.

Symptoms of *Leptospira* infection occur within 7-12 days following exposure to the bacteria. Because the symptoms can be nonspecific, most people who have antibodies to *Leptospira* do not remember having had an illness. Eighty-five to 90% of the cases are not serious and clear up on their own. Symptoms of the first stage of leptospirosis last three to seven days and are: fever (100-105°F [37.8-40.6°C]), severe **headache,** muscle **pain,** stomach pain, chills, nausea, vomiting, back pain, joint pain, neck stiffness, and extreme exhaustion. **Cough** and body rash sometimes occur.

Following the first stage of disease, a brief symptom-free period occurs for most patients. The symptoms of the second stage vary in each patient. Most patients have a low grade fever, headache, vomiting, and rash. Aseptic meningitis is common in the second stage, symptoms of which include headache and **photosensitivity** (sensitivity of the eye to light). *Leptospira* can affect the eyes and make them cloudy and yellow to orange colored. Vision may be blurred.

Ten percent of the persons infected with *Leptospira* develop a serious disease called Weil's syndrome. The symptoms of Weil's syndrome are more severe than those described above and there is no distinction between the first and second stages of disease. The hallmark of Weil's syndrome is liver, kidney, and blood vessel disease. The signs of severe disease are apparent after 3-7 days of illness. In addition to those listed above, symptoms of Weil's syndrome include **jaundice** (yellow skin and eyes), decreased or no urine output, **hypotension** (low blood pressure), rash, anemia (decreased number of red blood cells), **shock,** and severe mental status changes. Red spots on the skin, "blood shot" eyes, and bloody sputum signal that blood vessel damage and hemorrhage have occurred.

Diagnosis

Leptospirosis can be diagnosed and treated by doctors who specialize in infectious diseases. During the bacteremic phase of the disease, the symptoms are relatively nonspecific. This often causes an initial misdiagnosis because many diseases have similar symptoms to leptospirosis. The later symptoms of jaundice and kidney failure together with the bacteremic phase symptoms suggest leptospirosis. Blood samples will be tested to look for antibodies to *Leptospira interrogans*. Blood samples taken over a period of a few days would show an increase in the number of antibodies. Isolating *Leptospira* bacteria from blood, cerebrospinal fluid (performed by spinal tap), and urine samples is diagnostic of leptospirosis. It make take six weeks for *Leptospira* to grow in laboratory media. Most insurance companies would cover the diagnosis and treatment of this infection.

Treatment

Leptospirosis is treated with **antibiotics,** penicillin (Bicillin, Wycillin), doxycycline (Monodox), ibramycin, or erythromycin (E-mycin, Ery-Tab). As of early 1998, the timing of antibiotic treatment is controversial. It is generally agreed that antibiotic treatment during the first few days of illness is helpful. However, leptospirosis is often not diagnosed until the later stages of illness. The benefit of antibiotic treatment in the later stages of disease is controversial. A rare complication of antibiotic therapy for leptospirosis is the occurrence of the Jarisch-Herxheimer reaction, which is characterized by fever, chills, headache, and muscle pain.

Patients with severe illness will require hospitalization for treatment and monitoring. Medication or other treatment for pain, fever, vomiting, fluid loss, bleeding, mental changes, and low blood pressure may be provided. Patients with kidney failure will require hemodialysis to remove waste products from the blood.

Prognosis

The majority of patients infected with *Leptospira interrogans* experience a complete recovery. Ten percent of the patients will develop eye inflammation (**uveitis**) up to one year after the illness. In the United States, about one out of every 100 patients will die from leptospirosis. **Death** is usually caused by kidney failure, but has also been caused by **myocarditis** (inflammation of heart tissue), **septic shock** (reduced blood flow to the organs because of the bacterial infection), organ failure, and/or poorly functioning lungs.

Prevention

Persons who are at an extremely high risk (such as soldiers who are training in wetlands) can be pretreated with 200 mg of doxycycline once a week. As of early 1998, there were no vaccines available to prevent leptospirosis.

There are many ways to decrease the chances of being infected by *Leptospira*. These include:

- Avoid swimming or wading in freshwater ponds and slowly moving streams, especially those located near farms.

- Do not conduct canoe or kayak capsizing drills in freshwater ponds. Use a swimming pool instead.

- Boil or chemically treat pond or stream water before drinking it or cooking with it.

- Control rats and mice around the home.

- Have pets and farm animals vaccinated against *Leptospira*.

- Wear protective clothing (gloves, boots, long pants, and long-sleeved shirts) when working with wet soil or plants.

Resources

BOOKS

Cook, G.C. *Manson's Tropical Diseases,* 20th ed. London: W.B. Saunders Company, 1996.

Gorbach, Samuel L., John G. Bartlett, and Neil R. Blacklow. *Infectious Diseases,* 2nd ed. Philadelphia: W.B. Saunders Company, 1998.

PERIODICALS

Farr, R. Wesley. ''Leptospirosis.'' *Clinical Infectious Diseases* 21 (1995): 1-8.

OTHER

Centers for Disease Control and Prevention. 1998. http://www.cdc.gov (20 April 1998).

Mayo Health Oasis. 1998. http://www.mayohealth.org (5 March 1998).

Belinda M. Rowland

Lesch-Nyhan Syndrome

Definition

Lesch-Nyhan syndrome is a severe hereditary disorder that leads to physical and **mental retardation,** and is often associated with self-destructive biting of the hands and lips.

Description

Lesch-Nyhan syndrome affects 1 in 400,000 live births. Only male children are affected, but women can be asymptomatic carriers and pass the mutation on to their offspring.

Children with Lesch-Nyhan frequently injure themselves due to muscle spasms. They also show aggressiveness toward themselves and others. The most dramatic symptom of Lesch-Nyhan syndrome is the compulsive biting of the lips, tongue, and finger tips which can lead to serious injury and scarring. Over time, serious injury to the kidneys may develop as a result of the excessive uric acid in the blood.

Causes & symptoms

Lesch-Nyhan is caused by a mutation in the gene for the enzyme named hypoxanthine-guanine phosphoribosyltransferase (HPRT). HPRT catalyzes a reaction which is necessary to prevent the buildup of uric acid. Mutation in the HPRT gene leads to an absence of enzyme activity which, in turn, leads to markedly elevated uric acid levels in the blood (hyperuricemia) with further consequences that include urinary tract stones and severe developmental impact on the brain. The disease known as **gout** is caused by a less damaging mutation in the same gene, leading to reduced—but not eliminated—HPRT activity.

KEY TERMS

Amniocentesis—A procedure for sampling fetal cells from the amniotic fluid surrounding the fetus in the womb.

Chorionic villus sampling—A procedure for sampling fetal cells which is performed through the mother's vagina and cervix or through the abdomen.

Palsy—Uncontrollable tremors.

Spasticity—A spastic condition or state characterized by the sudden, involuntary contraction of one or more groups of muscles.

The HPRT gene is located on the X chromosome. Males have only one X chromosome, so any male who inherits the defective X will develop the disease. Women, however, have two X chromosomes. Because the mutant gene is recessive, a woman would need to inherit two defective copies in order to develop the disease. This is impossible because male Lesch-Nyhan patients are not capable of fathering children. As a result, all victims of Lesch-Nyhan syndrome are male. There is a 50% probability that any male child of a carrier will inherit the defective gene.

At birth, patients appear completely normal and often develop normally for the first few months. Often the earliest sign is the presence of sand-like crystals of uric acid in the diapers. The baby may be unusually irritable. The first symptom of nervous system impairment is inability to lift the head at an appropriate age of four to six months. By the end of the first year, writhing motions (athetosis), and spasmodic movements of the limbs and facial muscles (chorea) are clear evidence of defective motor development. Spasticity and palsy are terms used to describe the poor motor coordination of the victims.

Diagnosis

Diagnosis is based initially on the distinctive pattern of symptoms and is confirmed by DNA testing.

Prenatal diagnosis is possible by DNA testing of fetal tissue drawn by **amniocentesis** or **chorionic villus sampling.** Because Lesch-Nyhan is quite rare, not every fetus should be tested. Fetuses should be tested if the mother is a carrier of the defective HPRT gene. Women who carry a defective HPRT gene and are therefore at risk of bearing an affected fetus can readily be detected by a simple blood test. Any woman related to a HPRT patient should be tested to determine if she is a carrier.

Treatment

There are no known treatments for the neurological defects of Lesch-Nyhan. The gout medication allopurinol can lower blood uric acid levels and prevent damage to the kidneys. It is important that patients receive adequate fluid intake and that they be restrained when self-destructive behavior occurs.

Prognosis

With strong supportive care, infants born with Lesch-Nyhan can live into adulthood with symptoms continuing throughout life.

Prevention

At present, there are no preventive measures for Lesch-Nyhan syndrome. However, recent studies have indicated that this genetic disorder may be a good candidate for treatment with gene replacement therapy. Unfortunately, the technology neccessary to implement this therapy has not yet been perfected.

Resources

PERIODICALS

Lesch, M., and W. L. Nyhan. "A Familial Disorder of Uric Acid Metabolism and Central Nervous System Function." *American Journal of Medicine* 36(1964): 561-570.

ORGANIZATIONS

Alliance of Genetic Support Groups. (This service provides referals to specific disease support organizations.) 4301 Connecticut Ave. NW, Suite 404, Washington, DC 20008. (202) 966-5557. (800) 336-4363.

National Organization for Rare Disorders. P.O. Box 8923, New Fairfield, CT 06812-1783. (800) 999-6673.

OTHER

The National Institutes of Health maintain the following web page with information about Lesch-Nyhan syndrome: www.ninds.nih.gov/healinfo/disorder/lesch-nyhan/lesch-nyhan.htm

G. Victor Leipzig

Letterer-Siwe disease *see* **Histiocytosis X**

KEY TERMS

Bone marrow—The spongy tissue inside large bones where blood cells are formed.

Buffy coat—The thin layer of concentrated white blood cells that forms when a tube of blood is spun in a centrifuge.

Leukemia—Any of several cancers of the bone marrow characterized by the abnormal increase of a type of blood cell.

Leukemia stains—Special stains added to smears of blood or bone marrow, performed to diagnose and classify leukemia.

Leukemia stains

Definition

Leukemia stains are laboratory tests done on bone marrow or blood samples to help diagnose specific types of leukemia.

Purpose

Leukemia stains are done to diagnose and classify leukemia. Blood contains red cells, several varieties of white cells, and platelets. Cancerous overproduction of any one type of cell produces one of many types of leukemia. A patient's specific type of leukemia must be classified in order to provide the best treatment and most accurate prognosis.

The type and maturity of the cells involved are identified by analyzing blood and bone marrow under a microscope. Often, however, the abnormality or immatu-

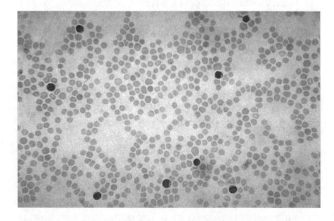

A magnified stain of chronic lymphocytic leukemia cells.
(Custom Medical Stock Photo. Reproduced by permission.)

rity of the cells make it difficult to identify the cell types with certainty. Special leukemia stains help to distinguish one cell type from another.

Description

Special stains are added to bone marrow or blood that has been smeared on a microscope slide. Cell types react differently to the chemicals in the stains.

If the patient has few white cells, a buffy coat smear is made. A tube of blood is spun in a centrifuge. Red cells fall, plasma rises, and white cells settle in a thin middle layer called the buffy coat. The smear is made from this layer.

Sudan black B stain

This stain distinguishes between acute lymphoblastic leukemia (cells stain positive) and acute myeloblastic leukemia (cells stain negative).

Periodic acid-Schiff stain (PAS)

The PAS stain is primarily used to identify erythroleukemia, a leukemia of immature red blood cells. These cells stain a bright fuchsia.

Terminal deoxynucleotidyl transferase stain (TdT)

The TdT stain differentiates between acute lymphoblastic leukemia (cells stain positive) and acute myelogenous leukemia (cells stain negative).

Leukocyte alkaline phosphatase (LAP)

The LAP stain is used to determine if an increase of cells is due to chronic myelogenous leukemia or a noncancerous reaction to an infection or similar conditions. Cells from a noncancerous reaction stain positive with many intense blue granules; cells from chronic myelogenous leukemia have few blue granules.

Tartrate-resistant acid phosphatase stain (TRAP)

The TRAP stain is primarily used to identify **hairy cell leukemia** cells. These cells stain with purple to dark red granules.

Myeloperoxidase stain

The myeloperoxidase stain distinguishes between the immature cells in acute myeloblastic leukemia (cells stain positive) and those in acute lymphoblastic leukemia (cells stain negative).

Leukocyte specific esterase

This stain identifies granulocytes, which show red granules.

Leukocyte nonspecific esterase

Nonspecific esterase stain identifies monocytes and immature platelets (megakaryocytes), which show positive black granules.

Preparation

Leukemia stains are done on smears of blood or bone marrow. To collect blood, a healthcare worker draws blood from a vein in the inner elbow region. Collection of the sample takes only a few minutes.

When bone marrow is needed, the person is given **local anesthesia.** Then the physician inserts a needle through the skin and into the bone—usually the breast bone or hip bone—and 0.5-2 mL of bone marrow is withdrawn. This procedure takes approximately 30 minutes.

Aftercare

Patients sometimes feel discomfort or bruising at the puncture site after blood collection. They may also become dizzy or faint. Pressure to the puncture site until the bleeding stops reduces bruising. Warm packs to the puncture site relieve discomfort.

Collection of bone marrow is done under a physician's supervision. The patient is asked to rest after the procedure and is watched for weakness and signs of bleeding.

Normal results

A normal blood or bone marrow smear shows no evidence of leukemic cells. The expected reaction of cells varies with the type of stain.

Abnormal results

Leukemia stain results that help diagnosis and classify leukemia are supported by the results of other laboratory tests and the person's clinical condition.

Resources

BOOKS

Fischbach, Francis. *Manual of Laboratory and Diagnostic Tests.* Philadelphia: Lippincott, 1996.

Nancy J. Nordenson

Leukemias, acute

Definition

Leukemia is a **cancer** that starts in the organs that make blood, namely the bone marrow and the lymph system. Depending on their characteristics, leukemias can be divided into two broad types. Acute leukemias are the rapidly progressing leukemias, while the **chronic leukemias** progress more slowly. The vast majority of the childhood leukemias are of the acute form.

Description

The cells that make up blood are produced in the bone marrow and the lymph system. The bone marrow is the spongy tissue found in the large bones of the body. The lymph system includes the spleen (an organ in the upper abdomen), the thymus (a small organ beneath the breastbone), and the tonsils (an organ in the throat). In addition, the lymph vessels (tiny tubes that branch like blood vessels into all parts of the body) and lymph nodes (pea-shaped organs that are found along the network of lymph vessels) are also part of the lymph system. The lymph is a milky fluid that contains cells. Clusters of lymph nodes are found in the neck, underarm, pelvis, abdomen, and chest.

The cells found in the blood are the red blood cells (RBCs), which carry oxygen and other materials to all tissues of the body; white blood cells (WBCs) that fight infection; and the platelets, which play a part in the clotting of the blood. The white blood cells can be further subdivided into three main types: granulocytes, monocytes, and lymphocytes.

The granulocytes, as their name suggests, have particles (granules) inside them. These granules contain special proteins (enzymes) and several other substances that can break down chemicals and destroy microorganisms, such as bacteria. Monocytes are the second type of white blood cell. They are also important in defending the body against pathogens.

The lymphocytes form the third type of white blood cell. There are two main types of lymphocytes: T lymphocytes and B lymphocytes. They have different functions within the immune system. The B cells protect the body by making "antibodies." Antibodies are proteins that can attach to the surfaces of bacteria and viruses. This "attachment" sends signals to many other cell types to come and destroy the antibody-coated organism. The T cells protect the body against viruses. When a virus enters a cell, it produces certain proteins that are projected onto the surface of the infected cell. The T cells recognize these proteins and make certain chemicals that are capa-

ble of destroying the virus-infected cells. In addition, the T cells can destroy some types of cancer cells.

The bone marrow makes stem cells, which are the precursors of the different blood cells. These stem cells mature through stages into either RBCs, WBCs, or platelets. In acute leukemias, the maturation process of the white blood cells is interrupted. The immature cells (or "blasts") proliferate rapidly and begin to accumulate in various organs and tissues, thereby affecting their normal function. This uncontrolled proliferation of the immature cells in the bone marrow affects the production of the normal red blood cells and platelets as well.

Acute leukemias are of two types: acute lymphocytic leukemia and acute myelogenous leukemia. Different types of white blood cells are involved in the two leukemias. In acute lymphocytic leukemia (ALL), it is the T or the B lymphocytes that become cancerous. The B cell leukemias are more common than T cell leukemias. Acute myelogenous leukemia, also known as acute nonlymphocytic leukemia (ANLL), is a cancer of the monocytes and/or granulocytes.

Leukemias account for 2% of all cancers. Because leukemia is the most common form of childhood cancer, it is often regarded as a disease of childhood. However, leukemias affect nine times as many adults as children. Half of the cases occur in people who are 60 years of age or older. The incidence of acute and chronic leukemias is about the same. According to the estimates of the American Cancer Society (ACS), approximately 29,000 new cases of leukemia will be diagnosed in 1998.

Causes & symptoms

Leukemia strikes both sexes and all ages. The human T-cell leukemia virus (HTLV-I) is believed to be the causative agent for some kinds of leukemias. However, the cause of most leukemias is not known. Acute lymphoid leukemia (ALL) is more common among Caucasians than among African-Americans, while acute myeloid leukemia (AML) affects both races equally. The

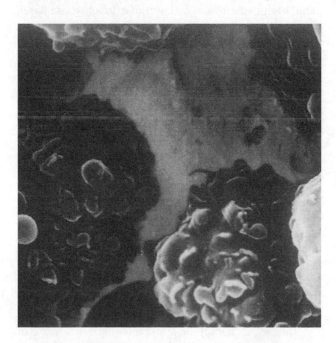

An enhanced scanning electron microscopy (SEM) image of acute myelogenous leukemia cells. *(Photograph by Robert Becker, Ph.D., Custom Medical Stock Photo. Reproduced by permission.)*

incidence of acute leukemia is slightly higher among men than women. People with Jewish ancestry have a higher likelihood of getting leukemia. A higher incidence of leukemia has also been observed among persons with **Down syndrome** and some other genetic abnormalities.

Exposure to ionizing radiation and to certain organic chemicals, such as benzene, is believed to increase the risk of getting leukemia. Having a history of diseases that damage the bone marrow, such as **aplastic anemia,** or a history of cancers of the lymphatic system puts people at a high risk for developing acute leukemias. Similarly, the use of anticancer medications, immunosuppressants, and the antibiotic chloramphenicol are also considered risk factors for developing acute leukemias.

The symptoms of leukemia are generally vague and non-specific. A patient may experience all or some of the following symptoms:

- Weakness or chronic fatigue
- **Fever of unknown origin**
- Weight loss that is not due to dieting or **exercise**
- Frequent bacterial or viral infections
- **Headaches**
- Skin rash
- Non-specific bone **pain**
- Easy bruising
- Bleeding from gums or nose
- Blood in urine or stools
- Enlarged lymph nodes and/or spleen
- Abdominal fullness.

Diagnosis

Like all cancers, acute leukemias are best treated when found early. There are no screening tests available.

If the doctor has reason to suspect leukemia, he or she will conduct a very thorough **physical examination** to look for enlarged lymph nodes in the neck, underarm, and pelvic region. Swollen gums, enlarged liver or spleen, **bruises,** or pinpoint red **rashes** all over the body are some of the signs of leukemia. Urine and blood tests may be ordered to check for microscopic amounts of blood in the urine and to obtain a complete differential **blood count.** This count will give the numbers and percentages of the different cells found in the blood. An abnormal blood test might suggest leukemia; however, the diagnosis has to be confirmed by more specific tests.

The doctor may perform a bone marrow biopsy to confirm the diagnosis of leukemia. During the biopsy, a cylindrical piece of bone and marrow is removed. The tissue is generally taken out of the hipbone. These sam-

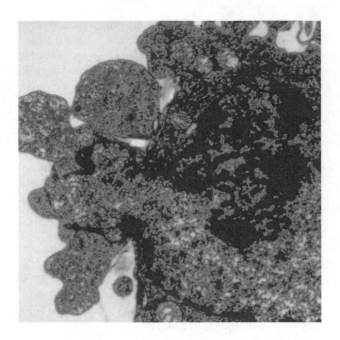

An enhanced transmission electron microscopy (TEM) image of acute myelogenous leukemia cells. *(Photograph by Robert Becker, Ph.D., Custom Medical Stock Photo. Reproduced by permission.)*

ples are sent to the laboratory for examination. In addition to diagnosis, the biopsy is also repeated during the treatment phase of the disease to see if the leukemia is responding to therapy.

A spinal tap (lumbar puncture) is another procedure that the doctor may order to diagnose leukemia. In this procedure, a small needle is inserted into the spinal cavity in the lower back to withdraw some cerebrospinal fluid and to look for leukemic cells.

Standard imaging tests, such as x rays, **computed tomography scans** (CT scans), and **magnetic resonance imaging** (MRI) may be used to check whether the leukemic cells have invaded other areas of the body, such as the bones, chest, kidneys, abdomen, or brain. A gallium scan or bone scan is a test in which a radioactive chemical is injected into the body. This chemical accumulates in the areas of cancer or infection, allowing them to be viewed with a special camera.

Treatment

There are two phases of treatment for leukemia. The first phase is called "induction therapy." As the name suggests, during this phase, the main aim of the treatment is to reduce the number of leukemic cells as far as possible and induce a remission in the patient. Once the patient shows no obvious signs of leukemia (no leukemic cells are detected in blood tests and bone marrow biopsies), the patient is said to be in remission. The

second phase of treatment is then initiated. This is called continuation or maintenance therapy, and the aim in this case is to kill any remaining cells and to maintain the remission for as long as possible.

Chemotherapy is the use of drugs to kill cancer cells. It is usually the treatment of choice and is used to relieve symptoms and achieve long-term remission of the disease. Generally, combination chemotherapy, in which multiple drugs are used, is more efficient than using a single drug for the treatment. Some drugs may be administered intravenously through a vein in the arm; others may be given by mouth in the form of pills. If the cancer cells have invaded the brain, then chemotherapeutic drugs may be put into the fluid that surrounds the brain through a needle in the brain or back. This is known as intrathecal chemotherapy.

Because leukemia cells can spread to all the organs via the blood stream and the lymph vessels, surgery is not considered an option for treating leukemias.

Radiation therapy, which involves the use of x rays or other high-energy rays to kill cancer cells and shrink tumors, may be used in some cases. For acute leukemias, the source of radiation is usually outside the body (external radiation therapy). If the leukemic cells have spread to the brain, radiation therapy can be given to the brain.

Bone marrow transplantation is a process in which the patient's diseased bone marrow is replaced with healthy marrow. There are two ways of doing a bone marrow transplant. In an allogeneic bone marrow transplant, healthy marrow is taken from a donor whose tissue is either the same as or very closely resembles the patient's tissues. The donor may be a twin, a brother or sister (sibling), or a person who is not related at all. First, the patient's bone marrow is destroyed with very high doses of chemotherapy and radiation therapy. Healthy marrow from the donor is then given to the patient through a needle in a vein to replace the destroyed marrow.

In the second type of bone marrow transplant, called an autologous bone marrow transplant, some of the patient's own marrow is taken out and treated with a combination of **anticancer drugs** to kill all the abnormal cells. This marrow is then frozen to save it. The marrow remaining in the patient's body is destroyed with high-dose chemotherapy and radiation therapy. The marrow that was frozen is then thawed and given back to the patient through a needle in a vein. This mode of bone marrow transplant is currently being investigated in clinical trials.

Biological therapy or immunotherapy is a mode of treatment in which the body's own immune system is harnessed to fight the cancer. Substances that are routinely made by the immune system (such as growth factors, hormones, and disease-fighting proteins) are either synthetically made in a laboratory or their effectiveness is boosted and they are then put back into the patient's body. This treatment mode is also being investigated in clinical trials all over the country at major cancer centers.

Prognosis

Like all cancers, the prognosis for leukemia depends on the patient's age and general health. According to statistics, more than 60% of the patients with leukemia survive for at least a year after diagnosis. Acute myelocytic leukemia (AML) has a poorer prognosis rate than acute lymphocytic leukemias (ALL) and the chronic leukemias. In the last 15 to 20 years, the five-year survival rate for patients with ALL has increased from 38% to 57%.

Interestingly enough, since most childhood leukemias are of the ALL type, chemotherapy has been highly successful in their treatment. This is because chemotherapeutic drugs are most effective against actively growing cells. Due to the new combinations of anticancer drugs being used, the survival rates among children with ALL have improved dramatically. Eighty percent of the children diagnosed with ALL now survive for five years or more, as compared to 50% in the late 1970s.

Prevention

Most cancers can be prevented by changes in lifestyle or diet, which will reduce the risk factors. However, in leukemias, there are no such known risk factors. Therefore, at the present time, no way is known to prevent leukemias from developing. People who are at an increased risk for developing leukemia because of proven exposure to ionizing radiation or exposure to the toxic liquid benzene, and people with Down syndrome, should undergo periodic medical checkups.

Resources

BOOKS

Berkow, Robert, et al., eds. *Merck Manual of Diagnosis and Therapy*, 16th ed. Merck Research Laboratories, 1992.

Dollinger, Malin. *Everyone's Guide to Cancer Therapy.* Somerville House Books Limited, 1994.

Morra, Marion E. *Choices.* Avon Books, 1994.

Murphy, Gerald P. *Informed Decisions: The Complete Book of Cancer Diagnosis, Treatment and Recovery.* American Cancer Society, 1997.

ORGANIZATIONS

American Cancer Society. 1599 Clifton Road, N.E., Atlanta, Georgia 30329. (800) 227-2345. http://www.cancer.org.

Cancer Research Institute. 681 Fifth Avenue, New York, N.Y. 10022. (800) 992-2623. http://www.cancerresearch.org.

Leukemia Society of America, Inc. 600 Third Avenue, New York, NY 10016. (800) 955-4572. http://www.leukemia.org.

National Cancer Institute. 9000 Rockville Pike, Building 31, Room 10A16, Bethesda, Maryland, 20892. (800) 422-6237. http://wwwicic.nci.nih.gov.

Oncolink. University of Pennsylvania Cancer Center. http://cancer.med.upenn.edu

Lata Cherath

Leukemias, chronic

Definition

Chronic leukemia is a disease in which too many white blood cells are made in the bone marrow. Depending on the type of white blood cell that is involved, chronic leukemia can be classified as chronic lymphocytic leukemia or chronic myeloid leukemia.

Description

Chronic leukemia is a **cancer** that starts in the blood cells made in the bone marrow. The bone marrow is the spongy tissue found in the large bones of the body. The bone marrow makes precursor cells called ''blasts'' or ''stem cells'' that mature into different types of blood cells. Unlike **acute leukemias,** in which the process of maturation of the blast cells is interrupted, in chronic leukemias, the cells do mature and only a few remain as immature cells. However, even though the cells appear normal, they do not function as normal cells.

The different types of cells that are produced in the bone marrow are red blood cells (RBCs), which carry oxygen and other materials to all tissues of the body; white blood cells (WBCs), which fight infection; and platelets, which play a part in the clotting of the blood. The white blood cells can be further subdivided into three main types: the granulocytes, monocytes, and the lymphocytes.

The granulocytes, as their name suggests, have granules (particles) inside them. These granules contain special proteins (enzymes) and several other substances that can break down chemicals and destroy microorganisms such as bacteria.

Monocytes are the second type of white blood cell. They are also important in defending the body against pathogens.

The lymphocytes form the third type of white blood cell. There are two main types of lymphocytes: T lymphocytes and B lymphocytes. They have different functions within the immune system. The B cells protect the body by making "antibodies." Antibodies are proteins that can attach to the surfaces of bacteria and viruses. This attachment sends signals to many other cell types to come and destroy the antibody-coated organism. The T cell protects the body against viruses. When a virus enters a cell, it produces certain proteins that are projected onto the surface of the infected cell. The T cells can recognize these proteins and produce certain chemicals (cytokines) that are capable of destroying the virus-infected cells. In addition, the T cells can destroy some types of cancer cells.

Chronic leukemias develop very gradually. The abnormal lymphocytes multiply slowly, but in a poorly regulated manner. They live much longer and thus their numbers build up in the body. The two types of chronic leukemias can be easily distinguished under the microscope. Chronic lymphocytic leukemia (CLL) involves the T or B lymphocytes. B cell abnormalities are more common than T cell abnormalities. T cells are affected in only 5% of the patients. The T and B lymphocytes can be differentiated from the other types of white blood cells based on their size and by the absence of granules inside them. In chronic myelogenous leukemia (CML), the cells that are affected are the granulocytes.

Chronic lymphocytic leukemia (CLL) often has no symptoms at first and may remain undetected for a long time. Chronic myelogenous leukemia (CML), on the other hand, may progress to a more acute form.

Chronic leukemias account for 1.2% of all cancers. Because leukemia is the most common form of childhood cancer, it is often regarded as a disease of childhood. However, leukemias affect nine times as many adults as children. In chronic lymphoid leukemia, 90% of the cases are seen in people who are 50 years or older, with the average age at diagnosis being 65. The incidence of the disease increases with age. It is almost never seen in children. Chronic myeloid leukemias are generally seen in people in their mid-40s. It accounts for about 4% of childhood leukemia cases. According to the estimates of the American Cancer Society (ACS), approximately 29,000 new cases of leukemia will be diagnosed in 1998.

Causes & symptoms

Leukemia strikes both sexes and all ages. Although the cause is unknown, chronic leukemia is linked to genetic abnormalities and environmental factors. For example, exposure to ionizing radiation and to certain organic chemicals, such as benzene, is believed to increase the risks for getting leukemia. Chronic leukemia occurs in some people who are infected with two human retroviruses (HTLV-I and HTLV-II). An abnormal chromosome known as the Philadelphia chromosome is seen in 90% of those with CML. The incidence of chronic leukemia is slightly higher among men than women.

The symptoms of chronic leukemia are generally vague and non-specific. In chronic lymphoid leukemia (CLL), a patient may experience all or some of the following symptoms:

- Swollen lymph nodes
- An enlarged spleen, which could make the patient complain of abdominal fullness
- Chronic fatigue

- A general feeling of ill-health
- **Fever of unknown origin**
- Night sweats
- Weight loss that is not due to dieting or **exercise**
- Frequent bacterial or viral infections.

In the early stages of chronic myeloid leukemia (CML), the symptoms are more or less similar to CLL. In the later stages of the disease, the patient may experience these symptoms:

- Non-specific bone **pain**
- Bleeding problems
- Mucus membrane irritation
- Frequent infections
- A pale color due to a low red blood cell count (anemia)
- Swollen lymph glands
- **Fever**
- Night sweats.

Diagnosis

There are no screening tests available for chronic leukemias. The detection of these diseases may occur by chance during a routine **physical examination.**

If the doctor has reason to suspect leukemia, he or she will conduct a very thorough physical examination to look for enlarged lymph nodes in the neck, underarm, and pelvic region. Swollen gums, an enlarged liver or spleen, **bruises,** or pinpoint red **rashes** all over the body are some of the signs of leukemia. Urine and blood tests may be ordered to check for microscopic amounts of blood in the urine and to obtain a complete differential **blood count.** This count will give the numbers and percentages of the different cells found in the blood. An abnormal blood test might suggest leukemia; however, the diagnosis has to be confirmed by more specific tests.

The doctor may perform a bone marrow biopsy to confirm the diagnosis of leukemia. During the bone marrow biopsy, a cylindrical piece of bone and marrow is removed. The tissue is generally taken out of the hipbone. These samples are sent to the laboratory for examination. In addition to diagnosis, bone marrow biopsy is also done during the treatment phase of the disease to see if the leukemia is responding to therapy.

Standard imaging tests such as x rays, **computed tomography scans** (CT scans), and **magnetic resonance imaging** (MRI) may be used to check whether the leukemic cells have invaded other organs of the body, such as the bones, chest, kidneys, abdomen, or brain.

Treatment

The treatment depends on the specific type of chronic leukemia and its stage. In general, **chemotherapy** is the standard approach to both CLL and CML. **Radiation therapy** is occasionally used. Because leukemia cells can spread to all the organs via the blood stream and the lymph vessels, surgery is not considered an option for treating leukemias.

Bone marrow transplantation (BMT) is becoming the treatment of choice for CML because it has the possibility of curing the illness. BMT is generally not considered an option in treating CLL because CLL primarily affects older people, who are not considered to be good candidates for the procedure.

In BMT, the patient's diseased bone marrow is replaced with healthy marrow. There are two ways of doing a bone marrow transplant. In an allogeneic bone marrow transplant, healthy marrow is taken from another person (donor) whose tissue is either the same or very closely resembles the patient's tissues. The donor may be a twin, a sibling, or a person who is not related at all. First, the patient's bone marrow is destroyed with very high doses of chemotherapy and radiation therapy. To replace the destroyed marrow, healthy marrow from the donor is given to the patient through a needle in the vein.

In the second type of bone marrow transplant, called an autologous bone marrow transplant, some of the patient's own marrow is taken out and treated with a combination of **anticancer drugs** to kill all the abnormal cells. This marrow is then frozen to save it. The marrow remaining in the patient's body is then destroyed with high dose chemotherapy and radiation therapy. Following that, the patient's own marrow that was frozen is thawed and given back to the patient through a needle in the vein. This mode of bone marrow transplant is currently being investigated in clinical trials.

In chronic lymphoid leukemia (CLL), chemotherapy is generally the treatment of choice. Depending on the stage of the disease, single or multiple drugs may be given. Drugs commonly prescribed include steroids, chlorambucil, fludarabine, and cladribine. Low dose radiation therapy may be given to the whole body, or it may be used to alleviate the symptoms and discomfort due to an enlarged spleen and lymph nodes. The spleen may be removed in a procedure called a **splenectomy.**

In chronic myeloid leukemia (CML), the treatment of choice is bone marrow transplantation. During the slow progress (chronic phase) of the disease, chemotherapy may be given to try to improve the cell counts. Radiation therapy, which involves the use of x rays or other high-energy rays to kill cancer cells and shrink tumors, may be used in some cases to reduce the discomfort and pain due to an enlarged spleen. For chronic leukemias, the source of radiation is usually outside the body (external radiation therapy). If the leukemic cells have spread to the brain, radiation therapy can be directed at the brain. As the disease progresses, the spleen may be removed in an attempt to try to control the pain and to improve the blood counts.

In the acute phase of CML, aggressive chemotherapy is given. Combination chemotherapy, in which multiple drugs are used, is more efficient than using a single drug for the treatment. The drugs may either be administered intravenously through a vein in the arm or by mouth in the form of pills. If the cancer cells have invaded the central nervous system (CNS), chemotherapeutic drugs may be put into the fluid that surrounds the brain through a needle in the brain or back. This is known as intrathecal chemotherapy.

Biological therapy or immunotherapy is a mode of treatment in which the body's own immune system is harnessed to fight the cancer. Substances that are routinely made by the immune system (such as growth factors, hormones, and disease-fighting proteins) are either synthetically made in a laboratory, or their effectiveness is boosted and they are then put back into the patient's body. This treatment mode is also being investigated in clinical trials all over the country at major cancer centers.

Prognosis

The prognosis for leukemia depends on the patient's age and general health. According to statistics, in chronic lymphoid leukemia, the overall survival for all stages of the disease is nine years. Most of the **deaths** in people with CLL are due to infections or other illnesses that occur as a result of the leukemia.

In CML, if bone marrow transplantation is performed within one to three years of diagnosis, 50-60% of the patients survive three years or more. If the disease progresses to the acute phase, the prognosis is poor. Less than 20% of these patients go into remission.

Prevention

Most cancers can be prevented by changes in lifestyle or diet, which will reduce the risk factors. However, in leukemias, there are no known risk factors. Therefore, at the present time, there is no way known to prevent the leukemias from developing. People who are at an increased risk for developing leukemia because of proven exposure to ionizing radiation, the organic liquid benzene, or people who have a history of other cancers of the lymphoid system (Hodgkin's lymphoma) should undergo periodic medical checkups.

Resources

BOOKS

Berkow, Robert, et al., eds. *Merck Manual of Diagnosis and Therapy*, 16th ed. Merck Research Laboratories, 1992.

Dollinger, Malin. *Everyone's Guide to Cancer Therapy.* Somerville House Books Limited, 1994.

Morra, Marion E. *Choices*. Avon Books, 1994.

Murphy, Gerald P. *Informed Decisions: The Complete Book of Cancer Diagnosis, Treatment and Recovery.* American Cancer Society, 1997.

ORGANIZATIONS

American Cancer Society. 1599 Clifton Road, N.E., Atlanta, Georgia 30329. (800) 227-2345. http://www.cancer.org.

Cancer Research Institute. 681 Fifth Avenue, New York, N.Y. 10022. (800) 992-2623. http://www.cancerresearch.org.

Leukemia Society of America, Inc. 600 Third Avenue, New York, NY 10016. (800) 955 4572. http://www.leukemia.org.

National Cancer Institute. 9000 Rockville Pike, Building 31, Room 10A16, Bethesda, Maryland, 20892. (800) 422-6237. http://wwwicic.nci.nih.gov.

Oncolink. University of Pennsylvania Cancer Center. http://cancer.med.upenn.edu.

Lata Cherath

Leukocytosis

Definition

Leukocytosis is a condition characterized by an elevated number of white cells in the blood.

Description

Leukocytosis is a condition that affects all types of white blood cells. Other illnesses, such as neutrophilia, lymphocytosis, and granulocytosis, target specific types of white blood cells. Normal white blood cell counts are 4,300-10,800 white blood cells per microliter. Leukocyte or white blood cell levels are considered elevated when they are between 15,000-20,000 per microliter. The increased number of leukocytes can occur abnormally as a result of an infection, **cancer,** or drug intake; however, leukocytosis can occur normally after eating a large meal or experiencing **stress.**

Causes & symptoms

Leukemias can cause white blood cell counts to increase to as much as 100,000. Each kind of white cell can produce a leukemia. Apart from leukemias, nearly all

KEY TERMS

Biopsy—Surgical removal of tissue for examination.

Inflammation—Heat, swelling, redness, and pain caused by tissue injury.

Ketoacidosis—A severe stage of diabetes where acids and ketones accumulate in the body.

NSAID—Non-steroidal anti-inflammatory drug such as ibuprofen.

leukocytosis is due to one type of white blood cell, the polymorphonuclear leukocyte (PMN). These conditions are more accurately referred to as neutrophilia.

The most common and important cause of neutrophilia is infection, and most infections cause neutrophilia. The degree of elevation often indicates the severity of the infection. Tissue damage from other causes raises the white count for similar reasons. **Burns,** infarction (cutting off the blood supply to a region of the body so that it dies), crush injuries, inflammatory diseases, **poisonings,** and severe diseases, like kidney failure and diabetic ketoacidosis, all cause neutrophilia.

Counts almost as high occur in leukemoid (leukemia-like) reactions caused by infection and non-infectious inflammation.

Drugs can also cause leukocytosis. Cortisone-like drugs (prednisone), lithium, and NSAIDs are the most common offenders.

Non-specific stresses also cause white blood cells to increase in the blood. Extensive testing of medical students reveals that neutrophilia accompanies every examination. Vigorous **exercise** and intense excitement also cause elevated white blood cell counts.

Diagnosis

A complete **blood count** (CBC) is one of the first tests obtained in any medical setting. More than 11,000 white cells in a cubic millimeter of blood is considered high. Bone marrow biopsy may help clarify the cause.

Treatment

Relieving the underlying cause returns the count to normal.

Prognosis

By treating the underlying condition, white blood cell counts usually return to normal

Resources

BOOKS

Baehner, Robert L. "Neutrophilia." In *Nelson Textbook of Pediatrics,* edited by Waldo E. Nelson, et al. Philadelphia: W. B. Saunders, 1996.

Bennett, J. Claude and Fred Plum, ed. "Leukocytosis and Leukemoid Reactions." In *Cecil Textbook of Medicine* Philadelphia: W. B. Saunders, 1996.

Dale, David C. "Neutrophilia." In *Williams Hematology,* edited by Ernest Beutler, et al. New York: McGraw-Hill, Inc. 1995.

Holland, Steven M. and John I. Gallin. "Disorders of granulocytes and monocytes." In *Harrison's Principles of Internal Medicine,* edited by Kurt Isselbacher, et al. New York: McGraw-Hill, 1998.

J. Ricker Polsdorfer

Levodopa *see* **Antiparkinson drugs**

Levofloxacin *see* **Fluoroquinolones**

Levothyroxine *see* **Thyroid hormones**

LGV *see* **Lymphogranuloma venereum**

Lice infestation

Definition

Lice infestations (pediculosis) are infections of the skin, hair, or genital region caused by lice living directly on the body or in hats or other garments. Lice are small wingless insect-like parasites with sucking mouthparts that feed on human blood and lay their eggs on body hairs or in clothing. The name pediculosis comes from the Latin word for louse (singular) or lice (plural).

Description

Lice infestations are not dangerous infections by themselves. It is, however a serious public health problem because some lice can carry organisms that cause other diseases, including **relapsing fever, trench fever,** and epidemic **typhus.** Although trench fever is self-limiting, the other two diseases have mortality rates of 5%-10%. Pubic lice are often associated with other **sexually transmitted diseases** (STDs) but do not spread them.

Lice infestations are frequent occurrences in areas of overcrowding or inadequate facilities for bathing and laundry. They are often associated with homelessness in the general population or with military, refugee, or prisoner camps in war-torn areas. All humans are equally susceptible to louse infestation; the elderly, however, are more vulnerable to typhus and other diseases carried by lice.

Causes & symptoms

The symptoms of lice infestations vary somewhat according to body location, although all are characterized by intense **itching,** usually with injury to the skin caused

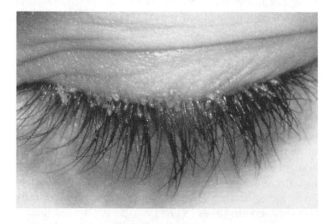

This woman's eyelashes are infested with nits, or eggs, of a body louse. *(Custom Medical Stock Photo. Reproduced by permission.)*

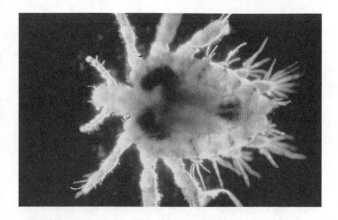

A close-up view of a body louse. *(Custom Medical Stock Photo. Reproduced by permission.)*

by scratching or scraping. The itching is an allergic reaction to a toxin in the saliva of the lice. Repeated bites can lead to a generalized skin eruption or inflammation.

Head lice

This type of infestation is caused by *Pediculosis humanus capitis*, the head louse. Head lice can be transmitted from one person to another by the sharing of hats, combs, or hair brushes. Epidemics of head lice are common among school-age children from all class backgrounds in all parts of the United States. The head louse is about 1/16 of an inch in length. The adult form may be visible on the patient's scalp, especially around the ears; or its grayish-white nits (eggs) may be visible at the base of the hairs close to the scalp. It takes between three and 14 days for the nits to hatch. After the nits hatch, the louse must feed on blood within a day or die.

Head lice can spread from the scalp to the eyebrows, eyelashes, and beard in adults, although they are more often limited to the scalp in children. The itching may be intense, and may be followed by bacterial infection of skin that has been scratched open. Another common complication is swelling or inflammation of the neck glands. Head lice do not spread typhus or other systemic diseases.

Body lice

Infestations of body lice are caused by *Pediculosis humanus corporis*, an organism that is similar in size to head lice. Body lice, however, are rarely seen on the skin itself because they come to the skin only to feed. They should be looked for in the seams of the patient's clothing. This type of infestation is associated by wearing the same clothing for long periods of time without laundering, as may happen in wartime or in cold climates; or with poor personal hygiene. It can be spread by close personal contact or shared bedding.

Patients with body lice often have intense itching with deep scratches around the upper shoulders, flanks, or neck. The bites first appear as small red pimples but may cause a generalized skin rash. If the infestation is not treated, the patient may develop complications that include **headache, fever,** and bacterial infection with scarring. Body lice can spread systemic typhus or other infections.

Pubic lice

Pubic lice are sometimes called "crabs." This type of infestation is caused by *Phthirus pubis* and is commonly spread by intimate contact. People can also get public lice from using the bedding, towels, or clothes of an infected person.

Pubic lice usually appear first on pubic hair, but may spread to other parts of the body, particularly if the patient is very hairy. Pubic lice are also sometimes seen on the eyelashes of children born to infected mothers. It is usually easier for the doctor to see marks from the patient's scratching than the bites from the lice, but pubic lice sometimes produce small bluish spots called maculae ceruleae on the patient's trunk or thighs. Pubic lice also sometimes leave small dark brown specks from their own excreted matter on the parts of the patient's underwear that cover the anal or genital areas.

Diagnosis

Doctors can diagnose lice infestations from looking closely at the parts of the body where the patient has been scratching. Lice are large enough to be easily seen with the naked eye or a magnifying glass. The eggs of pubic lice as well as head lice can often be found by looking at the base of the patient's hairs. Pediatricians are most likely to diagnose lice in school-age children.

It is important for doctors to rule out other diseases that can cause scratching and skin inflammation because the medications used to kill lice are very strong and can have bothersome side effects. The doctor will need to distinguish between head lice and dandruff; between body lice and **scabies** (a disease caused by skin mites); and between pubic lice and eczema. Blood tests or other laboratory tests are not useful in diagnosing lice infestations.

Treatment

Lice infestations are treated with externally applied medications that either kill the lice or prevent them from feeding. Cases of head lice are usually treated with shampoos or rinses containing either lindane (Kwell) or permethrin (Nix). Because lindane is absorbed through the skin, the person giving the application should wear rubber gloves and rinse the patient's hair or body completely after use. Following the treatment, nits should be removed from the hair with a fine-toothed comb or tweezers. Lindane is also effective for treating infestations of body or pubic lice, but it should not be used by pregnant women. In most cases one treatment is sufficient, but the medication can be reapplied a week later if living lice have reappeared.

Infestations of body lice can also be treated by washing the patient's clothes or bedding in boiling water, ironing seams with an iron on a high setting, or treating the clothes with 1% malathion powder or 10% DDT powder.

If the patient's eyelashes have been infested, the only safe treatments are either a thick coating of petroleum jelly (Vaseline) applied twice daily for eight days, or 1% yellow oxide of mercury applied four times a day for two weeks. Any remaining nits should be removed with tweezers.

Patients with pubic lice should be examined and tested for other STDs.

Alternative treatment

For pubic lice, some practitioners of holistic medicine recommend a mixture of 25% oil of pennyroyal (*Mentha pulegium*), 25% garlic (*Allium sativum*) oil, and 50% distilled water applied three times in a three-day period, followed by removal of dormant eggs to prevent reinfestation.

Prognosis

Lice can be successfully eradicated in almost all cases, although some cases of lindane-resistant lice have been reported. In general, patients are more at risk from typhus and other diseases spread by lice than from the lice themselves.

Prevention

There are no vaccines or skin treatments that will protect a person against lice prior to contact. In addition, lice infestation does not provide immunity against reinfection; recurrences are in fact quite common. Prevention depends on adequate personal hygiene at the individual level and the following public health measures:

• Teaching school-age children the basics of good personal hygiene, including the importance of not lending or borrowing combs, brushes, or hats.

• Notifying and treating an adult patient's close personal and sexual contacts.

• Examining homeless people, elderly patients incapable of self-care, and other high-risk individuals prior to hospital admission for signs of louse infestation. This measure is necessary to protect other hospitalized people from the spread of lice.

Resources

BOOKS

Berger, Timothy G. "Skin & Appendages." In *Current Medical Diagnosis & Treatment 1998,* edited by Lawrence M. Tierney, Jr., et al. Stamford, CT: Appleton & Lange, 1997.

"Dermatologic Disorders: Parasitic Infections of the Skin." In *The Merck Manual of Diagnosis and Therapy,* edited by Robert Berkow, et al. Rahway, NJ: Merck Research Laboratories, 1992.

"Lindane." In *Nurses Drug Guide 1995,* edited by Billie Ann Wilson, et al. Norwalk, CT: Appleton & Lange, 1995.

McCarthy, James S., and Thomas B. Nutman "Parasitic Diseases of the Skin." In *Conn's Current Therapy,* edited by Robert E. Rakel. Philadelphia: W. B. Saunders Company, 1997.

Millikin, Larry E. "Flies, Lice, Mites, and Bites." In *Current Diagnosis 9,* edited by Rex B. Conn, et al. Philadelphia: W. B. Saunders Company, 1997.

Morelli, Joseph G., and William L. Weston. "Skin." In *Current Pediatric Diagnosis & Treatment,* edited by William W. Hay, Jr., et al. Stamford, CT: Appleton & Lange, 1997.

"Permethrin." In *Nurses Drug Guide 1995,* edited by Billie Ann Wilson, et al. Norwalk, CT: Appleton & Lange, 1995.

Rebecca J. Frey

Lichen planus

Definition

Lichen planus is a skin condition of unknown origin that produces small, shiny, flat-topped, itchy pink or purple raised spots on the wrists, forearms or lower legs, especially in middle-aged patients.

Description

Lichen planus affects between 1-2% of the population, most of whom are middle-aged women. The condition is less common in the very young and the very old. The lesions are found on the skin, genitals, and in the mouth. Most cases resolve spontaneously within two years. Lichen planus is found throughout the world and is equally distributed among races.

Causes & symptoms

No one knows what causes lichen planus, although some experts suspect that it is an abnormal immune reaction following a viral infection, probably aggravated by **stress.** The condition is similar to symptoms caused by exposure to arsenic, bismuth, gold, or developers used in color photography. Occasionally, lichen planus in the mouth appears to be an allergic reaction to medications, filling material, dental hygiene products, chewing gum or candy.

Symptoms can appear suddenly, or they may gradually develop, usually on the arms or legs. The lesions on the skin may be preceded by a dryness and metallic taste or burning in the mouth.

Once the lesions appear, they change over time into flat, glistening, purple lesions marked with white lines or spots. Mild to severe **itching** is common. White, lacy lesions are usually painless, but eroded lesions often burn and can be painful. As the lesions clear up, they usually leave a brown discoloration behind, especially in dark skinned people.

Lichen planus in the mouth occurs in six different forms with a variety of symptoms, appearing as lacy-white streaks, white plaques, or eroded ulcers. Often the gums are affected, so that the surface of the gum peels off, leaving the gums red and raw.

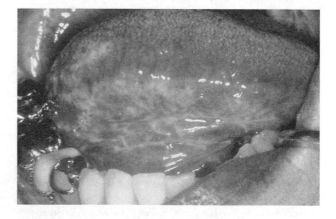

Lichen planus appearing under the tongue. *(Custom Medical Stock Photo. Reproduced by permission.)*

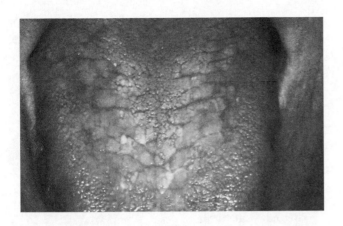

One example of lichen planus on the tongue. *(Custom Medical Stock Photo. Reproduced by permission.)*

Diagnosis

A doctor can probably diagnose the condition simply from looking at the characteristic lesions, but a **skin biopsy** may be needed to confirm the diagnosis.

Treatment

Treatment is aimed at easing symptoms. Itching can be treated with steroid creams and oral **antihistamines.** Severe lesions can be treated with **corticosteroids** by mouth, or combinations of photochemotherapy (PUVA) and griseofulvin.

Patients with lesions in the mouth may find that regular professional cleaning of the teeth and conscientious dental care improve the condition. Using milder toothpastes instead of tartar control products also seems to lessen the number of ulcers and makes them less sensitive.

Prognosis

While lichen planus can be annoying, it is usually fairly benign and clears up on its own. It may take months to reach its peak, but it usually clears up within 18 months.

Resources

BOOKS

Olbricht, Suzanne, Michael E. Bigby, and Kenneth Arndt. *Manual of Clinical Problems in Dermatology.* Boston: Little, Brown and Co., 1992.

PERIODICALS

Burkhart, N. W., E. J. Burkes, and E. J. Burker. "Meeting the Educational Needs of Patients with Oral Lichen Planus." *General Dentistry.* 45 (1997): 126-132.

OTHER

Lichen Planus Self-Help. http://www.tambcd.edu/lichen/lichen.htm.

Carol A. Turkington

Lichen simplex chronicus

Definition

Lichen simplex chronicus is a chronic inflammation of the skin (dermatitis) characterized by small, round itchy spots that thicken and become leathery as a result of scratching.

Description

Also termed neurodermatis, **lichen simplex** chronicus is the result of chronic skin irritation. It occurs in 4-5 out of every thousand people. Initial irritation causes **itching,** and in turn, itching causes scratching. Scratching leads to further irritation, which damages the skin. The possibility of infection is greatly increased when the outer layer of protective skin is broken. Skin usually repairs itself quickly; however, in the case of lichen simplex chronicus, healing skin causes more itching and more scratching causes a thickening of the skin (lichen). The small skin patches are usually 1–10 in (2.54–25.4 cm) in diameter.

Causes & symptoms

Lichen simplex chronicus is often caused by constant rubbing of the skin. The rubbing begins the chain of events that leads from itching to scratching and then to the presence of leather-like skin patches.

Symptoms are chronic itching which is often accompanied by nervous tension. The appearance of scratch marks and the leathery skin patches can be found anywhere on the body. A prolonged lichen simplex chronicus can result in brown-colored pigmentation at the site of irritation.

Diagnosis

A dermatologist, a physician specializing in the study and treatment of skin disorders, can make a diagnosis after a visual exam.

Treatment

Treatment of the itching is necessary to stop the scratching and resulting skin damage. There are a number of ways to stop itching. Perhaps the most important is to cut fingernails very short. Ice can substitute for the relief of scratching. Heat and fuzzy clothing worsen itching; cold and smooth clothing pacify it. If the itching is persistent, dressings may be applied to the affected areas.

Among the topical medications that relieve itching are a number of commercial preparations containing menthol, camphor, eucalyptus oil, and aloe. Topical cortisone is also available without a prescription. Some preparations also contain **antihistamines,** which penetrate intact skin poorly. All these medicines work better under occlusion, which means putting a waterproof barrier like a rubber glove or plastic wrap over them. For broken skin, **topical antibiotics** like bacitracin help prevent infection. These should be used early to forestall further damage to the skin.

Reducing the buildup of thick skin may require medicines that dissolve or melt keratin, the major chemical in skin's outer layer. These keratolytics include urea, lactic acid, and salicylic acid.

Resistant cases of lichen simplex chronicus will often respond to cortisone-like drugs injected directly into the lesions.

Sedatives or tranquilizers may be prescribed to combat the nervous tension and anxiety that often accompanies the condition.

Prognosis

Diligent adherence to treatment is usually rewarded with a resolution of the condition. The original cause of itching may be gone, or it may reappear. Preventive treatment in its early stages will arrest the process.

Prevention

Early, gentler substitutes for scratching can entirely prevent lichen simplex chronicus.

Resources

BOOKS

Habif, Thomas P. "Lichen Simplex Chronicus." In *Clinical Dermatology: A Color Guide to Diagnosis and Therapy.* St. Louis, MO: Mosby, 1995.

Parker, Frank. "Skin Diseases of General Importance." *Cecil Textbook of Medicine,* edited by J. Claude Bennett and Fred Plum. Philadelphia: W. B. Saunders, 1996.

Swerlick, Robert A. and Thomas J. Lawley. "Eczema, Psoriasis, Cutaneous Infections, Acne, and Other Common Skin Disorders." In *Harrison's Principles of Internal Medicine,* edited by Kurt Isselbacher, et al. New York: McGraw-Hill, 1998.

J. Ricker Polsdorfer

Lidocaine *see* **Antiarrhythmic drugs**

Light sensitivity *see* **Photosensitivity**

Light therapy *see* **Phototherapy**

Light treatment *see* **Ultraviolet light treatment**

Limb-girdle dystrophy *see* **Muscular dystrophy**

Lipase test

Definition

The lipase test is a blood test performed to determine the serum level of a specific protein (enzyme) involved in digestion. Lipase is an enzyme produced by the pancreas, which is a large gland situated near the stomach. Lipase works to break down a certain type of blood lipid (triglycerides) into fatty acids.

Lipase appears in the blood together with another enzyme called amylase following damage to or diseases affecting the pancreas. It was once thought that abnormally high lipase levels were associated only with diseases of the pancreas. Other conditions are now known to be associated with high lipase levels, especially kidney failure and intestinal obstruction. Diseases involving the pancreas, however, produce much higher lipase levels than diseases of other organs. Lipase levels in pancreatic disorders are often 5-10 times higher than normal.

Purpose

The lipase test is most often used in evaluating inflammation of the pancreas (**pancreatitis**), but it is also useful in diagnosing kidney failure, intestinal obstruction, **mumps,** and peptic **ulcers.** Doctors often order amylase and lipase tests at the same time to help distinguish pancreatitis from ulcers and other disorders in the abdomen. If the patient has acute (sudden onset) pancreatitis, the lipase level usually rises somewhat later than the amylase level—about 24-48 hours after onset of symptoms—and remains abnormally high for 5-7 days. Because the lipase level peaks later and remains elevated longer, its determination is more useful in late diagnosis of acute pancreatitis. Conversely, however, lipase levels are not as useful in diagnosing chronic pancreatic disease.

Precautions

Patients should be asked whether they are taking certain prescription drugs that can affect the accuracy of the lipase test. Drugs that can cause elevated lipase levels include bethanechol, cholinergics, codeine, indomethacin, meperidine, methacholine, and morphine. Drugs that may decrease levels include calcium ions.

Description

A lipase test is performed on a sample of the patient's blood, withdrawn from a vein into a vacuum tube. The procedure, which is called a venipuncture, takes about five minutes.

Preparation

The patient should have nothing to eat or drink for 12 hours before the lipase test.

Risks

Risks for this test are minimal, but may include slight bleeding from the puncture site, a small bruise or swelling in the area, **fainting,** or feeling lightheaded.

Normal results

Reference values for lipase determination are laboratory- and method-specific. In general, normal results are usually less than 200 units/L (triolein methods by titration or turbidimetry).

Abnormal results

Increased lipase levels are found in acute pancreatitis, chronic relapsing pancreatitis, and **pancreatic cancer.** High lipase levels also occur in certain liver diseases, kidney failure, bowel obstruction, peptic ulcer disease, and tumors or inflammation of the salivary glands.

Resources

BOOKS

Handbook of Diagnostic Tests, edited by Matthew Cahill. Springhouse, PA: Springhouse Corporation, 1995.

Jacobs, David S. *Laboratory Test Handbook,* Fourth Edition. Hudson, OH: Lexi-Comp Inc., 1996.

Mosby's Diagnostic and Laboratory Test Reference, edited by Kathleen Deska Pagana and Timothy James Pagana. St. Louis: Mosby-Year Book, Inc., 1998.

Janis O. Flores

Lipidoses

Definition

Lipidoses are heredity disorders, passed from parents to their children, characterized by defects of the digestive system that impair the way the body uses fat from the diet. When the body is unable to properly digest fats, lipids accumulate in body tissues in abnormal amounts.

KEY TERMS

Amniocentesis—A procedure where a needle is inserted through the abdomen into the uterus of a pregnant woman to remove a small amount of the fluid that surrounds the developing fetus. This test can be preformed at about week 16 of the pregnancy. Cells from the fetus can be tested for genetic defects.

Chorionic villi sampling—A procedure to remove a small tissue sample of the placenta, the sac that surrounds the developing fetus. This test can be performed as early as week 10 of the pregnancy. The tissue can be tested for genetic defects.

Lipids—Organic compounds not soluble in water, but soluble in fat solvents such as alcohol. Lipids are stored in the body as energy reserves and are also important components of cell membranes.

Recessive—Refers to an inherited characteristic or trait that is expressed only when two copies of the gene responsible for it are present.

X-linked—Refers to a gene carried on the X chromosome, one of the two sex chromosomes.

Description

The digestion, storage, and use of fats from foods is a complex process that involves hundreds of chemical reactions in the body. In most people, the body is already programmed by its genetic code to produce all of the enzymes and chemicals necessary to carry out these functions. These genetic instructions are passed from parents to their offspring during reproduction.

People with lipidoses are born without the genetic codes needed to tell their bodies how to complete a particular part of the fat digestion process. In most of these disorders, the body does not produce a certain enzyme or chemical. Over 30 different disorders of fat metabolism are related to genetic defects. Although the defects are passed from parents to children, the parents often do not have the disorders themselves.

The symptoms, available treatments, and long-term consequences of these conditions vary greatly. Some of the conditions become apparent shortly after the infant is born; in others, symptoms may not develop until adulthood. For most of the lipidoses, diagnosis is suspected based on the symptoms and family history. Blood tests, urine tests, and tissue tests can be used to confirm the diagnosis. **Genetic testing** can be used, in some cases, to identify the defective gene. Some of these disorders can be controlled with changes in the diet, medications, or enzyme supplements. For many, no treatment is available. Some may cause **death** in childhood or contribute to a shortened life expectancy. Some of the most common or most serious lipidoses are discussed below.

FABRY'S DISEASE

Causes & symptoms

Approximately 1 in every 40,000 males is born with Fabry's disease. This condition has an X-linked, recessive pattern of inheritance, meaning that the defective gene is carried on the X chromosome. A female who carries a defective recessive gene on one of her two X chromosomes has a 50% chance of passing the defective gene to her sons who will develop the disorder associated with the defective gene (a male receives one X chromosome from his mother and one Y chromosome from his father). She also has a 50% chance of passing the defective recessive gene to her daughters who will be carries of the disorder (like their mother). Some female carries of Fabry's disease show mild signs of the disorder, especially cloudiness of the cornea.

The gene that is defective in Fabry's disease causes a deficiency of the enzyme alpha-galactosidase A. Without this enzyme, fatty compounds starts to line the blood vessels. The collection of fatty deposits eventually affects blood vessels in the skin, heart, kidneys, and nervous system. The first symptoms in childhood are **pain** and discomfort in the hands and feet brought on by **exercise, fever, stress,** or changes in the weather. A raised rash of dark red-purple spots is common, especially on skin between the waistline and the knees. Other symptoms include a decreased ability to sweat and changes in the cornea or outer layer of the eye. Although the disease begins in childhood, it progresses very slowly. Kidney and heart problems develop in adulthood.

Diagnosis

The diagnosis can be confirmed by a blood test to measure for alpha-galactosidase A. Women who are carries of the defective gene can also be identified by a blood test.

Treatment

Treatment focuses on prevention of symptoms and long-term complications. Daily doses of diphenylhydantoin (Dilantin) or carbamazapine (Tegretol) can prevent or reduce the severity of pain in the hands and feet associated with the condition. A low sodium, low protein diet may be beneficial to those patients who have some kidney complications. If kidney problems progress, **kidney dialysis** or **kidney transplantation** may be required. Enzyme replacement therapy is currently being explored.

Prognosis

Although patients with Fabry's disease usually survive to adulthood, they are at increased risk for **stroke, heart attacks,** and kidney damage.

GAUCHER DISEASE

Causes & symptoms

Gaucher (pronounced go-shay) disease is the most common of the lipid storage disorders. It is found in populations all over the world (20,00 to 40,000 people have a type of the disease), and it occurs with equal frequency in males and females. **Gaucher disease** has a recessive pattern of inheritance, meaning that a person must inherit a copy of the defective gene from both parents in order to have the disease. The genetic defect causes a deficiency of the enzyme glucocerebrosidase that is responsible for breaking down a certain type of fat and releasing it from fat cells. These fat cells begin to crowd out healthy cells in the liver, spleen, bones, and nervous system. Symptoms of Gaucher disease can start in infancy, childhood, or adulthood.

Three types of Gaucher disease have been identified, but there are many variations in how symptoms develop. Type 1 is the most common and affects both children and adults. It occurs much more often in people of Eastern European and Russian Jewish (Ashkenazi) ancestry, affecting 1 out of every 450 live births. The first signs of the disease include an enlarged liver and spleen, causing the abdomen to swell. Children with this condition may be shorter than normal. Other symptoms include tiredness, pain, bone deterioration, broken bones, **anemia,** and increased bruising. Type 2 Gaucher disease is more serious, beginning within the first few months after birth. Symptoms, which are similar to those in Type 1, progress rapidly, but also include nervous system damage. Symptoms of Type 3 Gaucher disease begin during early childhood with symptoms like Type 1. Unlike Type 2, the progress of the disease is slower, although it also includes nervous system damage.

Diagnosis

Gaucher disease may be suspected based on symptoms and is confirmed with a blood test for levels of the enzyme. Samples of tissue from an affected area may also be used to confirm a diagnosis of the disease.

Treatment

The symptoms of Gaucher disease can be stopped and even reversed by treatment with injections of enzyme replacements. Two enzyme drugs currently available are alglucerase (Ceredase) and imiglucerase (Cerezyme).

Other treatments address specific symptoms such as anemia, broken bones, or pain.

Prognosis

The pain and deformities associated with symptoms can make coping with this illness very challenging for individuals and families. With treatment and control of symptoms, people with Type 1 Gaucher disease may lead fairly long and normal lives. Most infants with Type 2 die before the age of 2. Children with Type 3 Gaucher disease may survive to adolescence and early adulthood.

KRABBE'S DISEASE

Causes & symptoms

Krabbe's disease is caused by a deficiency of the enzyme galactoside beta-galactosidase. It has a recessive pattern of inheritance and is believed to occur in 1 of 40,000 births in the United States. This condition, which is also called globoid cell leukodystrophy or Krabbe leukodystrophy, is characterized by acute nervous system degeneration. It develops in early infancy with initial symptoms of irritability, vomiting and episodes of partial unconsciousness. Symptoms progress rapidly to seizures, difficulty swallowing, blindness, deafness, **mental retardation,** and **paralysis.**

Treatment

No treatment is available.

Prognosis

Children born with Krabbe's disease die in infancy.

NIEMANN-PICK DISEASE

Causes & symptoms

At least five different forms of Niemann-Pick disease (NPD) have been identified. The different types seem to be related to the activity level of the enzyme sphingomyelinase. In patients with Types A and B NPD, there is a build up of sphingomyelin in cells of the brain, liver, spleen, kidney and lung. Type A is the most common form of NPD and the most serious, with death usually occurring by the age of 18 months. Symptoms develop within the first few months of life and include poor appetite, failure to grow, enlarged liver and spleen, and the appearance of cherry red spots in the retina of the eye. Type B develops in infancy or childhood with symptoms of mild liver or spleen enlargement and lung problems. Some adults with this form (Type E) may also show a loss of muscle coordination. Types C or D NPD are related to cholesterol transfer out of cells. Children with Types C or D grow normally in early childhood, but eventually develop difficulty in walking and loss of muscle coordination. Ultimately, the nervous system becomes severely damaged and these patients die. Type C occurs in any population, while Type D has been identified only in patients from Nova Scotia, Canada.

Diagnosis

Diagnosis is confirmed by analyzing a sample of tissue. Prenatal diagnosis of Types A and B of NPD can be done with **amniocentesis** or **chorionic villus sampling.**

Treatment

Treatment consists of supportive care to deal with symptoms and the development of complications. **Bone marrow transplantation** is being investigated as a possible treatment. Low-cholesterol **diets** may be helpful for patients with Types C and D.

Prognosis

Patients with Type A NPD usually die within the first year and a half of life. Type B patients generally live to adulthood but suffer from significant liver and lung problems. With Types C and D NPD, there is significant nervous system damage leading to severe muscle spasms, seizures, and eventually, to **coma** and death. Some patients with Types C and D die in childhood, while less severely affected patients may survive to adulthood.

REFSUM'S DISEASE

Causes & symptoms

Refsum's disease has a recessive pattern of inheritance and affects populations from Northern Europe, particularly Scandinavians most frequently. It is due to a deficiency of phytanic acid hydroxylase, an enzyme that breaks down a fatty acid called phytanic acid. This condition affects the nervous system, eyes, bones, and skin. Symptoms, which usually appear by age 20, include vision problems [**retinitis pigmentosa** and rhythmic eye movements (**nystagmus**)], loss of muscle coordination, loss of sense of smell (**anosmia**), pain, numbness, and elevated protein in the cerebrospinal fluid.

Treatment

A diet free of phytanic acid (found in dairy products, tuna, cod, haddock, lamb, stewed beef, white bread, white rice, boiled potatoes, and egg yolk) can reduce some of the symptoms. **Plasmapheresis,** a process where whole blood is removed from the body, processed through a filtering system, and then return to the body, may be used to filter phytanic acid from the blood.

TAY-SACHS DISEASE

Causes & symptoms

Tay-Sachs disease (TSD) is a fatal condition caused by a deficiency of the enzyme hexosaminidase A (Hex-A). The defective gene that causes this disorder is found in roughly 1 in 250 people in the general population. However, certain populations have significantly higher rates of TSD. French-Canadians living near the St. Lawrence River and in the Cajun regions of Louisiana are at higher risk of having a child with TSD. The highest risk seems to be in people of Eastern European and Russian Jewish (Ashkenazi) descent. Tay-Sachs disease has a recessive pattern of inheritance, and approximately 1 in every 27 people of Jewish ancestry in the United States carries the TSD gene. Symptoms develop in infancy and are due to the accumulation of a fatty acid compound in the nervous system. Early symptoms include loss of vision and physical coordination, seizures, and mental retardation. Eventually, the child develops problems with breathing and swallowing. Blindness, paralysis, and death follow.

Diagnosis

Carriers of the Tay-Sachs related gene can be identified with a blood test. Amniocentesis or chorionic villi sampling can be used to determine if the fetus has Tay-Sachs disease.

Treatment

There is no treatment for Tay-Sachs disease. Parents who are identified as carriers may want to seek **genetic counseling.** If a fetus is identified as having TSD, parents may consider termination of the **pregnancy.**

Prognosis

Children born with Tay-Sachs disease become increasingly debilitated; most die by about age four.

WOLMAN'S DISEASE

Causes & symptoms

Wolman's disease is caused by a genetic defect (with a recessive pattern of inheritance) that results in deficiency of an enzyme that breaks down cholesterol. This causes large amounts of fat to accumulate in body tissues. Symptoms begin in the first few weeks of life and include an enlarged liver and spleen, adrenal calcification (hardening of adrenal tissue due to deposits of calcium salts), and fatty stools.

Treatment

No treatment is currently available.

Prognosis

Death generally occurs before six months of age.

Prevention

Couples who have family histories of genetic defects can undergo genetic testing and counseling to see if they are at risk for having a child with one of the lipidoses disorders. During pregnancy, cell samples can be collected from the fetus using amniocentesis or chorionic villi sampling. The results of these test can indicate if the developing fetus has a lipidosis disorder. Termination of the pregnancy may be considered in some cases.

Resources

BOOKS

"Lipid Storage Diseases." In *Internal Medicine*, edited by Jay H. Stein. 5th ed. St. Louis: Mosby, 1998.

McGovern, Margaret M., and Robert J. Desnick. "Lysosomal Storage Diseases." In *Cecil Textbook of Medicine*, edited by J. Claude Bennett and Fred Plum. 20th ed. Philadelphia: W.B. Saunders, 1996.

Valle, David L., ed. *The Metabolic and Molecular Bases of Inherited Disease.* 7th ed. New York: McGraw-Hill, 1994.

ORGANIZATIONS

International Center for Fabry Disease. Department of Human Genetics, Mount Sinai School of Medicine, Box 1497, Fifth Avenue and 100th Street, New York, NY 10029. (212) 241-6944. http://www.mssm.edu/crc/fabry/brochure.html.

National Institutes of Health. National Institute of Diabetes and Digestive and Kidney Diseases (NIDDK), 9000 Rockville Pike, Bethesda, MD 20892. (301) 496-3583.

National Institutes of Health. National Institute of Neurological Disorders and Stroke, 9000 Rockville Pike, Bethesda, MD 20892. (301) 496-5751. (800) 352-9424.

National Niemann-Pick Foundation. 3734 E. Olive Avenue, Gilbert, AZ 85234. (602) 497-6638.

National Organization for Rare Disorders (NORD). PO Box 8923, New Fairfield, CT 06812-8923. (203) 746-6518. (800) 999-6673.

National Tay-Sachs and Allied Diseases Association, Inc. 2001 Beacon Street, Brookline, MA 02146. (617) 277-4463. (800) 906-8723. http://mcrcr2.med.nyu.edu/murphp01/ntsad/t-sachs.htm.

OTHER

Gaucher Disease Treatment Program at Massachusetts General Hospital. http://neuro-www2.mgh.harvard.edu/gaucher/main.html.

Rare Genetic Diseases In Children: An Internet Resource Gateway. http://mcrcr2.med.nyu.edu/murphp01/homenew.htm.

Altha Roberts Edgren

Lipomas *see* **Skin lesions**

Lipoproteins test

Definition

Lipoproteins are the "packages" in which cholesterol and triglycerides travel throughout the body. Measuring the amount of cholesterol carried by each type of lipoprotein helps determine a person's risk for cardiovascular disease (disease that affects the heart and blood vessels, also called CVD).

Purpose

Cholesterol and triglycerides are fat-like substances called lipids. Cholesterol is used to build cell membranes and hormones. The body makes cholesterol and gets it from food. Triglycerides provide a major source of energy to the body tissues. Both cholesterol and triglycerides are vital to body function, but an excess of either one, especially cholesterol, puts a person at risk of cardiovascular disease.

Because cholesterol and triglycerides can't dissolve in watery liquid, they must be transported by something that can dissolve in blood serum. Lipoproteins contain cholesterol and triglycerides at the core and an outer layer of protein, called apolipoprotein.

There are four major classes of lipoproteins: chylomicrons, very low-density lipoproteins (VLDL), low-density lipoproteins (LDL), and high-density lipoproteins (HDL). There are also less commonly measured classes such as lipoprotein(a) and subtypes of the main classes. Each lipoprotein has characteristics that make the cholesterol it carries a greater or lesser risk. Measuring each type of lipoprotein helps determine a person's risk for cardiovascular disease more accurately than cholesterol measurement alone. When a person is discovered to be at risk, treatment by diet or medication can be started and his or her response to treatment monitored by repeated testing.

Description

Chylomicrons

Chylomicrons are made in the intestines from the triglycerides in food. They contain very little cholesterol. Chylomicrons circulate in the blood, getting smaller as they deposit the triglycerides in fatty tissue. Twelve hours after a meal, they are gone from circulation. Serum collected from a person directly after eating will form a

KEY TERMS

. . . .

Atherosclerosis—Disease of blood vessels caused by deposits of cholesterol on the inside walls of the vessels.

Cardiovascular disease—Disease that affects the heart and blood vessels.

Cholesterol—A fat-like substance called a lipid. It is used to build cell membranes and hormones. The body makes cholesterol and gets it from food.

Lipoproteins—The packages in which cholesterol and triglycerides travel throughout the body.

creamy layer on the top if left undisturbed and refrigerated overnight. This creamy layer is the chylomicrons.

Very low-density lipoproteins (VLDL)

VLDL are formed in the liver by the combination of cholesterol, triglycerides formed from circulating fatty acids, and apolipoprotein. This lipoprotein particle is smaller than a chylomicron, and contains less triglyceride but more cholesterol (10-15% of a person's total cholesterol). As the VLDL circulates in the blood, triglycerides are deposited and the particle gets smaller, eventually becoming a low-density lipoprotein (LDL). Serum from a person with a large amount of VLDL will be cloudy.

Low-density lipoproteins (LDL)

LDL, often called "bad" cholesterol, is formed primarily by the breakdown of VLDL. LDL contains little triglycerides and a large amount of cholesterol (60-70% of a person's total cholesterol). Although the particles are much smaller than chylomicrons and VLDL, LDL particles can vary in size and chemical structure. These variations represent subclasses within the LDL class. Serum from a person with a large amount of LDL will be clear.

LDL carries cholesterol in the blood and deposits it in body tissues and in the walls of blood vessels, a condition known as **atherosclerosis.** The amount of LDL in a person's blood is directly related to his or her risk of cardiovascular disease. The higher the LDL level, the greater the risk. LDL is the lipoprotein class most used to trigger and monitor cholesterol lowering therapy.

High-density lipoproteins (HDL)

HDL is often called "good" cholesterol. HDL removes excess cholesterol from tissues and vessel walls and carries it to the liver, where it is removed from the blood and discarded. The amount of HDL in a person's blood is inversely related to his or her risk of cardiovas-

cular disease. The lower the HDL level, the greater the risk; the higher the level, the lower the risk. The smallest lipoprotein, it contains 20-30% of a person's total cholesterol and can be separated into two major subclasses.

Lipoprotein(a)

Lipoprotein(a) is found in lower concentrations than other lipoproteins, yet it carries a unique and significant risk for cardiovascular disease. Because of its similarity to LDL, test methods often don't measure it separately, but include it within the LDL class. Testing specifically for this class may uncover why a person is not responding to standard cholesterol-lowering treatment. High lipoprotein(a) levels may not respond to treatment aimed at high LDL.

Measurement guidelines

The Expert Panel of the National Cholesterol Education Program (NCEP) sponsored by the National Institutes of Health has published guidelines for the detection of high cholesterol in adults. The NCEP panel recommends that adults over the age of 20 be tested for cholesterol and HDL every five years. If the cholesterol is high, the HDL is low (below 35 mg/dl), or other risk factors are present, a complete lipoprotein profile that includes total cholesterol, triglycerides, HDL, and calculated LDL should be done.

Measurement methods

There are a variety of methods to measure the lipoprotein classes. All require separation of the classes before they can be measured. One way to separate them is by spinning serum (the yellow, watery liquid that separates from the cells when blood clots) for a long time in a high-speed centrifuge (called ultracentrifugation). The most dense classes will settle towards the bottom, the least dense towards the top. Following centrifugation, the most complete measurement of all the lipoprotein classes is done using electrophoresis. This procedure measures the quantity of each lipoprotein class based on its movement in an electrical field.

Other, less extensive procedures are also used. For example, if only HDL is to be measured, a chemical is added to the serum that will clump the other classes, leaving HDL free in the serum to be measured by a chemical method. LDL often is not measured directly but its level is calculated based on the measurements of total cholesterol, HDL, and triglycerides. The formula is called the Friedewald formula: LDL = total cholesterol - HDL - (triglycerides/5). The calculated result will be inaccurate in a person with high triglycerides. Results are usually available the same or following day.

Preparation

The patient must fast for 12 hours before the test, eating nothing and drinking only water. The person should not have alcohol for 24 hours before the test. There should be a stable diet and no illnesses occurring in the preceding two weeks.

A lipoproteins test requires 5 mL (milliliters) of blood. A person's physical position while having blood collected affects the results. Values from blood drawn while a person is sitting may be different from those while the person is standing. If repeated testing is done, the person should be in same position each time.

Aftercare

Discomfort or bruising may occur at the puncture site or the person may feel dizzy or faint. Pressure to the puncture site until the bleeding stops reduces bruising. Warm packs to the puncture site relieve discomfort.

Normal results

People with HDL levels between 45 mg/dl and 59 mg/dl carry an average risk for cardiovascular disease. People with HDL levels above 60 mg/dl have a negative risk factor and appear to be protected from cardiovascular disease.

LDL levels below 130 mg/dl are desirable.

Some people have normal variations in their lipoprotein and total cholesterol levels. Repeat testing may be necessary, especially if a value is at a borderline risk category point.

Abnormal results

People with HDL levels 36-44 mg/dl have a moderate risk of cardiovascular disease. HDL levels below 35 mg/dl are a major risk.

LDL levels 130-159 mg/dl place a person at a borderline high risk of cardiovascular disease; levels above 160 mg/dl place a person at high risk. Relative proportions between HDL and LDL are important also.

Resources

BOOKS

Bachorik, Paul S., Basil M. Rafkind, and Peter O. Kwiterovich. "Lipids and Dyslipoproteinemia." In *Clinical Diagnosis and Management by Laboratory Methods,* 19th ed., edited by John B. Henry. Philadelphia: W. B. Saunders Company, 1996.

Rifai, Nader, G. Russell Warnick, and Marek H. Dominiczak. *Handbook of Lipoprotein Testing.* Washington, D.C.: American Association of Clinical Chemistry (AACC) Press, 1997.

PERIODICALS

O'Brien, Timothy and Tu. T. Nguyen. "Lipids and Lipoproteins in Women." *Mayo Clinic Proceedings,* (March 1997): 235-244.

Stein, James H. and Robert S. Rosenson. "Lipoprotein Lp(a) Excess and Coronary Heart Disease." *Archives of Internal Medicine,* (June 9, 1997): 1170-1176.

ORGANIZATIONS

American Heart Association. 7272 Greenville Avenue, Dallas, TX, 75231-4596. 214-706-1220. http://www.amhrt.org/.

National Cholesterol Education Program. The National Heart, Lung, and Blood Institute. National Institutes of Health. PO Box 30105, Bethesda, MD, 20824-0105. 301-251-1222. http://www.nhlbi.nih.gov/nhbli/nhbli.htm.

OTHER

National Cholesterol Education Program: Second Report of the Expert Panel on Detection, Evaluation, and Treatment of High Blood Cholesterol In Adults. NIH Publication No. 93-3096, Bethesda, Maryland, August, 1996.

Nancy J. Nordenson

Liposuction

Definition

Liposuction, also known as lipoplasty or suction-assisted lipectomy, is **cosmetic surgery** performed to remove unwanted deposits of fat from under the skin. The doctor sculpts and recontours the patient's body by removing excess fat deposits that have been resistant to reduction by diet or **exercise.** The fat is permanently removed from under the skin with a suction device.

Purpose

Liposuction is intended to reduce and smooth the contours of the body and improve the patient's appearance. Its goal is cosmetic improvement. It is the most commonly performed cosmetic procedure in the United States.

Liposuction does not remove large quantities of fat and is not intended as a weight reduction technique. The average amount of fat removed is about a liter, or a quart. Although liposuction is not intended to remove cellulite (lumpy fat), some doctors believe that it improves the appearance of cellulite areas (thighs, hips, buttocks, abdomen, and chin).

A new technique called liposhaving shows more promise at reducing cellulite.

Precautions

Liposuction is most successful on patients who have firm, elastic skin and concentrated pockets of fat in cellultite areas. To get good results after fat removal, the skin must contract to conform to the new contours without sagging. Older patients have less elastic skin and therefore may not be good candidates for this procedure. Patients with generalized fat distribution, rather than localized pockets, are not good candidates.

Patients should be in good general health and free of heart or lung disease. Patients with poor circulation or who have had recent surgery at the intended site of fat reduction are not good candidates.

Description

Most liposuction procedures are performed under **local anesthesia** (loss of sensation without loss of consciousness) by the tumescent or wet technique. In this technique, large volumes of very dilute local anesthetic (a substance that produces anesthesia) are injected under the patient's skin, making the tissue swollen and firm. Epinephrine is added to the solution to reduce bleeding, and make possible the removal of larger amounts of fat.

The doctor first numbs the skin with an injection of local anesthetic. After the skin is desensitized, the doctor makes a series of tiny incisions, usually 0.12-0.25 in (3-6 mm) in length. The area is then flooded with a larger amount of local anesthetic. Fat is then extracted with suction through a long, blunt hollow tube called a cannula. The doctor repeatedly pushes the cannula through the fat layers in a radiating pattern creating tunnels, removing fat, and recontouring the area. Large quantities

of intravenous fluid (IV) is given during the procedure to replace lost body fluid. Blood **transfusions** are possible.

Some newer modifications to the procedure involve the use of a cutting cannula called a liposhaver, or the use of ultrasound to help break up the fat deposits. The patient is awake and comfortable during these procedures.

The length of time required to perform the procedure varies with the amount of fat that is to be removed and the number of areas to be treated. Most operations take from 30 minutes to 2 hours, but extensive procedures can take longer. The length of time required also varies with the manner in which the anesthetic is injected.

The cost of liposuction can vary depending upon the standardized fees in the region of the country where it is performed, the extent of the area being treated, and the person performing the procedure. Generally, small areas, such as the chin or knees, can be done for as little as $500, while more extensive treatment, such as when hips,

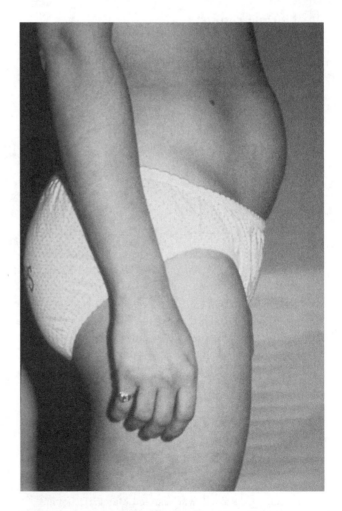

"Before" photo of patient undergoing liposuction.
(Photograph by I. Richard Toranto, M.D., Custom Medical Stock Photo. Reproduced by permission.)

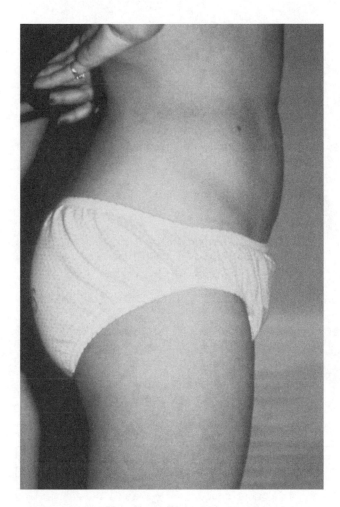

"After" photo of same patient following liposuction.
(Photograph by I. Richard Toranto, M.D., Custom Medical Stock Photo. Reproduced by permission.)

thighs, and abdomen are done simultaneously, can cost as much as $10,000. These procedures are cosmetic and are not covered by most insurance policies.

Preparation

The doctor will do a physical exam and may order blood work to determine clotting time and hemoglobin level for transfusions should the need arise. The patient may be placed on **antibiotics** immediately prior to surgery to ward off infection.

Aftercare

After the surgery, the patient will need to wear a support garment continuously for 2-3 weeks. If ankles or calves were treated, support hose will need to be worn for up to 6 weeks. The support garments can be removed during bathing 24 hours after surgery. A drainage tube, under the skin in the area of the procedure, may be inserted to prevent fluid build-up.

Mild side effects can include a burning sensation at the site of the surgery for up to one month. The patient should be prepared for swelling of the tissues below the operated site for 6-8 weeks after surgery. Wearing the special elastic garments will help reduce this swelling and help to achieve the desired final results.

The incisions involved in this procedure are tiny, but the surgeon may close them with stitches or staples. These will be removed the day after surgery. However, three out of eight doctors use no sutures. Minor bleeding or seepage through the incision site is common after this procedure. Wearing the elastic bandage or support garment helps reduce fluid loss.

This operation is virtually painless. However, for the first postoperative day, there may be some discomfort which will require light pain medication. Soreness or aching may persist for several days. The patient can usually return to normal activity within a week. Postoperative bruising will go away by itself within 10-14 days. Postoperative swelling begins to go down after a week. It may take 3-6 months for the final contour to be reached.

Risks

Liposuction under local anesthesia using the tumescent technique is exceptionally safe. A 1995 study of 15,336 patients showed no serious complications or **deaths.** Another study showed a 1% risk factor. However, as with any surgery, there are some risks and serious complications. Death is possible.

The main hazards associated with this surgery involve migration of a blood clot or fat globule to the heart, brain, or lungs. Such an event can cause a **heart attack, stroke,** or serious lung damage. However, this complication is rare and did not occur even once in the study of 15,336 patients. The risk of blood clot formation is reduced with the wearing of special girdle-like compression garments after the surgery, and with the resumption of normal mild activity soon after surgery.

Staying in bed increases the risk of clot formation, but not getting enough rest can result in increased swelling of the surgical area. Such swelling is a result of excess fluid and blood accumulation, and generally comes from not wearing the compression garments. If necessary, this excess fluid can be drained off with a needle in the doctor's office.

Infection is another complication, but this rarely occurs. If the physician is skilled and works in a sterile environment, infection should not be a concern.

If too much fat is removed, the skin may peel in that area. Smokers are at increased risk for shedding skin because their circulation is impaired. Another and more serious hazard of removing too much fat is that the patient may go into **shock.** Fat tissue has an abundant blood supply and removing too much of it at once can cause shock if the fluid is not replaced.

A rare complication is perforation or puncture of an organ. The procedure involves pushing a cannula vigorously through the fat layer. If the doctor pushes too hard or if the tissue gives way too easily under the force, the blunt hollow tube can go too far and injure internal organs.

Liposuction can damage superficial nerves. Some patients lose sensation in the area that has been suctioned, but feeling usually returns with time.

Normal results

The loss of fat cells is permanent, and the patient should have smoother, more pleasing body contours without excessive bulges. However, if the patient overeats, the remaining fat cells will grow in size. Although the patient may gain weight back, the body should retain the new proportions and the suctioned area should remain proportionally smaller.

Tiny scars about 0.25-0.5 in (6-12 mm) long at the site of incision are normal. The doctor usually makes the incisions in places where the scars are not likely to show.

In some instances, the skin may appear rippled, wavy, or baggy after surgery. Pigmentation spots may develop. The recontoured area may be uneven. This unevenness is common, occurring in 5-20% of the cases, and can be corrected with a second procedure that is less extensive than the first.

Resources

BOOKS

Hetter, Gregory P. *Lipoplasty: The Theory and Practice of Blunt Suction Lipectomy.* Little, Brown and Company, 1990.

Pitman, Gerald H. *Liposuction & Aesthetic Surgery.* Quality Medical Publishing, Inc., 1993.

Stegman, Samuel J., Theodore A. Tromovitch, and Richard G. Glogau. *Cosmetic Dermatologic Surgery.* Year Book Medical Publishers, Inc., 1990.

Wilson, Joleen. *The American Society of Plastic and Reconstructive Surgeon's Guide to Cosmetic Surgery.* Simon & Schuster, 1992.

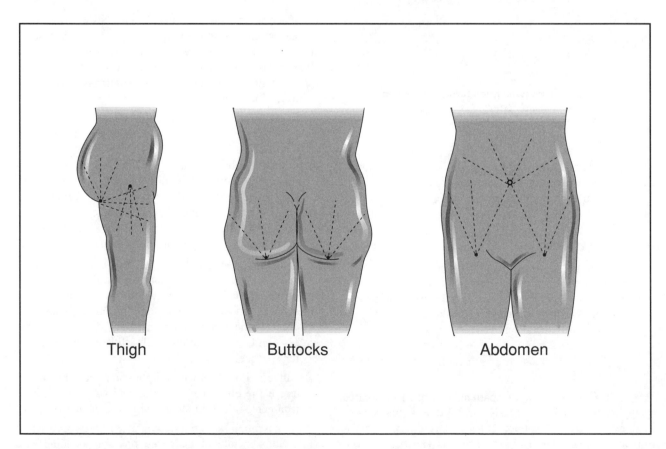

Common entry sites for liposuction procedures. *(Illustration by Electronic Illustrators Group.)*

Thigh Buttocks Abdomen

PERIODICALS

"Downsize Your Thighs." *Good Housekeeping* (May 1997): 69-75.

Hanke, C.W., G. Bernstein, and S. Bullock. "Safety of Tumescent Liposuction in 15,336 Patients." National Survey Results. *Dermatologic Surgery* 21 (May 1995): 459-462.

Murray, Louann. "Tumescent Liposuction Technique is Great Improvement." *Dermatology Times* (September 1995): 4.

Murray, Louann. "What is the Best Approach to Liposuction?" *Dermatology Times* (September 1995): 24-25.

"Sound Waves Help Break Up Fat." *USA Today* (October 1997): 15-16.

Taylor, Mia, Lloyd A. Hoffman, and Michael Lieberman. "Intestinal Perforation after Suction Lipoplasty: A Case Report and Review of the Literature." *Annals of Plastic Surgery* 38(2): 169-172.

Van Ness, David. "The Skinny on Liposuction." *Muscle and Fitness* (November 1997): 128-132, 201.

ORGANIZATIONS

American Society of Aesthetic Plastic Surgery. (888) 272-7711.

American Society of Plastic and Reconstructive Surgery. (800) 635-0635. http://:www.plasticsurgery.org.

Lipoplasty Society of North America. (800) 848-1991.

Louann W. Murray

Lisinopril *see* **Angiotensin-converting enzyme inhibitors**

Listeria monocytogenes infection *see* **Listeriosis**

Listeriosis

Definition

Listeriosis is an illness caused by the bacterium *Listeria monocytogenes* that is acquired by eating contaminated food. The organism can spread to the blood stream and central nervous system. During **pregnancy,** listeriosis often causes **miscarriage** or **stillbirth.**

Description

Listeriosis is caused by an infection with the bacterium *Listeria monocytogenes*. This bacteria can be carried by many animals and birds, and it has been found in soil, water, sewage, and animal feed. Five out of every

---

KEY TERMS

Abscess—An accumulation of pus caused by localized infection in tissues or organs. *Listeria monocytogenes* can cause abscesses in many organs including the brain, spleen, and liver.

Immunocompromised—To have a poor immune system due to disease or medication. Immunocompromised persons are at risk for developing infections because they can't fight off microorganisms like healthy persons can.

Macrophages—White blood cells whose job is to destroy invading microorganisms. *Listeria monocytogenes* avoids being killed and can multiply within the macrophage.

Meningitis—An inflammation of the tissues that surround the brain and spinal cord. It can be caused by a bacterial infection.

Sepsis—The presence of bacteria in the blood stream, a normally sterile environment.

---

100 people carry *Listeria monocytogenes* in their intestines. Listeriosis is considered a "food-borne illness" because most people are probably infected after eating food contaminated with *Listeria monocytogenes*. However, a woman can pass the bacteria to her baby during pregnancy. In addition, there have been a few cases where workers have developed *Listeria* skin infections by touching infected calves or poultry.

In the 1980s, the United States government began taking measures to decrease the occurrence of listeriosis. Processed meats and dairy products are now tested for the presence of *Listeria monocytogenes*. The Food and Drug Administration (FDA) and the Food Safety and Inspection Service (FSIS) can legally prevent food from being shipped, or order food recalls, if they detect any *Listeria* bacteria. These inspections, in combination with the public education regarding the proper handling of uncooked foods, appear to be working. In 1989, there were 1,965 cases of listeriosis with 481 **deaths.** In 1993, the numbers fell to 1,092 cases with 248 deaths.

In 1996, the Centers for Disease Control and Prevention (CDC) began a nationwide food-borne disease surveillance program called "FoodNet," in which seven states were participating by January 1997. Results from the program indicated that, in 1996, one person out of every 200,000 people got listeriosis. FoodNet also revealed that the hospitalization rate was higher for listeriosis (94%) than for any other food-borne illness. In addition, FoodNet found that the *Listeria* bacteria reached the blood and cerebrospinal fluid in 89% of cases, a higher percentage than in any other food-borne illness.

Persons at particular risk for listeriosis include the elderly, pregnant women, newborns, and those with a weakened immune system (called "immuno-compromised"). Risk is increased when a person suffers from diseases such as **AIDS, cancer,** kidney disease, **diabetes mellitus,** or by the use of certain medications. Infection is most common in babies younger than one month old and adults over 60 years of age. Pregnant women account for 27% of the cases and immunocompromised persons account for almost 70%. Persons with AIDS are 280 times more likely to get listeriosis than others.

Causes & symptoms

As noted, persons become infected with *Listeria monocytogenes* by eating contaminated food. *Listeria* has been found on raw vegetables, fish, poultry, raw (unpasteurized) milk, fresh meat, processed meat (such as deli meat, hot dogs, and canned meat), and certain soft cheeses. Listeriosis outbreaks in the United States since the 1980s have been linked to cole slaw, milk, Mexican-style cheese, undercooked hot dogs, undercooked chicken, and delicatessen foods. Unlike most other bacteria, *Listeria monocytogenes* does not stop growing when food is in the refrigerator — its growth is merely slowed. Fortunately, typical cooking temperatures and the pasteurization process do kill this bacteria.

Listeria bacteria can pass through the wall of the intestines, and from there they can get into the blood stream. Once in the blood stream, they can be transported anywhere in the body, but are commonly found the central nervous system (brain and spinal cord); and in pregnant women they are often found in the placenta (the organ which connects the baby's umbilical cord to the uterus). *Listeria monocytogenes* live inside specific white blood cells called macrophages. Inside macrophages, the bacteria can hide from immune responses and become inaccessible to certain **antibiotics.** *Listeria* bacteria are capable of multiplying within macrophages, and then may spread to other macrophages.

After consuming food contaminated with this bacteria, symptoms of infection may appear anywhere from 11-70 days later. Most people do not get any noticeable symptoms. Scientists are unsure, but they believe that *Listeria monocytogenes* can cause upset stomach and intestinal problems just like other food-borne illnesses. Persons with listeriosis may develop flu-like symptoms such as **fever, headache, nausea and vomiting,** tiredness, and **diarrhea.**

Pregnant women experience a mild, flu-like illness with fever, muscle aches, upset stomach, and intestinal problems. They recover, but the infection can cause mis-carriage, **premature labor,** early rupture of the birth sac, and stillbirth. Unfortunately, half of the newborns infected with *Listeria* will die from the illness.

There are two types of listeriosis in the newborn baby: early-onset disease and late-onset disease. Early-onset disease refers to a serious illness that is present at birth and usually causes the baby to be born prematurely. Babies infected during the pregnancy usually have a blood infection (**sepsis**) and may have a serious, whole body infection called granulomatosis infantisepticum. When a full-term baby becomes infected with *Listeria* during **childbirth,** that situation is called late-onset disease. Commonly, symptoms of late-onset listeriosis appear about two weeks after birth. Babies with late-term disease typically have **meningitis** (inflammation of the brain and spinal tissues); yet they have a better chance of surviving than those with early-onset disease.

Immunocompromised adults are at risk for a serious infection of the blood stream and central nervous system (brain and spinal cord). Meningitis occurs in about half of the cases of adult listeriosis. Symptoms of listerial meningitis occur about four days after the flu-like symptoms and include fever, personality change, uncoordinated muscle movement, **tremors,** muscle contractions, seizures, and slipping in and out of consciousness.

Listeria monocytogenes causes **endocarditis** in about 7.5% of the cases. Endocarditis is an inflammation of heart tissue due to the bacterial infection. Listerial endocarditis causes death in about half of the patients. Other diseases which have been caused by *Listeria monocytogenes* include **brain abscess,** eye infection, hepatitis (liver disease), **peritonitis** (abdominal infection), lung infection, joint infection, arthritis, heart disease, bone infection, and gallbladder infection.

Diagnosis

Listeriosis may be diagnosed and treated by infectious disease specialists and internal medicine specialists. The diagnosis and treatment of this infection should be covered by most insurance providers.

The only way to diagnose listeriosis is to isolate *Listeria monocytogenes* from blood, cerebrospinal fluid, or stool. A sample of cerebrospinal fluid is removed from the spinal cord using a needle and syringe. This procedure is commonly called a spinal tap. The amniotic fluid (the fluid which bathes the unborn baby) may be tested in pregnant women with listeriosis. This sample is obtained by inserting a needle through the abdomen into the uterus and withdrawing fluid. *Listeria* grows well in laboratory media and test results can be available within a few days.

Treatment

Listeriosis is treated with the antibiotics ampicillin (Omnipen) or sulfamethoxazole-trimethoprim (Bactrim, Septra). Because the bacteria live within macrophage cells, treatment may be difficult and the treatment periods may vary. Usually, pregnant women are treated for two weeks; newborns, two to three weeks; adults with mild disease, two to four weeks; persons with meningitis, three weeks; persons with brain abscesses, six weeks; and persons with endocarditis, four to six weeks.

Patients are often hospitalized for treatment and monitoring. Other drugs may be provided to relieve **pain** and fever and to treat other reactions to the infection.

Prognosis

The overall death rate for listeriosis is 26%. This high death rate is due to the serious illness suffered by newborns, the elderly, and immunocompromised persons. Healthy adults and older children have a low death rate. Complications of *Listeria* infection include: meningitis, sepsis, miscarriage, stillbirth, **pneumonia, shock,** endocarditis, **abscess** (localized infection) formation, and eye inflammation.

Prevention

The United States government has already done much to prevent listeriosis. Persons at extremely high risk (pregnant women, immunocompromised persons, etc.) must use extra caution. High risk persons should: avoid soft cheeses, such as Mexican cheese, feta, Brie, Camembert, and blue cheese (cottage cheese is safe), thoroughly cook leftovers and ready-to-eat foods (such as hot-dogs), and avoid foods from the deli.

For all people, the risk of listeriosis can be reduced by taking these precautions:

- Completely cook all meats and eggs.

- Carefully wash raw vegetables before eating.

- Keep raw meat away from raw vegetables and prepared foods. After cutting raw meat, wash the cutting board with detergent before using it for vegetables.

- Avoid drinking unpasteurized milk or foods made from such milk.

- Wash hands thoroughly after handling raw meat.

- Follow the instructions on food labels. Observe food expiration dates and storage conditions.

Resources

BOOKS

Gorbach, Samuel L., John G. Bartlett, and Neil R. Blacklow. *Infectious Diseases,* 2nd ed. Philadelphia: W.B. Saunders Company, 1998.

Lorber, Bennett. "Listeriosis." In *Infectious Diseases.* Philadelphia: Temple University School of Medicine and Hospital, 1996.

PERIODICALS

Calder, Jennifer. "Listeria Meningitis in Adults." *Lancet* 350 (1997): 307.

Farr, R. Wesley. "Leptospirosis." *Clinical Infectious Diseases* 21 (1995): 1-8.

Schlech, Walter F. "Listeria Gastroenteritis — Old Syndrome, New Pathogen." *New England Journal of Medicine* 336 (June 1997): 130-131.

OTHER

Centers for Disease Control and Prevention. Division of Bacterial and Mycotic Diseases. "Preventing Foodborne Illness: Listeriosis" http://www.cdc.gov/ncidad/diseases/foodborn/lister.htm.

HealthAnswers. "Listeriosis." http://housecall.orbisnews.com/databases/ami/convert/001380.html (12 April 1998).

USDA FSIS DHHS FDA. "Preventing Foodborne Listeriosis." http://www-micro.msb.le.ac.uk/FDA/vm.cfsan.fda.gov/~fsis/FSISLIST.html (12 April 1998).

Belinda M. Rowland

. . . .

Lithotripsy

Definition

Lithotripsy is the use of high-energy shock waves to fragment and disintegrate **kidney stones.** The shock wave, created by using a high-voltage spark or an electromagnetic impulse, is focused on the stone. This shock wave shatters the stone and this allows the fragments to pass through the urinary system. Since the shock wave is generated outside the body, the procedure is termed extracorporeal shock wave lithotripsy, or ESWL.

Purpose

ESWL is used when a kidney stone is too large to pass on its own, or when a stone becomes stuck in a ureter (a tube which carries urine from the kidney to the bladder) and will not pass. Kidney stones are extremely painful and can cause serious medical complications if not removed.

Precautions

ESWL should not be considered for patients with severe skeletal deformities, patients weighing over 300 lbs (136 kg), patients with abdominal **aortic aneurysms,**

KEY TERMS

Aneurysm—A dilation of the wall of an artery which causes a weak area prone to rupturing.

Bladder—Organ in which urine is stored prior to urination.

Bleeding disorder—Problems in the clotting mechanism of the blood.

Cardiologist—A physician who specializes in problems of the heart.

EKG—A tracing of the electrical activity of the heart.

ESWL (Extracorporeal shock wave lithotripsy)—The use of focused shock waves, generated outside the body, to fragment kidney stones.

Gravel—The debris which is formed from a fragmented kidney stone.

IVP (Intravenous pyelogram)—The use of a dye, injected into the veins, used to locate kidney stones. Also used to determine the anatomy of the urinary system.

Kidney stone—A hard mass that forms in the urinary tract and which can cause pain, bleeding, obstruction, or infection. Stones are primarily made up of calcium.

Stent—A plastic tube placed in the ureter prior to the ESWL procedure which facilitates the passage of gravel and urine

Ultrasound—Sound waves used to determine the internal structures of the body

Ureter—A tube which carries urine from the kidney to the bladder.

Urethra—A tube through which urine passes during urination.

Urologist—A physician who specializes in problems of the urinary system.

or patients with uncontrollable bleeding disorders. Patients who are pregnant should not be treated with ESWL. Patients with cardiac **pacemakers** should be evaluated by a cardiologist familiar with ESWL. The cardiologist should be present during the ESWL procedure in the event the pacemaker needs to be overridden.

Description

Lithotripsy uses the technique of focused shock waves to fragment a stone in the kidney or the ureter. The patient is placed in a tub of water or in contact with a water-filled cushion, and a shock wave is created which is focused on the stone. The wave shatters and fragments the stone. The resulting debris, called gravel, then passes through the remainder of the ureter, through the bladder, and through the urethra during urination. There is minimal chance of damage to skin or internal organs because biologic tissues are resilient, not brittle, and because the the shock waves are not focused on them.

Preparation

Prior to the lithotripsy procedure, a complete **physical examination** is done, followed by tests to determine the number, location, and size of the stone or stones. A test called an intravenous pyelogram, or IVP, is used to locate the stones. An IVP involves injecting a dye into a vein in the arm. This dye, which shows up on x ray, travels through the bloodstream and is excreted by the kidneys. The dye then flows down the ureters and into the bladder. The dye surrounds the stones, and x rays are then used to evaluate the stones and the anatomy of the urinary system. (Some people are allergic to the dye material, so it cannot be used. For these people, focused sound waves, called ultrasound, can be used to see where the stones are located.) Blood tests are done to determine if any potential bleeding problems exist. For women of childbearing age, a **pregnancy** test is done to make sure the patient isn't pregnant; and elderly patients have an EKG done to make sure no potential heart problems exist. Some patients may have a stent placed prior to the lithotripsy procedure. A stent is a plastic tube placed in the ureter which allows the passage of gravel and urine after the ESWL procedure is completed.

Aftercare

Most patients have a lot of blood in their urine after the ESWL procedure. This is normal and should clear after several days to a week or so. Lots of fluids should be taken to encourage the flushing of any gravel remaining in the urinary system. The patient should follow up with the urologist in about two weeks to make sure that everything is going as planned. If a stent has been inserted, it is normally removed at this time. Patients may return to work whenever they feel able.

Risks

Abdominal pain is not uncommon after ESWL, but it is usually not cause to worry. However, persistent or severe abdominal pain may imply unexpected internal injury. Colicky renal pain is very common as gravel is still passing. Other problems may include perirenal hematomas (blood clots near the kidneys) in 66% of the cases; nerve palsies; **pancreatitis** (inflammation of the pancreas); and obstruction by stone fragments. Occasionally, stones may not be completely fragmented during the

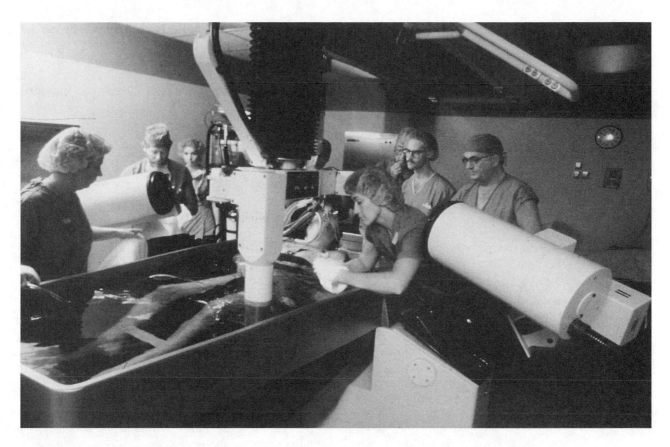

A lithotriptor in use by patient in tub. This noninvasive method crushes kidney stones through shock waves. *(Photo Researchers, Inc. Reproduced by permission.)*

first ESWL treatment and further ESWL procedures may be required.

Resources

BOOKS

Tanagho, Emil and Jack McAninch, eds. *Smith's General Urology,* 14th ed. Norwalk, CT: Appleton and Lange Publishers, 1995.

ORGANIZATIONS

American Urological Association. 1120 North Charles St., Baltimore, MD 21201-5559.

Joe Knight

Live cell therapy *see* **Cell therapy**

Liver biopsy

Definition

A liver biopsy is a medical procedure performed to obtain a small piece of liver tissue for diagnostic testing. The sample is usually examined under a microscope by a doctor who specializes in the effects of disease on body tissues (a pathologist) to check for any abnormalities of the liver. Liver biopsies are sometimes called percutaneous liver biopsies, because the tissue sample is obtained by going through the patient's skin.

Purpose

A liver biopsy is usually done to evaluate the extent of damage that has occurred to the liver because of chronic disease processes. Biopsies are often performed to identify abnormalities in liver tissues after imaging studies have failed to yield clear results.

A liver biopsy may be ordered to evaluate any of the following conditions or disorders:

- **Jaundice**

- **Cirrhosis**

- Repeated abnormal results from **liver function tests**

- Unexplained swelling or enlargement of the liver (hepatomegaly).

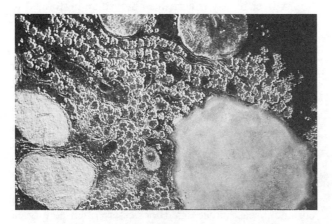

A false color image of hepatocyte cells of the liver that secrete bile. *(Custom Medical Stock Photo. Reproduced by permission.)*

- **Hemochromatosis,** which is a condition of excess iron in the liver

- Hepatitis

- **Abscesses** produced by infections, including **tuberculosis**

- Primary **cancers** of the liver, such as hepatomas, cholangiocarcinomas, and angiosarcomas

- Metastatic cancers of the liver. These are over 20 times as common in the United States as primary cancers.

Precautions

Some patients should not have percutaneous liver biopsies. They include patients with any of the following conditions:

- A **platelet count** below 100,000

- A prothrombin test time longer than 15 seconds

- A liver tumor with a large number of veins

- A large amount of abdominal fluid (**ascites**)

- A watery (hydatid) cyst

- A collection of pus (**empyema**) anywhere in the lungs, the linings of the lung cavity and the abdomen, the biliary tract, or the liver

- Benign tumors (angiomas) of the liver. These tumors consist mostly of enlarged or newly formed blood vessels and may bleed heavily.

Description

Percutaneous liver biopsy is sometimes called aspiration biopsy because it is done with a hollow needle attached to a suction syringe. The special needle that is used to perform a liver biopsy is called a Menghini needle. In many cases the biopsy is done by a doctor who specializes in x rays and imaging studies (a radiologist). The radiologist will use **computed tomography scan** (CT scan) or ultrasound to guide the choice of the site for the biopsy.

An hour or so before the biopsy, the patient will be given a sedative to help relaxation. He or she is then asked to lie on the back with the right elbow to the side and the right hand under the head. The patient is instructed to lie as still as possible during the procedure. He or she is warned to expect a sensation resembling a punch in the right shoulder when the needle passes a certain nerve (the phrenic nerve) but to hold still in spite of the momentary feeling.

Following these instructions to the patient, the doctor marks a spot on the skin where the needle will be inserted. The right side of the upper abdomen is thoroughly cleansed with an antiseptic solution, generally iodine. The patient is then given an anesthetic at the biopsy site.

The doctor prepares the Menghini needle by drawing sterile saline solution into a syringe. The syringe is then attached to the biopsy needle, which is inserted into the patient's chest wall. The doctor then draws the plunger of the syringe back to create a vacuum. At this point the patient is asked to take a deep breath and hold it. The needle is inserted into the liver and withdrawn quickly, usually within 2 seconds or less. The negative pressure in the syringe draws or pulls a sample of liver tissue into the biopsy needle. As soon as the needle is withdrawn, the patient can breathe normally. Pressure is applied at the biopsy site to stop any bleeding and a bandage will be placed over it. The liver tissue sample is placed in a cup with a 10% formalin solution and sent to the laboratory immediately. The entire procedure takes 10-15 minutes. Test results are usually available within a day.

Most patients experience minor discomfort during the procedure, but not severe **pain.** Mild medications of a non-**aspirin** type can be given after the biopsy if the pain lasts for several hours.

A liver biopsy generally costs between $400-$500. Insurance coverage for the test may vary, depending on the provider.

Preparation

Liver biopsies require some preparation of the patient. Since aspirin and ibuprofen (Advil, Motrin) are known to thin the blood and lessen clotting function, it is best to avoid these medications for at least a week before the biopsy. The doctor should check the patient's records to see whether he or she is taking any other medications that may affect blood clotting. Blood tests to check for clotting disorders are given to make sure that the patient's clotting factors are within the normal limits. The tests most commonly given to patients scheduled for a liver biopsy are platelet count tests and **prothrombin time** tests. The patient should limit food or drink for a period of four to eight hours before the biopsy.

Before the procedure, the patient or family member should sign a consent form. The patient will be checked for allergy to the local anesthetic and asked to empty the bladder so that he or she will be more comfortable during the procedure. His or her pulse rate, temperature, and breathing rate (vital signs) will be noted so that the doctor can tell during the procedure if he or she is having physical problems.

Aftercare

Liver biopsies are now considered outpatient procedures in most hospitals. Patients are usually discharged four to eight hours after the biopsy. At regular intervals, a nurse checks the patient's vital signs. If there are no complications, the patient is sent home.

Patients should arrange to have a friend or relative take them home after discharge. Bed rest for a day is recommended, followed by a week of avoiding heavy work or strenuous **exercise.** The patient can resume eating a normal diet.

Some mild soreness in the area of the biopsy is normal after the anesthetic wears off. Irritation of the muscle that lies over the liver can also cause mild discomfort in the shoulder for some patients. Tylenol can be taken for minor soreness, but aspirin and ibuprofen products are best avoided. The patient should, however, call the doctor if there is severe pain in the abdomen, chest or shoulder; difficulty breathing; or persistent bleeding. These signs may indicate that there has been leakage of bile into the abdominal cavity, or that air has been introduced into the cavity around the lungs.

Risks

The risks of a liver biopsy are usually very small. The most significant risk is prolonged internal bleeding. In about 0.4% of cases, a patient with **liver cancer** will develop a fatal hemorrhage from a percutaneous biopsy. These fatalities result because some liver tumors are supplied with a large number of blood vessels and bleed very easily. Other complications from percutaneous liver biopsies include the leakage of bile or the introduction of air into the chest cavity (**pneumothorax**). There is also a small chance that an infection may occur, or an internal organ such as the lung, gall bladder, or kidney could be punctured.

Normal results

After the biopsy, the liver sample is sent to the pathology laboratory and treated with special stains. A small piece of the treated tissue sample is placed on a slide and examined under the microscope by the pathologist. A normal (negative) result would find no evidence of malignancy in the tissue sample.

If the biopsy results indicate that there is an abnormality but that it is not cancerous, a laparotomy or **laparoscopy** may be ordered for further diagnostic study.

Abnormal results

Abnormal results include changes in liver tissue due to disease that are visible under the microscope. In cirrhosis, normal liver tissue has been replaced by fibrous scar tissue. In liver cancer, small dark malignant cells will be visible within the liver tissue.

Resources

BOOKS

''Hepatic and Biliary Disorders: Laboratory and Radiologic Evaluation.'' In *The Merck Manual of Diagnosis and Therapy,* edited by Robert Berkow, et al. Rahway, NJ: Merck Research Laboratories, 1992.

''Hepatobiliary Disorders: Introduction.'' In *Professional Guide to Diseases,* edited by Stanley Loeb, et al. Springhouse, PA: Springhouse Corporation, 1991.

Rudolph, Rebecca E., and Kris V. Kowdley. ''Cirrhosis of the Liver.'' In *Current Diagnosis 9,* edited by Rex B. Conn, et al. Philadelphia: W. B. Saunders Company, 1997.

Sobel, David S., and Tom Ferguson. *The People's Book of Medical Tests.* New York: Summit Books, 1985.

Springhouse Corporation. ''Percutaneous Liver Biopsy.'' In *Illustrated Guide to Diagnostic Tests.* Springhouse, PA: Springhouse Corporation, 1994.

ORGANIZATIONS

American Liver Foundation. 1425 Pompton Avenue, Cedar Grove, NJ 07009. (800)465-4837.

Lata Cherath

Liver cancer

Definition

Liver cancer is a form of **cancer** with a high mortality rate. Liver cancers can be classified into two types. They are either primary, when the cancer starts in the liver itself; or metastatic, when the cancer has spread to the liver from some other part of the body.

Description

Primary liver cancer

Primary liver cancer is a relatively rare disease in the United States, representing about 2% of all malignancies. It is, however, much more common in other parts of the world, representing from 10-50% of malignancies in Africa and parts of Asia. The American Cancer Society estimates that in 1998, at least 14,000 new cases of liver cancer will be diagnosed. It will also cause roughly 13,000 **deaths** in the United States in 1998.

TYPES OF PRIMARY LIVER CANCER

In adults, most primary liver cancers belong to one of two types: hepatomas, or hepatocellular carcinomas, which start in the liver tissue itself; and cholangiomas, or cholangiocarcinomas, which are cancers that develop in the bile ducts inside the liver. About 90% of primary liver

---

KEY TERMS

Aflatoxin—A substance produced by molds that grow on rice and peanuts. Exposure to aflatoxin is thought to explain the high rates of primary liver cancer in Africa and parts of Asia.

Alpha-fetoprotein—A protein in blood serum that is found in abnormally high concentrations in most patients with primary liver cancer.

Cirrhosis—A chronic degenerative disease of the liver, in which normal cells are replaced by fibrous tissue. Cirrhosis is a major risk factor for the later development of liver cancer.

Hepatitis—A viral disease characterized by inflammation of the liver cells (hepatocytes). People infected with hepatitis B or hepatitis C virus are at an increased risk for developing liver cancer.

Metastatic cancer—A cancer that has spread to an organ or tissue from a primary cancer located elsewhere in the body.

---

cancers are hepatomas. In the United States, about five persons in every 200,000 will develop a hepatoma; in Africa and Asia, over 40 persons in 200,000 will develop this form of cancer. Two rare types of primary liver cancer are mixed-cell tumors and Kupffer cell **sarcomas.**

There is one type of primary liver cancer that usually occurs in children younger than four years of age and between the ages of 12-15. This type of childhood liver cancer is called a hepatoblastoma. Unlike liver cancers in adults, hepatoblastomas have a good chance of being treated successfully. Approximately 70% of children

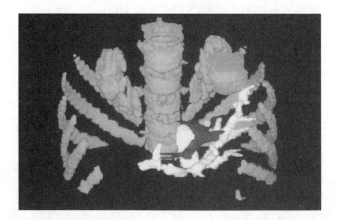

A three-dimensional computed tomography (CT) scan of a patient's abdomen showing a malignant tumor (bottom right of image) on the liver. *(Photo Researchers, Inc. Reproduced by permission.)*

with hepatoblastomas experience complete cures. If the tumor is detected early, the survival rate is over 90%.

Metastatic liver cancer

The second major category of liver cancer, metastatic liver cancer, is about 20 times as common in the United States as primary liver cancer. Because blood from all parts of the body must pass through the liver for filtration, cancer cells from other organs and tissues easily reach the liver, where they can lodge and grow into secondary tumors. Primary cancers in the colon, stomach, pancreas, rectum, esophagus, breast, lung, or skin are the most likely to spread (metastasize) to the liver. It is not unusual for the metastatic cancer in the liver to be the first noticeable sign of a cancer that started in another organ. After **cirrhosis,** metastatic liver cancer is the most common cause of fatal liver disease.

Causes & symptoms

Risk factors for primary liver cancer

The exact cause of primary liver cancer is still unknown. In adults, however, certain factors are known to place some individuals at higher risk of developing liver cancer. These factors include:

- Male sex. The male/female ratio for hepatoma is 4:1.

- Age over 60 years

- Exposure to substances in the environment that tend to cause cancer (carcinogens). These include a substance produced by a mold that grows on rice and peanuts (aflatoxin); thorium dioxide, which was used at one time as a contrast dye for x rays of the liver; and vinyl chloride, used in manufacturing plastics.

- Use of oral estrogens for birth control

- Hereditary **hemochromatosis.** Hemochromatosis is a disorder characterized by abnormally high levels of iron storage in the body. It often develops into cirrhosis.

- Cirrhosis. Hepatomas appear to be a frequent complication of cirrhosis of the liver. Between 30-70% of hepatoma patients also have cirrhosis. It is estimated that a patient with cirrhosis has 40 times the chance of developing a hepatoma than a person with a healthy liver.

- Exposure to **hepatitis B** (HBV) or **hepatitis C** (HBC) viruses. In Africa and most of Asia, exposure to hepatitis B is an important factor; in Japan and some Western countries, exposure to hepatitis C is connected with a higher risk of developing liver cancer. In the United States, nearly 25% of patients with liver cancer show evidence of HBV infection. Hepatitis is commonly found among intravenous drug abusers.

Symptoms of liver cancer

The early symptoms of primary, as well as metastatic, liver cancer are often vague and not unique to liver disorders. The long lagtime between the beginning of the tumor's growth and signs of illness is the major reason why the disease has such a high mortality rate. At the time of diagnosis, patients are often tired, with **fever,** abdominal **pain,** and loss of appetite. They may look emaciated and generally ill. As the tumor grows bigger, it stretches the membrane surrounding the liver (the capsule), causing pain in the upper abdomen on the right side. The pain may extend into the back and shoulder. Some patients develop a collection of fluid, known as **ascites,** in the abdominal cavity. Others may show signs of bleeding into the digestive tract. In addition, the tumor may block the ducts of the liver or the gall bladder, leading to **jaundice.** In patients with jaundice, the whites of the eyes and the skin may turn yellow, and the urine becomes dark-colored.

Diagnosis

Physical examination

If the doctor suspects a diagnosis of liver cancer, he or she will check the patient's history for risk factors and pay close attention to the condition of the patient's abdomen during the **physical examination.** Masses or lumps in the liver and ascites can often be felt while the patient is lying flat on the examination table. The liver is usually swollen and hard in patients with liver cancer; it may be sore when the doctor presses on it. In some cases, the patient's spleen is also enlarged. The doctor may be able to hear an abnormal sound (bruit) or rubbing noise (friction rub) if he or she uses a stethoscope to listen to the blood vessels that lie near the liver. The noises are caused by the pressure of the tumor on the blood vessels.

Laboratory tests

Blood tests may be used to test liver function or to evaluate risk factors in the patient's history. Between 50-75% of primary liver cancer patients have abnormally high blood serum levels of a particular protein (alpha-fetoprotein or AFP). The AFP test, however, cannot be used by itself to confirm a diagnosis of liver cancer, because cirrhosis or chronic hepatitis can also produce high alpha-fetoprotein levels. Tests for alkaline phosphatase, bilirubin, lactic dehydrogenase, and other chemicals indicate that the liver is not functioning normally. About 75% of patients with liver cancer show evidence of hepatitis infection. Again, however, abnormal liver function test results are not specific for liver cancer.

Imaging studies

Imaging studies are useful in locating specific areas of abnormal tissue in the liver. Liver tumors as small as an inch across can now be detected by ultrasound or **computed tomography scan** (CT scan). Imaging studies, however, cannot tell the difference between a hepatoma and other abnormal masses or lumps of tissue (nodules) in the liver. A sample of liver tissue for biopsy is needed to make the definitive diagnosis of a primary liver cancer. CT or ultrasound can be used to guide the doctor in selecting the best location for obtaining the biopsy sample.

Chest x rays may be used to see whether the liver tumor is primary or has metastasized from a primary tumor in the lungs.

Liver biopsy

Liver biopsy is considered to provide the definite diagnosis of liver cancer. A sample of the liver or tissue fluid is removed with a fine needle and is checked under a microscope for the presence of cancer cells. In about 70% of cases, the biopsy is positive for cancer. In most cases, there is little risk to the patient from the biopsy procedure. In about 0.4% of cases, however, the patient develops a fatal hemorrhage from the biopsy because some tumors are supplied with a large number of blood vessels and bleed very easily.

Laparoscopy

The doctor may also perform a **laparoscopy** to help in the diagnosis of liver cancer. A laparoscope is a small tube-shaped instrument with a light at one end. The doctor makes a small cut in the patient's abdomen and inserts the laparoscope. A small piece of liver tissue is removed and examined under a microscope for the presence of cancer cells.

Treatment

Treatment of liver cancer is based on several factors, including the type of cancer (primary or metastatic); stage (early or advanced); the location of other primary cancers or metastases in the patient's body; the patient's age; and other coexisting diseases, including cirrhosis. For many patients, treatment of liver cancer is primarily intended to relieve the pain caused by the cancer but cannot cure it.

Surgery

Few liver cancers in adults can be cured by surgery because they are usually too advanced by the time they are discovered. If the cancer is contained within one lobe of the liver, and if the patient does not have either cirrhosis, jaundice, or ascites, surgery is the best treatment option. Patients who can have their entire tumor removed have the best chance for survival. Unfortunately, only about 5% of patients with metastatic cancer (from primary tumors in the colon or rectum) fall into this group. If the entire visible tumor can be removed, about 25% of patients will be cured. The operation that is performed is called a partial hepatectomy, or partial removal of the liver. The surgeon will remove either an entire lobe of the liver (a lobectomy) or cut out the area around the tumor (a wedge resection).

Chemotherapy

Some patients with metastatic cancer of the liver can have their lives prolonged for a few months by **chemotherapy,** although cure is not possible. If the tumor cannot be removed by surgery, a tube (catheter) can be placed in the main artery of the liver and an implantable infusion pump can be installed. The pump allows much higher concentrations of the cancer drug to be carried to the tumor than is possible with chemotherapy carried through the bloodstream. The drug that is used for infusion pump therapy is usually floxuridine (FUDR), given for 14-day periods alternating with 14-day rests. Systemic chemotherapy can also be used to treat liver cancer. The medications usually used are 5-fluorouracil (Adrucil, Efudex) or methotrexate (MTX, Mexate). Systemic chemotherapy does not, however, significantly lengthen the patient's survival time.

Radiation therapy

Radiation therapy is the use of high-energy rays or x rays to kill cancer cells or to shrink tumors. Its use in liver cancer, however, is only to give brief relief from some of the symptoms. Liver cancers are not sensitive to radiation, and radiation therapy will not prolong the patient's life.

Liver transplantation

Removal of the entire liver (total hepatectomy) and **liver transplantation** are used very rarely in treating liver cancer as of 1998. This is because very few patients are eligible for this procedure, either because the cancer has spread beyond the liver or because there are no suitable donors. Further research in the field of transplant immunology may make liver transplantation a possible treatment method for more patients in the future.

Prognosis

Liver cancer has a very poor prognosis because it is often not diagnosed until it has metastasized. Fewer than 10% of patients survive three years after the initial diagnosis; the overall five-year survival rate for patients with hepatomas is around 4%. Most patients with primary liver cancer die within several months of diagnosis. Patients with liver cancers that metastasized from cancers in the colon live slightly longer than those whose cancers spread from cancers in the stomach or pancreas.

Prevention

There are no useful strategies at present for preventing metastatic cancers of the liver. Primary liver cancers, however, are 75-80% preventable. Current strategies focus on widespread **vaccination** for hepatitis B; early treatment of hereditary hemochromatosis; and screening of high-risk patients with alpha-fetoprotein testing and ultrasound examinations.

Lifestyle factors that can be modified in order to prevent liver cancer include avoidance of exposure to toxic chemicals and foods harboring molds that produce aflatoxin. Most important, however, is avoidance of alcohol and drug abuse. Alcohol abuse is responsible for 60-75% of cases of cirrhosis, which is a major risk factor for eventual development of primary liver cancer. Hepatitis is a widespread disease among persons who abuse intravenous drugs.

Resources

BOOKS

Dollinger, Malin. *Everyone's Guide to Cancer Therapy.* Kansas City: Somerville House Books Limited, 1994.

Friedman, Lawrence S. "Liver, Biliary Tract, & Pancreas." In *Current Medical Diagnosis & Treatment 1998,* edited by Lawrence M. Tierney, Jr., et al. Stamford, CT: Appleton & Lange, 1997.

"Hepatic and Biliary Disorders: Neoplasms of the Liver." In *The Merck Manual of Diagnosis and Therapy,* edited by Robert Berkow, et al. Rahway, NJ: Merck Research Laboratories, 1992.

"Liver Cancer." In *Professional Guide to Diseases,* edited by Stanley Loeb et al. Springhouse, PA: Springhouse Corporation, 1991.

Morra, Marion E. *Choices.* New York: Avon Books, October 1994.

Rudolph, Rebecca E., and Kris V. Kowdley. "Cirrhosis of the Liver." In *Current Diagnosis 9,* edited by Rex B. Conn, et al. Philadelphia: W. B. Saunders Company, 1997.

Way, Lawrence W. "Liver." In *Current Surgical Diagnosis & Treatment,* edited by Lawrence W. Way. Stamford, CT: Appleton & Lange, 1994.

ORGANIZATIONS

American Cancer Society. 1599 Clifton Road, N.E., Atlanta, GA 30329. (800)227-2345.

American Liver Foundation. 1425 Pompton Avenue, Cedar Grove, NJ 07009. (800)465-4837.

Cancer Research Institute. 681 Fifth Avenue, New York, NY 10022. (800)992-2623.

National Cancer Institute (National Institutes of Health). 9000 Rockville Pike, Bethesda, MD 20892. (800)422-6237.

Rebecca J. Frey

Liver cirrhosis *see* **Cirrhosis**

Liver encephalopathy

Definition

Liver encephalopathy is a potentially life-threatening disease in which toxic substances accumulate in the blood. Also known as hepatic encephalopathy or hepatic **coma,** this condition can cause confusion, disorientation, abnormal neurological signs, loss of consciousness, and **death.**

Description

A normally functioning liver metabolizes and detoxifies substances formed in the body during the digestive process. Impaired liver function allows substances like ammonia (formed when the body digests protein), some fatty acids, phenol, and mercaptans to escape into the bloodstream. From there, they may penetrate the blood-brain barrier, affect the central nervous system (CNS), and lead to hepatic coma.

Hepatic coma is most common in patients with chronic liver disease. It occurs in 50-70% of all those with **cirrhosis.**

Causes & symptoms

The cause of hepatic coma is unknown, but the condition is frequently associated with the following conditions:

- Acute or chronic liver disease
- Gastrointestinal bleeding
- Azotemia, the accumulation of nitrogen-containing compounds (such as urea) in the blood
- Inherited disorders that disrupt the process by which nitrogen is decomposed and excreted
- The use of shunts (devices implanted in the body to redirect the flow of fluid from one vessel to another)
- Electrolyte imbalances, including low levels of potassium (**hypokalemia**) and abnormally alkaline blood pH (alkalosis). These imbalances may result from the overuse of sedatives, **analgesics,** or **diuretics;** reduced lev-

KEY TERMS

Cirrhosis—A serious disease of the liver caused by chronic damage to its cells and the eventual formation of scar tissue (fibrosis).

Coma—A condition of deep unconsciousness from which the person cannot be aroused

Electrolytes—Substances that conduct electricity when they are in solution. In the body, electrolytes in the blood and tissues enable nerve impulses to flow normally.

Encephalopathy—A dysfunction of the brain. Hepatic encephalopathy is brain dysfunction that occurs because the liver isn't removing harmful substances from the blood.

els of oxygen (hypoxia), or withdrawal of excessive amounts of body fluid (hypovolemia)

• **Constipation,** which may increase the body's nitrogen load

• Surgery

• Infection

• Acute liver disease.

Binge drinking and acute infection are common causes of hepatic coma in patients with long-standing liver disease.

Symptoms of hepatic encephalopathy range from almost unnoticeable changes in personality, energy levels, and thinking patterns to deep coma.

Inability to reproduce a star or other simple design (apraxia) and deterioration of handwriting are common symptoms of early encephalopathy. Decreased brain function can also cause inappropriate behavior, lack of interest in personal grooming, mood swings, and uncharacteristically poor judgment.

The patient may be less alert than usual and develop new sleep patterns. Movement and speech may be slow and labored.

As the disease progresses, patients become confused, drowsy, and disoriented. The breath and urine acquires a sweet, musky odor. The hands shake, the outstretched arms flap (asterixis or ''liver flap''), and the patient may lapse into unconsciousness. As coma deepens, reflexes may be heightened (hyperreflexia). The toes sometimes splay when the sole of the foot is stroked (Babinski reflex).

Agitation occasionally occurs in children and in adults who suddenly develop severe symptoms. Seizures are uncommon.

Diagnosis

The absence of sensitive, reliable tests for encephalopathy make the physician's personal observations and professional judgment the most valuable diagnostic tools.

Confusion, disorientation, and other indications of impaired brain function strongly suggest encephalopathy in patients known to have liver disease. CAT scans and examination of spinal fluid don't provide diagnostic clues. Elevated arterial ammonia levels are almost always present in hepatic coma, but levels are not necessarily correlated with the severity or extent of the disease.

Magnetic resonance imaging (MRI) can show severe brain swelling that often occurs prior to coma, and **electroencephalography** (EEG) detects abnormal brain waves even in patients with early, mild symptoms. Blood and urine analyses can provide important information about the cause of encephalopathy in patients suspected of taking large quantities of sedatives or other drugs.

Treatment

This condition may disappear if the cause of symptoms is eliminated. In other cases, treatment is designed to improve liver function as much as possible; remove or relieve factors that worsen symptoms; and decrease the body's production of poisonous substances.

All non-essential medications are discontinued. Soft restraints are recommended in place of sedatives for patients who become agitated.

Enemas or **laxatives** are used to stimulate expulsion of toxic intestinal products. All or most protein is eliminated from the diet, and supplemental feeding may be necessary to replenish lost calories. Regular doses of neomycin (Neobiotic), taken orally or administered to comatose patients in liquid form through a tube, may be used to decrease production of protein-digesting bacteria in the bowel.

Lactulose, a synthetic sugar, changes the characteristics of intestinal bacteria, decreases the amount of ammonia accumulated in the body, and has laxative properties. The patient is given hourly doses of lactulose syrup until **diarrhea** occurs, then dosage is adjusted to maintain regular bowel function. Lactulose and dietary-protein restrictions may be used to control chronic encephalopathy.

Prognosis

Encephalopathy may be reversible if the responsible factor is identified and removed or treated. Patients whose condition is the result of chronic liver disease may recover completely after the underlying cause is corrected.

Despite intensive treatment, encephalopathy caused by acute liver inflammation (fulminant hepatitis) is fatal for as many as 80% of patients. Those with chronic liver failure often die in hepatic coma.

Resources

BOOKS

Bennet, J. Claude, and Fred Plum, eds. *Cecil Textbook of Medicine.* Philadelphia, PA: W.B. Saunders Co., 1996.

Berkow, Robert, ed. *The Merck Manual of Medical Information: Home Edition.* Whitehouse Station, NJ: Merck & Co., Inc., 1997.

Isselbacher, Kurt, J., et al., eds. *Harrison's Principles of Internal Medicine.* New York, NY: McGraw-Hill, Inc., 1994.

ORGANIZATIONS

American Liver Foundation. 1425 Pompton Avenue, Cedar Grove, NJ 07009. (800) GO-LIVER. http://www.liverfoundation.org/.

OTHER

Hepatic and Biliary Disorders. http://www.merck.com/!!tKNH50WVitKNRZ2qCQ/pubs/mmanual/html/hkfeqk.htm (12 May 1998).

Treatment of Hepatic Encephalopathy. http://www.ginet.com/papers/mpape.324.htm (12 May 1998).

Maureen Haggerty

Liver fluke infections *see* **Fluke infections**

. . . .

Liver function tests

Definition

Liver function tests, or LFTs, include tests for bilirubin, a breakdown product of hemoglobin, and ammonia, a protein byproduct that is normally converted into urea by the liver before being excreted by the kidneys. LFTs also commonly include tests to measure levels of several enzymes, which are special proteins that help the body break down and use (metabolize) other substances. Enzymes that are often measured in LFTs include gamma-glutamyl transferase (GGT); alanine aminotransferase (ALT or SGPT); aspartate aminotransferase (AST or SGOT); and alkaline phosphatase (ALP). LFTs also may include **prothrombin time** (PT), a measure of how long it takes for the blood to clot.

Purpose

Liver function tests are used to aid in the differential diagnosis of liver disease and injury, and to help monitor response to treatment.

Precautions

Bilirubin: Drugs that may cause increased blood levels of total bilirubin include anabolic steroids, **antibiotics,** antimalarials, ascorbic acid, Diabinese, codeine, **diuretics,** epinephrine, **oral contraceptives,** and vitamin A.

Ammonia: Muscular exertion can increase ammonia levels, while cigarette smoking produces significant increases within one hour of inhalation. Drugs that may cause increased levels include alcohol, **barbiturates,** narcotics, and diuretics. Drugs that may decrease levels include broad-spectrum antibiotics, levodopa, lactobacillus, and potassium salts.

ALT: Drugs that may increase ALT levels include **acetaminophen,** ampicillin, codeine, dicumarol, indomethacin, methotrexate, oral contraceptives, **tetracyclines,** and verapamil. Previous intramuscular injections may cause elevated levels.

GGT: Drugs that may cause increased GGT levels include alcohol, phenytoin, and phenobarbital. Drugs that may cause decreased levels include oral contraceptives.

Description

The liver is one of the most important organs in the body. As the body's "chemical factory," it regulates the levels of most of the main blood chemicals and acts with the kidneys to clear the blood of drugs and toxic substances. The liver metabolizes these products, alters their chemical structure, makes them water soluble, and excretes them in bile.

Liver function tests are used to determine if the liver has been damaged or its function impaired. Elevations of certain liver tests in relation to others aids in that determination. For example, aminotransferases (which include ALT and AST) are notably elevated in liver damage caused by liver cell disease (hepatocellular disease). However, in intrahepatic obstructive disease—which may be caused by some drugs or biliary **cirrhosis**—the alkaline phosphatases are most abnormal.

Alanine aminotransferase

Alanine aminotransferase (ALT), formerly called serum glutamate pyruvate transaminase, or SGPT, is an enzyme necessary for energy production. It is present in a number of tissues, including the liver, heart, and skeletal muscles, but is found in the highest concentration in the liver. Because of this, it is used in conjunction with other liver enzymes to detect liver disease, especially hepatitis or cirrhosis without **jaundice.** Additionally, in conjunction with the **aspartate aminotransferase test** (AST), it helps to distinguish between heart damage and liver tissue damage.

KEY TERMS

Cirrhosis—A serious disease of the liver caused by chronic damage to its cells and the eventual formation of scar tissue (fibrosis). The most common symptoms are mild jaundice, fluid collection in the tissues, mental confusion, and vomiting of blood. If left untreated, cirrhosis lead to liver failure and death.

Hemolytic disease of the newborn—Also known as erythroblastosis neonatorum, this is a condition in which a newborn's red blood cells are destroyed by antibodies that have crossed the placenta from the mother's blood. (Hemolytic disease begins in the fetus, in whom the disease is called erythroblastosis fetalis). Severe anemia caused by hemolytic disease is treated in the same way as other anemias, but when jaundice appears due to increased bilirubin, the jaundice is treated by exposing the infant to bright lights. In severe cases, exchange transfusion is required or brain damage may result.

Hepatic encephalopathy—Also called liver encephalopathy or hepatic coma, this is a disorder in which brain function deteriorates because toxic substances, which would normally be removed by the liver, accumulate in the bloodstream due to liver damage or disease. Early symptoms include subtle changes in logical thinking, personality and behavior. As the disorder progresses, signs of drowsiness and confusion increase until eventually the patient loses consciousness and lapses into coma.

Hepatitis—An inflammation of the liver, with accompanying liver cell damage or cell death, caused most frequently by viral infection, but also by certain drugs, chemicals, or poisons. May be either acute (of limited duration) or chronic (continuing). Symptoms include jaundice, nausea, vomiting, loss of appetite, tenderness in the right upper abdomen, aching muscles, and joint pain. In severe cases, liver failure may result.

Reye's syndrome—A rare disorder characterized by brain and liver damage following an upper respiratory tract infection, chickenpox, or influenza, almost entirely confined to children under age 15, and often related to aspirin ingestion for a viral infection. Symptoms include uncontrollable vomiting, often with lethargy, memory loss, disorientation, or delirium. Swelling of the brain may cause seizures, coma, and in severe cases, death.

Aspartate aminotransferase

Aspartate aminotransferase (AST), formerly called serum glutamic-oxaloacetic transaminase, or SGOT, is another enzyme necessary for energy production. It, too, may be elevated in liver and heart disease. In liver disease, the AST increase is usually less than the ALT increase. However, in liver disease caused by alcohol use, the AST increase may be two or three times greater than the ALT increase.

Alkaline phosphatase

Alkaline phosphatase (ALP) levels usually include two similar enzymes (isoenzymes) that mainly come from the liver and bone and from the placenta in pregnant women. In some cases, doctors may order a test to differentiate between the alkaline phosphatase that originates in the liver and the alkaline phosphatase originating in bone. If a person has elevated ALP, does not have bone disease and is not pregnant, he or she may have a problem with the biliary tract, the system that makes and stores bile. (Bile is made in the liver, then passes through ducts to the gall bladder, where it is stored.)

Gamma-glutamyl transferase

Gamma-glutamyl transferase (GGT), sometimes called gamma-glutamyl transpeptidase (GGPT), is an enzyme that is compared with ALP levels to distinguish between skeletal disease and liver disease. Because GGT is not increased in bone disorders, as is ALP, a normal GGT with an elevated ALP would indicate bone disease. Conversely, because the GGT is more specifically related to the liver, an elevated GGT with an elevated ALP would strengthen the diagnosis of liver or bile-duct disease. The GGT has also been used as an indicator of heavy and chronic alcohol use, but its value in these situations has been questioned recently. It is also commonly elevated in patients with **infectious mononucleosis**.

Bilirubin

Bilirubin, a breakdown product of hemoglobin, is the predominant pigment in a substance produced by the liver called bile. Excess bilirubin causes yellowing of body tissues (jaundice). There are two tests for bilirubin: direct-reacting (conjugated) and indirect-reacting (unconjugated). Differentiating between the two is important diagnostically, as elevated levels of indirect bilirubin are usually caused by liver cell dysfunction (e.g. hepatitis), while elevations of direct bilirubin typically result from obstruction either within the liver (intrahepatic) or a source outside the liver (e.g. **gallstones** or a tumor blocking the bile ducts). Bilirubin measurements are especially valuable in newborns, as extremely elevated levels of unconjugated bilirubin can accumulate in the brain, causing irreparable damage.

Ammonia

Analysis of blood ammonia aids in the diagnosis of severe liver diseases and helps to monitor the course of these diseases. Together with the AST and the ALT, ammonia levels are used to confirm a diagnosis of **Reye's syndrome** (a rare disorder usually seen in children and associated with **aspirin** intake), which is characterized by brain and liver damage following an upper respiratory tract infection, **chickenpox,** or **influenza.** Ammonia levels are also helpful in the diagnosis and treatment of hepatic encephalopathy, a serious brain condition caused by the accumulated toxins that result from liver disease and liver failure.

Preparation

Preparation requirements for all these tests vary from laboratory to laboratory, so it is generally considered best that the patient be in a **fasting** state (nothing to eat or drink) after midnight the day before the test(s).

Aftercare

Because many patients with liver disease have prolonged clotting times, it is important to monitor the puncture site for bleeding after blood is drawn (venipuncture).

Risks

Risks for this test are minimal, but may include slight bleeding from the blood-drawing site, **fainting** or feeling lightheaded after venipuncture, or hematoma (blood accumulating under the puncture site).

Normal results

Reference ranges vary from laboratory to laboratory and also depend upon the method used. However, normal values can generally be found within the following ranges, unless specified differently.

- ALT: 5-35 IU/L (values for the elderly may be slightly higher, and values also may be higher in men and in African-Americans)

- AST: 0-35 IU/L

- ALP: 30-120 IU/L

- GGT: Normal values for this test vary widely, depending on the laboratory performing the test, and the age and sex of the patient. For example, females less than 45 years old have lower values than both males and females over 45 years of age. Values in the newborn can be as much as five times higher than in adults.

- Bilirubin: (Adult, elderly, and child) Total bilirubin: 0.1-1.0 mg/dL; indirect bilirubin: 0.2-0.8 mg/dL; direct bilirubin: 0.1-0.3 mg/dL. (Newborn) Total bilirubin: 1-12 mg/dL. Note: critical values for adult: greater than 1.2 mg/dL. Critical values for newborn (requiring immediate treatment): greater than 15 mg/dL.

- Ammonia: Normal values for this test vary widely, depending upon the laboratory performing the test, the age of the patient, and the type of specimen. For example, values are somewhat higher in arterial than in venous blood.

- PT: 9-12 seconds.

Abnormal results

ALT: Values are significantly increased in cases of hepatitis, and moderately increased in cirrhosis, liver tumor, obstructive jaundice, and severe **burns.** Values are mildly increased in **pancreatitis, heart attack,** infectious mononucleosis, and **shock.** Most useful when compared with ALP levels.

- AST: High levels may indicate liver cell damage, hepatitis, heart attack, **heart failure,** or gall stones.

- ALP: Elevated levels occur in diseases that impair bile formation (**cholestasis**). ALP may also be elevated in many other liver disorders, as well as some **lung cancers** (bronchogenic carcinoma) and Hodgkin's lymphoma. However, elevated ALP levels may also occur in otherwise healthy people, especially among older people.

GGT: Increased levels are diagnostic of hepatitis, cirrhosis, liver tumor or metastasis, as well as injury from drugs toxic to the liver. Although the causes are unclear, GGT levels may increase with alcohol ingestion, heart attack, pancreatitis, infectious mononucleosis, and Reye's syndrome.

Bilirubin: Increased *indirect* or total bilirubin levels can indicate various serious **anemias,** including hemolytic disease of the newborn and **transfusion** reaction. Increased *direct* bilirubin levels can be diagnostic of bile duct obstruction, gallstones, cirrhosis, or hepatitis. It is important to note that if total bilirubin levels in the newborn reach or exceed critical levels, exchange transfusion is necessary to avoid kernicterus, a condition that causes brain damage.

Ammonia: Increased levels are seen in primary liver cell disease, Reye's syndrome, severe heart failure, hemolytic disease of the newborn, and hepatic encephalopathy.

PT: Elevated in acute liver injury, vitamin K deficiencies, and disorders with impair the absorption of vitamin K, including cholestasis.

Resources

BOOKS

Cahill, Matthew. *Handbook of Diagnostic Tests.* Springhouse Corporation, 1995.

Jacobs, David S. *Laboratory Test Handbook.* 4th ed. Lexi-Comp Inc., 1996.

Pagana, Kathleen Deska. *Mosby's Manual of Diagnostic and Laboratory Tests.* Mosby, Inc., 1998.

Janis O. Flores

Liver nuclear medicine scan

Definition

A liver scan is a diagnostic procedure to evaluate the liver for suspected disease. A radioactive substance which concentrates in the liver is injected intravenously and the image of its distribution in the body is analyzed to diagnose certain abnormalities.

Purpose

In the past, liver scans were used to evaluate the liver in a wide variety of situations. It was considered a useful study to detect abnormalities, but was often not able to establish a specific diagnosis. In the 1990s, radionuclide imaging of the liver (use of a radioactive form of cobalt or iodine) evolved into a more specialized study, used to identify individual diseases or conditions. This is accomplished by using different radioisotopes precisely designed to further evaluate a particular case. Isotopes are different forms of the same substance, such as radioactive iodine, that are injected into the body. This allows the physician to trace the process of the substance throughout the part of the body that is being tested for disease.

A liver scan is usually ordered after blood studies and other imaging procedures have shown a liver abnormality. It is most often used to further evaluate masses or tumors. These may be benign growths in the liver, or **cancer** which has developed in the liver or has spread (or metastasized) from another organ.

A liver scan may also be helpful in diagnosing specific disorders, by detecting features which are characteristic of a disorder, such as **cirrhosis** of the liver. This

study may also be part of the battery of tests used to evaluate potential candidates for liver transplant.

Precautions

Women who are pregnant or breast feeding should not have this test.

Description

This test can be performed in an outpatient setting or a hospital x-ray department. The patient usually lies down while a radioactive substance (radioactive isotope) which accumulates in the liver is injected through a vein in the arm. Scanning times may vary, depending on the specific radioisotope used. It most often begins within minutes after injection. The radionuclide scanner, sometimes called a gamma camera or scintillation camera, is positioned above the upper abdomen and may lightly touch the patient. It is important for the patient to lie quietly. Position changes and brief periods of breath holding may be required. The test usually takes approximately one hour.

A specialized liver scan used to assess blood flow is frequently used. It may be referred to as a radionuclide blood pool or volume study, a labeled red cell scintigram, or some combination of these terms. Other studies may be named for the radioisotope used. This test may also be called a liver-spleen scan.

Preparation

No physical preparation is required. A liver scan should be performed before doing any study that uses iodinated or barium-containing contrast agents, to prevent inaccurate results.

The patients should understand that there is no danger of radioactive exposure to themselves or others. Only small amounts of radionuclide are used. The total amount of radiation absorbed is often less than the dose received from ordinary x rays. The scanner does not emit any radiation, but detects and records it from the patient.

Aftercare

No special precautions are needed.

Normal results

A normal scan will show a liver of normal size, shape, and position.

Abnormal results

An abnormal liver scan may result from a mass. Depending on the radioisotope and technique used, the scan may identify particular types of tumors or certain cancers. Too much radioisotope in the spleen and bones, compared to the liver, can indicate potential **hypertension** or cirrhosis. Liver diseases such as cirrhosis or hepatitis may also cause an abnormal scan, but are rarely diagnosed from the information revealed by this study alone.

Resources

BOOKS

Vitti, Richard A., and Leon S. Malmud. "Gastrointestinal System." In *Nuclear Medicine,* edited by Donald R. Bernier, et al. St. Louis: Mosby, 1997.

PERIODICALS

Drane, Walter E. "Scintigraphic Techniques for Hepatic Imaging." *Radiologic Clinics of North America,* 36 (March 1998): 309-318.

Ellen S. Weber

Liver transplantation

Definition

Liver transplantation is a surgery that removes a diseased liver and replace it with a healthy donor liver.

Purpose

The liver is the body's principle chemical factory. It receives all nutrients, drugs, and toxins absorbed from the intestines and performs the final stages of digestion, converting food into energy and replacement parts for the body. The liver also filters the blood of all waste products, removes and detoxifies poisons and excretes many of these into the bile. It processes other chemicals for excretion by the kidneys. The liver is also an energy storage organ, changing food energy to a chemical called glycogen that can be rapidly converted to fuel.

As the liver fails, all of its functions diminish. Nutrition suffers, toxins build up, and waste products accumulate. Scar tissue builds up on the liver if disease is of long duration. As the liver scars, blood flow is progressively

restricted in the portal vein, which carries blood from the stomach and abdominal organs to the liver. The resulting high blood pressure (**hypertension**) causes swelling of and bleeding from the blood vessels of the esophagus. Severe **jaundice,** fluid accumulation in the abdomen (**ascites**), and deterioration of mental function, due to the build-up of toxins in the blood (**liver encephalopathy**), eventually occur, leading to **death.**

Among the many causes of liver failure that bring patients to transplant surgery are:

- Progressive hepatitis (mostly due to virus infection) accounts for more than a third.

- Alcohol damage brings in about 20%

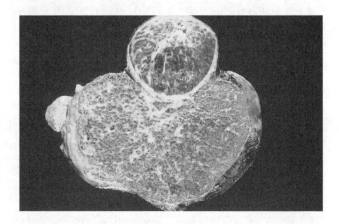

The diseased liver of a patient ready for transplantation.
(Custom Medical Stock Photo. Reproduced by permission.)

- Scarring or abnormality of the biliary system accounts for roughly another 20%.

- The remainder comes from selected **cancers,** other uncommon diseases, and a situation called fulminant liver failure.

Fulminant liver failure most commonly happens during acute viral hepatitis, but it is also the result of **mushroom poisoning** by *Amanita phalloides* and toxic reactions to some medicines, like an overdose of **acetaminophen.** This is a special category of candidates for liver transplant because of the speed of their disease and the immediate need of treatment.

The first human liver transplant was performed in 1963, and since then, thousands of liver transplants are done every year. Since the introduction of of cyclosporine (a drug that suppresses the immune response that rejects the donor organ), success rates for liver transplantation have reached 85%.

Precautions

Patients with advanced heart and lung disease, who are HIV positive, and who abuse drugs and alcohol are poor candidates for liver tranplantation. Their ability to survive the surgery and the difficult recovery period, as well as their longterm prognosis, is hindered by their conditions.

Description

There are three types of liver transplantation methods. They include:

- Orthotopic transplantation is the replacement of a whole diseased liver with a healthy donor liver.

- Heterotopic transplantation is the addition of a donor liver at another site, while the diseased liver is left intact.

- Reduced-size liver transplantation is the replacement of a whole diseased liver with a portion of a healthy donor liver. Reduced-size liver transplants are most often performed on children.

When an orthotopic transplantation is performed, a segment of the inferior vena cava attached to the liver is taken from the donor as well. The same parts are removed from the recipient and replaced by connecting the inferior vena cava, the hepatic artery, the portal vein and the bile ducts.

When there is a possibility that the afflicted liver may recover, a heterotopic tranplantation is performed. The donor liver is placed in a different site, but it still has to have the same connections. It is usually attached very near the original liver, and if the original liver recovers, the donor shrivels away. If the original liver does not recover, it will shrivel, leaving the donor in place.

Reduced-size liver transplantation tranplants part of a donor liver into a patient. It is possible to divide the liver into eight pieces, each supplied by a different set of blood vessels. Two of these pieces have been enough to save a patient in liver failure, especially if the patient is a child. It is therefore possible to transplant one liver into at least two patients and to transplant part of a liver from a living donor and have both donor and recipient survive. Liver tissue grows to accommodate its job so long as there is initially enough of the organ to use. Patients have survived with only 15-20% of their original liver, provided that 15-20% was healthy.

Availability of organs for transplant is a current crisis in the transplantation business. In October 1997, a national distribution system was established that gives priority to the sickest patients closest in location to the donor liver, but makes livers available nationally. It is now possible to preserve a liver out of the body for 10-20 hours by flushing it with cooled solutions of special chemicals and nutrients, so it can be transported across the country.

Preparation

Before transplantation takes place, the patient is first determined to be a good candidate for transplantation by going through rigorous medical examination. A suitable candidate boosts their nutritional intake in order to ensure that they are as healthy as possible before surgery. Drugs are administered that will decrease rejection after surgery. Consultation with the patient, as well as any family, is conducted to explain the surgery and its complications. Psychological counciling is recommended.

Aftercare

In order to prevent organ rejection, immunosuppressive drugs will be taken. Hospitalization ranges from four weeks to five months, depending on the rate of recovery.

Successfully receiving a transplanted liver is only the beginning of a life-long process. Patients with transplanted livers have to stay on **immunosuppressant drugs** for the rest of their lives to prevent organ rejection. Although many can reduce the dosage after the initial few months, virtually none can discontinue drugs altogether. Prednisone, azathioprine, and tacrolimus are often combined with cyclosporine for better results. Newer immunosuppressive agents are coming that promise even better results. In spite of immunosuppressants, rejection occurs most of the time and requires additional medication. In some cases it cannot be reversed, and retransplantation becomes necessary.

Risks

Early failure of the transplant occurs once in four surgeries and has to be repeated. Some transplants never work, some succumb to infection, and some suffer immune rejection. Primary failure is apparent within one or two days. Infections happen in half the patients and often appear during the first week. Rejection usually starts at the end of the first week. The surgery itself may need revision because of narrowing, leaking, or blood clots at the connections.

There are potential social and economic problems, psychological problems, and a vast array of possible medical and surgical complications. Close medical surveillance must continue for the rest of the patient's life. Infections are a constant risk while on immunosuppressive agents, because the immune system is supposed to prevent them. A way has not yet been devised to control rejection without hampering immune defenses against infections. Not only do ordinary infections pose a threat, but because of the impaired immunity, transplant patients are susceptible to the same "opportunistic" infections that threaten **AIDS** patients—**pneumocystis pneumonia,** herpes and **cytomegalovirus infections,** fungi, and a host of bacteria.

Immunosuppression also hinders the body's ability to resist cancer. All the drugs used to prevent rejection increase the risk of leukemias and lymphomas.

There is also a risk of the original disease returning. Hepatitis virus still inhabits the patient, as does the urge to drink alcohol. Newer **antiviral drugs** hold out promise for dealing with hepatitis, and Alcoholics Anonymous (AA) is the most effective treatment known for **alcoholism.**

Drug reactions are also a continuing threat. Every drug used to suppress the immune system has potential problems.

Resources

BOOKS

Dienstag, Jules. "Liver Transplantation." In *Harrison's Principles of Internal Medicine,* edited by Kurt Isselbacher, et al. New York: McGraw-Hill, 1998.

Gartner, J. Carleton. "Liver Transplantation." In *Nelson Textbook of Pediatrics,* edited by Waldo E. Nelson, et al. Philadelphia: W. B. Saunders, 1996.

Roberts, John P. "Liver Transplantation." In *Cecil Textbook of Medicine,* edited by J. Claude Bennett, and Fred Plum. Philadelphia: W. B. Saunders, 1996.

PERIODICALS

Butler, A and P. J. Friend. "Novel Strategies for Liver Support in Acute Liver Failure." *British Medical Bulletin* 53 (1997): 719-729.

Cao, S., C. O. Esquivel, and E. B. Keeffe. "New Approaches to Supporting the Failing Liver." *Annual Review of Medicine* 49 (1998): 85-94.

Lanza, R. P and D. K. Cooper "Xenotransplantation of Cells and Tissues: Application to a Range of Diseases, from Diabetes to Alzheimer's." *Molecular Medicine Today* 4 (January 1998): 39-45.

Luxon, B. A. "Liver Transplantation: Who Should Be Referred—And When?" *Postgraduate Medicine* 102 (December 1997): 103-108, 113.

Rao, V. K. "Posttransplant Medical Complications" *Surgical Clinics of North America* 78 (February 1998):113-132.

ORGANIZATIONS

American Liver Foundation. 1425 Pompton Avenue, Cedar Grove, NJ 07009. (800) 223-0179.

J. Ricker Polsdorfer

Liver ultrasound *see* **Abdominal ultrasound**

Liver-spleen scan *see* **Liver nuclear medicine scan**

Loaiasis *see* **Filariasis**

Lobectomy *see* **Lung surgery**

Lobotomy *see* **Psychosurgery**

Local anesthesia *see* **Anesthesia, local**

Localized scratch dermatitis *see* **Lichen simplex**

Lockjaw *see* **Tetanus**

Lomotil *see* **Antidiarrheal drugs**

Long-acting thyroid stimulator test *see* **Thyroid function tests**

Loperamide *see* **Antidiarrheal drugs**

Loratadine *see* **Antihistamines**

Lorazepam *see* **Benzodiazepines**

Lou Gehrig's disease *see* **Amyotrophic lateral sclerosis**

Louis-Bar syndrome *see* **Ataxia-telangiectasia**

Lovastatin *see* **Cholesterol-reducing drugs**

Low back pain

Definition

Low back pain is a common musculoskeletal symptom that may be either acute or chronic. It may be caused by a variety of diseases and disorders that affect the lumbar spine. Low back pain is often accompanied by **sciatica,** which is **pain** that involves the sciatic nerve and is felt in the lower back, the buttocks, and the backs of the thighs.

Description

Low back pain is a symptom that affects 80% of the general United States population at some point in life with sufficient severity to cause absence from work. It is the second most common reason for visits to primary care doctors, and is estimated to cost the American economy $75 billion every year.

Low back pain may be experienced in several different ways:

- Localized. In localized pain the patient will feel soreness or discomfort when the doctor palpates, or presses on, a specific surface area of the lower back.

- Diffuse. Diffuse pain is spread over a larger area and comes from deep tissue layers.

- Radicular. The pain is caused by irritation of a nerve root. Sciatica is an example of radicular pain.

- Referred. The pain is perceived in the lower back but is caused by inflammation elsewhere— often in the kidneys or lower abdomen.

Causes & Symptoms

Acute pain

Acute pain in the lower back that does not extend to the leg is most commonly caused by a sprain or muscle tear, usually occurring within 24 hours of heavy lifting or overuse of the back muscles. The pain is usually localized, and there may be muscle spasms or soreness when the doctor touches the area. The patient usually feels better when resting.

Chronic pain

Chronic low back pain has several different possible causes:

KEY TERMS

Ankylosing spondylitis—A type of arthritis that causes gradual loss of flexibility in the spinal column. It occurs most commonly in males between 16 and 35.

Cauda equina—The roots of the spinal nerves controlling movement and sensation in the legs. These nerve roots are located in the lower spine and resemble a horse's tail (*cauda equina* in Latin).

Chiropractic—A method of treatment based on the interactions of the spine and the nervous system. Chiropractors adjust or manipulate segments of the patient's spinal column in order to relieve pain.

Lumbar spine—The segment of the human spine above the pelvis that is involved in low back pain. There are five vertebrae, or bones, in the lumbar spine.

Radicular—Pain that is caused by the root of a nerve.

Referred pain—Pain that is experienced in one part of the body but originates in another organ or area. The pain is referred because the nerves that supply the damaged organ enter the spine in the same segment as the nerves that supply the area where the pain is felt.

Sciatica—Pain caused by irritation of the sciatic nerve. Sciatica is felt in the lower back, the buttocks, and the backs of the upper legs.

Spinal stenosis—A form of sciatica that is caused by a narrowing of the spinal canal in the lumbar vertebrae. The narrowing puts pressure on the roots of the sciatic nerve.

MECHANICAL

Chronic strain on the muscles of the lower back may be caused by **obesity; pregnancy;** or job-related stooping, bending, or other stressful postures.

MALIGNANCY

Low back pain at night that is not relieved by lying down may be caused by a tumor in the cauda equina (the roots of the spinal nerves controlling sensation in and movement of the legs), or a **cancer** that has spread to the spine from the prostate, breasts, or lungs. The risk factors for the spread of cancer to the lower back include a history of smoking, sudden weight loss, and age over 50.

ANKYLOSING SPONDYLITIS

Ankylosing spondylitis is a form of arthritis that causes chronic pain in the lower back. The pain is made worse by sitting or lying down and improves when the patient gets up. It is most commonly seen in males between 16 and 35. Ankylosing spondylitis is often confused with mechanical back pain in its early stages.

HERNIATED SPINAL DISK

Disk herniation is a disorder in which a spinal disk begins to bulge outward between the vertebrae. Herniated or ruptured disks are a common cause of chronic low back pain in adults.

PSYCHOGENIC

Back pain that is out of proportion to a minor injury, or that is unusually prolonged, may be associated with a somatoform disorder or other psychiatric disturbance.

Low back pain with leg involvement

Low back pain that radiates down the leg usually indicates involvement of the sciatic nerve. The nerve can be pinched or irritated by **herniated disks,** tumors of the cauda equina, **abscesses** in the space between the spinal cord and its covering, **spinal stenosis,** and compression **fractures.** Some patients experience numbness or weakness of the legs as well as pain.

Diagnosis

The diagnosis of low back pain can be complicated. Most cases are initially evaluated by primary care physicians rather than by specialists.

Initial workup

PATIENT HISTORY

The doctor will ask the patient specific questions about the location of the pain, its characteristics, its onset, and the body positions or activities that make it better or worse. If the doctor suspects that the pain is referred from other organs, he or she will ask about a history of diabetes, peptic **ulcers, kidney stones,** urinary tract infections, or **heart murmurs.**

PHYSICAL EXAMINATION

The doctor will examine the patient's back and hips to check for conditions that require surgery or emergency treatment. The examination includes several tests that involve moving the patient's legs in specific positions to test for nerve root irritation or disk herniation. The flexibility of the lumbar vertebrae may be measured to rule out ankylosing spondylitis.

Imaging studies

Imaging studies are not usually performed on patients whose history and **physical examination** suggest routine muscle strain or overuse. X rays are ordered for patients whose symptoms suggest cancer, infection, inflammation, pelvic or abdominal disease, or bone fractures. MRIs are usually ordered only for patients with certain types of masses or tumors.

It is important to know that the appearance of some abnormalities on imaging studies of the lower back does not necessarily indicate that they cause the pain. Many patients have minor deformities that do not create symptoms. The doctor must compare the results of imaging studies very carefully with information from the patient's history and physical examination.

Treatment

All forms of treatment of low back pain are aimed either at symptom relief or to prevent interference with the processes of healing. None of these methods appear to speed up healing.

Acute pain

Acute back pain is treated with nonsteroidal anti-inflammatory drugs (NSAIDs), such as ibuprofen, **muscle relaxants,** or **aspirin.** Applications of heat or cold compresses are also helpful to most patients. If the patient has not experienced some improvement after several weeks of treatment, the doctor will reinvestigate the cause of the pain.

Chronic pain

Patients with chronic back pain are treated with a combination of medications, physical therapy, and occupational or lifestyle modification. The medications given are usually NSAIDs, although patients with **hypertension,** kidney problems, or stomach ulcers should not take these drugs. Patients who take NSAIDs for longer than six weeks should be monitored periodically for complications.

Physical therapy for chronic low back pain usually includes regular **exercise** for fitness and flexibility, and **massage** or application of heat if necessary.

Lifestyle modifications include giving up smoking, weight reduction (if necessary), and evaluation of the patient's occupation or other customary activities.

Patients with herniated disks are treated surgically if the pain does not respond to medication.

Patients with chronic low back pain sometimes benefit from **pain management** techniques, including **biofeedback, acupuncture,** and **chiropractic** manipulation of the spine.

Psychotherapy is recommended for patients whose back pain is associated with a somatoform, **anxiety,** or depressive disorder.

Low back pain with leg involvement

Treatment of sciatica and other disorders that involve the legs may include NSAIDs. Patients with long-standing sciatica or spinal stenosis that do not respond to NSAIDs are treated surgically. Although some doctors use cortisone injections to relieve the pain, this form of treatment is still debated.

Alternative treatment

A thorough differential diagnosis is important before any treatment is considered. There are times when alternative therapies are the most beneficial, and other times when more invasive treatments are needed.

Chiropractic

Chiropractic treats patients by manipulating or adjusting sections of the spine. It is one of the most popular forms of alternative treatment in the United States for relief of back pain caused by straining or lifting injuries. Some osteopathic physicians, physical therapists, and naturopathic physicians also use spinal manipulation to treat patients with low back pain.

Traditional Chinese medicine

Practitioners of traditional Chinese medicine treat low back pain with acupuncture, *tui na* (push-and-rub) massage, and the application of herbal poultices.

Herbal medicine

Herbal medicine can utilize a variety of antispasmodic herbs in combination to help relieve low back pain due to spasm. Lobelia (*Lobelia inflata*) and myrrh (*Commiphora molmol*) are two examples of antispasmodic herbs.

Homeopathy

Homeopathic treatment for acute back pain consists of applications of *Arnica* oil to the sore area or oral doses of *Arnica* or *Rhus toxicodendron*. *Bellis perennis* is recommended for deep muscle injuries. Other remedies may be recommended based on the symptoms presented by the patient.

Body work and yoga

Massage and the numerous other body work techniques can be very effective in treating low back pain. Yoga, practiced regularly and done properly, can be most useful in preventing future episodes of low back pain.

Prognosis

The prognosis for most patients with acute low back pain is excellent. About 80% of patients recover completely in 4-6 weeks. The prognosis for recovery from chronic pain depends on the underlying cause.

Prevention

Low back pain due to muscle strain can be prevented by lifestyle choices, including regular physical exercise and weight control, avoiding smoking, and learning the proper techniques for lifting and moving heavy objects. Exercises designed to strengthen the muscles of the lower back, and chairs or car seats with lumbar supports are also recommended.

Resources

BOOKS

Esses, Stephen I. "Low Back Pain." In *Conn's Current Therapy,* edited by Robert E. Rakel. Philadelphia: W. B. Saunders Company, 1998.

Hellman, David B., "Arthritis & Musculoskeletal Disorders." In *Current Medical Diagnosis & Treatment 1998,* edited by Lawrence M. Tierney, Jr., et al. Stamford, CT: Appleton & Lange, 1998.

McKenzie, Robin. *Treat Your Own Back.* Waikanae, New Zealand: Spinal Publications New Zealand Ltd., 1997.

"Musculoskeletal and Connective Tissue Disorders: Low Back Pain and Sciatica." In *The Merck Manual of Diagnosis and Therapy,* edited by Robert Berkow, et al. Rahway, NJ: Merck Research Laboratories, 1992.

Theodosakis, Jason, et al. *The Arthritis Cure.* New York: St. Martin's Paperbacks, 1997.

Rebecca J. Frey

Low blood magnesium level *see* **Magnesium imbalance**

Low blood phosphate level *see* **Phosphorus imbalance**

Low blood pressure *see* **Hypotension; Orthostatic hypotension**

Low blood sugar *see* **Hypoglycemia**

Low calcium blood level *see* **Hypocalcemia**

Low potassium blood level *see* **Hypokalemia**

Low sodium blood level *see* **Hyponatremia**

Low-cholesterol diet *see* **Diets**

Lower esophageal ring

Definition

Lower esophageal ring is a condition in which there is a ring of tissue inside the lower part of the esophagus (the tube connecting the throat with the stomach). This tissue causes narrowing and partial blockage of the esophagus. Lower esophageal ring can also refer to the ring itself.

Description

Lower esophageal ring (also called Schatzki's ring and B-ring) affects about 10-14% of the population. Normally, the lower part of the esophagus, near where the esophagus meets the stomach, has an inside diameter of 1.5-2 inches. The diameter of this part of the esophagus is less when lower esophageal ring is present, and diameters as small as one-eighth inch have been seen. When the inside diameter is less than about three-fourths of an inch, intermittent difficulty with swallowing can result. About 96% of people with lower esophageal ring have no symptoms.

Causes & symptoms

Causes

Lower esophageal ring seems to result from infoldings of tissue near the bottom of the esophagus, but the underlying cause is unknown. Although some specialists speculate they are due to a congenital defect, most people do not develop symptoms until they reach their forties or later. Although lower esophageal ring is generally associated with hiatal **hernia,** and sometimes with **heartburn,** the cause/effect relationship is unclear.

Symptoms

Intermittent difficulty swallowing solid food is the primary symptom of this condition. The degree of difficulty in swallowing is directly related to the degree the esophagus is narrowed. Certain foods, especially tough or fibrous foods like meat, are more likely to cause swallowing difficulties.

Diagnosis

Gastroenterologists and internists are best equipped to diagnose and treat lower esophageal ring. The diagnosis is based on the patient's history of swallowing difficulties and a barium x ray of the upper gastrointestinal tract. For a barium x ray, the patient swallows a liquid containing barium, a substance that is opaque to x rays. Subsequent x-ray photography reveals the shape of the esophagus and any narrow regions present.

> ## KEY TERMS
>
> **Bougie**—A mercury-filled dilator in the shape of a cylinder or tapered cylinder. Bougies come in a range of different sizes.
>
> **Bougienage**—The procedure of dilating tubal organs, like the esophagus, with a bougie or bougies.
>
> **Congenital**—Existing at birth.
>
> **Dysphagia**—Difficulty swallowing.
>
> **Esophagoscopy (also esophagoendoscopy)**—Examination of the inside of the esophagus using a flexible tube that transmits video images.
>
> **Esophagus**—The tube connecting the throat to the stomach, which is about ten inches long in adults. It is coated with mucus and surrounded by muscles, and pushes food to the stomach by sequential waves of contraction. It functions to transport food from the throat to the stomach and to keep the contents of the stomach in the stomach.
>
> **Heartburn**—A burning sensation in the chest that can extend to the neck, throat, and face, caused by the movement of stomach acid into the esophagus.
>
> **Hiatal hernia**—A condition where part of the stomach extends through the diaphragm into the chest cavity.

The presence of a lower esophageal ring can also be shown with a test called an esophagoscopy. This procedure visualizes the inside of the esophagus with an inserted, thin, flexible tube. However, this test is less sensitive for lower esophageal ring and costs about five times as much as barium x ray. However, if the findings of a barium x ray are not definitive, esophagoscopy should be done. Biopsies can then be done on questionable areas.

Treatment

Dietary change

Swallowing difficulties due to lower esophageal ring can often be relieved by chewing food more thoroughly. Soft foods and liquids may also be recommended.

Dilation

Lower esophageal rings can be corrected by passing a bougie (a cylindrical, mercury-filled dilator) through the esophagus. This procedure, called bougienage, is effective most of the time, but may need to be repeated every few years. Complications and adverse reactions are extremely rare.

Surgery

If bougienage is unsuccessful, lower esophageal ring tissue can be surgically removed.

Prognosis

The probability of a favorable outcome is high. Swallowing difficulties can be alleviated in almost every case, and the rate of complications from bougienage or surgery is less than 1%.

Prevention

Since the cause of lower esophageal ring is not known, there are no definitive preventive measures. Nevertheless, anyone with lower esophageal ring who also suffers from heartburn would be wise to prevent or treat the heartburn. It is possible that the stomach acid in the esophagus associated with heartburn contributes to esophageal ring.

Resources

BOOKS

Castell, Donald O., ed. *The Esophagus,* 2nd ed. Boston: Little, Brown, 1995.

Groher, Michael E., ed. *Dysphagia: Diagnosis and Management,* 3rd ed. Boston: Butterworth-Heinemann, 1997.

ORGANIZATIONS

The American College of Gastroenterology (ACG). P.O. Box 3099, Alexandria, VA 22302. (703) 820-7400; (800) HRT-BURN. http://www.healthtouch.com.

The American Gastroenterological Association (AGA). 7910 Woodmont Avenue, 7th Floor, Bethesda, MD 20814. (310) 654-2055. http://www.gastro.org/index.html. aga001@aol.com.

American Society for Gastrointestinal Endoscopy. 13 Elm Street, Manchester, MA 01944. (508) 526-8330. http://www.asge.org/doc/201.

National Digestive Diseases Information Clearinghouse. 2 Information Way, Bethesda, MD 20892-3570. nddic@aerie.com. http://www.niddk.nih.gov/health/digest/nddic.htm.

Lorraine Lica

Lower GI exam *see* **Barium enema**

Low-fat diet *see* **Diets**

Low-salt diet *see* **Diets**

Lues *see* **Syphilis**

Lumbar puncture *see* **Cerebrospinal fluid (CSF) analysis**

Lumbar stenosis *see* **Spinal stenosis**

Lumbosacral radiculopathy *see* **Sciatica**

Lumpectomy

Definition

A lumpectomy is one type of surgery for **breast cancer.** The malignant tumor and a surrounding margin of normal breast tissue are removed. Lymph nodes in the armpit (axilla) may also be removed.

Purpose

Lumpectomy is a surgical treatment for newly diagnosed breast cancer. It is estimated that at least 50% of women with breast cancer are good candidates for this procedure. The location, size, and type of tumor are of primary importance when considering breast cancer surgery options. The size of the breast is another variable. The patient's psychological outlook, as well as her lifestyle choices, should also be taken into account when treatment decisions are made.

The severity of a **cancer** is evaluated or "staged" according to a fairly complex system. This considers the size of the tumor and whether the cancer has spread directly to adjacent tissues, such as the chest wall, the lymph nodes, and/or to distant parts of the body. Women with early stage breast cancers are usually better candidates for lumpectomy. In most cases, a course of **radiation therapy** after surgery is part of the treatment. **Chemotherapy** or hormone treatment may also be prescribed.

Many studies have compared the survival rates of women who have had removal of a breast (**mastectomy**) with those who have undergone lumpectomy and radiation therapy. The data is clear that for women with comparable stages of breast cancer, survival rates are equal between the two groups.

In some circumstances, a woman with later stage breast cancer may be able to have a lumpectomy. Chemotherapy can be administered before surgery to decrease tumor size and the chance of spread in selected cases.

Precautions

There are a number of factors that may prohibit a breast cancer patient from having a lumpectomy. The tumor itself may be too large or located in an area, such as near the nipple, where it would be difficult to remove with good cosmetic results. Sometimes several areas of cancer are found in one breast, so the tumor cannot be removed in a single mass of tissue. Tumors known to grow very rapidly would most likely not be treated with

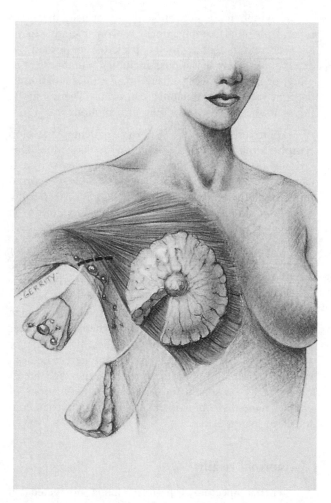

Lumpectomy is one form of breast cancer treatment in which the tumor and surrounding tissue is removed, thus preserving the breast. *(Illustration by Peg Gerrity, Custom Medical Stock Photo. Reproduced by permission.)*

lumpectomy. A cancer which has already attached itself to nearby structures, such as the skin or the chest wall, needs more extensive surgery.

Certain medical or physical circumstances may also eliminate lumpectomy as a treatment option. Sometimes lumpectomy may be attempted, but the surgeon is unable to remove the tumor with a sufficient amount of normal tissue surrounding it. This may be termed "persistently positive margins," or "lack of clear margins," referring to the margin of unaffected tissue around the tumor. Lumpectomy is not used for women who have had a previous lumpectomy and have a recurrence of the breast cancer.

Because of the need for radiation therapy after lumpectomy, this surgery may be medically unacceptable. A breast cancer discovered during **pregnancy** is not amenable to lumpectomy, due to the need for radiation therapy as part of the treatment. Radiation therapy cannot be administered to pregnant women, for fear of injuring the fetus. Women with collagen vascular disease, such as lupus erythematosus, or **scleroderma,** would experience scarring and damage to their connective tissue if exposed to radiation treatments. A woman who has already had therapeutic radiation to the chest area for other reasons cannot have additional exposure for breast cancer therapy.

Some women may choose not to have a lumpectomy for other reasons. They may strongly fear a recurrence of breast cancer, and may consider a lumpectomy too risky. Other women feel uncomfortable with a breast that has had a cancer, and they experience more peace of mind with the entire breast removed.

The need for radiation therapy may also be a barrier due to non-medical concerns. Some women simply fear this type of treatment and chose more extensive surgery so radiation will not be required. The commitment of time, usually five days a week for six weeks, may not be acceptable for others. This may be due to financial, personal, or job-related constraints. Finally, in geographically isolated areas, a course of radiation therapy may require lengthy travel, and perhaps unacceptable amounts of time away from the family and other responsibilities.

Description

Lumpectomy is an imprecise term. Any amount of tissue, from 1-50% of the breast, may be removed and called a lumpectomy. Other names are no more definite in their meaning, although some idea of the scope of tissue removal may be implied. Breast conservation surgery is a frequently used synonym for lumpectomy. Partial mastectomy, quadrantectomy, segmental excision, wide excision, and tylectomy are other names for this procedure.

A lumpectomy is typically done in a hospital setting, but specialized outpatient facilities are sometimes preferred. The surgery is usually done while the patient is under general anesthetic. Local anesthetic with additional sedation may be used for some patients. The tumor and surrounding margin of tissue is removed and sent to the pathologist. The surgical site is closed. If axillary lymph nodes were not removed before, a second incision is made in the armpit. The fat pad which contains lymph nodes is removed from this area and is also sent to the pathologist for analysis. This portion of the procedure is called an axillary node dissection; it is critical for determining the stage of the cancer. Typically, 10-15 nodes are removed, but the number may vary. Surgical drains may be left in place in either location to prevent fluid accumulation. The surgery may last from one to three hours.

The patient may stay in the hospital one or two days, or return home the same day. This generally depends on the extent of the surgery, the medical condition of the patient, and physician and patient preferences. A woman usually goes home with a small bandage. The inner part of the surgical site usually has dissolvable stitches. The skin may be sutured or stitched; or the skin edges may be held together with steristrips, which are special thin, clear pieces of tape.

Preparation

Routine preoperative preparations, such as taking nothing to eat or drink the night before surgery, are typically ordered for a lumpectomy. Information regarding expected outcomes and potential complications should also be part of preparation for lumpectomy, as for any surgical procedure. It is especially important that women know about sensations they might experience after the operation, so the sensations are not misinterpreted as signs of further cancer or poor healing.

If the tumor is not able to be felt (not palpable), a preoperative localization procedure is needed. A fine wire, or other device, is placed at the tumor site, using x ray or ultrasound for guidance. This is usually done in the radiology department of a hospital. The woman is most often sitting up and awake, although some sedation may be administered.

Aftercare

After a lumpectomy, patients are usually cautioned against lifting anything which weighs over five pounds for several days. Other activities may be restricted, according to individual needs. **Pain** is often enough to limit inappropriate motion. Women are often instructed to wear a well-fitting support bra both day and night for approximately one week after surgery.

Pain is usually well controlled with prescribed medication. If it is not, the patient should contact the surgeon, as severe pain may be a sign of a complication which needs medical attention. A return visit to the surgeon is normally scheduled approximately ten days to two weeks after the operation.

Radiation therapy is usually started as soon as feasible after lumpectomy. Other additional treatments, such as chemotherapy or hormone therapy, may also be prescribed. The timing of these is specific to each individual patient.

Risks

The risks are those which are common to any surgical procedure, including bleeding, infection, anesthesia reaction, or unexpected scarring. A lumpectomy may also cause loss of sensation in the breast. The size and shape of the breast will be affected by the operation. Fluid can accumulate in the area where tissue was removed, requiring drainage.

If lymph node dissection is performed, there are several potential complications. A woman may experience decreased feeling in the back of her armpit; or experience other sensations, including numbness, tingling, or increased skin sensitivity. An inflammation of the arm vein, called phlebitis, can occur. There may be injury to the nerves controlling arm motion.

Approximately 2-10% of patients develop **lymphedema** after axillary lymph node dissection. This swelling of the arm can range from mild to very severe. It can be treated with elastic bandages and specialized physical therapy, but it is a chronic condition, requiring continuing care. Lymphedema can arise at any time, even years after surgery.

A new technique that may eliminate the need for removing many axillary lymph nodes is being tested. The term "sentinel node biopsy" is most frequently used to refer to this method. It is based on the idea that the condition of the first lymph node in the network, which drains the affected area, can predict whether the cancer may have spread to the rest of the nodes. If this first, or sentinel, node is cancer-free, it is thought there is no need to look further. Many patients with early-stage breast cancers may be spared the risks and complications of axillary node dissection as the use of this approach continues to increase.

Normal results

When lumpectomy is performed, it is anticipated that it will be the definitive surgical treatment for breast cancer. Other forms of therapy, especially radiation, are often prescribed as part of the total treatment plan. The expected outcome is no recurrence of the breast cancer.

Resources

BOOKS

Love, Susan M., with Karen Lindsey. *Dr. Susan Love's Breast Book,* 2nd ed. Reading, MA: Addison-Wesley, 1995.

Robinson, Rebecca Y., and Jeanne A. Petrek. *A Step-by-Step Guide to Dealing With Your Breast Cancer.* New York: Carol Publishing Group, 1994.

PERIODICALS

Winchester, David P., and James D. Cox. "Standards for Diagnosis and Management of Invasive Breast Carcinoma." *CA-A Cancer Journal for Clinicians,* 48 (March/April 1998): 83-107.

ORGANIZATIONS

American Cancer Society. 1599 Clifton Rd. NE, Atlanta, GA 30329-4251. (800) 227-2345. http://www.cancer.org.

National Lymphedema Network. 2211 Post Street, Suite 404, San Francisco, CA 94115-3427. (800) 541-3259 or (415) 921-1306. http://www.wenet.net/~lymphnet/.

Ellen S. Weber

Lumpy breasts *see* **Fibrocystic condition of the breast**

Lumpy jaw *see* **Actinomycosis**

Lung abscess

Definition

Lung abscess is an acute or chronic infection of the lung, marked by a localized collection of pus, inflammation, and destruction of tissue.

Description

Lung abscess is the end result of a number of different disease processes ranging from fungal and bacterial infections to **cancer.** It can affect anyone at any age. Patients who are most vulnerable include those weakened by cancer and other chronic diseases; patients with a history of substance abuse, diabetes, epilepsy, or poor dental hygiene; patients who have recently had operations under anesthesia; and **stroke** patients. In children, the most vulnerable patients are those with weakened immune systems, **malnutrition,** or blunt injuries to the chest.

> **KEY TERMS**
>
> **Abscess**—An area of injured body tissue that fills with pus, as in lung abscess.
>
> **Anaerobe**—A type of bacterium that does not require air or oxygen to live. Anaerobic bacteria are frequent causes of lung abscess.
>
> **Aspiration**—Inhalation of fluid or foreign bodies into the airway or lungs. Aspiration often happens after vomiting.
>
> **Bronchoscope**—A lighted, flexible tube inserted into the windpipe to view the bronchi or withdraw fluid samples for testing. Bronchoscopy with a protected brush can be used in the diagnosis of lung abscess in severely ill patients.
>
> **Bronchus**—One of the two large tubes connecting the windpipe and the lungs.
>
> **Leukocytosis**—An increased level of white cells in the blood. Leukocytosis is a common reaction to infections, including lung abscess.
>
> **Necrotizing pneumonia**—Pneumonia that causes the death of lung tissue. It often precedes the development of lung abscess.
>
> **Sputum**—The substance that is brought up from the lungs and airway when a person coughs or spits. It is usually a mixture of saliva and mucus, but may contain blood or pus in patients with lung abscess or other diseases of the lungs.

Causes & symptoms

The immediate cause of most lung abscesses is infection caused by bacteria. About 65% of these infections are produced by anaerobes, which are bacteria that do not need air or oxygen to live. The remaining cases are caused by a mixture of anaerobic and aerobic (air breathing) bacteria. When the bacteria arrive in the lung, they are engulfed or eaten by special cells called phagocytes. The phagocytes release chemicals that contribute to inflammation and eventual necrosis, or death, of a part of the lung tissue. There are several different ways that bacteria can get into the lung.

Aspiration

Aspiration refers to the accidental inhalation of material from the mouth or throat into the airway and lungs. It is responsible for about 50% of cases of lung abscess. The human mouth and gums contain large numbers of anaerobic bacteria; patients with **periodontal** disease or poor **oral hygiene** have higher concentrations of these organisms. Aspiration is most likely to occur in patients who are unconscious or semi-conscious due to anesthesia, seizures, alcohol and drug abuse, or stroke. Patients who have problems swallowing or coughing, or who have nasogastric tubes in place are also at risk of aspiration.

Bronchial obstruction

The bronchi are the two branches of the windpipe that lead into the lungs. If they are blocked by tissue swelling, cancerous tumors, or **foreign objects,** a lung abscess may form from infection trapped behind the blockage.

Spread of infection

About 20% of cases of **pneumonia** that cause the death of lung tissue (necrotizing pneumonia) will develop into lung abscess. Lung abscess can also be caused by the spread of other infections from the liver, abdominal cavity, or open chest **wounds.** Rarely, **AIDS** patients can develop lung abscess from *Pneumocystis carinii* and other organisms that take advantage of a weakened immune system.

Lung abscess is usually slow to develop. It may take about two weeks after aspiration or bronchial obstruction for an **abscess** to produce noticeable symptoms. The patient may be acutely ill for two weeks to three months. In the beginning, the symptoms of lung abscess are difficult to distinguish from those of severe pneumonia. Adults will usually have moderate **fever** (101-102°F/38-39°C), chills, chest **pain,** and general weakness. Children may or may not have chest pain, but usually suffer weight loss and high fevers. As the illness progresses, about 75% of patients will cough up foul or musty-smelling sputum; some also cough up blood.

Lung abscess can lead to serious complications, including **emphysema,** spread of the abscess to other parts of the lung, hemorrhage, **adult respiratory distress syndrome,** rupture of the abscess, inflammation of the membrane surrounding the heart, or chronic inflammation of the lung.

Diagnosis

The diagnosis is made on the basis of the patient's medical history (especially recent operations under general anesthesia) and general health as well as imaging studies. Smears and cultures taken from the patient's sputum are not usually very helpful because they will be contaminated with bacteria from the mouth. The doctor will first use a bronchoscope (lighted tube inserted into the windpipe) to rule out the possibility of **lung cancer.** In some cases of serious infection, the doctor can use a fiberoptic bronchoscope with a protected specimen brush to take material directly from the patient's lungs, for

identification of the organism. This technique is time-consuming and expensive, and requires the patient to be taken off **antibiotics** for 48 hours. It is usually used only to evaluate severely ill patients with weakened immune systems.

In most cases, the doctor will use the results of a **chest x ray** to help distinguish lung abscess from **empyema,** cancer, **tuberculosis,** or cysts. In patients with lung abscess, the x ray will show a thick-walled unified clear space or cavity surrounded by solid tissue. There is often a visible air-fluid level. The doctor may also order a CT scan of the chest, in order to have a clearer picture of the exact location of the abscess.

Blood tests cannot be used to make a diagnosis of lung abscess, but they can be useful in ruling out other conditions. Patients with lung abscess usually have abnormally high white blood cell counts (leukocytosis) when their blood is tested, but this condition is not unique to lung abscess.

Treatment

Lung abscess is treated with a combination of antibiotic drugs, **oxygen therapy,** and surgery. The antibiotics that are usually given for lung abscess are penicillin G, penicillin V, and clindamycin. They are given intravenously until the patient shows signs of improvement, and then continued in oral form. The patient may need to take antibiotics for a month or longer, until the chest x ray indicates that the abscess is healing. Oxygen may be given to patients who are having trouble breathing.

Surgical treatment

Most patients with lung abscess will not need surgery. About 5% of patients—usually those who do not respond to antibiotics or are coughing up large amounts of blood (500 mL or more)—may have emergency surgery for removal of the diseased part of the lung or for insertion of a tube to drain the abscess. Antibiotic treatment is considered to have failed if fever and other symptoms continue after 10-14 days of treatment; if chest x rays indicate that the abscess is not shrinking; or if the patient has pneumonia that is spreading to other parts of the lung.

Supportive care

Because lung abscess is a serious condition, patients need quiet and bed rest. Hospital care usually includes increasing the patient's fluid intake to loosen up the secretions in the lungs, and physical therapy to strengthen the patient's breathing muscles.

Follow-up

Patients with lung abscess need careful follow-up care after the acute infection subsides. Follow-up usually includes a series of chest x rays to make sure that the infection has cleared up. Treatment with antibiotics may continue for as long as four months, to prevent recurrence.

Prognosis

About 95% of lung abscess patients can be treated successfully with antibiotics alone. Patients who need surgical treatment have a mortality rate of 10-15%.

Prevention

Some of the conditions that make people more vulnerable to lung abscess concern long-term lifestyle behaviors, such as substance abuse and lack of dental care. Others, however, are connected with chronic illness and hospitalization. Aspiration can be prevented with proper care of unconscious patients, which includes suctioning of throat secretions and positioning patients to promote drainage. Patients who are conscious can be given physical therapy to help them cough up material in their lungs and airways. Patients with weakened immune systems can be isolated from patients with pneumonia or fungal infections.

Resources

BOOKS

D'Esopo, Nicholas D. "Primary Lung Abscess." In *Conn's Current Therapy*, edited by Robert E. Rakel. Philadelphia: W. B. Saunders Company, 1997.

Larsen, Gary L., et al. "Respiratory Tract & Mediastinum." In *Current Pediatric Diagnosis & Treatment*, edited by William W. Hay, Jr., et al. Stamford, CT: Appleton & Lange, 1997.

Stauffer, John L. "Lung." In *Current Medical Diagnosis & Treatment 1998*, edited by Lawrence M. Tierney, Jr., et al. Stamford, CT: Appleton & Lange, 1997.

Turley, Kevin. "Thoracic Wall, Pleura, Mediastinum, & Lung." In *Current Surgical Diagnosis & Treatment*, edited by Lawrence W. Way. Stamford, CT: Appleton & Lange, 1994.

Vincent, Miriam T., and Stephan L. Kamholz. "Anaerobic Lung Infections." In *Current Diagnosis 9*, edited by Rex B. Conn, et al. Philadelphia: W. B. Saunders Company, 1997.

Rebecca J. Frey

Lung biopsy

Definition

Lung biopsy is a medical procedure performed to obtain a small piece of lung tissue for examination under a microscope. Biopsy examinations are usually performed by pathologists, who are doctors with special training in tissue abnormalities and other signs of disease.

Purpose

Lung biopsies are useful, first of all, in confirming a diagnosis of **cancer,** especially if malignant cells are detected in the patient's sputum. A lung biopsy may be ordered to examine other abnormalities that appear on **chest x rays,** such as lumps (nodules). It is also helpful in diagnosing symptoms such as coughing up bloody sputum, **wheezing** in the chest, or difficult breathing. In addition to evaluating lung tumors and their associated symptoms, lung biopsies can be used in the diagnosis of lung infections, especially tuberculosis, drug reactions, and such chronic diseases of the lung as **sarcoidosis.**

A lung biopsy can be used for treatment as well as diagnosis. **Bronchoscopy,** which is a type of lung biopsy performed with a long slender instrument called a bronchoscope, can be used to clear a patient's air passages of secretions and to remove blockages from the airways.

Precautions

As with any other biopsy, lung biopsies should not be performed on patients who have problems with blood clotting because of low **platelet counts.** Platelets are small blood cells that play a role in the blood clotting process. If the patient has a platelet count lower than 50,000/cubic mm, he or she can be given a platelet **transfusion** as a temporary relief measure, and a biopsy can then be performed.

Description

Overview

The lungs are a pair of cone-shaped organs that lie in the chest cavity. An area known as the mediastinum separates the right and the left lungs from each other. The heart, the windpipe (trachea), the lymph nodes, and the tube that brings the food to the stomach (the esophagus) lie in this mediastinal cavity. Lung biopsies may involve entering the mediastinum, as well as the lungs themselves.

KEY TERMS

Bronchoscopy—A medical test that enables the doctor to see the breathing passages and the lungs through a hollow, lighted tube.

Endotracheal tube—A hollow tube that is inserted into the windpipe to administer anesthesia.

Lymph nodes—Small, bean-shaped structures scattered along the lymphatic vessels which serve as filters. Lymph nodes retain any bacteria or cancer cells that are traveling through the system.

Mediastinoscopy—A medical procedure that allows the doctor to see the organs in the mediastinal space using a thin, lighted, hollow tube (a mediastinoscope).

Mediastinum—The area between the lungs, bounded by the spine, breastbone, and diaphragm.

Sputum—Mucus or phlegm that is coughed up from the passageways (bronchial tubes) in the lungs.

Types of lung biopsies

Lung biopsies can be performed using a variety of techniques. A bronchoscopy is ordered if a patch that looks suspicious on the x ray seems to be located deep in the chest. If the area lies close to the chest wall, a needle biopsy is often done. If both these methods fail to diagnose the problem, an open surgical biopsy may be carried out. If there are indications that the **lung cancer** has spread to the lymph nodes in the mediastinum, a **mediastinoscopy** is performed.

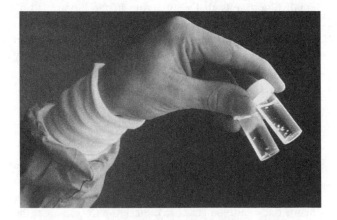

Surgeon's hand holding bottles containing lung tissue samples in saline solution. The sample was obtained by an endoscope. *(Photograph by James King-Holmes, Photo Researchers, Inc. Reproduced by permission.)*

NEEDLE BIOPSY

When a needle biopsy is to be done, the patient will be given a sedative about an hour before the procedure, to help relaxation. The patient sits in a chair with arms folded on a table in front of him or her. X rays are then taken to identify the location of the suspicious areas. Small metal markers are placed on the overlying skin to mark the biopsy site. The skin is thoroughly cleansed with an antiseptic solution, and a local anesthetic is injected to numb the area.

The doctor then makes a small cut (incision) about half an inch in length. The patient is asked to take a deep breath and hold it while the doctor inserts the special biopsy needle through the incision into the lung. When enough tissue has been obtained, the needle is withdrawn. Pressure is applied at the biopsy site and a sterile bandage is placed over the cut. The entire procedure takes between 30 and 45 minutes.

The patient may feel a brief sharp **pain** or some pressure as the biopsy needle is inserted. Most patients, however, do not experience severe pain.

OPEN BIOPSY

Open biopsies are performed in a hospital under general anesthesia. As with needle biopsies, patients are given sedatives before the procedure. An intravenous line is placed in the arm to give medications or fluids as necessary. A hollow tube, called an endotracheal tube, is passed through the throat, into the airway leading to the lungs. It is used to convey the general anesthetic.

Once the patient is under the influence of the anesthesia, the surgeon makes an incision over the lung area. Some lung tissue is removed and the cut closed with stitches. The entire procedure usually takes about an hour. A chest tube is sometimes placed with one end inside the lung and the other end protruding through the closed incision. Chest tube placement is done to prevent the lungs from collapsing by removing the air from the lungs. The tube is removed a few days after the biopsy.

A chest x ray is done following an open biopsy, to check for lung collapse. The patient may experience some grogginess for a few hours after the procedure. He or she may also experience tiredness and muscle aches for a day or two, because of the general anesthesia. The throat may be sore because of the placement of the hollow endotracheal tube. The patient may also have some pain or discomfort at the incision site, which can be relieved by medication.

MEDIASTINOSCOPY

The preparation for a mediastinoscopy is similar to that for an open biopsy. The patient is sedated and prepared for general anesthesia. The neck and the chest will be cleansed with an antiseptic solution.

After the patient has been put to sleep, an incision about two or three inches long is made at the base of the neck. A thin, hollow, lighted tube, called a mediastinoscope, is inserted through the cut into the space between the right and the left lungs. The doctor examines the space thoroughly and removes any lymph nodes or tissues that look abnormal. The mediastinoscope is then removed, and the incision stitched up and bandaged. A mediastinoscopy takes about an hour.

Preparation

Before scheduling any lung biopsy, the doctor will check to see if the patient is taking any prescription medications, if he or she has any medication **allergies,** and if there is a history of bleeding problems. Blood tests may be performed before the procedure to check for clotting problems and blood type, in case a transfusion becomes necessary.

If an open biopsy or a mediastinoscopy is being performed, the patient will be asked to sign a consent form. Since these procedures are done under general anesthesia, the patient will be asked to refrain from eating or drinking anything for at least 12 hours before the biopsy.

Aftercare

Needle biopsy

Following a needle biopsy, the patient is allowed to rest comfortably. He or she will be checked by a nurse at two-hour intervals. If there are no complications after four hours, the patient can go home. Patients are advised to rest at home for a day or two before resuming regular activities, and to avoid strenuous activities for a week after the biopsy.

Open biopsy or mediastinoscopy

After an open biopsy or a mediastinoscopy, patients are taken to a recovery room for observation. If no other complications develop, they are taken back to the hospital room. Stitches are usually removed after seven to 14 days.

If the patient has extreme pain, light-headedness, difficulty breathing, or develops a blue tinge to the skin after an open biopsy, the doctor should be notified immediately. The sputum may be slightly bloody for a day or two after the procedure. If, however, the bleeding is heavy or persistent, it should be brought to the attention of the doctor.

Risks

Needle biopsy

Needle biopsy is a less risky procedure than an open biopsy, because it does not involve general anesthesia. Very rarely, the lung may collapse because of air that leaks in through the hole made by the biopsy needle. If the lung collapses, a tube will have to be inserted into the chest to remove the air. Some coughing up of blood occurs in 5% of needle biopsies. Prolonged bleeding or infection may also occur, although these are very rare.

Open biopsy

Possible complications of an open biopsy include infection or lung collapse. **Death** occurs in about 1 in 3000 cases. If the patient has very severe breathing problems before the biopsy, breathing may be slightly impaired following the operation. If the person's lungs were functioning normally before the biopsy, the chances of any respiratory problems are very small.

Mediastinoscopy

Complications due to mediastinoscopy are rare; death occurs in fewer than 1 in 3000 cases. More common complications include lung collapse or bleeding caused by damage to the blood vessels near the heart. Injury to the esophagus or voice box (larynx) may sometimes occur. If the nerves leading to the larynx are injured, the patient may be left with a permanently hoarse voice. All of these complications are very rare.

Normal results

Normal results of a needle biopsy and an open biopsy include the absence of any evidence of infection in the lungs. No lumps or nodules will be detected in the lungs and the cells will not show any cancerous abnormalities. Normal results from the mediastinoscopy will show the lymph nodes to be free of cancer.

Abnormal results

Abnormal results may be associated with diseases other than cancer. Nodules in the lungs may be due to active infections such as tuberculosis, or may be scars from a previous infection. The lung cells on microscopic examination do not resemble normal cells, and show certain abnormalities that point to cancer. In a third of biopsies using a mediastinoscope, the lymph nodes that are biopsied prove to be cancerous. Abnormal results should always be considered in the context of the patient's medical history, **physical examination,** and other tests such as sputum examination, chest x rays, etc. before a final diagnosis is made.

Resources

BOOKS

"Bronchoscopy." In *The Merck Manual of Diagnosis and Therapy,* edited by Robert Berkow, et al. Rahway, NJ: Merck Research Laboratories, 1992.

Sobel, David S., and Tom Ferguson. *The People's Book of Medical Tests.* New York: Summit Books, 1985.

ORGANIZATIONS

American Cancer Society. 1599 Clifton Road, N.E., Atlanta, GA 30329. (800)227-2345.

American Lung Association. 1740 Broadway, New York, NY 10019-4374. (800)586-4872.

Cancer Research Institute. 681 Fifth Avenue, New York, NY 10022. (800)992-2623.

National Cancer Institute (National Institutes of Health). 9000 Rockville Pike, Bethesda, MD 20892. (800) 422-6237.

Lata Cherath

Lung cancer

Definition

Lung cancer is a disease in which the cells of the lung tissues grow uncontrollably and form tumors. It is the leading cause of **death** from **cancer** among both men and women in the United States. The American Cancer Society estimates that in 1998, at least 172,000 new cases of lung cancer will be diagnosed, and that lung cancer will account for 28% of all cancer deaths— approximately 160,000 people.

Description

Types of lung cancer

There are two kinds of lung cancers, primary and secondary. Primary lung cancer starts in the lung itself. Primary lung cancer is divided into small cell lung cancer and non-small cell lung cancer, depending on how the cells look under the microscope. Secondary lung cancer is cancer that starts somewhere else in the body (for example, the breast or colon) and spreads to the lungs.

Small cell cancer was formerly called oat cell cancer, because the cells resemble oats in their shape. About a fourth of all lung cancers are small cell cancers. This type is a very aggressive cancer and spreads to other organs within a short time. It is generally found in people who

---

KEY TERMS

Biopsy—The surgical removal and microscopic examination of living tissue for diagnostic purposes.

Bronchoscope—A thin, flexible, lighted tube that is used to view the air passages in the lungs.

Carcinogen—Any substance capable of causing cancer.

Chemotherapy—Treatment of cancer with synthetic drugs that destroy the tumor either by inhibiting the growth of cancerous cells or by killing them.

Lobectomy—Surgical removal of an entire lobe of the lung.

Pathologist—A doctor who specializes in the diagnosis of disease by studying cells and tissues under a microscope.

Pneumonectomy—Surgical removal of an entire lung.

Radiation therapy—Treatment using high energy radiation from X-ray machines, cobalt, radium, or other sources.

Sputum—Mucus or phlegm that is coughed up from the passageways of the lungs.

Stage—A term used to describe the size and extent of spread of cancer.

Wedge resection—Removal of only a small portion of a cancerous lung.

---

are heavy smokers. Non-small cell cancers account for the remaining 75% of lung cancers. They can be further subdivided into three categories.

Incidence of lung cancer

Lung cancer is rare among young adults. It is usually found in people who are 50 years of age or older, the average age at diagnosis being 60. While the incidence of the disease is decreasing among white men, it is steadily rising among African-American men, and among both white and African-American women. This change is probably due to the increase in the number of smokers in these groups. In 1987, lung cancer replaced **breast** cancer as the number one cancer killer among women.

Causes & symptoms

Causes

SMOKING

Tobacco smoking is the leading cause of lung cancer. Ninety percent of lung cancers can be prevented by giving up tobacco. Smoking marijuana cigarettes is considered yet another risk factor for cancer of the lung. These cigarettes have a higher tar content than tobacco cigarettes. In addition, they are inhaled very deeply— as a result, the smoke is held in the lungs for a longer time.

EXPOSURE TO ASBESTOS AND TOXIC CHEMICALS

Exposure to asbestos fibers, either at home or in the workplace, is also considered a risk factor for lung cancer. Studies show that compared to the general population, asbestos workers are seven times more likely to die from lung cancer. Asbestos workers who smoke increase their risk of getting lung cancer by 50-100 times. Besides asbestos, mining industry workers who are exposed to

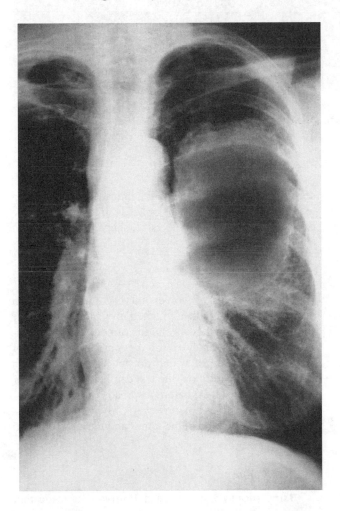

An x-ray image showing an oval-shaped carcinoma in the left lung (right of image). *(Custom Medical Stock Photo. Reproduced by permission.)*

coal products or radioactive substances such as uranium, and workers exposed to chemicals such as arsenic, vinyl chloride, mustard gas, and other carcinogens also have a higher than average risk of contracting lung cancer.

ENVIRONMENTAL CONTAMINATION

High levels of a radioactive gas (radon) that cannot be seen or smelled pose a risk for lung cancer. This gas is produced by the breakdown of uranium, and does not present any problem outdoors. In the basements of some houses that are built over soil containing natural uranium deposits, however, radon may accumulate to dangerous levels. Having one's house inspected for the presence of radon gas when buying or renting is a good idea. Other forms of environmental pollution (e.g., auto exhaust fumes) may also slightly increase the risk of lung cancer.

CHRONIC LUNG INFLAMMATION AND SCARRING

Inflammation and scar tissue are sometimes produced in the lung by diseases such as **silicosis** and **berylliosis,** which are caused by inhalation of certain **minerals; tuberculosis;** and certain types of **pneumonia.** This scarring may increase the risk of developing lung cancer.

FAMILY HISTORY

Although the exact cause of lung cancer is not known, people with a family history of lung cancer appear to have a slightly higher risk of contracting the disease.

Symptoms

Because lung cancers tend to spread very early, only 15% are detected in their early stages. The chances of early detection, however, can be improved by seeking medical care at once if any of the following symptoms appear:

- A **cough** that does not go away

- Chest **pain**

- **Shortness of breath**

- Persistent hoarseness

- Swelling of the neck and face

- Significant weight loss that is not due to dieting or vigorous **exercise;** fatigue and loss of appetite

- Bloody or brown-colored spit or phlegm (sputum)

- Unexplained **fever**

- Recurrent lung infections, such as **bronchitis** or pneumonia.

These symptoms may be caused by diseases other than lung cancer. It is vital, however, to consult a doctor to rule out the possibility that they are the first symptoms of lung cancer.

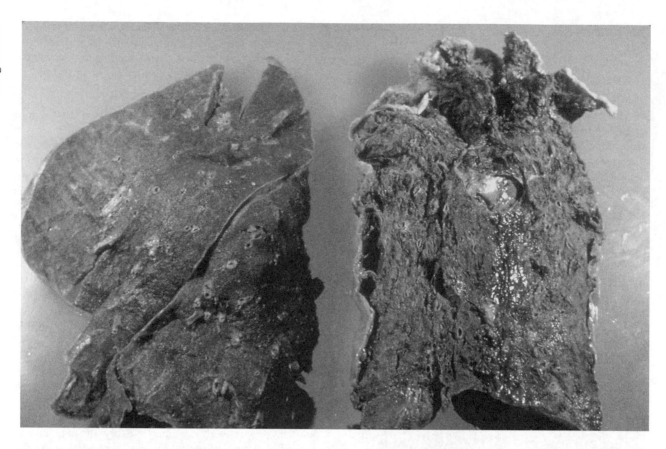

A normal lung (left) and the lung of a cigarette smoker (right). *(Photograph by A. Glauberman, Photo Researchers, Inc. Reproduced by permission.)*

If the lung cancer has spread to other organs, the patient may have other symptoms such as **headaches,** bone **fractures,** pain, bleeding, or blood clots. Early detection and treatment can increase the chances of a cure for some patients; for others, it can at least prolong life.

Diagnosis

Physical examination and initial tests

If the patient's doctor suspects lung cancer, he or she will take a detailed medical history to check all the symptoms and assess the risk factors. The history-taking will be followed by a complete **physical examination.** The doctor will examine the patient's throat to rule out other possible causes of hoarseness or coughing, and listen to the patient's breathing and the sounds made when the patient's chest and upper back are tapped (percussed). The physical examination, however, is not conclusive.

If the doctor has reason to suspect lung cancer— particularly if the patient has a history of heavy smoking or occupational exposure to substances that are known to irritate the lungs— he or she may order a chest x ray to see if there are any masses in the lungs. Special imaging techniques, such as CT scans or MRIs, may provide more precise information about the size, shape, and location of any tumors.

Sputum analysis

Sputum analysis involves microscopic examination of the cells that are either coughed up from the lungs, or are collected through a special instrument called a bronchoscope. Sputum analyses can diagnose at least 30% of lung cancers, some of which do not show up even on **chest x rays.** In addition, the test can help detect cancer in its very early stages, before it spreads to other regions. The sputum test does not, however, provide any information about the location of the tumor and must be followed by other tests.

Lung biopsy

Lung biopsy is the most definitive diagnostic tool for cancer. It can be performed in several different ways. The doctor can perform a **bronchoscopy,** which involves the insertion of a slender, lighted tube, called a bronchoscope, down the patient's throat and into the lungs. In addition to viewing the passageways of the lungs, the doctor can use the bronchoscope to obtain samples of the lung tissue. In another procedure known as a needle biopsy, the location of the tumor is first identified using a CT scan or MRI. The doctor then inserts a needle through the chest wall and collects a sample of tissue from the tumor. In the third procedure, known as surgical biopsy, the chest wall is opened up and a part of the tumor, or all of it, is removed. A doctor who specializes in the study of diseased tissue (a pathologist) examines the tumor samples to identify the cancer's type and stage.

Treatment

Treatment for lung cancer depends on the type of cancer, its location, and its stage. Staging is a process that tells the doctor if the cancer has spread and the extent of its spread. The patient's age, medical history, and general state of health are also taken into account. The most commonly used modes of treatment are surgery, **radiation therapy,** and **chemotherapy.**

Surgery

Surgery is not usually an option for small cell lung cancers, because they have usually spread beyond the lung by the time they are diagnosed. Because non-small cell lung cancers are less aggressive, however, surgery can be used to treat them. The surgeon will decide on the type of surgery, depending on how much of the lung is affected. Surgery may be the primary method of treatment, or radiation therapy and/or chemotherapy may be used to shrink the tumor before surgery is attempted.

There are three different types of surgical operations:

• Wedge resection. This procedure involves removing a small part of the lung. A wedge resection is done when the cancer is in a very small area and has not spread to any other chest tissues or other parts of the body.

• Lobectomy. A lobectomy is the removal of one lobe of the lung. The right lung has three lobes and the left lung has two lobes. If the cancer is limited to one part of the lung, the surgeon will perform a lobectomy.

• Pneumonectomy. A pneumonectomy is the removal of an entire lung. If the cancer cells have spread throughout the lung, and if the surgeon feels that removal of the entire lung is the best option for curing the cancer, a pneumonectomy will be performed.

The pain that follows surgery can be relieved by medications. A more serious side effect of surgery is the patient's increased vulnerability to bacterial and viral infections. The tendency of surgical stress to weaken the patient's immune system is treatable with **antibiotics,** anti-viral medicines, and vaccines.

Radiotherapy

Radiotherapy involves the use of high-energy rays to kill cancer cells. It is used either by itself or in combination with surgery or chemotherapy. Radiotherapy can be used to treat all types of cancer. The amount of radiation used depends on the size and the location of the tumor. There are two types of radiotherapy treatments: external beam radiation therapy; and internal (or interstitial) radiotherapy. In external radiation therapy, the radiation is delivered from a machine positioned outside the body. Internal radiotherapy uses a small pellet of radioactive materials placed inside the body in the area of the cancer.

Radiation therapy may produce such side effects as tiredness, skin **rashes,** upset stomach, and **diarrhea.** Dry or **sore throats,** difficulty in swallowing, and loss of hair in the treated area are all minor side effects of radiation. These may disappear either during the course of the treatment or after the treatment is over. The side effects should be discussed with the doctor.

Chemotherapy

Chemotherapy uses anti-cancer medications that are either given intravenously or taken by mouth. These drugs enter the bloodstream and travel to all parts of the body, killing cancer cells that have spread to different organs. Chemotherapy is used as the primary treatment for cancers that have spread beyond the lung and cannot be removed by surgery. It can also be used in addition to surgery or radiation therapy.

Chemotherapy is tailored to each patient's needs. It is dependent on the type of cancer, the extent of its spread, and the patient's general state of health. Most patients are given a combination of several different drugs. Besides killing the cancer cells, these drugs also harm normal cells. Hence, the dose has to be carefully adjusted to minimize damage to normal cells. Chemotherapy often has severe side effects, including nausea, vomiting, hair loss, anemia, weakening of the immune system, and sometimes **infertility.** Most of these side effects end when the treatment is over. Other medications can be given to lessen the unpleasant side effects of chemotherapy.

Prognosis

If the lung cancer is detected before it has had a chance to spread to other organs, and if it is treated appropriately, at least 49% of patients can survive five years or longer after the initial diagnosis. Only 15% of lung cancers, however, are found at this early stage.

Due to improvements in surgical technique and the development of new approaches to treatment, the one-year survival rate for lung cancer has improved considerably. As of 1998, approximately 40% of patients survive for at least a year after diagnosis, as opposed to 30% 20 years ago. The five-year survival rate for all stages of lung cancer is 14%.

Prevention

The best way to prevent lung cancer is not to smoke or to quit smoking if one has already started. Secondhand smoke from other people's tobacco should also be avoided. Appropriate precautions should be taken when working with cancer-causing substances (carcinogens). Eating well-balanced meals, testing houses for the presence of radon gas, and removing asbestos from buildings are also useful preventive strategies.

Resources

BOOKS

Dollinger, Malin, Ernest H. Rosenbaum, and Greg Cable. *Everyone's Guide to Cancer Therapy.* Kansas City, MO: Somerville House Books Limited, 1994.

Morra, Marion E., and Eve Potts. *Choices.* New York: Avon Books, 1994.

''Pulmonary Disorders: Tumors of the Lung.'' In *The Merck Manual of Diagnosis and Therapy,* edited by Robert Berkow, et al. Rahway, NJ: Merck Research Laboratories, 1992.

ORGANIZATIONS

American Cancer Society. 1599 Clifton Road, N.E., Atlanta, GA 30329. (800)227-2345.

American Lung Association. 1740 Broadway, New York, NY 10019-4374. (800)586-4872.

Cancer Research Institute. 681 Fifth Avenue, New York, NY 10022. (800)992-2623.

National Cancer Institute (National Institutes of Health). 9000 Rockville Pike, Bethesda, MD 20892. (800)422-6237.

Lata Cherath

....

Lung diseases due to gas or chemical exposure

Definition

Lung diseases due to gas or chemical exposure are conditions that can be acquired from indoor and outdoor air pollution and from ingesting tobacco smoke.

Description

The lungs are susceptible to many airborne poisons and irritants. Mucus present in the airways blocks foreign particles of a certain size, however it is unable to filter all

---

airborne particulates. There are hundreds of substances that can pollute air and harm lungs. Harmful gases and chemicals are just one type of airborne pollutant that can adversely effect the lungs. They include:

- Vehicle exhaust
- Localized pollutants such as arsenic, asbestos, lead, and mercury
- Outdoor pollutants caused by industry and intensified by weather conditions
- Household heating, such as wood-burning stoves
- Household chemical products
- Tobacco smoke.

Lungs respond to irritants in four ways, each of which can occur separately or, more often, trigger other responses.

- **Asthma** occurs when irritation causes the smooth muscles surrounding the airways to constrict.
- Increased mucus comes from irritated mucus glands lining the airway. Excess mucus clogs the airway and prevents air from circulating.
- Constriction of the lungs results from scarring when the supporting tissues are damaged.
- **Cancer** is caused by certain irritants, like asbestos and tobacco smoke.

The major categories that airborne irritants fall into are allergic, organic, inorganic, and poisonous, with many agents occupying more than one category.

- Allergic irritants bother only people who are sensitive to them. Cat hair, insect parts, and pollen are common allergens. Chemicals called sulfites, which are widely used as food preservatives, also cause asthma.
- There are many organic dusts that irritate the lungs. Most of them occur on the job and cause occupational lung disease. Grain dust causes silo filler's disease.

Cotton and other textile dusts cause **byssinosis.** Mold spores in hay cause farmer's lung.

- Inorganic dusts and aerosolized chemicals are also found mostly on the job. Classic among them are asbestos and coal dust. Many metals (cadmium, arsenic, chromium, and phosphorus), various other fine particles (cement, mica, rock), acid fumes, ammonia, ozone, and automobile and industrial emissions are part of a very long list.

- Most intentional poisons (cyanide, nerve gas) that enter through the lungs pass through and damage other parts of the body. Mustard gas, used during World War I and banned since, directly and immediately destroys lungs.

- Tobacco use scars the lungs and causes **emphysema** and **lung cancer.**

Causes & symptoms

Lung disease generates three major symptoms—coughing, wheezing, and **shortness of breath.** It also predisposes the lungs to infections such as **bronchitis** and **pneumonia.** Cancer is a late effect, requiring prolonged exposure to an irritant. In the case of tobacco, an average of a pack of cigarettes a day for forty years, or two packs a day for twenty years, will greatly increase the risk of lung cancer.

Diagnosis

A history of exposure combined with a **chest x ray** and lung function studies completes the diagnostic evaluation in most cases. Lung function measures the amount of air breathed in and out, the speed it moves, and the effectiveness of oxygen exchange with the blood. If the cause is still unclear, a **lung biopsy** reveals the answer.

Treatment

Eliminating the offending irritant and early **antibiotics** for infection are primary. There are many techniques available to remove excess mucus from the lungs. Respiratory therapists are experts in these methods. Finally, there are several machines available to enrich the oxygen content of breathed air.

A new surgical treatment called "lung reduction surgery" is just emerging from the experimental stage. It promises substantial return of lung function for selected patients with advanced emphysema.

Prognosis

Many of these diseases are progressive, because the irritants stay in the lungs forever. Others remain stable after the offensive agents are removed from the environment. Lungs do not heal from destructive damage, but

they can clean out infection and excess mucus, and function better.

Prevention

Industrial air filters, adequate ventilation, and respirators in polluted work sites are now mandatory. Tobacco smoke is the world's leading cause of lung disease and many other afflictions. Smoking cessation programs are widely available.

Resources

BOOKS

Beckett, William S., W. Morgan, and C. Keith. "Byssinosis and respiratory disease caused by vegetable dusts." In *Textbook of Pulmonary Diseases.* Edited by Gerald L. Baum, et al. Philadelphia: Lippincott-Raven, 1997.

Graham, David R. "Noxious gases and fumes." In *Textbook of Pulmonary Diseases.* Edited by Gerald L. Baum, et al. Philadelphia: Lippincott-Raven, 1997.

Kelley, Jason. "Occupational lung diseases caused by asbestos, silica, and other silicates." In *Textbook of Pulmonary Diseases.* Edited by Gerald L. Baum, et al. Philadelphia: Lippincott-Raven, 1997.

Looney, R. John and Mark J. Utell. "Occupational asthma and industrial bronchitis." In *Textbook of Pulmonary Diseases.* Edited by Gerald L. Baum, et al. Philadelphia: Lippincott-Raven, 1997.

Morgan, W. and C. Keith. "Occupational lung diseases: Coal workers' beryllium, and other pneumoconioses." In *Textbook of Pulmonary Diseases.* Edited by Gerald L. Baum, et al. Philadelphia: Lippincott-Raven, 1997,

PERIODICALS

Rogers, R.M., F.C. Sciurba, and R.J. Keenan. "Lung reduction surgery in chronic obstructive lung disease." *Medical Clinics of North America* 80 (May 1996): 623-44.

Sciurba, F.C. and R.M. Rogers. "Lung reduction surgery for emphysema." *Current Opinion In Pulmonary Medicine* 2 (March 1996): 97-103.

ORGANIZATIONS

American Lung Association. 1740 Broadway, New York, NY 10019. (212) 315-8700.

J. Ricker Polsdorfer

Lung fluke infections *see* **Fluke infections**

Lung function tests *see* **Pulmonary function tests**

Lung perfusion and ventilation scan

Definition

A lung perfusion scan is a nuclear medicine test that produces a picture of blood flow to the lungs. A lung ventilation scan measures the ability of the lungs to take in air and uses radiopharmaceuticals to produce a picture of how air is distributed in the lungs.

Purpose

Lung perfusion scans and lung ventilation scans are usually performed in the same session. They are done to detect **pulmonary embolisms,** determine how much blood is flowing to lungs, determine which areas of the lungs are capable of ventilation, and assess how well the lungs are functioning after surgery. These tests are called by different names, including perfusion lung scan, aerosol lung scan, radionucleotide ventilation lung scan, ventilation lung scan, xenon lung scan, ventilation/perfusion scanning (VPS), pulmonary scintiphotography, or, most commonly, V/Q scan.

Precautions

The amount of radioactivity a person is exposed to during these tests is very low and is not harmful. However, if the patient has had other recent radionuclear tests, it may be necessary to wait until other radiopharmaceuticals have been cleared from the body so that they do not interfere with these tests.

Description

In a lung perfusion scan, a small amount of the protein labeled with a radioisotope is injected into the patient's hand or arm vein. The patient is positioned under a special camera that can detect radioactive material, and a series of photographs are made of the chest. When these images are projected onto a screen (oscilloscope), they show how the radioactive protein has been distributed by the blood vessels running through the lungs.

In a lung ventilation scan, a mask is placed over the nose and mouth, and the patient is asked to inhale and exhale a combination of air and radioactive gas. Pictures are then taken that show the distribution of the gas in the lungs. Each test takes 15-30 minutes.

Preparation

There is little preparation needed for these tests. The patient may eat and drink normally before the procedure.

Tests to check for pulmonary embolism are often performed on an emergency basis.

Aftercare

No special aftercare is needed. The patient may resume normal activities immediately.

Risks

There are practically no risks associated with these tests.

Normal results

Normal results in both tests show an even distribution of radioactive material in all parts of the lungs.

Abnormal results

In the lung perfusion scan, an absence of radioactive marker material suggests decreased blood flow to that part of the lung, and possibly a pulmonary embolism. However, **pneumonia, emphysema,** or lung tumors can create readings on the lung perfusion scan that falsely suggest a pulmonary embolism is present.

In the lung ventilation scan, absence of marker material when the lung perfusion scan for the area is normal suggests lung disease.

Certain combinations of abnormalities in lung perfusion and ventilation scans suggest pulmonary embolism.

Resources

BOOKS

Pagana, Kathleen, and James Pagana. "Lung Scan." In *Mosby's Diagnostic and Laboratory Test Reference,* 2nd ed. St. Louis: Mosby, 1995, pp. 533-34.

"Scanning Tests." In *Illustrated Guide to Diagnostic Tests.* Springhouse: Springhouse Corp., 1996, pp. 679-82.

Zaret, Barry, ed. "Lung Scan." In *The Patient's Guide to Medical Tests.* New York: Houghton Mifflin, 1997, pp.138-40.

Tish Davidson

Lung surgery

Definition

Lung surgery includes a variety of procedures used to diagnose or treat diseases of the lungs. Biopsies are performed to extract a small amount of tissue for diagnosis, resections remove a portion of lung tissue, and other surgeries are aimed at reducing the volume of the lungs, removing cancerous tumors, or improving lung function.

Purpose

The type of lung surgery performed will depend upon the underlying disease or condition, as well as other factors.

- Pneumonectomy usually refers to the removal of a lung, or sometimes one or more lobes (sections containing lung tissue, air sacs, ducts, and respiratory bronchiole). It is most commonly indicated in certain forms and stages of **lung cancer.**

- Thoracotomy, or surgical incision of the chest wall, is used primarily as a diagnostic tool when other procedures have failed to provide adequate diagnostic information.

- Lobectomy is the term used to describe removal of one lobe of a lung. It is most commonly indicated for lung cancer, but may also be used for **cystic fibrosis** patients if other treatments have failed.

- Other surgical procedures include segmental resection or wedge resection. A resection is the removal of a part of the lung, often in order to remove a tumor. Wedge resection is removal of a wedge-shaped portion of lung tissue.

- Volume reduction surgery is a newer surgery used to help relieve **shortness of breath** and increase tolerance for **exercise** in patients with chronic obstructive pulmonary disease, such as **emphysema.**

- Other surgeries are continuously improved upon to make biopsy less invasive and surgery more effective, such as video-assisted lobectomy. Other purposes for lung surgery may include severe **abscess,** areas of long-term infection, or permanently enlarged or collapsed lung tissue.

Precautions

Thoracotomy should not be performed on patients whose general health status will not tolerate major surgery. Any surgery carries with it risks associated with general anesthesia and possibility of infection. Patients whose risk for these complications outweighs benefit may not be considered candidates for lung surgery. Each

individual patient's condition will be reviewed prior to the treatment decision.

Description

Lung surgery procedures will vary depending on the underlying cause of the surgical test or intervention. A patient will be placed under general anesthesia during the surgery. An incision is made to examine the lungs. Diseased tissue is removed and may be sent for biopsy. Following the surgery, drainage tubes may be placed in the chest to drain fluids, blood, and air from the chest cavity. Tubes will most likely remain in place for one to two days, depending on the surgery and the patient's condition. The chest cavity, ribs, and skin are closed and the incision will be sutured. Hospital stay averages from three to 10 days.

Pneumonectomy consists of removal of all of one lung. It may often be indicated only when a lobectomy does not successfully remove the cancerous or damaged tissue. Thoracotomy consists of reaching the lung tissue through incision and obtaining tissue for a biopsy. The biopsy is used to diagnose or stage cancer, and thoracotomy may be avoided until other less invasive methods have failed. Volume reduction surgery involves incision and removal of those parts of the lung or lungs which are the most destroyed, in order to allow for full function of the remaining lung structure. This procedure is still being studied.

Lobectomy is performed in the same general manner as other lung surgeries, but will involve removal of an entire lobe of the lung. Most patients with Stage I or II non-small cell lung cancer will receive this treatment for their disease, or a less extensive resection. Lobectomy may only be performed if a wedge or segmental resection is ineffective, but is generally preferred as treatment for primary lung cancer in any patient who can tolerate the procedure. Wedge and segmental resections are still major surgery, but remove less tissue and may be the first choice for some patients, such as those with Stage I and Stage II non-small cell lung cancer. Patients who do not have enough pulmonary function to undergo a lobectomy will receive a wedge or segmental resection instead. This may lead to a higher recurrence rate of cancer. In general, the surgery method chosen will depend on specific circumstances and consideration of benefit versus risk.

Preparation

Preparation for lung surgery is much like that for any major surgery. Patients will receive instructions from a physician concerning limit of food or water intake prior to the surgery, as well as risks and expected recovery. Patients should continue to follow treatment for the underlying condition, unless instructed otherwise by the physician, and should discuss medications and changes in condition with their physician prior to the surgery.

Aftercare

The chest tube inserted at the end of surgery will remain in place until the lung has fully expanded. Patients will be carefully monitored in the hospital for complications and infection. Deep breathing is recommended to help lessen the risk of **pneumonia** and infection. Breathing exercises will also help expand the lung. After discharge from the hospital, the patient may still receive some **pain** or infection-fighting medications and should recover within one to three months of the operation.

Risks

Risks of lung surgery follows those of any major surgery involving general anesthesia. These risks include reactions to anesthetics or medications, bleeding, infection, and problems restoring breathing. Lung surgery, in particular, offers the risk of pneumonia and blood clots. Thoracotomy, as a biopsy procedure, offers greater risk than most biopsy procedures.

Normal results

Outcome for any lung surgery depends on many factors and the severity of disease. In general, the predicted benefits, which justified the surgery, are normal expected results. Thoracotomy results in a definitive diagnosis in more than 90% of patients. Volume reduction surgery has been shown to result in relief of some symptoms and improvement in quality of life for selected patients with severe emphysema and have shown short-term promise.

Mortality from lung surgery improves as procedures move from the more complete pneumonectomy to lobectomy, and the lowest rate for segmental resection.

Resources

PERIODICALS

Norman, M., et al. "Improved Lung Function and Quality of Life Following Increased Elastic Recoil After Lung Volume Reduction Surgery in Emphysema." *Respiratory Medicine,* 92 (1998): 653-658.

ORGANIZATIONS

American Cancer Society. 1-800-ACS-2345. http://www.cancer.org.

American Lung Association. 1-800-LUNG-USA (1-800-586-4872). http://www.lungusa.org.

National Heart, Lung and Blood Institute. Building 31, Room 4A21, Bethesda, MD 20892. (301)496-4236. http://www.nhlbi.nih.gov.

Teresa G. Norris

Lung transplantation

Definition

Lung transplantation involves removal of one or both diseased lungs from a patient and the replacement of the lungs with healthy organs from a donor. Lung transplantation may refer to single, double, or even heart-lung transplantation.

Purpose

The purpose of lung transplantation is to replace a lung that no longer functions, or is cancerous, with a healthy lung. In order to qualify for lung transplantation, a patient must suffer from severe lung disease which limits activities of daily living. There should be potential for rehabilitated breathing function. Attempts at other medical treatments should be exhausted before transplantion is considered. Many candidates for this procedure have end-stage fibrotic lung disease, are dependent on **oxygen therapy,** and are likely to die of their disease in 12-18 months.

Patients with **emphysema** or chronic obstructive pulmonary disease (COPD) should be under 60 years of age, have a life expectancy without transplantation of two years or less, progressive deterioration, and emotional stability in order to be considered for lung transplantation. Young patients with end-stage **silicosis** (a progressive lung disease) may be candidates for lung or heart-lung transplantation. Patients with Stage III or Stage IV **sarcoidosis** (a chronic lung disease) with **cor pulmonale** should be considered as early as possible for lung transplantation. Other indicators of lung transplantation include pulmonary vascular disease and chronic pulmonary infection.

Precautions

Patients who have diseases or conditions which may make them more susceptible to organ rejection should not receive a lung transplant. This includes patients who are acutely ill and unstable; who have uncontrolled or untreatable pulmonary infection; significant dysfunction of other organs, particularly the liver, kidney, or central nervous system; and those with significant coronary disease or left ventricular dysfunction. Patients who actively smoke cigarettes or are dependent on drugs or alcohol may not be selected. There are a variety of protocols that are used to determine if a patient will be placed on a transplant recipient list, and criteria may vary depending on location.

Description

Once a patient has been selected as a possible organ recipient, the process of waiting for a donor organ match begins. The donor organ must meet clear requirements for tissue match in order to reduce the chance of organ rejection. It is estimated that it takes an average of one to two years to receive a suitable donor lung, and the wait is made less predictable by the necessity for tissue match. Patients on a recipient list must be available and ready to come to the hospital immediately when a donor match is found, since the life of the lungs outside the body is brief.

Single lung transplantation is performed via a standard thoracotomy (incision in the chest wall) with the patient under general anesthesia. Cardiopulmonary bypass (diversion of blood flow from the heart) is not always necessary for a single lung transplant. If bypass is necessary, it involves re-routing of the blood through tubes to a heart-lung bypass machine. Double lung transplantation involves implanting the lungs as two separate lungs, and cardiopulmonary bypass is usually required. The patient's lung or lungs are removed and the donor lungs are stitched into place. Drainage tubes are inserted into the chest area to help drain fluid, blood, and air out of the chest. They may remain in place for several days. Transplantation requires a long hospital stay and recovery can last up to six months.

Heart-lung transplants always require the use of cardiopulmonary bypass. An incision is made through the middle of the sternum. The heart, lung, and supporting structures are transplanted into the recipient at the same time.

Preparation

In addition to tests and criteria for selection as a candidate for transplantation, patients will be prepared by discussing the procedure, risks, and expected prognosis at length with their doctor. Patients should continue to follow all therapies and medications for treatment of the underlying disease unless otherwise instructed by their physician. Since lung transplantation takes place under general anesthesia, normal surgical and anesthesia preparation should be taken when possible. These include no food or drink from midnight before the surgery, discussion of current medications with the physician, and in forming the physician of any changes in condition while on the recipient waiting list.

Aftercare

Careful monitoring will take place in a recovery room immediately following the surgery and in the patient's hospital room. Patients must take immunosuppression, or anti-rejection, drugs to reduce the risk of rejection of the transplanted organ. The body considers the new organ an invader and will fight its presence. The anti-rejection drugs lower the body's immune function in order to improve acceptance of the new organs. This also makes the patient more susceptible to infection.

Frequent check-ups with a physician, including x ray and blood tests, will be necessary following surgery, probably for a period of several years.

Risks

Lung transplantation is a complicated and risky procedure, partly because of the organs and systems involved, and also because of the risk of rejection by the recipient's body. Acute rejection most often occurs within the first four months following surgery, but may occur years later. Infection is a substantial risk for organ recipients. An early complication of the surgery can be poor healing of the bronchial and tracheal openings created during the surgery. A late complication and risk is chronic rejection. This can result in inflammation of the bronchial tubes or in late infection from the prolonged use of **immunosuppressant drugs** to fight rejection.

NATIONAL TRANSPLANT WAITING LIST BY ORGAN TYPE (JUNE 1997)	
Organ Needed	*Number Waiting*
Kidney	36,148
Liver	8,447
Heart	3,777
Lung	2,452
Kidney-Pancreas	1,565
Pancreas	334
Heart-Lung	222
Intestine	85

Source: Colorado Health Net. http://www.coloradohealthnet. org/transplant/trans_main.html.

Overall, lung transplant recipients have demonstrated average one and two-year survival rates of more than 70%.

Normal results

The outcome of lung transplantation can be measured in survival rates, and also in improved quality of life for recipients. Studies have reported improved quality of life after lung and heart-lung transplants. One study showed that at the two-year follow-up period, 86% of studied recipients reported no limitation to their activity. Demonstration of normal results for patients may include quality of life measurements, as well as testing to ensure lack of infection and rejection.

Resources

BOOKS

Maurer, Janet R., Ronald F. Grossman, and Noel Zamel. ''Lung Transplantation.'' In *Textbook of Respiratory Medicine,* 2nd ed., edited by John F. Murray and Jay A. Nadel. Philadelphia: W. B. Saunders and Company, 1994.

ORGANIZATIONS

Children's Organ Transplant Association, Inc. 2501 COTA Drive, Bloomington, IN 47403. 800-366-2682. http://www.cota.org.

Second Wind Lung Transplant Association, Inc. 9030 West Lakeview Court, Crystal River, FL 34428. 888-222-2690. http://www.arthouse.com/secondwind.

Teresa G. Norris

Lupus erythematosus *see* **Systemic lupus erythematosus**

Luque rod instrumentation *see* **Spinal instrumentation**

Luteinizing hormone test

Definition

The luteinizing hormone (LH) test is a test of the blood or urine to measure the level of luteinizing hormone (lutropin). This hormone level is highest immediately before a woman ovulates during her menstrual cycle.

Purpose

The LH test is frequently used to determine the timing of ovulation. Couples who are trying to become

pregnant may use information about the timing of ovulation to improve their chance of conception. The LH test and other hormone tests may be used during **infertility** screening to chart a woman's menstrual cycle. It may also be used during preparation for **in vitro fertilization,** to determine when eggs are mature and ready to be removed from the ovary.

Description

Lutenizing hormone is a hormone released by the pituitary gland, a small gland at the base of the brain. The hormone stimulates the ovaries to produce and release eggs each month during the menstrual cycle. The level of LH in the blood is highest before ovulation. This increase in hormone level is sometimes called a ''surge.'' A urine or blood sample can be analyzed by a laboratory for the level of LH present. An LH test may be used as part of an infertility screening to determine if there is a hormonal imbalance that might make it difficult to become pregnant. If fertility drugs are given to stimulate ovulation, an LH test can help determine the best time for sexual intercourse. The LH test may also be used to determine when eggs are mature enough to be surgically removed from the ovary as part of the in vitro fertilization process. LH tests may also aid in the diagnoses of polycystic ovary disease, premature ovarian failure, and **menopause.**

A urine LH detection kit is also available for use at home. These are sometimes called ''ovulation tests'' and are similar to home **pregnancy** test kits. A sample of the woman's first morning urine is tested with the materials provided in the kit. These home tests are often used by women who want to become pregnant. By monitoring levels of LH and watching for the ''surge,'' they can time sexual intercourse to coincide with ovulation, increasing the chance that the egg will be fertilized.

Preparation

If a blood sample is taken, the skin around the vein where the needle will be inserted is swabbed with an antiseptic. No special preparation is necessary for collection of a urine sample.

Aftercare

No special aftercare is required. If the blood is tested, as with any blood sampling, the area where the needle was inserted should be kept clean.

Risks

There are no significant risks associated with either the blood or urine test for LH.

Normal results

The level of LH in the blood or urine will vary depending on when the sample was taken during the menstrual cycle. LH levels will be highest around the time of ovulation, about halfway between a woman's menstrual periods. Levels will be lower during the rest of the month. Women who have already experienced menopause will normally have lower LH levels.

Abnormal results

LH levels that remain low throughout the menstrual cycle may indicate a hormonal imbalance that could prevent ovulation. Additional testing may be required if this test is done as part of an infertility screening.

Resources

BOOKS

"Pituitary Disorders." In *The Merck Manual of Diagnosis and Therapy*, edited by Robert Berkow. Rahway, NJ: Merck Research Laboratories, 1992.

Sher, G., V.M. Davis, and J. Stoess. *In Vitro Fertilization: The A.R.T. of Making Babies.* New York, NY: Facts On File, 1995.

Zaret, Barry J. *The Patient's Guide to Medical Tests.* Boston, MA: Houghton Mifflin Company, 1997.

Altha Roberts Edgren

Lyme borreliosis *see* **Lyme disease**

. . . .

Lyme disease

Definition

Lyme disease is an infection transmitted by the bite of ticks carrying the spiral-shaped bacterium *Borrelia burgdorferi* (Bb). The disease was named for Lyme, Connecticut, the town where it was first diagnosed in 1975, after a puzzling outbreak of arthritis. The organism was named for its discoverer, Willy Burgdorfer. The

KEY TERMS

. . . .

Blood-brain barrier—A blockade of cells separating the circulating blood from elements of the central nervous system (CNS); it acts as a filter, preventing many substances from entering the central nervous system.

Cerebrospinal fluid—Clear fluid found around the brain and spinal cord and in the ventricles of the brain.

Vector-borne—Delivered from one host to another, as in an insect or tick bearing an organism causing an infectious disease.

effects of this disease can be long-term and disabling unless it is recognized and treated properly with **antibiotics.**

Description

Lyme disease is a vector-borne disease, which means it is delivered from one host to another. In this case, a tick bearing the Bb organism literally inserts it into a host's bloodstream when it bites the host to feed on its blood. It is important to note that neither Bb nor Lyme disease can be transmitted from one person to another.

In the United States, Lyme disease accounts for more than 90% of all reported vector-borne illnesses. It is a significant public health problem and continues to be diagnosed in increasing numbers. More than 99,000 cases were reported between 1982 and 1996. When the numbers for 1996 Lyme disease cases reported were tallied, there were 16,455 *new cases*, a record high following a drop in reported cases from 1994 (13,043 cases) to 1995 (11,700 cases). Controversy clouds the true incidence of Lyme disease because no test is definitively diagnostic for the disease, and the broad spectrum of Lyme disease's symptoms mimic those of so many other diseases. Originally, public health specialists thought Lyme disease was limited geographically in the United States to the East Coast. We now know it occurs in most states, with the highest number of cases in the eastern third of the country.

The risk for acquiring Lyme disease varies, depending on what stage in its life cycle a tick has reached. A tick passes through three stages of development—larva, nymph, and adult—each of which is dependent on a live host for food. In the United States, Bb is borne by ticks of several species in the genus *Ixodes*, which usually feed on the white-footed mouse and deer (and are often called deer ticks). In the summer, the larval ticks hatch from eggs laid in the ground and feed by attaching themselves

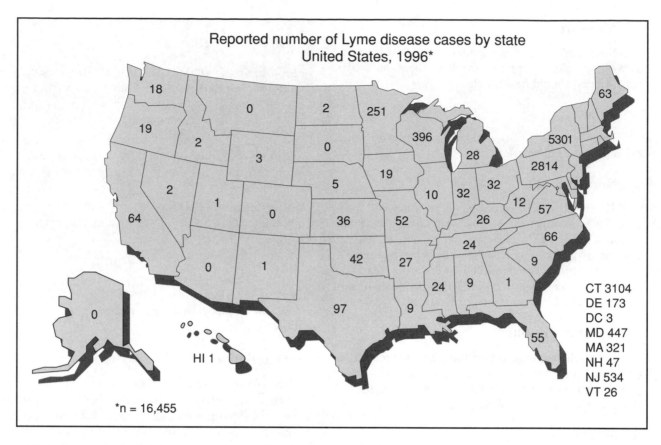

Reported number of Lyme disease cases by state
United States, 1996*

18

19

0

2

2

3

0

251

63

396

28

5301

2814

2

1

5

19

32

32

12

57

64

0

36

10

32

26

52

24

66

0

1

42

27

9

97

24

9

1

9

*n = 16,455

HI 1

0

9

55

CT 3104
DE 173
DC 3
MD 447
MA 321
NH 47
NJ 534
VT 26

Lyme disease accounts for more than 90% of all reported vector-borne illnesses in the United States. It is caused by an infection transmitted by the bite of ticks carrying the *Borrelia burgdorferi* bacterium. *(Data taken from the Centers for Disease Control. Illustration by Electronic Illustrators Group.)*

to small animals and birds. At this stage they are not a problem for humans. It is the next stage—the nymph—that causes most cases of Lyme disease. Nymphs are very active from spring through early summer, at the height of outdoor activity for most people. Because they are still quite small (less than 2 mm), they are difficult to spot, giving them ample opportunity to transmit Bb while feeding. Although far more adult ticks than nymphs carry Bb, the adult ticks are much larger, more easily noticed, and more likely to be removed before the 24 hours or more of continuous feeding needed to transmit Bb.

Causes & symptoms

Lyme disease is a collection of effects caused by Bb. Once Bb gains entry to the body through a tick bite, it can move through the bloodstream quickly. Only 12 hours after entering the bloodstream, Bb can be found in cerebrospinal fluid (which means it can affect the nervous system). Treating Lyme disease early and thoroughly is important because Bb can hide for long periods within the body in a clinically latent state. That ability explains why

symptoms can recur in cycles and can flare up after months or years, even over decades. It is important to note, however, that not everyone exposed to Bb develops the disease.

Lyme disease is usually described in terms of length of infection (time since the person was bitten by a tick infected with Bb) and whether Bb is localized or disseminated (spread through the body by fluids and cells carrying Bb). Furthermore, when and how symptoms of Lyme disease appear can vary widely from patient to patient. People who experience recurrent bouts of symptoms over time are said to have chronic Lyme disease.

Early, localized Lyme disease

The most recognizable indicator of Lyme disease is a rash around the site of the tick bite. Often, the tick exposure has not been recognized. The eruption might be warm or itch. The rash—erythema migrans (EM)—generally develops within 3-30 days and usually begins as a round, red patch that expands. Clearing may take place from the center out, leaving a bull's-eye effect; in some cases, the center gets redder instead of clearing. The rash may look like a bruise on people with dark skin. Of those who develop Lyme disease, about 50% notice the rash; about 50% notice flu-like symptoms, including fatigue, **headache,** chills and **fever,** muscle and joint **pain,** and lymph node swelling. However, a rash at the site can also be an allergic reaction to the tick saliva rather than an indicator of Lyme disease, particularly if the rash appears in *less* than 3 days and disappears only days later.

Late, disseminated disease and chronic Lyme disease

Weeks, months, or even years after an untreated tick bite, symptoms can appear in several forms, including:

- Fatigue, forgetfulness, confusion, mood swings, irritability, numbness

- Neurologic problems, such as pain (unexplained and not triggered by an injury), **Bell's palsy** (facial **paralysis,** usually one-sided but may be on both sides), and a mimicking of the inflammation of brain membranes known as **meningitis;** (fever, severe headache, stiff neck)

- Arthritis (short episodes of pain and swelling in joints) and other musculoskeletal complaints.

Less common effects of Lyme disease are heart abnormalities (such as irregular rhythm or cardiac block) and eye abnormalities (such as swelling of the cornea, tissue, or eye muscles and nerves).

Diagnosis

A clear diagnosis of Lyme disease can be difficult, and relies on information the patient provides and the doctor's clinical judgment, particularly through elimination of other possible causes of the symptoms. Lyme disease may mimic other conditions, including **chronic fatigue syndrome** (CFS), **multiple sclerosis** (MS), and other diseases with many symptoms involving multiple body systems. Differential diagnosis (distinguishing Lyme disease from other diseases) is based on clinical evaluation with laboratory tests used for clarification, when necessary. A two-test approach is common to confirm the results. Because of the potential for misleading results (false-positive and false-negative), laboratory tests alone cannot establish the diagnosis.

Doctors generally know which disease-causing organisms are common in their geographic area. The most helpful piece of information is whether a tick bite or rash was noticed and whether it happened locally or while traveling. Doctors may not consider Lyme disease if it is rare locally, but will take it into account if a patient mentions vacationing in an area where the disease is commonly found.

Treatment

The treatment for Lyme disease is antibiotic therapy; however, overprescribing of antibiotics can lead to serious problems, so the decision to treat must be made with care. Disease organisms can develop resistance to families of medications over time, rendering the drugs useless. Furthermore, testing and treatments can be expensive. If a patient has strong indications of Lyme disease (symptoms and medical history), the doctor will probably begin treatment on the presumption of this disease. The American College of Physicians recommends treatment for a patient with a rash resembling EM or who has arthritis, a history of an EM-type rash, and a previous tick bite.

The benefits of treating early must be weighed against the risks of overtreatment. The longer a patient is ill with Lyme disease before treatment, the longer the course of therapy must be, and the more aggressive the treatment. The development of opportunistic organisms may produce other symptoms. For example, after long-term antibiotic therapy, patients can become more susceptible to yeast infections. Treatment may also be associated with adverse drug reactions. Another concern is that insurance coverage for long-term antibiotic therapy may be limited by the insurer or by law in some states.

For most patients, oral antibiotics (doxycycline or amoxicillin) are prescribed for 21 days. When symptoms indicate nervous system involvement or a severe episode of Lyme disease, intravenous antibiotic (ceftriaxone) may be given for 14-30 days. Some physicians consider intravenous ceftriaxone the best therapy for any late manifestation of disease, but this is controversial. **Corticosteroids** (oral) may be prescribed if eye abnormalities occur, but they should not be used without first consulting an eye doctor.

The doctor may have to adjust the treatment regimen or change medications based on the patient's response. Treatment can be difficult because Bb comes in several strains (some may react to different antibiotics than others) and may even have the ability to switch forms during the course of infection. Also, Bb can shut itself up in cell niches, allowing it to hide from antibiotics. Finally, antibiotics can kill Bb only while it is active rather than dormant.

Therapy will not be effective, no matter which drugs are chosen, unless the doctor's instructions are followed. Medication must be taken in the correct amounts at the times indicated, alcohol consumption should be avoided during treatment, and the patient should rest regularly, preferably before the onset of fatigue.

Alternative treatment

Supportive therapies may minimize symptoms of LD or improve the immune response. These include vitamin and nutritional supplements, mostly for chronic fatigue and increased susceptibility to infection. For example, yogurt and *Lactobacillus acidophilus* preparations help fight yeast infections, which are common in people on long-term antibiotic therapy. In addition, botanical medicine and homeopathy can be considered to help bring the body's systems back to a state of health and well being. A western herb, spilanthes (*Spilanthes* spp.), may be effective in treating diseases like LD that are caused by spirochetes (spiral-shaped bacteria).

Prognosis

If aggressive antibiotic therapy is given early, and the patient cooperates fully and sticks to the medication schedule, recovery should be complete. Only a small percentage of Lyme disease patients fail to respond or relapse (have recurring episodes). Most long-term effects of the disease result when diagnosis and treatment is delayed or missed. Co-infection with other infectious organisms spread by ticks in the same areas as Bb (**babesiosis** and **ehrlichiosis,** for instance) may be responsible for treatment failures or more severe symptoms. Lyme disease has been responsible for deaths, but that is rare.

Prevention

An approved vaccine may be available quite soon. Two vaccines are being tested and are similar in that they both require three injections, the first two given a month apart; a third injection given a year later. In 1997, the early results from a very large study of 10,000 adults in many locations showed strong promise of a safe, effective vaccine. Until then, the best prevention strategy is through minimizing risk of exposure to ticks and using personal protection precautions. There is also research into **vaccination** against the tick vector to prevent the tick from feeding long enough to transmit the infection.

Minimize risk of exposure

Precautions to avoid contact with ticks include moving leaves and brush away from living quarters. Most important are personal protection techniques when outdoors, such as:

- Using repellents containing DEET
- Wearing light-colored clothing to maximize ability to see ticks
- Tucking pant legs into socks or boot top
- Checking children frequently for ticks.

In highly tick-populated areas, each individual should be inspected at the end of the day to look for ticks.

Minimize risk of disease

The two most important factors are removing the tick quickly and carefully, and seeking a doctor's evaluation at the first sign of symptoms of Lyme disease. When in an area that may be tick-populated:

- Check for ticks, particularly in the area of the groin, underarm, behind ears, and on the scalp
- Stay calm and grasp the tick as near to the skin as possible, using a tweezer
- To minimize the risk of squeezing more bacteria into the bite, pull straight back steadily and slowly
- Do not try to make the tick back out by using vaseline, alcohol, or a lit match
- Place the tick in a closed container (for species identification later, should symptoms develop) or dispose of it by flushing
- See a physician for any sort of rash or patchy discoloration that appears 3-30 days after a tick bite.

Medical studies to date do not support the preventative use of antibiotics after a tick bite, even if the tick has been identified as a deer tick. The risk of Lyme disease after a deer tick exposure appears to be quite low.

Resources

BOOKS

Territo, J., and D.V. Lang. *Coping With Lyme Disease: A Practical Guide to Dealing With Diagnosis and Treatment.* Henry Holt, 1997.

Vanderhoof-Forschne, K. *Everything You Need to Know About Lyme Disease and Other Tick-Borne Disorders.* New York: John Wiley & Sons, 1997.

PERIODICALS

"Breakthrough of the Year: The Runners-Up." *Science* 278(December 19, 1997): 2039.

Eckman, M.H., et. al. "Cost Effectiveness of Oral as Compared with Intravenous Antibiotic Therapy for Patients with Early Lyme Disease or Lyme Arthritis." *The New England Journal of Medicine* Special Report. (July 31, 1997).

Feder, H.M., Jr., and M.S. Hunt. "Pitfalls in the Diagnosis and Treatment of Lyme Disease in Children." *Journal of the American Medical Association* 274(July 5, 1995): 66-8.

Sigal, L.H. "Lyme Disease Controversy: Social and Financial Costs of Misdiagnosis and Mismanagement." *Archives of Internal Medicine* (July 22, 1996): 1493-1500.

Walker, D.H., et.al. "Emerging Bacterial Zoonotic and Vector-Borne Diseases. Ecological and Epidemiological Factors." *Journal of the American Medical Association* 275(1996): 463-9.

ORGANIZATIONS

American Lyme Disease Foundation, Inc. Mill Pond Offices, 293 Route 100, Suite 204, Somers, NY 10589. 800-876-LYME. http://www.w2.com/docs2/d5/lyme.html.

Centers for Disease Control, Washington, D.C. Lyme Disease Information Voice Information System. (404) 332-4555. Online Information Services, http://www.cdc.gov/ncidod/dvbid/lymeinfo.htm.

The Lyme Disease Network of NJ, Inc. 43 Winton Road, East Brunswick, NJ 08816. http://www.lymenet.org.

Jill S. Lasker

Lymph node angiogram *see*
Lymphangiography

Lymph node biopsy

Definition

Lymph node biopsy is a procedure in which a sample of lymph node tissue is removed for microscopic examination. Lymph nodes are the lumps of tissue found along the lymphatic system.

Purpose

The lymphatic system is like a road system with interchanges throughout the body, secondary to circulating blood. The lymph system carries fluids and cells between tissue and the blood. The lymph nodes are lumps of tissue along the lymphatic system into which fluids drain. Via the lymphatic system, infectious organisms can travel throughout the body and **cancer** cells can spread (metastasize). Lymph nodes also serve as a battle station. They swell in response to invaders, like infections and cancer cells. Lymph nodes produce white blood cells (lymphocytes) to fight the invader.

Swollen lymph nodes (swollen glands) are only a signal of an immune response. A lymph node biopsy is used to determine the cause. Microscopic examination of biopsy tissue taken from a lymph node is used to detect several forms of cancer, like **head and neck cancers,** lymphocytic leukemia, and **Hodgkin's disease.** Lymph node biopsy can be used to determine whether cancer cells have spread from a nearby tumor or lesion. The procedure can also be used to identify certain infectious

---

diseases, like **tuberculosis** and **infectious mononucleosis.**

Description

Biopsy of a lymph node can be done by withdrawing cells through a fine needle (needle aspiration) or by surgically removing one node or a colony of nodes (excision). The sample is examined by a pathologist who then provides the primary doctor with a written report. The results generally are available in a day or two and will help determine future treatment. If an infection is present, cell cultures and histopathological examination will help determine the origin and appropriate treatment.

Until recently, removal of several lymph nodes in the area of a tumor was common. A major advance was made with the new concept of using a 'sentinel' lymph node (SLN) biopsy for patients suspected to have cancer. The node *nearest* a tumor acts as the filter through which the tumor drains. To identify which node is the sentinel (gatekeeper) for the tumor, a surgeon injects the tumor with a small amount of dye or a radioactive tracer. The tracer travels through the lymphatic system and is only absorbed by the first (or sentinel) node in the cluster of lymph nodes. This sentinel can then be located by a probe that measures radioactivity. If the sentinel does not contain tumor cells, no further surgery is needed. If cancer cells are found in the sentinel, all nearby lymph nodes are removed. This procedure is called therapeutic lymph node dissection. It is done to assess and contain the spread of cancer cells. The results will also be used to help determine future therapy.

Recent studies have shown that in almost every case, SLN biopsy provides the same information as removing the entire colony of lymph nodes. SLN biopsy is performed as an outpatient procedure with minimal discomfort for the patient. The procedure is less invasive, produces less **pain** and discomfort for the patient, and has fewer surgical complications. SLN biopsy also decreases the risk of leg or arm swelling caused by accumulated lymph fluid (**lymphedema**).

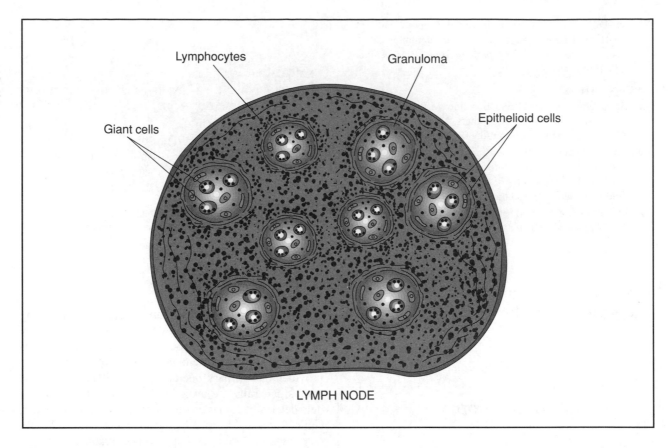

Lymphocytes

Granuloma

Giant cells

Epithelioid cells

LYMPH NODE

Lymph node biopsy is a procedure in which a sample of lymph node tissue is removed for laboratory analysis. It is generally performed on an outpatient basis. *(Illustration by Electronic Illustrators Group.)*

Preparation

Lymph node biopsies are generally done as outpatient procedures. Preparation for a biopsy depends on the type of procedure and the location of the nodes. Usually a local anesthetic is used, but **general anesthesia** may be needed. Patients are likely to experience only minor discomfort (associated with swelling) for a day or so.

Resources

BOOKS

Everything You Need to Know about Medical Tests, edited by Michael Shaw. PA: Springhouse Corporation, 1996.

ORGANIZATIONS

American Cancer Society. 1599 Clifton Rd. NE, Atlanta, GA 30329. (800) ACS-2345.

Cancer Information Service sponsored by the National Cancer Institute. (800) 422-6237.

Jill S. Lasker

Lymphadenitis

Definition

Lymphadenitis is the inflammation of a lymph node. It is often a complication of a bacterial infection of a wound, although it can also be caused by viruses or other disease agents. Lymphadenitis may be either generalized, involving a number of lymph nodes; or limited to a few nodes in the area of a localized infection. Lymphadenitis is sometimes accompanied by lymphangitis, which is the inflammation of the lymphatic vessels that connect the lymph nodes.

Description

Lymphadenitis is marked by swollen lymph nodes that are painful, in most cases, when the doctor touches them. If the lymphadenitis is related to an infected wound, the skin over the nodes may be red and warm to the touch. If the lymphatic vessels are also infected, there will be red streaks extending from the wound in the direction of the lymph nodes. In most cases, the infectious organisms are hemolytic *Streptococci* or *Staphylococci*. Hemolytic means that the bacteria produce a toxin that destroys red blood cells.

The extensive network of lymphatic vessels throughout the body and their relation to the lymph nodes helps to explain why bacterial infection of the nodes can spread rapidly to or from other parts of the body. Lymphadenitis in children often occurs in the neck area because these lymph nodes are close to the ears and throat, which are frequent locations of bacterial infections in children.

Causes & symptoms

Streptococcal and staphylococcal bacteria are the most common causes of lymphadenitis, although viruses, protozoa, rickettsiae, fungi, and the **tuberculosis** bacillus can also infect the lymph nodes. Diseases or disorders that involve lymph nodes in specific areas of the body include rabbit fever (**tularemia**), **cat-scratch disease, lymphogranuloma venereum, chancroid, genital her-**

pes, infected **acne,** dental **abscesses,** and bubonic **plague.** In children, **tonsillitis** or bacterial **sore throats** are the most common causes of lymphadenitis in the neck area. Diseases that involve lymph nodes throughout the body include mononucleosis, **cytomegalovirus infection, toxoplasmosis,** and **brucellosis.**

The early symptoms of lymphadenitis are swelling of the nodes caused by a buildup of tissue fluid and an increased number of white blood cells resulting from the body's response to the infection. Further developments include fever, often as high as 101-102°F (38-39°C) together with chills, loss of appetite, heavy perspiration, a rapid pulse, and general weakness.

Diagnosis

Physical examination

The diagnosis of lymphadenitis is usually based on a combination of the patient's history, the external symptoms, and laboratory cultures. The doctor will press (palpate) the affected lymph nodes to see if they are sore or tender. Swollen nodes without soreness are often caused by cat-scratch disease. In children, the doctor will need to rule out **mumps,** tumors in the neck region, and congenital cysts that resemble swollen lymph nodes.

Although lymphadenitis is usually diagnosed in lymph nodes in the neck, arms, or legs, it can also occur in lymph nodes in the chest or abdomen. If the patient has acutely swollen lymph nodes in the groin, the doctor will need to rule out a **hernia** in the groin that has failed to reduce (incarcerated inguinal hernia). Hernias occur in

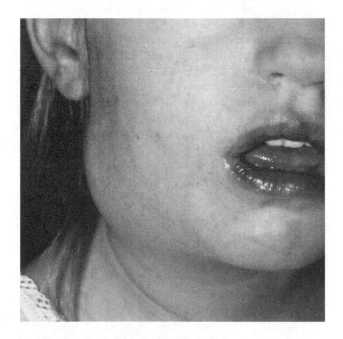

Swollen lymph nodes glands in a young girl's neck.
(Custom Medical Stock Photo. Reproduced by permission.)

1% of the general population; 85% of patients with hernias are male.

Laboratory tests

The most significant tests are a white blood cell count (WBC) and a **blood culture** to identify the organism. A high proportion of immature white blood cells indicates a bacterial infection. Blood cultures may be positive, most often for a species of staphylococcus or streptococcus. In some cases, the doctor may order a biopsy of the lymph node.

Treatment

Medications

The medications given for lymphadenitis vary according to the bacterium or virus that is causing it. If the patient also has lymphangitis, he or she will be treated with **antibiotics**, usually penicillin G (Pfizerpen, Pentids), nafcillin (Nafcil, Unipen), or **cephalosporins**. Erythromycin (Eryc, E-Mycin, Erythrocin) is given to patients who are allergic to penicillin.

Supportive care

Supportive care of lymphadenitis includes resting the affected limb and treating the area with hot moist compresses.

Surgery

Cellulitis associated with lymphadenitis should *not* be treated surgically because of the risk of spreading the infection. Pus is drained only if there is an abscess and usually after the patient has been started on antibiotic treatment. In some cases, a biopsy of an inflamed lymph node is necessary if no diagnosis has been made and no response to treatment has occurred.

Prognosis

The prognosis for recovery is good if the patient is treated promptly with antibiotics. In most cases, the infection can be brought under control in three or four days. Patients with untreated lymphadenitis may develop blood poisoning (septicemia), which is sometimes fatal.

Prevention

Prevention of lymphadenitis depends on prompt treatment of bacterial and viral infections.

Resources

BOOKS

Berman, Stephen, and Ken Chan. "Ear, Nose, & Throat." In *Current Pediatric Diagnosis & Treatment,* edited by William W. Hay, Jr., et al. Stamford, CT: Appleton & Lange, 1997.

Grossi, Carlo E., and Peter M. Lydyard. "Lymph Nodes." In *Encyclopedia of Immunology,* vol. II, edited by Ivan M. Roitt, and Peter J. Delves. London: Academic Press, 1992.

Hall, Joseph G. "Lymphatic System." In *Encyclopedia of Immunology,* vol. II, edited by Ivan M. Roitt, and Peter J. Delves. London: Academic Press, 1992.

"Infectious Disease: Superficial Infections." In *The Merck Manual of Diagnosis and Therapy,* vol. I, edited by Robert Berkow, et al. Rahway, NJ: Merck Research Laboratories, 1992.

Tierney, Lawrence M., Jr. "Blood Vessels & Lymphatics." In *Current Medical Diagnosis & Treatment 1998,* edited by Lawrence M. Tierney, Jr., et al. Stamford, CT: Appleton & Lange, 1997.

Rebecca J. Frey

Lymphangiography

Definition

Lymphangiography, or lymph node angiogram, is a test which utilizes x-ray technology, along with the injection of a contrast agent, to view lymphatic circulation and lymph nodes for diagnostic purposes.

Purpose

The lymphatic system is a one way circulation that channels tissue fluid back into the heart. The watery fluid called lymph seeps out of the blood into tissues, and while journeying back to the heart, it picks up germs, **cancer** cells, and some waste products. Lymph passes through the lymph nodes, which are major arsenals of immune defense that attack germs carried in the lymph. Cancer cells are also subject to attack in lymph nodes.

Cancers of the lymph system, such as **Hodgkin's disease** and non-Hodgkin's lymphomas, spread throughout the body. Treatment often depends upon finding all the disease and directing radiation to each location. Planning other kinds of treatment, such as surgery or **chemotherapy,** may also require that the full extent of the disease be known.

The lymphatic circulation may become clogged by infection, injury, or several other types of cancer that

KEY TERMS

Contrast agent—A substance that makes shadows on x rays.

Filariasis—A tropical disease caused by worms that live in lymph channels.

Hodgkin's disease—A cancer of the lymphatic system.

Lymphoma—A type of lyphatic cancer.

have spread through lymphatic channels. Swelling, sometimes massive, can result from blocked lymphatics. The most outstanding example of this is the tropical disease **filariasis,** which results in the swelling of the legs termed elephangiasis.

Lymphangiography gives precise information on the extent and location of lymph vessels and lymph nodes. Oftentimes, it is performed to evaluate the extent of a lymphatic cancer. Rarely, it is a tool, which aids surgeons attempting to reconstruct the lymphatics.

Precautions

Lymphangiography should not be performed on patients with dye or shellfish **allergies** or on patients with chronic lung disease, kidney disease, heart disease, or liver disease.

Description

A lymphangiogram begins by injecting a blue dye into a hand or foot. The lymph system picks up dye, which in turn will highlight the lymph vessels. This process may take a full day. When the lymphatic channel is clearly visible, the radiologist will insert an even tinier needle into that vessel and inject a contrast agent. X rays outline the journey of the contrast agent as it travels to the heart through lymph vessels and nodes.

Preparation

Unless a dye allergy is suspected, no special preparation is need. If an allergy is suspected, a non-ionic contrast agent can be administered instead.

Aftercare

Prior to suture removal seven to 10 days after the procedure, the patient should watch for any sign of infection around the site.

Risks

Lipid **pneumonia** can occur if the contrast agent penetrates the thoracic duct. An allergic reaction to the contrast agent is possible, causing a range of symptoms that can range from innocuous to life threatening.

Resources

BOOKS

Merrill, Vinta. "Lymphangiography." In *Atlas of roentgenographic positions and standard radiologic procedures.* Saint Louis, MO: The C.V. Mosby Company, 1975, pp.939-944.

J. Ricker Polsdorfer

Lymphangiomas *see* **Birthmarks**

Lymphedema

Definition

Lymphedema is the swelling of tissues (**edema),** usually the feet and legs, due to lymphatic obstruction.

Description

Lymphatic fluid seeps out of the blood circulation into the tissues. It returns to the heart through separate channels called lymphatics, carrying waste products and germs. On its way to the heart, it passes through lymph nodes, where infecting germs (including some **cancers**) are attacked by the body's defense mechanisms.

If lymphatic channels are obstructed or inadequate, fluid backs up and causes edema. Tissue fluid can also return to the circulation through tissues, without using the lymphatics, but gravity hinders this flow. So lymphedema is usually confined to the feet and legs.

Causes & symptoms

There are several types of congenital abnormalities associated with other **birth defects** of the lymphatics, which cause this condition. One in 10,000 people have this type of lymphedema.

Lymphatics can be damaged or obstructed by many different agents. Repeated bouts of blood poisoning can scar the vessels. Surgery to remove cancerous lymph nodes or **radiation therapy** can damage them. Cancer itself, as it invades the lymph system, as well as several other infectious and inflammatory conditions, can result in blockage of lymph flow. The most common worldwide cause of lymphedema is a group of worms known as

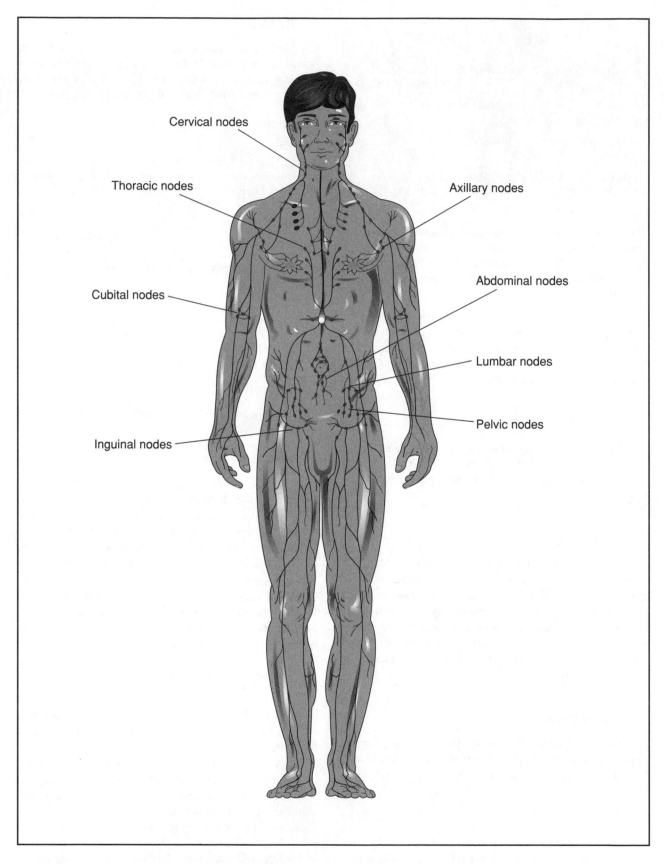

The lymphatic system. *(Illustration by Electronic Illustrators Group.)*

filaria. Filaria can be found in most of the developing regions of the world. They enter humans through insect bites, mostly mosquitoes, and take up residence in lymphatic channels, irritating them enough to scar them and impair their ability to carry lymph. Long-standing lymphatic **filariasis** can cause massive swelling of the legs, earning the name **elephantiasis**.

Diagnosis

Since other types of swelling may look similar to lymphedema, precise diagnostic tools must be used. Ultrasound, **computed tomography scans** (CT), and **magnetic resonance imaging** (MRI) scans may help with diagnosis. **Lymphangiography** may be needed to clarify the cause.

Treatment

Physical activity can pump some of the fluid out of the tissues. Compression stockings are of some value, as are devices that actively squeeze fluid out of tissues. **Diuretics** may alleviate some of the edema. Because the ability of the skin to defend itself is hampered by the swelling, infections are more common. It is therefore important to care for **wounds** and to treat infections early.

When caused by infection, lymphedema can be treated by eliminating the underlying infection with **antibiotics**.

Reconstructing lymphatic channels using microvascular surgery has recently achieved some success.

Prognosis

If congenital, lymphedema is a progressive and lifelong condition. If secondary or caused by an underlying disease or infection, lymphedema can be treated by treating the disease.

Prevention

When traveling in regions known to have filaria, avoidance of insect bites is crucial. Prompt and effective treatment of the infection will prevent the consequences.

Resources

BOOKS

Creager, Mark A. and Victor A. Dzau. "Vascular diseases of the extremities." In *Harrison's Principles of Internal Medicine*. Edited by Kurt Isselbacher, et al. New York: McGraw-Hill, 1998, pp.1405-1406.

Kontos, Hermes A. "Vascular diseases of the limbs." In *Cecil Textbook of Medicine*. Edited by J. Claude Bennett and Fred Plum. Philadelphia: W. B. Saunders, 1996, pp.357.

Nutman, Thomas B. and Peter F. Weller. "Filariasis and related infections." In *Cecil Textbook of Medicine*. Edited by J. Claude Bennett and Fred Plum. Philadelphia: W. B. Saunders, 1996.

J. Ricker Polsdorfer

Lymphocyte typing

Definition

Lymphocyte typing focuses on identifying the numbers and relative percentages of lymphocytes in an individual's bloodstream. Lymphocytes, primarily T cells and B cells, are types of white blood cells, the underlying supports of the immune system in the bloodstream.

Purpose

Determining the numbers and relative percentages of T cells and B cells provides information on the state of a person's immune system. By comparing these values to normal numbers and percentages, the presence of disease and the side effects of certain drugs can be revealed. Lymphocyte typing can also show whether a person has been exposed to certain poisonous substances.

Description

To do a white blood cell count, a small amount of blood is drawn from a vein. The total number of white blood cells is calculated, either through microscopic examination of a blood smear or by using automated counting equipment. For a white blood cell count with differential, 100 white blood cells are counted and the proportion of each type is calculated. Since T cells and B cells have similar appearances, a differential can only give the proportion of lymphocytes in the blood, not the proportion of specific lymphocyte types.

For more specific information on B cells and T cells, it is necessary to divide the blood into its separate components. In this procedure, a tube of blood is placed in a centrifuge, a piece of equipment that spins the tube in circles at high speed. The force generated by the spinning causes the various elements in the bloodstream to settle at different levels of the tube.

The lymphocytes are extracted from the tube and treated with special dyes, or stains. Each stain is equipped with an antibody portion that adheres to a specific type of lymphocyte, such as a B cell or a T cell. The stains make the cells visible to an automated counting machine, called a flow cytometer. Based on the number of times the machine detects a particular stain, it can calculate the number of the associated cell type. This procedure can also be used to classify T cells and B cells into their subtypes.

Preparation

If possible, a person should avoid eating a heavy meal within hours of the test or engaging in strenuous **exercise** for the 24 hours preceding the blood test.

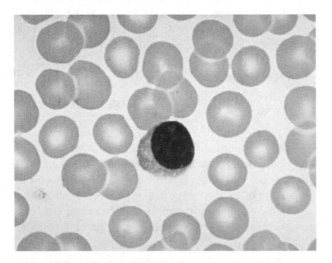

A lymphocyte cell. *(Photograph by Lester V. Bergman, Corbis Images. Reproduced by permission.)*

Normal results

In general, normal levels of white blood cells vary slightly by age and gender. Normal values are lower in children under the age of 15 and in young adults between the ages of 20 and 30. After age 30, men have slightly higher levels of white blood cells than women.

Normal adult levels of white blood cells are 4,500-11,000 cells per microliter of blood. Lymphocytes account for approximately 25-45% of the total white blood cell count; the normal range is 1,000-4,800 lymphocytes per microliter of blood. Of the total lymphocytes, 60-80% are T cells and approximately 15% are B cells. (There are two other types of lymphocytes; natural killer and K-type; that constitute a minor proportion of the total lymphocyte numbers.)

Abnormal results

A higher-than-normal level of lymphocytes is called lymphocytosis. Lymphocytosis occurs if a person has a viral, bacterial, or other type of infection. It can also occur with certain blood disorders, such as leukemia.

Lower-than-normal levels of lymphocytes is called lymphopenia. Lymphopenia can be an indicator of certain **cancers,** bone marrow failure, or immune system deficiency. Medical treatments, such as **chemotherapy** and **radiation therapy,** can also deplete the body's supply of lymphocytes, as can exposure to poisonous substances.

Resources

BOOKS

Corbett, Jane Vincent. *Laboratory Tests & Diagnostic Procedures with Nursing Diagnoses,* 4th ed. Stamford, CT: Appleton & Lange, 1996.

Janeway, Charles A., and Paul Travers. *Immunobiology: The Immune System in Health and Disease,* 2nd ed. New York: Garland Publishing, Inc., 1996.

Malarkey, Louise M., and Mary Ellen McMorrow. *Nurse's Manual of Laboratory Tests and Diagnostic Procedures.* Philadelphia: W.B. Saunders Company, 1996.

Turgeon, Mary Louise. *Immunology & Serology in Laboratory Medicine.* St. Louis: Mosby-Year Book, Inc., 1996.

Julia Barrett

Lymphocytic choriomeningitis

Definition

Lymphocytic choriomeningitis (LCM) is a viral infection of the membranes surrounding the brain and spinal cord and of the cerebrospinal fluid.

Description

Lymphocytic choriomeningitis virus infection is relatively rare and recovery usually occurs spontaneously within a couple of weeks. Many cases are probably not even identified because the symptoms range from extremely mild to those resembling severe flu. A few patients develop symptoms of **meningitis.** In some rare cases, the LCM viral infection can spread throughout the central nervous system, and may even be fatal.

Causes & symptoms

LCM is caused by an arenavirus, which is an RNA virus and is a mild cousin in the family containing the much more threatening arenaviruses that cause hemmorrhagic fever. Humans acquire LCM virus from infected rodents by coming in contact with the animals or their excretions. Exposure to the virus is not as unlikely to occur as it seems, because the viral hosts can be common house mice and even pets, such as hamsters and chinchillas. Most cases of LCM occur in fall and winter, when mice seek warmth inside dwellings. Food and dust can become contaminated by the excretions of rodents infected with LCM virus. In 1997, French scientists alerted physicians to suspect LCM viral infection in people who had contact with Syrian hamsters.

The symptoms of LCM occur in two phases. The first (prodrome) stage can produce fever, chills, muscle aches, **cough,** and vomiting. In the second phase, characteristic meningitis symptoms of **headache,** stiff neck, listlessness, and **nausea and vomiting** may occur. In adults, complications are rare and recovery may even occur before the second phase.

The virus is not spread from person to person, except through **pregnancy.** LCM virus is one of the few viruses that can cross the placenta from mother to child during pregnancy and may be an underrecognized cause of congenital infection in newborns. Infection with cytomegalovirus, *Toxoplasma gondii,* or LCM virus can appear similar enough in infants to be confused when diagnosed. In cases that have been recognized among infants, LCM viral infection has a high mortality rate (about one-third of the babies studied died).

Diagnosis

LCM can be distinguished from bacterial meningitis by the history of prodrome symptoms and the period of time before meningitis symptoms begin, which is about 15-21 days for LCM.

Treatment

No antiviral agents exist for LCM virus. Treatment consists of supporting the patient and treating the symptoms until the infection subsides, generally within a few weeks.

Jill S. Lasker

Lymphocytic leukemia, acute *see*
Leukemias, acute

Lymphocytic leukemia, chronic *see*
Leukemias, chronic

Lymphocytopenia

Definition

Lymphocytopenia is a condition marked by an abnormally low level of lymphocytes in the blood. Lymphocytes are a specific type of white blood cell with important functions in the immune system.

Description

Lymphocytes normally account for 15-40% of all white cells in the bloodstream. They help to protect the body from infections caused by viruses or fungi. They also coordinate the activities of other cells in the immune system. In addition, lymphocytes fight **cancer** and develop into antibody-producing cells that neutralize the effect of foreign substances in the blood.

Lymphocytopenia is the result of abnormalities in the way lymphocytes are produced, make their way through the bloodstream, or are lost or destroyed. These conditions can result from congenital or drug-induced

---

KEY TERMS

Prodrome—Symptom(s) experienced prior to the onset of a disease. For example, visual disturbances may precede and signal the onset of a migraine headache.

KEY TERMS

B lymphocyte—A type of lymphocyte that circulates in the blood and lymph and produces antibodies when it encounters specific antigens. B lymphocytes are also called B cells.

Lymph—A clear yellowish fluid circulated by the lymphatic system. The lymph carries mostly lymphocytes and fats.

Lymphocyte—A specific type of white blood cell that is important in the production of antibodies.

decreases in the body's ability to recognize and attack invaders.

Causes & symptoms

Lymphocytopenia has a wide range of possible causes:

* **AIDS** and other viral, bacterial, and fungal infections

* Chronic failure of the right ventricle of the heart. This chamber of the heart pumps blood to the lungs.

* **Hodgkin's disease** and cancers of the lymphatic system

* A leak or rupture in the thoracic duct. The thoracic duct removes lymphatic fluid from the legs and abdomen.

* Leukemia

* Side effects of prescription medications

* **Malnutrition. Diets** that are low in protein and overall calorie intake may cause lymphocytopenia.

* **Radiation therapy**

* High **stress** levels

* Trauma.

The symptoms of lymphocytopenia vary. Lymphocytes constitute only a fraction of the body's white blood cells, and a decline in their number may not produce any symptoms. A patient who has lymphocytopenia may have symptoms of the condition responsible for the depressed level of lymphocytes.

Diagnosis

Lymphocytopenia is most often detected when blood tests are performed to diagnose other diseases.

Treatment

Treatment for lymphocytopenia is designed to identify and correct the underlying cause of the condition.

Drug-depressed lymphocyte levels usually return to normal a few days after the patient stops taking the medication.

A deficiency of B lymphocytes, which mature into antibody-producing plasma cells, can result in abnormally low lymphocyte levels. When the number of B lymphocytes is low, the patient may be treated with **antibiotics,** antifungal medications, antiviral agents, or a substance containing a high concentration of antibodies (gamma globulin) to prevent infection.

It is not usually possible to restore normal lymphocyte levels in AIDS patients. Drugs like AZT (azidothymidine, sold under the trade name Retrovir) can increase the number of helper T cells, which help other cells wipe out disease organisms.

Prognosis

Very low levels of lymphocytes make patients vulnerable to life-threatening infection. Researchers are studying the effectiveness of transplanting bone marrow and other cells to restore normal lymphocyte levels. **Gene therapy,** which uses the body's own resources or artificial substances to counter diseases or disorders, is also being evaluated as a treatment for lymphocytopenia.

Resources

BOOKS

Cecil Textbook of Medicine, edited by J. Claude Bennett, and Fred Plum. Philadelphia: W. B. Saunders Company, 1996.

Merck Manual of Medical Information: Home Edition, edited by Robert Berkow, et al. Whitehouse Station, NJ: Merck Research Laboratories, 1997.

Maureen Haggerty

Lymphogranuloma venereum

Definition

Lymphogranuloma venereum (LGV) is a sexually transmitted systemic disease (STD) caused by a parasitic organism closely related to certain types of bacteria. It affects the lymph nodes and rectal area, as well as the genitals, in humans. The name comes from two Latin words that mean a swelling of granulation tissue in the lymph nodes resulting from sexual intercourse. Granulation tissue is tissue that forms during wound or ulcer healing that has a rough or lumpy surface.

KEY TERMS

Anogenitorectal syndrome—Another name for third-stage LGV.

Aspiration—A procedure in which pus or other fluid is removed from a body cavity through a hollow needle connected to a syringe.

Bubo—An inflamed swelling inside a lymph node, characteristic of second-stage LGV.

Elephantiasis—Abnormal enlargement of the legs and groin area caused by blockage of the lymphatic system, as a complication of LGV.

Fistula—A passageway formed by a disease or injury that drains fluid from an infected area to the outside or to other parts of the body.

Lymph—A clear yellowish fluid that circulates throughout the body, carrying white blood cells and fats. The system that produces and circulates lymph is called the lymphatic system; it includes lymph vessels, lymph nodes, the thymus gland, and the spleen.

Proctitis—Inflammation of the anus and rectum.

Stricture—An abnormal narrowing or tightening of a body passage. LGV can cause strictures to form in the patient's rectum, or in the vagina of female patients.

Description

Although LGV is easily treated in its early stages, it can produce serious complications in its later stages. LGV is most likely to occur among people living in tropical or subtropical countries and among military personnel or tourists in countries or large cities with high rates of the disease. Prostitutes play a major role in carrying and transmitting LGV, as was documented during an outbreak in Florida in the late 1980s. There are about 1000 documented cases of LGV in the United States in an average year.

Causes & symptoms

LGV is caused by *Chlamydia trachomatis*, a globe-shaped parasitic organism that reproduces only inside of living cells. *C. trachomatis* has 17 subtypes and is responsible for a wide range of infections in both men and women; however, only subtypes L1, L2, and L3 cause lymphogranuloma venereum. The parasite has a two-part lifecycle. In the first stage, it is inert and can survive outside of cells. In its second stage, it lacks a cell wall and actively reproduces after gaining entry to a cell. As the chlamydia organism reproduces inside the cell, it pushes the nucleus aside and forms an inclusion that can be identified with tissue staining. LGV differs from other diseases caused by *C. trachomatis* in that it affects the body's lymphatic system and not just the moist tissues of the genital region. In humans, the chlamydia organism is transmitted through vaginal or anal intercourse, oral sex, or contact with fluid from open ulcers or infected tissues.

Lymphogranuloma venereum has three stages. In its primary stage, the disease is more likely to be detected in men; it may go unnoticed in women. After an incubation period of four to 30 days, a small painless ulcer or blister develops in the genital area. Second-stage LGV develops between one and six weeks later. In this stage, the infection spreads to the lymphatic system, forming buboes (swellings) in the lymph nodes of the groin area. The buboes often merge, soften, and rupture, forming sinuses and fistulas (hollow passages and ducts) that carry an infectious bloody discharge to the outside of the body. Patients with second-stage LGV may also have **fever,** nausea, **headaches,** pains in their joints, skin **rashes,** and enlargement of the spleen or liver. Third-stage LGV, which is sometimes called anogenitorectal syndrome, develops in about 25% of patients. In men, this stage is usually seen in homosexuals. Third-stage LGV is marked by rectal pain, **constipation,** a discharge containing pus or bloody mucus, and the development of strictures (nar-

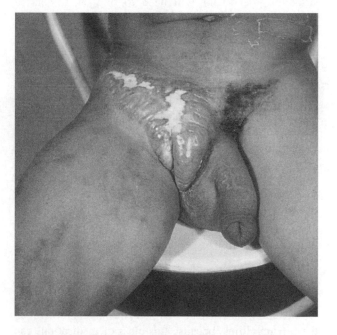

This man suffers from lymphogranuloma venereum, a venereal disease that is caused by the bacterium *Chlamydia trachomatis.* (Photograph by Milton Reisch, M.D., Corbis Images. Reproduced by permission.)

rowing or tightening of a body passage) in the rectum or vagina.

LGV can have a number of serious complications. *C. trachomatis* infections of any subtype are associated with long-term fertility problems in women. Strictures in the rectum can completely close off the lower bowel, producing eventual rupture of the bowel and inflammation of the abdominal cavity. The patient can develop chronic **abscesses** or fistulae in the anal area or in the vagina in women. Long-term blockages in the lymph nodes can produce **elephantiasis,** a condition in which the patient's upper legs and groin area become greatly enlarged. Patients with chronic LGV infection have a higher risk of developing **cancer** in the inflamed areas.

Chronic LGV can be reactivated in patients who become infected with the **AIDS** virus. These patients develop open ulcers in the groin that are difficult to treat.

Diagnosis

The diagnosis of LGV is usually made on the basis of the patient's history, careful examination of the genital area and lymph nodes, and blood tests or cultures to confirm the diagnosis. In the early stages of the disease, the doctor will need to distinguish between LGV and such other STDs as **syphilis** and herpes. If the patient has developed buboes, the doctor will need to rule out **tuberculosis, cat-scratch disease,** bubonic **plague,** or **tularemia** (a disease similar to plague that is carried by rabbits and squirrels). If the patient has developed rectal strictures, the doctor will need to rule out tumors or colitis.

There are several blood tests that can be used to confirm the diagnosis of LGV. The most commonly used are the complement fixation (CF) test and the microimmunofluorescence (micro-IF) tests. Although the micro-IF test is considered more sensitive than the CF test, it is less widely available. An antibody titer (concentration) of 1:64 or greater on the CF test or 1:512 or greater on the micro-IF test is needed to make the diagnosis of LGV. In some cases, the diagnosis can be made from culturing *C. trachomatis* taken from samples of tissue fluid from ulcers or buboes, or from a tissue sample from the patient's rectum.

Treatment

LGV is treated with oral **antibiotics,** usually tetracycline or doxycycline for 10-20 days, or erythromycin or trimethoprim sulfamethoxazole for 14 days. Pregnant women are usually treated with erythromycin rather than the **tetracyclines,** because this class of medications can harm the fetus.

Patients who have developed second- and third-stage complications may need surgical treatment. The doctor can treat buboes by withdrawing fluid from them through a hollow needle into a suction syringe. This procedure is called aspiration. Fistulas and abscesses also can be treated surgically. Patients who develop elephantiasis are usually treated by plastic surgeons. Patients with rectal strictures may need surgery to prevent bowel obstruction and rupture into the abdomen.

Prognosis

The prognosis for recovery for most patients is good, with the exception of AIDS patients. Prompt treatment of the early stages of LGV is essential to prevent transmission of the disease as well as fertility problems and other serious complications of the later stages.

Prevention

Prevention of lymphogranuloma venereum has four important aspects:

• Avoidance of casual sexual contacts, particularly with prostitutes, in countries with high rates of the disease.

• Observance of proper safeguards by health professionals. Doctors and other healthcare workers should wear gloves when touching infected areas of the patient's body or handling soiled dressings and other contaminated items. All contaminated materials and instruments should be double-bagged before disposing.

• Tracing and examination of an infected person's recent sexual contacts.

• Monitoring the patient for recurring symptoms for a period of six months after antibiotic treatment.

Resources

BOOKS

Chambers, Henry F. "Infectious Diseases: Bacterial & Chlamydial." In *Current Medical Diagnosis & Treatment 1998,* edited by Lawrence M. Tierney, Jr., et al. Stamford, CT: Appleton & Lange, 1997.

Chapel, Thomas A., and Johanna Chapel. "Lymphogranuloma Venereum." In *Conn's Current Therapy,* edited by Robert E. Rakel. Philadelphia: W. B. Saunders Company, 1997.

Hill, Edward C. "Gynecology." In *Current Surgical Diagnosis & Treatment,* edited by Lawrence W. Way. Stamford, CT: Appleton & Lange, 1994.

"Infectious Disease: Sexually Transmitted Diseases." In *The Merck Manual of Diagnosis and Therapy,* vol. I, edited by Robert Berkow, et al. Rahway, NJ: Merck Research Laboratories, 1992.

Thomas, Isabelle, et al. ''Lymphogranuloma Venereum.'' In *Current Diagnosis 9,* edited by Rex B. Conn, et al. Philadelphia: W. B. Saunders Company, 1997.

Rebecca J. Frey

Lymphomas *see* **Hodgkin's disease; Malignant lymphomas**

Lymphopenia *see* **Lymphocytopenia**

Lymphosarcomas *see* **Malignant lymphomas**

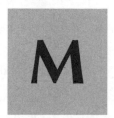

Macular degeneration

Definition

Macular degeneration is the progressive deterioration of a critical region of the retina called the macula. The macula is a 3-5 mm area in the retina that is responsible for central vision. This disorder leads to irreversible loss of central vision, although peripheral vision is retained. In the early stages, vision may be gray, hazy, or distorted.

Description

Macular degeneration is the most common cause of legal blindness in people over 60, and accounts for approximately 11.7% of blindness in the United States. About 28% of the population over age 74 is affected by this disease.

Age-related macular degeneration (ARMD) is the most common form of macular degeneration. It is also known as age-related maculopathy (ARM), aged macular degeneration, and senile macular degeneration. Approximately 10 million Americans have some vision loss that is due to ARMD.

ARMD is subdivided into a dry (atrophic) and a wet (exudative) form. The dry form is more common and accounts for 70-90% of cases of ARMD. It progresses more slowly than the wet form and vision loss is less severe. In the dry form, the macula thins over time as part of the aging process and the pigmented retinal epithelium (a dark-colored cell layer at the back of the eye) is gradually lost. Words may appear blurred or hazy and colors may appear dim or gray.

In the wet form of ARMD, new blood vessels grow underneath the retina and distort the retina. These blood vessels can leak, causing scar tissue to form on the retina. The wet form may cause visual distortion and make straight lines appear wavy. A central blind spot develops. The wet type progresses more rapidly and vision loss is

more pronounced. Treatments are available for some, but not most, cases of the wet form.

Other less common forms of macular degeneration include:

• Cystoid macular degeneration. Loss of vision in the macula due to fluid-filled areas (cysts) in the macular

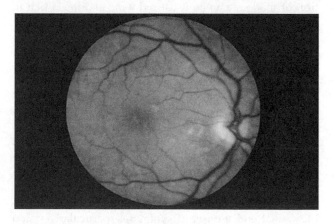

A slit-lamp view showing macular degeneration of the eye. (Custom Medical Stock Photo. Reproduced by permission.)

region. This may be a result of other disorders, such as aging, inflammation, or high **myopia.**

• Diabetic macular degeneration. Deterioration of the macula due to diabetes.

• Senile disciform degeneration (also known as Kuhnt-Junius macular degeneration). A specific and severe type of the wet form of ARMD that involves leaking blood vessels (hemorrhaging) in the macular region. It usually occurs in people over 40 years old.

Causes & symptoms

Age-related macular degeneration is part of the aging process. There may be a hereditary component. Having a family member with ARMD increases a person's risk for developing it. There is a slightly higher incidence in females. Whites and Asians are more susceptible to developing ARMD than blacks, in whom the disorder is rare.

ARMD is thought to be caused by hardening and blocking of the arteries (arteriosclerosis) in the blood vessels supplying the retina. Some of the same things that are bad for the heart are thought to contribute to the development of macular degeneration. These risk factors include smoking and a diet that is rich in saturated fat. Smokers have a risk of developing ARMD that is approximately 2.4-3 times that of non-smokers. Smoking increases the risk of developing wet-type ARMD, and may increase the risk of developing dry-type as well. Dietary fat also increase the risk. In one study of older (age 45-84) Americans, signs of early ARMD were 80% more common in the group who ate the most saturated fat compared to those who ate the least. Low consumption of antioxidants, such as foods rich in vitamin A, is associated with a higher risk for developing ARMD. Consumption of moderate amounts of red wine and foods rich in vitamin A is associated with a lower risk. It is generally believed that exposure to ultraviolet (UV) light may contribute to disease development, but this has not been proven.

The main symptom of macular degeneration is a change in central vision. The patient may notice blurred central vision or a blank spot on the page when reading. The patient may notice visual distortion such as bending of straight lines. Images may appear smaller. Some patients notice a change in color perception and some experience abnormal light sensations. These symptoms may come on suddenly and become progressively more troublesome. Sudden onset of symptoms, particularly vision distortion, is an indication for immediate evaluation by an ophthalmologist.

Diagnosis

To make the diagnosis of macular degeneration, the doctor dilates the pupil with eye drops and examines the interior of the eye, looking at the retina for the presence of yellow bumps called drusen and for gross changes in the macula such as thinning. The doctor also administers a visual field test, looking for blank spots in the central vision. The doctor may call for fluorescein **angiography** (intravenous injection of fluorescent dye followed by visual examination and photography of the back of the eye) to determine if blood vessels in the retina are leaking.

A central visual field test called an Amsler grid is usually given to patients who are suspected of having ARMD. It is a grid printed on a sheet of paper (so it is easy to take home). When looking at a central dot on the page, the patient should call the doctor right away if any of the lines appear to be wavy or missing. This may be an indication of fluid and the onset of wet ARMD. Patients may also be asked to come in for more frequent checkups.

Treatment

While loss of vision cannot be reversed, early detection is important because treatments are available that may halt or slow the progression of the wet form of ARMD. Treatment for the dry form is not available as of 1998, but cell transplantation studies are under study.

In wet-type ARMD and in senile disciform macular degeneration, new capillaries grow in the macular region and leak. This leaking of blood and fluid causes a portion of the retina to detach. Blood vessel growth, called neovascularization, can be treated with laser photocoagulation in some cases, depending upon the location and extent of the growth. Argon or krypton lasers can destroy the new tissue and flatten the retina. This treatment is effective in about half the cases but results may be temporary. A concern with laser therapy is that the laser also destroys the photoreceptors in the treated area. If the blood vessels have grown into the fovea (a region of the macula responsible for fine vision), treatment may not be possible. Because capillaries can grow very quickly, this form of macular degeneration should be handled as an emergency and treated quickly. Patients who are experiencing visual distortion should seek help immediately.

Another form of treatment for the wet form of ARMD is **radiation therapy** with either x rays or a proton beam. Blood vessels that are proliferating (growing) are sensitive to treatment with low doses of ionizing radiation. Nerve cells in the retina are not growing and are insensitive, so they are not harmed by this treatment. External beam radiation treatment has shown promising results at slowing progression in limited, early trials. An alternative treatment is internal beam radiation therapy. For this treatment, the patient is given a local anesthetic and an applicator containing strontium 90 is inserted into the affected eye. This brief and localized radiation therapy prevents the growth of blood vessels.

Other therapies that are under study include treatment with alpha-interferon, thalidomide, and other drugs that slow the growth of blood vessels. Subretinal surgery also has shown promise in rapid-onset cases of wet ARMD. This surgery carries the risk of **retinal detachment,** hemorrhage, and acceleration of cataract formation. Other experimental treatments include photodynamic therapy (PDT). For this treatment, a photosensitizing dye is injected, followed by irradiation of the area of new blood vessel growth with a special, low-intensity diode laser. This treatment damages the cells in the blood vessel walls and causes them to stop growing.

A controversial treatment called rheotherapy involves pumping the patient's blood through a device that removes some proteins and fats. As of 1998, this had not been proven to be safe or effective.

Alternative treatment

Consumption of a diet rich in antioxidants (beta carotene and the mixed carotenoids that are precursors of vitamin A, **vitamins** C and E, selenium, and zinc), or taking antioxidant nutritional supplements, may help prevent macular degeneration, particularly if started early in life. Good dietary sources of antioxidants include citrus fruits, cauliflower, broccoli, nuts, seeds, orange and yellow vegetables, cherries, blackberries, and blueberries. Research has shown that nutritional therapy can prevent ARMD or slow its progression once established. Some doctors recommend taking beta carotene and zinc as a precautionary measure. Some vitamins are marketed specifically for the eyes.

Prognosis

The dry form of ARMD is self-limiting and eventually stabilizes. The loss of vision is permanent. The vision of patients with the wet form of ARMD often stabilizes or improves even without treatment, at least temporarily. However, after a few years, patients with the wet form of ARMD are usually left with only coarse peripheral vision remaining.

Many patients with macular degeneration lose their central vision permanently and may become legally blind. However, macular degeneration rarely causes total loss of vision. Peripheral vision is retained. The patient can compensate, to some extent, for the loss of central vision, even though macular degeneration may render them legally blind. Improved lighting and special low-vision aids may help even if sharpness of vision (visual

acuity) is poor. Vision aids include special magnifiers that allow the patient to read and telescopic aids for long-distance vision. The use of these visual aids plus the retained peripheral vision usually allow the patient to remain independent. Registration as a legally blind person will enable a patient to obtain special services and considerations.

Prevention

Avoiding the risk factors for macular degeneration may help prevent it. This includes avoiding tobacco smoke and eating a diet low in saturated fat. Some other behaviors that may help reduce the risk of wet-type ARMD are eating a diet rich in green, leafy vegetables and yellow vegetables such as carrots, sweet potatoes, and winter squash; drinking moderate amounts of alcohol, such as one or two glasses of red wine a day; and taking an antioxidant vitamin supplement, especially vitamin A. Some vitamins may be toxic in large doses, so patients should speak with their doctors. Vitamins C and E have not been shown to reduce risk, nor did selenium in one large study. The use of zinc is controversial: some studies showed a benefit, others showed no benefit, and one actually showed an increased risk of ARMD with increased levels of zinc in the blood. Some doctors suggest that wearing UV-blocking sunglasses reduces risk. Use of estrogen in postmenopausal women is associated with a lower risk of developing ARMD.

Resources

BOOKS

Caird, F.I., and John Williamson. *The Eye and Its Disorders in the Elderly.* Bristol, U.K.: Wright, 1986.

Current Medical Diagnosis and Treatment, 37th Edition, edited by Lawrence M. Tierney, Jr., Stephen J. McPhee, and Maxine A. Papadakis. Stamford, CT: Appleton and Lange, 1998.

Eden, John. *The Physician's Guide to Cataracts, Glaucoma, and Other Eye Problems.* Yonkers, New York: Consumer Reports Books, a division of Consumers Union, 1992.

Norris, June, ed. *Professional Guide to Diseases,* Fifth Edition. Springhouse, PA: Springhouse Corporation, 1995.

PERIODICALS

"All the Better to See You." *Harvard Health Letter* 21 (3)(January, 1996): 8.

"Macular Degeneration." *Mayo Clinic Health Letter* 15 (6)(June, 1997): 4.

O'Shea, John. "Age-related Macular Degeneration: A Leading Cause of Blindness." *Medical Journal of Australia* 165 (10)(November 18, 1996): 561-4.

ORGANIZATIONS

American Academy of Ophthalmology (National Eyecare Project). P.O. Box 429098, San Francisco CA. 94142-9098. (800)222-EYES. http://www.eyenet.org.

American Optometric Association. 243 North Lindbergh Blvd., St. Louis, MO 63141. (314) 991-4100. http://www.aoanet.org.

Prevent Blindness America. 500 East Remington Road, Schaumburg, IL 60173. (800) 331-2020. http://www.prevent-blindness.org.

Louann W. Murray

Macule *see* **Skin lesions**

Mad cow disease *see* **Creutzfeldt-Jakob disease**

Madura foot *see* **Mycetoma**

Maduromycosis *see* **Mycetoma**

Magnesium hydroxide *see* **Antacids**

Magnesium imbalance

Definition

A mineral found in the fluid that surrounds cells, magnesium (Mg) is an essential component of more than 300 enzymes that regulate many body functions. Imbalances occur when the blood contains more or less magnesium than it should.

Description

Magnesium is necessary for the formation and functioning of healthy bones, teeth, muscles, and nerves. It converts food into energy, builds proteins, and is instrumental in maintaining adequate levels of calcium in the blood. Magnesium helps prevent cardiovascular disease and irregular heartbeat, reduces the risk of bone loss (**osteoporosis**), and increases an individual's chance of surviving a **heart attack.** It may also help prevent **stroke** and lessen the effects of existing osteoporosis.

Fish, dairy products, leafy green vegetables, legumes, nuts, seeds, and grains are especially good sources of magnesium, but varying amounts of this mineral are found in all foods. Some is stored in the kidneys, and excess amounts are excreted in the urine or stools.

Magnesium deficiency (hypomagnesemia) or excess (hypermagnesemia) is rare, but either condition can be serious.

Causes & symptoms

Hypomagnesemia

Magnesium deficiency most often occurs in people who have been fed intravenously for a long time, whose diet doesn't contain enough magnesium, or who are unable to absorb and excrete the mineral properly.

Secreting too much aldosterone (the hormone that regulates the body's salt-fluid balance), ADH (a hormone that inhibits urine production), or thyroid hormone can cause hypomagnesemia.

Other factors associated with hypomagnesemia include:

- Loss of body fluids as a result of stomach suctioning or chronic **diarrhea**
- Cisplatin (a **chemotherapy** drug)
- Long-term diuretic therapy
- **Hypercalcemia** (abnormally high levels of calcium in the blood)
- Diabetic acidosis (a condition in which the body's tissues have a higher-than-normal acid content)
- Complications of bowel surgery
- Chronic **alcoholism**
- **Malnutrition**
- **Starvation**
- Severe **dehydration.**

People who have hypomagnesemia usually experience loss of weight and appetite, bloating, and muscle **pain,** and they pass stools that have a high fat content. Also, they may be listless, disoriented, confused, and very irritable. Other symptoms of hypomagnesemia are:

- Nausea
- Vomiting
- Muscle weakness
- Tremor

• Irregular heart beat

• **Delusions** and **hallucinations**

• Leg and foot cramps

• Muscle twitches

• Changes in blood pressure.

Severe magnesium deficiency can cause seizures, especially in children.

Neonatal hypomagnesemia can occur in premature babies and in infants who have genetic parathyroid disorders or who have had blood **transfusions.** This condition also occurs in babies born to magnesium-deficient mothers or to women who have:

• **Diabetes mellitus.**

• **Hyperparathyroidism** (overactive parathyroid glands)

• Toxemia (a pregnancy-related condition characterized by high blood pressure and fluid retention).

Hypermagnesemia

Hypermagnesemia is most common in patients whose kidneys cannot excrete the magnesium they derive from food or take as medication. This condition can also develop in patients who take magnesium salts, or in healthy people who use large quantities of magnesium-containing **antacids, laxatives,** or **analgesics** (pain relievers).

Magnesium poisoning can cause severe diarrhea in young people, and mask the symptoms of other illnesses. Very high overdoses can lead to **coma.** The risk of complications of magnesium poisoning is greatest for:

• Elderly people with inefficient kidney function

• Patients with kidney problems or intestinal disorders

• People who use **antihistamines, muscle relaxants,** or narcotics.

Severe dehydration or an overdose of supplements taken to counteract hypomagnesemia can also cause this condition.

People who have hypermagnesemia may feel flushed and drowsy, perspire heavily, and have diarrhea. Breathing becomes shallow, reflexes diminish, and the patient becomes unresponsive. Muscle weakness and hallucinations are common. The patient's heart beat slows dramatically and blood pressure plummets. Extreme toxicity, which can lead to coma and cardiac arrest, can be fatal.

Diagnosis

Blood tests are used to measure magnesium levels.

Treatment

The goal of treatment is to identify and correct the cause of the imbalance. Oral magnesium supplements or injections are usually prescribed to correct mild magnesium deficiency. If the deficiency is more severe or does not respond to treatment, magnesium sulfate or magnesium chloride may be administered intravenously.

Doctors usually prescribe **diuretics** (urine-producing drugs) for patients with hypermagnesemia and advise them to drink more fluids to flush the excess mineral from the body. Patients whose magnesium levels are extremely high may need mechanical support to breathe and to circulate blood throughout their bodies.

Intravenously administered calcium gluconate may reverse damage caused by excess magnesium. Intravenous furosemide (Lasix) or ethacrynic acid (Edecrin) can increase magnesium excretion in patients who get enough fluids and whose kidneys are functioning properly.

In an emergency, dialysis can provide temporary relief for patients whose kidney function is poor or who are unable to excrete excess **minerals.**

Prognosis

Because imbalances may recur if the underlying condition is not eliminated, monitoring of magnesium levels should continue after treatment has been completed.

Prevention

Most people consume adequate amounts of magnesium in the food they eat. Dietary supplements can be used safely, but should only be used under a doctor's supervision.

Resources

BOOKS

The Editors of Time-Life Books. *The Medical Advisor: The Complete Guide to Alternative & Conventional Treatments.* Alexandria, VA: Time-Life, Inc., 1996.

Shaw, Michael, ed. *Everything You Need to Know About Diseases.* Springhouse, PA: Springhouse Corporation, 1996.

Slupnik, Ramona, ed. *American Medical Association Complete Guide to Women's Health.* New York: Random House, Inc., 1996.

OTHER

The Merck Manual: Hypermagnesemia. http://www.merck.com/!!uYwVO15ELuYWVO15Elu/pubs/mmanual/html. (2 May 1998).

The Merck Manual: Hypomagnesemia Etiology and Pathogenesis. http://www.merck.com/!!uYwVO15ELuYwV015E4/pubs/mmanual/html/khihhe.htm. (1 May 1998)

Mineral Guide. http://www.cnn.com/HEALTH/indepth.food/
vitamins.minerals.faqs.minerals.html. (2 May 1998).

Report Says Excessive Antacid Use Can Cause Poisoning.
http://cnn.com/HEALTH/9508/magnesium/index.html. (2
May 1998).

Maureen Haggerty

Magnetic field therapy

Definition

Magnetic field therapy is the use of magnets and electrical devices to treat and diagnose many medical conditions, including **cancer,** rheumatoid disease, stress-related illness, and **pain.**

Purpose

Magnetic field therapy (MFT) is an alternative treatment for a wide variety of symptoms, most notably for pain. While the use of magnets for healing has a centuries-old history, only recently have some controlled studies been done which demonstrate the effectiveness of magnetic field therapy.

The human body is surrounded by magnetic fields present on the earth, and the body is full of magnetic materials. Magnetic fields penetrate the body easily, because it is 70% water and offers no resistance. A strong magnet held on one side of the hand can easily affect the needle on a compass on the other side of the same hand. Measurements show that tissue that has been exposed to a magnet will keep enhanced magnetic signals for sometime afterwards. Different types of magnets can produce these effects, including flat magnetic pads and electromagnets, such as **magnetic resonance imaging** (MRI) machines and nerve conduction testing devices.

The mechanism of action of MFT is not understood. Possible explanations of its beneficial effect on the body include its ability to increase blood flow, change the alignment of bodily electromagnetic fields, and interact with **acupuncture** points and meridians on the body. Certainly the placebo effect, in which a treatment is helpful because the patient thinks it is, may be acting in some cases. However, MFT has also been used successfully in treating pain in horses, where the placebo effect presumably is not a factor.

Claims of successful treatment have been made for many more conditions, including cancer, arthritis, **headache, sleep disorders,** neurological disease, stress-related conditions, and **osteoporosis.**

KEY TERMS

Double-blind study—A scientific investigation in which in which neither the subject nor the investigator knows what treatment, if any, the subject is receiving.

Magnet—A body that has the ability to attract particles of iron and that, when it is freely suspended, assumes a definite direction between the magnetic poles of the earth.

Meridian—In Chinese medicine, a network of pathways running throughout the body, carrying energy from organ to organ, and connecting every cell of the body.

Placebo—An inactive substance given to satisfy a patient's demands or desires.

Some double-blind scientific studies have shown varying results in the use of MFT to reduce pain associated with hip replacement and heel pain. Another small investigation demonstrated improvement in the healing of leg ulcers.

Precautions

MFT is not approved by the Food and Drug Administration as a treatment for any medical condition, and magnetic therapy products are not registered medical devices. Those with cardiac **pacemakers** or other implanted devices should not use magnets. Marketers of MFT devices warn against use during **pregnancy** or on open **wounds,** and state that magnets may cause pain, toxin release, medication interactions, digestive difficulties, seizures, **insomnia,** hyperactivity, and tumor growth.

Description

Magnetic therapy can be applied in many ways, from the use of small, simple magnets to a large machine. Small magnets, either embedded in flexible plastic or wrapped in cloth, are strapped over the area to be treated, and left in place for variable lengths of time. They can also be carried in a person's pocket or placed in a shoe. Magnetic blankets and mattress pads also are available. Large machines that can generate high levels of field strength are used for treating **fractures** that are slow to heal, and in pseudoarthritis, a joint disease caused by nerve breakdown.

Risks

In the limited studies of MFT, no adverse effects have been reported. Since the body's electromagnetic fields are easily altered, magnetic therapy should be practiced under the supervision of an experienced professional.

Normal results

MFT seems to be effective, according to the literature, for relief of some types of pain and in healing leg ulcers. Further study is needed to confirm its effectiveness in treating other conditions.

Resources

BOOKS

The Burton Goldberg Group. *Alternative Medicine: The Definitive Guide.* Fife, WA: Future Medicine Publishing, 1995.

PERIODICALS

Caselli M.A. et al. "Evaluation of Magnetic Foil and PPT Insoles in the Treatment of Heel Pain." *Journal of American Podiatry Medical Association* 87 (1)(January 1997): 11-6.

Kenkre J.E., et al. "A Randomized Controlled Trial of Electromagnetic Therapy in the Primary Care Management of Venous Leg Ulceration." *Family Practice* 13 (3)(June 1996): 236-41.

Konrad K., et al. "Therapy with Pulsed Electromagnetic Fields in Aseptic Loosening of Total Hip Prostheses: A Prospective Study." *Clinical Rheumatology* 15 (4)(July 1996): 325-8.

Vallbona, C., et al. "Response of Pain to Static Magnetic Fields in Postpolio Patients: A Double-Blind Pilot Study." *Archives of Physical Medicine and Rehabilitation* 78 (11)(November 1997): 1200-3.

OTHER

"Health Technologies." http://www.healthtechnologies.com/magnets/magresearch3.html. (1998).

"Magnetic Products." http://hre.com/totalhealth/magnet.html. (1998).

Magnetic resonance angiography *see*
Magnetic resonance imaging

Magnetic resonance imaging

Definition

Magnetic resonance imaging (MRI) is the newest, and perhaps most versatile, medical imaging technology available. Doctors can get highly refined images of the body's interior without surgery, using MRI. By using strong magnets and pulses of radio waves to manipulate the natural magnetic properties in the body, this technique makes better images of organs and soft tissues than those of other scanning technologies. MRI is particularly

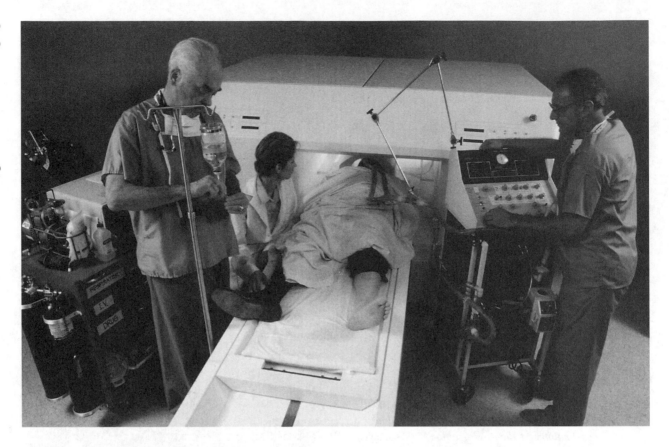

A patient undergoing a magnetic resonance imaging test. *(FPG International. Reproduced by permission.)*

useful for imaging the brain and spine, as well as the soft tissues of joints and the interior structure of bones. The entire body is visible to the technique, which poses few known health risks.

Purpose

MRI was developed in the 1980s. The latest additions to MRI technology are **angiography** (MRA) and spectroscopy (MRS). MRA was developed to study blood flow, while MRS can identify the chemical composition of diseased tissue and produce color images of brain function. The many advantages of MRI include:

- Detail. MRI creates precise images of the body based on the varying proportions of magnetic elements in different tissues. Very minor fluctuations in chemical composition can be determined. MRI images have greater natural contrast than standard x rays, **computed tomography scan** (CT scan), or ultrasound, all of which depend on the differing physical properties of tissues. This sensitivity lets MRI distinguish fine variations in tissues deep within the body. It also is particularly useful for spotting and distinguishing diseased tissues (tumors and other lesions) early in their development.

Often, doctors prescribe an MRI scan to more fully investigate earlier findings of the other imaging techniques.

- Scope. The entire body can be scanned, from head to toe and from the skin to the deepest recesses of the brain. Moreover, MRI scans are not obstructed by bone, gas, or body waste, which can hinder other imaging techniques. (Although the scans can be degraded by motion such as breathing, heartbeat, and normal bowel activity.) The MRI process produces cross-sectional images of the body that are as sharp in the middle as on the edges, even of the brain through the skull. A close series of these two-dimensional images can provide a three-dimensional view of a targeted area.

- Safety. MRI does not depend on potentially harmful ionizing radiation, as do standard x-ray and CT scans. There are no known risks specific to the procedure, other than for people who might have metal objects in their bodies.

Given all the advantages, doctors would undoubtedly prescribe MRI as frequently as ultrasound scanning, but the MRI process is complex and costly. The process requires large, expensive, and complicated equipment; a highly trained operator; and a doctor specializing in radiology. Generally, MRI is prescribed only when serious symptoms and/or negative results from other tests indicate a need. Many times another test is appropriate for the type of diagnosis needed.

Doctors may prescribe an MRI scan of different areas of the body.

- Brain and head. MRI technology was developed because of the need for brain imaging. It is one of the few imaging tool that can see through bone (the skull) and deliver high quality pictures of the brain's delicate soft tissue structures. MRI may be needed for patients with symptoms of a **brain tumor, stroke,** or infection (like **meningitis**). MRI also may be needed when cognitive and/or psychological symptoms suggest brain disease (like Alzheimer's or **Huntington's diseases,** or **multiple sclerosis**), or when developmental retardation suggests a birth defect. MRI can also provide pictures of the sinuses and other areas of the head beneath the face.

- Spine. Spinal problems can create a host of seemingly unrelated symptoms. MRI is particularly useful for identifying and evaluating degenerated or herniated spinal discs. It can also be used to determine the condition of nerve tissue within the spinal cord.

- Joint. MRI scanning is most commonly used to diagnose and assess joint problems. MRI can provide clear images of the bone, cartilage, ligament, and tendon that comprise a joint. MRI can be used to diagnose joint injuries due to sports, advancing age, or arthritis. MRI can also be used to diagnose shoulder problems, like a torn rotator cuff. MRI can also detect the presence of an otherwise hidden tumor or infection in a joint, and can be used to diagnose the nature of developmental joint abnormalities in children.

- Skeleton. The properties of MRI that allow it to see though the skull also allow it to view the inside of bones. It can be used to detect bone **cancer,** inspect the marrow for leukemia and other diseases, assess bone loss (**osteoporosis**), and examine complex **fractures.**

- The rest of the body. While CT and ultrasound satisfy most chest, abdominal, and general body imaging needs, MRI may be needed in certain circumstances to provide better pictures or when repeated scanning is required. The progress of some therapies, like **liver cancer** therapy, needs to be monitored, and the effect of repeated x-ray exposure is a concern.

Precautions

MRI scanning should not be used when there is the potential for an interaction between the strong MRI magnet and metal objects that might be imbedded in a pa-
tient's body. The force of magnetic attraction on certain types of metal objects (including surgical steel) could move them within the body and cause serious injury. Metal may be imbedded in a person's body for several reasons.

- Medical. People with implanted cardiac **pacemakers,** metal aneurysm clips, or who have had broken bones repaired with metal pins, screws, rods, or plates must tell their radiologist prior to having an MRI scan. In some cases (like a metal rod in a reconstructed leg) the difficulty may be overcome.

- Injury. Patients must tell their doctors if they have bullet fragments or other metal pieces in their body from old **wounds.** The suspected presence of metal, whether from an old or recent wound, should be confirmed before scanning.

- Occupational. People with significant work exposure to metal particles (working with a metal grinder, for example) should discuss this with their doctor and radiologist. The patient may need prescan testing—usually a single, regular x ray of the eyes to see if any metal is present.

Chemical agents designed to improve the picture and/or allow for the imaging of blood or other fluid flow during MRA may be injected. In rare cases, patients may be allergic to or intolerant of these agents, and these patients should not receive them. If these chemical agents are to be used, patients should discuss any concerns they have with their doctor and radiologist.

The potential side effects of magnetic and electric fields on human health remain a source of debate. In particular, the possible effects on an unborn baby are not well known. Any woman who is, or may be, pregnant should carefully discuss this issue with her doctor and radiologist before undergoing a scan.

As with all medical imaging techniques, **obesity** greatly interferes with the quality of MRI.

Description

In essence, MRI produces a map of hydrogen distribution in the body. Hydrogen is the simplest element known, the most abundant in biological tissue, and one that can be magnetized. It will align itself within a strong magnetic field, like the needle of a compass. The earth's magnetic field is not strong enough to keep a person's hydrogen atoms pointing in the same direction, but the superconducting magnet of an MRI machine can. This comprises the "magnetic" part of MRI.

Once a patient's hydrogen atoms have been aligned in the magnet, pulses of very specific radio wave frequencies are used to knock them back out of alignment. The hydrogen atoms alternately absorb and emit radio wave energy, vibrating back and forth between their resting (magnetized) state and their agitated (radio pulse) state. This comprises the "resonance" part of MRI.

The MRI equipment records the duration, strength, and source location of the signals emitted by the atoms as they relax and translates the data into an image on a television monitor. The state of hydrogen in diseased tissue differs from healthy tissue of the same type, making MRI particularly good at identifying tumors and other lesions. In some cases, chemical agents such as gadolinium can be injected to improve the contrast between healthy and diseased tissue.

A single MRI exposure produces a two-dimensional image of a slice through the entire target area. A series of these image slices closely spaced (usually less than half an inch) makes a virtual three-dimensional view of the area.

Magnetic resonance spectroscopy (MRS) is different from MRI because MRS uses a continuous band of radio wave frequencies to excite hydrogen atoms in a variety of chemical compounds other than water. These compounds absorb and emit radio energy at characteristic frequencies, or spectra, which can be used to identify them. Generally, a color image is created by assigning a color to each distinctive spectral emission. This comprises the "spectroscopy" part of MRS. MRS is still experimental and is available in only a few research centers.

Doctors primarily use MRS to study the brain and disorders, like epilepsy, **Alzheimer's disease,** brain tumors, and the effects of drugs on brain growth and metabolism. The technique is also useful in evaluating metabolic disorders of the muscles and nervous system.

Magnetic resonance angiography (MRA) is another variation on standard MRI. MRA, like other types of angiography, looks specifically at fluid flow within the blood (vascular) system, but does so without the injection of dyes or radioactive tracers. Standard MRI cannot make a good picture of flowing blood, but MRA uses specific radio pulse sequences to capture usable signals. The technique is generally used in combination with MRI to obtain images that show both vascular structure and flow within the brain and head in cases of stroke, or when a blood clot or aneurysm is suspected.

Regardless of the exact type of MRI planned, or area of the body targeted, the procedure involved is basically the same and occurs in a special MRI suite. The patient lies back on a narrow table and is made as comfortable as possible. Transmitters are positioned on the body and the cushioned table that the patient is lying on moves into a long tube that houses the magnet. The tube is as long as an average adult lying down, and the tube is narrow and open at both ends. Once the area to be examined has been properly positioned, a radio pulse is applied. Then a two-dimensional image corresponding to one slice through the area is made. The table then moves a fraction of an inch and the next image is made. Each image exposure takes several seconds and the entire exam will last anywhere from 30-90 minutes. During this time, the patient is not allowed to move. If the patient moves during the scan, the picture will not be clear.

Depending on the area to be imaged, the radio-wave transmitters will be positioned in different locations.

• For the head and neck, a helmet-like hat is worn.

• For the spine, chest, and abdomen, the patient will be lying on the transmitters.

• For the knee, shoulder, or other joint, the transmitters will be applied directly to the joint.

Additional probes will monitor vital signs (like pulse, respiration, etc.).

The process is very noisy and confining. The patient hears a thumping sound for the duration of the procedure. Since the procedure is noisy, music supplied via earphones is often provided. Some patients get anxious or panic because they are in the small, enclosed tube. This is why vital signs are monitored and the patient and medical team can communicate between each other. If the chest or abdomen are to be imaged, the patient will be asked to hold his/her breath as each exposure is made. Other instructions may be given to the patient, as needed. In many cases, the entire examination will be performed by an MRI operator who is not a doctor. However, the supervising radiologist should be available to consult as necessary during the exam, and will view and interpret the results sometime later.

Preparation

In some cases (such as for MRI brain scanning or an MRA), a chemical designed to increase image contrast may be given by the radiologist immediately before the exam. If a patient suffers from **anxiety** or claustrophobia, drugs may be given to help the patient relax.

The patient must remove all metal objects (watches, jewelry, eye glasses, hair clips, etc). Any magnetized objects (like credit and bank machine cards, audio tapes, etc.) should be kept far away from the MRI equipment because they can be erased. The patient cannnot bring their wallet or keys into the MRI machine. The patient may be asked to wear clothing without metal snaps, buckles, or zippers, unless a medical gown is worn during the procedure. The patient may be asked to remove any hair spray, hair gel, or cosmetics that may interfere with the scan.

Aftercare

No aftercare is necessary, unless the patient received medication or had a reaction to a contrast agent. Normally, patients can immediately return to their daily activities. If the exam reveals a serious condition that requires more testing and/or treatment, appropriate information and counseling will be needed.

Risks

MRI poses no known health risks to the patient and produces no physical side effects. Again, the potential effects of MRI on an unborn baby are not well known. Any woman who is, or may be, pregnant, should carefully discuss this issue with her doctor and radiologist before undergoing a scan.

Normal results

A normal MRI, MRA, or MRS result is one that shows the patient's physical condition to fall within normal ranges for the target area scanned.

Abnormal results

Generally, MRI is prescribed only when serious symptoms and/or negative results from other tests indicate a need. There often exists strong evidence of a condition that the scan is designed to detect and assess. Thus, the results will often be abnormal, confirming the earlier diagnosis. At that point, further testing and appropriate medical treatment is needed. For example, if the MRI indicates the presence of a brain tumor, an MRS may be prescribed to determine the type of tumor so that aggressive treatment can begin immediately without the need for a surgical biopsy.

Resources

BOOKS

Edelman, Robert R., et al., eds. *Clinical Magnetic Resonance Imaging.* Philadelphia, PA: Saunders, 1990.

Haaga, John R., et al., eds. *Computed Tomography and Magnetic Resonance Imaging of the Whole Body.* St. Louis, MO: Mosby, 1994.

Kevles, Bettyann Holtzmann. *Naked to the Bone: Medical Imaging in the Twentieth Century.* New Brunswick, NJ: Rutgers University Press, 1997.

Shtasel, Philip. *Medical Tests and Diagnostic Procedures: A Patient's Guide to Just What the Doctor Ordered.* New York: Harper & Row, 1990.

Zaret, Barry L., et al., eds. *The Patient's Guide to Medical Tests.* Boston: Houghton Mifflin Company, 1997.

PERIODICALS

Doria, John J. "A Primer on Imaging." *Alcohol Health & Research World* 19 (December 1995): 261-265.

Fein, George, Dieter J. Meyerhoff, and Michael W. Weiner. "Magnetic Resonance Spectroscopy of the Brain in Alcohol Abuse." *Alcohol Health & Research World* 19 (December 1995): 306-314.

Kevles, Bettyann. "Body Imaging." *Newsweek* (Winter 97/ 98 Extra Millennium Issue): 74-76.

ORGANIZATIONS

American College of Radiology. 1891 Preston White Dr., Reston, VA 22091. (703) 648-8900. http://www.acr.org.

American Society of Radiologic Technologists. 15000 Central Ave. SE, Albuquerque, NM 87123-3917. (505) 298-4500. http://www.asrt.org.

Center for Devices and Radiological Health. United States Food and Drug Administration. 1901 Chapman Ave., Rockville, MD 20857. (301) 443-4109. http://www.fda.gov/cdrh.

Kurt Richard Sternlof

Magnetic resonance spectroscopy *see* **Magnetic resonance imaging**

Major depression *see* **Depressive disorders**

Major tranquilizers *see* **Antipsychotic drugs**

Malabsorption syndrome

Definition

Malabsorption syndrome is an alteration in the ability of the intestine to absorb nutrients adequately into the bloodstream.

Causes & symptoms

Protein, fats, and carbohydrates (macronutrients) normally are absorbed in the small intestine; the small bowel also absorbs about 80% of the eight to ten liters of fluid ingested daily. There are many different conditions that affect fluid and nutrient absorption by the intestine. A fault in the digestive process may result from failure of the body to produce the enzymes needed to digest certain foods. Congenital structural defects or diseases of the pancreas, gall bladder, or liver may alter the digestive process. Inflammation, infection, injury, or surgical removal of portions of the intestine may also result in absorption problems; reduced length or surface area of intestine available for fluid and nutrient absorption can result in malabsorption. **Radiation therapy** may injure the mucosal lining of the intestine, resulting in **diarrhea** that may not become evident until several years later. The use of some **antibiotics** can also affect the bacteria that normally live in the intestine and affect intestinal function.

KEY TERMS

Anemia—A decrease in the number of red blood cells in the bloodstream, characterized by pallor, loss of energy, and generalized weakness.

Atrophy—A wasting away of a tissue or organ, often because of insufficient nutrition.

Biopsy—A tissue sample removed from the body for examination under the microscope.

Cystic fibrosis—A hereditary genetic disorder that occurs most often in Caucasians. Thick, sticky secretions from mucus-producing glands cause blockages in the pancreatic ducts and the airways.

Edema—From the Greek word meaning swelling, an excessive accumulation of fluid in the tissue spaces. Excessive generalized edema may also be referred to as ascites.

Gluten enteropathy—A hereditary malabsorption disorder caused by sensitivity to gluten, a protein found in wheat, rye, barley, and oats. Also called non-tropical sprue or celiac disease.

Intestines—The intestines, also known as the bowels, are divided into the large and small intestines. They extend from the stomach to the anus.

Short bowel syndrome—A condition in which the bowel is not as long as normal, either because of surgery or because of a congenital defect. Because the bowel has less surface area to absorb nutrients, it can result in malabsorption syndrome.

Steatorrhea—An excessive amount of fat in the stool.

Risk factors for malabsorption syndrome include:

• Family history of malabsorption or **cystic fibrosis**

• Use of certain drugs, such as mineral oil or other **laxatives**

• Travel to foreign countries

• Intestinal surgery

• Excess alcohol consumption.

The most common symptoms of malabsorption include:

• Anemia, with weakness and fatigue due to inadequate absorption of vitamin B_{12}, iron, and folic acid

• Diarrhea, steatorrhea (excessive amount of fat in the stool), and abdominal distention with cramps, bloating, and gas due to impaired water and carbohydrate absorp-

tion, and irritation from unabsorbed fatty acids. The individual may also report explosive diarrhea with greasy, foul-smelling stools.

• **Edema** (fluid retention in the body's tissues) due to decreased protein absorption

• **Malnutrition** and weight loss due to decreased fat, carbohydrate, and protein absorption. Weight may be 80-90% of usual weight despite increased oral intake of nutrients.

• Muscle cramping due to decreased vitamin D, calcium, and potassium levels

• Muscle wasting and atrophy due to decreased protein absorption and metabolism

• Perianal skin burning, **itching,** or soreness due to frequent loose stools.

Irregular heart rhythms may also result from inadequate levels of potassium and other electrolytes. Blood clotting disorders may occur due to a **vitamin K deficiency.** Children with malabsorption syndrome often exhibit a failure to grow and thrive.

Several disorders can lead to malabsorption syndrome, including cystic fibrosis, chronic **pancreatitis,** lactose intolerance, and gluten enteropathy (non-tropical sprue.)

Tropical sprue is a malabsorptive disorder that is uncommon in the United States, but seen more often in people from the Caribbean, India, or southeast Asia. Although its cause is unknown, it is thought to be related to environmental factors, including infection, intestinal parasites, or possibly the consumption of certain food toxins. Symptoms often include a sore tongue, anemia, weight loss, along with diarrhea and passage of fatty stools.

Whipple's disease is a relatively rare malabsorptive disorder, affecting mostly middle-aged men. The cause is thought to be related to bacterial infection, resulting in nutritional deficiencies, chronic low-grade **fever,** diarrhea, joint **pain,** weight loss, and darkening of the skin's pigmentation. Other organs of the body may be affected, including the brain, heart, lungs, and eyes.

Short bowel syndromes—which may be present at birth (congenital) or the result of surgery—reduce the surface area of the bowel available to absorb nutrients and can also result in malabsorption syndrome.

Diagnosis

The diagnosis of malabsorption syndrome and identification of the underlying cause can require extensive diagnostic testing. The first phase involves a thorough medical history and **physical examination** by a physician, who will then determine the appropriate laboratory studies and x rays to assist in diagnosis. A 72-hour stool collection may be ordered for fecal fat measurement; increased fecal fat in the stool collected indicates malabsorption. A biopsy of the small intestine may be done to assist in differentiating between malabsorption syndrome and small bowel disease. Ultrasound, **computed tomography scan** (CT scan), **magnetic resonance imaging** (MRI), **barium enema,** or other x rays to identify abnormalities of the gastrointestinal tract and pancreas may also be ordered.

Laboratory studies of the blood may include:

- Serum cholesterol. May be low due to decreased fat absorption and digestion.

- Serum sodium, potassium, and chloride. May be low due to electrolyte losses with diarrhea.

- Serum calcium. May be low due to vitamin D and amino acid malabsorption.

- Serum protein and albumin. May be low due to protein losses.

- Serum vitamin A and carotene. May be low due to bile salt deficiency and impaired fat absorption.

- D-xylose test. Decreased excretion may indicate malabsorption.

- Schilling test. May indicate malabsorption of vitamin B_{12}.

Treatment

Fluid and nutrient monitoring and replacement is essential for any individual with malabsorption syndrome. Hospitalization may be required when severe fluid and electrolyte imbalances occur. Consultation with a dietitian to assist with nutritional support and meal planning is helpful. If the patient is able to eat, the diet and supplements should provide bulk and be rich in carbohydrates, proteins, fats, **minerals,** and **vitamins.** The patient should be encouraged to eat several small, frequent meals throughout the day, avoiding fluids and foods that promote diarrhea. Intake and output should be monitored, along with the number, color, and consistency of stools.

The individual with malabsorption syndrome must be monitored for **dehydration,** including dry tongue, mouth and skin; increased thirst; low, concentrated urine output; or feeling weak or dizzy when standing. Pulse and blood pressure should be monitored, observing for increased or irregular pulse rate, or **hypotension** (low blood pressure). The individual should also be alert for signs of nutrient, vitamin, and mineral depletion, including nausea or vomiting; fissures at corner of mouth; fatigue or weakness; dry, pluckable hair; easy bruising; tingling in fingers or toes; and numbness or burning sensation in legs or feet. Fluid volume excess, as a result of diminished protein stores, may require fluid intake restrictions. The physician should also be notified of any **shortness of breath.**

Other specific medical management for malabsorption syndrome is dependent upon the cause. Treatment for tropical sprue consists of folic acid supplements and long-term antibiotics. Depending on the severity of the disorder, this treatment may be continued for six months or longer. Whipple's disease also may require long-term use of antibiotics, such as tetracycline. Management of some individuals with malabsorption syndrome may require injections of vitamin B_{12} and oral iron supplements. The doctor may also prescribe enzymes to replace missing intestinal enzymes, or antispasmodics to reduce abdominal cramping and associated diarrhea. People with cystic fibrosis and chronic pancreatitis require pancreatic supplements. Those with lactose intolerance or gluten enteropathy (non-tropical sprue) will have to modify their **diets** to avoid foods that they cannot properly digest.

Prognosis

The expected course for the individual with malabsorption syndrome varies depending on the cause. The onset of symptoms may be slow and difficult to diagnose. Treatment may be long, complicated, and changed often for optimal effectiveness. Patience and a positive attitude are important in controlling or curing the disorder. Careful monitoring is necessary to prevent additional illnesses cause by nutritional deficiencies.

Resources

BOOKS

Brunner, Lillian, and Doris Suddarth. *The Lippincott Manual of Nursing Practice.* Philadelphia: J.B. Lippincott Company, 1991.

Doughty, Dorothy. *Gastrointestinal Disorders.* St. Louis: Mosby-Yearbook, Inc., 1993.

Griffith, H. Winter. *Complete Guide to Pediatric Symptoms, Illness and Medications.* New York: Putnam Berkley Group, Inc., 1989.

Monahan, Frances, and Marianne Neighbors. *Medical-Surgical Nursing: Foundations for Clinical Practice.* Philadelphia: W. B. Saunders Company, 1998.

OTHER

Ask the Mayo Dietitian. http://www.mayohealth.com. (24April1998).

Malabsorption. http://www.thriveonline.com. (24April1998).

Kathleen Dredge Wright

Malaria

Definition

Malaria is a serious, infectious disease spread by certain mosquitoes. It is most common in tropical climates. It is characterized by recurrent symptoms of chills, **fever,** and an enlarged spleen. The disease can be treated with medication, but it often recurs. Malaria is endemic (occurs frequently in a particular locality) in many third world countries. Isolated, small outbreaks sometimes occur within the boundaries of the United States.

Description

Malaria is not a serious problem in the United States. Within the last 10 years, only about 1200 cases have been reported each year in this country, mostly by people who were infected elsewhere. Locally transmitted malaria has occurred in California, Florida, Texas, Michigan, New Jersey, and New York City. While malaria can be transmitted in blood, the American blood supply is not screened for malaria. Widespread malarial epidemics are far less likely to occur in the United States, but small, localized epidemics could return to the western world.

The picture is far more bleak outside the territorial boundaries of the United States. A recent government panel warned that disaster looms over Africa from the disease. Malaria infects between 300 and 500 million people every year in Africa, India, southeast Asia, the Middle East, Oceania, and Central and South America. About 2 million of the infected die each year. Most of the cases and almost all of the **deaths** occur in sub-Saharan Africa. At the present time, malaria kills about twice as many people as does **AIDS.** As many as half a billion people worldwide are left with chronic anemia due to malaria infection. In some parts of Africa, people battle up to 40 or more separate episodes of malaria in their lifetimes. The spread of malaria is becoming even more serious as the parasites that cause malaria develop resistance to the drugs used to treat the condition.

Causes & symptoms

Human malaria is caused by four different species of a parasite called plasmodium: *Plasmodium falciparum* (the most deadly), *P.vivax, P. malariae,* and *P. ovale.* The last two are fairly uncommon. Many animals can get malaria but human malaria does not spread to animals. In turn, animal malaria does not spread to humans.

A person gets malaria when bitten by a female mosquito who is looking for a blood meal and is infected with the malaria parasite. The parasites enter the blood stream and travel to the liver, where they multiply. When

KEY TERMS

Arteminisinins—An antimalarial family of products derived from an ancient Chinese herbal remedy. Two of the most popular varieties are artemether and artesunate, used mainly in southeast Asia in combination with mefloquine.

Chloroquine—This antimalarial drug was first used in the 1940s, until the first evidence of quinine resistance appeared in the 1960s. It is now ineffective against falciparum malaria almost everywhere. However, because it is inexpensive, it is still the antimalarial drug most widely used in Africa. Native individuals with partial immunity may have better results with chloroquine than a traveler with no previous exposure.

Mefloquine—An antimalarial drug that was developed by the United States Army in the early 1980s. Today, malaria resistance to this drug has become a problem in some parts of Asia (especially Thailand and Cambodia).

Quinine—One of the first treatments for malaria, quinine is a natural product made from the bark of the Cinchona tree. It was popular until being superseded by the development of chloroquine in the 1940s. In the wake of widespread chloroquine resistance, however, it has become popular again. It or its close relative quinidine can be given intravenously to treat severe falciparum malaria.

Sulfadoxone/pyrimethamine (Fansidar)—This antimalarial drug developed in the 1960s is the first drug tried in some parts of the world where chloroquine resistance is widespread. It has been associated with severe allergic reactions due to its sulfa component.

they re-emerge into the blood, symptoms appear. By the time a patient shows symptoms, the parasites have reproduced very rapidly, clogging blood vessels and rupturing blood cells.

Malaria cannot be casually transmitted directly from one person to another. Instead, a mosquito bites an infected person and then passes the infection on to the next human it bites. It is also possible to spread malaria via contaminated needles or in blood **transfusions.** This is why all blood donors are carefully screened with questionnaires for possible exposure to malaria.

The amount of time between the mosquito bite and the appearance of symptoms varies, depending on the strain of parasite involved. The incubation period is usually between 8 and 12 days for falciparum malaria, but it

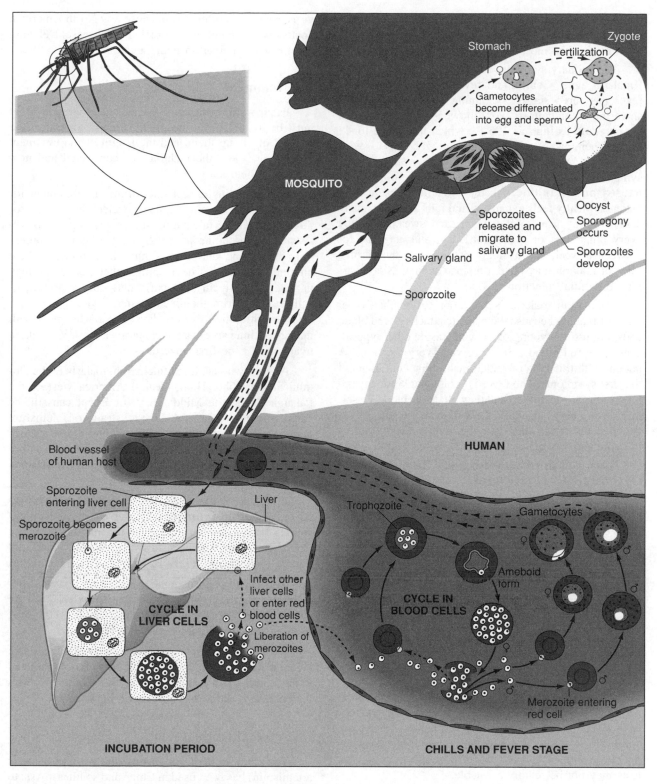

Stomach

Zygote

Fertilization

Gametocytes become differentiated into egg and sperm

Sporozoites released and migrate to salivary gland

Oocyst

Sporogony occurs

Sporozoites develop

MOSQUITO

Salivary gland

Sporozoite

Blood vessel of human host

HUMAN

Sporozoite entering liver cell

Liver

Trophozoite

Gametocytes

Sporozoite becomes merozoite

Infect other liver cells or enter red blood cells

Liberation of merozoites

Ameboid form

CYCLE IN LIVER CELLS

CYCLE IN BLOOD CELLS

Merozoite entering red cell

INCUBATION PERIOD

CHILLS AND FEVER STAGE

The life cycle of *Plasmodium vivax*, the parasite that causes malaria. *(Illustration by Hans & Cassady, Inc.)*

can be as long as a month for the other types. Symptoms from some strains of *P.vivax* may not appear until 8–10 months after the mosquito bite occurred.

The primary symptom of all types of malaria is the "malaria ague" (chills and fever). In most cases, the fever has three stages, beginning with uncontrollable shivering for an hour or two, followed by a rapid spike in temperature (as high as 106°F), which lasts three to six hours. Then, just as suddenly, the patient begins to sweat profusely, which will quickly bring down the fever. Other symptoms may include fatigue, severe **headache,** or **nausea and vomiting.** As the sweating subsides, the patient typically feels exhausted and falls asleep. In many cases, this cycle of chills, fever, and sweating occurs every other day, or every third day, and may last for between a week and a month. Those with the chronic form of malaria may have a relapse as long as 50 years after the initial infection.

Falciparum malaria is far more severe than other types of malaria because the parasite attacks all red blood cells, not just the young or old cells, as do other types. It causes the red blood cells to become very "sticky." A patient with this type of malaria can die within hours of the first symptoms. The fever is prolonged. So many red blood cells are destroyed that they block the blood vessels in vital organs (especially the kidneys), and the spleen becomes enlarged. There may be brain damage, leading to **coma** and convulsions. The kidneys and liver may fail.

Malaria in **pregnancy** can lead to premature delivery, **miscarriage,** or **stillbirth.**

Certain kinds of mosquitoes (called anopheles) can pick up the parasite by biting an infected human. (The more common kinds of mosquitoes in the United States do not transmit the infection.) This is true for as long as that human has parasites in his/her blood. Since strains of malaria do not protect against each other, it is possible to be reinfected with the parasites again and again. It is also possible to develop a chronic infection without developing an effective immune response.

Diagnosis

Malaria is diagnosed by examining blood under a microscope. The parasite can be seen in the blood smears on a slide. These blood smears may need to be repeated over a 72-hour period in order to make a diagnosis. Antibody tests are not usually helpful because many people developed antibodies from past infections, and the tests may not be readily available.

Anyone who becomes ill with chills and fever after being in an area where malaria exists must see a doctor and mention their recent travel to endemic areas. A person with the above symptoms who has been in a high-risk area should insist on a blood test for malaria. The doctor may believe the symptoms are just the common flu virus. Malaria is often misdiagnosed by North American doctors who are not used to seeing the disease. Delaying treatment of falciparum malaria can be fatal.

Treatment

Falciparum malaria is a medical emergency that must be treated in the hospital. The type of drugs, the method of giving them, and the length of the treatment depend on where the malaria was contracted and how sick the patient is.

For all strains except falciparum, the treatment for malaria is usually chloroquine (Aralen) by mouth for three days. Those falciparum strains suspected to be resistant to chloroquine are usually treated with a combination of quinine and tetracycline. In countries where quinine resistance is developing, other treatments may include clindamycin (Cleocin), mefloquin (Lariam), or sulfadoxone/pyrimethamine (Fansidar). Most patients receive an antibiotic for seven days. Those who are very ill may need intensive care and intravenous (IV) malaria treatment for the first three days.

Anyone who acquired falciparum malaria in the Dominican Republic, Haiti, Central America west of the Panama Canal, the Middle East, or Egypt can still be cured with chloroquine. Almost all strains of falciparum malaria in Africa, South Africa, India, and southeast Asia are now resistant to chloroquine. In Thailand and Cambodia, there are strains of falciparum malaria that have some resistance to almost all known drugs.

A patient with falciparum malaria needs to be hospitalized and given **antimalarial drugs** in different combinations and doses depending on the resistance of the strain. The patient may need IV fluids, red blood cell transfusions, **kidney dialysis,** and assistance breathing.

A drug called primaquine may prevent relapses after recovery from *P. vivax* or *P. ovale*. These relapses are caused by a form of the parasite that remains in the liver and can reactivate months or years later.

Another new drug, halofantrine, is available abroad. While it is licensed in the United States, it is not marketed in this country and it is not recommended by the Centers for Disease Control and Prevention in Atlanta.

Alternative treatment

The Chinese herb qiinghaosu (the western name is artemisinin) has been used in China and southeast Asia to fight severe malaria, and became available in Europe in 1994. Because this treatment often fails, it is usually combined with another antimalarial drug (mefloquine) to boost its effectiveness. It is not available in the United States and other parts of the developed world due to fears of its toxicity, in addition to licensing and other issues.

A western herb called wormwood (*Artemesia annua*) that is taken as a daily dose can be effective against malaria. Protecting the liver with herbs like goldenseal (*Hydrastis canadensis*), Chinese goldenthread (*Coptis chinensis*), and milk thistle (*Silybum marianum*) can be used as preventive treatment. Preventing mosquitoes from biting you while in the tropics is another possible way to avoid malaria.

Prognosis

If treated in the early stages, malaria can be cured. Those who live in areas where malaria is epidemic, however, can contract the disease repeatedly, never fully recovering between bouts of acute infection.

Prevention

Several researchers are currently working on a malarial vaccine, but the complex life cycle of the malaria parasite makes it difficult. A parasite has much more genetic material than a virus or bacterium. For this reason, a successful vaccine has not yet been developed.

Malaria is an especially difficult disease to vaccinate against because the parasite goes through several separate stages. One recent, promising vaccine appears to have protected up to 60% of people exposed to maleria. This was evident during field trials for the drug that were conducted in South America and Africa. It is not yet commercially available.

The World Health Association (WHO) has been trying to eliminate malaria for the past 30 years by controlling mosquitoes. Their efforts were successful as long as the pesticide DDT killed mosquitoes and antimalarial drugs cured those who were infected. Today, however, the problem has returned a hundredfold, especially in Africa. Because both the mosquito and parasite are now extremely resistant to the insecticides designed to kill them, governments are now trying to teach people to take antimalarial drugs as a preventive medicine and avoid getting bitten by mosquitoes.

Travelers to high-risk areas should use insect repellant containing DEET for exposed skin. Because DEET is toxic in large amounts, children should not use a concentration higher than 35%. DEET should not be inhaled. It should not be rubbed onto the eye area, on any broken or irritated skin, or on children's hands. It should be thoroughly washed off after coming indoors.

Those who use the following preventive measures get fewer infections than those who do not:

- Between dusk and dawn, remain indoors in well-screened areas.
- Sleep inside pyrethrin or permethrin repellent-soaked mosquito nets.

- Wear clothes over the entire body.

Anyone visiting endemic areas should take antimalarial drugs starting a day or two before they leave the United States. The drugs used are usually chloroquine or mefloquine. This treatment is continued through at least four weeks after leaving the endemic area. However, even those who take antimalarial drugs and are careful to avoid mosquito bites can still contract malaria.

International travelers are at risk for becoming infected. Most Americans who have acquired falciparum malaria were visiting sub-Saharan Africa; travelers in Asia and South America are less at risk. Travelers who stay in air conditioned hotels on tourist itineraries in urban or resort areas are at lower risk than backpackers, missionaries, and Peace Corps volunteers. Some people in western cities where malaria does not usually exist may acquire the infection from a mosquito carried onto a jet. This is called airport or runway malaria.

Resources

BOOKS

Desowitz, Robert S. *The Malaria Capers: More Tales of Parasites and People, Research and Reality.* New York: W.W. Norton, 1993.

Stoffman, Phyllis. *The Family Guide to Preventing and Treating 100 Infectious Illnesses.* New York: John Wiley & Sons, 1995.

PERIODICALS

Kristof, Nicholas D. "Malaria Makes a Comeback, Deadlier Than Ever." *The New York Times* (Jan. 8, 1997).

Mack, Alison. "Collaborative Efforts Under Way to Combat Malaria." *The Scientist* 10 (May 12, 1997): 1, 6.

Shell, Ellen Ruppel. "Resurgence of a Deadly Disease." *The Atlantic Monthly* 280 (August 1997).

ORGANIZATIONS

Centers for Disease Control Malaria Hotline. (770) 332-4555.

Centers for Disease Control Travelers Hotline. (770) 332-4559.

OTHER

Malaria Foundation. http://www.malaria.org.

Carol A. Turkington

Malayan filariasis *see* **Elephantiasis**

Male breast enlargement *see* **Gynecomastia**

Male infertility *see* **Infertility**

Male pattern baldness *see* **Alopecia**

Malignant giant cell tumor *see* **Sarcomas**

Malignant lymphomas

Definition

Lymphomas are a group of **cancers** in which cells of the lymphatic system become abnormal and start to grow uncontrollably. Because there is lymph tissue in many parts of the body, lymphomas can start in almost any organ of the body.

Description

The lymph system is made up of ducts or tubules that carry lymph to all parts of the body. Lymph is a milky fluid that contains the lymphocytes or white blood cells. These are the infection- fighting cells of the blood. Small pea-shaped organs are found along the network of lymph vessels. These are called the lymph nodes, and their main function is to make and store the lymphocytes. Clusters of lymph nodes are found in the pelvis region, underarm, neck, chest, and abdomen. The spleen (an organ in the upper abdomen), the tonsils, and the thymus (a small organ found beneath the breastbone) are part of the lymphatic system.

The lymphocyte is the main cell of the lymphoid tissue. There are two main types of lymphocytes: the T lymphocyte and the B lymphocyte. Lymphomas develop from these two cell types. B cell lymphomas are more common among adults, while among children, the incidence of T and B cell lymphomas are almost equal.

The T and the B cell perform different jobs within the immune system. When an infectious bacterium enters the body, the B cell makes proteins called "antibodies." These antibodies attach themselves to the bacteria, and flag them for destruction by other immune cells. The T cells help protect the body against viruses. When a virus enters the cell, it generally produces certain proteins that are projected on the surface of the infected cell. T cells recognize these proteins and produce certain substances (cytokines) that destroy the infected cells. Some of the cytokines made by the T cells attract other cell types, which are capable of digesting the virus-infected cell. The T cells can also destroy some types of cancerous cells.

Lymphomas can be divided into two main types: Hodgkin's lymphoma or **Hodgkin's disease,** and non-Hodgkin's lymphomas. There are at least 10 types of non-Hodgkin's lymphomas. They are grouped (staged) by how aggressively they grow; slow growing (low

grade), intermediate growing, and rapidly growing (high grade); and how far they spread.

A majority of non-Hodgkin's lymphomas begin in the lymph nodes. About 20% start in other organs, such as the lungs, liver or the gastrointestinal tract. Malignant lymphocytes multiply uncontrollably and do not perform their normal functions. Hence, the body's ability to fight infections is affected. In addition, these malignant cells may crowd the bone marrow, and, depending on the stage, prevent the production of normal red blood cells, white blood cells, and platelets. A low red blood cell count causes anemia, while a reduction in the number of platelets makes the person susceptible to excessive bleeding. Cancerous cells can also invade other organs through the circulatory system of the lymph, causing those organs to malfunction.

Causes & symptoms

The exact cause of non-Hodgkin's lymphomas is not known. However, the incidence has increased significantly in the recent years. Part of the increase is due to the

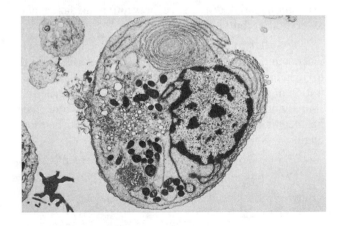

A malignant lymph cell. (*Custom Medical Stock Photo. Reproduced by permission.*)

AIDS epidemic. Individuals infected with the AIDS virus have a higher likelihood of developing non-Hodgkin's lymphomas. In general, males are at a higher risk for having non-Hodgkin's lymphomas than are females. The risk increases with age. Though it can strike people as young as 40, people between the ages of 60 and 69 are at the highest risk.

People exposed to certain pesticides and ionizing radiation have a higher than average chance of developing this disease. For example, an increased incidence of lymphomas has been seen in survivors of the atomic bomb explosion in Hiroshima, and in people who have undergone aggressive **radiation therapy.** People who suffer from immune-deficient disorders, as well as those who have been treated with immune suppressive drugs for heart or kidney transplants, and for conditions such as **rheumatoid arthritis** and autoimmune diseases, are at an increased risk for this disease.

There have been some studies that have shown a loose association between retroviruses, such as HTLV-I, and some rare forms of lymphoma. The Epstein-Barr virus has been linked to Burkitt's lymphoma in African countries. However, a direct cause-and-effect relationship has not been established.

The symptoms of lymphomas are often vague and non-specific. Patients may experience loss of appetite, weight loss, nausea, vomiting, abdominal discomfort, and **indigestion.** The patient may complain of a feeling of fullness, which is a result of enlarged lymph nodes in the abdomen. Pressure or **pain** in the lower back is another symptom. In the advanced stages, the patient may have bone pain, **headaches,** constant coughing, and abnormal pressure and congestion in the face, neck, and upper chest. Some may have **fevers** and night sweats. In most cases, patients go to the doctor because of the presence of swollen glands in the neck, armpits, or groin area. Since all the symptoms are common to many other illnesses, it is essential to seek medical attention if any of the conditions persist for two weeks or more. Only a qualified physician can correctly diagnose if the symptoms are due to lymphoma or some other ailment.

Diagnosis

Like all cancers, lymphomas are best treated when found early. However, it is often difficult to diagnose lymphomas. There are no screening tests available, and, since the symptoms are non-specific, lymphomas are rarely recognized in their early stages. Detection often occurs by chance during a routine **physical examination.**

When the doctor suspects lymphoma, a complete medical history is taken, and a thorough physical examination is performed. Enlargement of the lymph nodes, liver, or spleen may suggest lymphomas. Blood tests will determine the cell counts and obtain information on how well the organs, such as the kidney and liver, are functioning.

A biopsy of the enlarged lymph node is the most definitive diagnostic tool for staging purposes. The doctor may perform a bone marrow biopsy. During the biopsy, a cylindrical piece of bone and marrow fluid is removed. They are generally taken out of the hipbone. These samples are sent to the laboratory for examination. In addition to diagnosis, the biopsy may also be repeated during the treatment phase of the disease to see if the lymphoma is responding to therapy.

Once the exact form of lymphoma is known, it is then staged to determine how aggressive it is, and how far it has spread. Staging is necessary to plan appropriate treatment.

Conventional imaging tests, such as x rays, **computed tomography scans** (CT scans), **magnetic resonance imaging,** and abdominal sonograms, are used to determine the extent of spread of the disease.

Lymphangiograms are x rays of the lymphatic system. In this procedure, a special dye is injected into the lymphatic channels through a small cut (incision) made in each foot. The dye is injected slowly over a period of three to four hours. This dye clearly outlines the lymphatic system and allows it to stand out. Multiple x rays are then taken and any abnormality, if present, is revealed.

Rarely, a lumbar puncture or a spinal tap is performed to check if malignant cells are present in the fluid surrounding the brain. In this test, the physician inserts a needle into the epidural space at the base of the spine and collects a small amount of spinal fluid for microscopic examination.

Treatment

Treatment options for lymphomas depend on the type of lymphoma and its present stage. In most cases, treatment consists of **chemotherapy,** radiotherapy, or a combination of the two methods.

Chemotherapy is the use of anti-cancer drugs to kill cancer cells. In non-Hodgkin's lymphomas, combination therapy, which involves the use of multiple drugs, has been found more effective than single drug use. The treatment may last about six months, but in some cases may last as long as a year. The drugs may either be administered intravenously (through a vein) in the arm or given orally in the form of pills. If cancer cells have invaded the central nervous system, then chemotherapeutic drugs may be instilled, through a needle in the brain or back, into the fluid that surrounds the brain. This procedure is known as intrathecal chemotherapy.

Radiation therapy, where high-energy ionizing rays are directed at specific portions of the body, such as the upper chest, abdomen, pelvis, or neck, is often used for treatment of lymphomas. External radiation therapy, where the rays are directed from a source outside the body, is the most common mode of radiation treatment.

Bone marrow transplantation is used in cases where the lymphomas do not respond to conventional therapy, or in cases where the patient has had a relapse or suffers from recurrent lymphomas.

There are two ways of doing bone marrow transplantation. In a procedure called "allogeneic bone marrow transplant," a donor is found whose marrow matches that of the patient. The donor can be a twin (best match), a sibling, or a person who is not related at all. High-dose chemotherapy or radiation therapy is given to eradicate the lymphoma. The donor marrow is then given to replace the marrow destroyed by the therapy.

In "autologous bone marrow transplantation," some of the patient's own bone marrow is harvested, chemically purged, and frozen. High-dose chemotherapy and radiation therapy are given. The marrow that was harvested, purged, and frozen is then thawed and put back into the patient's body to replace the destroyed marrow.

A new treatment option for patients with lymphoma is known as "peripheral stem cell transplantation." In this treatment approach, cells that normally circulate in the blood are collected when the patient has normal **blood counts** taken, and these cells are saved via a process called "pheresis." Researchers are exploring whether these cells can be used to restore the normal function and development of blood cells, rather than using a bone marrow transplant.

Prognosis

Like all cancers, the prognosis for lymphoma depends on the stage of the cancer, and the patient's age and general health. When all the different types and stages of lymphoma are considered together, only 50% of patients survive 5 years or more after initial diagnosis. This is because some types of lymphoma are more aggressive than others.

The survival rate among children is definitely better than among older people. About 90% of the children diagnosed with early stage disease survive 5 years or more, while only 60-70% of adults diagnosed with low grade lymphomas survive for 5 years or more. The survival rate for children with the more advanced stages is about 75-85%, while among adults it is 40-60%.

Prevention

Although many cancers may be prevented by making diet and life style changes which reduce risk factors, there is currently no known way to prevent lymphomas. Protecting oneself from developing AIDS, which may be a risk factor for lymphomas, is the only preventive measure that can be practiced.

At present, there are no special tests that are available for early detection of non-Hodgkin's lymphomas. Paying prompt attention to the signs and symptoms of this disease, and seeing a doctor if the symptoms persist, are the best strategies for an early diagnosis of lymphoma. Early detection affords the best chance for a cure.

Resources

BOOKS

Berkow, Robert, et al., eds. *Merck Manual of Diagnosis and Therapy,* 16th ed. St. Louis: Merck Research Laboratories, 1992.

Dollinger, Malin. *Everyone's Guide to Cancer Therapy.* Kansas City, MO: Somerville House Books Limited, 1994.

Morra, Marion E. *Choices.* NY: Avon Books, October 1994.

Murphy, Gerald P. *Informed Decisions: The Complete book of Cancer Diagnosis, Treatment and Recovery.* NY: American Cancer Society, 1997.

ORGANIZATIONS

American Cancer Society (National Headquarters). 1599 Clifton Road, N.E. Atlanta, GA 30329. (800) 227-2345. http://www.cancer.org.

Cancer Research Institute (National Headquarters). 681 Fifth Avenue, New York, NY 10022. (800) 992-2623. http://www.cancerresearch.org.

Leukemia Society of America, Inc. 600 Third Avenue, New York, NY 10016 (800) 955 4572. http://www.leukemia.org.

Lymphoma Research Foundation. 8800 Venice Boulevard, Suite 207, Los Angeles, CA 90034. (310) 204 7040.

National Cancer Institute. 9000 Rockville Pike, Building 31, room 10A16, Bethesda, MD 20892. (800) 422-6237. http://wwwicic.nci.nih.gov.

Oncolink. University of Pennsylvania Cancer Center. http://cancer.med.upenn.edu.

OTHER

1998 Cancer facts and figures. American Cancer Society.

Hodgkin's disease and non-Hodgkin's lymphoma. Leukemia Society of America.

NCI/PDQ Patient Statement, "Adults non-Hodgkin's lymphoma." National Cancer Institute.

NCI/PDQ Patient Statement, "Childhood non-Hodgkin's lymphoma." National Cancer Institute.

Lata Cherath

Malignant melanoma

Definition

Malignant melanoma is a type of skin tumor that is characterized by the cancerous growth of melanocytes, which are cells that produce a dark pigment called melanin.

Description

Overview

Cancer of the skin is the most common type of cancer and continues to grow in incidence. Skin cancer starts in the top layer of skin (the epidermis) but can grow down into the lower layers, the dermis and the subcutaneous layer. There are three main types of cells located in the epidermis, each of which can become cancerous. Melanocytes are the pigmented cells that are scattered throughout the skin, providing protection from ultraviolet (UV) light. Basal cells rest near the bottom of the epidermis and the layer of cells that continually grow to replace skin. The third type of epidermal cell is the squamous cells which make up most of the cells in human skin.

Melanoma

Malignant melanoma is the most serious type of skin cancer. It develops from the melanocytes. Although melanoma is the least common skin cancer, it is the most aggressive. It spreads (metastasizes) to other parts of the body— especially the lungs and liver— as well as invading surrounding tissues. Melanomas in their early stages resemble **moles.** In Caucasians, melanomas appear most often on the trunk, head, and neck in men and on the arms and legs in women. Melanomas in African Americans, however, occur primarily on the palms of the hand, soles of the feet, and under the nails. Melanomas appear only rarely in the eyes, mouth, vagina, or digestive tract. Although melanomas are associated with exposure to the sun, the greatest risk factor for developing melanoma

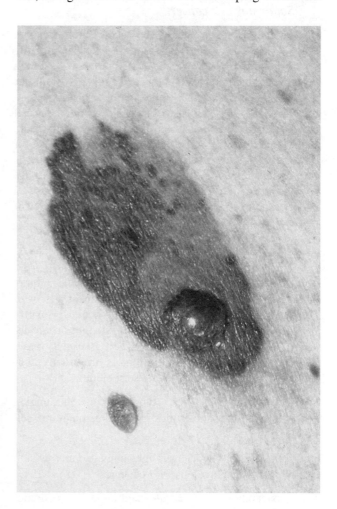

A close-up image of a malignant melanoma on a patient's back. *(Custom Medical Stock Photo. Reproduced by permission.)*

KEY TERMS

Biopsy—Removal of a small piece of tissue for examination. This is done under local anesthesia and removed by either using a scalpel or a punch, which removes a small cylindrical portion of tissue.

Cryosurgery—The use of extreme cold to destroy tissue in treating skin cancer.

Epidermis—The outermost layer of skin.

Interferon—A group of proteins that have an effect on immune function and appear to have an antitumor effect in some patients.

Melanin—A dark pigment that is found in certain skin cells and helps to protect the skin from ultraviolet light.

Melanocyte—A specialized skin cell that produces melanin.

Metastasis—The movement of cancer cells from one area of the body to another through the blood or the lymph vessels.

Staging—The process of classifying and evaluating the progression of a cancer.

TNM staging—A staging system for classifying cancers developed by the American Joint Committee on Cancer. The initials stand for tumor, nodes, and metastasis.

may be genetic. People who have a first-degree relative with melanoma have an increased risk up to eight times greater of developing the disease.

Basal cell cancer

Basal cell cancer is the most common type of skin cancer, accounting for about 75% of all skin cancers. It occurs primarily on the parts of the skin exposed to the sun and is most common in people living in equatorial regions or areas of high ozone depletion. Light-skinned people are more at risk of developing basal cell cancer than dark-skinned people. This form of skin cancer is primarily a disease of adults; it appears most often after age 30, peaking around age 70. Basal cell cancer grows very slowly; if it is not treated, however, it can invade deeper skin layers and cause disfigurement. This type of cancer can appear as a shiny, translucent nodule on the skin or as a red, wrinkled and scaly area.

Squamous cell cancer

Squamous cell cancer is the second most frequent type of skin cancer. It arises from the outer keratinizing layer of skin, so named because it contains a tough protein called keratin. Squamous cell cancer grows faster than basal cell cancer; it is more likely to metastasize to the lymph nodes as well as to distant sites. Squamous cell cancer most often appears on the arms, head, and neck. Fair-skinned people of Celtic descent are at high risk for developing squamous cell cancer. This type of cancer is rarely life-threatening but can cause serious problems if it spreads and can also cause disfigurement. Squamous cell cancer usually appears as a scaly, slightly elevated area of damaged skin.

Other skin cancers

Besides the three major types of skin cancer, there are a few other relatively rare forms. The most serious of these is **Kaposi's sarcoma** (KS), which occurs primarily in **AIDS** patients or older males of Mediterranean descent. When KS occurs with AIDS it is usually more aggressive. Other types of skin tumors are usually non-malignant and grow slowly. These include:

- Bowen's disease. This is a type of skin inflammation (**dermatitis**) that sometimes looks like squamous cell cancer.

- Solar keratosis. This is a sunlight-damaged area of skin that sometimes develops into cancer.

- Keratoacanthoma. A keratoacanthoma is a dome-shaped tumor that can grow quickly and appear like squamous cell cancer. Although it is usually benign, it should be removed.

Risk factors

SUN EXPOSURE

Most skin cancers are associated with the amount of time that a person spends in the sun and the number of **sunburns** received, especially if they occurred at an early age. Skin cancer typically does not appear for 10-20 years after the sun damage has occurred. Because of this time lag, skin cancer rarely occurs before **puberty** and occurs more frequently with age.

MOLES

The number of moles (nevi) on a person's skin is related to the likelihood of developing melanoma. There are three types of nevi: not cancerous (benign); atypical (dysplastic); or birthmark (congenital). All three types of nevi have been associated with a higher risk of developing melanoma. Sometimes the moles themselves can become cancerous; usually, however, the cancer is a new growth that occurs on normal skin.

HEREDITY

The tendency to develop skin cancer also tends to run in families. As has already been mentioned, there appears to be a significant genetic factor in the development of melanoma.

Causes & symptoms

Skin cancer begins to develop when a change or mutation occurs in one of the cells of the skin, causing it to grow without control. This mutation can be caused by ultraviolet (UV) light; most skin cancers are thought to be caused by overexposure to UV light from the sun. The incidence of severe, blistering sunburns is particularly closely related to skin cancer, more so when these **burns** occur during childhood. Exposure to ionizing radiation, arsenic, or polycyclic hydrocarbons in the workplace also appears to stimulate the development of skin cancers. The use of psoralen for treatment of **psoriasis** may be associated with the development of squamous cell cancer. Skin cancers are also more common in immunocompromised patients, such as AIDS patients or those who have undergone organ transplants.

The first sign of skin cancer is usually a change in an existing mole, the presence of a new mole, or a change in a specific area of skin. Any change in a mole or skin lesion, including changes in color, size, or shape, tenderness, scaliness, or **itching** should be suspected of being skin cancer. Areas that bleed or are ulcerated may be signs of more advanced skin cancer. By doing a monthly self-examination, a person can identify abnormal moles or areas of skin and seek evaluation from a qualified health professional. The ABCD rule provides an easy way to remember the important characteristics of moles when one is examining the skin:

- Asymmetry. A normal mole is round, whereas a suspicious mole is unevenly shaped.

- Border. A normal mole has a clear-cut border with the surrounding skin, whereas the edges of a suspect mole are often irregular.

- Color. Normal moles are uniformly tan or brown, but cancerous moles may appear as mixtures of red, white, blue, brown, purple, or black.

- Diameter. Normal moles are usually less than 5 millimeters in diameter. A skin lesion greater than 1/4 inch across may be suspected as cancerous.

There are two systems used in staging melanomas— Clark's and the American Joint Committee on Cancer's. The second system is sometimes called the TNM system, which stands for tumor-nodes-metastasis, after the three major phases in cancer progression.

Diagnosis

A person who has a suspicious-looking mole or area of skin should consult a doctor. In many cases, the patient's primary care physician will refer him or her to a doctor who specializes in skin diseases (a dermatologist). The dermatologist will carefully examine the lesion for the characteristic features of skin cancer. If further testing seems necessary, the doctor will perform a **skin biopsy** by removing the lesion under local anesthesia. Because melanomas tend to grow in diameter, as well as downwards into the epidermis and fatty layers of skin, a biopsy sample that is larger than the mole will be taken. This tissue is then analyzed under a microscope by a specialist in diseased organs and tissues (a pathologist). The pathologist makes the diagnosis of cancer and determines how far the tumor has grown into the skin. The evaluation of the progression of the cancer is called staging. Staging refers to how advanced the cancer is and is determined by the thickness and size of the tumor. Additional tests will also be done to determine if the cancer has moved into the lymph nodes or other areas of the body. These tests might include chest x ray, **computed tomography scan** (CT scan), **magnetic resonance imaging** (MRI), and blood tests.

Treatment

Surgery

The primary treatment for skin cancer is to cut out (excise) the tumor or diseased area of skin. Surgery usually involves a simple excision using a scalpel to remove the lesion and a small amount of normal surrounding tissue. A procedure known as microscopically controlled excision can be used to examine each layer of skin as it is removed to ensure that the proper amount is taken. Depending on the amount of skin removed, the cut is either closed with stitches or covered with a skin graft. When surgical excision is performed on visible areas, such as the face, cosmetic surgery may also be performed to minimize the scar. Other techniques for removing skin tumors include burning, freezing with dry ice (cryosurgery), or **laser surgery.** For skin cancer that is localized and has not spread to other areas of the body, excision may be the only treatment needed.

Nonsurgical approaches

Although **chemotherapy** is the normal course of therapy for most other types of advanced cancer, it is not usually effective and not usually used for advanced skin cancer. For advanced melanoma that has moved beyond the original tumor site, the local lymph nodes may be surgically removed. Immunotherapy in the form of interferon or interleukin is being used more often with success for advanced melanoma. There is growing evidence that **radiation** therapy may be useful for advanced melanoma. Other treatments under investigation for melanoma include **gene therapy** and **vaccination.** Recent studies have shown that the use of a vaccine prepared from the patient's own cancer cells may be useful in treating advanced melanoma. For people previously diagnosed with skin cancers, the chances of getting additional skin cancers are high. Therefore, regular monthly self-examination, as well as frequent examinations by a dermatologist, are essential.

Alternative treatment

There are no established alternative treatments for skin cancer. Immunotherapy, which strengthens the immune system, is an approach that may prove valuable in the future. Preventive measures that can be helpful include a diet high in antioxidants and supplementation with antioxidant nutrients.

Prognosis

The prognosis for skin cancer depends on several factors, the most important of which are the invasiveness of the tumor and its location. The prognosis is good for localized skin cancers that are diagnosed and treated early. For basal cell cancer and squamous cell cancer, the cure rate is close to 100%, although most of these patients will have recurrent skin cancer. For localized melanoma, the cure rate is approximately 95%. The prognosis worsens with larger tumors. Melanoma that has spread to the lymph nodes has a 5-year survival rate of 54%; advanced melanoma has a survival rate of only 13%. When melanoma has spread to other parts of the body, it is generally considered incurable; the median length of survival is six months.

Prevention

Prevention is the best way to deal with skin cancer. Avoiding unnecessary sun exposure— including sun lamps and tanning salons— is relatively simple. Parents of small children should protect them against the risk of sunburn. Precautions include avoiding high sun, when the rays of the sun are most intense (between 11 A.M. and 1 P.M.) In addition, persons living at high elevations need to take extra precautions because the intensity of UV radiation increases by 4% with every 1000-foot rise above sea level.

There is presently some debate about the ability of sunscreen to protect against skin cancer. Some scientists believe that gradual exposure to the sun, in order to develop a mild tan, may offer the best protection from skin cancer. Skin cancer has also been related to **diets** that are high in fat. Decreasing the amount of fat consumed may also help to decrease the risk of skin cancer.

Resources

BOOKS

Friedman, R.J., et al. ''Basal Cell and Squamous Cell Carcinoma of the Skin.'' In *American Cancer Society Textbook of Clinical Oncology,* edited by G. P. Murphy, et al. Atlanta, GA: American Cancer Society, 1995.

Haynes, H.A., et al. ''Cancer of the Skin.'' In *Cancer Manual,* 9th ed. Boston: American Cancer Society, 1996.

Reed, W.P., et al. ''Cutaneous Melanoma.'' In *Cancer Manual,* 9th ed. Boston: American Cancer Society, 1996.

Urist, M.M., et al. ''Malignant Melanoma.'' In *American Cancer Society Textbook of Clinical Oncology,* edited by G.P. Murphy, et al. Atlanta, GA: American Cancer Society, 1995.

PERIODICALS

''Melanoma: Sunscreens May Not Protect Against Skin Cancer.'' *Cancer Weekly Plus* (March 2, 1998): 1.

''Radiation Therapy Effective in Treating Advanced Stages of Skin Cancer.'' *Cancer Weekly Plus* (October 27, 1997): 21.

''Vaccine Treatment Prolongs Survival in Patients.'' *Cancer Weekly Plus* (September 8, 1997): 24.

ORGANIZATIONS

American Academy of Dermatology. 930 N. Meacham Rd., Schaumburg, IL, 60168-4014. (847) 330-0230.

American Cancer Society. 1599 Clifton Rd. NE, Atlanta, GA 30329. (800) ACS-2345. http://www.cancer.org.

National Cancer Institute, Cancer Information Service. (800) 4-CANCER.

Skin Cancer Foundation. P.O. Box 561, New York, NY 10156. (800) 754-6490.

OTHER

Cancer Care News. http://www.cancercarinc.org.

Cindy L. Jones

Malignant otitis externa *see* **Otitis externa**

Malignant plasmacytoma *see* **Multiple myeloma**

. . . .

Malingering

Definition

In the context of medicine, malingering is the act of intentionally feigning or exaggerating physical or psychological symptoms for personal gain.

Description

People may feign physical or psychological illness for any number of reasons. Faked illness can get them out of work, military duty, or criminal prosecution. It can also help them obtain financial compensation through insurance claims, lawsuits, or workers' compensation. Feigned symptoms may also be a way of getting the doctor to prescribe certain drugs.

According to the American Psychiatric Association, patients who malinger are different from people who invent symptoms for sympathy (factitious diseases). Patients who malinger clearly have something tangible to gain. People with factitious diseases appear to have a need to play the ''sick'' role. They may feign illness for attention or sympathy.

Malingering may take the form of complaints of chronic **whiplash pain** from automobile accidents. Whiplash claims are controversial. Although some people clearly do suffer from whiplash injury, others may be exaggerating the pain for insurance claims or lawsuits. Some intriguing scientific studies have shown that chronic whiplash pain after automobile accidents is almost nonexistent in Lithuania and Greece. In these countries, the legal systems do not encourage personal injury lawsuits or financial settlements. The psychological symptoms experienced by survivors of disaster (**post-traumatic stress disorder**) are also faked by malingerers.

Causes & symptoms

People malinger for personal gain. The symptoms may vary. Generally malingerers complain of psychological disorders such as **anxiety.** They may also complain of chronic pain for which objective tests such as x rays can find no physical cause. Because it is often impossible to determine who is malingering and who is not, it is impossible to know how frequently malingering occurs.

KEY TERMS

Antisocial personality—A personality characterized by attitudes and behaviors at odds with society's customs and moral standards, including illegal acts.

Factitious diseases—Conditions in which symptoms are deliberately manufactured by patients in order to gain attention and sympathy. Patients with factitious diseases do not fake symptoms for obvious financial gain or to evade the legal system.

Post traumatic stress disorder (PTSD)—A disorder that occurs among survivors of severe environmental stress such as a tornado, an airplane crash, or military combat. Symptoms include anxiety, insomnia, flashbacks, and nightmares. Patients with PTSD are unnecessarily vigilant; they may experience survivor guilt, and they sometimes cannot concentrate or experience joy.

Diagnosis

Malingering may be suspected:

• When a patient is referred for examination by an attorney

• When the onset of illness coincides with a large financial incentive, such as a new disability policy

• When objective medical tests do not confirm the patient's complaints

• When the patient does not cooperate with the diagnostic work-up or prescribed treatment

• When the patient has antisocial attitudes and behaviors (antisocial personality).

The diagnosis of malingering is a challenge for doctors. On the one hand, the doctor does not want to overlook a treatable disease. On the other hand, he or she does not want to continue ordering tests and treatments if the symptoms are faked. Malingering is difficult to distinguish from certain legitimate **personality disorders,** such as factitious diseases or post-traumatic distress syndrome. In legal cases, malingering patients may be referred to a psychiatrist. Psychiatrists use certain written tests to try to determine whether the patient is faking the symptoms.

Treatment

In a sense, malingering cannot be treated because the American Psychiatric Association does not recognize it as a personality disorder. Patients who are purposefully faking symptoms for gain do not want to be cured. Often, the malingering patient fails to report any improvement with treatment, and the doctor may try many treatments without success.

Resources

BOOKS

American Psychiatric Association. *Diagnostic and Statistical Manual of Mental Disorders,* 4th ed. Washington, DC, American Psychiatric Association, 1994.

Resnick, Phillip J. "Malingered Psychosis." In *Clinical Assessment of Malingering and Deception,* 2nd ed., edited by Richard Rogers. New York: Gilford Publications, 1997.

PERIODICALS

Klass, Peri. "How Sick Is It to Want to Be Sick?" *Discover* 78 (January 1986): 20-21.

Resnick, Phillip J. "Defrocking the Fraud." *Israel Journal of Psychiatry and Related Sciences* 30 (1993): 93-101.

Schrader, H., D. Oblienne, G. Bovim, D. Surkiene, D. Micheviciene, and I. Miseviciene. "Natural Evolution of Late Whiplash Syndrome Outside the Medicolegal Context." *The Lancet* 347 (May 4, 1996): 1207-1211.

"Two New Studies Question Basis for Whiplash Claims." *The Back Letter* 12 (December 1997): 133-34.

ORGANIZATIONS

American Psychiatric Association. 1400 K Street, N.W., Washington, DC 20005. (202) 682-6000. http://www.psych.org.

Robert Scott Dinsmoor

Mallory-Weiss syndrome

Definition

Mallory-Weiss syndrome is bleeding from an arterial blood vessel in the upper gastrointestinal tract, caused by a mucosal gastric tear at or near the point where the esophagus and stomach join.

Description

Mallory-Weiss syndrome causes about 5% of all upper gastrointestinal bleeding. The condition was originally diagnosed in alcoholics and is associated with heavy alcohol use, although it can also be found in patients who are not alcoholics. Earlier episodes of heavy hiccupping, vomiting, and retching are reported by about half the patients who are diagnosed with Mallory-Weiss syndrome. It is thought that the tear or laceration occurs when there is a sudden increase in intra-abdominal pres-

KEY TERMS

Electrolytes—Salts and minerals that can conduct electrical impulses in the body. Common human electrolytes are sodium chloride, potassium, calcium, and sodium bicarbonate. Electrolytes control the fluid balance of the body and are important in muscle contraction, energy generation, and almost every major biochemical reaction in the body.

Endoscopy—A procedure in which an instrument containing a camera and a light source is inserted into the gastrointestinal tract so that the doctor can visually inspect the gastrointestinal system.

Esophageal varix—An enlarged vein of the esophagus. (Plural: esophageal varices.)

Portal hypertension—High blood pressure in the portal vein, which carries blood from the abdominal organs to the liver.

sure. Patients with increased pressure in the vein leading into the liver (portal **hypertension**) are more likely to bleed heavily from an esophageal laceration than those whose blood pressure is normal.

Causes & symptoms

In Mallory-Weiss syndrome, a tear occurs in the gastric mucosa, near where the esophagus and stomach join. About 10% of the tears are in the esophagus. Most are either right at the junction of the esophagus and stomach or in the stomach just slightly below the junction.

Bleeding from the tear causes a disruption in fluid and electrolyte balance of the body. The patient often produces vomit tinged with either fresh blood or older, blackish blood. Blood loss can be considerable.

Diagnosis

A Mallory-Weiss syndrome tear is not visible on standard upper gastrointestinal x rays. A tear about one-eighth to one and one-half inches long (0.5-4 cm) is revealed by endoscopy. Endoscopy also shows that in 35% of patients there is another potential cause for gastrointestinal bleeding, such as peptic **ulcer,** erosive **gastritis,** or esophageal varices.

Treatment

The patient is resuscitated and stabilized with blood **transfusions** and intravenous fluids to restore the fluid and electrolyte balance. Most of the time, esophageal bleeding stops spontaneously. When bleeding does not stop, patients are treated with an injection of epinephrine (adrenaline) and/or the bleeding artery is cauterized with heat. If these treatments fail, surgery is performed to stop the bleeding.

Prognosis

In 90-95% of patients whose bleeding does not stop spontaneously, cauterization without surgery will stop the bleeding. Patients at highest risk for a recurrence of bleeding are those with portal hypertension.

Prevention

Mallory-Weiss syndrome is associated with **alcoholism.** Limiting alcohol intake may help prevent the disorder.

Resources

BOOKS

''Esophageal Laceration and Rupture.'' In *The Merck Manual of Diagnosis and Therapy,* 16th ed., edited by Robert Berkow. Rahway, NJ: Merck Research Laboratories, 1992.

''Mallory-Weiss Syndrome.'' In *Current Medical Diagnosis & Treatment 1998,* edited by Lawrence Tierney, Jr., Stephen McPhee, and Maxine Papadakis. Stamford, CT: Appleton & Lange, 1998.

Tish Davidson

Malnutrition

Definition

Malnutrition is the condition that develops when the body does not get the right amount of the **vitamins, minerals,** and other nutrients it needs to maintain healthy tissues and organ function.

Description

Undernutrition

Malnutrition occurs in people who are either undernourished or over-nourished. Undernutrition is a consequence of consuming too few essential nutrients or using or excreting them more rapidly than they can be replaced.

Infants, young children, and teenagers need additional nutrients. So do women who are pregnant or breastfeeding. Nutrient loss can be accelerated by **diarrhea,** excessive sweating, heavy bleeding (hemorrhage), or kidney failure. Nutrient intake can be restricted by age-related illnesses and conditions, excessive dieting, severe injury, serious illness, a lengthy hospitalization, or substance abuse.

The leading cause of death in children in developing countries is **protein-energy malnutrition.** This type of malnutrition is the result of inadequate intake of calories from proteins, vitamins, and minerals. Children who are already undernourished can suffer from protein-energy malnutrition when rapid growth, infection, or disease increases the need for protein and essential minerals.

Overnutrition

In the United States, nutritional deficiencies have generally been replaced by dietary imbalances or excesses associated with many of the leading causes of **death** and disability. Overnutrition results from eating too much, eating too many of the wrong things, not exercising enough, or taking too many vitamins or other dietary replacements.

Risk of overnutrition is also increased by being more than 20% overweight, consuming a diet high in fat and salt, and taking high doses of:

- Nicotinic acid (niacin) to lower elevated cholesterol levels
- Vitamin B_6 to relieve **premenstrual syndrome**
- Vitamin A to clear up skin problems
- Iron or other trace minerals not prescribed by a doctor.

Nutritional disorders can affect any system in the body and the senses of sight, taste, and smell. Malnutrition begins with changes in nutrient levels in blood and tissues. Alterations in enzyme levels, tissue abnormalities, and organ malfunction may be followed by illness and death.

Causes & symptoms

Poverty and lack of food are the primary reasons why malnutrition occurs in the United States. Ten percent of all members of low income households do not always have enough healthful food to eat, and malnutrition affects one in four elderly Americans. Protein-energy malnutrition occurs in 50% of surgical patients and in 48% of all other hospital patients.

There is an increased risk of malnutrition associated with chronic diseases, especially disease of the intestinal tract, kidneys, and liver. Patients with chronic diseases like cancer, AIDS, and intestinal disorders may lose weight rapidly and become susceptible to undernourishment because they cannot absorb valuable vitamins, calories, and iron.

People with drug or alcohol dependencies are also at increased risk of malnurtrition. These people tend to maintain inadequate diets for long periods of time and

their ability to absorb nutrients is impaired by the alcohol or drug's affect on body tissues, particularly the liver, pancreas, and brain.

Unintentionally losing 10 pounds or more may be a sign of malnutrition. People who are malnourished may be skinny or bloated. Their skin is pale, thick, dry, and **bruises** easily. **Rashes** and changes in pigmentation are common.

Hair is thin, tightly curled, and pulls out easily. Joints ache and bones are soft and tender. The gums bleed. The tongue may be swollen or shriveled and cracked. Visual disturbances include night blindness and increased sensitivity to light and glare.

Other symptoms of malnutrition include:

- Anemia
- Diarrhea
- Disorientation
- **Goiter** (enlarged thyroid gland)
- Loss of reflexes and lack of coordination
- Muscle twitches
- Scaling and cracking of the lips and mouth.

Malnourished children may be short for their age, thin, listless, and have weakened immune systems.

Diagnosis

Overall appearance, behavior, body-fat distribution, and organ function can alert a family physician, internist, or nutrition specialist to the presence of malnutrition. Patients may be asked to record what they eat during a specific period. X rays can determine bone density and reveal gastrointestinal disturbances, and heart and lung damage.

Blood and urine tests are used to measure levels of vitamins, minerals, and waste products. Nutritional status can also be determined by:

- Comparing a patient's weight to standardized charts
- Calculating body mass index (BMI) according to a formula that divides height into weight
- Measuring skin-fold thickness or the circumference of the upper arm.

Treatment

Normalizing nutritional status starts with a nutritional assessment. This process enables a clinical nutritionist or registered dietician to confirm the presence of malnutrition, assess the effects of the disorder, and formulate **diets** that will restore adequate nutrition.

Patients who cannot or will not eat, or who are unable to absorb nutrients taken by mouth, may be fed intravenously (parenteral nutrition) or through a tube inserted into the gastrointestinal (GI) tract (enteral nutrition).

Tube feeding is often used to provide nutrients to patients who have suffered **burns** or who have inflammatory bowel disease. This procedure involves inserting a thin tube through the nose and carefully guiding it along the throat until it reaches the stomach or small intestine. If long-term tube feeding is necessary, the tube may be placed directly into the stomach or small intestine through an incision in the abdomen.

Tube feeding cannot always deliver adequate nutrients to patients who:

• Are severely malnourished

• Require surgery

• Are undergoing **chemotherapy** or radiation treatments

• Have been seriously burned

• Have persistent diarrhea or vomiting

• Whose gastrointestinal tract is paralyzed.

Intravenous feeding can supply some or all of the nutrients these patients need.

Prognosis

Up to 10% of a person's body weight can be lost without side effects, but if more than 40% is lost, the situation is almost always fatal. Death usually results from heart failure, electrolyte imbalance, or low body temperature. Patients with semiconsciousness, persistent diarrhea, jaundice, or low blood sodium levels have a poorer prognosis.

Some children with protein-energy malnutrition recover completely. Others have many health problems throughout life, including mental retardation and the inability to absorb nutrients through the intestinal tract. Prognosis for all patients with malnutrition seems to be dependent on the age of the patient, and the length and severity of the malnutrition, with young children and the elderly having the highest rate of long-term complications and death.

Prevention

Breastfeeding a baby for at least six months is considered the best way to prevent early-childhood malnutrition. The United States Department of Agriculture and Health and Human Service recommend that all Americans over the age of two:

• Consume plenty of fruits, grains, and vegetables

• Eat a variety of foods that are low in fats and cholesterols and contain only moderate amounts of salt, sugars, and sodium

• Engage in moderate physical activity for at least 30 minutes, at least several times a week

• Achieve or maintain their ideal weight

• Use alcohol sparingly or avoid it altogether.

Every patient admitted to a hospital should be screened for the presence of illnesses and conditions that could lead to protein-energy malnutrition. Patients with higher-than-average risk for malnutrition should be more closely assessed and reevaluated often during long-term hospitalization or nursing-home care.

Resources

BOOKS

Andersen, Jean and Barbara Deskins. *The Nutrition Bible.* New York, NY: William Morrow and Company, 1995.

Bennett, J. Claude, and Fred Plum, eds. *Cecil Textbook of Medicine.* Philadelphia, PA: W.B. Saunders Company, 1996.

Berkow, Robert, ed. *The Merck Manual of Medical Information: Home Edition.* Whitehouse Station, NJ: Merck Research Laboratories, Inc., 1997.

The Surgeon General's Report on Nutrition and Health. Rocklin, CA: Prima Publishing and Communications, 1988.

ORGANIZATIONS

American College of Nutrition. 722 Robert E. Lee Drive, Wilmington, NC 20412-0927. (919) 452-1222.

American Institute of Nutrition. 9650 Rockville Pike, Bethesda, MD 20814-3990. (301) 530-7050.

Food and Nutrition Information Center. 10301 Baltimore Boulevard, Room 304, Beltsville, MD 20705-2351. http://www.nalusda.gov/fnic/.

OTHER

Malnutrition. http://www.nutrition.uu.se/malnutrition/malnutr.html. (3 May 1998).

New Dietary Guidelines for Americans. http://www.mayohealth.org/mayo/9602.htm/dietguid.htm. (3 May 1998).

Mary K. Fyke

Malocclusion

Definition

Malocclusion is a problem in the way the upper and lower teeth fit together in biting or chewing. The word malocclusion literally means "bad bite." The condition may also be referred to as an irregular bite, crossbite, or overbite.

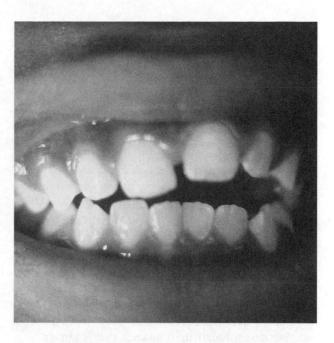

This patient's teeth are misarranged because of excessive thumb sucking. *(Custom Medical Stock Photo. Reproduced by permission.)*

Description

Malocclusion may be seen as crooked, crowded, or protruding teeth. It may affect a person's appearance, speech, and/or ability to eat.

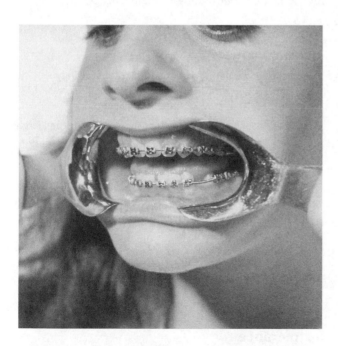

Orthodontia treatments usually include the use of braces and retainers. *(Photograph by Lester V. Bergman, Corbis Images. Reproduced by permission).*

Causes & symptoms

Malocclusions are most often inherited, but may be acquired. Inherited conditions include too many or too few teeth, too much or too little space between teeth, irregular mouth and jaw size and shape, and atypical formations of the jaws and face, such as a cleft palate. Malocclusions may be acquired from habits like finger or thumb sucking, tongue thrusting, premature loss of teeth from an accident or dental disease, and medical conditions such as enlarged tonsils and adenoids that lead to mouth breathing.

Malocclusions may be symptomless or they may produce **pain** from increased stress on the oral structures. Teeth may show abnormal signs of wear on the chewing surfaces or decay in areas of tight overlap. Chewing may be difficult.

Diagnosis

Malocclusion is most often found during a routine dental examination. A dentist will check a patient's occlusion by watching how the teeth make contact when the patient bites down normally. The dentist may ask the patient to bite down with a piece of coated paper between the upper and lower teeth; this paper will leave colored marks at the points of contact. When malocclusion is suspected, photographs and x rays of the face and mouth may be taken for further study. To confirm the presence and extent of malocclusion, the dentist makes plaster, plastic, or artificial stone models of the patient's teeth from impressions. These models duplicate the fit of the teeth and are very useful in treatment planning.

Treatment

Malocclusion may be remedied by orthodontic treatment; orthodontics is a specialty of dentistry that manages the growth and correction of dental and facial structures. Braces are the most commonly used orthodontic appliances in the treatment of malocclusion. At any given time, approximately 4 million people in the United States are wearing braces, including 800,000 adults.

Braces apply constant gentle force to slowly change the position of the teeth, straightening them and properly aligning them with the opposing teeth. Braces consist of brackets cemented to the surface of each tooth and wires of stainless steel or nickel titanium alloy. When the wires are threaded through the brackets, they exert pressure against the teeth, causing them to gradually move.

Braces are not removable for daily tooth brushing, so the patient must be especially diligent about keeping the mouth clean and removing food particles which become easily trapped, to prevent **tooth decay.** Foods that are crunchy should be avoided to minimize the risk of breaking the appliance. Hard fruits, vegetables, and breads must be cut into bite-sized pieces before eating. Foods that are sticky, including chewing gum, should be avoided because they may pull off the brackets or weaken the cement. Carbonated beverages may also weaken the cement, as well as contribute to tooth decay. Teeth should be brushed immediately after eating sweet foods. Special floss threaders are available to make flossing easier.

If overcrowding is creating malocclusion, one or more teeth may be extracted (surgically removed), giving the others room to move. If a tooth has not yet erupted or is prematurely lost, the orthodontist may insert an appliance called a space maintainer to keep the other teeth from moving out of their natural position. In severe cases of malocclusion, surgery may be necessary and the patient would be referred to yet another specialist, an oral or maxillofacial surgeon.

Once the teeth have been moved into their new position, the braces are removed and a retainer is worn until the teeth stabilize in that position. Retainers do not move teeth, they only hold them in place.

Orthodontic treatment is the only effective treatment for malocclusion not requiring surgery. However, depending on the cause and severity of the condition, an orthodontist may be able to suggest other appliances as alternatives to braces.

Alternative treatment

There are some techniques of craniosacral therapy that can alter structure. This therapy may allow correction of some cases of malocclusion. If surgery is required, pre- and post-surgical care with homeopathic remedies, as well as vitamin and mineral supplements, can enhance recovery. Night guards are sometimes recommended to ease the strain on the jaw and to limit teeth grinding.

Prognosis

Depending on the cause and severity of the malocclusion and the appliance used in treatment, a patient may expect correction of the condition to take 2 or more years. Patients typically wear braces 18-24 months and a retainer for another year. Treatment is faster and more successful in children and teens whose teeth and bones are still developing. The length of treatment time is also affected by how well the patient follows orthodontic instructions.

Prevention

In general, malocclusion is not preventable. It may be minimized by controlling habits such as finger or thumb sucking. An initial consultation with an orthodontist before a child is 7 years old may lead to appropriate management of the growth and development of the child's dental and facial structures, circumventing many of the factors contributing to malocclusion.

Resources

ORGANIZATIONS

American Association of Oral and Maxillofacial Surgeons. 9700 West Bryn Mawr Avenue, Rosemont, IL 60018-5701. (847) 678-6200. http://www.aaoms.org.

American Association of Orthodontists. 401 North Lindbergh Boulevard, St. Louis, MO 63141-7816. (314) 993-1700. http://www.aaortho.org.

OTHER

OrthoFind. (310) 328-2020. http://www.orthofind.com.

Bethany Thivierge

Malta fever *see* **Brucellosis**

Maltose intolerance *see* **Carbohydrate intolerance**

Mammogram screening *see* **Mammography**

Mammography

Definition

Mammography is the study of the breast using x ray. The actual test is called a mammogram. It is an x ray of the breast which shows the soft tissue and internal structures. There are two types of mammograms. A screening mammogram is ordered for women who have no problems with their breasts. It consists of two x-ray views of each breast. A diagnostic mammogram is for evaluation of abnormalities. Additional x rays from other angles, or special views of certain areas are taken.

Purpose

The purpose of screening mammography is **breast cancer** detection. A screening test, by definition, is used for patients without any signs or symptoms, in order to detect disease as early as possible. Many studies have shown that having regular mammograms increases a woman's chances of finding breast cancer in an early stage, when it is more likely to be curable. It has been estimated that a mammogram may find a **cancer** as much as two or three years before it can be felt. As of March 1997, American Cancer Society (ACS) guidelines recommended an annual screening mammogram for every woman of average risk beginning at age 40. There is some controversy between government and physician groups about the usefulness of screening women between the ages of 40-50.

Some women are at increased risk for developing breast cancer, such as those with multiple relatives with the disease. Beginning screening mammography at a younger age may be recommended for these women.

Diagnostic mammography is used to evaluate an existing problem, such as a lump, discharge from the nipple, or unusual tenderness in one area. The cause of the problem may be definitively diagnosed from this study or further investigation using other methods may be necessary. This test is also used to evaluate findings from screening mammography tests.

Precautions

Screening mammograms are not usually recommended for women under age 40 who have no special risk factors and a normal physical breast examination. A mammogram may be useful if a lump or other problem is discovered in a woman aged 30-40. Below age 30, breasts tend to be ''radiographically dense,'' which means it is difficult to see many details. Mammograms for this age group are controversial.

Description

A mammogram may be offered in a variety of settings. Hospitals, outpatient clinics, physician's offices, or other facilities may have mammography equipment. In the United States, since October 1, 1994, only places certified by the Food and Drug Administration (FDA) are

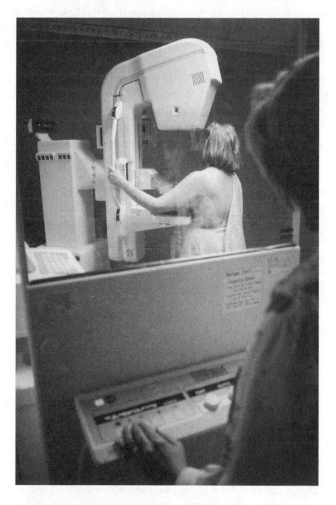

Mammography is very effective in the early detection of breast cancer. (Photograph by Ron Chapple, FPG International. Reproduced by permission.)

legally permitted to perform, interpret, or develop mammograms.

In addition to the usual paperwork, a woman will be asked to fill out a form asking for information relevant to her risk of breast cancer. Beyond her personal and family history of cancer, details about menstruation, child bearing, birth control, and **hormone replacement therapy** are significant. Information about Breast Self Examination (BSE) and other breast health issues is usually available at no charge.

At some centers, a technologist may perform a **physical examination** of the breasts before the mammogram. Whether or not this is done, it is essential for the patient to tell the technologist about any lumps, nipple discharge, breast **pain,** or other concerns.

Clothing from the waist up is removed and a hospital gown or similar covering is put on. The woman stands facing the mammography machine. The technologist exposes one breast and places it on a plastic or metal film holder about the size of a placemat. The breast is compressed as flat as possible between the film holder and a rectangle of plastic (called a paddle), which presses down onto the breast from above. The compression should only last a few seconds, just enough to take the x ray. Good compression can be uncomfortable, but it is necessary to ensure the clearest view of all breast tissues.

Next, the woman is positioned with her side towards the mammography unit. The film holder is tilted so the outside of the breast rests against it, and a corner is touching the armpit. The paddle again holds the breast firmly as the x ray is taken. This procedure is repeated for the other breast. A total of four x rays, two of each breast, are taken for a screening mammogram. Additional x rays, using special paddles, different breast positions, or other techniques may be taken for a diagnostic mammogram.

The mammogram may be seen and interpreted by a radiologist right away, or it may not be reviewed until later. If there is any questionable area or abnormality, extra x rays may be recommended. These may be taken during the same appointment. More commonly, especially for screening mammograms, the woman is called back on another day for these additional films.

A screening mammogram usually takes approximately 15-30 minutes. A woman having a diagnostic mammogram can expect to spend up to an hour for the procedure.

The cost of mammography varies widely. Many mammography facilities accept "self referral". This means women can schedule themselves without a physician's referral. However, some insurance policies do require a doctor's prescription to ensure payment. As of January 1, 1998, Medicare will pay for annual screening mammograms for all women over age 39.

Preparation

The compression or squeezing of the breast necessary for a mammogram is a concern of many women. Mammograms should be scheduled when a woman's breasts are least likely to be tender. One to two weeks after the first day of the menstrual period is usually best. Some women with sensitive breasts also find that stopping or decreasing **caffeine** intake from coffee, tea, colas, and chocolate for a week or two before the examination decreases any discomfort. Over-the-counter pain relievers are also recommended an hour before the mammogram appointment, if pain is a significant problem.

Women should not put deodorant, powder, or lotion on their upper body on the day the mammogram is performed. Particles from these products can get on the breast or film holder and may look like abnormalities on the mammogram film.

Aftercare

No special aftercare is required.

Risks

The risk of radiation exposure from a mammogram is considered virtually nonexistent. Experts are unanimous that any negligible risk is by far outweighed by the potential benefits of mammography.

Some breast cancers do not show up on mammograms, or "hide" in dense breast tissue. A normal (or negative) study is not a guarantee that a woman is cancer-free. The "false-negative" rate is estimated to be 10-15%.

"False positive" readings are also possible. Breast biopsies may be recommended on the basis of a mammogram, and find no cancer. In 1996, it was estimated that 75-80% of all breast biopsies resulted in benign (no cancer present) findings. This is considered an acceptable rate, because recommending fewer biopsies would result in too many missed cancers.

Normal results

A mammography report describes details about the x ray appearance of the breasts. It also rates the mammogram according to standardized categories, as part of the Breast Imaging Reporting and Data System (BIRADS) created by the American College of Radiology (ACR). A normal mammogram may be rated as BIRADS 1 or negative, which means no abnormalities were seen. A normal mammogram may also be rated as BIRADS 2 or benign findings. This means there are one or more abnormalities but they are clearly benign (not cancerous), or variations of normal. Some kinds of calcification, lymph nodes in the breast, or obvious cysts might generate a BIRADS 2 rating.

Abnormal results

Many mammograms are considered borderline or indeterminate in their findings. BIRADS 3 means an abnormality is seen and is probably (but not definitely) benign. A follow-up mammogram within a short interval of three to six months is suggested. This helps to ensure that the abnormality is not changing, or is "stable." This stability in the abnormality indicates that a cancer is probably not present. If the abnormality was a cancer, it would have grown in the interval between mammograms. Some women are uncomfortable or anxious about waiting, and may want to consult with their doctor about a having a biopsy. BIRADS 4 means suspicious for cancer. A biopsy is usually recommended in this case. BIRADS 5 means an abnormality is highly suggestive of cancer. A biopsy or other appropriate action should be taken.

Resources

BOOKS

Baron-Faust, Rita. *Breast Cancer: What Every Woman Should Know.* New York, NY: Hearst Books, 1995.

Love, Susan with Lindsey, Karen. *Dr. Susan Love's Breast Book,* 2nd edition. Reading, MA: Addison-Wesley, 1995.

PERIODICALS

Letich, A., et al. "American Cancer Society Guidelines for the Early Detection of Breast Cancer: Update 1997." *CA: A Cancer Journal for Clinicians* 47 (May/June 1997): 150-153.

"The Mammography Muddle." *Harvard Women's Health Watch.* 7 (March 1997): 4-5.

Weber, Ellen. "Questions and Answers About Breast Cancer Diagnosis." *American Journal of Nursing* (October 1997): 34-38.

ORGANIZATIONS

American Cancer Society. 1599 Clifton Rd., Atlanta, GA 30329.(ACS) 1 800-ACS-2345 (1-800-227-2345) http://www.cancer.org.

Federal Drug Administration. 5600 Fishers lane, Rockville, MD 20857. (FDA) 1-800- 532-4440. http://www.fda.gov.

National Cancer Institute. Office of Cancer Communications, Bldg. 31, Room 10A16, Bethesda, MD 20892. (NCI/Cancer Information Service (CIS) 1-800-4-CANCER (1-800-422-6237). http://cancernet.nci.nih.gov.

Ellen S. Weber

Mandelamine *see* **Urinary anti-infectives**

Manganese deficiency *see* **Mineral deficiency**

Manganese excess *see* **Mineral toxicity**

··

Mania

Definition

Mania is an abnormally elated mental state, typically characterized by feelings of euphoria, lack of inhibitions, racing thoughts, diminished need for sleep, talkativeness, risk taking, and irritability. In extreme cases, mania can induce **hallucinations** and other psychotic symptoms.

Description

Mania typically occurs as a symptom of **bipolar disorder** (a mood disorder characterized by both manic and depressive episodes). Individuals experiencing a manic episode often have feelings of self-importance, elation, talkativeness, sociability, and a desire to embark on goal-oriented activities, coupled with the less desirable characteristics of irritability, impatience, impulsiveness, hyperactivity, and a decreased need for sleep. (Note: Hypomania is a term applied to a condition resembling mania. It is characterized by persistent or elevated expansive mood, hyperactivity, inflated self esteem, etc., but of less intensity than mania.) Severe mania may have psychotic features.

Causes & symptoms

Mania can be induced by the use or abuse of stimulant drugs such as cocaine and amphetamines. It is also the predominant feature of bipolar disorder, or manic depression, an affective mental illness that causes radical emotional changes and mood swings.

The Diagnostic and Statistical Manual of Mental Disorders, Fourth Edition (*DSM-IV*), the diagnostic standard for mental health professionals in the U.S., describes a manic episode as an abnormally elevated mood lasting at least one week that is distinguished by at least three of the following symptoms: inflated self-esteem, decreased need for sleep, talkativeness, racing thoughts, distractibility, increase in goal-directed activity, or excessive involvement in pleasurable activities that have a high potential for painful consequences. If the mood of the patient is irritable and not elevated, four of these symptoms are required.

KEY TERMS

Hypomania—A less severe form of elevated mood state that is a characteristic of bipolar type II disorder.

Mixed mania—A mental state in which symptoms of both depression and mania occur simultaneously.

Diagnosis

Mania is usually diagnosed and treated by a psychiatrist and/or a psychologist in an outpatient setting. However, most severely manic patients require hospitalization. In addition to an interview, several clinical inventories or scales may be used to assess the patient's mental status and determine the presence and severity of mania. An assessment commonly includes the Young Mania Rating Scale (YMRS). The Mini-Mental State Examination (MMSE) may also be given to screen out other illnesses such as **dementia.**

Treatment

Mania is primarily treated with drugs. The following mood-stabilizing agents are commonly prescribed to regulate manic episodes:

• Lithium (Cibalith-S, Eskalith, Lithane) is one of the oldest and most frequently prescribed drugs available for the treatment of mania. Because the drug takes four to seven days to reach a therapeutic level in the bloodstream, it is sometimes prescribed in conjunction with neuroleptics (**antipsychotic drugs**) and/or **benzodiazepines** (tranquilizers) to provide more immediate relief of mania.

• Carbamazepine (Tegretol, Atretol) is an anticonvulsant drug usually prescribed in conjunction with other mood-stabilizing agents. The drug is often used to treat bipolar patients who have not responded well to lithium therapy. As of early 1998, carbamazepine was not approved for the treatment of mania by the FDA.

• Valproate (divalproex sodium, or Depakote; valproic acid, or Depakene) is an anticonvulsant drug prescribed alone or in combination with carbamazepine and/or lithium. For patients experiencing "mixed mania," or mania with features of depression, valproate is preferred over lithium.

Clozapine (Clozaril) is an atypical antipsychotic medication used to control manic episodes in patients who have not responded to typical mood-stabilizing agents. The drug has also been a useful preventative treatment in some bipolar patients. Other new anticonvulsants (lamotrigine, gubapentin) are being investigated for treatment of mania and bipolar disorder.

Prognosis

Patients experiencing mania as a result of bipolar disorder will require long-term care to prevent recurrence; bipolar disorder is a chronic condition that requires lifelong observation and treatment after diagnosis. Data show that almost 90% of patients who experience one manic episode will go on to have another.

Prevention

Mania as a result of bipolar disorder can only be prevented through ongoing pharmacologic treatment. Patient education in the form of therapy or self-help groups is crucial for training patients to recognize signs of mania and to take an active part in their treatment program. Psychotherapy is an important adjunctive treatment for patients with bipolar disorder.

Resources

BOOKS

American Psychiatric Association. *Diagnostic and Statistical Manual of Mental Disorders,* 4th ed. Washington, DC: American Psychiatric Press, Inc., 1994.

Maxmen, Jerrold S., and Nicholas G. Ward. "Mood Disorders." In *Essential Psychopathology and Its Treatment,* 2nd ed. New York: W.W. Norton, 1995.

Whybrow, Peter C. *A Mood Apart.* New York: HarperCollins, 1997.

PERIODICALS

Biederman, Joseph A. "Is There a Childhood Form of Bipolar Disorder?" *Harvard Mental Health Letter* 13 (March 1997): 8.

Daly, Ian. "Seminar: Mania." *The Lancet* 349 (1997): 1157-60.

ORGANIZATIONS

American Psychiatric Association (APA). Office of Public Affairs. 1400 K Street NW, Washington, DC 20005. (202) 682-6119. http://www.psych.org/.

National Alliance for the Mentally Ill (NAMI). 200 North Glebe Road, Suite 1015, Arlington, VA 22203-3754. (800) 950-6264. http://www.nami.org.

National Depressive and Manic-Depressive Association (NDMDA). 730 N. Franklin St., Suite 501, Chicago, IL 60610. (800) 826-3632. http://www.ndmda.org.

National Institute of Mental Health (NIMH). 5600 Fishers Lane, Rm. 7C-02, Bethesda, MD 20857. (301) 443-4513. http://www.nimh.nih.gov/.

OTHER

Bowden, Charles L. "Choosing the Appropriate Therapy for Bipolar Disorder." *Medscape Mental Health* 2, no. 8 (1997). http://www.medscape.com.

Sachs, Gary. ''Adolescent Mania: Underdiagnosed and Undertreated.'' Reported by Deborah Carver. *Online Coverage from the 150th Annual Meeting of the American Psychiatric Association—Medscape Mental Health.* (May 1997). http://www.medscape.com.

Paula Anne Ford-Martin

Manic depression *see* **Bipolar disorder**

Manic episode *see* **Mania**

MAO inhibitors *see* **Monoamine oxidase inhibitors**

Marasmus *see* **Protein-energy malnutrition**

Marble bones *see* **Osteopetroses**

Marburg virus infection *see* **Hemorrhagic fevers**

Marfan syndrome

Definition

Marfan syndrome (or Marfan's syndrome) is an inherited disease that affects the connective tissue within the body. This results in a variety of skeletal deformities, as well as problems with the heart and the blood vessels (the cardiovascular system).

Description

Marfan syndrome is known to be a dominant genetic disorder, which means that a person needs to inherit only one defective gene in order to actually have the syndrome. In addition to those cases of Marfan's which are clearly inherited, 20% of all Marfan's patients have no family history of the syndrome. It is believed that these patients have undergone a spontaneous genetic mutation leading to the syndrome. Interestingly, one risk factor for Marfan syndrome (in a family where Marfan's is not already an inherited disorder) is an elderly father. Marfan syndrome is said to have variable expression, meaning that either all, or only a few, of the classic signs of Marfan syndrome may occur in any given patient.

The biochemical problem which results in Marfan syndrome has not been well defined. The group of tissues affected by Marfan syndrome are called the connective tissues. These are tissues that are made of fibrous compo-

nents, and they provide structural support for other body tissues. Included in the group called connective tissues are bone, cartilage, fat tissue, lymph tissue, and blood. The current belief is that the affected gene results in an abnormality in a protein called microfibrillin; and this protein is responsible for certain structural characteristics of connective tissue throughout the body.

Causes & symptoms

Typically, a person with Marfan syndrome appears quite tall and thin, particularly when compared with other

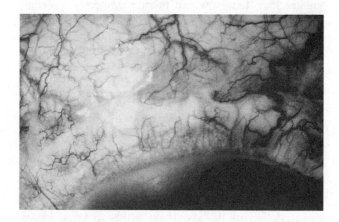

Marfan's syndrome often causes circulatory defects in the sclera of the eye, as shown above. *(Custom Medical Stock Photo. Reproduced by permission.)*

members of the same family. The patient's arms are proportionally quite long, compared to their stature, and their fingers are also long and thin, termed "arachnodactyly" (*arachno* means spider-like, while *dactyly* refers to fingers). The patient's chest wall may protrude out, or be sunken in, while the spine often has an abnormal curvature. The patient's joints are usually loose, and may be able to be bent in the wrong direction (double-jointedness). Muscles are often smaller than normal, and **hernias** (protrusions of internal organs through weak areas in muscle) are frequent in Marfan's patients. Several lung problems are common, including the tendency to spontaneously suffer a collapsed lung (**pneumothorax**).

A variety of eye abnormalities usually accompany Marfan syndrome, with extreme nearsightedness and dislocation of the lens the most common manifestations. **Glaucoma, cataracts,** and **retinal detachment** also occur more frequently than normal.

The most serious and potentially life-threatening complications of Marfan syndrome occur due to the involvement of the heart and blood vessels. The mitral valve (the gateway out of the heart for all the blood entering the body's circulation) is frequently abnormal, resulting in a heart murmur. The wall of the aorta (the major artery leaving the heart) is prone to stretching (dilation). Over time, the aorta becomes increasingly weak, leading to bulging (called an aneurysm) and possible rupture. Such ruptures lead to heavy, uncontrollable bleeding into the body (severe hemorrhage), and almost certain **death.**

Diagnosis

There are no laboratory tests to aid in the diagnosis of Marfan syndrome, so diagnosis relies on the identification of some cluster of the classic signs of Marfan's occurring in a particular patient. Of course, suspicion is greater in a family where other members are already known to have Marfan syndrome. The particular type of lens dislocation common in Marfan syndrome is so rare outside of Marfan's, that this finding alone should lead to a high degree of suspicion. Diagnosis is crucial, because an individual with Marfan syndrome must receive regular, careful evaluation of the cardiovascular system (especially the aorta), in order to avoid the potentially fatal complication of a ruptured aneurysm.

Treatment

There is no treatment for Marfan syndrome itself that can reverse the overall connective tissue defects. Each manifestation of the syndrome needs to be addressed individually (braces and physical therapy for the spinal curvature, occasional lens removal for the lens dislocations, etc.). For girls who have grown quite tall, and have cosmetic concerns about any further height, hormonal medications have been given to initiate an early **puberty,** so that growth stops sooner and adult height is closer to normal.

As stated previously, the most important problems to follow closely are those affecting the heart and aorta. Some medications seem to be somewhat useful in slowing the stretching of the aorta, although surgical replacement of part of the aorta is sometimes necessary, as may be replacement of the defective mitral valve.

Prognosis

Careful monitoring of Marfan's patients, along with advice to avoid **stress** (physical, emotional, and the stress of **pregnancy**) has helped to increase the expected life span of Marfan's patients well beyond the age of 30 or 40 years, which was once the typical age of death.

Prevention

While prevention is not totally possible, it is important that any couple who is aware of a family history of Marfan's receive careful **genetic counseling** prior to having a baby. Counseling should provide such a couple with information on which to base their child-bearing decisions, including the fact that the child of a parent with Marfan syndrome has a 50% chance of having Marfan's.

Resources

BOOKS

Cecil Essentials of Medicine, edited by Thomas E. Andreoli. Philadelphia: W.B. Saunders Company, 1997.

Procknop, Darwin J., et al. "Marfan Syndrome." In *Harrison's Principles of Internal Medicine,* edited by Anthony S. Fauci, et al. New York: McGraw-Hill, 1998.

ORGANIZATIONS

National Marfan Foundation. 382 Main Street, Port Washington, NY 11050. (800) 8-MARFAN. http://www.marfan.org.

Rosalyn S. Carson-DeWitt

Marie-Strümpell disease *see* **Ankylosing spondylitis**

Marriage counseling

Definition

Marriage counseling is a type of psychotherapy for a married couple or established partners that tries to resolve problems in the relationship. Typically, two people attend counseling sessions together to discuss specific issues.

Purpose

Marriage counseling is based on research that shows that individuals and their problems are best handled within the context of their relationships. Marriage counselors are trained in psychotherapy and family systems, and focus on understanding their clients' symptoms and the way their interactions contribute to problems in the relationship.

Description

Marriage counseling is usually a short-term therapy that may take only a few sessions to work out problems in the relationship. Typically, marriage counselors ask questions about the couple's roles, patterns, rules, goals, and beliefs. Therapy often begins as the couple analyzes the good and bad aspects of the relationship. The marriage counselor then works with the couple to help them understand that, in most cases, both partners are contributing to problems in the relationship. When this is understood, the two can then learn to change how they interact with each other to solve problems. The partners may be encouraged to draw up a contract in which each partner describes the behavior he or she will be trying to maintain.

Marriage is not a requirement for two people to get help from a marriage counselor. Anyone person wishing to improve his or her relationships can get help with behavioral problems, relationship issues, or with mental or emotional disorders. Marriage counselors also offer treatment for couples before they get married to help them understand potential problem areas. A third type of marriage counseling involves postmarital therapy, in which divorcing couples who share children seek help in working out their differences. Couples in the midst of a divorce find that marriage therapy during separation can help them find a common ground as they negotiate interpersonal issues and child custody.

Choosing a therapist

A marriage counselor is trained to use different types of therapy in work with individuals, couples, and groups. American Association of Marriage and Family Therapy (AAMFT) training includes supervision by experienced therapists, a minimum of a master's degree (including specific training in marriage and **family therapy**), and specific graduate training in marriage and family therapy.

When looking for a marriage counselor, a couple should find out the counselor's training and educational background, professional associations, such as AAMFT, and state licensure, and whether the person has experience in treating particular kinds of problem. Also, questions should be asked concerning fees, insurance coverage, the average length of therapy, and so on.

Normal results

Marriage counseling helps couples learn to deal more effectively with problems, and can help prevent small problems from becoming serious. Research shows that marriage counseling, when effective, tends to improve a person's physical as well as mental health, in addition to improving the relationship.

Resources

PERIODICALS

Johnson, S.M. and E. Talitman. "Predictors of Success in Emotionally- Focused Marital Therapy." *Journal of Marital and Family Therapy* 23 (1997): 135-152.

Lee, M. "A Study of Solution-Focused Brief Family Therapy: Outcomes and Issues." *The American Journal of Family Therapy* 25 (1997): 3-17.

ORGANIZATIONS

American Association of Marriage and Family Therapy. 1133 Fifteenth St. NW, Ste. 300, Washington, DC 20005. (202) 452-0109.

American Psychological Association. 750 First St. NE, Washington, DC 20002. (202) 336-5500.

Carol A. Turkington

Marshall-Marchetti-Krantz procedure

Definition

The Marshall-Marchetti-Krantz procedure surgically reinforces the bladder neck in order to prevent unintentional urine loss.

Purpose

The Marshall-Marchetti-Krantz procedure is performed to correct stress incontinence in women, a common result of **childbirth** and/or **menopause.** Incontinence also occurs when an individual involuntarily loses urine after pressure is placed on the abdomen

KEY TERMS

Biofeedback—Biofeedback training monitors temperature and muscle contractions in the vagina to help incontinent patients control their pelvic muscles.

Bladder training—A behavioral modification program used to treat stress incontinence. Bladder training involves putting the patient on a toilet schedule, and gradually increasing the time interval between urination.

Catheter—A long, thin, flexible tube. A catheter is used to drain the bladder of urine during a Marshall-Marchetti-Krantz procedure.

Kegel exercises—Exercises that tighten the pelvic floor muscles. Kegel exercises can assist some women in controlling their stress incontinence.

Urethra—The narrow tube, leading from the bladder that drains the body's urine.

(like during **exercise,** sexual activity, sneezing, coughing, laughing, or hugging).

Precautions

In some women, stress incontinence may be controlled through nonsurgical means, such as:

- Kegel exercises (exercises that tighten pelvic muscles)
- **Biofeedback** (monitors temperature and muscle contractions in the vagina to help incontinent patients control their pelvic muscles)
- **Bladder training** (behavioral modification program used to treat stress incontinence)
- Medication
- Inserted incontinence devices.

Each patient should undergo a full diagnostic workup to determine the best course of treatment.

Description

The Marshall-Marchetti-Krantz procedure, also known as retropubic suspension or bladder neck suspension surgery, is performed by a surgeon in a hospital setting. The patient is placed under general anesthesia, and a long, thin, flexible tube (catheter) is inserted into the bladder through the narrow tube (urethra) that drains the body's urine. An incision is made across the abdomen, and the bladder is exposed. The bladder is separated from surrounding tissues. Stitches (sutures) are placed in these tissues near the bladder neck and urethra. The urethra is then lifted, and the sutures are attached to the pubic bone itself, or to tissue (fascia) behind the pubic bone. The sutures support the bladder neck, helping the patient gain control over urine flow.

Preparation

A complete evaluation to determine the cause of incontinence is critical to proper treatment. A thorough medical history and general **physical examination** should be performed on candidates for the Marshall-Marchetti-Krantz procedure. Diagnostic testing may include x rays, ultrasound, urine tests, and examination of the pelvis. It may also include a series of urodynamic testing exams that measure bladder pressure and capacity, and urinary flow.

Patients undergoing a Marshall-Marchetti-Krantz procedure must not eat or drink for eight hours prior to the surgery.

Aftercare

Recovery from a Marshall-Marchetti-Krantz procedure requires two to six days of hospitalization. The catheter will be removed from the patient's bladder once normal bladder function resumes. Patients are advised to refrain from heavy lifting for four to six weeks after the procedure.

Patients should contact their physician immediately if they experience **fever, dizziness,** or extreme nausea, or if their incision site becomes swollen, red, or hard.

Risks

The Marshall-Marchetti-Krantz procedure is an invasive surgical procedure and, as such, it carries risks of infection, internal bleeding, and hemorrhage. There is also a possibility of permanent damage to the bladder or urethra. The urethra may become scarred, causing a permanent narrowing, or stricture.

Normal results

Approximately 85% of women who undergo the Marshall-Marchetti-Krantz procedure are cured of their stress incontinence.

Resources

BOOKS

Blaivas, Jerry. *Conquering Bladder and Prostate Problems: The Authoritative Guide for Men and Women.* New York: Plenum, 1998.

ORGANIZATIONS

American Foundation for Urologic Disease. 1128 North Charles Street, Baltimore, MD 21201. (800)242-2383. http://www.afud.org/.

National Association for Continence. 2650 East Main Street, Spartanburg, SC 29307. (800) 252-3337. http://www.nafc.org/.

National Kidney and Urologic Diseases Information Clearinghouse (NKUDIC). 3 Information Way, Bethesda, MD 20892-3508. (800) 891-5388. http://www.niddk.nih.gov/health/urolog/pubs/kuorg/kuorg.htm/.

Paula Anne Ford-Martin

Massage

Definition

Massage is a manual means of rubbing and kneading soft tissues of the body to stimulate circulation and promote relaxation of muscles. There are many forms of massage in use throughout the world, including Swedish, deep tissue, Tui Na, Hawaiian, and others. For the most part, this article discusses the form most commonly used in sports medicine in the United States, a derivation of Swedish massage.

Purpose

Massage helps the muscles relax by stimulating a reflex response of the nervous system. The application of smooth, steady, rhythmical massage can relieve tension and soothe sore muscles. This decrease in muscle tension causes the muscle to become more relaxed and elastic. Also, massage's effect on the circulatory system is beneficial for the healing of soft tissue injuries.

Massage's ability to aid in the recovery from soft tissue injuries, such as **sprains and strains,** is an important use of massage. Many soft tissue injuries are not serious enough to cause a visit to the doctor or hospital for treatment. Therefore, many injuries are treated with first aid; but they still may cause some discomfort and disability long after the initial injury. Massage can speed and improve the rate of recovery and reduce discomfort from such mishaps.

To understand how massage helps healing in cases of soft tissue injury, it is important to understand the inflammatory process. Inflammation begins because blood circulates to the injured area to bring important chemicals essential for healing. After a period of time, the initial inflammation stops. If applied at this point, massage will help again increase circulation, and thus promote healing, as the increased blood flow brings additional oxygen and nutrients to the injured area. In this way, massage helps bridge the gap between common neglect of injury and major expensive medical intervention.

Massage can also help stimulate the flow of lymph, the fluid that helps the body remove waste products. Massage helps facilitate the flow of lymph to areas where **pain** has slowed down the ability of this natural cleanser to remove the waste products of the injury.

Massage can affect muscles directly by stimulating inactive muscles whose inactivity is due to illness or injury. Deep continuous massage can relieve muscle tension and help prevent painful muscle spasms, which are common following injury. Also, massage can stretch and break down fibrous scar tissue that is not healing properly because it is not aligned to the adjoining muscle fibers.

Massage affects pain through the central nervous system. In one particular theory of pain called the ''gate theory,'' messages of pain which normally travel from the injury to the brain, are blocked before reaching the centers responsible for interpreting pain. Massage helps stimulate and close the so-called gate of pain messages. As a result, the intensity of the pain perceived by the brain is decreased.

Psychosomatic studies show how **stress** factors can cause migraines, **hypertension,** depression, some peptic **ulcers,** etc. Some researchers have estimated that 80% of disease is stress related. Soothing and relaxing massage therapy can help reduce illness by counteracting stress effects.

Precautions

Massage usually is not recommended for individuals with a circulatory problem; it could produce complications in individuals with high blood pressure or a history of heart trouble. Injury to bone can occur if massage is performed too soon after injury over an area of advanced **osteoporosis** or bone fracture. Also, in cases of **cancer,** massage is contra-indicted because an increase in circulation might help the cancer spread more rapidly. Severe diabetes, skin infection, tubercular joints, **burns,** or abrasions may also be indications that massage should be avoided.

When selecting a massage therapist, it is important to check his or her credentials, including whether he or she has graduated from a school approved by a credible accrediting agency, such as the Commission for Massage Training Accreditation (COMTA). Also one could check whether the therapist is a member of AMTA (American Massage Therapy Association).

Description

Massage is a valuable tool in the management of many musculoskeletal disorders. While there are many forms of massage in use around the world, Swedish type massage is the type most commonly used in sports medicine in the United States. Sports medicine massage can be separated into five basic categories.

Effluerage

Effleurage is primarily a stroking technique that is divided into light and deep methods. Light stroking methods are used to sedate, while deeper stroking provides a method to compress the soft tissue and encourage circulation.

Petrissage

Petrissage is a kneading procedure used on loose, heavy tissues found in larger muscle groups of the body. This kneading action wrings out the muscle, which results in loosening adhesions left from the healing process, and squeezing out unwanted waste materials, thus facilitating movement of these waste products back into the circulatory system.

Friction massage

Friction massage is a useful method applied around joints and other areas where tissues are thin and more resilient. This includes scars and adhesions — the goal being to stretch underlying tissues and exert friction on the area. Friction massage is also utilized to increase circulation, especially around a joint.

Tapotement

In the massage technique termed tapotement, a portion of the body is tapped in a rhythmic manner with the fingers or sides of the hands, using short, rapid repetitive movements. This method can be performed by several techniques including cupping with the hands to create a dull hollow sound, or hacking, using the little finger side of the hand to strike the surface of the skin and rhythmically tapping with the finger tips.

Vibration

Vibration produces a quivering or trembling in the muscle and soft tissue. It is used primarily to soothe and promote relaxation. Vibration may be produced either manually or with the aid of a electrical vibrator machine.

Preparation

The client will undress and lie, totally draped, on a massage table. Only the area being massaged will be undraped. Since the client may have to be helped to relax prior to the massage, coaching the subject to feel at ease becomes an important aspect of the preparation. Then, in many instances, heat or ice may be applied prior to the massage. Heat is helpful to enhance relaxation and circulation. Cold, in the form of ice, can be helpful for pain reduction if the area is slightly tender.

Aftercare

During the final portion of the massage, light stroking methods are used to help relax tissues that may have been previously stimulated from more aggressive kneading techniques. The individual is often shown stretching **exercises** he may use to help continue the benefits the massage has produced in muscle flexibility and pain reduction.

Risks

Massage can have adverse effects if not used properly, or if used over inappropriate areas. Massage will also have a negative effect if applied over an area that is infected. Massage over a recent injury may increase the inflammation and possibly cause additional soft tissue injury.

Normal results

If massage is applied properly and under the correct conditions, muscle relaxation occurs along with increased circulation resulting in the enhancement of the healing process for the individual.

Abnormal results

If an individual has poor circulation, abnormal results are possible, such as a decrease or unwanted fluctuation in blood supply to critical areas of the body. As noted, massage can produce abnormal blood flow in individuals with high blood pressure or a history of heart trouble. Injury to bone can occur if massage is performed too soon over a bone fracture, or over an area of advanced osteoporosis.

Resources

BOOKS

Hertling, Darlene, and Randolph M. Kessler. *Management of Common Musculoskeletal Disorders: Physical Therapy Principles and Methods.* Philadelphia, PA: J.B. Lippincott Company, 1990.

PERIODICALS

Larson, Jeffrey P. "Massage as a Modality in Trauma and Sports Medicine." *Trauma* 35(Dec. 1993): 81-94.

ORGANIZATIONS

American Massage Therapy Association. 820 Davis Street, Suite 100, Evanston, Illinois 60201-4444.

Jeffrey Peter Larson

Mastectomy

Definition

Mastectomy is the surgical removal of the breast for the treatment or prevention of **breast cancer.**

Purpose

The size, location, and type of tumor are very important when choosing the best surgery to treat a woman's breast cancer. The size of the breast is also an important factor. A woman's psychological concerns, and her lifestyle choices should also be considered when decisions are made.

The severity of a **cancer** is evaluated according to a complex system called staging. This takes into account the size of the tumor, and whether it has spread to the lymph nodes, adjacent tissues, and/or distant parts of the body. A mastectomy is usually the recommended surgery for more advanced breast cancers. Women with earlier stage breast cancers, who could have breast conserving surgery (**lumpectomy**), may decide to have a mastectomy.

There are many factors that make a mastectomy the treatment of choice for a patient. A large tumor is often an indication of a later stage of breast cancer, when the removal of the entire breast is recommended. In addition, large tumors are difficult to remove with good cosmetic results. This is especially true if the woman has small breasts. Very rapidly growing breast cancers are usually treated with a mastectomy. Sometimes multiple areas of cancer are found in one breast, making removal of the whole breast necessary. A cancer that has already attached itself to nearby tissues, such as the skin or chest wall, is most likely to be removed with a mastectomy.

Breast conserving surgery may be attempted, but prove unsuccessful. The surgeon is sometimes unable to remove the tumor with a sufficient amount, or margin, of normal tissue surrounding it. The entire breast needs to be removed in this situation. Recurrence of breast cancer after a lumpectomy is another indication for mastectomy.

Radiation therapy is almost always recommended following a lumpectomy. If a woman is unable to have radiation, a mastectomy is the treatment of choice. Pregnant women cannot have radiation therapy, for fear of harming the fetus. A woman with certain collagen vascular diseases, such as **systemic lupus erythematosus** or **scleroderma,** would experience unacceptable scarring and damage to her connective tissue from radiation exposure. Any woman who has had therapeutic radiation to the chest area for other reasons cannot tolerate additional exposure for breast cancer therapy. Diminished lung capacity due to other disease also makes a woman a poor candidate for radiation therapy.

The need for radiation therapy after breast conserving surgery may make mastectomy more appealing for nonmedical reasons. Some women fear radiation, and choose the more extensive surgery, so radiation treatment will not be required. The commitment of time, usually five days a week, for six weeks, may not be acceptable for other women. This may be due to financial, personal, or job-related factors. In geographically isolated areas, a course of radiation therapy may require lengthy travel, and perhaps unacceptable amounts of time away from family or other responsibilities.

Some women choose mastectomy because they strongly fear recurrence of the breast cancer, and lumpectomy seems too risky. Keeping a breast that has contained cancer may feel uncomfortable for some patients. They prefer mastectomy, so the entire breast will be removed.

The issue of prophylactic mastectomy, or removal of the breast to prevent future breast cancer, is controversial. Women with a strong family history of breast cancer and/ or who test positive for a known cancer-causing gene may choose this option. Patients who have had certain types of breast cancers that are more likely to recur may elect to have the unaffected breast removed. Although there is some evidence that this procedure can decrease the chances of developing breast cancer, it is not a guarantee. It is not possible to be certain that all breast tissue has been removed. There have been cases where breast cancers have occurred after both breasts have been removed.

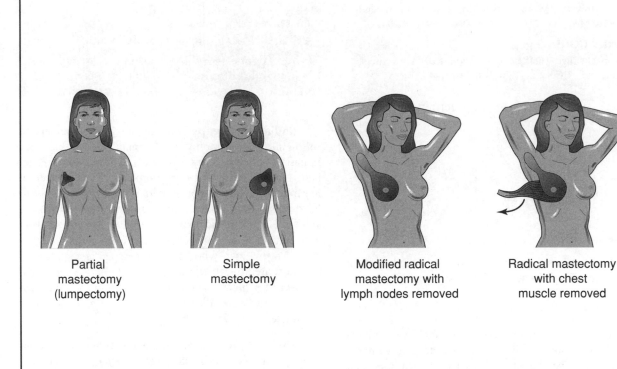

Partial
mastectomy
(lumpectomy)

Simple
mastectomy

Modified radical
mastectomy with
lymph nodes removed

Radical mastectomy
with chest
muscle removed

There are four types of mastectomies: partial mastectomy, or lumpectomy, in which the tumor and surrounding tissue is removed; simple mastectomy, where the entire breast and some axillary lymph nodes are removed; modified radical mastectomy, in which the entire breast and all axillary lymph nodes are removed; and the radical mastectomy, where the entire breast, axillary lymph nodes, and chest muscles are removed. *(Illustration by Electronic Illustrators Group.)*

Precautions

The decision to have mastectomy or lumpectomy should be carefully considered. It is important that the woman be fully informed of all the potential risks and benefits of different surgical treatments before making a choice.

Description

There are several types of mastectomies. The radical mastectomy, also called the Halsted mastectomy, is very rarely performed today. It was developed in the late 1800s, when it was thought that more extensive surgery was most likely to cure cancer. A radical mastectomy involves removal of the breast, all surrounding lymph nodes up to the collarbone, and the underlying chest muscle. Women were often left disfigured and disabled, with a large defect in the chest wall and significantly decreased arm sensation and motion. Unfortunately, and inaccurately, it is still the operation many women picture, when the word mastectomy is mentioned.

Surgery that removes breast tissue and some axillary or underarm lymph nodes and leaves the chest muscle intact is usually called a modified radical mastectomy. This is the most common type of mastectomy performed in the 1990s. The surgery leaves a woman with a more normal chest shape than the older radical mastectomy procedure, and a scar which is not visible in most clothing. It also allows for immediate or delayed **breast reconstruction.**

In a simple mastectomy, only the breast itself is removed. If a few of the axillary lymph nodes closest to the breast are also taken out, the surgery may be called an extended simple mastectomy.

There are other variations on the term mastectomy. A skin-sparing mastectomy uses special techniques that preserve the patient's breast skin for use in reconstruction. Total mastectomy is a confusing expression, as it may be used to refer to a modified radical mastectomy or a simple mastectomy.

A mastectomy is typically performed in a hospital setting, but specialized outpatient facilities are sometimes used. The surgery is done under general anesthesia. The type and location of the incision may vary according to plans for reconstruction or other factors, such as old scars. As much breast tissue as possible is removed. Axillary lymph nodes are taken out if they were not removed with biopsy. Approximately 10-15 nodes are usually removed. All tissue is sent to the pathology laboratory for analysis. If no immediate reconstruction is planned, surgical drains are left in place to prevent fluid accumulation. The skin is sutured, and bandages are applied.

The surgery may take from two to five hours. Women usually stay at least one night in the hospital, although some surgeons advocate outpatient mastectomy for selected patients. The cost is approximately $2,600-$3,200 or more for a simple mastectomy. Charges for a modified radical mastectomy with axillary node removal range from $4,500-$8,000. Insurance usually covers the cost of mastectomy. If immediate reconstruction is performed, the length of stay, recovery period, insurance reimbursement, and fees will vary from mastectomy alone.

Preparation

Routine preoperative preparations, such as nothing to eat or drink the night before surgery, are typically ordered for a mastectomy. Information regarding expected outcomes and potential complications should also be a part of preparation for a mastectomy, as for any surgical procedure. It is especially important that women know about sensations they might experience after surgery, so they are not misinterpreted as a sign of poor wound healing or recurrent cancer.

Aftercare

In the past, women often stayed in the hospital at least several days. Now many patients go home within a day or two after their mastectomies. Visits from home care nurses can sometimes be arranged, but patients need to learn how to care for themselves before discharge from the hospital.

The woman may need to learn to change her bandages, and/or care for the incision. The surgical drains must be attended to properly. This includes emptying the drain, measuring the fluid output, moving clots through the drain, and identifying problems that need attention from the doctor or nurse. If the drain becomes blocked, fluid or blood may collect at the surgical site. Left untreated, this accumulation may cause infection and/or delayed wound healing.

After a mastectomy, activities such as driving may be restricted according to individual needs. **Pain** is usu-ally well controlled with prescribed medication. Severe pain may be a sign of complications, and should be reported to the physician. A return visit to the surgeon is usually scheduled 7-10 days after the procedure.

Exercises to maintain shoulder and arm mobility may be prescribed as early as 24 hours after surgery. These are very important in restoring strength and promoting good circulation. The specific exercises will change as healing progresses. Physical therapy is an integral part of care after a mastectomy, aiding in the overall recovery process.

Emotional care is another important aspect of recovery from a mastectomy. Patients are often advised to seek counseling and/or support groups. Assistance in dealing with the psychological effects of the breast cancer diagnosis, as well as the surgery, can be invaluable for women.

Measures to prevent injury or infection to the affected arm should be taken, especially if axillary lymph nodes were removed. There are a number of specific instructions, all directed toward avoiding pressure or constriction of the arm. Extra care must be exercised to avoid injury, treat it properly if it occurs, and seek medical attention promptly when appropriate.

Additional treatment for breast cancer may be necessary after a mastectomy. Depending on the type of tumor, lymph node status, and other factors, **chemotherapy,** radiation therapy, and/or hormone therapy may be prescribed.

Risks

Risks that are common to any surgical procedure include bleeding, infection, anesthesia reaction, or unexpected scarring. After mastectomy and axillary lymph node dissection, a number of complications are possible. A woman may experience decreased feeling in the back of her armpit, or other sensations including numbness, tingling, or increased skin sensitivity. Some women report phantom breast symptoms, experiencing **itching,** aching, or other sensations in the breast that has been removed. There may be injury to the nerves controlling arm motion, resulting in decreased arm mobility.

Approximately 2-10% of patients develop **lymphedema** after axillary lymph node removal. This swelling of the arm, caused by faulty lymph drainage, can range from mild to very severe. It can be treated with elevation, elastic bandages, and specialized physical therapy. Lymphedema is a chronic condition, which requires continuing treatment. This complication can arise at any time, even years after surgery. A new technique called sentinel node biopsy, which may eliminate the need for removing many lymph nodes, is being tested.

Normal results

A mastectomy is performed as the definitive surgical treatment for breast cancer. The expected outcome is no recurrence of the breast cancer.

Resources

BOOKS

Love, Susan M. with Karen Lindsey. *Dr. Susan Love's Breast Book.* 2nd edition. Reading, MA: Addison-Wesley, 1995.

Robinson, Rebecca Y. and Jeanne A. Petrek. *A Step-by-Step Guide to Dealing With Your Breast Cancer.* New York: Carol Publishing Group, 1994.

PERIODICALS

Lynden, Patricia. ''Your Breasts or Your Life.'' *American Health for Women* 16 (June 1997): 29-31.

ORGANIZATIONS

American Cancer Society. 1599 Clifton Rd., NE, Atlanta, GA 30329-4251. (800) 227-2345. http://www.cancer.org.

National Lymphedema Network. 2211 Post Street, Suite 404, San Francisco, CA 94115-3427. (800) 541-3259 or (415) 921-1306. http://www.wenet.net/~lymphnet/.

Y-ME National Organization for Breast Cancer Information and Support. 18220 Harwood Ave., Homewood, IL 60430. Hotlines: (800) 221-2141 or (708) 799-8228 (available 24 hours).

Ellen S. Weber

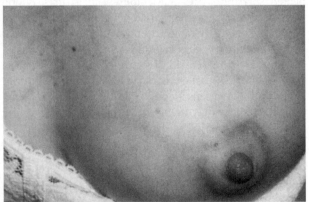

Mastitis is usually caused by a bacterial infection through a nipple damaged during breast feeding. *(Photograph by Dr. P. Marazzi, Photo Researchers, Inc. Reproduced by permission.)*

Mastitis

Definition

Mastitis is an infection of the breast. It usually only occurs in women who are breastfeeding their babies.

Description

Breastfeeding is the act of allowing a baby to suckle at the breast, in order to drink the mother's milk. In the process, unaccustomed to the vigorous pull and tug of the infant's suck, the nipples may become sore, cracked, or slightly abraded. This creates a tiny opening in the breast, through which bacteria can enter. The presence of milk, with high sugar content, gives the bacteria an excellent source of nutrition. Under these conditions, the bacteria are able to multiply, until they are plentiful enough to cause an infection within the breast.

Mastitis usually begins more than two to four weeks after delivery of the baby. It is a relatively uncommon complication of breastfeeding mothers, occurring in only approximately 2% of women.

Causes & symptoms

The most common bacteria causing mastitis is called *Staphylococcus aureus*. In 25-30% of people, this bacteria is present on the skin lining normal, uninfected nostrils. It is probably this bacteria, clinging to the baby's nostrils, that is available to create infection when an opportunity (crack in the nipple) presents itself.

Usually, only one breast is involved. An area of the affected breast becomes swollen, red, hard, and painful. Other symptoms of mastitis include **fever,** chills, and increased heart rate.

Diagnosis

Diagnosis involves obtaining a sample of breast milk from the infected breast. The milk is cultured, allowing colonies of bacteria to grow. The causative bacteria can then be specially prepared for identification under a microscope. At the same time, tests can be performed to determine what type of antibiotic would be most effective against that particular bacteria.

Treatment

The **antibiotics** dicloxacillin and erythromycin are both used to treat mastitis. Breastfeeding should be continued, because the rate of **abscess** formation (an abscess is a persistent pocket of pus) in the infected breast goes up steeply among women who stop breastfeeding during a bout with mastitis. Most practitioners allow women to take **acetaminophen** while nursing, to relieve both fever and **pain.** As always, breastfeeding women need to make sure that any medication they take is also safe for the baby, since almost all drugs they take appear in the breastmilk. Warm compresses applied to the affected breast can be soothing.

Prognosis

Prognosis for uncomplicated mastitis is excellent. About 10% of women with mastitis will end up with an abscess within the affected breast. An abscess is a collection of pus within the breast. This complication will require a surgical procedure to drain the pus.

Prevention

The most important aspect of prevention involves good handwashing to try to prevent the infant from acquiring the *Staphylococcus aureus* bacteria in the first place.

Resources

BOOKS

Current Obstetric & Gynecologic Diagnosis & Treatment, edited by Alan H. DeCherney. Norwalk, CT: Appleton & Lange, 1994.

Williams Obstetrics, edited by F. Gary Cunningham, et al. Stamford, CT: Appleton & Lange, 1997.

ORGANIZATIONS

LaLeche League International. 1400 N. Meacham Rd., Schaumburg, IL 60173-4048. (847) 519-7730 or (800) LALECHE. http://www.lalecheleague.org.

Rosalyn S. Carson-DeWitt

Mastocytosis

Definition

Mastocytosis is a disease characterized by the presence of too many mast cells in various organs and tissues.

Description

The body has a variety of free-roaming cell populations that function as immunogenic agents. Most immunogenic cells fall into the category of white blood cells, but some remain in tissues and are not found in the blood. Mast cells are such a group.

Mast cells are found primarily in the skin and digestive system, including the liver and spleen, and produce histamine, a chemical most famous for its ability to cause **itching.** Histamine also causes acid indigestion,

diarrhea, flushing, heart pounding, **headaches,** and can even cause the blood pressure to drop suddenly.

Mastocytosis comes in three forms. Most cases produce symptoms but do not shorten life expectancy. The three forms are:

- Mastocytoma, a benign skin tumor.
- Urticaria pigmentosa, small collections of mast cells in the skin that manifest as salmon or brown-colored patches.
- Systemic mastocytosis, the collection of mast cells in the skin, lymph nodes, liver, spleen, gastrointestinal tract, and bones.

Causes & symptoms

The cause of mastocytosis is unknown. People with systemic mastocytosis have bone and joint pain. Peptic **ulcers** are frequent because of the increased stomach acid stimulated by histamine. Many patients with systemic mastocytosis also develop urticaria pigmentosa. These skin lesions itch when stroked and may become fluid-filled.

Diagnosis

A biopsy of the skin patches aids diagnosis. An elevated level of histamine in the urine or blood is also indicative of mastocytosis.

Treatment

Mastocytoma usually occurs in childhood and clears-up on its own. Urticaria pigmentosa (present alone without systemic disease) also dramatically clears or improves as adolescence approaches.

Several medications are helpful in relieving symptoms of systemic mastocytosis. **Antihistamines** and drugs that reduce stomach acid are frequently needed. Headaches respond to migraine treatment. A medicine called cromolyn helps with the bowel symptoms. Several other standard and experimental medications have been used.

Prognosis

Mastocytoma and urticaria pigmentosa rarely if ever, develop into systemic mastocytosis, and both spontaneously improve over time. Systemic mastocytosis is only symptomatically treated. There is no known treatment that decreases the number of mast cells within tissue.

Resources

BOOKS

Austen, K. Frank. "Diseases of immediate type hypersensitivity." In *Harrison's Principles of Internal Medicine,* edited by Anthony S. Fauci, et al. New York: McGraw-Hill, 1998, pp.1866-1867.

Metcalfe, Dean D. "Mastocytosis." In *Cecil Textbook of Medicine,* edited by J. Claude Bennett and Fred Plum. Philadelphia: W. B. Saunders, 1996, pp.1435-1437.

J. Ricker Polsdorfer

Mastoidectomy

Definition

Mastoidectomy is a surgical procedure to remove an infected portion of the bone behind the ear when medical treatment is not effective. This surgery is rarely needed today because of the widespread use of **antibiotics.**

Purpose

Mastoidectomy is performed to remove infected air cells within the mastoid bone caused by **mastoiditis,** ear infection, or an inflammatory disease of the middle ear (cholesteatoma). The cells are open spaces containing air that are located throughout the mastoid bone. They are connected to a cavity in the upper part of the bone, which is in turn connected to the middle ear. As a result, infections in the middle ear can sometimes spread through the mastoid bone. When antibiotics can't clear this infection, it may be necessary to remove the infected air cells by surgery. Mastoidectomies are also performed sometimes to repair paralyzed facial nerves.

Description

Mastoidectomy is performed less often today because of the widespread use of antibiotics to treat ear infections.

There are several different types of mastoidectomy:

• Simple (or closed). The operation is performed through the ear or through a cut (incision) behind the ear. The surgeon opens the mastoid bone and removes the in-

fected air cells. The eardrum is cut (incised) to drain the middle ear. **Topical antibiotics** are then placed in the ear.

• Radical mastoidectomy. The eardrum and most middle ear structures are removed, but the innermost small bone (the stapes) is left behind so that a hearing aid can be used later to offset the **hearing loss.**

• Modified radical mastoidectomy. The eardrum and the middle ear structures are saved, which allows for better hearing than is possible after a radical operation.

The wound is then stitched up around a drainage tube, which is removed a day or two later. The procedure usually takes between two and three hours.

Preparation

The doctor will give the patient a thorough ear, nose, and throat examination as well as a detailed hearing test before surgery. Patients are given an injection before surgery to make them drowsy.

Aftercare

Painkillers are usually needed for the first day or two after the operation. The patient should drink fluids freely. After the stitches are removed, the bulky mastoid dressing can be replaced with a smaller dressing if the ear is still draining. The patient is given antibiotics for several days.

The patient should tell the doctor if any of the following symptoms occur:

• Bright red blood on the dressing.

• Stiff neck or disorientation. These may be signs of **meningitis.**

• Facial **paralysis,** drooping mouth, or problems swallowing.

Risks

Complications don't often occur, but they may include:

• Persistent ear drainage.

• Infections, including meningitis or **brain abscesses.**

• Hearing loss.

• Facial nerve injury. This is a rare complication.

• Temporary **dizziness.**

• Temporary loss of taste on the side of the tongue.

Resources

BOOKS

Turkington, Carol A. *The Hearing Loss Sourcebook.* New York: Plume/Signet, 1997.

ORGANIZATIONS

American Academy of Otolaryngology-Head and Neck Surgery. 1 Prince St., Alexandria, VA 22316. (703) 836-4444.

American Hearing Research Foundation. 55 E. Washington St., Ste. 2022, Chicago, IL 60602. (312) 726-9670.

Better Hearing Institute. PO Box 1840, Washington, DC 20013. (800) EAR-WELL.

Carol A. Turkington

Mastoiditis

Definition

Mastoiditis is an infection of the spaces within the mastoid bone. It is almost always associated with **otitis media,** an infection of the middle ear. In the most serious cases, the bone itself becomes infected.

Description

The mastoid is a part of the side (temporal bone) of the skull. It can be felt as a bony bump just behind and slightly above the level of the earlobe. The mastoid has been described as resembling a "honeycomb" of tiny partitioned-off airspaces. The mastoid is connected with the middle ear, so that when there is a collection of fluid in the middle ear, there is usually also a slight collection of fluid within the airspaces of the mastoid.

Mastoiditis can range from a simple case of some fluid escaping into the mastoid air cells during a middle ear infection, to a more complex infection which penetrates through to the lining of the mastoid bone, to a very

---

severe and destructive infection of the mastoid bone itself.

Causes & symptoms

Mastoiditis is caused by the same types of bacteria which cause middle ear infections (*Streptococcus pneumoniae* and *Haemophilus influenzae*), as well as by a variety of other bacteria (*Staphylococcus aureus, Pseuodomonas aeruginosa, Klebsiella, Escherichia coli, Proteus, Prevotella, Fusobacterium, Porphyromonas,* and *Bacteroides*). Mastoiditis may occur due to the progression of an untreated, or undertreated, middle ear infection.

Symptoms of mastoiditis may at first be the same as symptoms of an early middle ear infection. With progression, however, the swollen mastoid may push the outer ear slightly forward and away from the head. The area behind the ear will appear red and swollen, and will be very sore. There may be drainage of pus from the infected ear. In some cases, the skin over the mastoid may develop an opening through which pus drains. **Fever** is common.

Diagnosis

Mastoiditis is usually suspected when a severe middle ear infection is accompanied by redness, swelling, and **pain** in the mastoid area. A **computed tomography scan** (CT scan) will show inflammation and fluid within the airspaces of the mastoid, as well as the erosion of the little walls of bone that should separate the air spaces. If there is any fluid draining from the ear or mastoid, this can be collected and processed in a laboratory to allow identification of the causative organism. If there is no fluid available, a tiny needle can be used to obtain a sample of the fluid which has accumulated behind the eardrum.

Treatment

Identification of the causative organism guides the practitioner's choice of antibiotic. Depending on the severity of the infection, the antibiotic can be given initially through a needle in the vein (intravenously or IV), and then (as the patient improves) by mouth.

In the case of a very severe infection of the mastoid bone itself, with a collection of pus (**abscess**), an operation to remove the mastoid part of the temporal bone is often necessary (**mastoidectomy**).

Prognosis

With early identification of mastoiditis, the prognosis is very good. When symptoms are not caught early enough, however, a number of complications can occur. These include an infection of the tissues covering the brain and spinal cord (**meningitis**), a pocket of infection within the brain (abscess), or an abscess within the muscles of the neck. All of these complications have potentially more serious prognoses.

Prevention

Prevention of mastoiditis involves careful and complete treatment of any middle ear infections.

Resources

BOOKS

Duran, Marlene, et al. "Infections of the Upper Respiratory Tract." In *Harrison's Principles of Internal Medicine,* edited by Anthony S. Fauci, et al. New York: McGraw-Hill, 1998.

"Otitis Media and its Complications." In *Nelson Textbook of Pediatrics,* edited by Richard Behrman. Philadelphia: W.B. Saunders Co., 1996.

Ray, C. George. "Eye, Ear, and Sinus Infections." In *Sherris Medical Microbiology: An Introduction to Infectious Diseases,* edited by Kenneth J. Ryan. Norwalk, CT: Appleton and Lange, 1994.

ORGANIZATIONS

American Academy of Otolaryngology-Head and Neck Surgery. One Prince Street, Alexandria VA 22314-3357. (703) 836-4444.

Rosalyn S. Carson-DeWitt

Maternal serum alpha-fetoprotein test *see* **Alpha-fetoprotein test**

Mathematics disorder *see* **Learning disorders**

McArdle's disease *see* **Glycogen storage diseases**

MCS syndrome *see* **Multiple chemical sensitivity**

MD *see* **Muscular dystrophy**

Measles

Definition

Measles is an infection, caused by a virus, which causes an illness displaying a characteristic skin rash. Measles is also sometimes called rubeola, 5-day measles, or hard measles.

Description

Measles infections appear all over the world. Prior to the current effective immunization program, large-scale measles outbreaks occurred on a two to three-year cycle, usually in the winter and spring. Smaller outbreaks occurred during the off-years. Babies up to about eight months of age are usually protected from contracting measles, due to immune cells they receive from their mothers in the uterus. Once someone has had measles infection, he or she can never get it again.

Causes & symptoms

Measles is caused by a type of virus called a paramyxovirus. It is an extremely contagious infection, spread through the tiny droplets that may spray into the air when an individual carrying the virus sneezes or **coughs.** About 85% of those people exposed to the virus will become infected with it. About 95% of those people infected with the virus will develop the illness called measles. Once someone is infected with the virus, it takes about 7-18 days before he or she actually becomes ill. The most contagious time period is the three to five days before symptoms begin through about four days after the characteristic measles rash has begun to appear.

The first signs of measles infection are **fever,** extremely runny nose, red, runny eyes, and a cough. A few days later, a rash appears in the mouth, particularly on the mucous membrane which lines the cheeks. This rash consists of tiny white dots (like grains of salt or sand) on a reddish bump. These are called Koplik's spots, and are unique to measles infection. The throat becomes red, swollen, and sore.

A couple of days after the appearance of the Koplik's spots, the measles rash begins. It appears in a characteristic progression, from the head, face, and neck, to the trunk, then abdomen, and next out along the arms and legs. The rash starts out as flat, red patches, but eventually develops some bumps. The rash may be somewhat itchy. When the rash begins to appear, the fever usually

KEY TERMS

Antibodies—Cells made by the immune system which have the ability to recognize foreign invaders (bacteria, viruses), and thus stimulate the immune system to kill them.

Antigens—Markers on the outside of such organisms as bacteria and viruses, which allow antibodies to recognize foreign invaders.

Encephalitis—Swelling, inflammation of the brain.

Koplik's spots—Tiny spots occurring inside the mouth, especially on the inside of the cheek. These spots consist of minuscule white dots (like grains of salt or sand) set onto a reddened bump. Unique to measles.

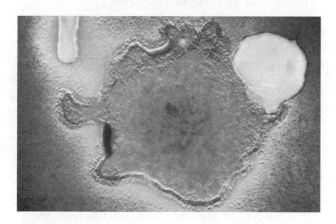

A transmission electron microscopy (TEM) image of a single measles virion. *(Custom Medical Stock Photo. Reproduced by permission.)*

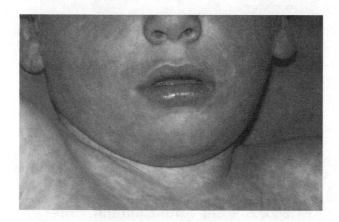

Measles on child's face. *(Custom Medical Stock Photo. Reproduced by permission.)*

climbs higher, sometimes reaching as high as 105°F (40.5°C). There may be nausea, vomiting, **diarrhea,** and multiple swollen lymph nodes. The cough is usually more problematic at this point, and the patient feels awful. The rash usually lasts about five days. As it fades, it turns a brownish color, and eventually the affected skin becomes dry and flaky.

Many patients (about 5-15%) develop other complications. Bacterial infections, such as ear infections, sinus infections, and **pneumonia** are common, especially in children. Other viral infections may also strike the patient, including **croup, bronchitis, laryngitis,** or viral pneumonia. Inflammation of the liver, appendix, intestine, or lymph nodes within the abdomen may cause other complications. Rarely, inflammations of the heart or kidneys, a drop in platelet count (causing episodes of difficult-to-control bleeding), or reactivation of an old **tuberculosis** infection can occur.

An extremely serious complication of measles infection is swelling of the brain. Called **encephalitis,** this can occur up to several weeks after the basic measles symptoms have resolved. About one out of every 1,000 patients develops this complication, and about 10-15% of these patients die. Symptoms include fever, **headache,** sleepiness, seizures, and **coma.** Long-term problems following recovery from measles encephalitis may include seizures and **mental retardation.**

A very rare complication of measles can occur up to 10 years following the initial infection. Called **subacute sclerosing panencephalitis,** this is a slowly progressing, smoldering swelling and destruction of the entire brain. It is most common among people who had measles infection prior to the age of two years. Symptoms include changes in personality, decreased intelligence with accompanying school problems, decreased coordination, involuntary jerks and movements of the body. The disease progresses so that the individual becomes increasingly dependent, ultimately becoming bedridden and unaware of his or her surroundings. Blindness may develop, and the temperature may spike (rise rapidly) and fall unpredictably as the brain structures responsible for temperature regulation are affected. **Death** is inevitable.

Diagnosis

Measles infection is almost always diagnosed based on its characteristic symptoms, including Koplik's spots, and a rash which spreads from central body structures out towards the arms and legs. If there is any doubt as to the diagnosis, then a specimen of body fluids (mucus, urine) can be collected and combined with fluorescent-tagged measles virus antibodies. Antibodies are produced by the body's immune cells that can recognize and bind to markers (antigens) on the outside of specific organisms, in this case the measles virus. Once the fluorescent antibodies have attached themselves to the measles antigens in the specimen, the specimen can be viewed under a special microscope to verify the presence of measles virus.

Treatment

There are no treatments available to stop measles infection. Treatment is primarily aimed at helping the patient to be as comfortable as possible, and watching carefully so that **antibiotics** can be started promptly if a bacterial infection develops. Fever and discomfort can be treated with **acetaminophen.** Children with measles should never be given **aspirin,** as this has caused the fatal disease **Reye's syndrome** in the past. A cool-mist vaporizer may help decrease the cough. Patients should be given a lot of liquids to drink, in order to avoid **dehydration** from the fever.

Some studies have shown that children with measles encephalitis benefit from relatively large doses of vitamin A.

Alternative treatment

Botanical immune enhancement (with echinacea, for example) can assist the body in working through this viral infection. Homeopathic support also can be effective throughout the course of the illness. Some specific alternative treatments to soothe patients with measles include the Chinese herbs bupleurum (*Bupleurum chinense*) and peppermint (*Mentha piperita*), as well as a preparation made from empty cicada (*Cryptotympana atrata*) shells. The itchiness of the rash can be relieved with witch hazel (*Hamamelis virginiana*), chickweed (*Stellaria media*), or oatmeal baths. The eyes can be soothed with an eyewash made from the herb eyebright (*Euphrasia officinalis*). Practitioners of **ayurvedic medicine** recommend ginger or clove tea.

Prognosis

The prognosis for an otherwise healthy, well-nourished child who contracts measles is usually quite good. In developing countries, however, death rates may reach 15-25%. Adolescents and adults usually have a more difficult course. Women who contract the disease while pregnant may give birth to a baby with hearing impairment. Although only 1 in 1,000 patients with measles will develop encephalitis, 10-15% of those who do will die, and about another 25% will be left with permanent brain damage.

Prevention

Measles is a highly preventable infection. A very effective vaccine exists, made of live measles viruses which have been treated so that they cannot cause actual infection. The important markers on the viruses are intact, however, which causes an individual's immune system to react. Immune cells called antibodies are produced, which in the event of a future infection with measles virus will quickly recognize the organism, and kill it off. Measles vaccines are usually given at about 15 months of age; because prior to that age, the baby's immune system is not mature enough to initiate a reaction strong enough to insure long-term protection from the virus. A repeat injection should be given at about 10 or 11 years of age. Outbreaks on college campuses have occurred among unimmunized or incorrectly immunized students.

Resources

BOOKS

Gershon, Anne. "Measles (Rubeola)." In *Harrison's Principles of Internal Medicine,* edited by Anthony S. Fauci, et al. New York: McGraw-Hill, 1998.

Ray, C. George. "Pathogenic Viruses." In *Sherris Medical Microbiology: An Introduction to Infectious Diseases,* edited by Kenneth J. Ryan. Norwalk, CT: Appleton and Lange, 1994.

Stoffman, Phyllis. *The Family Guide to Preventing and Treating 100 Infectious Diseases.* New York: John Wiley and Sons, Inc., 1995.

PERIODICALS

Borton, Dorothy. "Keeping Measles at Bay: Use These Four Techniques to Stop the Spread." *Nursing* 27, 12 (December 1997): 26.

Chavez, Gilberto F., and Arthur A. Ellis. "Pediatric Hospital Admissions for Measles: Lessons from the 1990 Epidemic." *The Western Journal of Medicine* 165, 1-2 (July/August 1996): 20 + .

Hussey, Greg. "Managing Measles: Integrated Case Management Reduces Disease Severity." *British Medical Journal* 314, 7077 (February 1, 1997): 316 + .

Klass, Perri. "Rash Decision." *American Health* 14, 4 (May 1995): 102 + .

"Progress Toward Global Measles Control and Elimination, 1990-1996." *The Journal of the American Medical Association* 278, 17 (November 5, 1997): 1396 + .

Ramsey, Alison. "Childhood Diseases Are Back." *Reader's Digest* 148, 886 (February 1996): 73 + .

ORGANIZATIONS

Centers for Disease Control and Prevention. (404) 332-4559. http://www.cdc.gov.

Rosalyn S. Carson-DeWitt

Mebendazole *see* **Antihelminthic drugs**

Mechanical debridement *see* **Debridement**

Mechanical ventilation *see* **Inhalation therapies**

Meckel's diverticulum

Definition

Meckel's diverticulum is a congenital pouch (diverticulum) about two inches long located at the lower end of the small intestine.

Description

At the beginning of its development, the digestive tract is a single cell. As it grows, the separate parts differentiate and gradually assume their proper places. There is a lot of twisting and bending involved in its development. Near the junction between the small and large intestines is an important embryonic attachment that was part of the yolk sac that nourished the early embryo. It is supposed to disappear as the digestive system develops. If it does not, it turns into a small pouch. Furthermore, since it formed from very early embryonic tissue, it could end up being a piece of any part of the system—upper small intestine, large intestine, stomach, or even pancreas. It can be found near the appendix in the right side of the lower abdomen.

Even though it is in the distal small intestine, a piece of stomach can produce acid. The acid causes peptic **ulcers** in the small intestine next to it. Diverticula that are not errant stomach tissue can still be involved in mechanical obstruction. This can happen in two ways. The pouch may turn inside out and be dragged into the bowel, or it may twist on a ligament attached to the abdominal wall. The first situation is called intussusception, and the second volvulus.

Causes & symptoms

This developmental defect is present in about 2% of people, but causes symptoms in fewer than that. It is not hereditary.

Symptoms usually occur in children under 10 years old. There may be bleeding from the rectum, **pain** and vomiting, or simply tiredness and weakness from unnoticed blood loss. It is not unusual for a Meckel's diverticulum to be mistaken for the much more common disease, **appendicitis.** If there is obstruction, the abdomen will distend and there will be cramping pain and vomiting.

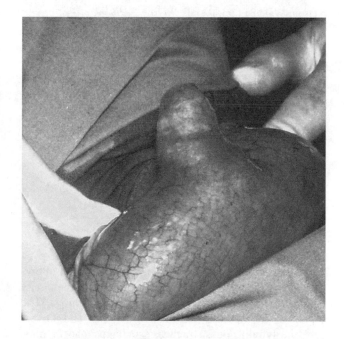

A close-up image of a patient's small intestine with a protruding sac. This condition, called Meckel's diverticulum, is a congenital abnormality occurring in 2% of the population, usually males. *(Custom Medical Stock Photo. Reproduced by permission.)*

Diagnosis

The situation may be so acute that surgery is needed as an emergency. It is often the case with bowel obstruction, heavy bleeding, or severe pain that, whatever the cause, surgery is the cure. The finer points of diagnosis can be accomplished when the abdomen is open for inspection. This situation is called an acute abdomen.

If there is more time, the best way to diagnose Meckel's diverticulum is with a nuclear scan. A radioactive isotope injected into the bloodstream will accumulate at sites of bleeding or in stomach tissue. If a piece of stomach tissue or a pool of blood shows up in the lower intestine, Meckel's diverticulum is indicated.

Treatment

A Meckel's diverticulum that is causing trouble must be removed surgically. This procedure is nearly as simple as an **appendectomy.** The outcome is equally excellent.

Resources

BOOKS

Hay, William W., et al., ed. *Current Pediatric Diagnosis and Treatment.* Stamford, CT: Appleton & Lange, 1997.

Isselbacher, Kurt J. and Alan Epstein. "Diverticular, Vascular, and Other Disorders of the Intestine and Peritoneum." In *Harrison's Principles of Internal Medicine,* edited by Anthony S. Fauci, et al. New York: McGraw-Hill, 1998.

Nelson, Waldo E., et al., eds. *Nelson Textbook of Pediatrics.* Philadelphia: W. B. Saunders, 1996.

J. Ricker Polsdorfer

Median nerve entrapment *see* **Carpal tunnel syndrome**

Mediastinoscopy

Definition

Mediastinoscopy is a surgical procedure that allows physicians to view areas of the mediastinum, the cavity behind the breastbone that lies between the lungs. The organs in the mediastinum include the heart and its vessels, the lymph nodes, trachea, esophagus, and thymus.

Mediastinoscopy is most commonly used to detect or stage **cancer.** It is also ordered to detect infection, and to confirm diagnosis of certain conditions and diseases of the respiratory organs. The procedure involves insertion

---

of an endotracheal (within the trachea) tube, followed by a small incision in the chest. A mediastinoscope is inserted through the incision. The purpose of this equipment is to allow the physician to directly see the organs inside the mediastinum, and to collect tissue samples for laboratory study.

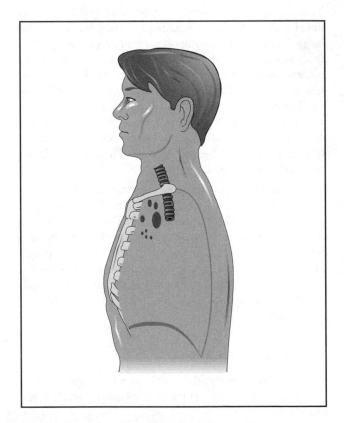

Mediastinoscopy is a surgical procedure used to detect or stage lymphoma or lung cancer. In this procedure, the surgeon makes an incision below the neck and inserts a mediastinoscope (a narrow, hollow tube with an attached light) through it to reach the area behind the breastbone. The surgeon can then insert tools through the scope to collect tissue for laboratory analysis. *(Illustration by Electronic Illustrators Group.)*

Purpose

Mediastinoscopy is often the diagnostic method of choice for detecting lymphoma, including **Hodgkin's disease.** Diagnosis of **sarcoidosis** (a chronic lung disease) and the staging of **lung cancer** can also be accomplished through mediastinoscopy. Lung cancer staging involves the placement of the cancer's progression into stages, or levels. These stages help a physician study cancer and provide consistent definition levels of cancer and corresponding treatments. The lymph nodes in the mediastinum are likely to show if lung cancer has spread beyond the lungs. Mediastinoscopy allows a physician to observe and extract a sample from the nodes for further study. Involvement of these lymph nodes indicates diagnosis and stages of lung cancer.

Mediastinoscopy may also be ordered to verify a diagnosis that was not clearly confirmed by other methods, such as certain radiographic and laboratory studies. Mediastinoscopy may also aid in certain surgical biopsies of nodes or cancerous tissue in the mediastinum. In fact, the surgeon may immediately perform a surgical procedure if a malignant tumor is confirmed while the patient is undergoing mediastinoscopy, thus combining the diagnostic exam and surgical procedure into one operation when possible.

Precautions

Since mediastinoscopy is a surgical procedure, it should only be performed when the benefits of the exam's findings outweigh the risks of surgery and anesthesia. Patients who previously had mediastinoscopy should not receive it again if there is scarring present from the first exam.

Description

Mediastinoscopy is usually performed in a hospital under general anesthesia. An endotracheal tube is inserted first, after local anesthesia is applied to the throat. Once the patient is under general anesthesia, a small incision is made usually just below the neck. The surgeon may clear a path and feel the patient's lymph nodes first to evaluate any abnormalities within the nodes. Next, the physician will insert the mediastinoscope through the incision. The scope is a narrow, hollow tube with an attached light, which allows the surgeon to see inside the area. The surgeon can insert tools through the hollow tube to help perform the exam. A sample of tissue from the lymph nodes or one of the organs can be extracted and sent for study under a microscope or on to a laboratory for further testing.

In some cases, analysis of the tissue sample which shows malignancy will suggest the need for immediate surgery while the patient is already prepared and under anesthesia. In other cases, the surgeon will complete the visual study and tissue extraction and stitch the small incision closed. The patient will remain in the surgery recovery area until it is determined that the effects of anesthesia have lessened and it is safe for the patient to leave the area. The entire procedure should take about an hour, not counting preparation and recovery time. Studies have shown that mediastinoscopy is a thorough and cost-effective diagnostic tool with less risk than some other procedures.

Preparation

Patients are asked to sign a consent form after having reviewed the risks of mediastinoscopy and known risks or reactions to anesthesia. The physician will normally instruct the patient to fast from midnight before the test until after the procedure is completed. A physician may also prescribe a sedative the night before the exam and before the procedure. Often a local anesthetic will be applied to the throat to prevent discomfort during placement of the endotracheal tube.

Aftercare

Following mediastinoscopy, patients will be carefully monitored to watch for changes in vital signs or indications of complications of the procedure or the anesthesia. A patient may have a **sore throat** from the endotracheal tube and temporary chest **pain,** soreness, or tenderness at the site of incision.

Risks

Complications from the actual mediastinoscopy procedure are relatively rare. It is possible that damage to organs or nerves in the area could occur, such as puncture of the esophagus or trachea. Infection and hemorrhage are other rare complications. The usual risks associated with general anesthesia apply to this procedure.

Normal results

In the majority of procedures performed to diagnose cancer, a normal result would involve evidence of normal lymph nodes and no tumors. In the case of lung cancer staging, results are related to the severity and progression of the cancer.

Abnormal results

If the lymph nodes are malignant, this will probably indicate that cancer such as lymphoma (including Hodgkin's disease), lung cancer, or **esophageal cancer** are present.

Resources

BOOKS

Springhouse Corporation. *Illustrated Guide to Diagnostic Tests.* Springhouse, PA: Springhouse Corporation, 1997.

ORGANIZATIONS

American Lung Association. 1740 Broadway, New York, NY 10019-4374. 1-800-LUNG-USA (1-800-586-4872). http://www.lungusa.org

American Cancer Society. 1599 Clifton Rd. NE, Atlanta, GA 30329. 1-800-ACS-2345. http://www.cancer.org

Teresa G. Norris

Meditation

Definition

Meditation is a discipline or practice of contemplation or awareness found in most of the world's major religions. It is not a treatment in the usual medical sense. Meditation is, however, frequently recommended by mainstream medical practitioners as well as alternative therapists because of its demonstrated healing effects on the central nervous system, heart rate, and level of muscular tension. It is also reputed to have benefits for the entire person: physical, mental, emotional, and spiritual.

Purpose

The purposes of meditation have been variously defined as increased awareness, greater ability to live in the moment, freedom from the ego, spiritual growth, or union with God or the universe. It is important to understand that although better health is a frequent side effect of meditation, it is not the goal or focus of meditation practice. The paradox of meditation as an approach to treatment of diseases and disorders is that it asks the patient to put aside immediate concerns with health or wellness.

Precautions

Meditation is suitable for most people who are not vulnerable to psychotic episodes. Some teachers of meditation warn against extended periods of breathing exercises unless the person has a teacher or spiritual guide, on the grounds that some people may experience **hallucinations** or dissociative episodes. The other major precaution concerns the patient's expectations. Most persons beginning a meditation practice will not find it easy; they are often disturbed by the distractions of their mental processes or the physical discomfort of sitting still for a period of time.

KEY TERMS

Dissociation—In psychology, a defense mechanism in which a group of memories or mental processes are separated from the rest of a person's mental processes to avoid emotional distress.

Hallucination—A sense perception without a source in the external world; the sensation of seeing or hearing something which is not actually there.

Mantra—A name of God or sacred formula, repeated over and over as a way of focusing the mind during meditation.

Transcendental meditation (TM)—A meditation technique based on Hindu practices that is centered on the use of a mantra. TM attracted considerable attention in the United States in the late 1960s and early 1970s, but was frequently criticized because of its commercialization of meditation.

Visualization—A technique of devotional meditation that involves the formation of mental images or pictures, usually of God or a holy person. It has been adapted for use in the treatment of cancer, AIDS, and other chronic or terminal illnesses.

Description

The form of meditation with which most Westerners are familiar involves sitting quietly in a chair or on the floor for a period of time with eyes closed in order to concentrate or focus the mind. There are, however, a variety of approaches to meditation practice.

Concentrating the mind

The goal of all forms of meditation is single-mindedness — to let go of all distractions and focus on one object of attention or devotion. There are several techniques that meditators use to help them achieve this level of concentration. Most people will find that some techniques work better for them than others. Teachers of meditation advise beginners to use the approach that they find most congenial.

BREATHING EXERCISES

Breathing exercises are often recommended to beginners because breathing is a natural function that does not have to be consciously "learned." Meditation on the breath does not require changing one's breathing in any way, but only paying attention to it — to the feel of the air as it enters or leaves the nostrils without following it into the lungs. This narrowness of focus helps to develop the meditator's ability to concentrate. When the person becomes aware that his or her attention has wandered, he or she simply returns to focusing on the breath again.

A variation of this approach is focusing on body sensations. This technique is sometimes called body scanning. The meditator simply focuses attention on the sensations in each part of his or her body in turn. Sometimes body scanning is combined with a breathing exercise; the meditator imagines breathing into and out of each part of the body as he or she attends to its sensations.

MANTRAS

A mantra is a name of God or other sacred phrase that the meditator repeats over and over in order to focus the mind. The repetition of a mantra is the basic technique of transcendental meditation, or TM. TM was introduced to the West in the 1960s by the Maharishi Mahesh Yogi and helped to make meditation acceptable to mainstream medical doctors. People initiated into TM are given individual mantras by their teachers.

There is some disagreement as to the importance of the mantra's content. Some persons think that any word or phrase is as effective as any other in focusing the mind. Others, however, maintain that the mantra must have some connection to the sacred in order to fully release the human mind from its own preoccupations. Examples of religious mantras include the Jesus prayer of Christian tradition, the holy Name of God in Judaism, or the Om mantra of Tibetan Buddhism.

DEVOTION

Devotional meditation has an interpersonal quality in that the meditator focuses on a being who represents the divine or some quality of holiness for him or her. This approach also allows the meditator to integrate feelings of love or gratitude with his or her mental focus.

Devotional meditation can take the form of chanting hymns that use the names of God, or visualizing the person or being that represents God to the meditator. Meditation in the Christian tradition sometimes includes visualizing Jesus or certain events in his life. Visualization is a useful approach to meditation for people who are sensitive to visual stimuli.

Visualization meditation has also been used in the treatment of **cancer** and **AIDS** and other disease processes. In visualization therapy, the patient visualizes the inner workings of his or her body, with healthy cells fighting off the cancer or AIDS virus or rebalancing what is out of alignment with health.. Another visualization technique asks the patient to imagine the affected parts of his or her body being surrounded by healing light or filled with energy. The patient can combine visualizations with breathing exercises by imagining that the breath is sending healing energy to the body. Patients with any illness can use devotional visualization as a way of integrating religious beliefs with visualization therapy.

Moving meditation

Meditation is a holistic practice that regards the body's positioning or activity as an important dimension of concentration. If the meditator is sitting, he or she is usually instructed to sit upright and wear loose or comfortable clothing in order to be alert as well as relaxed. Some forms of meditation, however, use body motion or postures as an intentional technique of concentration.

WALKING MEDITATION

In this form of meditation, the person slows down the pace of walking in order to focus on each movement of his or her legs or feet. Walking meditation is often done inside in a large room or without a particular destination, in order to keep the focus on the body movements themselves rather than on the goal of getting to a specific place or covering distance. Sometimes meditators repeat the words "lifting," "moving," and "placing" as they lift each foot, move the leg forward, and place the foot on the ground.

HATHA YOGA

The asanas or postures that a person assumes in the course of **yoga** practice can be used as a form of meditation. Breathing exercises are also an important part of yoga instruction. In addition, the changes in the body's position affect the meditator's energy flow in different ways. Many people find that regular yoga practice makes them more aware of their body's processes, needs, and signals, and thus better able to recognize minor symptoms before they become major health problems.

SUFI WALKING

Sufi walking (or dancing) is a form of moving meditation that developed in medieval Islam. The person walks in a rhythmic fashion, usually chanting, in order to focus the mind on a specific quality of God. For example, a Sufi walker who wishes to focus on strength and courage would walk with forceful steps, arms swinging, and chant an Arabic phrase that means "O king of kings."

Preparation

Teaching or instruction

People can learn to meditate in a variety of ways. There are many fine self-help books written from a variety of religious and philosophical perspectives that explain the basic techniques of meditation. Most people, however, can benefit from an experienced teacher or spiritual guide. A spiritual director who knows the apprentice meditator can guide him or her to the forms of meditation that are most likely to be beneficial, and offer advice about possible pitfalls or unexpected experiences.

Basics of meditation practice

The following guidelines are recommended for beginners in meditation:

• Regularity of practice. A minimum of 10-20 minutes daily is recommended for beginners, at the same time each day if at all possible.

• Quiet and privacy. Meditators should select a room or other location where they will not be disturbed by other people or the telephone. Setting aside a specific place as well as time for regular practice is ideal.

• Posture. The meditator should sit upright in a chair or on the floor with eyes closed. Good posture helps to maintain the flow of energy during breathing exercises.

• Proper breathing. Meditators should breathe deeply from the diaphragm rather than from the upper chest.

Aftercare

Teachers of meditation advise people to return to their normal activities gently and gradually following their meditation practice, rather than making abrupt or hurried transitions.

Risks

The major risk associated with meditation is the emergence of energy states or spiritual phenomena that are startling or worrisome to most Westerners. In most cases these experiences are byproducts of the attitudinal or behavioral changes that result from regular meditation practice. They do not indicate that the meditator is psychotic. One advantage of practicing meditation under the guidance of a spiritual director or teacher is his or her experience in dealing with these phenomena.

Normal results

As has been previously mentioned, meditation is the opposite of result-oriented treatments. Persons who practice meditation on a regular basis, however, usually experience the specific benefits of lowered blood pressure, more restful sleep, and relief from such physical effects of **stress** as **ulcers, headaches,** chronic muscle **pain,** and skin **rashes.** Therapeutic visualization has been shown to extend the survival time and quality of life of terminally ill patients.

Resources

BOOKS

Adair, Margo, and Lynn Johnson. "Applied Meditations for Healing." In *Psychoimmunity & the Healing Process: A Holistic Approach to Immunity & AIDS,* edited by Jason Serinus. Berkeley, CA: Celestial Arts, 1986.

Borysenko, Joan. *Minding the Body, Mending the Mind.* Reading, MA: Addison-Wesley Publishing Company, Inc., 1987.

Dass, Ram. *Journey of Awakening: A Meditator's Guidebook.* New York: Bantam Books, 1978.

de Mello, Anthony. *Sadhana, A Way to God: Christian Exercises in Eastern Form.* Garden City, NY: Image Books, 1978.

Goldstein, Joseph, and Jack Kornfield. *Seeking the Heart of Wisdom: The Path of Insight Meditation.* Boston and London: Shambhala, 1987.

Inglis, Brian, and Ruth West. *The Alternative Health Guide.* New York: Alfred A. Knopf, 1983.

Kabat-Zinn, Jon. *Full Catastrophe Living: Using the Wisdom of Your Body and Mind to Face Stress, Pain, and Illness.* New York: Bantam Doubleday Dell Publishing Group, Inc., 1990.

A Visual Encyclopedia of Unconventional Medicine, edited by Ann Hill. New York: Crown Publishers, Inc., 1979.

PERIODICALS

Kamenetz, Rodger. "Unorthodox Jews Rummage Through the Orthodox Tradition." *The New York Times Magazine* (December 7, 1997): 84-86.

Rebecca J. Frey

Mediterranean anemia *see* **Thalassemia**

. . . .

Medullary sponge kidney

Definition

Medullary sponge kidney is a congenital defect of the kidneys where the kidneys fill with pools of urine.

Description

One of every 100 to 200 people have some form of this disease. The kidneys filter urine from the blood and direct it down tiny collecting tubes toward the ureters (ducts that carry urine from the kidney to the bladder). These tiny tubes gradually join together until they reach the renal pelvis, where the ureters begin. As the tubes join, they are supposed to get progressively bigger as they get fewer in number. In medullary sponge kidney, the tubes are irregular in diameter, forming pools of urine

KEY TERMS

Congenital—Present at birth.

Intravenous pyelogram—X rays of the upper urinary system using a contrast agent that is excreted by the kidneys into the urine.

Thiazide diuretic—A particular class of medication that encourages urine production.

along the way. These pools encourage stone formation and infection.

Causes & symptoms

Although some cases of this disorder seem to be inherited, usually the cause is not known.

The symptoms associated with medullary sponge kidney are those related to infection and stone passage. Infection causes **fever;** back and flank **pain;** cloudy, frequent, and burning urine; and general discomfort. Stones cause pain in the flank or groin as they pass. They usually cause some bleeding. The bleeding may not be visible in the urine, but it is apparent under a microscope.

Diagnosis

Recurring kidney infections, bleeding, or stones will prompt x rays of the kidneys. The appearance of medullary sponge kidney on an intravenous pyelogram (x rays of the upper urinary system) is characteristic.

Treatment

Many people never have trouble with this disorder. For those that do, infections and stones will need periodic treatment. Infections should be treated with **antibiotics** early in order to prevent kidney damage. Stones may need to be surgically removed. Often, removal can be accomplished without an incision but rather by reaching up with instruments through the lower urinary tract to grab the stones. There is also a new method of stone treatment called shock wave **lithotripsy.** A special machine delivers a focused blast of shock waves that breaks stones into sand so that they will pass out naturally. It is considered reasonably safe and usually effective.

Prognosis

Ignoring symptoms can result in progressive damage to the kidneys and ultimate kidney failure, but attentive early treatment will preserve kidney function.

Prevention

Diligent monitoring for infection at regular intervals and at the first symptom will give the best long-term results. By drinking extra liquids, most stones can be prevented. The most common kind of stones, calcium stones, can be deterred by regularly taking a medication that encourages urine production (thiazide diuretic).

Resources

BOOKS

Asplin, John R. and Frederic L. Coe. "Hereditary Tubular Disorders." In *Harrison's Principles of Internal Medicine,* edited by Anthony S. Fauci, et al. New York: McGraw-Hill, 1998.

Martin, Thomas V. and R. Earnest Sosa. "Shock Wave Lithotripsy." In *Campbell's Urology,* edited by Patrick C. Walsh, et al. Philadelphia: W. B. Saunders, 1998.

PERIODICALS

Saklayen, M.G. "Medical Management of Nephrolithiasis." *Medical Clinics of North America* 81 (May 1997): 785-799.

ORGANIZATIONS

American Association of Kidney Patients. 111 South Parker Street, Suite 405, Tampa, Florida 33606. 800-749-2257.

American Kidney Foundation. 6110 Executive Boulevard, #1010, Rockville, Maryland 20852. 800-638-8299.

The National Kidney Foundation. 30 East 33rd Street, New York, NY 10016. 800-622-9010.

J. Ricker Polsdorfer

Medulloblastoma *see* **Brain tumor**

Mefloquine *see* **Antimalarial drugs**

Megalencephaly *see* **Congenital brain defects**

Melanoma *see* **Malignant melanoma**

Melioidosis

Definition

Melioidosis is an infectious disease of humans and animals caused by a gram-negative bacillus found in soil and water. It has both acute and chronic forms.

Description

Melioidosis, which is sometimes called *Pseudomonas pseudomallei* infection, is endemic (occur-

KEY TERMS

Osteomyelitis—An inflammation of bone or bone marrow, often caused by bacterial infections. Chronic melioidosis may cause osteomyelitis.

Septicemia—Bacterial infection of the bloodstream. One form of melioidosis is an acute septicemic infection.

ring naturally and consistently) in Southeast Asia, Australia, and parts of Africa. It was rare in the United States prior to recent immigration from Southeast Asia. Melioidosis is presently a public health concern because it is most common in **AIDS** patients and intravenous drug users.

Causes & symptoms

Melioidosis is caused by *Pseudomonas pseudomallei,* a bacillus that can cause disease in sheep, goats, pigs, horses, and other animals, as well as in humans. The organism enters the body through skin abrasions, **burns,** or **wounds** infected by contaminated soil; inhalation of dust; or by eating food contaminated with *P. pseudomallei.* Person-to-person transmission is unusual. Drug addicts acquire the disease from shared needles. The incubation period is two to three days.

Chronic melioidosis is characterized by **osteomyelitis** (inflammation of the bone) and pus-filled **abscesses** in the skin, lungs, or other organs. Acute melioidosis takes one of three forms: a localized skin infection that may spread to nearby lymph nodes; an infection of the lungs associated with high **fever** (102°F/38.9°C), **headache,** chest **pain,** and coughing; and septicemia (blood poisoning) characterized by disorientation, difficulty breathing, severe headache, and an eruption of pimples on the head or trunk. The third form is most common among drug addicts and may be rapidly fatal.

Diagnosis

Melioidosis is usually suspected based on the patient's history, especially travel, occupational exposure to infected animals, or a history of intravenous drug. Diagnosis must then be confirmed through laboratory tests. *P. pseudomallei* can be cultured from samples of the patient's sputum, blood, or tissue fluid from abscesses. Blood tests, including complement fixation (CF) tests and hemagglutination tests, also help to confirm the diagnosis. In acute infections, **chest x rays** and **liver function tests** are usually abnormal.

Treatment

Patients with mild or moderate infections are given a course of trimethoprim-sulfamethoxazole (TMP/SMX) and ceftazidime by mouth. Patients with acute melioidosis are given a lengthy course of ceftazidime followed by TMP/SMX. In patients with acute septicemia, a combination of **antibiotics** is administered intravenously, usually tetracycline, chloramphenicol, and TMP/SMX.

Prognosis

The mortality rate in acute cases of pulmonary melioidosis is about 10%; the mortality rate for the septicemic form is significantly higher (slightly above 50%). The prognosis for recovery from mild infections is excellent.

Prevention

There is no form of immunization for melioidosis. Prevention requires prompt cleansing of scrapes, burns, or other open wounds in areas where the disease is common and avoidance of needle sharing among drug addicts.

Resources

BOOKS

"Bacterial Diseases: Melioidosis." In *The Merck Manual of Diagnosis and Therapy,* vol. I, edited by Robert Berkow, et al. Rahway, NJ: Merck Research Laboratories, 1992.

"Ceftazidime." In *Nurses Drug Guide 1995,* edited by Billie Ann Wilson, et al. Norwalk, CT: Appleton & Lange, 1995.

Pollock, Matthew. "Infections Due to *Pseudomonas* Species and Related Organisms." In *Harrison's Principles of Internal Medicine,* edited by Anthony S. Fauci, et al. New York: McGraw-Hill, 1998.

"Trimethoprim-sulfamethoxazole." In *Nurses Drug Guide 1995,* edited by Billie Ann Wilson, et al. Norwalk, CT: Appleton & Lange, 1995.

Rebecca J. Frey

Melphalan *see* **Anticancer drugs**

Membranoproliferative glomerulopathy *see* **Nephrotic syndrome**

Membranous glomerulopathy *see* **Nephrotic syndrome**

Memory loss *see* **Amnesia**

Meniere's disease

Definition

Meniere's disease is a condition characterized by recurring vertigo (**dizziness**), **hearing loss,** and **tinnitus** (a roaring, buzzing or ringing sound in the ears).

Description

Meniere's disease was named for the French physician Prosper Meniere who first described the illness in 1861. It is an abnormality within the inner ear. A fluid called endolymph moves in the membranous labyrinth or semicircular canals within the bony labyrinth inside the inner ear. When the head or body moves, the endolymph moves, causing nerve receptors in the membranous labyrinth to send signals to the brain about the body's motion. A change in the volume of the endolymph fluid, or swelling or rupture of the membranous labyrinth is thought to result in Meniere's disease symptoms.

Causes & symptoms

The cause of Meniere's disease is unknown; however, scientists are studying several possible causes including noise pollution, viral infections, or other biological factors. The symptoms are associated with a change in fluid volume within the labyrinth of the inner ear.

Symptoms include severe dizziness or vertigo, tinnitus, hearing loss, and the sensation of **pain** or pressure in the affected ear. Symptoms appear suddenly, last up to several hours, and can occur as often as daily to as infrequently as once a year. A typical attack includes vertigo, tinnitus and hearing loss; however, some individuals with Meniere's disease may experience a single symptom, like an occasional bout of slight dizziness or periodic, intense ringing in the ear. Attacks of severe vertigo can force the sufferer to have to sit or lie down, and may be accompanied by **headache,** nausea, vomiting, or **diarrhea.** Hearing tends to recover between attacks, but becomes progressively worse over time.

Meniere's disease usually starts between the ages of 20 and 50 years and affects men and women in equal numbers. In most patients, only one ear is affected, but in about 15% of patients, both ears are involved.

Diagnosis

An estimated 3 to 5 million people in the United States have Meniere's disease, and almost 100,000 new cases are diagnosed each year. Diagnosis is based on medical history, **physical examination,** hearing and balance tests, and medical imaging with **magnetic resonance imaging** (MRI).

Several types of tests may be used to diagnose the disease and to evaluation the extent of hearing loss. In patients with Meniere's disease, audiometric tests (hearing tests) usually indicate a sensory type of hearing loss in the affected ear. Speech discrimination or the ability to distinguish between words that sound alike is often diminished. In about 50% of patients, the balance function is reduced in the affected ear. An electronystagnograph (ENG) may be used to evaluate balance. Since the eyes and ears work together through the nervous system to coordinate balance, measurement of eye movements can be used to test the balance system. For this test, the patient is seated in a darkened room and recording electrodes, similar to those used with a heart monitor, are placed near the eyes. Warm and cool water or air are gently introduced into the each ear canal and eye movements are recorded.

Another test that may be used is an electrocochleograph (EcoG), which can measure increased inner ear fluid pressure.

Treatment

There is no cure for Meniere's disease, but medication, surgery, and dietary and behavioral changes, can help control or improve the symptoms.

Medications

Symptoms of Meniere's disease may be treated with a variety of oral or injectable medications. **Antihistamines,** like diphenhydramine, meclizine, and cyclizine can be prescribed to sedate the vestibular system. A barbiturate medication like pentobarbital may be used to completely sedate the patient and relieve the vertigo. Anticholinergic drugs, like atropine or scopolamine, can help minimize **nausea and vomiting.** Diazepam has been found to be particularly effective for relief of vertigo and nausea in Meniere's disease.

There have been some reports of successful control of vertigo after **antibiotics** (gentamicin or streptomycin) or a steroid medication (dexamethasone) are injected directly into the inner ear. This procedure is done in the doctor's office and is less expensive and less invasive than a surgical procedure.

Surgical procedures

Surgical procedures may be recommended if the vertigo attacks are frequent, severe, or disabling and cannot be controlled by other treatments. The most common surgical treatment is insertion of a small tube or shunt to drain some of the fluid from the canal. This treatment usually preserves hearing and controls vertigo in about one-half to two-thirds of cases, but it is not a permanent cure in all patients.

The vestibular nerve leads from the inner ear to the brain and is responsible for conducting nerve impulses related to balance. A vestibular neurectomy is a procedure where this nerve is cut so the distorted impulses causing dizziness no longer reach the brain. This procedure permanently cures the majority of patients and hearing is preserved in most cases. There is a slight risk that hearing or facial muscle control will be affected.

A labyrinthectomy is a surgical procedure in which the balance and hearing mechanism in the inner ear are destroyed on one side. This procedure is considered when the patient has poor hearing in the affected ear. Labyrinthectomy results in the highest rates of control of vertigo attacks, however, it also causes complete deafness in the affected ear.

Alternative treatment

Changes in diet and behavior are sometimes recommended. Eliminating **caffeine,** alcohol, and salt may relieve the frequency and intensity of attacks in some people with Meniere's disease. Reducing **stress** levels and eliminating tobacco use may also help.

Prognosis

Meniere's disease is a complex and unpredictable condition for which there is no cure. The vertigo associated with the disease can generally be managed or eliminated with medications and surgery. Hearing tends to become worse over time, and some of the surgical procedures recommended, in fact, cause deafness.

Prevention

Since the cause of Meniere's disease is unknown, there are no current strategies for its prevention. Research continues on the environmental and biological factors that may cause Meniere's disease or induce an attack, as well as on the physiological components of the fluid and labyrinth system involved in hearing and balance. Preventive strategies and more effective treatment should become evident once these mechanisms are better understood.

Resources

BOOKS

''Meniere's Disease.'' In *The Merck Manual of Diagnosis and Therapy,* 16th ed., edited by Robert Berkow. Rahway, NJ: Merck & Co., 1992.

PERIODICALS

Cohen H., L.R. Ewell, and H.A. Jenkins. ''Disability in Meniere's Disease.'' *Archives of Otolaryngology, Head and Neck Surgery* 121 (January 1995): 29-33.

Driscoll, C.L., et al. ''Low-Dose Gentamicin and the Treatment of Meniere's Disease: Preliminary Results.'' *Laryngoscope* 107 (January 1997): 83-89.

Filipo, R., and M. Barbara. ''Natural Course of Meniere's Disease in Surgically-Selected Patients.'' *Ear, Nose & Throat Journal* 73 (April 1994): 254-257.

ORGANIZATIONS

American Academy of Otolaryngology-Head and Neck Surgery. One Prince Street, Alexandria, VA 22314. (703) 836-4444.

The Meniere's Network. 2000 Church Street, P.O. Box 111, Nashville, TN 37236. (800) 545-HEAR. http://www.healthy.net/pan/cso/cioi/mn.htm.

On-Balance, A Support Group for People with Meniere's Disease. http://www.midwestear.com/onbal.htm.

Vestibular Disorders Association. P.O. Box 4467, Portland, OR 97208-4467. (800)837-8428.

Altha Roberts Edgren

Meningioma *see* **Brain tumor**

Meningitis

Definition

Meningitis is a potentially fatal inflammation of the meninges, the thin, membranous covering of the brain and the spinal cord. Meningitis is most commonly caused by infection (by bacteria, viruses, or fungi), although it can also be caused by bleeding into the meninges, **cancer,** diseases of the immune system, and an inflammatory response to certain types of **chemotherapy** or other chemical agents. The most serious and difficult-to-treat types of meningitis tend to be those caused by bacteria.

Description

Meningitis is a particularly dangerous infection because of the very delicate nature of the brain. Brain cells are some of the only cells in the body that, once killed, will not regenerate themselves. Therefore, if enough

KEY TERMS

. . . .

Blood-brain barrier—An arrangement of cells within the blood vessels of the brain that prevents the passage of toxic substances, including infectious agents, from the blood and into the brain. It also makes it difficult for certain medications to pass into brain tissue.

Cerebrospinal fluid (CSF)—Fluid made in chambers within the brain which then flows over the surface of the brain and spinal cord. CSF provides nutrition to cells of the nervous system, as well as providing a cushion for the nervous system structures. It may accumulate abnormally in some disease processes, causing pressure on and damage to brain structures.

Lumbar puncture (LP)—A medical test in which a very narrow needle is inserted into a specific space between the vertebrae of the lower back in order to draw off a sample of CSF for further examination.

Meninges—The three-layer membranous covering of the brain and spinal cord, composed of the dura, arachnoid, and pia. It provides protection for the brain and spinal cord, as well as housing many blood vessels and participating in the appropriate flow of CSF.

brain tissue is damaged by an infection, serious, life-long handicaps will remain.

In order to learn about meningitis, it is important to have a basic understanding of the anatomy of the brain. The meninges are three separate membranes, layered together, which encase the brain and spinal cord:

- The dura is the toughest, outermost layer, and is closely attached to the inside of the skull.

- The middle layer, the arachnoid, is important because of its involvement in the normal flow of the cerebrospinal fluid (CSF), a lubricating and nutritive fluid that bathes both the brain and the spinal cord.

- The innermost layer, the pia, helps direct blood vessels into the brain.

- The space between the arachnoid and the pia contains CSF, which helps insulate the brain from trauma. Many blood vessels course through this space.

CSF, produced within specialized chambers deep inside the brain, flows over the surface of the brain and spinal cord. This fluid serves to cushion these relatively delicate structures, as well as supplying important nutrients for brain cells. CSF is reabsorbed by blood vessels

located within the meninges. A careful balance between CSF production and reabsorption is important to avoid the accumulation of too much CSF.

Because the brain is enclosed in the hard, bony case of the skull, any disease that produces swelling will be damaging to the brain. The skull cannot expand at all, so when the swollen brain tissue pushes up against the skull's hard bone, the brain tissue becomes damaged and may ultimately die. Furthermore, swelling on the right side of the brain will not only cause pressure and damage to that side of the brain, but by taking up precious space within the tight confines of the skull, the left side of the brain will also be pushed up against the hard surface of the skull, causing damage to the left side of the brain as well.

Another way that infections injure the brain involves the way in which the chemical environment of the brain changes in response to the presence of an infection. The cells of the brain require a very well-regulated environment. Careful balance of oxygen, carbon dioxide, sugar (glucose), sodium, calcium, potassium, and other substances must be maintained in order to avoid damage to brain tissue. An infection upsets this balance, and brain damage can occur when the cells of the brain are either deprived of important nutrients or exposed to toxic levels of particular substances.

The cells lining the brain's tiny blood vessels (capillaries) are specifically designed to prevent many substances from passing into brain tissue. This is commonly referred to as the blood-brain barrier. The blood-brain barrier prevents various substances that could be poisonous to brain tissue (toxins), as well as many agents of infection, from crossing from the blood stream into the brain tissue. While this barrier is obviously an important protective feature for the brain, it also serves to complicate treatment in the case of an infection by making it difficult for medications to pass out of the blood and into the brain tissue where the infection is located.

Causes & symptoms

The most common infectious causes of meningitis vary according to an individual's age, habits, living environment, and health status. While nonbacterial types of meningitis are more common, bacterial meningitis is the more potentially life-threatening. Three bacterial agents are responsible for about 80% of all bacterial meningitis cases. These bacteria are *Haemophilus influenzae* type b, *Neisseria meningitidis* (causing meningococcal meningitis), and *Streptococcus pneumoniae* (causing pneumococcal meningitis).

In newborns, the most common agents of meningitis are those that are contracted from the newborn's mother, including Group B streptococci (becoming an increasingly common infecting organism in the newborn period), *Escherichia coli*, and *Listeria monocytogenes*. The highest incidence of meningitis occurs in babies under a month old, with an increased risk of meningitis continuing through about two years of age.

Older children are more frequently infected by the bacteria *Haemophilus influenzae*, *Neisseria meningitidis*, and *Streptococci pneumoniae*.

Adults are most commonly infected by either *S. pneumoniae* or *N. meningitidis*, with pneumococcal meningitis the more common. Certain conditions predispose to this type of meningitis, including **alcoholism** and chronic upper respiratory tract infections (especially of the middle ear, sinuses, and mastoids).

N. meningitidis is the only organism that can cause epidemics of meningitis. In particular, these have occurred when a child in a crowded day-care situation or a military recruit in a crowded training camp has fallen ill with meningococcal meningitis.

Viral causes of meningitis include the herpes simplex virus, the **mumps** and **measles** viruses (against which most children are protected due to mass immunization programs), the virus that causes chicken pox, the **rabies** virus, and a number of viruses that are acquired through the bites of infected mosquitoes.

A number of medical conditions predispose individuals to meningitis caused by specific organisms. Patients with **AIDS** (acquired immunodeficiency syndrome) are more prone to getting meningitis from fungi, as well as from the agent that causes **tuberculosis.** Patients who have had their spleens removed, or whose spleens are no longer functional (as in the case of patients with sickle cell disease) are more susceptible to other infections, including meningococcal and pneumococcal meningitis.

The majority of meningitis infections are acquired by blood-borne spread. A person may have another type of infection (of the lungs, throat, or tissues of the heart) caused by an organism that can also cause meningitis. If this initial infection is not properly treated, the organism will continue to multiply, find its way into the blood stream, and be delivered in sufficient quantities to invade past the blood brain barrier. Direct spread occurs when an organism spreads to the meninges from infected tissue next to or very near the meninges. This can occur, for example, with a severe, poorly treated ear or sinus infection.

Patients who suffer from skull **fractures** possess abnormal openings to the sinuses, nasal passages, and middle ears. Organisms that usually live in the human respiratory system without causing disease can pass through openings caused by such fractures, reach the meninges, and cause infection. Similarly, patients who undergo surgical procedures or who have had foreign bodies surgically placed within their skulls (such as tubes to drain abnormal amounts of accumulated CSF) have an increased risk of meningitis.

Organisms can also reach the meninges via an uncommon but interesting method called intraneural spread. This involves an organism invading the body at a considerable distance away from the head, spreading along a nerve, and using that nerve as a kind of ladder into the skull, where the organism can multiply and cause meningitis. Herpes simplex virus is known to use this type of spread, as is the rabies virus.

The most classic symptoms of meningitis (particularly of bacterial meningitis) include **fever, headache,** vomiting, sensitivity to light (photophobia), irritability, severe fatigue (lethargy), stiff neck, and a reddish purple rash on the skin. Untreated, the disease progresses with seizures, confusion, and eventually **coma.**

A very young infant may not show the classic signs of meningitis. Early in infancy, a baby's immune system is not yet developed enough to mount a fever in response to infection, so fever may be absent. Some infants with meningitis have seizures as their only identifiable symptom. Similarly, debilitated elderly patients may not have fever or other identifiable symptoms of meningitis.

Damage due to meningitis occurs from a variety of phenomena. The action of infectious agents on the brain tissue is one direct cause of damage. Other types of damage may be due to the mechanical effects of swelling and compression of brain tissue against the bony surface of the skull. Swelling of the meninges may interfere with the normal absorption of CSF by blood vessels, causing accumulation of CSF and damage from the resulting pressure on the brain. Interference with the brain's carefully regulated chemical environment may cause damaging amounts of normally present substances (carbon dioxide, potassium) to accumulate. Inflammation may cause the blood-brain barrier to become less effective at preventing the passage of toxic substances into brain tissue.

Diagnosis

A number of techniques are used when examining a patient suspected of having meningitis to verify the diagnosis. Certain manipulations of the head (lowering the head, chin towards chest, for example) are difficult to perform and painful for a patient with meningitis.

The most important test used to diagnose meningitis is the lumbar puncture (commonly called a spinal tap). Lumbar puncture (LP) involves the insertion of a thin needle into a space between the vertebrae in the lower back and the withdrawal of a small amount of CSF. The CSF is then examined under a microscope to look for bacteria or fungi. Normal CSF contains set percentages of glucose and protein. These percentages will vary with bacterial, viral, or other causes of meningitis. For example, bacterial meningitis causes a greatly lower than normal percentage of glucose to be present in CSF, as the bacteria are essentially "eating" the host's glucose, and using it for their own nutrition and energy production. Normal CSF should contain no infection-fighting cells (white blood cells), so the presence of white blood cells in CSF is another indication of meningitis. Some of the withdrawn CSF is also put into special lab dishes to allow growth of the infecting organism, which can then be identified more easily. Special immunologic and serologic tests may also be used to help identify the infectious agent.

In rare instances, CSF from a lumbar puncture cannot be examined because the amount of swelling within the skull is so great that the pressure within the skull (intracranial pressure) is extremely high. This pressure is always measured immediately upon insertion of the LP needle. If it is found to be very high, no fluid is withdrawn because doing so could cause herniation of the brain stem. Herniation of the brain stem occurs when the part of the brain connecting to the spinal cord is thrust through the opening at the base of the skull into the spinal canal. Such herniation will cause compression of those structures within the brain stem that control the most vital functions of the body (breathing, heart beat, consciousness). **Death** or permanent debilitation follows herniation of the brain stem.

Treatment

Antibiotic medications (forms of penicillin and **cephalosporins,** for example) are the most important element of treatment against bacterial agents of meningitis. Because of the effectiveness of the blood-brain barrier in preventing the passage of substances into the brain, medications must be delivered directly into the patient's veins (intravenously, or by IV), at very high doses. **Antiviral drugs** (acyclovir) may be helpful in shortening the course of viral meningitis, and antifungal medications are available as well.

Other treatments for meningitis involve decreasing inflammation (with steroid preparations) and paying careful attention to the balance of fluids, glucose, sodium, potassium, oxygen, and carbon dioxide in the patient's system. Patients who develop seizures will require medications to halt the seizures and prevent their return.

Prognosis

Viral meningitis is the least severe type of meningitis, and patients usually recover with no long-term effects from the infection. Bacterial infections, however, are much more severe, and progress rapidly. Without very rapid treatment with the appropriate antibiotic, the infection can swiftly lead to coma and death in less than a day's time. While death rates from meningitis vary de-

pending on the specific infecting organism, the overall death rate is just under 20%.

The most frequent long-term effects of meningitis include deafness and blindness, which may be caused by the compression of specific nerves and brain areas responsible for the senses of hearing and sight. Some patients develop permanent **seizure disorders,** requiring life-long treatment with anti-seizure medications. Scarring of the meninges may result in obstruction of the normal flow of CSF, causing abnormal accumulation of CSF. This may be a chronic problem for some patients, requiring the installation of shunt tubes to drain the accumulation regularly.

Prevention

Prevention of meningitis primarily involves the appropriate treatment of other infections an individual may acquire, particularly those that have a track record of seeding to the meninges (such as ear and sinus infections). Preventive treatment with **antibiotics** is sometimes recommended for the close contacts of an individual who is ill with meningococcal or *H. influenzae* type b meningitis. A meningococcal vaccine exists, and is sometimes recommended to individuals who are traveling to very high risk areas. A vaccine for *H. influenzae* type b is now given to babies as part of the standard array of childhood immunizations.

Resources

BOOKS

Ray, C. George. "Central Nervous System Infections." In *Sherris Medical Microbiology: An Introduction to Infectious Diseases*, edited by Kenneth J. Ryan. Norwalk, CT: Appleton and Lange, 1994.

Stoffman, Phyllis. *The Family Guide to Preventing and Treating 100 Infectious Diseases.* New York: John Wiley and Sons, Inc., 1995.

Swartz, Morton N. "Bacterial Meningitis." In *Cecil Textbook of Medicine*, edited by J. Claude Bennett and Fred Plum. Philadelphia: W.B. Saunders, 1996.

PERIODICALS

Meissner, Judith W. "Caring for Patients With Meningitis." *Nursing,* (July 1995): 50+.

Schuchat, Anne, et al. "Bacterial Meningitis in the United States in 1995." *New England Journal of Medicine,* (October 2, 1997).

ORGANIZATIONS

American Academy of Neurology. 1080 Montreal Avenue, St. Paul, MN 55116. (612) 695-1940. http://www.aan.com.

Meningitis Foundation of America. 7155 Shadeland Station, Suite 190, Indianapolis, IN 46256-3922. (800) 668-1129. http://www.musa.org/welcome.htm.

Rosalyn S. Carson-DeWitt

Meningocele *see* **Spina bifida**

Meningococcemia

Definition

Meningococcemia is the presence of meningococcus in the bloodstream. Meningococcus, a bacteria formally called *Neisseria meningitidis*, can be one of the most dramatic and rapidly fatal of all infectious diseases.

Causes & symptoms

Meningococcemia, a relatively rare infection, occurs most commonly in children and young adults. In susceptible people, it can cause a very severe illness that can kill within hours. The bacteria, which can spread from person to person, usually first causes a colonization in the upper airway, but no symptoms. From there, it can penetrate into the bloodstream to the central nervous system and cause **meningitis** or develop into a full-blown bloodstream infection (meningococcemia). Fortunately in most colonized people, this does not happen and the result of this colonization is long-lasting immunity against the particular strain.

After colonization is established, symptoms can develop within one day to one to two weeks. After a short period of time (one hour up to one to two days) when the patient complains of **fever** and muscle aches, more severe symptoms can develop. Unfortunately during this early stage, a doctor cannot tell this illness from any other illness, such as a viral infection like **influenza.** Unless the case is occurring in a person known to have been exposed to or in the midst of an epidemic of meningococcal disease, there may be no specific symptoms or signs found that help the doctor diagnose the problem. Rarely, a low-grade bloodstream infection called chronic meningococcemia can occur.

After this initial period, the patient will often complain of continued fever, shaking chills, overwhelming weakness, and even a feeling of impending doom. The organism is multiplying in the bloodstream, unchecked by the immune system. The severity of the illness and its dire complications are caused by the damage the organism does to the small blood vessel walls. This damage is called a **vasculitis,** inflammation of a blood vessel. Dam-

age to the small vessels causes them to leak. The first signs of the infection's severity are small bleeding spots seen on the skin (petechiae). A doctor should always suspect meningococcemia when he/she finds an acutely ill patient with fever, chills, and petechiae.

Quickly (within hours), the blood vessel damage increases and large bleeding areas on the skin (purpura) are seen. The same changes are taking place in the affected person's internal organs. The blood pressure is often low and there may be signs of bleeding from other organs (like coughing up blood, nose bleeds, blood in the urine). The organism not only damages the blood vessels by causing them to leak, but also causes clotting inside the

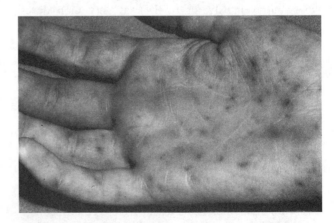

A close-up of a person's hand with meningococcemia. This disease is caused by the presence of meningococcus (*Neisseria meningitidis***) in the bloodstream. The organism can cause multiple illnesses and can damage small blood vessels.** *(Custom Medical Stock Photo. Reproduced by permission.)*

vessels. If this clotting occurs in the larger arteries, it results in major tissue damage. Essentially, large areas of skin, muscle, and internal organs die from lack of blood and oxygen. Even if the disease is quickly diagnosed and treated, the patient has a high risk of dying.

Diagnosis

The diagnosis of meningococcemia can be made by the growth of the organism from **blood cultures.** Treatment should begin when the diagnosis is suspected and should not be delayed waiting for positive cultures. Obtaining fluid from a pectechial spot and staining it in the laboratory can assist in quickly seeing the organism.

Treatment

Immediate treatment of a suspected case of meningococcemia begins with **antibiotics** that work against the organism. Possible choices include penicillin G, ceftriaxone (Rocephin), cefotaxime (Claforan), or trimethoprim/sulfamethoxazole (Bactrim, Septra). If the patient is diagnosed in a doctor's office, antibiotics should be given immediately if possible, even before transfer to the hospital and even if cultures cannot be obtained before treatment. It is most likely that the speed of initial treatment will affect the ultimate outcome.

Prognosis

As many as 15-20% of patients with meningococcemia will die as a result of the acute infection. A significant percentage of the survivors will have tissue damage that requires surgical treatment. This treatment may consist of skin grafts, or even partial or full **amputations** of an arm or leg. Certain people with immune system defects (particularly those with defects in the complement system) may have recurrent episodes of meningococcemia. These patients, however, seem to have a less serious outcome.

Prevention

Although a vaccine is available for meningococcus, it is still difficult at this time to produce a vaccine for the type B organism, the most common one in the U.S. Because of this and the short time that the vaccine seems to offer protection, the product is not commonly used in the U.S. It can be used for travelers going to areas where meningococcal disease is more common or is epidemic.

It is, however, recommended that all people take certain antibiotics if they have had contact (like at home or in a daycare) with a person who has meningococcal infection. The most common antibiotics given are rifampin (Rifadin) or ciprofloxacin (Cipro). These medicines are usually taken by mouth twice a day for two days. This treatment will decrease the risk of infection in these people who have been exposed. However, the overall risk to people who have been exposed, even without antibiotic use, is probably no more than 1-2%.

Resources

PERIODICALS

Centers for Disease Control. "Recommendation of the Immunization Practices Advisory Committee (ACIP): Meningococcal Vaccines." *Morbidity and Mortality Weekly Report* 34(May 10, 1985): 255-259.

Devine, L. F., et al. "Rifampin: Effect of Two-Day Treatment on the Meningococcal Carrier State and the Relationship to the Levels of Drug in Sera and Saliva." *American Journal of the Medical Sciences* 261(February 1971): 79-83.

McCormick, Joseph B., and John V. Bennett. "Public Health Considerations in the Management of Meningococcal Disease." *Annals of Internal Medicine* 83(December 1975): 883-886.

Salzman, Mark B., and Lorry G. Rubin. "Meningococcemia." *Infectious Disease Clinics of North America* 10(December 1996): 709-725.

Larry I. Lutwick

Meningomyelocele *see* **Spina bifida**

Menkes' syndrome *see* **Mineral deficiency**

Menopause

Definition

Menopause represents the end of menstruation. While technically it refers to the final period, it is not an abrupt event, but a gradual process. Menopause is not a disease that needs to be cured, but a natural life-stage transition. However, women have to make important decisions about "treatment," including the use of **hormone replacement therapy** (HRT).

Description

Many women have irregular periods and other problems of "pre-menopause" for years. It's not easy to predict when menopause begins, although doctors agree it is complete when a woman has not had a period for a year. Eight out of every hundred women stop menstruating before age 40. At the other end of the spectrum, five out of every 100 continue to have periods until they are almost 60. The average age of menopause is 51.

There's no mathematical formula to figure out when the ovaries will begin to scale back either, but a woman

KEY TERMS

Endometrium—The lining of the uterus, which is shed with each menstrual period.

Estrogen—Female hormone produced by the ovaries and released by the follicles as they mature. Responsible for female sexual characteristics, estrogen stimulates and triggers a response from at least 300 tissues, and may help some types of breast cancer to grow. After menopause, the production of the hormone gradually stops.

Estrogen replacement therapy (ERT)—A treatment for menopause in which estrogen is given in pill, patch, or cream form.

Follicle-stimulating hormone (FSH)—The pituitary hormone that stimulates the ovary to mature egg capsules (follicles). It is linked with rising estrogen production throughout the cycle. An elevated FSH (above 40) indicates menopause.

Hormone—A chemical messenger secreted by a gland that is released into the blood, and that travels to distant cells where it exerts an effect.

Hormone replacement therapy (HRT)—The use of estrogen and progesterone to replace hormones that the ovary no longer supplies.

Hot flash—A wave of heat that is one of the most common perimenopausal symptoms, triggered by the hypothalamus' response to estrogen withdrawal.

Hysterectomy—Surgical removal of the uterus.

Ovary—One of the two almond-shaped glands in the female reproductive system responsible for producing eggs and the hormones estrogen and progesterone.

Ovulation—The monthly release of an egg from the ovary.

Pituitary gland—The "master gland" at the base of the brain that secretes a number of hormones responsible for growth, reproduction, and other activities. Pituitary hormones stimulate the ovaries to release estrogen and progesterone.

Progesterone—The hormone that is produced by the ovary after ovulation to prepare the uterine lining for a fertilized egg.

Testosterone—Male hormone produced by the testes and (in small amounts) in the ovaries. Testosterone is responsible for some masculine secondary sex characteristics such as growth of body hair and deepening voice.

Uterus—The female reproductive organ that contains and nourishes a fetus from implantation until birth. Also known as the womb.

Vagina—The tube-like passage from the vulva (a woman's external genital structures) to the cervix (the portion of the uterus that projects into the vagina).

can get a general idea based on her family history, body type, and lifestyle. Women who began menstruating early will not necessarily stop having periods early as well. It is true that a woman will likely enter menopause at about the same age as her mother. Menopause may occur later than average among smokers.

Causes & symptoms

Once a woman enters **puberty,** each month her body releases one of the more than 400,000 eggs that are stored in her ovaries, and the lining of the womb (uterus) thickens in anticipation of receiving a fertilized egg. If the egg isn't fertilized, progesterone levels drop and the uterine lining sheds and bleeds.

By the time a woman reaches her late 30s or 40s, her ovaries begin to shut down, producing less estrogen and progesterone and releasing eggs less often. The gradual decline of estrogen causes a wide variety of changes in tissues that respond to estrogen—including the vagina, vulva, uterus, bladder, urethra, breasts, bones, heart,

blood vessels, brain, skin, hair, and mucous membranes. Over the long run, the lack of estrogen can make a woman more vulnerable to **osteoporosis** (which can begin in the 40s) and heart disease.

As the levels of hormones fluctuate, the menstrual cycle begins to change. Some women may have longer periods with heavy flow followed by shorter cycles and hardly any bleeding. Others will begin to miss periods completely. During this time, a woman also becomes less able to get pregnant.

The most common symptom of menopause is a change in the menstrual cycle, but there are a variety of other symptoms as well, including:

- Hot flashes
- Night sweats
- **Insomnia**
- Mood swings/irritability
- Memory or concentration problems
- Vaginal dryness

- Heavy bleeding
- Fatigue
- Depression
- Hair changes
- **Headaches**
- Heart **palpitations**
- Sexual disinterest
- Urinary changes
- Weight gain.

Diagnosis

The clearest indication of menopause is the absence of a period for one year. It is also possible to diagnose menopause by testing hormone levels. One important test measures the levels of follicle-stimulating hormone (FSH), which rise steadily as a woman ages.

However, as a woman first enters menopause, her hormones often fluctuate wildly from day to day. For example, if a woman's estrogen levels are high and progesterone is low, she may have mood swings, irritability, and other symptoms similar to **premenstrual syndrome** (PMS). As hormone levels shift and estrogen level falls, hot flashes occur. Because of these fluctuations, a normal hormone level when the blood is tested may not necessarily mean the levels were normal the day before or will be the day after.

If it has been at least three months since a woman's last period, an FSH test might be more helpful in determining whether menopause has occurred. Most doctors believe that the FSH test alone can't be used as proof that a woman has entered early menopause. A better measure of menopause is a test that checks the levels of estrogen, progesterone, testosterone and other hormones at midcycle, in addition to FSH.

Treatment

When a woman enters menopause, her levels of estrogen drop and annoying symptoms (such as hot flashes and vaginal dryness) begin. Hormone replacement therapy can treat these symptoms by boosting the estrogen levels enough to suppress symptoms while also providing protection against heart disease and osteoporosis, which causes the bones to weaken. Experts disagree on whether HRT increases or decreases the risk of developing **breast cancer.** A Harvard study concluded that short-term use of hormones carries little risk, while HRT used for more than five years among women 55 and over seems to increase the risk of breast cancer.

There are two types of hormone treatments: hormone replacement therapy (HRT) and estrogen replacement therapy (ERT). HRT is the administration of estrogen and progesterone; ERT is the administration of estrogen alone. Only women who have had a **hysterectomy** (removal of the uterus) can take estrogen alone, since taking this "unopposed" estrogen can cause uterine **cancer.** The combination of progesterone and estrogen in HRT eliminates the risk of uterine cancer.

Most physicians don't recommend HRT until a woman's periods have stopped completely for one year. This is because women in early menopause who still have an occasional period are still producing estrogen; HRT would then provide far too much estrogen.

Most doctors believe that every woman (except those with certain cancers) should take hormones as they approach menopause because of the protection against heart disease, osteoporosis, and uterine cancer and the relatively low risk of breast cancer. Heart disease and osteoporosis are two of the leading causes of disability and **death** among post-menopausal women.

Critics say the benefit of taking hormonal drugs to ease symptoms isn't worth the risk of breast cancer. Since menopause isn't a disease, critics argue, women shouldn't take hormones to cure what is actually a natural process of aging. Advocates of HRT contend that the purpose of taking hormones is not to "treat" menopause but to prevent the development of other diseases.

There are risks with HRT, and there are risks without it. In order to decide whether to take HRT, a woman should balance her risk of getting breast cancer against her risk of getting heart disease, and decide how annoying her menopause symptoms are. Most doctors agree that short-term use of estrogen for those women with annoying symptoms of hot flashes or night sweats is a sensible choice as long as they don't have a history of breast cancer.

For a woman who has no family history of cancer and a high risk of dying from heart disease, for example, the low risk of cancer might be worth the protective benefit of avoiding heart disease. Certainly, for white women aged 50 to 94, the risk of dying from heart disease is far greater than the risk of dying of breast cancer.

Women are poor candidates for hormone replacement therapy if they:

- Have ever had breast or **endometrial cancer**
- Have a close relative (mother, sister, grandmother) who died of breast cancer or have two relatives who got breast cancer before age 40
- Have had endometrial cancer
- Have had gallbladder or liver disease
- Have blood clots or phlebitis.

(Some women with liver or gallbladder disease, or who have clotting problems, may be able to go on HRT if they use a patch to administer the hormones through the skin, bypassing the liver).

Women would make a good candidate for HRT if they:

• Need to prevent osteoporosis

• Have had their ovaries removed

• Need to prevent heart disease

• Have significant symptoms.

Taking hormones can almost immediately eliminate hot flashes, vaginal dryness, **urinary incontinence** (depending on the cause), insomnia, moodiness, memory problems, heavy irregular periods, and concentration problems. But side effects of treatment include bloating, breakthrough bleeding, headaches, vaginal discharge, fluid retention, swollen breasts, or nausea. Up to 20% of women who try hormone replacement stop within nine months because of these side effects. However, some side effects can be lessened or prevented by changing the HRT regimen.

The decision should be made by a woman and her doctor after taking into consideration her medical history and situation. Women who choose to take hormones should have an annual mammogram, breast exam, and pelvic exam and should report any unusual vaginal bleeding or spotting (a sign of possible uterine cancer).

Anti-estrogens

A new type of hormone therapy offers some of the same protection against heart disease and bone loss as estrogen, but without the increased risk of breast cancer. This new class of drugs, known as ''anti-estrogens,'' may be available in the late 1990s.

The best known of these anti-estrogens is raloxifene, which mimics the effects of estrogen in the bones and blood, but blocks some of its negative effects elsewhere. It's called an anti-estrogen because for a long time these drugs had been used to counter the harmful effects of estrogen that caused breast cancer. Oddly enough, in other parts of the body these drugs mimic estrogen, protecting against heart disease and osteoporosis without putting a woman at risk for breast cancer.

Like estrogen, raloxifene works by attaching to an estrogen ''receptor,'' much like a key fits into a lock. When raloxifene clicks into the estrogen receptors in the breast and uterus, it blocks estrogen at these sites. This is the secret of its cancer-fighting property. (Many tumors in the breast are fueled by estrogen; if the estrogen can't get in, then the cancer can't grow.)

Women may prefer to take raloxifene instead of hormone replacement because the new drug doesn't boost the breast cancer risk and doesn't have side effects like uterine bleeding, bloating, or breast soreness. Unfor-

tunately, the drug may worsen hot flashes. Raloxifene is basically a treatment to prevent osteoporosis. It doesn't help with common symptoms and it is unclear if it has the same protective effect against heart disease as estrogen does.

Testosterone replacement

The ovaries also produce a small amount of male hormones, which decreases slightly as a woman enters menopause. The vast majority of women never need testosterone replacement, but it can be important if a woman has declining interest in sex. Testosterone can improve the libido, and decrease **anxiety** and depression; adding testosterone especially helps women who have had hysterectomies. Testosterone also eases breast tenderness and helps prevent bone loss.

However, testosterone does have side effects. Some women experience mild **acne** and some facial hair growth, but because only small amounts of testosterone are prescribed, most women don't appear to have extreme masculine changes.

Birth control pills

Women who are still having periods but who have annoying menopausal symptoms may take low-dose birth control pills to ease the problems; this treatment has been approved by the FDA for perimenopausal symptoms in women under age 55. HRT is the preferred treatment for menopause, however, because it uses lower doses of estrogen.

Alternative treatment

Some women also report success in using natural remedies to treat the unpleasant symptoms of menopause. Not all women need estrogen and some women can't take it. Many doctors don't want to give hormones to women who are still having their periods, however erratically. Indeed, only a third of menopausal women in the United States try HRT and of those who do, eventually half of them drop the therapy. Some are worried about breast cancer, some can't tolerate the side effects, some don't want to medicate what they consider to be a natural occurrence.

Herbs

Herbs have been used to relieve menopausal symptoms for centuries. In general, most herbs are considered safe, and there is no substantial evidence that herbal products are a major source of toxic reactions. But because herbal products aren't regulated in the United States, contamination or accidental overdose is possible. Herbs should be bought from a recognized company or through a qualified herbal practitioner.

Women who choose to take herbs for menopausal symptoms should learn as much as possible about herbs and work with a qualified practitioner (an herbalist, a traditional Chinese doctor, or a naturopathic physician). Pregnant women should avoid herbs because of unknown effects on a developing fetus.

The following list of herbs include those that herbalists most often prescribe to treat menstrual complaints:

- Black cohosh (*Cimicifuga racemosa*): hot flashes and other menstrual complaints

- Black currant: breast tenderness

- Chaste tree/chasteberry (*Vitex agnus-castus*): hot flashes, excessive menstrual bleeding, fibroids, and moodiness

- Evening primrose oil (*Oenothera biennis*): mood swings, irritability, and breast tenderness

- Fennel (*Foeniculum vulgare*): hot flashes, digestive gas, and bloating

- Flaxseed (linseed): excessive menstrual bleeding, breast tenderness, and other symptoms, including dry skin and vaginal dryness

- Gingko (*Gingko biloba*): memory problems

- Ginseng (*Panax ginseng*): hot flashes, fatigue and vaginal thinning.

- Hawthorn (*Crataegus laevigata*): memory problems, fuzzy thinking

- Lady's mantle: excessive menstrual bleeding

- Mexican wild yam (*Dioscorea villosa*) root: vaginal dryness, hot flashes and general menopause symptoms

- Motherwort (*Leonurus cardiaca*): night sweats, hot flashes

- Oat (*Avena sativa*) straw: mood swings, anxiety

- Red clover (*Trifolium pratense*): hot flashes

- Sage (*Salvia officinalis*): mood swings, headaches, night sweats

- Valerian (*Valeriana officinalis*): insomnia.

Natural estrogens (phytoestrogens)

Proponents of plant estrogens (including soy products) believe that plant estrogens are better than synthetic estrogen, but science has not yet proven this. The results of smaller preliminary trials suggest that the estrogen compounds in soy products can indeed relieve the severity of hot flashes and lower cholesterol. But no one yet has proven that soy can provide all the benefits of synthetic estrogen without its negative effects.

It is true that people in other countries who eat foods high in plant estrogens (especially soy products) have lower rates of breast cancer and report fewer "symptoms" of menopause. While up to 80% of menopausal women in the United States complain of hot flashes, night sweats, and vaginal dryness, only 15% of Japanese women have similar complaints. When all other things are equal, a soy-based diet may make a difference (and soy is very high in plant estrogens).

The study of phytoestrogens is so new that there aren't very many recommendations on how much a woman can consume. Herbal practitioners recommend a dose based on a woman's history, body size, lifestyle, diet, and reported symptoms. In one study at Bowman-Gray Medical School in North Carolina, women were able to ease their symptoms by eating a large amount of fruits, vegetables, and whole grains, together with four ounces of tofu four times a week.

What concerns some critics of other alternative remedies is that many women think that "natural" or "plant-based" means "harmless." In large doses, phytoestrogens can promote the abnormal growth of cells in the uterine lining. Unopposed estrogen of any type can lead to endometrial cancer, which is why women on conventional estrogen-replacement therapy usually take progesterone (progestin) along with their estrogen. However, a plant-based progesterone product can sometimes be effective alone, without estrogen, in assisting the menopausal woman in rebalancing her hormonal action throughout this transition time.

Yoga

Many women find that **yoga** (the ancient meditation/ **exercise** developed in India 5,000 years ago) can ease menopausal symptoms. Yoga focuses on helping women unite the mind, body, and spirit to create balance. Because yoga has been shown to balance the endocrine system, some experts believe it may affect hormone-related problems. Studies have found that yoga can reduce **stress,** improve mood, boost a sluggish metabolism, and slow the heart rate. Specific yoga positions deal with particular problems, such as hot flashes, mood swings, vaginal and urinary problems, and other **pains.**

Exercise

Exercise helps ease hot flashes by lowering the amount of circulating FSH and LH and by raising endorphin levels (which drop while you're having a hot flash). Even exercising 20 minutes three times a week can significantly reduce hot flashes.

Elimination

Regular, daily bowel movements to eliminate waste products from the body can be crucial in maintaining balance through menopause. The bowels are where circulating hormones are gathered and eliminated, keeping the body from recycling them and causing an imbalance.

Acupuncture

This ancient Asian art involves placing very thin needles into different parts of the body to stimulate the system and unblock energy. It is usually painless and has been used for many menopausal symptoms, including insomnia, hot flashes, and irregular periods. Practitioners believe that **acupuncture** can facilitate the opening of blocked energy channels, allowing the life force energy (chi) to flow freely. This allows the menopausal woman to keep her energy moving. Blocked energy usually increases the symptoms of menopause.

Acupressure and massage

Therapeutic **massage** involving **acupressure** can bring relief from a wide range of menopause symptoms by placing finger pressure at the same meridian points on the body that are used in acupuncture. There are more than 80 different types of massage, including foot **reflexology,** Shiatsu massage, or Swedish massage, but they are all based on the idea that boosting the circulation of blood and lymph benefits health.

Biofeedback

Some women have been able to control hot flashes through **biofeedback,** a painless technique that helps a person train her mind to control her body. A biofeedback machine provides information about body processes (such as heart rate) as the woman relaxes her body. Using this technique, it is possible to control the body's temperature, heart rate, and breathing.

Prognosis

Menopause is a natural condition of aging. Some women have no problems at all with menopause, while others notice significant unpleasant symptoms. A wide array of treatments, from natural to hormone replacement, mean that no woman needs to suffer through this time of her life.

Prevention

Menopause is a natural part of the aging process and not a disease that needs to be prevented. Most doctors recommend HRT for almost all post-menopausal women, usually for a few years. When HRT is then stopped, symptoms should be mild or non existent. But HRT is not only useful in lessening the symptoms of menopause; it also protects against heart disease and osteoporosis.

Resources

BOOKS

Carlson, Karen J., Stephanie Eisenstat, and Terra Ziporyn. *The Harvard Guide to Women's Health.* Cambridge, MA: Harvard University Press, 1996.

Jacobowitz, Ruth S. *150 Most-Asked Questions About Menopause.* New York: William Morrow, 1993.

Notelovitz, Morris, and Diana Tonnessen. *Estrogen: Yes or No?* New York: St. Martin's Press, 1993.

Notelovitz, Morris, and Diana Tonnessen. *Menopause and Midlife Health.* New York: St. Martin's Press, 1993.

Perry, Susan, and Kate O'Hanlan. *Natural Menopause: The Complete Guide.* Reading, MA: Addison-Wesley, 1997.

Sachs, Judith. *What Women Should Know About Menopause.* New York: Dell Publishing, 1991.

Teaff, Nancy Lee, and Kim Wright Wiley. *Perimenopause: Preparing for the Change.* Prima Publishing, 1996.

Turkington, Carol A. *The Perimenopause Sourcebook.* New York: Contemporary Books, 1998.

PERIODICALS

Adami, H.O., and I. Persson. ''Hormone Replacement and Breast Cancer: A Remaining Controversy?'' *Journal of the American Medical Association* 274 (1995): 178-9.

Nash, J. Madeleine. ''Early Flash Points: Beset by Symptoms Caused by Ebbing Hormones, Women in Midlife Turn to Herbs and Health Foods to Smooth Out the Rocky Road to Menopause.'' *Time* 146 (April 21, 1997).

Seachrist, Lia. ''What Risk Hormones? Conflicting Studies Reveal Problems in Pinning Down Breast Cancer Risks.'' *Science News* 148 (Aug. 5, 1995): 94-95.

Shute, Nancy. ''Menopause is No Disease.'' *U.S. News & World Report* 122 (March 24, 1997): 71.

Stampfer, M.J, et al. ''Postmenopausal Estrogen Therapy and Cardiovascular Disease: Ten Year Follow Up From the Nurses' Health Study.'' *New England Journal of Medicine* 325 (Sept. 12, 1991): 756-762.

Stanford, J.L., N.S. Weiss, et al. ''Combined Estrogen and Progestin Hormone Replacement Therapy in Relation to Risk of Breast Cancer.'' *Journal of the American Medical Association* 274 (July 12, 1995): 137-142.

Wallis, Claudia. ''The Estrogen Dilemma.'' *Time* 145 (June 26, 1995).

Wright, Karen, ''Menopause, Naturally.'' *Health* (Jan./Feb. 1996): 75-79.

ORGANIZATIONS

American Menopause Foundation, Inc. Empire State Bldg., 350 Fifth Ave., Ste. 2822, New York, NY 10118. (212) 714-2398.

Federation of Feminist Women's Health Centers. 633 East 11th Ave., Eugene, OR 97401. (503) 344-0966.

Hysterectomy Educational Resources and Services Foundation (HERS), 422 Bryn Mawr Ave., Bala Cynwyd, PA 19004. (215) 667-7757.

National Women's Health Network. 1325 G St. NW, Washington, DC 20005. (202) 347-1140.

North American Menopause Society. PO Box 94527, Cleveland, OH 44101. (216) 844-8748. http:www.menopause.org/.

Resources for Midlife and Older Women. 226 E. 70 St., Ste. 1C, New York, NY 10021. (212) 439-1913.

OTHER

Menopause. http://www.howdyneighbor.com/menopaus/.

Menopause Online. http://www.menopause-online.com/links.htm.

Meno Times. http://www.aimnet.com/~hyperion/meno/menotimes.index.html.

Power Surge Reading Room. http://members.aol.com/dearest/news.htm.

Women's Health. http://women.shn.net/index.html.

Women's Health Initiative. http://www.nih.gov/od/odp/whi.

Carol A. Turkington

Menorrhagia *see* **Dysfunctional uterine bleeding**

Menstrual disorders *see* **Dysfunctional uterine bleeding; Dysmenorrhea; Oligomenorrhea**

Menstrual pain *see* **Dysmenorrhea**

Mental retardation

Definition

Mental retardation is a developmental disability that first appears in children under the age of 18. It is defined as an intellectual functioning level (as measured by standard tests for intelligence quotient) that is well below average and significant limitations in daily living skills (adaptive functioning).

Description

Mental retardation occurs in 2.5-3% of the general population. About 6-7.5 million mentally retarded individuals live in the United States alone. Mental retardation begins in childhood or adolescence before the age of 18. In most cases, it persists throughout adulthood. A diagnosis of mental retardation is made if an individual has an intellectual functioning level well below average and significant limitations in two or more adaptive skill areas. Intellectual functioning level is defined by standardized tests that measure the ability to reason in terms of mental age (intelligence quotient or IQ). Mental retardation is defined as IQ score below 70-75. Adaptive skills are the skills needed for daily life. Such skills include the ability to produce and understand language (communication); home-living skills; use of community resources; health, safety, leisure, self-care, and social skills; self-direction; functional academic skills (reading, writing, and arithmetic); and work skills.

In general, mentally retarded children reach developmental milestones such as walking and talking much later than the general population. Symptoms of mental retardation may appear at birth or later in childhood. Time of onset depends on the suspected cause of the disability. Some cases of mild mental retardation are not diagnosed before the child enters preschool. These children typically have difficulties with social, communication, and functional academic skills. Children who have a neurological disorder or illness such as **encephalitis** or **meningitis** may suddenly show signs of cognitive impairment and adaptive difficulties.

Mental retardation varies in severity. *The Diagnostic and Statistical Manual of Mental Disorders,* Fourth Edition (*DSM-IV*) is the diagnostic standard for mental healthcare professionals in the United States. The *DSM-IV* classifies four different degrees of mental retardation: *mild, moderate, severe,* and *profound.* These categories are based on the functioning level of the individual.

Mild mental retardation

Approximately 85% of the mentally retarded population is in the mildly retarded category. Their IQ score ranges from 50-75, and they can often acquire academic skills up to the 6th grade level. They can become fairly self-sufficient and in some cases live independently, with community and social support.

Moderate mental retardation

About 10% of the mentally retarded population is considered moderately retarded. Moderately retarded individuals have IQ scores ranging from 35-55. They can carry out work and self-care tasks with moderate supervision. They typically acquire communication skills in childhood and are able to live and function successfully within the community in a supervised environment such as a group home.

Severe mental retardation

About 3-4% of the mentally retarded population is severely retarded. Severely retarded individuals have IQ scores of 20-40. They may master very basic self-care skills and some communication skills. Many severely retarded individuals are able to live in a group home.

KEY TERMS

Amniocentesis—A test usually done between 16 and 20 weeks of pregnancy to detect any abnormalities in the development of the fetus. A small amount of the fluid surrounding the fetus (amniotic fluid) is drawn out through a needle inserted into the mother's womb. Laboratory analysis of this fluid can detect various genetic defects, such as Down syndrome, or neural tube defects.

Developmental delay—The failure to meet certain developmental milestones, such as sitting, walking, and talking, at the average age. Developmental delay may indicate a problem in development of the central nervous system.

Down syndrome—A disorder caused by an abnormality at the 21st chromosome. One symptom of Down syndrome is mental retardation.

Extensive support—Ongoing daily support required to assist an individual in a specific adaptive area, such as daily help with preparing meals.

Hib disease—An infection caused by *Haemophilus influenza* type b (Hib). This disease mainly affects children under the age of five. In that age group, it is the leading cause of bacterial meningitis, pneumonia, joint and bone infections, and throat inflammations.

Inborn error of metabolism—A rare enzyme deficiency; children with inborn errors of metabolism do not have certain enzymes that the body requires to maintain organ functions. Inborn errors of metabolism can cause brain damage and mental retardation if left untreated. Phenylketonuria is an inborn error of metabolism.

Limited support—A predetermined period of assistance required to deal with a specific event, such as training for a new job.

Phenylketonuria (PKU)—An inborn error in metabolism that prevents the body from using phenylalanine, an amino acid necessary for normal growth and development.

Trisomy—An abnormality in chromosomal development. Chromosomes are the structures within a cell that carry its genetic information. They are organized in pairs. Humans have 23 pairs of chromosomes. In a trisomy syndrome, an extra chromosome is present so that the individual has three of a particular chromosome instead of the normal pair. An extra chromosome 18 (trisomy 18) causes mental retardation.

Ultrasonography—A process that uses the reflection of high-frequency sound waves to make an image of structures deep within the body. Ultrasonography is routinely used to detect fetal abnormalities.

Profound mental retardation

Only 1-2% of the mentally retarded population is classified as profoundly retarded. Profoundly retarded individuals have IQ scores under 20-25. They may be able to develop basic self-care and communication skills with appropriate support and training. Their retardation is often caused by an accompanying neurological disorder. The profoundly retarded need a high level of structure and supervision.

The American Association on Mental Retardation (AAMR) has developed another widely accepted diagnostic classification system for mental retardation. The AAMR classification system focuses on the capabilities of the retarded individual rather than on the limitations. The categories describe the level of support required. They are: *intermittent support, limited support, extensive support*, and *pervasive support*. To some extent, the AAMR classification mirrors the *DSM-IV* classification. Intermittent support, for example, is support needed only occasionally, perhaps during times of **stress** or crisis. It is

the type of support typically required for most mildly retarded individuals. At the other end of the spectrum, pervasive support, or life-long, daily support for most adaptive areas, would be required for profoundly retarded individuals.

Causes & symptoms

Low IQ scores and limitations in adaptive skills are the hallmarks of mental retardation. Aggression, self-injury, and **mood disorders** are sometimes associated with the disability. The severity of the symptoms and the age at which they first appear depend on the cause. Children who are mentally retarded reach developmental milestones significantly later than expected, if at all. If retardation is caused by chromosomal or other genetic disorders, it is often apparent from infancy. If retardation is caused by childhood illnesses or injuries, learning and adaptive skills that were once easy may suddenly become difficult or impossible to master.

In about 35% of cases, the cause of mental retardation cannot be found. Biological and environmental factors that can cause mental retardation include:

Genetics

About 5% of mental retardation is caused by hereditary factors. Mental retardation may be caused by an inherited abnormality of the genes, such as **fragile X syndrome.** Fragile X, a defect in the chromosome that determines sex, is the most common inherited cause of mental retardation. Single gene defects such as **phenylketonuria** (PKU) and other inborn errors of metabolism may also cause mental retardation if they are not found and treated early. An accident or mutation in genetic development may also cause retardation. Examples of such accidents are development of an extra chromosome 18 (trisomy 18) and **Down syndrome.** Down syndrome, also called mongolism or trisomy 21, is caused by an abnormality in the development of chromosome 21. It is the most common genetic cause of mental retardation.

Prenatal illnesses and issues

Fetal alcohol syndrome affects one in 600 children in the United States. It is caused by excessive alcohol intake in the first twelve weeks (trimester) of **pregnancy.** Some studies have shown that even moderate alcohol use during pregnancy may cause learning disabilities in children. Drug abuse and cigarette smoking during pregnancy have also been linked to mental retardation.

Maternal infections and illnesses such as glandular disorders, **rubella, toxoplasmosis,** and **cytomegalovirus infection** may cause mental retardation. When the mother has high blood pressure (**hypertension**) or blood poisoning (toxemia), the flow of oxygen to the fetus may be reduced, causing brain damage and mental retardation.

Birth defects that cause physical deformities of the head, brain, and central nervous system frequently cause mental retardation. Neural tube defect, for example, is a birth defect in which the neural tube that forms the spinal cord does not close completely. This defect may cause children to develop an accumulation of cerebrospinal fluid on the brain (**hydrocephalus**). Hydrocephalus can cause learning impairment by putting pressure on the brain.

Childhood illnesses and injuries

Hyperthyroidism, whooping cough, chickenpox, measles, and Hib disease (a bacterial infection) may cause mental retardation if they are not treated adequately. An infection of the membrane covering the brain (meningitis) or an inflammation of the brain itself (encephalitis) cause swelling that in turn may cause brain damage and mental retardation. Traumatic brain injury caused by a blow or a violent shake to the head may also cause brain damage and mental retardation in children.

Environmental factors

Ignored or neglected infants who are not provided the mental and physical stimulation required for normal development may suffer irreversible learning impairments. Children who live in poverty and suffer from **malnutrition,** unhealthy living conditions, and improper or inadequate medical care are at a higher risk. Exposure to lead can also cause mental retardation. Many children have developed **lead poisoning** by eating the flaking lead-based paint often found in older buildings.

Diagnosis

If mental retardation is suspected, a comprehensive **physical examination** and medical history should be done immediately to discover any organic cause of symptoms. Conditions such as hyperthyroidism and PKU are treatable. If these conditions are discovered early, the progression of retardation can be stopped and, in some cases, partially reversed. If a neurological cause such as brain injury is suspected, the child may be referred to a neurologist or neuropsychologist for testing.

A complete medical, family, social, and educational history is compiled from existing medical and school records (if applicable) and from interviews with parents. Children are given intelligence tests to measure their learning abilities and intellectual functioning. Such tests include the **Stanford-Binet Intelligence Scale,** the Wechsler Intelligence Scales, the Wechsler Preschool and Primary Scale of Intelligence, and the Kaufmann Assessment Battery for Children. For infants, the Bayley Scales of Infant Development may be used to assess motor, language, and problem-solving skills. Interviews with parents or other caregivers are used to assess the child's daily living, muscle control, communication, and social skills. The Woodcock-Johnson Scales of Independent Behavior and the Vineland Adaptive Behavior Scale (VABS) are frequently used to test these skills.

Treatment

Federal legislation entitles mentally retarded children to free testing and appropriate, individualized education and skills training within the school system from ages 3-21. For children under the age of three, many states have established early intervention programs that assess, recommend, and begin treatment programs. Many day schools are available to help train retarded children in basic skills such as bathing and feeding themselves. Extracurricular activities and social programs are also important in helping retarded children and adolescents gain self-esteem.

Training in independent living and job skills is often begun in early adulthood. The level of training depends on the degree of retardation. Mildly retarded individuals can often acquire the skills needed to live independently and hold an outside job. Moderate to profoundly retarded individuals usually require supervised community living.

Family therapy can help relatives of the mentally retarded develop coping skills. It can also help parents deal with feelings of guilt or anger. A supportive, warm home environment is essential to help the mentally retarded reach their full potential.

Prognosis

Individuals with mild to moderate mental retardation are frequently able to achieve some self-sufficiency and to lead happy and fulfilling lives. To reach these goals, they need appropriate and consistent educational, community, social, family, and vocational supports. The outlook is less promising for those with severe to profound retardation. Studies have shown that these individuals have a shortened life expectancy. The diseases that are usually associated with severe retardation may cause the shorter life span. People with Down syndrome will develop the brain changes that characterize **Alzheimer's disease** in later life and may develop the clinical symptoms of this disease as well.

Prevention

Immunization against diseases such as measles and Hib prevents many of the illnesses that can cause mental retardation. In addition, all children should undergo routine developmental screening as part of their pediatric care. Screening is particularly critical for those children who may be neglected or undernourished or may live in disease-producing conditions. Newborn screening and immediate treatment for PKU and hyperthyroidism can usually catch these disorders early enough to prevent retardation.

Good prenatal care can also help prevent retardation. Pregnant women should be educated about the risks of drinking and the need to maintain good nutrition during pregnancy. Tests such as **amniocentesis** and ultrasonography can determine whether a fetus is developing normally in the womb.

Resources

BOOKS

American Psychiatric Association. *Diagnostic and Statistical Manual of Mental Disorders.* 4th ed. Washington, DC: American Psychiatric Press, Inc., 1994.

Batshaw, Mark L. and Bruce K. Shapiro. "Mental Retardation." In *Children with Disabilities,* edited by Mark L. Batshaw. 4th edition. Baltimore: Paul H. Brookes, 1997.

Maxmen, Jerrold S. and Nicholas G. Ward. "Disorders Usually First Diagnosed in Infancy, Childhood, or Adolescence." In *Essential Psychopathology and Its Treatment.* 2nd ed. New York: W.W. Norton, 1995.

PERIODICALS

Martin, Barry A. "Primary Care of Adults with Mental Retardation Living in the Community." *American Family Physician* 56(August 1997): 485-494.

ORGANIZATIONS

American Association on Mental Retardation (AAMR). 444 North Capitol Street, NW, Suite 846, Washington, D.C. 20001-1512 (800)424-3688. http://www.aamr.org.

The Arc of the United States (formerly Association for Retarded Citizens of the United States). 500 East Border Street, Suite 300, Arlington, TX 76010. (817)261-6003. http://Thearc.org.

OTHER

U.S. Department of Justice. Americans With Disabilities Act (ADA) Homepage. http://www.usdoj.gov/crt/ada/adahom1.htm.

Paula Anne Ford-Martin

Meperidine *see* **Analgesics, opioid**

Metabolic acidosis

Definition

Metabolic acidosis is a pH imbalance in which the body has accumulated too much acid and does not have enough bicarbonate to effectively neutralize the effects of the acid.

Description

Metabolic acidosis, as a disruption of the body's acid/base balance, can be a mild symptom brought on by a lack of insulin, a **starvation** diet, or a gastrointestinal disorder like vomiting and **diarrhea.** Metabolic acidosis can indicate a more serious problem with a major organ like the liver, heart, or kidneys. It can also be one of the first signs of **drug overdose** or **poisoning.**

Causes & symptoms

Metabolic acidosis occurs when the body has more acid than base in it. Chemists use the term "pH" to describe how acidic or basic a substance is. Based on a scale of 14, a pH of 7.0 is neutral. A pH below 7.0 is an acid; the lower the number, the stronger the acid. A pH above 7.0 is a base; the higher the number, the stronger

KEY TERMS

Diabetic ketoacidosis—A condition caused by low insulin levels where the amount of sugar and ketones in the blood is high.

pH—A measurement of the acidity or alkalinity of a solution based on the amount of hydrogen ions available. Based on a scale of 14, a pH of 7.0 is neutral. A pH below 7.0 is an acid; the lower the number, the stronger the acid. A pH above 7.0 is a base; the higher the number, the stronger the base. Blood pH is slightly alkaline (basic) with a normal range of 7.36-7.44.

the base. Blood pH is slightly basic (alkaline), with a normal range of 7.36-7.44.

Acid is a natural by-product of the breakdown of fats and other processes in the body; however, in some conditions, the body does not have enough bicarbonate, an acid neutralizer, to balance the acids produced. This can occur when the body uses fats for energy instead of carbohydrates. Conditions where metabolic acidosis can occur include chronic **alcoholism, malnutrition,** and diabetic ketoacidosis. Consuming a diet low in carbohydrates and high in fats can also produce metabolic acidosis. The disorder may also be a symptom of another condition like kidney failure, liver failure, or severe diarrhea. The build up of lactic acid in the blood due to such conditions as **heart failure, shock,** or **cancer,** induces metabolic acidosis. Some poisonings and overdoses (**aspirin,** methanol, or ethylene glycol) also produce symptoms of metabolic acidosis.

In mild cases of metabolic acidosis, symptoms include **headache,** lack of energy, and sleepiness. Breathing may become fast and shallow. Nausea, vomiting, diarrhea, **dehydration,** and loss of appetite are also associated with metabolic acidosis. Diabetic patients with symptoms of metabolic acidosis may also have breath that smells fruity. The patient may lose consciousness or become disoriented. Severe cases can produce **coma** and **death.**

Diagnosis

Metabolic acidosis is suspected based on symptoms, but is usually confirmed by laboratory tests on blood and urine samples. Blood pH below 7.35 confirms the condition. Levels of other blood components, including potassium, glucose, ketones, or lactic acid, may also be above normal ranges. The level of bicarbonate in the blood will be low, usually less than 22 mEq/L. Urine pH may fall below 4.5 in metabolic acidosis.

Treatment

Treatment focuses first on correcting the acid imbalance. Usually, sodium bicarbonate and fluids will be injected into the blood through a vein. An intravenous line may be started to administer fluids and allow for the quick injection of other drugs that may be needed. If the patient is diabetic, insulin may be administered. Drugs to regulate blood pressure or heart rate, to prevent seizures, or to control **nausea and vomiting** might be given. Vital signs like pulse, respiration, blood pressure, and body temperature will be monitored. The underlying cause of the metabolic acidosis must also be diagnosed and corrected.

Prognosis

If the metabolic acidosis is recognized and treated promptly, the patient may have no long-term complications, however, the underlying condition that caused the acidosis needs to be corrected or managed. Severe metabolic acidosis that is left untreated will lead to coma and death.

Prevention

Diabetic patients need to routinely test their urine for sugar and acetone, strictly follow their appropriate diet, and take any medications or insulin to prevent metabolic acidosis. Patients receiving **tube feedings** or intravenous feedings must be monitored to prevent dehydration or the accumulation of ketones or lactic acid.

Resources

BOOKS

''Acid-Base Disturbances.'' In *Cecil Textbook of Medicine.* 20th ed. Philadelphia: W.B. Saunders Company, 1996.

DuBose, Thomas D., Jr. ''Acidosis and Alkalosis.'' In *Harrison's Principles of Internal Medicine.* 14th ed. New York: McGraw-Hill, 1998.

''Fluid, Electrolyte, and Acid-Base Disorders.'' In *Family Medicine Principles and Practices.* 5th ed. New York: Springer-Verlag, 1998.

''Fluid & Electrolyte Disorders.'' In *Current Medical Diagnosis & Treatment 1998.* 37th ed. Stamford, CT: Appleton & Lange, 1998.

Altha Roberts Edgren

Metabolic alkalosis

Definition

Metabolic alkalosis is a pH imbalance in which the body has accumulated too much of an alkaline substance, such as bicarbonate, and does not have enough acid to effectively neutralize the effects of the alkali.

Description

Metabolic alkalosis, as a disturbance of the body's acid/base balance, can be a mild condition, brought on by vomiting, the use of steroids or diuretic drugs, or the overuse of **antacids** or **laxatives.** Metabolic alkalosis can also indicate a more serious problem with a major organ such as the kidneys.

Causes & symptoms

Metabolic alkalosis occurs when the body has more base than acid in the system. Chemists use the term ''pH'' to decribe how acidic or alkaline (also called basic) a substance is. Based on a scale of 14, a pH of 7.0 is neutral. A pH below 7.0 is an acid; the lower the number, the stronger the acid. A pH above 7.0 is alkaline; the higher the number, the stronger the alkali. Blood pH is slightly alkaline, with a normal range of 7.36-7.44. Conditions that lead to a reduced amount of fluid in the body, like vomiting or excessive urination due to use of diuretic drugs, change the balance of fluids and salts. The blood levels of potassium and sodium can decrease dramatically, causing symptoms of metabolic alkalosis.

In cases of metabolic alkalosis, slowed breathing may be an initial symptom. The patient may have episodes of apnea (not breathing) that may go on 15 seconds or longer. **Cyanosis,** a bluish or purplish discoloration of the skin, may also develop as a sign of inadequate oxygen intake. Nausea, vomiting, and **diarrhea** may also occur. Other symptoms can include irritability, twitching, confusion, and picking at bedclothes. Rapid heart rate, irregular heart beats, and a drop in blood pressure are also

symptoms. Severe cases can lead to convulsions and **coma.**

Diagnosis

Metabolic alkalosis may be suspected based on symptoms, but often may not be noticeable. The condition is usually confirmed by laboratory tests on blood and urine samples. Blood pH above 7.45 confirms the condition. Levels of other blood components, including salts like potassium, sodium, and chloride, fall below normal ranges. The level of bicarbonate in the blood will be high, usually greater than 29 mEq/L. Urine pH may rise to about 7.0 in metabolic alkalosis.

Treatment

Treatment focuses first on correcting the imbalance. An intravenous line may be started to administer fluids (generally normal saline, a salt water solution) and allow for the quick injection of other drugs that may be needed. Potassium chloride will be administered. Drugs to regulate blood pressure or heart rate, or to control **nausea and vomiting** might be given. Vital signs like pulse, respiration, blood pressure, and body temperature will be monitored. The underlying cause of the metabolic alkalosis must also be diagnosed and corrected.

Prognosis

If metabolic alkalosis is recognized and treated promptly, the patient may have no long-term complications; however, the underlying condition that caused the alkalosis needs to be corrected or managed. Severe metabolic alkalosis that is left untreated will lead to convulsions, **heart failure,** and coma.

Prevention

Patients receiving **tube feedings** or intravenous feedings must be monitored to prevent an imbalance of fluids and salts, particularly potassium, sodium, and chloride. Overuse of some drugs, including **diuretics,** laxatives, and antacids, should be avoided.

Resources

BOOKS

''Acid-Base Disturbances.'' In *Cecil Textbook of Medicine.* 20th ed. Philadelphia: W.B. Saunders Company, 1996.

DuBose, Thomas D., Jr. ''Acidosis and Alkalosis.'' In *Harrison's Principles of Internal Medicine.* 14th ed. New York: McGraw-Hill, 1998.

''Fluid, Electrolyte, and Acid-Base Disorders.'' In *Family Medicine Principles and Practices.* 5th ed. New York: Springer-Verlag, 1998.

"Fluid & Electrolyte Disorders." In *Current Medical Diagnosis & Treatment 1998*. 37th ed. Stamford, CT: Appleton & Lange, 1998.

Altha Roberts Edgren

Metabolic encephalopahty *see* **Delirium**

Metaproterenol *see* **Bronchodilators**

Methocarbamol *see* **Muscle relaxants**

Methotrexate *see* **Anticancer drugs**

Methyl salicylate *see* **Antiseptics**

Methylphenidate *see* **Central nervous system stimulants**

Metoprolol *see* **Beta blockers**

Metronidazole *see* **Antiprotozoal drugs**

Metrorrhagia *see* **Dysfunctional uterine bleeding**

Micronazole *see* **Antifungal drugs, topical**

Middle ear infection *see* **Otitis media**

Migraine headache

Definition

Migraine is a type of **headache** marked by severe head **pain** lasting several hours or more.

Description

Migraine is an intense, often debilitating type of headache. Migraines affect as many as 24 million people in the United States, and are responsible for billions of dollars in lost work, poor job performance, and direct medical costs. Approximately 18% of women and 6% of men experience at least one migraine attack per year. More than three million women and one million men have one or more severe headaches every month. Migraines often begin in adolescence, and are rare after age 60.

Two types of migraine are recognized. Eighty percent of migraine sufferers experience "migraine without

aura," formerly called common migraine. In "migraine with aura," formerly called classic migraine, pain is preceded or accompanied by visual or other sensory disturbances, including **hallucinations,** partial obstruction of the visual field, numbness or tingling, or a feeling of heaviness. Symptoms are often most prominent on one side of the body, and may begin as early as 72 hours before the onset of pain.

Causes & symptoms

Causes

The physiological basis of migraine has proved difficult to uncover. Genetics appear to play a part for many, but not all, people with migraine. There are a multitude of potential triggers for a migraine attack, and recognizing one's own set of triggers is the key to prevention.

PHYSIOLOGY

The most widely accepted hypothesis of migraine suggests that a migraine attack is precipitated when pain-sensing nerve cells in the brain (called nociceptors) release chemicals called neuropeptides. At least one of the neurotransmitters, substance P, increases the pain sensitivity of other nearby nociceptors.

Other neuropeptides act on the smooth muscle surrounding cranial blood vessels. This smooth muscle regulates blood flow in the brain by relaxing or contracting, thus dilating (enlarging) or constricting the enclosed blood vessels. At the onset of a migraine **headache,** neuropeptides are thought to cause muscle relaxation, allowing vessel dilation and increased blood flow. Other neuropeptides increase the leakiness of cranial vessels, allowing fluid leak, and promote inflammation and tissue swelling. The pain of migraine is though to result from this combination of increased pain sensitivity, tissue and vessel swelling, and inflammation. The aura seen during a migraine may be related to constriction in the blood vessels that dilate in the headache phase.

GENETICS

Susceptibility to migraine may be inherited. A child of a migraine sufferer has as much as a 50% chance of developing migraine. If both parents are affected, the chance rises to 70%. However, the gene or genes responsible have not been identified, and many cases of migraine have no obvious familial basis. It is likely that whatever genes are involved set the stage for migraine, and that full development requires environmental influences as well.

TRIGGERS

A wide variety of foods, drugs, environmental cues, and personal events are known to trigger migraines. It is not known how most triggers set off the events of mi-

Phase 1 (The Prodrome): up to 24 hours prior to the headache
Roughly half of all migraine sufferers experience this stage, which is characterized by symptoms of heightened or dulled perception, irritability or withdrawal, and food cravings.

Phase 2 (The Aura): up to 1 hour prior to the headache
One out of five migraine sufferers experience this stage of visual disturbances. There may be flashing lights, shimmering zig-zag lines, and luminous blind spots, as well as non-visual sensations like numbness and pins and needles in the hands.

Phase 3 (The Headache): 4-72 hours long
Characterized by:
• Severe aching, often pulsating or throbbing pain on one or both sides of the head

• Intolerance of light (photophobia)

• Intolerance of noise (phonophobia)

• Nausea and vomiting

• Sensitivity to movement

• And less commonly, speech difficulties

Phase 4 (The Postdrome): up to 24 hours after the headache
Most migraine sufferers experience aching muscles and feel tired and drained after the headache, although some few go through a period of euphoria.

The phases of a typical migraine headache. (*Illustration by Hans & Cassady, Inc.*)

graine, nor why individual migraine sufferers are affected by particular triggers but not others.

Common food triggers include:

• Cheese
• Alcohol
• **Caffeine** products, and caffeine withdrawal
• Chocolate
• Intensely sweet foods
• Dairy products
• Fermented or pickled foods
• Citrus fruits
• Nuts
• Processed foods, especially those containing nitrites, sulfites, or monosodium glutamate (MSG).

Environmental and event-related triggers include:

• **Stress** or time pressure
• Menstrual periods, **menopause**
• Sleep changes or disturbances, oversleeping
• Prolonged overexertion or uncomfortable posture

• Hunger or **fasting**
• Odors, smoke, or perfume
• Strong glare or flashing lights.

Drugs which may trigger migraine include:

• **Oral contraceptives**
• Estrogen replacement therapy
• Nitrates
• Theophylline
• Reserpine
• Nifedipine
• Indomethicin
• Cimetidine
• Decongestant overuse
• Analgesic overuse
• Benzodiazepine withdrawal.

Symptoms

Migraine without aura may be preceded by elevations in mood or energy level for up to 24 hours before the attack. Other pre-migraine symptoms may include fatigue, depression, and excessive yawning.

Aura most often begins with shimmering, jagged arcs of white or colored light progressing over the visual field in the course of 10-20 minutes. This may be preceded or replaced by dark areas or other visual disturbances. **Numbness and tingling** is common, especially of the face and hands. These sensations may spread, and may be accompanied by a sensation of weakness or heaviness in the affected limb.

The pain of migraine is often present only on one side of the head, although it may involve both, or switch sides during attacks. The pain is usually throbbing, and may range from mild to incapacitating. It is often accompanied by nausea or vomiting, painful sensitivity to light and sound, and intolerance of food or odors. Blurred vision is common.

Migraine pain tends to intensify over the first 30 minutes to several hours, and may last from several hours to a day or longer. Afterward, the affected person is usually weary, and sensitive to sudden head movements.

Diagnosis

Migraine is diagnosed by a careful medical history. Lab tests and imaging studies such as **computed tomography** (CT scan) or **magnetic resonance imaging** (MRI) scans have not been useful for identifying migraine. However, for some patients, those tests may be needed to rule out a **brain tumor** or other structural causes of migraine headache.

Treatment

Once a migraine begins, the person will usually seek out a dark, quiet room to lessen painful stimuli. Several drugs may be used to reduce the pain and severity of the attack.

Nonsteroidal anti-inflammatory drugs (NSAIDs) are helpful for early and mild headache. NSAIDs include **acetaminophen,** ibuprofen, naproxen, and others. A recent study concluded that a combination of acetaminophen, **aspirin,** and caffeine could effectively relieve symptoms for many migraine patients. One such over-the-counter preparation is available as Exedrin Migraine.

More severe or unresponsive attacks may be treated with drugs that act on serotonin receptors in the smooth muscle surrounding cranial blood vessels. Serotonin, also known as 5-hydroxytryptamine, constricts these vessels, relieving migraine pain. Drugs that mimic serotonin and bind to these receptors have the same effect. The oldest of them is ergotamine, a derivative of a common grain fungus. Ergotamine and dihydroergotamine are used for both acute and preventive treatment. Derivatives with fewer side effects have come onto the market in the past

decade, including sumatriptan (Imitrex). Some of these drugs are available as nasal sprays, intramuscular injections, or rectal suppositories for patients in whom vomiting precludes oral administration. Other drugs used for acute attacks include meperidine and metoclopramide.

Continued use of some anti-migraine drugs can lead to "rebound headache," marked by frequent or chronic headaches, especially in the early morning hours. Rebound headache is avoided by using anti-migraine drugs under a doctor's supervision, with the minimum dose necessary to treat symptoms. Patients with frequent migraines may need preventive therapy.

Alternative treatments

Alternative treatments are aimed at prevention of migraine. Migraine headaches are often linked with food allergies or intolerances. Identification and elimination of the offending food or foods can decrease the frequency of migraines and/or alleviate these headaches altogether. Herbal therapy with feverfew (*Chrysanthemum parthenium*) may lessen the frequency of attacks. Learning to increase the flow of blood to the extremities through **biofeedback** training may allow a patient to prevent some of the vascular changes once a migraine begins. During a migraine, keep the lights low; put the feet in a tub of hot water and place a cold cloth on the occipital region (the back of the head). This draws the blood to the feet and decreases the pressure in the head.

Prognosis

Most people with migraines can bring their attacks under control through recognizing and avoiding triggers, and by use of appropriate drugs when migraine occurs. Some people with severe migraines do not respond to preventive or drug therapy. Migraines usually wane in intensity by age 60 and beyond.

Prevention

The frequency of migraine may be lessened by avoiding triggers. It is useful to keep a headache journal, recording the particulars and noting possible triggers for each attack. Specific measures which may help include:

• Eating at regular times, and not skipping meals

• Reducing the use of caffeine and pain-relievers

• Restricting physical exertion, especially on hot days

• Keeping regular sleep hours, but not oversleeping

• Managing time to avoid stress at work and home.

Some drugs can be used for migraine prevention, including specific members of these drug classes:

• **Beta blockers**

• **Tricyclic antidepressants**

• **Calcium channel blockers**

• Anticonvulsants

• Prozac

• **Monoamine oxidase inhibitors** (MAO)

• Serotonin antagonists.

For most patients, preventive drug therapy is not an appropriate option, since it requires continued use of powerful drugs. However, for women whose migraines coincide with the menstrual period, limited preventive treatment may be effective. Since these drugs are appropriate for patients with other medical conditions, the decision to prescribe them for migraine may be influenced by expected benefit elsewhere.

Resources

BOOKS

The American Council on Headache Education. *Migraine: The Complete Guide.* New York: Dell, 1994.

Sacks, O. *Migraine.* University of California Press, 1992.

PERIODICALS

"Drug Treatment of Migraine: Part I." *American Family Physician* (November 15, 1997): 2039-2048.

"Drug Treatment of Migraine: Part II." *American Family Physician* (December, 1997): 2279-2286.

"Guidelines for the Diagnosis and Management of Migraine in Clinical Practice." *Canadian Medical Association Journal* 156 (May 1, 1997): 1273-1287.

OTHER

American Medical Association. *Migraine.* www.ama-assn.org/special/migraine/.

Miliaria *see* **Prickly heat**

Milk of magnesia *see* **Antacids**

Miner's asthma *see* **Black lung disease**

Mineral deficiency

Definition

The term mineral deficiency means a condition where the concentration of any one of the **minerals** essential to human health is abnormally low in the body. In some cases, an abnormally low mineral concentration is defined as that which leads to an impairment in a function dependent on the mineral. In other cases, the

convention may be to define an abnormally low mineral concentration as a level lower than that found in a specific healthy population.

The mineral nutrients are defined as all the inorganic elements or inorganic molecules that are required for life. As far as human nutrition is concerned, the inorganic nutrients include water, sodium, potassium, chloride, calcium, phosphate, sulfate, magnesium, iron, copper, zinc, manganese, iodine, selenium, and molybdenum. Some of the inorganic nutrients, such as water, do not occur as single atoms, but occur as molecules. Other inorganic nutrients that are molecules include phosphate, sulfate, and selenite. Phosphate contains an atom of phosphorus. Sulfate contains an atom of sulfur. We do not need to eat sulfate, since the body can acquire all the sulfate it needs from protein. Selenium occurs in foods as selenite and selenate.

There is some evidence that other inorganic nutrients, such as chromium and boron, play a part in human health, but their role is not well established. Fluoride has been proven to increase the strength of bones and teeth, but there is little or no reason to believe that is needed for human life.

The mineral content of the body may be measured by testing samples of blood plasma, red blood cells, or urine. In the case of calcium and phosphate deficiency, the diagnosis may also involve taking x rays of the skeleton. In the case of iodine deficiency, the diagnosis may include examining the patient's neck with the eyes and hands. In the case of iron deficiency, the diagnosis may include the performance of a stair-stepping test by the patient. Since all the minerals serve strikingly different functions in the body, the tests for the corresponding deficiency are markedly different from each other.

Description

Laboratory studies with animals have revealed that severe deficiencies in any one of the inorganic nutrients can result in very specific symptoms, and finally in **death,** due to the failure of functions associated with that nutrient. In humans, deficiency in one nutrient may occur less often than deficiency in several nutrients. A patient suffering from **malnutrition** is deficient in a variety of nutrients. In the United States, malnutrition is most often found among severe alcoholics. In part, this is because the alcohol consumption may supply half of the energy requirement, resulting in a mineral and vitamin intake of half the expected level. Deficiencies in one nutrient do occur, for example, in human populations living in iodine-poor regions of the world, and in iron deficient persons who lose excess iron by abnormal bleeding.

Inorganic nutrients have a great variety of functions in the body. Water, sodium, and potassium deficiencies are most closely associated with abnormal nerve action and cardiac **arrhythmias.** Deficiencies in these nutrients tend to result not from a lack of content in the diet, but from excessive losses due to severe **diarrhea** and other causes. Iodine deficiency is a global public health problem. It occurs in parts of the world with iodine-deficient soils, and results in **goiter,** which involves a relatively harmless swelling of the neck, and cretinism, a severe birth defect. The only use of iodine in the body is for making thyroid hormone. However, since thyroid hormone has a variety of roles in development of the embryo, iodine deficiency during **pregnancy** results in a number of **birth defects.**

Calcium deficiency due to lack of dietary calcium occurs only rarely. However, calcium deficiency due to **vitamin D deficiency** can be found among certain populations. Vitamin D is required for the efficient absorption of calcium from the diet, and hence vitamin D deficiency in growing infants and children can result in calcium deficiency.

Dietary phosphate deficiency is rare because phosphate is plentiful in plant and animal foods, but also because phosphate is efficiently absorbed from the diet into the body. Iron deficiency causes anemia (lack of red blood cells), which results in tiredness and **shortness of breath.**

Dietary deficiencies in the remaining inorganic nutrients tend to be rare. Magnesium deficiency is uncommon, but when it occurs it tends to occur in chronic alcoholics, in persons taking diuretic drugs, and in those suffering from severe and prolonged diarrhea. Magnesium deficiency tends to occur with the same conditions that provoke deficiencies in sodium and potassium. Zinc deficiency is rare, but it has been found in impoverished populations in the Middle East, who rely on unleavened whole wheat bread as a major food source. Copper deficiency is also rare, but dramatic and health-threatening changes in copper metabolism occur in two genetic diseases, **Wilson's disease** and Menkes' disease.

Selenium deficiency may occur in regions of the world where the soils are poor in selenium. Low-selenium soils can produce foods that are also low in selenium. Premature infants may also be at risk for selenium deficiency. Manganese deficiency is very rare. Experimental studies with humans fed a manganese deficient diet have revealed that the deficiency produces a scaly, red rash on the skin of the upper torso. Molybdenum deficiency has probably never occurred, but indirect evidence suggests that if molybdenum deficiency could occur, it would result in **mental retardation** and death.

Causes & symptoms

Sodium deficiency (**hyponatremia**) and water deficiency are the most serious and widespread deficiencies in the world. These deficiencies tend to arise from excessive losses from the body, as during prolonged and severe diarrhea or vomiting. Diarrheal diseases are a major world health problem, and are responsible for about a quarter of the 10 million infant deaths that occur each year. Nearly all of these deaths occur in impoverished parts of Africa and Asia, where they result from contamination of the water supply by animal and human feces.

The main concern in treating diarrheal diseases is **dehydration,** that is, the losses of sodium and water which deplete the fluids of the circulatory system (the heart, veins, arteries, and capillaries). Severe losses of the fluids of the circulatory system result in **shock.** Shock nearly always occurs when dehydration is severe enough to produce a 10% reduction in body weight. Shock, which is defined as inadequate supply of blood to the various tissues of the body, results in a lack of oxygen to all the cells of the body. Although diarrheal fluids contain a number of electrolytes, the main concern in avoiding shock is the replacement of sodium and water.

Sodium deficiency and potassium deficiency also frequently result during treatment with drugs called **diuretics.** Diuretics work because they cause loss of sodium from the body. These drugs are used to treat high blood pressure (**hypertension**), where the resulting decline in blood pressure reduces the risk for cardiovascular disease. However, diuretics can lead to sodium deficiency, resulting in low plasma sodium levels. A side effect of some diuretics is excessive loss of potassium, and low plasma potassium (**hypokalemia**) may result.

Iodine deficiency tends to occur in regions of the world where the soil is poor in iodine. Where soil used in agriculture is poor in iodine, the foods grown in the soil will also be low in iodine. An iodine intake of 0.10-0.15 mg/day is considered to be nutritionally adequate, while iodine deficiency occurs at below 0.05 mg/day. Goiter, an enlargement of the thyroid gland (located in the neck), results from iodine deficiency. Goiter continues to be a problem in eastern Europe, parts of India and South America, and in Southeast Asia. Goiter has been eradicated in the United States because of the fortification of foods with iodine. Iodine deficiency during pregnancy results in cretinism in the newborn. Cretinism involves mental retardation, a large tongue, and sometimes deafness, muteness, and lameness.

Iron deficiency occurs due to periods of dietary deficiency, rapid growth, and excessive loss of the body's iron. Human milk and cow milk both contains low levels of iron. Infants are at risk for acquiring iron deficiency because their rapid rate of growth needs a corresponding increased supply of dietary iron, for use in making blood and muscles. Human milk is a better source of iron than cow milk, since about half of the iron in human breast milk is absorbed by the infant's digestive tract. In contrast, only 10% of the iron in cow milk is absorbed by the infant. Surveys of lower-income families in the United States have revealed that about 6% of the infants are anemic indicating a deficiency of iron in their diets. Blood loss that occurs with menstruation in women, as well as with a variety of causes of intestinal bleeding is a major cause of iron deficiency. The symptoms of iron deficiency are generally limited to anemia, and the resulting tiredness, weakness, and a reduced ability to perform physical work.

Calcium and phosphate are closely related nutrients. About 99% of the calcium and 85% of the phosphate in the body occur in the skeleton, where they exist as crystals of solid calcium phosphate. Both of these nutrients occur in a great variety of foods. Milk, eggs, and green, leafy vegetables are rich in calcium and phosphate. Whole cow milk, for example, contains about 1.2 g calcium and 0.95 g phosphorus per kg of food. Broccoli contains 1.0 g calcium and 0.67 g phosphorus per kg food. Eggs supply about one third of the calcium and phosphate of the overall population of the United States. Dietary deficiencies in calcium (**hypocalcemia**) or phosphate are extremely rare throughout the world. Vitamin D deficiency can be found among young infants, the elderly, and others who may be shielded from sunshine for prolonged periods of time. Vitamin D deficiency impairs the absorption of calcium from the diet, and in this way can provoke calcium deficiency even when the diet contains adequate calcium.

Zinc deficiency has been found among peasant populations in rural areas of the Middle East. Unleavened whole wheat bread can account for 75% of the energy intake in these areas. This diet, which does not contain meat, does contain zinc, but it also contains phytic acid at a level of about 3 g/day. The phytic acid, which naturally occurs in wheat, inhibits zinc absorption. The yeast used to leaven bread produces enzymes that inactivate the phytic acid. Unleavened bread does not contain yeast, and therefore, contains intact phytic acid. The symptoms of zinc deficiency include lack of sexual maturation, lack of pubic hair, and small stature. The amount of phytic acid in a typical American diet cannot provoke zinc deficiency.

Zinc deficiency is relatively uncommon in the United States, but it may occur in adults with **alcoholism** or intestinal malabsorption problems. Low plasma zinc has been found in patients with alcoholic **cirrhosis, Crohn's disease,** and **celiac disease.** Experimental studies with humans have shown that the signs of zinc deficiency are detectable after two to five weeks of consumption of the zinc-free diet. The signs include a rash and diarrhea. The rash occurs on the face, groin, hands, and feet. These symptoms can easily be reversed by administering zinc. An emerging concern is that increased calcium intake can interfere with zinc absorption or retention. Hence, there is some interest in the question of whether persons taking calcium to prevent **osteoporosis** should also take zinc supplements.

Severe alterations in copper metabolism occur in two genetic diseases, Wilson's disease and Menkes' disease. Both of these diseases are rare and occur in about one in 100,000 births. Both diseases involve mutations in copper transport proteins, that is, in special channels that allow the passage of copper ions through cell membranes. Menkes' disease is a genetic disease involving mental retardation and death before the age of three years. The disease also results in steely or kinky hair. The hair is tangled, grayish, and easily broken. Menkes' disease involves a decrease in copper levels in the serum, liver, and brain, and increases in copper in the cells of the intestines and kidney.

Selenium deficiency may occur in premature infants, since this population naturally tends to have low levels of plasma selenium. Full term infants have plasma selenium levels of about 0.001-0.002 mM, while premature infants may have levels about one third this amount. Whether these lower levels result in adverse consequences is not clear. Selenium deficiency occurs in regions of the world containing low-selenium soils. These regions include Keshan Province in China, New Zealand, and Finland. In Keshan Province, a disease (Keshan disease) occurs which results in deterioration of regions of the heart and the development of fibers in these regions. Keshan disease, which may be fatal, is thought to result from a combination of selenium deficiency and a virus.

Diagnosis

The diagnosis of deficiencies in water, sodium, potassium, iron, calcium, and phosphate involve chemical testing of the blood plasma, urine, and red blood cells.

Iodine deficiency can be diagnosed by measuring the concentration of iodine in the urine. A urinary level greater than 0.05 mg iodine per gram creatinine means adequate iodine status. Levels under 0.025 mg iodine/g creatinine indicate a serious risk.

Normal blood serum magnesium levels are 1.2-2.0 mM. Magnesium deficiency results in hypomagnesemia, which is defined as serum magnesium levels below 0.8 mM. Magnesium levels below 0.5 mM provoke a decline in serum calcium levels. Hypomagnesemia can also result in low serum potassium. Some of the symptoms of hypomagnesemia, which include twitching and convulsions, actually result from the hypocalcemia. Other symptoms of hypomagnesemia, such as cardiac arrhythmias, result from the low potassium levels.

There is no reliable test for zinc deficiency. When humans eat diets containing normal levels of zinc (16 mg/day), the level of urinary zinc is about 0.45 mg/day, while humans consuming low-zinc diets (0.3 mg/day) may have urinary levels of about 0.150 mg/day. Plasma zinc levels tend to be maintained during a dietary deficiency in zinc. Plasma and urinary zinc levels can be influenced by a variety of factors, and for this reason cannot provide a clear picture of zinc status.

Selenium deficiency may be diagnosed by measuring the selenium in plasma (70 ng/mL) or red blood cells (90 ng/mL), where the normal values are indicated. There is also some interest in measuring the activity of an enzyme in blood platelets, in order to assess selenium status. This enzyme is glutathione peroxidase. Platelets are small cells of the bloodstream which are used mainly to allow the clotting of blood after an injury.

Treatment

The treatment of deficiencies in sodium, potassium, calcium, phosphate, and iron usually involves intravenous injections of the deficient mineral.

Iodine deficiency can be easily prevented and treated by fortifying foods with iodine. Table salt is fortified with 100 mg potassium iodide per kg sodium chloride. Goiter was once common in the United States in areas from Washington State to the Great Lakes region, but this problem has been eliminated by iodized salt. Public health programs in impoverished countries have involved injections of synthetic oils containing iodine. Goiter is reversible but, cretinism is not.

Magnesium deficiency can be treated with a magnesium rich diet. If magnesium deficiency is due to a prolonged period of depletion, treatment may include injections of magnesium sulfate (2.0 mL of 50% $MgSO_4$). Where magnesium deficiency is severe enough to provoke convulsions, magnesium needs to be administered by injections or infusions. For infusion, 500 mL of a 1% solution (1 gram/100 mL) of magnesium sulfate is gradually introduced into a vein over the course of about five hours.

Zinc deficiency and copper deficiency are quite rare, but when they are detected or suspected, they can be treated by consuming zinc or copper, on a daily basis, at levels defined by the RDA.

Selenium deficiency in adults can be treated by eating 100 mg selenium per day for a week, where the selenium is supplied as selenomethionine. The incidence of Keshan disease in China has been reduced by supplementing children with 1.0 mg sodium selenite per week.

Prognosis

In iodine deficiency, the prognosis for treating goiter is excellent, however cretinism cannot be reversed. The effects of iron deficiency are not life-threatening and can be easily treated. The prognosis for treating magnesium deficiency is excellent. The symptoms may be relieved promptly or, at most, within two days of starting treatment. In cases of zinc deficiency in Iran and other parts of the Middle East, supplementation of affected young adults with zinc has been found to provoke the growth of pubic hair and enlargement of genitalia to a normal size within a few months.

Prevention

In the healthy population, all mineral deficiencies can be prevented by the consumption of inorganic nutrients at levels defined by the Recommended Dietary Allowances (RDA). Where a balanced diet is not available, government programs for treating individuals, or for fortifying the food supply, may be used. Government sponsored programs for the prevention of iron deficiency and iodine deficiency are widespread throughout the world. Selenium treatment programs have been used in parts of the world where selenium deficiency exists. Attention to potassium status, and to the prevention of potassium deficiency, is an issue mainly in patients taking diuretic drugs. In many cases of mineral deficiency, the deficiency occurs because of disease, and individual medical attention, rather than preventative measures, is used. The prevention of calcium deficiency is generally not an issue or concern, however calcium supplements are widely used with the hope of preventing osteoporosis. The prevention of deficiencies in magnesium, zinc, copper, manganese, or molybdenum are not major health issues in the United States. Ensuring an adequate intake of these minerals, by eating a balanced diet or by taking mineral supplements, is the best way to prevent deficiencies.

Resources

BOOKS

Brody, Tom. *Nutritional Biochemistry.* San Diego, CA: Academic Press, 1998.

Food and Nutrition Board. *Recommended Dietary Allowances.* 10th ed. Washington, DC: National Academy Press, 1989.

Tom Brody

Mineral excess *see* **Mineral toxicity**

Mineral toxicity

Definition

The term mineral toxicity means a condition where the concentration in the body of any one of the **minerals** is abnormally high, and where there is an adverse effect on health.

Description

In general, mineral toxicity results when there is an accidental consumption of too much of any mineral, as with drinking ocean water (sodium toxicity) or with overexposure to industrial pollutants, household chemicals, or certain drugs. Mineral toxicity may also apply to toxicity that can be the result of certain diseases or injuries. For example, **hemochromatosis** leads to iron toxicity; **Wilson's disease** results in copper toxicity; severe trauma can lead to **hyperkalemia** (potassium toxicity).

The mineral nutrients are defined as all the inorganic elements or inorganic molecules that are required for life. As far as human nutrition is concerned, the inorganic nutrients include water, sodium, potassium, chloride, calcium, phosphate, sulfate, magnesium, iron, copper, zinc, manganese, iodine, selenium, and molybdenum.

The mineral content of the body may be measured by testing samples of blood plasma, red blood cells, and urine.

Causes & symptoms

An increase in the concentrations of sodium in the bloodstream can be toxic. The normal concentration of sodium in the blood plasma is 136-145 mM, while levels over 152 mM can result in seizures and **death.** Increased plasma sodium, which is called **hypernatremia,** causes various cells of the body, including those of the brain, to shrink. Shrinkage of the brain cells results in confusion, **coma, paralysis** of the lung muscles, and death. Death has occurred where table salt (sodium chloride) was accidently used, instead of sugar, for feeding infants. Death due to sodium toxicity has also resulted when baking soda (sodium bicarbonate) was used during attempted therapy of excessive **diarrhea** or vomiting. Although a variety of processed foods contain high levels of sodium chloride, the levels used are not enough to result in sodium toxicity.

The normal level of potassium in the bloodstream is in the range of 3.5-5.0 mM, while levels of 6.3-8.0 mM (severe **hyperkalemia**) result in cardiac **arrhythmias** or even death due to cardiac arrest. Potassium is potentially quite toxic, however toxicity or death due to potassium poisoning is usually prevented because of the vomiting reflex. The consumption of food results in mild increases in the concentration of potassium in the bloodstream, but levels of potassium do not become toxic because of the uptake of potassium by various cells of the body, as well as by the action of the kidneys transferring the potassium ions from the blood to the urine. The body's regulatory mechanisms can easily be overwhelmed, however, when potassium chloride is injected intravenously, as high doses of injected potassium can easily result in death.

Iodine toxicity can result from an intake of 2.0 mg of iodide per day. The toxicity results in impairment of the creation of thyroid hormone, resulting in lower levels of thyroid hormone in the bloodstream. The thyroid gland enlarges, as a consequence, and **goiter** is produced. This enlargement is also called **hyperthyroidism.** Goiter is usually caused by iodine deficiency. In addition to goiter, iodine toxicity produces ulcers on the skin. This condition has been called "kelp acne," because of its association with eating kelp, an ocean plant, which contains high levels of iodine. Iodine toxicity occurs in Japan, where large amounts of seaweed are consumed.

Iron toxicity is not uncommon, due to the wide distribution of iron pills. A lethal dose of iron is in the range of 200-250 mg iron/kg body weight. Hence, a child who accidently eats 20 or more iron tablets may die as a result of iron toxicity. Within six hours of ingestion, iron toxicity can result in vomiting, diarrhea, abdominal **pain,** seizures, and possibly **coma.** A latent period, where the symptoms appear to improve, may occur but it is followed by **shock,** low blood glucose, liver damage, convulsions, and death, occuring 12-48 hours after toxic levels of iron are ingested.

Nitrite poisoning should be considered along with iron toxicity, since nitrite produces its toxic effect by reacting with the iron atom of hemoglobin. Hemoglobin is an iron-containing protein that resides within the red blood cells. This protein is responsible for the transport of nearly all of the oxygen, acquired from the lungs, to various tissues and organs of the body. Hemoglobin accounts for the red color of our red blood cells. A very small fraction of our hemoglobin spontaneously oxidizes per day, producing a protein of a slightly different structure, called methemoglobin. Normally, the amount of methemoglobin constitutes less than 1% of the total hemoglobin. Methemoglobin can accumulate in the blood as a result of nitrite poisoning. Infants are especially susceptible to poisoning by nitrite.

Nitrate, which is naturally present in green leafy vegetables and in the water supply is rapidly converted to nitrite by the naturally occurring bacteria residing on our tongue, as well as in the intestines, and then absorbed into the bloodstream. The amount of nitrate that is supplied by leafy vegetables and in drinking water is generally about 100-170 mg/day. The amount of nitrite supplied by a typical diet is much less, that is, than 0.1 mg nitrite/day. Poisoning by nitrite, or nitrate after its conversion to nitrite, results in the inability of hemoglobin to carry oxygen throughout the body. This condition can be seen by the blue color of the skin. Adverse symptoms occur when over 30% of the hemoglobin has been converted to methemoglobin, and these symptoms include cardiac arrhythmias, **headache, nausea and vomiting,** and in severe cases, seizures.

Calcium and phosphate are closely related nutrients. Calcium toxicity is rare, but overconsumption of calcium supplements may lead to deposits of calcium phosphate in the soft tissues of the body. Phosphate toxicity can occur with overuse of **laxatives** or **enemas** that contain phosphate. Severe phosphate toxicity can result in **hypocalcemia,** and in various symptoms resulting from low plasma calcium levels. Moderate phosphate toxicity, occurring over a period of months, can result in the deposit of calcium phosphate crystals in various tissues of the body.

Zinc toxicity is rare, but it can occur in metal workers who are exposed to fumes containing zinc. Excessive dietary supplements of zinc can result in nausea, vomiting, and diarrhea. The chronic intake of excessive zinc supplements can result in copper deficiency, as zinc inhibits the absorption of copper.

Severe alterations in copper metabolism occur in two genetic diseases, Wilson's disease and Menkes' disease. Both of these diseases are rare and occur in about one in 100,000 births. Both diseases involve mutations in the proteins that transport copper, that is, in special channels that allow the passage of copper ions through cell membranes. Wilson's disease tends to occur in teenagers and in young adults, and then remain for the lifetime. Copper accumulates in the liver, kidney, and brain, resulting in damage to the liver and nervous system. Wilson's disease can be successfully controlled by lifelong treatment with d-penicillamine. Treatment also involves avoiding foods that are high in copper, such as liver, nuts, chocolate, and mollusks. After an initial period of treatment with penicillamine, Wilson's disease may be treated with zinc (150 mg oral Zn/day). The zinc inhibits the absorption of dietary copper.

Selenium toxicity occurs in regions of the world, including some parts of China, where soils contain high levels of selenium. A daily intake of 0.75-5.0 mg selenium may occur in these regions, due to the presence of selenium in foods and water. Early signs of selenium toxicity include nausea, weakness, and diarrhea. With continued intake of selenium, changes in fingernails and hair loss results, and damage to the nervous system occurs. The breath may acquire a garlic odor, as a result of the increased production of dimethylselenide in the body, and its release via the lungs.

Manganese toxicity occurs in miners in manganese mines, where men breath air containing dust bearing manganese at a concentration of 5-250 mg/cubic meter. Manganese toxicity in miners has been documented in Chile, India, Japan, Mexico, and elsewhere. Symptoms of manganese poisoning typically occur within several months or years of exposure. These symptoms include a mental disorder resembling **schizophrenia,** as well as hyperirritability, violent acts, **hallucinations,** and difficulty in walking.

Diagnosis

The initial diagnosis of mineral toxicity involves questioning the patient in order to determine any unusual aspects of the diet, unusual intake of drugs and chemicals, and possible occupational exposure. Diagnosis of mineral toxicities also involves measuring the metal concentration in the plasma or urine. Concentrations that are above the normal range can confirm the initial, suspected diagnosis.

Treatment

Iron toxicity is treated by efforts to remove remaining iron from the stomach, by use of a solution of 5% sodium bicarbonate. Where plasma iron levels are above 0.35 mg/dL, the patient is treated with deferoxamine. Treatment of manganese toxicity involves removal of the patient from the high manganese environment, as well as lifelong doses of the drug L-dopa. The treatment is only partially successful. Treatment of nitrite or nitrate toxicity involves inhalation of 100% oxygen for several hours. If oxygen treatment is not effective, then methylene blue may be injected, as a 1.0% solution, in a dose of 1.0 mg methylene blue/kg body weight.

Prognosis

The prognosis for treating toxicity due to sodium, potassium, calcium, and phosphate is usually excellent. Toxicity due to the deposit of calcium phosphate crystals is not usually reversible. The prognosis for treating iodine toxicity is excellent. For any mineral overdose that causes coma or seizures, the prognosis for recovery is often poor, and death results in a small fraction of patients. For any mineral toxicity that causes nerve damage, the prognosis is often fair to poor.

Prevention

When mineral toxicity results from the excessive consumption of mineral supplements, toxicity can be prevented by not using supplements. In the case of manganese, toxicity can be prevented by avoiding work in manganese mines. In the case of iodine, toxicity can be prevented by avoiding overconsumption of seaweed or kelp. In the case of selenium toxicity that arises due to high-selenium soils, toxicity can be prevented by relying on food and water acquired from a low-selenium region.

Resources

BOOKS

Brody, Tom. *Nutritional Biochemistry.* San Diego, CA: Academic Press, 1998.

Food and Nutrition Board. *Recommended Dietary Allowances.* 10th ed. Washington, DC: National Academy Press, 1989.

O'Dell, B. and Sunde, R.A. *Handbook of Nutritionally Essential Mineral Elements.* New York, NY: Marcel Dekker, 1997.

PERIODICALS

Johnson, C., et al. "Fatal Outcome of Methemoglobinemia in an Infant." *Journal of the American Medical Association,* 257 (1987): 2796-2797.

Tom Brody

. . . .

Minerals

Definition

The minerals (inorganic nutrients) that are relevant to human nutrition include water, sodium, potassium, chloride, calcium, phosphate, sulfate, magnesium, iron, copper, zinc, manganese, iodine, selenium, and molybdenum. Cobalt is a required mineral for human health, but it is supplied by vitamin B_{12}. Cobalt appears to have no other function, aside from being part of this vitamin. There is some evidence that chromium, boron, and other inorganic elements play some part in human nutrition, but the evidence is indirect and not yet convincing. Fluoride seems not to be required for human life, but its presence in the diet contributes to long term dental health. Some of the minerals do not occur as single atoms, but occur as molecules. These include water, phosphate, sulfate, and selenite (a form of selenium). Sulfate contains an atom of sulfur. We do not need to eat sulfate, since the body can acquire all the sulfate it needs from protein.

The statement that various minerals, or inorganic nutrients, are required for life means that their continued supply in the diet is needed for growth, maintenance of body weight in adulthood, and for reproduction. The amount of each mineral that is needed to support growth during infancy and childhood, to maintain body weight and health, and to facilitate **pregnancy** and **lactation,** are listed in a table called the Recommended Dietary Allowances (RDA). This table was compiled by the Food and Nutrition Board, a committee that serves the United States government. All of the values listed in the RDA indicate the daily amounts that are expected to maintain health throughout most of the general population. The actual levels of each inorganic nutrient required by any given individual is likely to be less than that stated by the RDA. The RDAs are all based on studies that provided the exact, minimal requirement of each mineral needed to maintain health. However, the RDA values are actually greater than the minimal requirement, as determined by studies on small groups of healthy human subjects, in order to accomodate the variability expected among the general population.

The RDAs for adult males are 800 mg of calcium, 800 mg of phosphorus, 350 mg of magnesium, 10 mg of iron, 15 mg of zinc, 0.15 mg of iodine, and 0.07 mg of selenium. The RDA for sodium is expressed as a range (0.5-2.4 g/day). The minimal requirement for chloride is about 0.75 g/day, and the minimal requirement for potassium is 1.6-2.0 g/day, though RDA values have not been set for these nutrients. The RDAs for several other minerals has not been determined, and here the estimated safe and adequate daily dietary intake has been listed by the Food and Nutrition Board. These values are listed for copper (1.5-3.0 mg), manganese (2-5 mg), fluoride (1.5-4.0 mg), molybdenum (0.075-0.25 mg), and chromium (0.05-0.2 mg). In noting the appearance of chromium in this list, one should note that the function of chromium is essentially unknown, and evidence for its necessity exists only for animals, and not for human beings. In considering the amount of any mineral used for treating **mineral deficiency,** one should compare the recommended level with the RDA for that mineral. Treatment at a level that is one tenth of the RDA might not be expected to be adequate, while treatment at levels ranging from 10-1,000 times the RDA might be expected to exert a toxic effect, depending on the mineral. In this way, one can judge whether any claim of action, for a specific mineral treatment, is likely to be adequate or appropriate.

Purpose

People are treated with minerals for several reasons. The primary reason is to relieve a mineral deficiency, when a deficiency has been detected. Chemical tests suitable for the detection of all mineral deficiencies are available. The diagnosis of the deficiency is often aided by tests that do not involve chemical reactions, such as the

hematocrit test for the red blood cell content in blood for iron deficiency, the visual examination of the neck for iodine deficiency, or the examination of bones by densitometry for calcium deficiency. Mineral treatment is conducted after a test and diagnosis for iron-deficiency anemia, in the case of iron, and after a test and diagnosis for hypomagnesemia, in the case of magnesium, to give two examples.

A second general reason for mineral treatment is to prevent the development of a possible or expected deficiency. Here, minerals are administered when tests for possible mineral deficiency are not given. Examples include the practice of giving young infants iron supplements, and of the food industry's practice of supplementing infant formulas with iron. The purpose here is to reduce the risk for **iron deficiency anemia.** Another example is the practice of many women of taking calcium supplements, with the hope of reducing the risk of **osteoporosis.**

Most minerals are commercially available at supermarkets, drug stores, and specialty stores. There is reason to believe that the purchase and consumption of most of these minerals is beneficial to health for some, but not all, of the minerals. Potassium supplements are useful for reducing blood pressure, in cases of persons with high blood pressure. The effect of potassium varies from person to person. The consumption of calcium supplements is likely to have some effect on reducing the risk for osteoporosis. The consumption of selenium supplements is expected to be of value only for residents of Keshan Province, China, because of the established association of selenium deficiency in this region with "Keshan disease."

Precautions

During emergency treatment of sodium deficiency (**hyponatremia**), potassium deficiency (**hypokalemia**), and calcium deficiency (**hypocalcemia**) with intravenous injections, extreme caution must be taken to avoid producing toxic levels of each of these minerals (**hypernatremia, hyperkalemia,** and **hypercalcemia**), as mineral toxicity can be life-threatening in some instances. The latter three conditions can be life threatening. Selenium is distinguished among most of the nutrients in that dietary intakes at levels only ten times that of the RDA can be toxic. Hence, one must guard against any overdose of selenium. Calcium and zinc supplements, when taken orally, are distinguished among most of the other minerals in that their toxicity is relatively uncommon.

Description

Minerals are used in treatments by three methods, namely, by replacing a poor diet with a diet that supplies the RDA, by consuming oral supplements, or by injections or infusions. Injections are especially useful for infants, for mentally disabled persons, or where the physician wants to be totally sure of compliance. Infusions, as well as injections, are essential for medical emergencies, as during mineral deficiency situations like hyponatremia, hypokalemia, hypocalcemia, and hypomagnesemia. Oral mineral supplements are especially useful for mentally alert persons who otherwise cannot or will not consume food that is a good mineral source, such as meat. For example, a vegetarian who will not consume meat may be encouraged to consume oral supplements of iron, as well as supplements of vitamin B_{12}.

Iron treatment is used for young infants, given as supplements of 7 mg of iron per day to prevent anemia. Iron is also supplied to infants via the food industry's practice of including iron at 12 mg/L in cow milk-based infant formulas, as well as adding powdered iron at levels of 50 mg iron per 100 g dry infant cereal.

Calcium supplements, along with estrogen and calcitonin therapy, are commonly used in the prevention and treatment of osteoporosis. Estrogen and calcitonin are naturally occurring hormones. Bone loss occurs with diets supplying under 400 mg Ca/day. Bone loss can be minimized with the consumption of the RDA for calcium. There is some thought that all postmenopausal women should consume 1,000–1,500 mg of calcium per day. These levels are higher than the RDA. There is some evidence that such supplementation can reduce bone losses in some bones, such as the elbow (ulna), but not in other bones. Calcium absorption by the intestines decreases with aging, especially after the age of 70. The regulatory mechanisms of the intestines that allow absorption of adequate calcium (500 mg Ca/day or less) may be impaired in the elderly. Because of these changes, there is much interest in increasing the RDA for calcium for older women.

Fluoride has been proven to reduce the rate of **tooth decay.** When fluoride occurs in the diet, it is incorporated into the structure of the teeth, and other bones. The optimal range of fluoride in drinking water is 0.7-1.2 mg/L. This level results in a reduction in the rate of tooth decay by about 50%. The American Dental Association recommends that persons living in areas lacking fluoridated water take fluoride supplements. The recommendation is 0.25 mg F/day from the ages of 0-2 years, 0.5 mg F/day for 2-3 years, and 1.0 mg F/day for ages 3-13 years.

Magnesium is often used to treat a dangerous condition, called eclampsia, that occasionally occurs during pregnancy. In this case, magnesium is used as a drug, and not to relieve a deficiency. High blood pressure is a fairly common disorder during pregnancy, affecting 1-5% of pregnant mothers. **Hypertension** during pregnancy can result in increased release of protein in the urine. In pregnancy, the combination of hypertension with increased urinary protein is called preeclampsia. Preeclampsia is a concern during pregnancies as it may lead to eclampsia. Eclampsia involves convulsions and possibly **death** to the mother. Magnesium sulfate is the drug of choice for preventing the convulsions of eclampsia.

Treatment with cobalt, in the form of vitamin B_{12}, is used for relieving the symptoms of **pernicious anemia.** Pernicious anemia is a relatively common disease which tends to occur in persons older than 40 years. Free cobalt is never used for the treatment of any disease.

Preparation

Evaluation of a patient's mineral levels requires a blood sample, and the preparation of plasma or serum from the blood sample. An overnight fast is usually recommended as preparation prior to drawing the blood and chemical analysis. The reason for this is that any mineral present in the food consumed at breakfast may artificially boost the plasma mineral content beyond the normal fasting level, and thereby mask a mineral deficiency. In some cases, red blood cells are used for the mineral status assay.

Aftercare

The healthcare provider assesses the patient's response to mineral treatment. A positive response confirms that the diagnosis was correct. Lack of response indicates that the diagnosis was incorrect, that the patient had failed to take the mineral supplement, or that a higher dose of mineral was needed. The response to mineral treatment can be monitored by chemical tests, by an examination of red blood cells or white blood cells, or by physiological tests, depending on the exact mineral deficiency.

Risks

There are few risks associated with mineral treatment. In treating emergency cases of hyponatremia, hypokalemia, or hypocalcemia by intravenous injections, there exists a very real risk that giving too much sodium, potassium, or calcium, can result in hypernatremia, hyperkalemia, or hypercalcemia, respectively. Risk for toxicity is rare where treatment is by dietary means. This is because the intestines act as a barrier, and absorption of any mineral supplement is gradual. The gradual passage of any mineral through the intestines, especially when the mineral supplement is taken with food, allows the various organs of the body to acquire the mineral. Gradual passage of the mineral into the bloodstream also allows the

kidneys to excrete the mineral in the urine, should levels of the mineral rise to toxic levels in the blood.

Resources

BOOKS

Brody, Tom. *Nutritional Biochemistry.* San Diego, CA: Academic Press, 1998.

Food and Nutrition Board. *Recommended Dietary Allowances.* 10th ed. Washington, DC: National Academy Press, 1989.

PERIODICALS

Sibai, B.M. "Treatment of Hypertension in Pregnant Women." *New England Journal of Medicine,* 335 (1996): 227-265.

Tom Brody

Minimal change disease *see* **Nephrotic syndrome**

Minor tranquilizers *see* **Antianxiety drugs**

. . . .

Miscarriage

Definition

Miscarriage means loss of an embryo or fetus before the 20th week of **pregnancy.** Most miscarriages occur during the first 14 weeks of pregnancy. The medical term for miscarriage is spontaneous abortion.

Description

Miscarriages are very common. Approximately 20% of pregnancies (one in five) end in miscarriage. The most common cause is a genetic abnormality of the fetus. Not all women realize that they are miscarrying and others may not seek medical care when it occurs.

A miscarriage is often a traumatic event for both partners, and can cause feelings similar to the loss of a child or other member of the family. Fortunately, 90% of women who have had one miscarriage subsequently have a normal pregnancy and healthy baby; 60% are able to have a healthy baby after two miscarriages. Even a woman who has had three miscarriages in a row still has more than a 50% chance of having a successful pregnancy the fourth time.

Causes & symptoms

There are many reasons why a woman's pregnancy ends in miscarriage. Often the cause is not clear. How-

KEY TERMS

Diethylstilbestrol (DES)—This is a synthetic estrogen drug that is used to treat a number of hormonal conditions. However, it causes problems in developing fetuses and should not be taken during pregnancy. From about 1938 to 1971, DES was given to pregnant women because it was thought to prevent miscarriage. Children of women who took the drug during pregnancy are at risk for certain health problems.

Dilation and curettage (D&C)—A procedure in which the neck of the womb (cervix) is expanded and the lining of the uterus is scraped to remove pregnancy tissue or abnormal tissue.

Embryo—An unborn child in the first eight weeks after conception. After the eighth week until birth, the baby is called a fetus.

ever, more than half the miscarriages that occur in the first eight weeks of pregnancy involve serious chromosomal abnormalities or **birth defects** that would make it impossible for the baby to survive. These are different from inherited genetic diseases. They probably occur during development of the specific egg or sperm, and therefore are not likely to occur again.

In about 17% of cases, miscarriage is caused by an abnormal hormonal imbalance that interferes with the ability of the uterus to support the growing embryo. This is known as luteal phase defect. In another 10% of cases, there is a problem with the structure of the uterus or cervix. This can especially occur in women whose mothers used diethylstilbestrol (DES) when pregnant with them.

The risk of miscarriage is increased by:

• Smoking (up to a 50% increased risk)

• Infection

• Exposure to toxins (such as arsenic, lead, formaldehyde, benzene, and ethylene oxide)

• **Multiple pregnancy**

• Poorly-controlled diabetes.

The most common symptom of miscarriage is bleeding from the vagina, which may be light or heavy. However, bleeding during early pregnancy is common and is not always serious. Many women have slight vaginal bleeding after the egg implants in the uterus (about 7-10 days after conception), which can be mistaken for a threatened miscarriage. A few women bleed at the time of their monthly periods through the pregnancy. However, any bleeding in the first three months of pregnancy (first trimester) is considered a threat of miscarriage.

Women should not ignore vaginal bleeding during early pregnancy. In addition to signaling a threatened miscarriage, it could also indicate a potentially life-threatening condition known as **ectopic pregnancy.** In an ectopic pregnancy, the fetus implants at a site other than the inside of the uterus. Most often this occurs in the fallopian tube.

Cramping is another common sign of a possible miscarriage. The cramping occurs because the uterus attempts to push out the pregnancy tissue. If a pregnant woman experiences both bleeding and cramping the possibility of miscarriage is more likely than if only one of these symptoms is present.

If a woman experiences any sign of impending miscarriage, she should be examined by a practitioner. The doctor or nurse will perform a pelvic exam to check if the cervix is closed as it should be. If the cervix is open, miscarriage is inevitable and nothing can preserve the pregnancy. Symptoms of an inevitable miscarriage may include dull relentless or sharp intermittent **pain** in the lower abdomen or back. Bleeding may be heavy. Clotted material and tissue (the placenta and embryo) may pass from the vagina.

A situation in which only some of the products in the uterus have been expelled is called an incomplete miscarriage. Pain and bleeding may continue and become severe. An incomplete miscarriage requires medical attention.

A "missed abortion" occurs when the fetus has died but neither the fetus nor placenta is expelled. There may not be any bleeding or pain, but the symptoms of pregnancy will disappear. The physician may suspect a missed abortion if the uterus does not continue to grow. The physician will diagnose a missed abortion with an ultrasound examination.

A woman should contact her doctor if she experiences any of the following:

• Any bleeding during pregnancy.

• Pain or cramps during pregnancy.

• Passing of tissue.

• **Fever** and chills during or after miscarriage.

Diagnosis

If a woman experiences any sign of impending miscarriage she should see a doctor or nurse for a pelvic examination to check if the cervix is closed, as it should be. If the cervix is open, miscarriage is inevitable.

An ultrasound examination can confirm a missed abortion if the uterus has shrunk and the patient has had continual spotting with no other symptoms.

Treatment

Threatened miscarriage

For women who experience bleeding and cramping, bed rest is often ordered until symptoms disappear. Women should not have sex until the outcome of the threatened miscarriage is determined. If bleeding and cramping are severe, women should drink fluids only.

Miscarriage

Although it may be psychologically difficult, if a woman has a miscarriage at home she should try to collect any material she passes in a clean container for analysis in a laboratory. This may help determine why the miscarriage occurred.

An incomplete miscarriage or missed abortion may require the removal of the fetus and placenta by a D&C (**dilatation and curettage**). In this procedure the contents of the uterus are scraped out. It is performed in the doctor's office or hospital.

After miscarriage, a doctor may prescribe rest or **antibiotics** for infection. There will be some bleeding from the vagina for several days to two weeks after miscarriage. To give the cervix time to close and avoid possible infection, women should not use tampons or have sex for at least two weeks. Couples should wait for one to three normal menstrual cycles before trying to get pregnant again.

Prognosis

A miscarriage that is properly treated is not life-threatening, and usually does not affect a woman's ability to deliver a healthy baby in the future.

Feelings of grief and loss after a miscarriage are common. In fact, some women who experience a miscarriage suffer from major depression during the six months after the loss. This is especially true for women who don't have any children or who have had depression in the past. The emotional crisis can be similar to that of a woman whose baby has died after birth.

Prevention

The majority of miscarriages cannot be prevented because they are caused by severe genetic problems determined at conception. Some doctors advise women who have a threatened miscarriage to rest in bed for a day and avoid sex for a few weeks after the bleeding stops. Other experts believe that a healthy woman (especially early in the pregnancy) should continue normal activities instead of protecting a pregnancy that may end in miscarriage later on, causing even more profound distress.

If miscarriage was caused by a hormonal imbalance (luteal phase defect), this can be treated with a hormone called progesterone to help prevent subsequent miscarriages. If structural problems have led to repeated miscarriage, there are some possible procedures to treat these problems. Other possible ways to prevent miscarriage are to treat genital infections, eat a well-balanced diet, and refrain from smoking and using recreational drugs.

Resources

BOOKS

Allen, Marie and Shelly Marks. *Miscarriage: Women Sharing From the Heart.* New York: John Wiley & Sons, 1993.

Friedman, Lynn, Irene Daria, and Laurie Abkemeier. *A Woman Doctor's Guide to Miscarriage.* New York: Hyperion, 1996.

Hinton, Clara H. *Silent Grief; Miscarriage—Finding Your Way Through the Darkness.* Green Forest, AK: New Leaf Press, 1998.

Ingram, Kristen J. and Christine O. Lafser. *Always Precious in our Memory: Reflections After Miscarriage, Stillbirth, or Neonatal Death.* Anaheim, CA: Acta Publications, 1997.

Lachelin, Gillian C.L. *Miscarriage: The Facts.* New York: Oxford Medical Publications, 1996.

Vredevelt, Pam W. *Empty Arms: Emotional Support for Those Who Have Suffered Miscarriage or Stillbirth.* New York: Questar Publications, 1995.

PERIODICALS

"Aftermath of Loss." *U.S. News and World Report* 122/6(Feb. 17, 1997): 66.

Bennetts, L. "Preventing Miscarriage." *Parents* 69/2(February 1994): 64-66.

Petterson, S. "Miscarriage Myths." *Your Health* 33/2(Jan. 25, 1994): 23-24.

ORGANIZATIONS

American College of Obstetricians and Gynecologists. 600 Maryland Ave. SW, Ste. 30, Washington, DC 20024. (202) 638-5577.

Hygeia. PO Box 3943, Amity Station, New Haven, CT 06525. http://www.hygeia.org

Carol A. Turkington

Mitral incompetence *see* **Mitral valve insufficiency**

Mitral regurgitation *see* **Mitral valve insufficiency**

Mitral stenosis *see* **Mitral valve stenosis**

Mitral valve insufficiency

Definition

Mitral valve insufficiency is a term used when the valve between the upper left chamber of the heart (atrium) and the lower left chamber (ventricle) doesn't close well enough to prevent back flow of blood when the ventricle contracts. Mitral valve insufficiency is also known as mitral valve regurgitation or mitral valve incompetence.

Description

Normally, blood enters the left atrium of the heart from the lungs and is pumped through the mitral valve into the left ventricle. The left ventricle contracts to pump the blood forward into the aorta. The aorta is a large artery that sends oxygenated blood through the circulatory system to all of the tissues in the body. If the mitral valve is leaky due to mitral valve insufficiency, it allows some blood to get pushed back into the atrium. This extra blood creates an increase in pressure in the atrium, which then increases blood pressure in the vessels that bring the blood from the lungs to the heart. Increased pressure in these vessels can result in increased fluid buildup in the lungs.

Causes & symptoms

In the past, **rheumatic fever** was the most common cause of mitral valve insufficiency. However, the increased use of **antibiotics** for **strep throat** has made rheumatic fever rare in developed countries. In these countries, mitral valve insufficiency caused by rheumatic fever is seen mostly in the elderly. In countries with less developed health care, rheumatic fever is still common and is often a cause of mitral valve insufficiency.

Heart attacks that damage the structures that support the mitral valve are a common cause of mitral valve insufficiency. Myxomatous degeneration can cause a "floppy" mitral valve that leaks. In other cases, the valve simply deteriorates with age and becomes less efficient.

People with mitral valve insufficiency may not have any symptoms at all. It is often discovered during a doctor's visit when the doctor listens to the heart sounds.

Both the left atrium and left ventricle tend to get a little bigger when the mitral valve does not work properly. The ventricle has to pump more blood so it gets bigger to increase the force of each beat. The atrium gets bigger to hold the extra blood. An enlarged ventricle can cause **palpitations.** An enlarged atrium can develop an erratic rhythm (atrial fibrillation), which reduces its efficiency and can lead to blood clots forming in the atrium.

Diagnosis

When the doctor listens to the heart sounds, mitral valve insufficiency is generally recognized by the sound the blood makes as it leaks backward. It sounds like a regurgitant murmur. The next step is generally a **chest x ray** and an electrocardiogram (ECG) to see if the heart is enlarged. The most definitive noninvasive test is **echocardiography,** a test that uses sound waves to make an image of the heart. This test gives a picture of the valve in action and shows the severity of the problem.

Treatment

A severely impaired valve needs to be repaired or replaced. Either option will require surgery. Repairing the valve can fix the problem completely or reduce it enough to make it bearable and prevent damage to the heart. Valves can be replaced with either a mechanical valve or one that is partly mechanical and partly from a pig's heart.

Mechanical valves are effective but can increase the incidence of blood clots. To prevent blood clots from forming, the patient will need to take drugs that prevent abnormal blood clotting (anticoagulants). The valves made partly from a pigs heart don't have as great a risk of blood clots but don't last as long as fully mechanical valves. If a valve wears out, it must be replaced again.

Damaged heart valves are easily infected. Anytime a procedure is contemplated that might allow infectious organisms to enter the blood, the person with mitral valve insufficiency should take antibiotics to prevent possible infection.

Prognosis

The diagnostic, medical and surgical procedures available to the person with mitral valve insufficiency are all likely to produce good results.

Prevention

The only possible way to prevent mitral valve insufficiency is to prevent rheumatic fever. This can be done by evaluating **sore throats** for the presence of the bacteria that causes strep throat. Strep throat is easily treated with antibiotics.

Resources

BOOKS

McGoon, Michael D., *Mayo Clinic Heart Book: The Ultimate Guide to Heart Health.* New York: William Morrow and Company, Inc., 1993.

PERIODICALS

Ling, Lieng H., et al. ''Clinical Outcome of Mitral Regurgitation Due to Flail Leaflet.'' *New England Journal of Medicine* 335 (November 7, 1996): 1417+

ORGANIZATIONS

American Heart Association, 7320 Greenville Avenue, Dallas, TX 75231, 1-800-889-7943.

OTHER

Merck online. http://www.merck.com.

Dorothy Elinor Stonely

Mitral valve prolapse

Definition

Mitral valve prolapse (MVP) is a ballooning of the support structures of the mitral heart valve into the left upper collection chamber of the heart.

Description

Other names for MVP include floppy valve and Barlow's syndrome. The mitral valve is located on the left side of the heart between the top chamber (left atrium) and the bottom chamber (left ventricle). The valve opens and closes according to the heartbeat and the pressure that is exerted upon it from the blood in both chambers.

The valve has supporting structures that attach to the heart muscle to help it open and close properly. When these structures weaken or lengthen abnormally, the valve may balloon into the left atrium. Sometimes this can cause the mitral valve to leak blood backward.

This condition may be inherited and occurs in approximately 10% of the population. It affects more women than men and often peaks after the age of 40.

KEY TERMS

Heart murmur—Sound during the heartbeat caused by a heart valve that does not close properly.

Rheumatic heart disease—A condition caused by a streptococcus infection which can result in permanent heart damage.

Causes & symptoms

MVP may occur due to rheumatic heart disease but is usually found in healthy people. Changes that occur in the valve are caused by rapid multiplication of cells in the middle layer that presses on the outer layer. The outer layer weakens, causing a prolapse of the valve toward the left atrium.

Most persons do not have symptoms. Those that do may experience sharp, left-sided chest **pain.** Some complain of fatigue, or a pounding feeling in the chest. Others can have an irregular heart beat and even pass out. Some persons may experience difficulty breathing, ankle swelling and fluid in the lungs. Other symptoms may include **anxiety, headaches,** morning tiredness and constantly cold hands and feet. **Death** from this condition is rare.

Diagnosis

The diagnosis of MVP is based on symptoms and physical exam. During the exam, the physician may hear a click and/or heart murmur with a stethoscope.

The best diagnostic test for MVP is the echocardiogram. The test reflects sound waves through the chest wall to give two-dimensional color flow pictures of the heart, its size, position, motion, chambers, and valves. Unfortunately, during the early 1980s, this diagnosis was often made excessively from faulty echocardiographic criteria prevalent at that time.

Any person with symptoms or family history of MVP should consider having an echocardiogram. The test takes 15-20 minutes and is done in doctor's offices and hospitals. It is performed by trained technicians and is read by cardiologists. Family physicians, internists, cardiologists, and nurse practitioners can treat MVP. Echocardiograms are recommended periodically depending on the extent of valve leakage.

Treatment

Persons who experience certain types of an irregular heartbeat with MVP should be treated. Propranolol (Inderal) or other **beta blockers** or digoxin (Lanoxin) are often helpful. Persons who develop moderate to severe

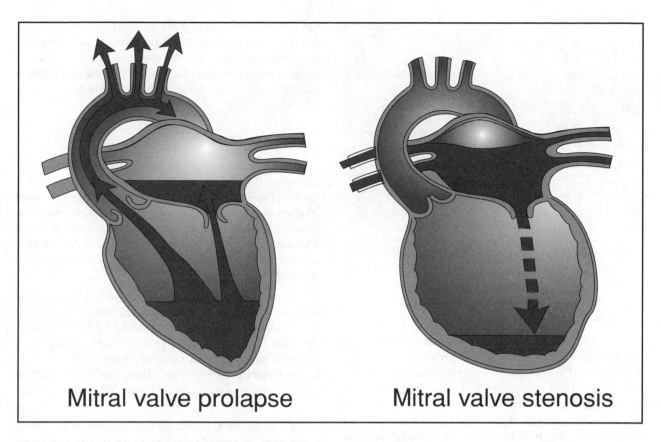

Mitral valve prolapse

Mitral valve stenosis

Mitral valve prolapse occurs when the mitral valve does not open and close properly. When this happens, the valve may balloon into the left atrium of the heart, causing the mitral valve to leak blood backward. Mitral valve stenosis refers to the narrowing of the mitral valve, in which the flow of blood from the atrium to the ventricle becomes restricted. (*Illustration by Electronic Illustrators Group.*)

symptoms with a leaky mitral valve may require repair or replacement of the mitral valve with an artificial heart valve. Persons with MVP and a leaky valve need to protect themselves from heart or heart valve infections. **Antibiotics** should be taken before any surgical, dental or oral procedures according to the American Heart Association recommendations.

Other treatments include drinking lots of fluids during strenuous activity and hot weather. Water pills, **caffeine** and donating blood may aggravate the symptoms of MVP.

Prognosis

MVP is usually not a serious condition. However, dangerous, untreated irregular heartbeats may rarely cause sudden death. These persons should be carefully monitored.

Resources

BOOKS

LeDoux, Denise."Acquired Valvular Heart Disease." In *Cardiac Nursing,* edited by Susan Woods, et al. Philadelphia.: J.B. Lippincott Co., 1995.

PERIODICALS

McGrath, Dicey. "Mitral Valve Prolapse." *American Journal of Nursing* (May 1997): 40-41.

Lisa A. Papp

Mitral valve stenosis

Definition

The term stenosis means an abnormal narrowing of an opening. Mitral valve stenosis refers to a condition in the heart in which one of the valve openings has become

KEY TERMS

· ·

Atrium—One of the two upper chambers of the heart.

Beta blocker—A drug that can be used to reduce blood pressure.

Rheumatic fever—An illness which sometimes follows a streptococcal infection of the throat.

Ventricle—One of the two lower chambers of the heart.

narrow and restricts the flow of blood from the upper left chamber (left atrium) to the lower left chamber (left ventricle).

Description

In the heart, the valve that regulates the flow of blood between the left atrium and the left ventricle is called the mitral valve. If the mitral valve is abnormally narrow, due to disease or birth defect, blood flow from the atrium to the ventricle is restricted. This restricted flow leads to an increase in the pressure of blood in the left atrium. Over a period of time, this back pressure causes fluid to leak into the lungs. It can also lead to an abnormal heart rhythm (atrial fibrillation), which further decreases the efficiency of the pumping action of the heart.

Causes & symptoms

Mitral valve stenosis is almost always caused by **rheumatic fever.** As a result of rheumatic fever, the leaflets that form the opening of the valve are partially fused together. Mitral valve stenosis can also be present at birth. Babies born with this problem usually require surgery if they are to survive. Sometimes, growths or tumors can block the mitral valve, mimicking mitral valve stenosis.

If the restriction is severe, the increased blood pressure can lead to **heart failure.** The first symptoms of heart failure, which are fatigue and **shortness of breath,** usually appear only during physical activity. As the condition gets worse, symptoms may also be felt even during rest. A person may also develop a deep red coloring in the cheeks.

Diagnosis

Mitral valve stenosis is usually detected by a physician listening to heart sounds. Normal heart valves open silently to permit the flow of blood. A stenotic valve makes a snapping sound followed by a ''rumbling'' murmur. The condition can be confirmed with a **chest x** ray and an electrocardiogram, both of which will show an enlarged atrium. **Echocardiography,** which produces images of the heart's structure, is also helpful in making the diagnosis. If surgery is necessary, **cardiac catheterization** may be done to fully evaluate the heart before the operation.

Treatment

Drug therapy may help to slow the heart rate, strengthen the heart beat, and control abnormal heart rhythm. Drugs such as **beta blockers, calcium channel blockers,** and digoxin may be prescribed. A drug that prevents abnormal blood clotting (anticoagulant) called warfarin (Coumadin) may be recommended. If drug therapy does not produce satisfactory results, valve repair or replacement may be necessary.

Repair can be accomplished in two ways. In the first method, **balloon valvuloplasty,** the doctor will try to stretch the valve opening by threading a thin tube (catheter) with a balloon tip through a vein and into the heart. Once the catheter is positioned in the valve, the balloon is inflated, separating the fused areas. The second method involves opening the heart and surgically separating the fused areas.

If the valve is damaged beyond repair, it can be replaced with a mechanical valve or one that is partly mechanical and partly made from a pig's heart.

Prognosis

Procedures available to treat mitral valve stenosis, whether medical or surgical, all produce effective results.

Prevention

The only possible way to prevent mitral valve stenosis is to prevent rheumatic fever. This can be done by evaluating **sore throats** for the presence of the bacteria that causes **strep throat.** Strep throat is easily treated with **antibiotics.**

Resources

BOOKS

McGoon, Michael D., editor-in-chief. *Mayo Clinic Heart Book: The Ultimate Guide to Heart Health* New York: William Morrow and Company, Inc., 1993

PERIODICALS

''Opening Mitral Valves Without Surgery.'' *Harvard Heart Letter* 6 (November 1995):5 + .

ORGANIZATIONS

American Heart Association, 7320 Greenville Avenue, Dallas, TX 75231, 1-800-889-7943

OTHER

Merck online. http://www.merck.com.

Dorothy Elinor Stonely

Molar pregnancy *see* **Hydatidiform mole**

Moles

Definition

A mole (nevus) is a pigmented (colored) spot on the outer layer of the skin (epidermis).

Description

Moles can be round, oval, flat, or raised. They can occur singly or in clusters on any part of the body. Most moles are brown, but colors can range from pinkish flesh tones to yellow, dark blue, or black.

Everyone has at least a few moles. They generally appear by the time a person is 20 and look, at first, like freckles. A mole's color and shape don't usually change. Changes in hormone levels that occur during **puberty** and **pregnancy** can make moles larger and darker. New moles may also appear during this period.

A mole usually lasts about 50 years before beginning to fade. Some moles disappear completely, and some never lighten at all. Some moles develop stalks that raise them above the skin's surface; these moles eventually drop off.

Types of moles

About 1-3% of all babies have one or more moles when they are born. Moles that are present at birth are called congenital nevi.

Other types of moles include:

• Junctional moles, which are usually brown and may be flat or slightly raised.

• Compound moles, which are slightly raised, range in color from tan to dark brown, and involve pigment-producing cells (melanocytes) in both the upper and lower layers of the skin (epidermis and dermis).

• Dermal moles, which range from flesh-color to brown, are elevated, most common on the upper body, and may contain hairs.

• Sebaceous moles, which are produced by over-active oil glands and are yellow and rough-textured.

> ## KEY TERMS
>
> **Malignant melanoma**—Most moles are benign, but atypical moles (called dysplastic nevi) may develop into malignant melanoma, a potentially fatal form of skin cancer. Atypical moles are usually hereditary. Most are bigger than a pencil eraser, and the shape and pigmentation are irregular.

• Blue moles, which are slightly raised, colored by pigment deep within the skin, and most common on the head, neck, and arms of women.

Most moles are benign, but atypical moles (dysplastic nevi) may develop into **malignant melanoma,** a potentially fatal form of skin **cancer.** Atypical moles are usually hereditary. Most are bigger than a pencil eraser, and the shape and pigmentation are irregular.

Congenital nevi are more apt to become cancerous than moles that develop after birth, especially if they are more than eight inches in diameter. Lentigo maligna (melanotic freckle of Hutchinson), most common on the face and after the age of 50, first appears as a flat spot containing two or more shades of tan. It gradually becomes larger and darker. One in three of these moles develop into a form of skin cancer known as lentigo maligna melanoma.

Causes & symptoms

The cause of moles is unknown, although atypical moles seem to run in families and result from exposure to sunlight.

Diagnosis

Only a small percentage of moles require medical attention. A mole that has the following symptoms should be evaluated by a dermatologist (a physician spealizing in skin diseases).

• Appears after the age of 20

• Bleeds

• Itches

• Looks unusual or changes in any way.

A doctor who suspects skin cancer will remove all or part of the mole for microscopic examination. This procedure, which is usually performed in a doctor's office, is simple, relatively painless, and doesn't take more than a few minutes. It does leave a scar.

Treatment

If laboratory analysis confirms that a mole is cancerous, the dermatologist will remove the rest of the mole. Patients should realize that slicing off a section of a malignant mole will not cause the cancer to spread.

Removing a mole for cosmetic reasons involves numbing the area and using scissors or a scalpel to remove the elevated portion. The patient is left with a flat mole the same color as the original growth. Cutting out parts of the mole above and beneath the surface of the skin can leave a scar more noticeable than the mole.

Scissors or a razor can be used to temporarily remove hair from a mole. Permanent hair removal requires electrolysis or surgical removal of the mole.

Prognosis

Moles are rarely cancerous and, once removed, unlikely to recur. A dermatologist should be consulted if a mole reappears after being removed.

Prevention

Wearing a sunscreen and limiting sun exposure may prevent some moles. Anyone who has moles should examine them every month and see a dermatologist if changes in size, shape, color, or texture occur or if new moles appear.

Anyone with a family history of melanoma should see a dermatologist for an annual skin examination. Everyone should know the ABCDs of melanoma:

- A: Asymmetry, which occurs when the two halves of the mole are not identical
- B: Borders that are irregular or indistinct
- C: Color that varies in a single mole
- D: Diameter, which should be no larger than the eraser on a pencil.

A mole exhibiting any of these characteristics should be evaluated by a dermatologist.

Resources

BOOKS

Harrison's Principles of Internal Medicine, edited by Anthony Fauci. 14th ed. New York: McGraw-Hill, 1998.

ORGANIZATIONS

American Academy of Dermatology. P.O. Box 681069, Schaumburg, IL 60618-4014. (703) 330-0230. http://www.aad.org/.

Nevus Outreach, Inc. 1616 Alpha Street, Lansing, MI 48910. (517) 487-2306. http://www.nevus.org.

OTHER

Atypical Moles. http://www.skinsite.com/info_atypical moles.htm (8 April 1998).

Moles. http://www.aad.org/aadpamphrework/Moles.html (7 April 1998).

Moles. http://www.skinsite.com/info_moles.htm (8 April 1998).

Maureen Haggerty

Molybdenum deficiency *see* **Mineral deficiency**

Mometasone *see* **Corticosteroids**

Monocytic ehrlichiosis *see* **Ehrlichiosis**

Mongolism *see* **Down syndrome**

Moniliasis *see* **Candidiasis**

Monkeypox

Definition

Certain African squirrels and primates carry a virus that causes monkeypox in humans. This virus is related to the **smallpox** virus, but it usually produces a less severe illness with fewer fatalities. However, symptoms are similar: **fever,** pus-filled blisters all over the body, and respiratory problems.

Description

Most monkeypox cases have been diagnosed in remote areas of central and west Africa. Contact with infected animals is unusual because they are isolated in forests, away from humans. However, between February 1996 and October 1997, there were 511 suspected cases of monkeypox in the Democratic Republic of the Congo (DRC, formerly Zaire). This outbreak, the largest ever, raised fears that the virus had mutated and become more infectious.

In late 1997, the U.S. Centers for Disease Control and Prevention (CDC) and the World Health Organization (WHO) announced that this relatively large outbreak was likely due to human behavior, rather than virus mutation. During the outbreak, the DRC was embroiled in civil war. Food shortages increased reliance on hunting and raised chances that people would come into contact with infected animals.

Monkeypox is less severe than smallpox and can sometimes be confused with **chickenpox.** It seems partly preventable with smallpox **vaccination,** but vaccination programs were discontinued in the late 1970s. (Barring

KEY TERMS

Antiviral—Refers to a drug that can destroy viruses and help treat illnesses caused by them.

Mutation—A change in an organism's genetic code that causes it to develop new characteristics.

Symptomatic—Refers to treatment that addresses the symptoms of an illness, but not its underlying cause.

samples stored in laboratories, smallpox has been eradicated.) People under the age of 16—those born after smallpox vaccination ended—seem the most susceptible to monkeypox. During the 1996-97 outbreak, approximately 85% of the cases were in this age group.

This outbreak also seemed to indicate high person-to-person transmission. Initial reports claimed as many as 78% of suspected cases were transmitted person to person rather than animal to person . However, according to WHO and the CDC, further study revealed that about 8% of cases were transmitted this way.

Causes & symptoms

The monkeypox virus is transmitted to humans through an infected animal's blood or by its bite. Initial symptoms are a fever and a bodywide rash of pus-filled blisters. These symptoms can be accompanied by **diarrhea,** swollen lymph nodes, a **sore throat,** and mouth sores. In some cases, a victim may experience trouble breathing. Symptoms are at their worst for 3-7 days, after which the fever lessens and blisters begin to form crusts.

Diagnosis

Since the symptoms resemble other pox diseases, definitive diagnosis may require laboratory testing to uncover the virus or evidence that it is present.

Treatment

Like most viruses, monkeypox cannot be resolved with medication. The only treatment option is symptomatic—that is, patients are made as comfortable as possible. In March 1998, the U.S. Army Medical Research Institute for Infectious Diseases reported that an antiviral drug called cidofovir may combat monkeypox infection. The drug has worked successfully in primates, but further research is needed to determine its effectiveness in humans.

Prognosis

Children are more likely to contract the disease and have the highest **death** rate. Monkeypox is not as lethal as smallpox, but the death rate among young children may reach 2-10%. In some cases, hospitalization is required. Recovery is good among survivors, although some scarring may result from the blisters.

Prevention

Although smallpox vaccination may protect against monkeypox, experts do not generally recommend getting a smallpox vaccine simply to guard against monkeypox. This vaccine carries risks, including severe, potentially fatal complications. For most people, the risk posed by the smallpox vaccine far outweighs the odds that they might come in contact with the monkeypox virus.

Resources

BOOKS

Fenner, Frank. "Human Monkeypox, a Newly Discovered Virus Disease." In *Emerging Viruses,* edited by Stephen S. Morse. Oxford University Press, 1993.

PERIODICALS

Cohen, Jon. "Is an Old Virus Up to New Tricks?" *Science* 277(July 18, 1997): 312.

OTHER

Outbreak An on-line information service about emerging diseases. http://www.outbreak.org/.

The World Health Organization, Division of Control of Tropical Diseases. http://www.who.ch/ctd/html/homepage.html.

Julia Barrett

Monoamine oxidase inhibitors

Definition

Monoamine oxidase inhibitors (MAO inhibitors) are medicines that relieve certain types of mental depression.

Purpose

MAO inhibitors are a type of antidepressant and are used to treat mental depression. Like other **antidepressant drugs,** MAO inhibitors help reduce the extreme sadness, hopelessness, and lack of interest in life that are typical in people with depression. MAO inhibitors are especially useful in treating people whose depres-

KEY TERMS

Anxiety—Worry or tension in response to real or imagined stress, danger, or dreaded situations. Physical reactions, such as fast pulse, sweating, trembling, fatigue, and weakness may accompany anxiety.

Central nervous system—The brain and spinal cord.

Depression—A mental condition in which people feel extremely sad and lose interest in life. People with depression may also have sleep problems and loss of appetite and may have trouble concentrating and carrying out everyday activities.

Neurotransmitter—A chemical that carries messages from one nerve cell to another.

Phobia—An intense, abnormal, or illogical fear of something specific, such as heights or open spaces.

Withdrawal symptoms—A group of physical or mental symptoms that may occur when a person suddenly stops using a drug to which he or she has become dependent.

sion is combined with other problems such as **anxiety,** panic attacks, **phobias,** or the desire to sleep too much.

Description

Discovered in the 1950s, MAO inhibitors work by correcting chemical imbalances in the brain. Normally, natural chemicals called neurotransmitters carry signals from one brain cell to another. Some neurotransmitters, such as serotonin and norepinephrine, play important roles in controlling mood. But other substances in the brain may interfere with mood control by breaking down these neurotransmitters. Researchers believe that MAO inhibitors work by blocking the chemicals that break down serotonin and norepinephrine. This gives the neurotransmitters more time to do their important work.

Because MAO inhibitors also affect other chemicals throughout the body, these drugs may produce many unwanted side effects. They can be especially dangerous when taken with certain foods, beverages and medicines. Anyone taking these drugs should ask his or her physician or pharmacist for a list of products to avoid.

MAO inhibitors are available only with a physician's prescription. They are sold in tablet form. Some commonly used MAO inhibitors are isocarboxazid (Marplan), phenelzine (Nardil), and tranylcypromine (Parnate).

Recommended dosage

The recommended dosage depends on the type of MAO inhibitor and the type of depression for which it is being taken. Dosages may be different for different patients. Check with the physician who prescribed the drug or the pharmacist who filled the prescription for the correct dosage.

Always take MAO inhibitors exactly as directed by your physician. Never take larger or more frequent doses, and do not take the drug for longer than directed. See the physician regularly while taking this medicine, especially in the first few months of treatment. The physician will check to make sure the medicine is working as it should and will note unwanted side effects. The physician may also need to adjust the dosage during this period.

Several weeks may be needed for the effects of this medicine to be felt. Be sure to keep taking it as directed, even if it does not seem to be helping.

Do not stop taking this medicine suddenly. Tapering the dose may be necessary to reduce the chance of withdrawal symptoms. If it is necessary to stop taking the drug, check with the physician who prescribed it for instructions on how to stop.

MAO inhibitors may be taken with or without food, on a full or empty stomach. Check package directions or ask the physician or pharmacist for instructions on how to take the medicine. Remember that some foods and beverages must be avoided during treatment with MAO inhibitors.

Precautions

The effects of this medicine may continue for 2 weeks or more after patients stop taking it. All precautions should be observed during this period, as well as throughout treatment with MAO inhibitors.

MAO inhibitors may cause serious and possibly life-threatening reactions, such as sudden high blood pressure, when taken with certain foods, beverages, or medicines. The dangerous reactions may not begin until several hours after consuming these things. Aged cheeses, red wines, smoked or pickled meats, chocolate, caffeinated beverages, and foods containing monosodium glutamate (MSG) are among the foods and drinks to be avoided. Be sure to get a complete list from the physician who prescribed the medicine or the pharmacist who filled the prescription.

Do not drink any alcoholic beverages or reduced-alcohol or alcohol-free beer or wine while taking this medicine.

Anyone who is taking MAO inhibitors should not use any other medicine unless it has been approved or prescribed by a physician who knows that they are taking MAO inhibitors. This includes nonprescription (over-the-counter) medicines such as sleep aids; medicines for colds, **cough,** hay fever, or **asthma** (including nose drops or sprays); medicines to increase alertness or keep from falling asleep; and appetite control products.

Because MAO inhibitors work on the central nervous system, they may add to the effects of alcohol and other drugs that slow down the central nervous system, such as **antihistamines,** cold medicine, allergy medicine, sleep aids, medicine for seizures, tranquilizers, some **pain** relievers, and **muscle relaxants.** Anyone taking MAO inhibitors should check with his or her physician before taking any of the above.

MAO inhibitors may interact with medicines used during surgery, dental procedures, or emergency treatment. These interactions could increase the chance of side effects. Anyone who is taking MAO inhibitors should be sure to tell the health care professional in charge before having any surgical or dental procedures or receiving emergency treatment.

Some people feel drowsy, dizzy, lightheaded, or less alert when using MAO inhibitors. The drugs may also cause blurred vision. For these reasons, anyone who takes these drugs should not drive, use machines or do anything else that might be dangerous until they have found out how the drugs affect them.

These medicines also make some people feel lightheaded, dizzy, or faint when they get up after sitting or lying down. To lessen the problem, get up gradually and hold onto something for support if possible.

Older people may be especially sensitive to the effects of MAO inhibitors. This may increase the chance of side effects, such as **dizziness** or lightheadedness.

Special conditions

People with certain medical conditions or who are taking certain other medicines can have problems if they take MAO inhibitors. Before taking these drugs, be sure to let the physician know about any of these conditions:

ALLERGIES

Anyone who has had unusual reactions to MAO inhibitors in the past should let his or her physician know before taking the drugs again. The physician should also be told about any **allergies** to foods, dyes, preservatives, or other substances.

PREGNANCY

Studies suggest that taking MAO inhibitors during **pregnancy** may increase the risk of **birth defects** or problems in the newborn after birth. Women who are pregnant or who may become pregnant should check with their physicians before using MAO inhibitors.

BREASTFEEDING

MAO inhibitors may pass into breast milk, but no problems have been reported in nursing babies whose mothers took the medicine. Women who are breastfeeding their babies should check with their physicians before using this medicine.

DIABETES

MAO inhibitors may affect blood sugar levels. Persons with diabetes who are taking this medicine and notice changes in their blood or urine tests should check with their physicians.

ANGINA

MAO inhibitors may make people feel unusually energetic and healthy. People with **angina** (chest pain) should be careful not to overexert themselves and should check with their physicians before increasing their levels of activity or **exercise.**

OTHER MEDICAL CONDITIONS

Before using MAO inhibitors, people with any of these medical problems should make sure their physicians are aware of their conditions:

• Alcohol abuse

• High blood pressure

• Recent **heart attack** or **stroke**

• Heart or blood vessel disease

• Liver disease

• Kidney disease

• Frequent or severe **headaches**

• Epilepsy

• **Parkinson's disease**

• Current or past mental illness

• Asthma or **bronchitis**

• Overactive thyroid

• **Pheochromocytoma** (a tumor of the adrenal gland).

USE OF CERTAIN MEDICINES

Taking MAO inhibitors with certain other drugs may affect the way the drugs work or may increase the chance of side effects.

Side effects

The most common side effects are dizziness, lightheadedness, drowsiness, tiredness, weakness, blurred vision, shakiness or trembling, restlessness, sleep problems or twitching during sleep, increased appetite (especially for sweets), weight gain, decreased sexual ability, decreased amount of urine, and mild headache. These problems usually go away as the body adjusts to the drug and do not require medical treatment unless they interfere with normal activities.

More serious side effects may occur. If any of the following side effects occur, stop taking the medicine and get emergency medical attention immediately:

* Severe chest pain

* Severe headache

* Stiff, sore neck

* Enlarged pupils

* Increased sensitivity of eyes to light

* Fast or slow heartbeat

* Sweating, with or without **fever** or cold, clammy skin

* **Nausea and vomiting.**

Other side effects may occur. Anyone who has unusual or troublesome symptoms after taking MAO inhibitors should get in touch with his or her physician.

Interactions

MAO inhibitors may interact with many other medicines. When this happens, the effects of one or both of the drugs may change or the risk of side effects may be greater. *Anyone who takes MAO inhibitors must check with his or her physician before taking any other prescription or nonprescription (over-the-counter) medicine.* Among the drugs that may interact with MAO inhibitors are:

* Central nervous system (CNS) depressants such as medicine for allergies, colds, hay fever, and asthma; sedatives; tranquilizers; prescription pain medicine; muscle relaxants; medicine for seizures; sleep aids; **barbiturates;** and anesthetics.

* Medicine for high blood pressure

* Other antidepressants, including **tricyclic antidepressants** (such as Tofranil and Norpramin), antidepressants that raise serotonin levels (such as Prozac and Zoloft), and bupropion (Wellbutrin)

* Diabetes medicines taken by mouth

* Insulin

* Water pills (**diuretics**).

The list above does not include every drug that may interact with MAO inhibitors. Check with a physician or pharmacist before combining MAO inhibitors with any other prescription or nonprescription (over-the-counter) medicine.

Nancy Ross-Flanigan

Mononucleosis *see* **Infectious mononucleosis**

Montezuma's revenge *see* **Traveler's diarrhea**

. . . .

Mood disorders

Definition

Mood disorders are mental disorders characterized by periods of depression, sometimes alternating with periods of elevated mood.

Description

While many people go through sad or elated moods from time to time, people with mood disorders suffer from severe or prolonged mood states that disrupt their daily functioning. Among the general mood disorders classified in the fourth edition (1994) of the *Diagnostic and Statistical Manual of Mental Disorders* (*DSM-IV*) are major depressive disorder, **bipolar disorder,** and dysthymia.

In classifying and diagnosing mood disorders, doctors determine if the mood disorder is unipolar or bipolar. When only one extreme in mood (the depressed state) is experienced, this type of depression is called unipolar. Major depression refers to a single severe period of depression, marked by negative or hopeless thoughts and physical symptoms like fatigue. In major depressive disorder, some patients have isolated episodes of depression. In between these episodes, the patient does not feel depressed or have other symptoms associated with depression. Other patients have more frequent episodes.

Bipolar depression or bipolar disorder (sometimes called manic depression) refers to a condition in which people experience two extremes in mood. They alternate between depression (the ''low'' mood) and **mania** or hypomania (the ''high'' mood). These patients go from depression to a frenzied, abnormal elevation in mood. Mania and hypomania are similar, but mania is usually more severe and debilitating to the patient.

Dysthymia is a recurrent or lengthy depression that may last a lifetime. It is similar to major depressive disorder, but dysthymia is chronic, long-lasting, persistent, and mild. Patients may have symptoms that are not as severe as major depression, but the symptoms last for many years. It seems that a mild form of the depression is always present. In some cases, people may also experience a major depressive episode on top of their

---

dysthymia, a condition sometimes referred to as a "double depression."

Causes & symptoms

Mood disorders tend to run in families. These disorders are associated with imbalances in certain chemicals that carry signals between brain cells (neurotransmitters). These chemicals include serotonin, norepinephrine, and dopamine. Women are more vulnerable to unipolar depression than are men. Major life stressors (like divorce, serious financial problems, **death** of a family member, etc.) will often provoke the symptoms of depression in susceptible people.

Major depression is more serious than just feeling "sad" or "blue." The symptoms of major depression may include:

• Loss of appetite

• A change in the sleep pattern, like not sleeping (**insomnia**) or sleeping too much

• Feelings of worthlessness, hopelessness, or inappropriate guilt

• Fatigue

• Difficulty in concentrating or making decisions

• Overwhelming and intense feelings of sadness or grief

• Disturbed thinking. The person may also have physical symptoms like stomachaches or **headaches.**

Bipolar disorder includes mania or hypomania. Mania is an abnormal elevation in mood. The person may be excessively cheerful, have grandiose ideas, and may sleep less. They may talk nonstop for hours, have unending enthusiasm, and demonstrate poor judgement. Sometimes the elevation in mood is marked by irritability and hostility rather than cheerfulness. While the person may at first seem normal with an increase in energy, others who know the person well see a marked difference in behavior. The patient may seem to be in a frenzy and will often make poor, bizarre, or dangerous choices in his/her personal and professional lives. Hypomania is not as severe as mania and does not cause the level of impairment in work and social activities that mania can.

Diagnosis

Doctors diagnose mood disorders based on the patient's description of the symptoms as well as the patient's family history. The length of time the patient has had symptoms is also important. Generally patients are diagnosed with dysthymia if they feel depressed more days than not for at least two years. The depression is mild but long lasting. In major depressive disorder, the patient is depressed almost all day nearly every day of the week for at least two weeks. The depression is severe. Sometimes laboratory tests are performed to rule out other causes for the symptoms (like thyroid disease). The diagnosis may be confirmed when a patient responds well to medication.

Treatment

The most effective treatment for mood disorders is a combination of medication and psychotherapy. The four different classes of drugs used in mood disorders are:

• Heterocyclic antidepressants (HCAs), like amitriptyline (Elavil)

• **Selective serotonin reuptake inhibitors** (SSRI inhibitors), like fluoxetine (Prozac), paroxetine (Paxil), and sertraline (Zoloft)

• **Monoamine oxidase inhibitors** (MAOI inhibitors), like phenelzine sulfate (Nardil) and tranylcypromine sulfate (Parnate)

• Mood stabilizers, like lithium carbonate (Eskalith) and valproate, often used in people with bipolar mood disorders.

A number of psychotherapy approaches are useful as well. Interpersonal psychotherapy helps the patient recognize the interaction between the mood disorder and interpersonal relationships. **Cognitive-behavioral therapy** explores how the patient's view of the world may be affecting his or her mood and outlook.

When depression fails to respond to treatment or when there is a high risk of suicide, **electroconvulsive therapy** (ECT) is sometimes used. ECT is believed to affect neurotransmitters like the medications do. Patients are anesthetized and given **muscle relaxants** to minimize discomfort. Then low-level electric current is passed through the brain to cause a brief convulsion. The most common side effect of ECT is mild, short-term memory loss.

Alternative treatment

There are many alternative therapies that may help in the treatment of mood disorders, including **acupuncture,** botanical medicine, homeopathy, **aromatherapy,** constitutional **hydrotherapy,** and light therapy. The therapy used is an individual choice. Short-term clinical studies have shown that the herb St. John's wort (*Hypericum perforatum*) can effectively treat some types of depression. Though it appears very safe, the herb may have some side effects and its long-term effectiveness has not been proven. It has not been tested in patients with bipolar disorder. St. John's wort and **antidepressant drugs** should not be taken simultaneously, so patients should tell their doctor if they are taking St. John's wort.

Prognosis

Most cases of mood disorders can be successfully managed if properly diagnosed and treated.

Prevention

People can take steps to improve mild depression and keep it from becoming worse. They can learn **stress** management (like relaxation training or breathing exercises), **exercise** regularly, and avoid drugs or alcohol.

Resources

BOOKS

Gold, Mark S. *The Good News About Depression: Cures and Treatments in the New Age of Psychiatry.* New York: Bantam Books, 1995.

Kramer, Peter D. *Listening to Prozac: A Psychiatrist Explores Antidepressants and the Remaking of Self.* New York: Viking Penguin, 1993.

"Mood Disorders." In *Diagnostic and Statistical Manual of Mental Disorders.* 4th ed. Washington, DC: American Psychiatric Association, 1994.

PERIODICALS

Jamison, Kay Redfield. "Manic-Depressive Illness and Creativity." *Scientific American* (February 1995): 62-67.

Michels, Robert, and Peter M. Marzuk. "Progress in Psychiatry." *The New England Journal of Medicine* 329(August 26, 1993): 628-38.

Price, Lawrence H., and George R. Heninger. "Lithium in the Treatment of Mood Disorders." *The New England Journal of Medicine* 331(September 1, 1994): 591-98.

Whybrow, Peter C. "Making Sense of Mania & Depression." *Psychology Today* (May/June 1997): 35-38, 71-72.

ORGANIZATIONS

American Psychiatric Association. 1400 K St. NW, Washington, DC 20005. (202) 682-6000. http://www.psych.org.

National Depressive and Manic Depressive Association. 730 N. Franklin St., Suite 501, Chicago, IL 60610. (312) 642-0049.

National Institute of Mental Health, Mental Health Public Inquiries. 5600 Fishers Lane, Room 15C-05, Rockville, MD 20857. (301) 443-4513 or (888) 826-9438. http://www.nimh.nih.gov.

Robert Scott Dinsmoor

Morphine *see* **Analgesics, opioid**

Morquio's syndrome *see* **Mucopolysaccharidoses**

Motion sickness

Definition

Motion sickness is the uncomfortable **dizziness,** nausea, and vomiting that people experience when their sense of balance and equilibrium is disturbed by constant motion. Riding in a car, aboard a ship or boat, or riding on a swing all cause stimulation of the vestibular system and visual stimulation that often leads to discomfort. While motion sickness can be bothersome, it is not a serious illness, and can be prevented.

Description

Motion sickness is a common problem with nearly 80% of the population enduring its affects at one time in their lives. While it may occur at any age, motion sickness most often afflicts children over the age of two, with the majority outgrowing this susceptibility.

When looking at why motion sickness occurs, it is helpful to understand the role of the sensory organs. The sensory organs control a body's sense of balance by telling the brain what direction the body is pointing, the direction it is moving, and if it is standing still or turning. These messages are relayed by the inner ears (or labyrinth); the eyes; the skin pressure receptors, such as in those in the feet; the muscle and joint sensory receptors, which track what body parts are moving; and the central nervous system (the brain and spinal cord), which is responsible for processing all incoming sensory information.

KEY TERMS

Acupressure—Often described as acupuncture without needles, acupressure is a traditional Chinese medical technique based on theory of *qi* (life energy) flowing in energy meridians or channels in the body. Applying pressure with the thumb and fingers to acupressure points can relieve specific conditions and promote overall balance and health.

Acupuncture—Based on the same traditional Chinese medical foundation as acupressure, acupuncture uses sterile needles inserted at specific points to treat certain conditions or relieve pain.

Neurological system—The tissue that initiates and transmits nerve impulses including the brain, spinal cord, and nerves.

Optokinetic—A reflex that causes a person's eyes to move when their field of vision moves.

Vertigo—The sensation of moving around in space, or objects moving around a person. It is a disturbance of equilibrium.

Vestibular system—The brain and parts of the inner ear that work together to detect movement and position.

Motion sickness and its symptoms surface when conflicting messages are sent to the central nervous system. An example of this is reading a book in the back seat of a moving car. The inner ears and skin receptors sense the motion, but the eyes register only the stationary pages of the book. This conflicting information may cause the usual motion sickness symptoms of dizziness, **nausea and vomiting.**

Causes & symptoms

While all five of the body's sensory organs contribute to motion sickness, excess stimulation to the vestibular system within the inner ear (the body's "balance center") has been shown to be one of the primary reasons for this condition. Balance problems, or vertigo, are caused by a conflict between what is seen and how the inner ear perceives it, leading to confusion in the brain. This confusion may result in higher heart rates, rapid breathing, nausea and sweating, along with dizziness and vomiting.

Pure optokinetic motion sickness is caused solely by visual stimuli, or what is seen. The optokinetic system is the reflex that allow the eyes to move when an object moves. Many people suffer when what they view is rotating or swaying, even if they are standing still.

Additional factors that may contribute to the occurrence of motion sickness include:

• Poor ventilation.

• **Anxiety** or fear. Both have been found to lower a person's threshold for experiencing motion sickness symptoms.

• Food. It is recommended that a heavy meal of spicy and greasy foods be avoided before and during a trip.

• Alcohol. A drink is often thought to help calm the nerves, but in this case it could upset the stomach further. A hangover for the next morning's trip may also lead to motion sickness.

• Genetic predisposition. Research suggests that some people are predisposed to motion sickness symptoms partly due to a hereditary link.

Often viewed as a minor annoyance, some travelers are temporarily immobilized by motion sickness, and a few continue to feel its effects for hours and even days after a trip (the "mal d'embarquement" syndrome).

Diagnosis

Most cases of motion sickness are mild and self-treatable disorders. If symptoms such as dizziness become chronic, a doctor may be able to help alleviate the discomfort by looking further into a patient's general health. Questions regarding medications, head injuries, recent infections, and other questions about the ear and neurological system will be asked. An examination of the ears, nose, and throat, as well as tests of nerve and balance function, may also be completed.

Severe cases of motion sickness symptoms, and those that become progressively worse, may require additional, specific tests. Diagnosis in these situations deserves the attention and care of a doctor with specialized skills in diseases of the ear, nose, throat, equilibrium, and neurological system.

Treatment

There are a variety of medications to help ease the symptoms of motion sickness, and most of these are available without a prescription. Known as over-the-counter (OTC) medications, it is recommended that these be taken 30-60 minutes before traveling to prevent motion sickness symptoms, as well as during an extended trip.

Drugs

The following OTC drugs consist of ingredients that have been considered safe and effective for the treatment of motion sickness by the Food and Drug Administration:

• Marezine (and others). Includes the active ingredient cyclizine and is not for use in children under age 6.

• Benadryl (and others). Includes the active ingredient diphenhydramine and is not for use in children under age 6.

• Dramamine (and others). Includes the active ingredient dimenhydrinate and is not for use in children under age 2.

• Bonine (and others). Includes the active ingredient meclizine and is not for use in children under age 12.

Each of the active ingredients listed above are **antihistamines** whose main side effect is drowsiness. Caution should be used when driving a vehicle or operating machinery, and alcohol should be avoided when taking any drug for motion sickness. Large doses of OTC drugs for motion sickness may also cause **dry mouth** and occasional blurred vision.

The Food and Drug Administration recommends that people with **emphysema,** chronic **bronchitis,** glaucoma, or difficulty urinating due to an **enlarged prostate** do not use OTC drugs for motion sickness unless directed by their doctor.

Longer trips may require a prescription medication called scopolamine (Transderm Scop). Formerly used in the transdermal skin patch (now discontinued), travelers must now ask their doctor to prescribe it in the form of a gel. In gel form, scopolamine is most effective when smeared on the arm or neck and covered with a bandage.

Alternative treatment

Alternative treatments for motion sickness have become widely accepted as a standard means of care. Ginger (*Zingiber officinale*) in its various forms is often used to calm the stomach, and it is now known that the oils it contains (gingerols and shogaols) appear to relax the intestinal tract in addition to mildly depressing the central nervous system. Some of the most effective forms of ginger include the powdered, encapsulated form; ginger tea prepared from sliced ginger root; or candied pieces. All forms of ginger should be taken on an empty stomach.

Placing manual pressure on the Neiguan or Pericardium-6 **acupuncture** point (located about three fingerwidths above the wrist on the inner arm), either by acupuncture, **acupressure,** or a mild, electrical pulse, has shown to be effective against the symptoms of motion sickness. Elastic wristbands sold at most drugstores are also used as a source of relief due to the pressure it places

in this area. Pressing the small intestine 17 (just below the earlobes in the indentations behind the jawbone) may also help in the functioning of the ear's balancing mechanism.

There are several homeopathic remedies that work specifically for motion sickness. They include *Cocculus, Petroleum,* and *Tabacum.*

Prognosis

While there is no cure for motion sickness, its symptoms can be controlled or even prevented. Most people respond successfully to the variety of treatments, or avoid the unpleasant symptoms through prevention methods.

Prevention

Because motion sickness is easier to prevent than treat once it has begun, the best treatment is prevention. The following steps may help deter the unpleasant symptoms of motion sickness before they occur:

• Avoid reading while traveling, and do not sit in a backward facing seat.

• Always ride where the eyes may see the same motion that the body and inner ears feel. Safe positions include the front seat of the car while looking at distant scenery; the deck of a ship where the horizon can be seen; and sitting by the window of an airplane. The least motion on an airplane is in a seat over the wings.

• Maintain a fairly straight-ahead view.

• Eat a light meal before traveling, or if already nauseated, avoid food altogether.

• Avoid watching or talking to another traveler who is having motion sickness.

• Take motion sickness medicine at least 30-60 minutes before travel begins, or as recommended by a physician.

• Learn to live with the condition. Even those who frequently endure motion sickness can learn to travel by anticipating the conditions of their next trip. Research also suggests that increased exposure to the stimulation that causes motion sickness may help decrease its symptoms on future trips.

Resources

BOOKS

Blakely, Brian W., and Mary-Ellen Siegel. ''Peripheral Vestibular Disorders.'' In *Feeling Dizzy: Understanding and Treating Dizziness, Vertigo, and Other Balance Disorders.* New York: Macmillan, 1995.

''Motion Sickness.'' In *The Medical Advisor: The Complete Guide to Alternative & Conventional Treatments.* Richmond, VA: Time-Life, Inc., 1996.

PERIODICALS

"Acupuncture Effective In Combating Nausea." *Executive Health's Good Health Report* 33(June 1997): 5.

Brown, Edwin W. "Ginger Not Just For Ale And Cookies." *Medical Update* 20(December 1996): 5.

Farley, Dixie. "Taming Tummy Turmoil." *FDA Consumer* (June 1995).

Gannon, Robert. "How To Prevent Motion Sickness." *Popular Science* 246(March 1995): 98.

Mowrey, Daniel B. "Ginger Root—A Blessing For The Gastrointestinal Tract." *Health News & Review* (Spring 1995): 18.

Munson, Marty and Greg Gutfeld with Beth Higbee and Teresa Yeykal. "A Soothing Shock: A Little Electricity Helps Ease Nausea." *Prevention* (January 1994): 26.

Purcell, Lauren. "How To Cure Motion Sickness." *Health* 11(January 1997): 26.

"Traveler's Advisory: A Glob Of Scop Is Good News For The Nauseated." *Prevention* 49(August 1997): 22.

ORGANIZATIONS

Vestibular Disorders Association. PO Box 4467, Portland, OR 97208-4467. (800) 837-8428. http://www.teleport.com/veda.

Beth A. Kapes

Motofen *see* **Antidiarrheal drugs**

Mountain sickness *see* **Altitude sickness**

Mouth cancer *see* **Head and neck cancer**

Movement disorders

Definition

Movement disorders are a group of diseases and syndromes affecting the ability to produce and control movement.

Description

Though it seems simple and effortless, normal movement in fact requires an astonishingly complex system of control. Disruption of any portion of this system can cause a person to produce movements that are too weak, too forceful, too uncoordinated, or too poorly controlled for the task at hand. Unwanted movements may occur at rest. Intentional movement may become impossible. Such conditions are called movement disorders.

Abnormal movements themselves are symptoms of underlying disorders. In some cases, the abnormal move-

ments are the only symptoms. Disorders causing abnormal movements include:

- **Parkinson's disease**
- Parkinsonism caused by drugs or poisons
- Parkinson-plus syndromes (**progressive supranuclear palsy,** multiple system atrophy, and cortical-basal ganglionic degeneration)
- **Huntington's disease**
- **Wilson's disease**
- Inherited ataxias (**Friedreich's ataxia,** Machado-Joseph disease, and spinocerebellar ataxias)
- **Tourette syndrome** and other tic disorders
- Essential tremor
- Restless leg syndrome
- Dystonia
- **Stroke**
- **Cerebral palsy**
- Encephalopathies
- Intoxication
- **Poisoning** by carbon monoxide, cyanide, methanol, or manganese.

Causes & symptoms

Causes

Movement is produced and coordinated by several interacting brain centers, including the motor cortex, the cerebellum, and a group of structures in the inner portions of the brain called the basal ganglia. Sensory information provides critical input on the current position and velocity of body parts, and spinal nerve cells (neurons) help prevent opposing muscle groups from contracting at the same time.

To understand how movement disorders occur, it is helpful to consider a normal voluntary movement, such as reaching to touch a nearby object with the right index finger. To accomplish the desired movement, the arm must be lifted and extended. The hand must be held out to align with the forearm, and the forefinger must be extended while the other fingers remain flexed.

THE MOTOR CORTEX

Voluntary motor commands begin in the motor cortex located on the outer, wrinkled surface of the brain. Movement of the right arm is begun by the left motor cortex, which generates a large volley of signals to the involved muscles. These electrical signals pass along upper motor neurons through the midbrain to the spinal cord. Within the spinal cord, they connect to lower motor neurons, which convey the signals out of the spinal cord

KEY TERMS

Botulinum toxin—Any of a group of potent bacterial toxins or poisons produced by different strains of the bacterium *Clostridium botulinum*. The toxins cause muscle paralysis, and thus force the relaxation of a muscle in spasm.

Cerebral palsy—A movement disorder caused by a permanent brain defect or injury present at birth or shortly after. It is frequently associated with premature birth. Cerebral palsy is not progressive.

Computed tomography (CT)—An imaging technique in which cross-sectional x rays of the body are compiled to create a three-dimensional image of the body's internal structures.

Encephalopathy—An abnormality in the structure or function of tissues of the brain.

Essential tremor—An uncontrollable (involuntary) shaking of the hands, head, and face. Also called familial tremor because it is sometimes inherited, it can begin in the teens or in middle age. The exact cause is not known.

Fetal tissue transplantation—A method of treating Parkinson's and other neurological diseases by grafting brain cells from human fetuses onto the basal ganglia. Human adults cannot grow new brain cells but developing fetuses can. Grafting fetal tissue stimulates the growth of new brain cells in affected adult brains.

Hereditary ataxia—One of a group of hereditary degenerative diseases of the spinal cord or cerebellum. These diseases cause tremor, spasm, and wasting of muscle.

Huntington's disease—A rare hereditary condition that causes progressive chorea (jerky muscle movements) and mental deterioration that ends in dementia. Huntington's symptoms usually appear in patients in their 40s. There is no effective treatment.

Levodopa (L-dopa)—A substance used in the treatment of Parkinson's disease. Levodopa can cross the blood-brain barrier that protects the brain. Once in the brain, it is converted to dopamine and thus can replace the dopamine lost in Parkinson's disease.

Magnetic resonance imaging (MRI)—An imaging technique that uses a large circular magnet and radio waves to generate signals from atoms in the body. These signals are used to construct images of internal structures.

Parkinson's disease—A slowly progressive disease that destroys nerve cells in the basal ganglia and thus causes loss of dopamine, a chemical that aids in transmission of nerve signals (neurotransmitter). Parkinson's is characterized by shaking in resting muscles, a stooping posture, slurred speech, muscular stiffness, and weakness.

Positron emission tomography (PET)—A diagnostic technique in which computer-assisted x rays are used to track a radioactive substance inside a patient's body. PET can be used to study the biochemical activity of the brain.

Progressive supranuclear palsy—A rare disease that gradually destroys nerve cells in the parts of the brain that control eye movements, breathing, and muscle coordination. The loss of nerve cells causes palsy, or paralysis, that slowly gets worse as the disease progresses. The palsy affects ability to move the eyes, relax the muscles, and control balance.

Restless legs syndrome—A condition that causes an annoying feeling of tiredness, uneasiness, and itching deep within the muscle of the leg. It is accompanied by twitching and sometimes pain. The only relief is in walking or moving the legs.

Tourette syndrome—An abnormal condition that causes uncontrollable facial grimaces and tics and arm and shoulder movements. Tourette sydnrome is perhaps best known for uncontrollable vocal tics that include grunts, shouts, and use of obscene language (coprolalia).

Wilson's disease—An inborn defect of copper metabolism in which free copper may be deposited in a variety of areas of the body. Deposits in the brain can cause tremor and other symptoms of Parkinson's disease.

to the surface of the muscles involved. Electrical stimulation of the muscles causes contraction, and the force of contraction pulling on the skeleton causes movement of the arm, hand, and fingers.

Damage to or death of any of the neurons along this path causes weakness or **paralysis** of the affected muscles.

ANTAGONISTIC MUSCLE PAIRS

This picture of movement is too simple, however. One important refinement to it comes from considering the role of opposing, or antagonistic, muscle pairs. Contraction of the biceps muscle, located on the top of the upper arm, pulls on the forearm to flex the elbow and bend the arm. Contraction of the triceps, located on the opposite side, extends the elbow and straightens the arm. Within the spine, these muscles are normally wired so that willed (voluntary) contraction of one is automatically accompanied by blocking of the other. In other words, the command to contract the biceps provokes another command within the spine to prevent contraction of the triceps. In this way, these antagonist muscles are kept from resisting one another. Spinal cord or brain injury can damage this control system and cause involuntary simultaneous contraction and spasticity, an increase in resistance to movement during motion.

THE CEREBELLUM

Once the movement of the arm is initiated, sensory information is needed to guide the finger to its precise destination. In addition to sight, the most important source of information comes from the ''position sense'' provided by the many sensory neurons located within the limbs (proprioception). Proprioception is what allows you to touch your nose with your finger even with your eyes closed. The balance organs in the ears provide important information about posture. Both postural and proprioceptive information are processed by a structure at the rear of the brain called the cerebellum. The cerebellum sends out electrical signals to modify movements as they progress, ''sculpting'' the barrage of voluntary commands into a tightly controlled, constantly evolving pattern. Cerebellar disorders cause inability to control the force, fine positioning, and speed of movements (ataxia). Disorders of the cerebellum may also impair the ability to judge distance so that a person under- or over-reaches the target (dysmetria). Tremor during voluntary movements can also result from cerebellar damage.

THE BASAL GANGLIA

Both the cerebellum and the motor cortex send information to a set of structures deep within the brain that help control involuntary components of movement (basal ganglia). The basal ganglia send output messages to the motor cortex, helping to initiate movements, regulate repetitive or patterned movements, and control muscle tone.

Circuits within the basal ganglia are complex. Within this structure, some groups of cells begin the action of other basal ganglia components and some groups of cells block the action. These complicated feedback circuits are not entirely understood. Disruptions of these circuits are known to cause several distinct movement disorders. A portion of the basal ganglia called the substantia nigra sends electrical signals that block output from another structure called the subthalamic nucleus. The subthalamic nucleus sends signals to the globus pallidus, which in turn blocks the thalamic nuclei. Finally, the thalamic nuclei send signals to the motor cortex. The substantia nigra, then, begins movement and the globus pallidus blocks it.

This complicated circuit can be disrupted at several points. For instance, loss of substantia nigra cells, as in Parkinson's disease, increases blocking of the thalamic nuclei, preventing them from sending signals to the motor cortex. The result is a loss of movement (motor activity), a characteristic of Parkinson's.

In contrast, cell loss in early Huntington's disease decreases blocking of signals from the thalamic nuclei, causing more cortex stimulation and stronger but uncontrolled movements.

Disruptions in other portions of the basal ganglia are thought to cause tics, **tremors,** dystonia, and a variety of other movement disorders, although the exact mechanisms are not well understood.

Some movement disorders, including Huntington's disease and inherited ataxias, are caused by inherited genetic defects. Some disease that cause sustained muscle contraction limited to a particular muscle group (focal dystonia) are inherited, but others are caused by trauma. The cause of most cases of Parkinson's disease is unknown, although genes have been found for some familial forms.

Symptoms

Abnormal movements are broadly classified as either hyperkinetic—too much movement—and hypokinetic—too little movement. Hyperkinetic movements include:

• Dystonia. Sustained muscle contractions, often causing twisting or repetitive movements and abnormal postures. Dystonia may be limited to one area (focal) or may affect the whole body (general). Focal dystonias may affect the neck (cervical dystonia or **torticollis),** the face (one-sided or hemifacial spasm, contraction of the eyelid or blepharospasm, contraction of the mouth and jaw or oromandibular dystonia, simultaneous spasm of the chin and eyelid or Meige syndrome), the vocal cords (laryngeal dystonia), or the arms and legs (writer's cramp, occupational cramps). Dystonia may be painful as well as incapacitating.

• Tremor. Uncontrollable (involuntary) shaking of a body part. Tremor may occur only when muscles are relaxed or it may occur only during an action or holding an active posture.

• Tics. Involuntary, rapid, nonrhythmic movement or sound. Tics can be controlled briefly.

• Myoclonus. A sudden, shock-like muscle contraction. Myoclonic jerks may occur singly or repetitively. Unlike tics, myoclonus cannot be controlled even briefly.

• Chorea. Rapid, nonrhythmic, usually jerky movements, most often in the arms and legs.

• Ballism. Like chorea, but the movements are much larger, more explosive and involve more of the arm or leg. This condition, also called ballismus, can occur on both sides of the body or on one side only (hemiballismus).

• Akathisia. Restlessness and a desire to move to relieve uncomfortable sensations. Sensations may include a feeling of crawling, **itching,** stretching, or creeping, usually in the legs.

• Athetosis. Slow, writhing, continuous, uncontrollable movement of the arms and legs.

Hypokinetic movements include:

• Bradykinesia. Slowness of movement.

• Freezing. Inability to begin a movement or involuntary stopping of a movement before it is completed.

• Rigidity. An increase in muscle tension when an arm or leg is moved by an outside force.

• Postural instability. Loss of ability to maintain upright posture caused by slow or absent righting reflexes.

Diagnosis

Diagnosis of movement disorders requires a careful medical history and a thorough physical and neurological examination. Brain imaging studies are usually performed. Imaging techniques include **computed tomography scan** (CT scan), **positron emission tomography (PET),** or **magnetic resonance imaging** (MRI) scans. Routine blood and urine analyses are performed. A lumbar puncture (spinal tap) may be necessary. Video recording of the abnormal movement is often used to analyze movement patterns and to track progress of the disorder and its treatment. **Genetic testing** is available for some forms of movement disorders.

Treatment

Treatment of a movement disorder begins with determining its cause. Physical and occupational therapy may help make up for lost control and strength. Drug therapy can help compensate for some imbalances of the basal ganglionic circuit. For instance, levodopa (L-dopa) or related compounds can substitute for lost dopamine-producing cells in Parkinson's disease. Conversely, blocking normal dopamine action is a possible treatment in some hyperkinetic disorders, including tics. Oral medications can also help reduce overall muscle tone. Local injections of botulinum toxin can selectively weaken overactive muscles in dystonia and spasticity. Destruction of peripheral nerves through injection of phenol can reduce spasticity. All of these treatments may have some side effects.

Surgical destruction or inactivation of basal ganglionic circuits has proven effective for Parkinson's disease and is being tested for other movement disorders. Transplantation of fetal cells into the basal ganglia has produced mixed results in Parkinson's disease.

Alternative treatment

There are several alternative therapies that can be useful when treating movement disorders. The progress made will depend on the individual and his/her condition. Among the therapies that may be helpful are **acupuncture** and **biofeedback.**

Prognosis

The prognosis for a patient with a movement disorder depends on the specific disorder.

Prevention

Prevention depends on the specific disorder.

Resources

BOOKS

Martini, Frederic. *Fundamentals of Anatomy and Physiology.* Englewood Cliffs, NJ: Prentice Hall, 1989.

Watts, Ray L. and William C. Koller, eds. *Movement Disorders: Neurologic Principles and Practice.* New York: McGraw-Hill, 1997.

PERIODICALS

Movement Disorders. Lippincott-Raven Publishers, 12107 Insurance Way, Hagerstown, MD 21740.

ORGANIZATIONS

WE MOVE. 1 Gustave L. Levy Place, Box 1052, New York, NY 10029. (800) 437-MOV2. http://www.wemove.org.

Movement therapy

Definition

Movement therapy is the utilization of body movement to affect physiological functioning. It includes stabile bodywork such as muscle and tissue manipulation,

KEY TERMS

. . . .

Imbalance—The condition of being out of balance or equilibrium.

Kinesthetic—A feeling in the muscles, tendons, and joints stimulated by body movement.

Organic disease—A disease associated with changes in one or more bodily organs.

Stabile bodywork—Work performed while the body is stationary or not moving.

education and awareness, breathing and emotional expression, as well as specific movement patterns.

Purpose

Movement therapy is used to enhance an individual's mind/body awareness and insure a healthier lifestyle.

Precautions

All movement therapies are safe when taught by a properly trained instructor. Those involving deep muscle **massage** should be avoided by individuals with organic disease or inflammation of the joints, nerves, or muscles.

Description

Movement therapies work on the premise that by repatterning muscle relationships, one can overcome discomfort and experience a heightened sense of the body and its relationship to the environment. Most therapies were developed by individuals who sought relief from chronic **pain** or saw others who needed therapeutic relief. Neuromuscular reeducation is integral to the process of movement therapy. Some therapies involve deep muscle massage which acts as a first step in releasing tension. The field of movement therapy can be broken down into specific theories and techniques.

Aston patterning is a deep muscle manipulation technique used in conjunction with neuromuscular reeducation. It is particularly beneficial for individuals with chronic pain such as **tennis elbow** and for people with postural problems. It differs from other techniques in that the patient receives long term relief. Reeducation is essential to the technique for one must consciously change the movement patterns that caused the pain.

The **Alexander technique** was developed by F. Mathias Alexander, an Australian actor who suffered severe vocal difficulties and studied his own habits of movement to determine what might be causing them. He discovered a habit of tensing his neck muscles with the intake of each breath that resulted in distortion of the head-neck-spine relationship and a consequent interference with natural coordination. He named this head-neck-spine relationship the ''primary control'' and promoted a system of movement reeducation to bring increased awareness to anatomical design and an enlightened cooperation with inherent patterns of coordination. This technique results in a sense of kinesthetic lightness where thinking becomes clearer, sensations livelier, and movement more pleasurable.

The **Feldenkrais method** deals with structural integration of the mind and the body, using movement training, gentle touch, and verbal dialogue. Moshe Feldenkrais was a physicist who suffered a sports related injury which drove him to explore his own movement patterns. He succeeded in overcoming his handicap and in the process developed sequences of movements designed to replace old negative habits with new structurally integrated ones. He developed two approaches: *awareness through movement,* which uses group sessions, and *functional integration,* which specializes in individualized gentle touch. Results include improved posture, better flexibility, coordination, and less pain and tension.

Hellerwork combines deep tissue massage, guided verbal dialogue, and movement education. The purpose is to structurally realign the body, release tension, and enhance mind/body awareness. The technique involves deep massage along with dialogue on how to move properly and how to change habits and lifestyle in order to reduce tension. Results are improved posture, relief of common aches and pains and increased awareness of emotional problems contributing to physical disabilities.

The Pilates method is a system of physical conditioning and **rehabilitation.** Pilates works from the inside out, beginning with pelvic stabilization, intense concentration, patience, body alignment, breathing, and intelligence. Joseph Pilates was a gymnast and bodybuilder born in 1880. During World War I, he devised a series of **exercises** to aid rehabilitation of wounded soldiers using springs attached to a hospital bed. He moved to New York City in 1923 and began to use the wooden bed, now called the universal reformer, to recondition dancers and athletes. Pilates later added other apparatus to his system, such as the chair, the trapeze table, and the barrel, as well as an extensive series of mat exercises. Deep breathing and abdominal support are important ingredients in the technique. Results are strength, control, lengthening through the spine, and correction of imbalance and faulty neuromuscular patterning.

Trager work is a method of gentle, rhythmical touch combined with movement reeducation. As the individual lies on a table, a certified practitioner uses gentle, non intrusive touch to loosen muscles and joints. These gentle movements trigger a sense of sensory motor feedback between the mind and body, which in turn produces psychophysical integration. After the manipulation session, the patient is introduced to a series of movements to maintain a sense of lightness and awareness called *mentastics*. Trager work is beneficial for sever neuromuscular disturbances and produces increased body awareness.

Movement therapy has proven beneficial for all individuals who seek not only relief from chronic pain, but for those who want to enjoy movement as a part of daily life.

Preparation

Most movement or body therapies require the practitioner receive proper training before entering the field. The patient, in turn, should be thoroughly educated in the principles of the proposed therapy for the best results.

Risks

When taught by a qualified teacher in the proper setting, there are no risks.

Normal results

The patient feels a release of tension and relief from muscular pain, while experiencing a heightened awareness of his or her own body and its relationship to the environment.

Resources

BOOKS

Bradford, Nikki, ed. *Alternative Medicine*. San Diego, CA: Thunder Bay Press, 1997.

Stillerman, Elaine. *Encyclopedia of Body Work*. New York: Facts on File, Inc., 1996.

Thompson, Robert. *Grosset Encyclopedia of Natural Medicine*. New York: Grosset & Dunlap, 1980.

Carol D. Halsted

MR *see* **Magnetic resonance imaging**

MRA *see* **Magnetic resonance imaging**

MRI *see* **Magnetic resonance imaging**

MRS *see* **Magnetic resonance imaging**

MS *see* **Multiple sclerosis**

Mucopolysaccharidoses

Definition

Mucopolysaccharidosis (MPS) is a general term for a number of inherited diseases in which the accumulation of mucopolysaccharide leads to developmental abnormalities. Other names for the MPS diseases include Hunter, Hurler, Scheie, Morquio, Sanfilippo, Sly, and Maroteaux-Lamy syndromes.

Description

In all forms of MPS, the symptoms include a variety of developmental abnormalities, both physical and mental. The range of severity of symptoms is wide, from very mild to deadly. Most forms of MPS are caused by the absence of a specific enzyme that is necessary for the normal processing of a particular mucopolysaccharide. When an enzyme is missing its "target," mucopolysaccharide accumulates in the body. At least 10 different enzymes are associated with these diseases.

Causes & symptoms

Each type of MPS is an inherited deficiency of an enzyme involved in the metabolism of molecules known as mucopolysaccharides or glycosaminoglycans (GAGs). Each enzyme is necessary for the normal processing of a specific GAG. In the absence of the enzyme, the GAG is not processed normally and therefore accumulates. The excess GAG may be partially excreted in the urine, but still builds up to damaging levels in tissues throughout the body.

Accumulation within the brain is responsible for **mental retardation.** Accumulation in numerous other tissues accounts for the wide array of symptoms. The accumulating material is stored in cellular structures called lysosomes, and these disorders are therefore also known as lysosomal storage diseases.

All types of MPS (except Hunter syndrome) are autosomal recessive genetic disorders. This means that the defective gene causing the disorder is located on one of the 22 non-sex chromosomes and that a person must receive a copy of this gene from each parent in order to have the syndrome. Hunter syndrome is an X-linked recessive genetic disorder. This means that the defective gene is carried on the X chromosome, one of the two human sex chromosomes. Since a male has only one X chromosome, he will have the disease if the X chromosome inherited from his mother carries the defective gene.

KEY TERMS

Autosomal gene—In humans, a gene found on one of the 22 pairs of non-sex chromosomes.

Enzyme—A protein that catalyzes chemical reactions in the body.

Kyphosis—A hunchback condition caused by flexure of the spine.

Lysosome—A cellular structure involved in the process of localized, intracellular digestion.

Mucopolysaccharides—A group of carbohydrates.

Recessive gene—A gene that must be present in both copies of the gene pair to control expression of a trait.

X-linked gene—A gene carried on the X chromosome, one of the two sex chromosomes in humans. The other sex chromosome is the Y chromosome.

Hurler syndrome (MPS type I H)

Hurler syndrome is caused by a deficiency of the enzyme iduronidase. Patients have a characteristic pattern of facial features described as gargoylism. Skeletal abnormalities include dwarfism, **kyphosis,** and a broad hand with short fingers. Movement at the joints can be limited. Airway obstruction and respiratory infections are common. Other common symptoms include structural abnormalities of the heart, enlarged spleen and liver, and clouding of the cornea. Mental development is usually normal in the first few years of childhood, but by later childhood severe **learning disorders** are seen in many patients. **Death** due to heart or lung failure usually occurs by age 10.

Scheie syndrome (MPS type I S)

This syndrome, also caused by a deficiency of the enzyme iduronidase, can be considered a mild form of Hurler syndrome. At one time, it was designated MPS type V. Patients often survive through adulthood. Common problems include heart abnormalities and orthopedic difficulties of the hand and back. Conditions of intermediate severity are now referred to as Hurler/Scheie or MPS I H/S.

Hunter syndrome (MPS type II)

Hunter syndrome is caused by a deficiency of the enzyme iduronate sulphate sulphatase. Most patients are severely affected with airway problems similar to those of MPS I. Although dwarfism and kyphosis are common, skeletal abnormalities are generally not as severe as in Hurler syndrome. Neurological degeneration causes death by the mid-teens. These patients are all male, because the responsible gene is X-linked.

Sanfilippo syndrome (MPS type III)

This is the most common form of MPS and it is highly variable. Mental retardation is often severe and associated with behavioral disorders. The four subtypes, A through D, are caused by four different enzyme deficiencies, but lead to similar symptoms.

Morquio syndrome (MPS type IV)

Morquio syndrome, caused by a deficiency of the enzymes galactosamine-6-sulphatase and beta-galactosidase, is one of the less common types of MPS. It is also highly variable in severity. Intelligence is often completely normal. In severe cases, skeletal abnormalities can be extreme and include dwarfism, kyphosis, enlarged sternum, and knock-knees. The earliest symptom of this condition is often an abnormal gait noticed as the child learns to walk. In mild cases, limb stiffness and joint **pain** are the primary symptoms.

Maroteaux-Lamy syndrome (MPS type VI)

This syndrome, another uncommon type of MPS, is caused by a deficiency of the enzyme N-acetylglucosamine-4-sulphatase. No impact on the nervous system or intelligence is seen. Airway obstruction, however, can be a serious problem.

Sly syndrome (MPS type VII)

This extremely rare syndrome is cause by a deficiency of the enzyme beta-glucuronidase. It is also highly variable, but symptoms are generally similar to those of Hurler syndrome.

Many MPS patients have a problem with constriction of the airway. This constriction may be so serious as to create significant difficulties in administering general anesthesia. Therefore, it is recommended that surgical procedures be performed under local anesthesia whenever possible.

Diagnosis

Diagnosis for each type of MPS is often made on the basis of visible symptoms described above. Biochemical testing can confirm the specific enzyme deficiency and therefore the specific disease type. Detailed DNA analysis can be performed to pinpoint exactly the mutation responsible for a given genetic defect.

Treatment

No true cure is available for inherited diseases like MPS. Treatment for the relief of symptoms is available in some cases. For MPS, as for many other genetic diseases, research is underway that may someday allow gene replacement therapy (the insertion of normal copies of a gene into the cells of patients whose gene copies are defective).

Prevention

No specific preventative measures are available for genetic diseases of this type. For some of the MPS diseases, biochemical tests are available that will identify healthy individuals who are carriers of the defective gene, allowing them to make informed reproductive decisions. In some cases, testing also allows detection of affected fetuses.

Resources

PERIODICALS

Wraith, J.E. ''The Mucopolysaccharidoses: A Clinical Review and Guide to Management.''*Archives of Disease in Childhood* 72(1995): 263-267.

ORGANIZATIONS

National MPS Society. 4441 New York Ave., Island Park, NY 11558. (516) 432-1797. http://members.AOL.com/mpssociety.

G. Victor Leipzig

Mucormycosis

Definition

Mucormycosis is a rare but often fatal disease caused by certain fungi. It is sometimes called zygomycosis or phycomycosis. Mucormycosis is an opportunistic infection that typically develops in patients with weakened immune systems, diabetes, kidney failure, organ transplants, or **chemotherapy.**

Description

In the United States, mucormycosis is most likely to develop in the patient's nasal area or in the lungs.

Rhinocerebral mucormycosis

Rhinocerebral mucormycosis is an infection of the nose, eyes, and brain. The fungus destroys the tissue of the nasal passages, sinuses, or hard palate, producing a black discharge and visible patches of dying tissue. The

---

> **KEY TERMS**
>
> **Amphotericin B**—An antibiotic used to treat mucormycosis and other severe fungal infections.
>
> **Opportunistic infection**—An infection that develops only when a person's immune system is weakened.
>
> **Orbit**—The bony cavity or socket surrounding the eye.
>
> **Zygomycosis**—Another term for mucormycosis. The fungi that cause mucormycosis belong to a group called Zygomycetes.

---

fungus then invades the tissues around the eye socket and eventually the brain.

Pulmonary mucormycosis

Most patients with the pulmonary form of the disease are being treated for leukemia. The fungus enters the patient's lungs, where it eventually invades a major blood vessel, causing the patient to **cough** up blood or hemorrhage into the lungs.

Causes & symptoms

Mucormycosis is caused by fungi of several different species, including *Mucor*, *Rhizopus*, *Absidia*, and *Rhizomucor*. When these organisms gain access to the mucous membranes of the patient's nose or lungs, they multiply rapidly and invade the nearby blood vessels. The fungi destroy soft tissue and bone, as well as the walls of blood vessels.

The early symptoms of rhinocerebral mucormycosis include **fever,** sinus **pain, headache,** and **cellulitis.** As the fungus reaches the eye tissues, the patient develops dilated pupils, drooping eyelids, a bulging eye, and eventually hemorrhage of the blood vessels in the brain—causing convulsions, partial **paralysis,** and **death.**

The symptoms of pulmonary mucormycosis include fever and difficulty breathing, with eventual bleeding from the lungs.

Diagnosis

Diagnosis is usually based on a combination of the patient's medical history and a visual examination of the nose and throat. The doctor will take a tissue sample for biopsy, or a PAS, potassium hydroxide (KOH), or Calcofluor stain in order to make a tentative diagnosis. Confirmation requires a laboratory culture.

Imaging studies are not needed to make the diagnosis. If the patient has mucormycosis, however, **magnetic** resonance imaging (MRI) and computed tomography scans (CT scans) will usually show the destruction of soft tissue or bone in patients with advanced disease. Chest x rays will sometimes show a cavity in the lung or an area filled with tissue fluid if the patient has pulmonary mucormycosis.

Treatment

Treatment is usually begun without waiting for laboratory reports because of the rapid spread and high mortality rate of the disease. It includes intravenous amphotericin B (Fungizone); surgical removal of infected tissue; and careful monitoring of the disorder or condition that is responsible for the patient's vulnerability.

Prognosis

The prognosis for recovery from mucormycosis is poor. The mortality rate is 30%-50% of patients with the rhinocerebral form, and even higher for patients with pulmonary mucormycosis. The disease is almost 100% fatal for patients with AIDS.

Prevention

Prevention depends on protecting high-risk patients from contact with sugary foods, decaying plants, moldy bread, manure, and other breeding grounds for fungi.

Resources

BOOKS

Beavis, Kathleen G. "Systemic Mycoses." In *Current Diagnosis 9,* edited by Rex B. Conn, et al. Philadelphia: W. B. Saunders Company, 1997.

Hamill, Richard J. "Infectious Diseases: Mycotic." In *Current Medical Diagnosis & Treatment 1998,* edited by Lawrence M. Tierney Jr., et al. Stamford, CT: Appleton & Lange, 1997.

"Infectious Disease: Systemic Fungal Diseases." In *The Merck Manual of Diagnosis and Therapy.* vol. II, edited by Robert Berkow, et al. Rahway, NJ: Merck Research Laboratories, 1992.

Jackler, Robert K., and Michael J. Kaplan. "Ear, Nose, & Throat." In *Current Medical Diagnosis & Treatment 1998,* edited by Lawrence M. Tierney, Jr., et al. Stamford, CT: Appleton & Lange, 1997.

Rebecca J. Frey

Mucoviscidosis *see* **Cystic fibrosis**

MUGA scan *see* **Multiple-gated acquisition (MUGA) scan**

Multiple chemical sensitivity

Definition

Multiple chemical sensitivity, also known as MCS syndrome or simply MCS, is a disorder in which a person develops symptoms from exposure to chemicals in the environment. With each incidence of exposure, lower levels of the chemical will trigger a reaction and the person becomes increasingly vulnerable to reactions triggered by other chemicals.

Description

Multiple chemical sensitivity typically begins with one high-dose exposure to a chemical, but it may also develop with long-term exposure to a low level of a chemical. Chemicals most often connected with MCS include: formaldehyde; pesticides; solvents; petrochemical fuels such as diesel, gasoline, and kerosene; waxes, detergents, and cleaning products; latex; tobacco smoke; perfumes and fragrances; and artificial colors, flavors, and preservatives. People who develop MCS are commonly exposed in one of the following situations: on the job as an industrial worker; residing or working in a poorly ventilated building; or living in conditions of high air or water pollution. Others may be exposed in unique incidents.

Because MCS is difficult to diagnose, estimates vary as to what percentage of the population develops MCS. However, most MCS patients are female. The median age of MCS patients is 40 years old, and most experienced symptoms before they were 30 years old.

Causes & symptoms

Chemical exposure is often a result of indoor air pollution. Buildings which are tightly sealed for energy conservation may cause a related illness called sick building syndrome, in which people develop symptoms from chronic exposure to airborne environmental chemicals such as formaldehyde from the furniture, carpet glues, and latex caulking. A person moving into a newly constructed building, which has not had time to degas, may experience the initial high-dose exposure that leads to MCS.

The symptoms of MCS vary from person to person and are not chemical-specific. Symptoms are not limited to one physiological system, but primarily affect the respiratory and nervous systems. Symptoms commonly reported are **headache,** fatigue, weakness, difficulty concentrating, short-term memory loss, **dizziness,** irritability and depression, **itching,** numbness, burning sensation, congestion, **sore throat,** hoarseness, **shortness of breath, cough,** and stomach **pains.**

KEY TERMS

Degas—To release and vent gases. New building materials often give off gases and odors and the air should be well circulated to remove them.

Sick building syndrome—An illness related to MCS in which a person develops symptoms in response to chronic exposure to airborne environmental chemicals found in a tightly sealed building.

Diagnosis

Multiple chemical sensitivity is a twentieth-century disorder, becoming more prevalent as more man-made chemicals are introduced into the environment in greater quantities. It is especially difficult to diagnose because it presents no consistent or measurable set of symptoms and has no single diagnostic test or marker. Physicians are often unaware of MCS as a condition. They may be unable to diagnose it, or may misdiagnose it as another degenerative disease, or may label it as a psychosomatic illness (a physical illness that is caused by emotional problems). Their lack of understanding generates frustration, **anxiety,** and distrust in patients already struggling with MCS. However, a new specialty of medicine is evolving to address MCS and related illnesses: occupational and environmental medicine. A physician looking for MCS will take a complete patient history and try to identify chemical exposures.

Treatment

While doctors may recommend **antihistamines, analgesics,** and other medications to combat the symptoms, the most effective treatment is to avoid those chemicals which trigger the symptoms. This becomes increasingly difficult as the number of offending chemicals increases, and people with MCS often remain at home where they are able to control the chemicals in their environment. This **isolation** often limits their abilities to work and socialize, so supportive counseling may also be appropriate.

Alternative treatment

Some MCS patients find relief with detoxification programs of **exercise** and sweating, and chelation of heavy metals. Others support their health with nutritional regimens and immunotherapy vaccines. Some undergo food-allergy testing and testing for accumulated pesticides in the body to learn more about their condition and what chemicals to avoid. Homeopathy and **acupuncture** can give added support to any treatment program for MCS patients. Botanical medicine can help to support the liver and other involved organs.

Prognosis

Once MCS sets in, sensitivity continues to increase and a person's health continues to deteriorate. Strictly avoiding exposure to triggering chemicals for a year or more may improve health.

Prevention

Multiple chemical sensitivity is difficult to prevent because even at high-dose exposures, different people react differently. Ensuring adequate ventilation in situations with potential for acute high-dose or chronic low-dose chemical exposure, as well as wearing the proper protective equipment in industrial situations, will minimize the risk.

Resources

BOOKS

Hu, Howard, and Frank E. Speizer. "Specific Environmental and Occupational Hazards." In *Harrison's Principles of Internal Medicine*, 14th ed., edited by Anthony S. Fauci, et al. New York: McGraw-Hill, 1998.

PERIODICALS

Sparks, P.J., et al. "Multiple Chemical Sensitivity Syndrome: A Clinical Perspective." *Journal of Occupational Medicine* 36(1994): 718.

ORGANIZATIONS

American Academy of Environmental Medicine. P.O. Box CN 1001-8001, New Hope, PA 18938. (215) 862-4544.

Bethany Thivierge

Multiple endocrine adenomatosis *see*
Multiple endocrine neoplasia syndromes

Multiple endocrine neoplasia syndromes

Definition

The multiple endocrine neoplasia (MEN) syndromes are three related disorders affecting the thyroid and other hormonal (endocrine) glands of the body. MEN has previously been known as familial endocrine adenomatosis.

Description

The three forms of MEN are MEN1 (Wermer's syndrome), MEN2A (Sipple syndrome), and MEN2B (previously known as MEN3). Each is an autosomal dominant genetic condition which predisposes to hyperplasia (excessive growth of cells) and tumor formation in a number of endocrine glands.

Causes & symptoms

MEN1 patients experience hyperplasia or tumors of several endocrine glands, including the parathyroids, the pancreas, and the pituitary. The most frequent symptom of MEN1 is **hyperparathyroidism.** Overgrowth of the parathyroid glands leads to over secretion of parathyroid hormone, which leads to elevated blood calcium levels, **kidney stones,** weakened bones, and nervous system depression. Almost all MEN1 patients show parathyroid symptoms by age 40.

Tumors of the pancreas known as **gastrinomas** are also common in MEN1. Excessive secretion of gastrin (a hormone secreted into the stomach to aid in digestion) by these tumors can cause upper gastrointestinal **ulcers.** The anterior pituitary and the adrenal glands can also be affected. Unlike MEN2, the thyroid gland is rarely involved in MEN1 symptoms.

Patients with MEN2A and MEN2B experience two main symptoms, medullary **thyroid cancer** (MTC) and a tumor of the adrenal gland medulla known as **pheochromocytoma.** MTC is a slow-growing **cancer,** but one that can be cured in less than 50% of cases. Pheochromocytoma is usually a benign tumor that causes excessive secretion of adrenal hormones, which, in turn, can cause life-threatening **hypertension** and cardiac arrhythmia.

The two forms of MEN2 are distinguished by additional symptoms. MEN2A patients have a predisposition to increase in size (hypertrophy) and to develop tumors of the parathyroid gland. Although similar to MEN1, less than 20% of MEN2A patients will show parathyroid involvement.

MEN2B patients show a variety of additional conditions: a characteristic facial appearance with swollen lips; tumors of the mucous membranes of the eye, mouth, tongue, and nasal cavity; enlarged colon; and skeletal abnormalities. Symptoms develop early in life (often under five years of age) in cases of MEN2B and the tumors are more aggressive. MEN2B is about ten-fold less common than MEN2A.

MEN1 is caused by mutation at the PYGM gene. PYGM is one of a group of genes known as tumor suppressor genes. A patient who inherits one defective copy of a tumor suppressor gene from either parent has a strong predisposition to the disease because of the high probability of incurring a second mutation in at least one dividing cell. That cell no longer possesses even one normal copy of the gene. When both copies are defective, tumor suppression fails and tumors develop.

Both types of MEN2 are caused by mutations in another gene, known as RET. A mutation in only one copy of the RET gene is sufficient to cause disease. A number of different mutations can lead to MEN2A, but only one specific genetic alteration leads to MEN2B.

For all types of MEN, the children of an affected individual have a 50% chance of inheriting the defective gene.

Diagnosis

Classical diagnosis of MEN is based on clinical features and on testing for elevated hormone levels. For MEN1, the relevant hormone is parathyroid hormone. For both types of MEN2, the greatest concern is development of medullary thyroid cancer. MTC can be detected by measuring levels of the thyroid hormone, calcitonin. Numerous other hormone levels can be measured to assess the involvement of the various other endocrine glands.

Diagnosis of MEN2B can be made by **physical examination** alone. However, MEN2A shows no distinct physical features and must be identified by measuring hormone levels or by finding endocrine tumors.

Since 1994, genetic screening using DNA technology has been available for both MEN1 and MEN2. This new methodology allows diagnosis prior to the onset of symptoms.

In the past, there was no way of definitively identifying which children had inherited the defective gene. As a result, all children had to be considered at risk. In the case of MEN2A and MEN2B, children would undergo frequent calcitonin testing. Molecular techniques now

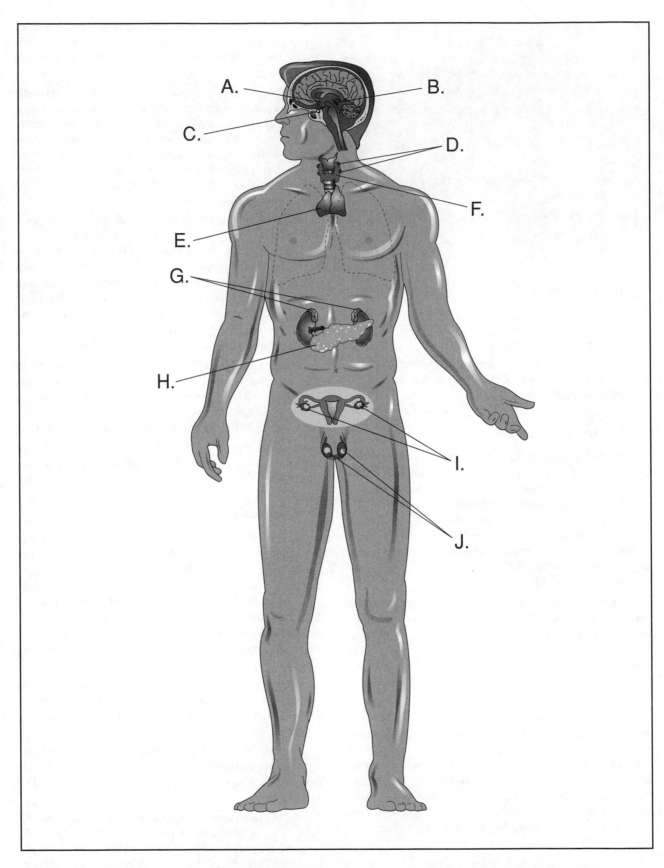

The human endocrine system: A. Hypothalamus. B. Pineal. C. Pituitary. D. Parathyroid. E. Thymus. F. Thyroid. G. Adrenals. H. Pancreas. I. Ovaries (female). J. Testes (male). *(Illustration by Electronic Illustrators Group.)*

allow a positive distinction to be made between children who are and are not actually at risk.

Children who are identified as carriers of the RET gene can be offered total **thyroidectomy** on a preventative (prophylactic) basis to prevent the development of MTC.

Treatment

No comprehensive treatment is available for genetic conditions such as MEN. However, some of the consequences of MEN can be symptomatically treated.

Pheochromocytoma in both types of MEN 2 can be cured by surgical removal of this slow growing tumor.

Treatment of MTC is by surgical removal of the thyroid, although doctors may disagree at what stage to remove the thyroid. After thyroidectomy, the patient will receive normal levels of thyroid hormone orally or by injection.

Even when surgery is performed early, metastatic spread of the cancer may have already occurred. Since this cancer is slow growing, metastasis may not be obvious. Metastasis is very serious in MTC because **chemotherapy** and **radiation therapy** are not effective in controlling its spread.

Prognosis

Diagnosed early, the prognosis for the MEN diseases is reasonably good, even for MEN2B, the most dangerous of the three forms. Even in the absence of treatment, a few individuals with MEN2A mutations will never show any symptoms at all. Analysis of at-risk family members using molecular genetic techniques will lead to earlier treatment and improved outcomes.

Prevention

One of the most serious consequences of MEN is MTC, which can be prevented by thyroidectomy. There is no preventive measure to block the occurrence of genetic mutations such as those that cause MEN.

Resources

PERIODICALS

Gardner, David G. "Recent Advances in Multiple Endocrine Neoplasia Syndromes." *Advances in Internal Medicine* (1997): 597-625.

Moley, Jeffrey F. "The Molecular Genetics of Multiple Endocrine Neoplasia Type 2A and Related Syndromes." *Annual Review of Medicine* 48(1997): 409-420.

ORGANIZATIONS

Canadian MEN Society. P.O. Box 100, Meola, Saskatchewan SOM 1XO. (306) 892-2080.

G. Victor Leipzig

Multiple myeloma

Definition

Multiple myeloma is a disorder in which plasma cells are produced in an uncontrolled and invasive (malignant) fashion.

Description

Plasma cells develop from lymphocytes, a type of white blood cell. They are found primarily in the bone marrow and lymph nodes. The marrow is located in spaces within the bones, especially within the sternum (breast bone), spine, ribs, skull, pelvic bones, and the long bone of the thigh. Bone marrow is a very active tissue that is responsible for producing the different cells that circulate in blood. These include red blood cells, platelets, and the many types of white blood cells.

Plasma cells are responsible for helping the body fight infection. They produce substances called antibodies (also called immunoglobulins). Antibodies circulate within the blood and recognize markers, called antigens, on the cells of invading organisms (like bacteria). These antibodies have a variety of functions, all of which ultimately serve the purpose of defending the body against invading organisms.

Multiple myeloma occurs when the plasma cells in the bone marrow begin reproducing uncontrollably. While normal bone marrow contains less than 5% plasma cells, bone marrow in a patient with multiple myeloma contains over 10% plasma cells.

Multiple myeloma tends to be a disease of the elderly. The average patient is 68 years old when diagnosed. During the last 10 years, doctors have seen an increase in cases of multiple myeloma occurring at younger ages, but patients are usually over age 40. Men have a slightly increased chance of having multiple myeloma, and African-Americans are twice as likely as caucasians to develop the disease. Worldwide, the disease rates are about the same, with approximately four people in 100,000 developing multiple myeloma.

Although the exact cause of multiple myeloma has not been determined, researchers believe that there may be a link between exposure to certain environmental substances and the development of multiple myeloma. This is based on several observations:

• About 20 years after World War II, there was an increased incidence in multiple myeloma among people who had been exposed to the radiation in nuclear warheads.

KEY TERMS

Anemia—Any condition where the oxygen-carrying capacity of the red blood cells is reduced; symptoms often include fatigue.

Electrophoresis—A procedure during which an electrical current is applied to a solution of blood or urine. Because proteins have an electrical charge, the electrical current causes the proteins to move. Specific proteins can be identified by virtue of the distance moved in response to the current.

Malignant—Refers to certain abnormal characteristics of a cell, including uncontrollable growth and duplication, and an ability to invade nearby tissue.

Osteolysis—Softening, absorption, and destruction of bone tissue.

Osteoporosis—A condition where bones lose their mineral content (especially calcium). The bones then become weak and porous.

Plasma cells—A type of white blood cell (infection-fighting cell) produced within the bone marrow. Plasma cells produce antibodies.

Platelets—Blood cells produced within the bone marrow; involved in the clotting process.

White blood cells—The infection-fighting cells of the body produced within the bone marrow.

- There is an increased incidence of multiple myeloma among people who farm, and among those who work with wood, leather, and petroleum products.

Causes & symptoms

Bone **pain** is an extremely common symptom among patients with multiple myeloma. About 70% of all patients will report bone pain as their first symptom. This pain is due to several different processes. Plasma cells grow in number within the bone marrow, replacing normal marrow and putting pressure on the bone containing the marrow. Plasma cells also produce chemicals called osteoclast activating factors (OAF). OAF encourage special cells called osteoclasts to break down bone. This is a normal process, which should be balanced by the building up of new bone by cells called osteoblasts. In multiple myeloma, however, excess OAF are produced, upsetting the normal process called bone remodeling. Bone is eaten away by these overly active osteoclasts. Bones become weak (causing **osteoporosis**) and may even break (causing pathologic **fractures**).

The antibodies that are over produced in multiple myeloma function abnormally. Furthermore, other types of antibodies are under produced. Destruction of circulating antibodies also increases. This results in an increased chance of developing serious bacterial infections. The most common types of infections include **pneumonia** and kidney infections (**pyelonephritis**).

Abnormalities in the structure and function of kidney cells are extremely common in multiple myeloma. About half of all patients have these types of kidney problems. These problems occur because of several reasons, including:

- High levels of calcium in the blood (due to bone breaking down)

- Increased kidney infections

- **Amyloidosis,** a disease where protein deposits build up in organs and tissues in the body

- Increased circulating uric acid

- Exposure of kidney structures to very large amounts of the broken down products of antibodies. Furthermore, the blood in multiple myeloma may become thick and sludgy (referred to as hyperviscosity) due to the large amount of circulating protein from antibodies. This sludge may clog the delicate tubal system within the kidneys, causing damage or kidney failure.

A number of other problems are common in multiple myeloma. Because plasma cells take up space within the bone marrow, other cells normally produced there de-

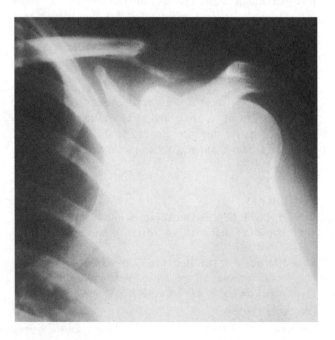

This x ray of the patient's left clavicle indicates an occurrence of myelomas in the bone. *(Custom Medical Stock Photo. Reproduced by permission.)*

crease and are sometimes defective in shape and function. Red blood cells decrease, resulting in anemia in about 80% of all people with multiple myeloma. Circulating antibodies may interfere with clotting, resulting in an increased risk of bleeding. The abnormally thick blood may interfere with blood circulation anywhere in the body, resulting in Raynaud's phenomenon. This circulation problem is particularly common in the fingers, toes, ears, and nose. Hyperviscosity may also cause **headache,** fatigue, and vision problems. Excess calcium in the blood may cause patients to feel weak, depressed, and confused. Sometimes, the plasma cells create a tumor called a plasmacytoma. Plasmacytomas may press on bone, causing fractures. Fractured bones may place unusual pressure on nearby nerves, resulting in nerve damage, pain, burning, tingling, and weakness of the affected muscle.

Diagnosis

Diagnosis of multiple myeloma involves examination of blood, urine, bone marrow, and bones.

Blood tests will reveal a number of abnormalities, including anemia with abnormal red blood cells. Blood calcium will be high in about 33% of all patients. A very specialized test called electrophoresis can be used to show an increased amount of circulating antibodies. This same type of test can be performed on urine to demonstrate that an increased amount of circulating antibodies is also present in urine. The technique of electrophoresis is based on the fact that proteins (including antibodies) have electrical charges. When electricity is applied to the blood or urine, different types of antibodies (with different electrical charges) will move different distances. This allows a healthcare professional to determine the type and the quantity of the various antibodies present in blood or urine. In both blood and urine electrophoresis, an increase in certain antibodies will give a result called an M-spike, indicative of multiple myeloma.

Examination of the bone marrow will require a test called a bone marrow aspiration. An extremely thin long needle is placed into the hip, and a sample of bone marrow is withdrawn. In multiple myeloma, bone marrow will have a significantly increased percentage of plasma cells, usually well over 10%.

X rays will show bone breakdown, including osteoporosis and the punched-out appearance of osteolysis. Pathologic fractures may also be identified.

Treatment

Because the treatments for multiple myeloma can be very damaging, and because the disease often progresses slowly, many patients are not treated until measurements of antibodies in the blood reach a particularly high level. **Chemotherapy** agents used in multiple myeloma include melphalan, cyclophosphamide, chlorambucil, and prednisone. These may be given over four to seven days in four to six week intervals. Chemotherapy may be given for several years. The disease usually recurs within a year after treatment has stopped. Chemotherapy can be given again, but each time the disease relapses it is less responsive to treatment.

Bone pain is often treated with radiation directed at the problem area. High blood levels of calcium may respond to treatment with prednisone. High blood levels of uric acid may improve with allopurinol. When anemia causes symptoms, blood **transfusions** may be necessary. It is important that patients with multiple myeloma drink large amounts of fluid to balance the effects of hyperviscous blood. In the case of kidney failure, a special procedure called **plasmapheresis** is very helpful. In this procedure, blood is filtered through a machine that is capable of removing the large amount of protein present. Infections will require prompt treatment with **antibiotics.**

Alternative treatment

One general recommendation for alternative **cancer** treatment includes dietary supplementation with beta-carotene, vitamin B_6, vitamin C, vitamin E, selenium, and zinc as antioxidant protection. There are also many herbs, including ginseng and astragalus, that are useful in treating cancer. Other recommendations include reducing **stress** through techniques like **biofeedback** training, **guided imagery,** and **meditation.** These same techniques are useful for pain relief.

Prognosis

The prognosis for patients with multiple myeloma varies. About 15% of all patients die within three months of diagnosis. About 60% of all patients respond to treatment and go on to live for an average of two and a half to three years after diagnosis. About 23% of all patients die of other illnesses associated with advanced age (including **stroke, heart attack,** lung disease, and diabetes).

Resources

BOOKS

Longo, Dan L. ''Plasma Cell Disorders.'' In *Harrison's Principles of Internal Medicine,* edited by Anthony S. Fauci, et al. New York: McGraw-Hill, 1998.

Malpas, James S. *Myeloma: Biology and Management.* Oxford: Oxford University Press, 1998.

PERIODICALS

Bataille, Regis, and Jean-Luc Harousseau. ''Multiple Myeloma.'' *The New England Journal of Medicine* 336,23(June 5, 1997): 960 + .

McCarthy, Michael. "Clinical Notes from American Society of Haematology." *The Lancet* 346(December 16, 1995): 1621.

Singer, Charles R. J. "Multiple Myeloma and Related Conditions." *The New England Journal of Medicine* 336(June 5, 1997): 1657+.

ORGANIZATIONS

International Myeloma Foundation. 2120 Stanley Hills Dr., Los Angeles, CA 90046. (800) 452-CURE.

Rosalyn S. Carson-DeWitt

Multiple personality disorder

Definition

Multiple personality disorder, or MPD, is a mental disturbance classified as one of the **dissociative disorders** in the fourth edition of the *Diagnostic and Statistical Manual of Mental Disorders* (*DSM-IV*). It has been renamed dissociative identity disorder (DID). MPD or DID is defined as a condition in which "two or more distinct identities or personality states" alternate in controlling the patient's consciousness and behavior. Note: "Split personality" is not an accurate term for DID and should not be used as a synonym for **schizophrenia.**

Description

The precise nature of DID (MPD) as well as its relationship to other mental disorders is still a subject of debate. Some researchers think that DID may be a relatively recent development in western society. It may be a culture-specific syndrome found in western society, caused primarily by both childhood abuse and unspecified long-term societal changes. Unlike depression or **anxiety disorders,** which have been recognized, in some form, for centuries, the earliest cases of persons reporting DID symptoms were not recorded until the 1790s. Most were considered medical oddities or curiosities until the late 1970s, when increasing numbers of cases were reported in the United States. Psychiatrists are still debating whether DID was previously misdiagnosed and underreported, or whether it is currently over-diagnosed. Because childhood trauma is a factor in the development of DID, some doctors think it may be a variation of **post-traumatic stress disorder** (PTSD). DID and PTSD are conditions where dissociation is a prominent mechanism. The female to male ratio for DID is about 9:1, but the reasons for the gender imbalance are unclear. Some have attributed the imbalance in reported cases to higher rates of abuse of female children; and some to the

---

KEY TERMS

Alter—An alternate or secondary personality in a patient with DID.

Amnesia—A general medical term for loss of memory that is not due to ordinary forgetfulness. Amnesia can be caused by head injuries, brain disease, or epilepsy as well as by dissociation.

Depersonalization—A dissociative symptom in which the patient feels that his or her body is unreal, is changing, or is dissolving.

Derealization—A dissociative symptom in which the external environment is perceived as unreal.

Dissociation—A psychological mechanism that allows the mind to split off traumatic memories or disturbing ideas from conscious awareness.

Dissociative identity disorder (DID)—Term that replaced Multiple Personality Disorder (MPD). A condition in which two or more distinctive identities or personality states alternate in controlling a person's consciousness and behavior.

Hypnosis—An induced trance state used to treat the amnesia and identity disturbances that occur in dissociative identity disorder (DID).

Multiple personality disorder (MPD)—The former, though often still used, term for dissociative identity disorder (DID).

Primary personality—The core personality of an DID patient. In women, the primary personality is often timid and passive, and may be diagnosed as depressed.

Trauma—A disastrous or life-threatening event that can cause severe emotional distress. DID is associated with trauma in a person's early life or adult experience.

---

possibility that males with DID are underreported because they might be in prison for violent crimes.

The most distinctive feature of DID is the formation and emergence of alternate personality states, or "alters." Patients with DID experience their alters as distinctive individuals possessing different names, histories, and personality traits. It is not unusual for DID patients to have alters of different genders, sexual orientations, ages, or nationalities. Some patients have been reported with alters that are not even human; alters have been animals, or even aliens from outer space. The average DID patient has between two and 10 alters, but some have been reported with over one hundred.

Causes & symptoms

The severe dissociation that characterizes patients with DID is currently understood to result from a set of causes:

- An innate ability to dissociate easily
- Repeated episodes of severe physical or sexual abuse in childhood
- The lack of a supportive or comforting person to counteract abusive relative(s)
- The influence of other relatives with dissociative symptoms or disorders

The relationship of dissociative disorders to childhood abuse has led to intense controversy and lawsuits concerning the accuracy of childhood memories. The brain's storage, retrieval, and interpretation of childhood memories are still not fully understood.

The major dissociative symptoms experienced by DID patients are amnesia, depersonalization, derealization, and identity disturbances.

Amnesia

Amnesia in DID is marked by gaps in the patient's memory for long periods of their past, in some cases, their entire childhood. Most DID patients have amnesia, or "lose time," for periods when another personality is "out." They may report finding items in their house that they can't remember having purchased, finding notes written in different handwriting, or other evidence of unexplained activity.

Depersonalization

Depersonalization is a dissociative symptom in which the patient feels that his or her body is unreal, is changing, or is dissolving. Some DID patients experience depersonalization as feeling to be outside of their body, or as watching a movie of themselves.

Derealization

Derealization is a dissociative symptom in which the patient perceives the external environment as unreal. Patients may see walls, buildings, or other objects as changing in shape, size, or color. DID patients may fail to recognize relatives or close friends.

Identity disturbances

Identity disturbances in DID result from the patient's having split off entire personality traits or characteristics as well as memories. When a stressful or traumatic experience triggers the reemergence of these dissociated parts, the patient switches — usually within seconds — into an alternate personality. Some patients have histories of erratic performance in school or in their jobs caused by the emergence of alternate personalities during examinations or other stressful situations. Patients vary with regard to their alters' awareness of one another.

Diagnosis

The diagnosis of DID is complex and some physicians believe it is often missed, while others feel it is over-diagnosed. Patients have been known to have been treated under a variety of other psychiatric diagnoses for a long time before being re-diagnosed with DID. The average DID patient is in the mental health care system for six to seven years before being diagnosed as a person with DID. Many DID patients are misdiagnosed as depressed because the primary or "core" personality is subdued and withdrawn, particularly in female patients. However, some core personalities, or alters, may genuinely be depressed, and may benefit from antidepressant medications. One reason misdiagnoses are common is because DID patients may truly meet the criteria for **panic disorder** or somatization disorder.

Misdiagnoses include schizophrenia, borderline personality disorder, and, as noted, somatization disorder and panic disorder. DID patients are often frightened by their dissociative experiences, which can include losing awareness of hours or even days of time, meeting people who claim to know them by another name, or feeling "out of body." Persons with the disorder may go to emergency rooms or clinics because they fear they are going insane.

When a doctor is evaluating a patient for DID, he or she will first rule out physical conditions that sometimes produce amnesia, depersonalization, or derealization. These conditions include head injuries; brain disease, especially seizure disorders; side effects from medications; substance abuse or intoxication; **AIDS dementia** complex; or recent periods of extreme physical stress and sleeplessness. In some cases, the doctor may give the patient an electroencephalograph (EEG) to exclude epilepsy or other seizure disorders. The physician also must consider whether the patient is **malingering** and/or offering fictitious complaints.

If the patient appears to be physically normal, the doctor will next rule out psychotic disturbances, including schizophrenia. Many patients with DID are misdiagnosed as schizophrenic because they may "hear" their alters "talking" inside their heads. If the doctor suspects DID, he or she can use a screening test called the Dissociative Experiences Scale (DES). If the patient has a high score on this test, he or she can be evaluated further with the Dissociative Disorders Interview Schedule (DDIS) or the Structured Clinical Interview for *DSM-IV* Dissociative Disorders (SCID-D). The doctor may also use the

Hypnotic Induction Profile (HIP) or a similar test of the patient's hypnotizability.

Treatment

Treatment of DID may last for five to seven years in adults and usually requires several different treatment methods.

Psychotherapy

Ideally, patients with DID should be treated by a therapist with specialized training in dissociation. This specialized training is important because the patient's personality switches can be confusing or startling. In addition, many patients with DID have hostile or suicidal alter personalities. Most therapists who treat DID patients have rules or contracts for treatment that include such issues as the patient's responsibility for his or her safety. Psychotherapy for DID patients typically has several stages: an initial phase for uncovering and "mapping" the patient's alters; a phase of treating the traumatic memories and "fusing" the alters; and a phase of consolidating the patient's newly integrated personality.

Most therapists who treat multiples, or DID patients, recommend further treatment after personality integration, on the grounds that the patient has not learned the social skills that most people acquire in adolescence and early adult life. In addition, **family therapy** is often recommended to help the patient's family understand DID and the changes that occur during personality reintegration.

Many DID patients are helped by group as well as individual treatment, provided that the group is limited to people with dissociative disorders. DID patients sometimes have setbacks in mixed therapy groups because other patients are bothered or frightened by their personality switches.

Medications

Some doctors will prescribe tranquilizers or antidepressants for DID patients because their alter personalities may have **anxiety** or **mood disorders.** However, other therapists who treat DID patients prefer to keep medications to a minimum because these patients can easily become psychologically dependent on drugs. In addition, many DID patients have at least one alter who abuses drugs or alcohol, substances which are dangerous in combination with most tranquilizers.

Hypnosis

While not always necessary, **hypnosis** is a standard method of treatment for DID patients. Hypnosis may help patients recover repressed ideas and memories. Further, hypnosis can also be used to control problematic behaviors that many DID patients exhibit, such as self-mutilation, or eating disorders like **bulimia nervosa.** In the later stages of treatment, the therapist may use hypnosis to "fuse" the alters as part of the patient's personality integration process.

Alternative treatment

Alternative treatments that help to relax the body are often recommended for DID patients as an adjunct to psychotherapy and/or medication. These treatments include **hydrotherapy,** botanical medicine (primarily herbs that help the nervous system), therapeutic **massage,** and **yoga.** Homeopathic treatment can also be effective for some people. Art therapy and the keeping of journals are often recommended as ways that patients can integrate their past into their present life. **Meditation** is usually discouraged until the patient's personality has been reintegrated.

Prognosis

Some therapists believe that the prognosis for recovery is excellent for children and good for most adults. Although treatment takes several years, it is often ultimately effective. As a general rule, the earlier the patient is diagnosed and properly treated, the better the prognosis.

Prevention

Prevention of DID requires intervention in abusive families and treating children with dissociative symptoms as early as possible.

Resources

BOOKS

"Dissociative Disorders." In *Diagnostic and Statistical Manual of Mental Disorders.* 4th ed. Washington, DC: The American Psychiatric Association, 1994.

Eisendrath, Stuart J. "Psychiatric Disorders." In *Current Medical Diagnosis & Treatment 1998*, edited by Lawrence M. Tierney, Jr., et al. Stamford, CT: Appleton & Lange, 1997.

Napier, Nancy J. *Getting Through The Day: Strategies for Adults Hurt as Children.* New York: W. W. Norton & Company, 1994.

Nemiah, John C. "Psychoneurotic Disorders." In *The New Harvard Guide to Psychiatry*, edited by Armand M. Nicholi, Jr. Cambridge, MA: The Belknap Press of Harvard University Press, 1988.

Noll, Richard. *The Encyclopedia of Schizophrenia and the Psychotic Disorders.* New York: Facts On File, 1992.

Pascuzzi, Robert M., and Mary C. Weber. "Conversion Disorders, Malingering, and Dissociative Disorders." In *Current Diagnosis 9*, edited by Rex B. Conn, et al. Philadelphia: W. B. Saunders Company, 1997.

van der Kolk, Bessel A., and Onno van der Hart. "The Intrusive Past: The Flexibility of Memory and the Engraving of Trauma." In *Trauma: Explorations in Memory*, edited by Cathy Caruth. Baltimore: The Johns Hopkins University Press, 1995.

Rebecca J. Frey

Multiple pregnancy

Definition

Multiple pregnancy is a **pregnancy** where more than one fetus develops in the womb.

Description

Twins happen naturally about one in every 100 births. There are two types of twinning—identical and fraternal. Identical twins represent the splitting of a single fertilized zygote (union of two gametes or male/female sex cells that produce a developing fetus) into two separate individuals. They usually, but not always, have identical genes. When they do not separate completely, the result is Siamese (or conjoined) twins. Fraternal twins are three times as common as identical twins. They occur when two eggs are fertilized by separate sperm. Each has a different selection of its parents' genes. The natural incidence of multiple pregnancy has been upset by advances in fertility treatments, resulting in higher rates of multiple births in the U.S. All these children are fraternal; they each arose from a separate egg and a separate sperm. Cloning produces identical twins.

The human female is designed to release one egg every menstrual cycle. A hormone called progesterone, released by the first egg to be produced, prevents any other egg from maturing during that cycle. When this control fails, fertilization of more than one egg is possible. Fertility drugs inhibit these controls, allowing multiple pregnancy to occur. Multiple pregnancy is more difficult and poses more health risks than single pregnancy. Premature birth is greater with each additional fetus.

The problem with multiple births is that there is only so much room in even the most accommodating womb (uterus). Babies need to reach a certain size and gestational age before they can survive outside the uterus. **Prematurity** is the constant threat of multiple pregnancies. Twins have five times the **death** rate of single births. Triplets and higher die even more often. The principle threat of prematurity is that the lungs are not fully developed. A disease called hyaline membrane

disease afflicts premature infants. Their lungs do not stay open after their first breath because they lack a chemical called surfactant. Survival of premature infants was greatly improved when surfactant was finally synthesized in a form that could be of benefit to premature babies. Tiny babies also have trouble regulating their body temperature.

Causes & symptoms

Fertility drugs prevent the normal process of single ovulation by permitting more than one egg at a time to mature and ovulate (move from the ovary to the uterus in anticipation of fertilization). This happens naturally to produce fraternal twins. The first drug to accomplish this was clomiphene. Subsequently, two natural hormones—follicle stimulating hormone and chorionic gonadotrophin—were developed and used.

Diagnosis

Multiple pregnancies cause the uterus to grow faster than usual. Obstetricians can detect this unusually rapid growth as the pregnancy progresses. Before birth, an ultrasound will also detect multiple babies in the uterus. After birth, physical appearance or a careful examination of the placenta and amniotic membranes will usually reveal whether the babies were in the same water bag or separate ones. One bag means identical twins.

Treatment

Mothers generally do well with multiple births. The babies often remain hospitalized, where their breathing can be assisted and their temperature controlled in an incubator. Extremely premature babies will need artificial ventilation until their lungs mature. These babies are fragile in many other ways, but modern methods of intensive care have successfully stabilized babies as small as one pound.

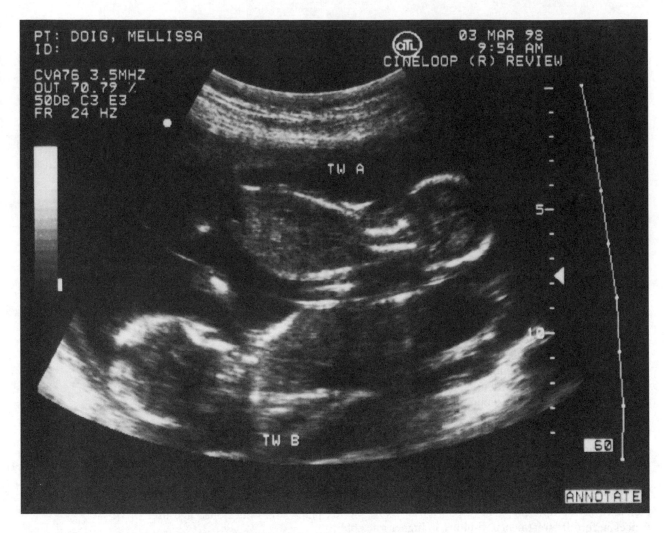

An ultrasound image of identical twin male fetuses. The distortion is due to "twin B" being closer to the transducer. *(Courtesy of Melissa Walsh Doig. Reproduced by permission.)*

Alternative treatment

There are no specific treatments to alleviate medical difficulties caused by multiple pregnancies, however there are supportive measures that may help both mother and children recover from the birthing process. There are treatments to encourage breast milk production and to combat postpartum difficulties. Various homeopathic remedies and **massage** can be helpful to both mother and children during the early adjustment period after birth.

Prognosis

With modern medical advances and excellent prenatal care, many multiple pregnancies reach fruition without difficulties. If the babies are born prematurely, immediate medical care increases the chance of survival without any complications.

Resources

BOOKS

Cunningham, F. Gary, et al., eds. *Williams Obstetrics*. Stamford, CT: Appleton & Lange, 1997.

PERIODICALS

Doyle, P. "The Outcome of Multiple Pregnancy." *Human Reprodtion* 11(December 1996): 110-120.

Evans, M.I., et al. "Selective Reduction For Multifetal Pregnancy. Early Opinions Revisited." *Journal of Reproductive Medicine* 42(December 1997): 771-777.

Evans, M.I., et al. "What Are The Ethical And Technical Problems Associated With Multifetal Pregnancy Reduction." *Clinical Obstetrics and Gynecology* 41(March 1998): 46-54.

Hecht, B.R., and M.W. Magoon. "Can The Epidemic Of Iatrogenic Multiples Be Conquered?" *Clinical Obstetrics and Gynecology* 41(March 1998): 126-137.

Kok, J.H., et al. "Outcome Of Very Preterm Small For Gestational Age Infants: The First Nine Years Of Life." *British Journal of Obstetrics and Gynaecology* 105(February 1998): 162-168.

Kousta, E., D.M. White, and S. Franks. "Modern Use Of Clomiphene Citrate In Induction Of Ovulation." *Human Reproduction Update* 3(July 1997): 359-365.

Styrcula, L. "Code Seven: The Birth Of The Septuplets." *Nursing Spectrum* 9(February 1998):14-15.

J. Ricker Polsdorfer

Multiple sclerosis

Definition

Multiple sclerosis (MS) is a chronic **autoimmune disorder** affecting movement, sensation, and bodily functions. It is caused by destruction of the myelin insulation covering nerve fibers (neurons) in the central nervous system (brain and spinal cord).

Description

MS is a nerve disorder caused by destruction of the insulating layer surrounding neurons in the brain and spinal cord. This insulation, called myelin, helps electrical signals pass quickly and smoothly between the brain and the rest of the body. When the myelin is destroyed, nerve messages are sent more slowly and less efficiently. Patches of scar tissue, called plaques, form over the affected areas, further disrupting nerve communication. The symptoms of MS occur when the brain and spinal cord nerves no longer communicate properly with other parts of the body. MS causes a wide variety of symptoms and can affect vision, balance, strength, sensation, coordination, and bodily functions.

Multiple sclerosis affects more than a quarter of a million people in the United States. Most people have their first symptoms between the ages of 20 and 40; symptoms rarely begin before 15 or after 60. Women are almost twice as likely to get MS as men, especially in their early years. People of northern European heritage are more likely to be affected than people of other racial backgrounds, and MS rates are higher in the United States, Canada, and Northern Europe than in other parts of the world. MS is very rare among Asians, North and South American Indians, and Eskimos.

KEY TERMS

Evoked potentials—Tests that measure the brain's electrical response to stimulation of sensory organs (eyes or ears) or peripheral nerves (skin). These tests may help confirm the diagnosis of multiple sclerosis.

Myelin—A layer of insulation that surrounds the nerve fibers in the brain and spinal cord.

Plaque—Patches of scar tissue that form where the layer of myelin covering the nerve fibers is destroyed by the multiple sclerosis disease process.

Primary progressive—A pattern of symptoms of multiple sclerosis in which the disease progresses without remission, or with occasional plateaus or slight improvements.

Relapsing-remitting—A pattern of symptoms of multiple sclerosis in which symptomatic attacks occur that last 24 hours or more, followed by complete or almost complete improvement.

Secondary progressive—A pattern of symptoms of multiple sclerosis in which there are relapses and remissions, followed by more steady progression of symptoms.

Causes & symptoms

Causes

Multiple sclerosis is an autoimmune disease, meaning its cause is an attack by the body's own immune system. For unknown reasons, immune cells attack and destroy the myelin sheath that insulates neurons in the brain and spinal cord. This myelin sheath, created by other brain cells called glia, speeds transmission and prevents electrical activity in one cell from short-circuiting to another cell. Disruption of communication between the brain and other parts of the body prevent normal passage of sensations and control messages, leading to the symptoms of MS. The demyelinated areas appear as plaques, small round areas of gray neuron without the white myelin covering. The progression of symptoms in MS is correlated with development of new plaques in the portion of the brain or spinal cord controlling the affected areas. Because there appears to be no pattern in the appearance of new plaques, the progression of MS can be unpredictable.

Despite considerable research, the trigger for this autoimmune destruction is still unknown. At various times, evidence has pointed to genes, environmental factors, viruses, or a combination of these.

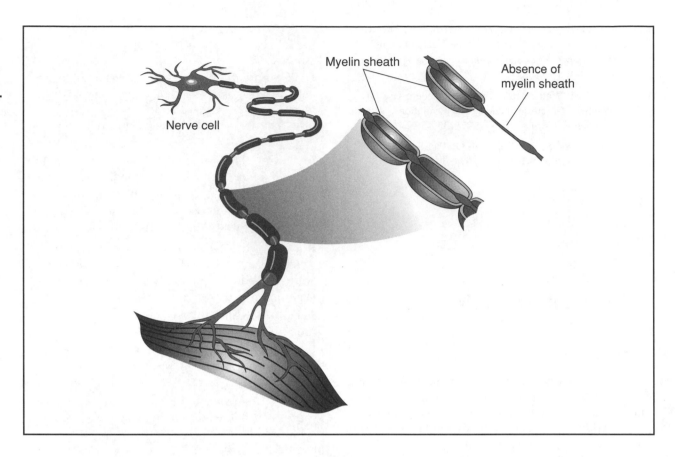

Multiple sclerosis (MS) is an autoimmune disease in which immune cells attack and destroy the myelin sheath which stimulates neurons in the brain and spinal cord. When the myelin is destroyed, nerve messages are sent more slowly and less efficiently. Scar tissue then forms over the affected areas, disrupting nerve communication. MS symptoms occur when the brain and spinal cord nerves cease to communicate properly with other parts of the body. *(Illustration by Electronic Illustrators Group.)*

The risk of developing MS is higher if another family member is affected, suggesting the influence of genetic factors. In addition, the higher prevalence of MS among people of northern European background suggests some genetic susceptibility.

The role of an environmental factor is suggested by studies of the effect of migration on the risk of developing MS. Age plays an important role in determining this change in risk—young people in low-risk groups who move into countries with higher MS rates display the risk rates of their new surroundings, while older migrants retain the risk of their original home country. One interpretation of these studies is that an environmental factor, either protective or harmful, is acquired in early life; the risk of disease later in life reflects the effects of the early environment.

These same data can be used to support the involvement of a slow-acting virus, one that is acquired early on but begins its destructive effects much later. Slow viruses are known to cause other diseases, including **AIDS.** In addition, viruses have been implicated in other autoimmune diseases. Many claims have been made for the role of viruses, slow or otherwise, as the trigger for MS, but as of 1997, no strong candidate has emerged.

How a virus could trigger the autoimmune reaction is also unclear. There are two main models of virally-induced autoimmunity. The first suggests the immune system is actually attacking a virus (one too well-hidden for detection in the laboratory), and the myelin damage is an unintentional consequence of fighting the infection. The second model suggests the immune system mistakes myelin for a viral protein, one it encountered during a prior infection. Primed for the attack, it destroys myelin because it resembles the previously-recognized viral invader.

Either of these models allows a role for genetic factors, since certain genes can increase the likelihood of autoimmunity. Environmental factors as well might change the sensitivity of the immune system or interact with myelin to provide the trigger for the secondary immune response. Possible environmental triggers that have been invoked in MS include viral infection, trauma, electrical injury, and chemical exposure, although controlled studies do not support a causative role.

Symptoms

The symptoms of multiple sclerosis may occur in one of three patterns:

- The most common pattern is the "relapsing-remitting" pattern, in which there are clearly defined symptomatic attacks lasting 24 hours or more, followed by complete or almost complete improvement. The period between attacks may be a year or more at the beginning of the disease, but may shrink to several months later on. This pattern is especially common in younger people who develop MS.

- In the "primary progressive" pattern, the disease progresses without remission or with occasional plateaus or slight improvements. This pattern is more common in older people.

- In the "secondary progressive" pattern, the person with MS begins with relapses and remissions, followed by more steady progression of symptoms.

Between 10–20% of people have a benign type of MS, meaning their symptoms progress very little over the course of their lives.

Because plaques may form in any part of the central nervous system, the symptoms of MS vary widely from person-to-person and from stage-to-stage of the disease. Initial symptoms often include:

- Muscle weakness, causing difficulty walking
- Loss of coordination or balance
- Numbness, "pins and needles," or other abnormal sensations
- Visual disturbances, including blurred or double vision.
  Later symptoms may include:
- Fatigue
- Muscle spasticity and stiffness
- **Tremors**
- **Paralysis**
- **Pain**
- Vertigo
- Speech or swallowing difficulty
- Loss of bowel and bladder control
- Incontinence, **constipation**
- **Sexual dysfunction**
- Cognitive changes.

Weakness in one or both legs is common, and may be the first symptom noticed by a person with MS. Muscle spasticity, or excessive tightness, is also common and may be more disabling than weakness.

Double vision or eye tremor (**nystagmus**) may result from involvement of the nerve pathways controlling movement of the eye muscles. Visual disturbances result from involvement of the optic nerves (optic neutritis) and may include development of blind spots in one or both eyes, changes in color vision, or blindness. Optic neuritis usually involves only one eye at a time and is often associated with movement of the effected eye.

More than half of all people affected by MS have pain during the course of their disease, and many experience chronic pain, including pain from spasticity. Acute pain occurs in about 10% of cases. This pain may be a sharp, stabbing pain especially in the face, neck, or down the back. Facial numbness and weakness are also common.

Cognitive changes, including memory disturbances, depression, and personality changes, are found in people affected by MS, though it is not entirely clear whether these changes are due primarily to the disease or to the psychological reaction to it. Depression may be severe enough to require treatment in up to 25% of those with MS. A smaller number of people experience disease-related euphoria, or abnormally elevated mood, usually after a long disease duration and in combination with other psychological changes.

Symptoms of MS may be worsened by heat or increased body temperature, including **fever,** intense physical activity, or exposure to sun, hot baths, or showers.

Diagnosis

There is no single test that confirms the diagnosis of multiple sclerosis, and there are a number of other diseases with similar symptoms. While one person's diagnosis may be immediately suggested by her symptoms and history, another's may not be confirmed without multiple tests and prolonged observation. The distribution of symptoms is important: MS affects multiple areas of the body over time. The pattern of symptoms is also critical, especially evidence of the relapsing- remitting pattern, so a detailed medical history is one of the most important parts of the diagnostic process. A thorough search to exclude other causes of a patient's symptoms is especially important if the following features are present: 1) family history of neurologic disease, 2) symptoms and findings attributable to a single anatomic location, 3) persistent back pain, 4) age of onset over 60 or under 15 years of age, or 5) progressively worsening disease.

In addition to the medical history and a standard neurological exam, several lab tests are used to help confirm or rule out a diagnosis of MS:

- **Magnetic resonance imaging** (MRI) can reveal plaques on the brain and spinal cord. Gadolinium enhancement can distinguish between old and new plaques, allowing a correlation of new plaques with new symptoms. Plaques may be seen in several other diseases as well, including encephalomyelitis, neurosarcoidosis, and cerebral lupus. Plaques on MRI may be difficult to distinguish from small **strokes,** areas of decreased blood flow, or changes seen with trauma or normal aging.

- A lumbar puncture, or spinal tap, is done to measure levels of immune proteins, which are usually elevated in the cerebrospinal fluid of a person with MS. This test may not be necessary if other tests are diagnostic.

- Evoked potential tests, electrical tests of conduction speed in the nerves, can reveal reduced speeds consistent with the damage caused by plaques. These tests may be done with small electrical charges applied to the skin (somatosensory evoked potential), with light patterns flashed on the eyes (visual evoked potential), or with sounds presented to the ears (auditory evoked potential).

The clinician making the diagnosis, usually a neurologist, may classify the disease as ''definite MS,'' meaning the symptoms and test results all point toward MS as the cause. ''Probable MS'' and ''possible MS'' reflect less certainty and may require more time to pass to observe the progression of the disease and the distribution of symptoms.

Treatment

As of 1997, there are three drugs approved for the treatment of multiple sclerosis which have been shown to affect the course of the disease. None of these drugs is a cure, but they can slow disease progression in many patients.

Avonex and Betaseron are forms of the immune system protein beta interferon, while Copaxone is glatiramer acetate (formerly called copolymer-1). All three have been shown to reduce the rate of relapses in the relapsing-remitting form of MS. Different measurements from tests of each have demonstrated other benefits as well: Avonex may slow the progress of physical impairment, Betaseron may reduce the severity of symptoms, and Copaxone may decrease disability. All three drugs are administered by injection—Copaxone daily, Betaseron every other day, and Avonex weekly. Betaseron, at least, has led to the development of neutralizing antibodies, which reduce the effectiveness of treatment.

Immunosuppressant drugs have been used for many years to treat acute exacerbations (relapses). Drugs used include **corticosteroids** such as prednisone and methylprednisone; the hormone adrenocorticotropic hormone (ACTH); and azathioprine. Recent studies indicate that several days of intravenous methylprednisone may be more effective than other immunosuppressant treatments for acute symptoms. This treatment may require hospitalization.

MS causes a large variety of symptoms, and the treatments for these are equally diverse. Most symptoms can be treated and complications avoided with good care and attention from medical professionals. Good health and nutrition remain important preventive measures. **Vaccination** against **influenza** can prevent respiratory complications, and contrary to earlier concerns, is not associated with worsening of symptoms. Preventing complications such as **pneumonia,** bed sores, injuries from falls, or urinary infection requires attention to the primary problems which may cause them. Shortened life spans with MS are almost always due to complications rather than primary symptoms themselves.

Physical therapy helps the person with MS to strengthen and retrain affected muscles; to maintain range of motion to prevent muscle stiffening; to learn to use assistive devices such as canes and walkers; and to learn safer and more energy-efficient ways of moving, sitting, and transferring. **Exercise** and stretching programs are usually designed by the physical therapist and taught to the patient and caregivers for use at home. Exercise is an important part of maintaining function for the person with MS. Swimming is often recommended, not only for its low-impact workout, but also because it allows strenuous activity without overheating.

Occupational therapy helps the person with MS adapt to her environment and adapt the environment to her. The occupational therapist suggests alternate strategies and assistive devices for activities of daily living, such as dressing, feeding, and washing, and evaluates the home and work environment for safety and efficiency improvements that may be made.

Training in bowel and bladder care may be needed to prevent or compensate for incontinence. If the urge to urinate becomes great before the bladder is full, some drugs may be helpful, including propantheline bromide (Probanthine), oxybutynin chloride (Ditropan), or imipramine (Tofranil). Baclofen (Lioresal) may relax the sphincter muscle, allowing full emptying. Intermittent catheterization is effective in controlling bladder dysfunction. In this technique, a catheter is used to periodically empty the bladder.

Spasticity can be treated with oral medications, including baclofen and diazepam (Valium), or by injection with botulinum toxin (Botox). Spasticity relief may also bring relief from chronic pain. Other more acute types of pain may respond to carbamazepine (Tegretol) or diphenylhydantoin (Dilantin). **Low back pain** is common from increased use of the back muscles to compensate for weakened legs. Physical therapy and over-the-counter pain relievers may help.

Fatigue may be partially avoidable with changes in the daily routine to allow more frequent rests. Amantadine (Symmetrel) and pemoline (Cylert) may improve alertness and lessen fatigue. Visual disturbances often respond to corticosteroids. Other symptoms that may be treated with drugs include seizures, vertigo, and tremor.

Myloral, an oral preparation of bovine myelin, has recently been tested in clinical trials for its effectiveness in reducing the frequency and severity of relapses. Preliminary data indicate no difference between it and placebo.

Alternative treatment

Bee venom has been suggested as a treatment for MS, but no studies or objective reports support this claim.

In British studies, marijuana has been shown to have variable effects on the symptoms of MS. Improvements have been documented for tremor, pain, and spasticity, and worsening for posture and balance. Side effects have included weakness, **dizziness,** relaxation, and incoordination, as well as euphoria. As a result, marijuana is not recommended as an alternative treatment.

Some studies support the value of high doses of **vitamins, minerals,** and other dietary supplements for controlling disease progression or improving symptoms. Alpha-linoleic and linoleic acids, as well as selenium and vitamin E, have shown some effectiveness in the treatment of MS. The selenium and vitamin E act as antioxidants. In addition, the Swank diet (low in saturated fats), maintained over a long period of time, may retard the disease process.

Removal of mercury fillings has been touted as a possible cure, but is of no proven benefit.

Prognosis

It is difficult to predict how multiple sclerosis will progress in any one person. Most people with MS will be able to continue to walk and function at their work for many years after their diagnosis. The factors associated with the mildest course of MS are being female, having the relapsing-remitting form, having the first symptoms at a younger age, having longer periods of remission between relapses, and initial symptoms of decreased sensation or vision rather than of weakness or incoordination.

Less than 5% of people with MS have a severe progressive form, leading to **death** from complications within five years. At the other extreme, 10-20% have a benign form, with a very slow or no progression of their symptoms. The most recent studies show that about seven out of 10 people with MS are still alive 25 years after their diagnosis, compared to about nine out of 10 people of similar age without disease. On average, MS shortens the lives of affected women by about six years, and men by 11 years. Suicide is a significant cause of death in MS, especially in younger patients.

The degree of disability a person experiences five years after onset is, on average, about three-quarters of the expected disability at 10–15 years. A benign course for the first five years usually indicates the disease will not cause marked disability.

Prevention

There is no known way to prevent multiple sclerosis. Until the cause of the disease is discovered, this is unlikely to change. Good nutrition; adequate rest; avoidance of **stress,** heat, and extreme physical exertion; and good bladder hygiene may improve quality of life and reduce symptoms.

Resources

BOOKS
Holland, Nancy, T. Jock Murray, and Stephen Reingold. *Multiple Sclerosis: A Guide for the Newly Diagnosed.* Demos Vermande, 1996.
Matthews, Bryan. *Multiple Sclerosis: The Facts.* New York: Oxford University Press, 1993.
Sibley, William. *Therapeutic Claims in Multiple Sclerosis: A Guide to Treatments.* 4th ed. Demos Vermande, 1996.
Swank, R.L., and M.H. Pullen. *The Multiple Sclerosis Diet Book.* Garden City, NY: Doubleday, 1977.

ORGANIZATIONS
ABLEDATA Adaptive Equipment Center. 8455 Colesville Road, Suite 935, Silver Spring, MD 20910-3319. (800) 227-0216.
The National Multiple Sclerosis Society. 733 Third Avenue, New York, NY 10017. (800) FIGHT-MS (800-344-4867). http://www.nmss.org.

Multiple-gated acquisition (MUGA) scan

Definition

The multiple-gated acquisition (MUGA) scan is a non-invasive nuclear test that uses a radioactive isotope called technetium to evaluate the functioning of the heart's ventricles.

KEY TERMS

Ejection fraction—The fraction of all blood in the ventricle that is ejected at each heartbeat. One of the main advantages of the MUGA scan is its ability to measure ejection fraction, one of the most important measures of the heart's performance.

Electrocardiogram—A test in which electronic sensors called electrodes are placed on the body to record the heart's electrical activities.

Heart attack—A cardiac emergency that occurs when a clot blocks blood flow in one or more of the heart's arteries. Oxygen supply to the heart muscle is cut off, resulting in the death of heart tissue in the affected area.

Ischemia—A decreased supply of oxygenated blood to a body part or organ, often marked by pain and organ dysfunction, as in ischemic heart disease.

Non-invasive—A procedure that does not penetrate the body.

Radioactive isotope—One of two or more atoms with the same number of protons but a different number of neutrons with a nuclear composition. In nuclear scanning, radioactive isotopes are used as a diagnostic agent.

Techentium—A radioactive isotope frequently used in radionuclide scanning of the heart and other organs. It is produced during nuclear fission reactions.

Ventricles—The heart's lower chambers are called the left and right ventricles. They send blood to the lungs and throughout the body. The MUGA scan is performed to evaluate the ventricles.

Purpose

The MUGA scan is performed to determine if the heart's left and right ventricles are functioning properly and to diagnose abnormalities in the heart wall. It can be ordered in the following patients:

• With known or suspected **coronary artery disease,** to diagnose the disease and predict outcomes

• With lesions in their heart valves

• Who have recently had a **heart attack,** to assess damage to heart tissue and predict the likelihood of future cardiac events

• With congestive **heart failure**

• Who have undergone percutaneous transluminal coronary **angioplasty,** coronary artery bypass graft surgery, or medical therapy, to assess the efficacy of the treatment

• With low cardiac output after open-heart surgery

• Who are undergoing **chemotherapy.**

Precautions

Pregnant women and those who are breastfeeding should not be exposed to technetium.

Description

The MUGA scan measures the heart's function and the flow of blood through it. The strongest chamber in the heart is the left ventricle, which serves as the main pump of blood through the body. The left ventricular is assessed by measuring the amount of blood pumped with each heartbeat (the ejection fraction), ventricle filling, and the blood flow into the pumping chamber. A normal ejection fraction is 50% or more. The heart's ejection fraction is one of the most important measures of its performance. The right ventricle's ability to pump blood to the lungs is also assessed, and any abnormalities in the heart wall are identified. The MUGA scan is the most accurate, non-invasive test available to assess the heart's ventricles.

MUGA is a nuclear heart scan, which means that it involves the use of a radioactive isotope that targets the heart and a radionuclide detector that traces the absorption of the radioactive isotope. The isotope is injected into a vein and absorbed by healthy tissue at a known rate during a certain time period. The radionuclide detector, in this case a gamma scintillation camera, picks up the gamma rays emitted by the isotope.

During the MUGA scan, electrodes are placed on the patient's body so that an electrocardiogram (ECG) can be conducted. The imaging equipment and computer are synchronized with the ECG so that images of the heart can be recorded without motion or blur. Then a small amount of a mildly radioactive isotope called technetium Tc99m stannous pyrophosphate, usually called technetium, is injected, usually into an arm vein. While the patient lies motionless on the test table, a gamma scintillation camera follows the movement of the technetium through the blood circulating in the heart. The camera, which looks like an x-ray machine and is suspended above the table, moves back and forth over the patient. It displays multiple images of the heart in motion and records them on a computer for later analysis.

The MUGA scan is usually performed in a hospital's nuclear medicine department, but it can also be performed in an outpatient facility or at the patient's bedside if equipment is available. The scan is done immediately after injection of the technetium and usually takes about

30 minutes to one hour. It is also called multigated graft acquisition, multigated acquisition scan, cardiac blood-pool imaging, and equilibrium radionuclide angiography. Test results can be affected by patient movement during the test, electrocardiogram abnormalities, an irregular heartbeat, or long-acting nitrates.

The MUGA scan can be done with the patient at rest or exercising (called a stress MUGA). The stress MUGA is often performed in patients who have or are suspected of having coronary artery disease. The resting MUGA is compared to the stress MUGA and changes in the heart's pumping performance are analyzed. In some cases, the rest MUGA is compared to a nitroglycerin MUGA, in which a strong heart drug called nitroglycerin is administered to the patient before the scan. For the nitroglycerin MUGA, a cardiologist should be present.

The MUGA scan is not dangerous. The technetium is completely gone from the body within a few days of the test. The scan itself exposes the patient to about the same amount of radiation as a **chest x ray.** The patient can resume normal activities immediately after the test.

Normal results

If the patient's heart is normal, the technetium will appear to be evenly distributed in the scans. In a stress MUGA, patients with normal hearts will exhibit an increase in ejection fraction or no change.

Abnormal results

An uneven distribution of technetium in the heart indicates that the patient has coronary artery disease, a cardiomyopathy, or blood shunting within the heart. Abnormalities in a resting MUGA usually indicate a heart attack, while those that occur during **exercise** usually indicate **ischemia.** In a stress MUGA, patients with coronary artery disease may exhibit a decrease in ejection fraction.

Resources

BOOKS

DeBakey, Michael E. and Gotto, Antonio M., Jr. "Noninvasive Diagnostic Procedures." In *The New Living Heart.* Holbrook, MA: Adams Media Corporation, 1997, pp. 59-70.

"Radionuclide Angiography." In *Cardiac Stress Testing & Imaging,* edited by Thomas H. Marwick. New York: Churchill Livingstone, 1996, pp. 517-521.

Raizner, Albert E. "Nuclear Cardiology Testing." *Indications for Diagnostic Procedures: Topics in Clinical Cardilogy.* New York, Tokyo: Igaku-Shon, 1997, pp. 44-47.

Texas Heart Institute. "Diagnosing Heart Diseases." In *Texas Heart Institute Heart Owner's Handbook.* New York: John Wiley & Sons, 1996, p. 333.

ORGANIZATIONS

American Heart Association. National Center. 7272 Greenville Avenue, Dallas, TX 75231-4596. (214) 373-6300. http://www.medsearch.com/pf/profiles/amerh/.

Texas Heart Institute Heart Information Service. P.O. Box 20345, Houston, TX 77225-0345. (800) 292-2221. http://www.tmc.edu/thi/his.html.

OTHER

American Heart Association. *Tests To Diagnose Heart Disease.* (1997). http://www.amhrt.org/Heart_and_Stroke_A_Z_Guide/cat.html (13 Mar 1998).

Lori De Milto

. . . .

Mumps

Definition

Mumps is a relatively mild, short-term viral infection of the salivary glands that usually occurs during childhood. Typically, mumps is characterized by a painful swelling of both cheek areas, although the person could have swelling on one side or no perceivable swelling at all. The salivary glands are also called the parotid glands, therefore, mumps is sometimes referred to as an inflammation of the parotid glands (epidemic parotitis). The word mumps comes from an old English dialect, meaning lumps or bumps within the cheeks.

Description

Mumps is a very contagious infection that spreads easily in highly populated areas, such as schools. Although not as contagious as **measles** or **chickenpox,** mumps was once quite common. Prior to the release of a mumps vaccine in the United States in 1967, approximately 92% of all children had been exposed to mumps by the age of 15. In these pre-vaccine years, most children contracted mumps between the ages of four and seven. Mumps epidemics came in two to five year cycles. The greatest mumps epidemic was in 1941 when approximately 250 cases were reported for every 100,000 people. In 1968, the year after the live mumps vaccine was released, only 76 cases were reported for every 100,000 people. By 1985, less than 3,000 cases of mumps were reported throughout the entire United States, which works out to about 1 case per 100,000 people. The reason for the decline in mumps was the increased usage of the mumps vaccine. However, 1987 noted a five-fold increase in the incidence of the disease because of the reluctance of some states to adopt comprehensive school immunization laws. Since then, state-enforced school

KEY TERMS

Asymptomatic—Persons who carry a disease and may be capable of transmitting the disease but who do not exhibit symptoms of the disease are said to be asymptomatic.

Encephalitis—Inflammation of the brain.

Meningitis—Inflammation of the membranes covering the brain and spinal cord.

Orchitis—Inflammation or swelling of the scrotal sac containing the testicles.

Parotitis—Inflammation and swelling of the salivary glands.

Post-pubertal—After puberty, in males approximately after the age of 14 years.

entry requirements have achieved student immunization rates of nearly 100% in kindergarten and first grade. In 1996, the Centers for Disease Control and Prevention (CDC) reported only 751 cases of mumps nationwide, or, in other words, about one case for every five million people.

Causes & symptoms

The virus that causes mumps is harbored in the saliva and is spread by sneezing, coughing, and other direct contact with another person's infected saliva. Once the person is exposed to the virus, symptoms generally occur in 14-24 days. Initial symptoms include chills, **headache,** loss of appetite, and a lack of energy. However, an infected person may not experience these initial symptoms. Swelling of the salivary glands in the face (parotitis) generally occurs within 12-24 hours of the above symptoms. Accompanying the swollen glands is pain on chewing or swallowing, especially with acidic beverages, such as lemonade. A **fever** as high as 104°F (40°C) is also common. Swelling of the glands reaches a maximum on about the second day and usually disappears by the seventh day. Once a person has contracted mumps, they become immune to the disease, despite how mild or severe their symptoms may have been.

While the majority of cases of mumps are uncomplicated and pass without incident, some complications can occur. Complications are, however, more noticeable in adults who get the infection. In 15% of cases, the covering of the brain and spinal cord becomes inflamed (**meningitis**). Symptoms of meningitis usually develop within four or five days after the first signs of mumps. These symptoms include a stiff neck, headache, vomiting, and a lack of energy. Mumps meningitis is usually resolved within seven days, and damage to the brain is exceedingly rare.

The mumps infection can spread into the brain causing inflammation of the brain (**encephalitis**). Symptoms of mumps encephalitis include the inability to feel pain, seizures, and high fever. Encephalitis can occur during the parotitis stage or one to two weeks later. Recovery from mumps encephalitis is usually complete, although complications, such as **seizure disorders,** have been noted. Only about 1 in 100 with mumps encephalitis dies from the complication.

About one-quarter of all post-pubertal males who contract mumps can develop a swelling of the scrotum (orchitis) about seven days after the parotitis stage. Symptoms include marked swelling of one or both testicles, severe pain, fever, nausea, and headache. Pain and swelling usually subside after five to seven days, although the testicles can remain tender for weeks.

Diagnosis

When mumps reaches epidemic proportions, diagnosis is relatively easy, because swollen salivary glands are so characteristic of the infection. With so many people vaccinated today, a case of mumps must be properly diagnosed in the event the salivary glands are swollen for reasons other than viral infection. For example, in persons with poor **oral hygiene,** the salivary glands can be infected with bacteria. In these cases, **antibiotics** are necessary. Also in rare cases, the salivary glands can become blocked, develop tumors, or swell due to the use of certain drugs, such as iodine. A test can be performed to determine whether the person with swelling of the salivary glands actually has the mumps virus.

Treatment

When mumps does occurs, the illness is usually allowed to run its course. The symptoms, however, are treatable. Because of difficulty swallowing, the most important challenge is to keep the patient fed and hydrated. The individual should be provided a soft diet, consisting of cooked cereals, mashed potatoes, broth-based soups, prepared baby foods, or foods put through a home food processor. **Aspirin, acetaminophen,** or ibuprofen can relieve some of the pain due to swelling, headache, and fever. Avoid fruit juices and other acidic foods or beverages that can irritate the salivary glands. Avoid dairy products that can be hard to digest. In the event of complications, a physician should be contacted at once. For example, if orchitis occurs, a physician should be called. Also, supporting the scrotum in a cotton bed on an adhesive-tape bridge between the thighs can minimize tension. Ice packs are also helpful.

Alternative treatment

Acupressure can be used effectively to relieve pain caused by swollen glands. The patient can, by using the middle fingers, gently press the area between the jawbone and the ear for two minutes while breathing deeply.

A number of homeopathic remedies can be differentiated for the treatment of mumps. For example, belladonna may be useful for flushing, redness, and swelling. Bryonia (wild hops) may be useful for irritability, lack of energy, or thirst. Phytolacca (poke root) may be prescribed for extremely swollen glands. A homeopathic physician should always be consulted for appropriate doses for children, and remedies that do not work within one day should be stopped. A homeopathic preparation of the mumps virus can also be used prophylactically or as a treatment for the disease.

Several herbal remedies may be useful in helping the body recover from the infection or may help alleviate the discomfort associated with the disease. Echinacea (*Echinacea* spp.) can be used to boost the immune system and help the body fight the infection. Other herbs taken internally, such as cleavers (*Galium aparine*), calendula (*Calendula officinalis*), and phytolacca (poke root), target the lymphatic system and may help to enhance the activity of the body's internal filtration system. Since phytolacca can be toxic, it should only be used by patients under the care of a skilled practitioner. Topical applications are also useful in relieving the discomfort of mumps. A cloth dipped in a heated mixture of vinegar and cayenne (*Capsicum frutescens*) can be wrapped around the neck several times a day. Cleavers or calendula can also be combined with vinegar, heated, and applied in a similar manner.

Prognosis

When mumps is uncomplicated, prognosis is excellent. However, in rare cases, a relapse occurs after about two weeks. Complications can also delay complete recovery.

Prevention

A vaccine exists to protect against mumps. The vaccine preparation (MMR) is usually given as part of a combination injection that helps protect against measles, mumps, and **rubella.** MMR is a live vaccine administered in one dose between the ages of 12-15 months, 4-6 years, or 11-12 years. Persons who are unsure of their mumps history and/or mumps **vaccination** history should be vaccinated. Susceptible health care workers, especially those who work in hospitals, should be vaccinated. Because mumps is still prevalent throughout the world, susceptible persons over age one who are traveling abroad would benefit from receiving the mumps vaccine.

The mumps vaccine is extremely effective, and virtually everyone should be vaccinated against this disease. There are, however, a few reasons why people should NOT be vaccinated against mumps:

- Pregnant women who contract mumps during **pregnancy** have an increased rate of **miscarriage,** but not **birth defects.** As a result, pregnant women should not receive the mumps vaccine because of the possibility of damage to the fetus. Women who have had the vaccine should postpone pregnancy for three months after vaccination.

- Unvaccinated persons who have been exposed to mumps should not get the vaccine, as it may not provide protection. The person should, however, be vaccinated if no symptoms result from the exposure to mumps.

- Persons with minor fever-producing illnesses, such as an upper respiratory infection, should not get the vaccine until the illness has subsided.

- Because mumps vaccine is produced using eggs, individuals who develop **hives,** swelling of the mouth or throat, **dizziness,** or breathing difficulties after eating eggs should not receive the mumps vaccine.

- Persons with immune deficiency diseases and/or those whose immunity has been suppressed with anti-**cancer** drugs, **corticosteroids,** or radiation should not receive the vaccine. Family members of immunocompromised people, however, should get vaccinated to reduce the risk of mumps.

- The CDC recommends that all children infected with human **immunodeficiency** disease (HIV) who are asymptomatic should receive an the MMR vaccine at 15 months of age.

Resources

PERIODICALS

Immunization of Adolescents. November 22, 1996, Volume 45, RR-13. Can be purchased from Superintendent of Documents, U. S. Government Printing Office, Washington, DC 20402-9325. (202) 783-3238.

Recommended Childhood Immunization Schedules—United States, 1995. June 16, 1995, Volume 44, RR-5. Can be purchased from Superintendent of Documents, U. S. Government Printing Office, Washington, DC 20402-9325. (202) 783- 3238.

Update: Vaccine Side Effects, Adverse Reactions, Contraindications, and Precautions. September 6, 1996, Volume 45, RR-12. Can be purchased from Superintendent of Documents, U. S. Government Printing Office, Washington, DC 20402-9325. (202) 783-3238.

Ron D. Gasbarro

Munchausen syndrome

Definition

Munchausen syndrome is a psychiatric disorder that causes an individual to self-inflict injury or illness or to fabricate symptoms of physical or mental illness, in order to receive medical care or hospitalization. In a variation of the disorder, Munchausen by proxy (MSBP), an individual, typically a mother, intentionally causes or fabricates illness in a child or other person under her care.

Description

Munchausen syndrome takes its name from Baron Karl Friederich von Munchausen, an 18th century German military man known for his tall tales. The disorder first appeared in psychiatric literature in the early 1950s when it was used to describe patients who sought hospitalization by inventing symptoms and complicated medical histories, and/or inducing illness and injury in themselves. Categorized as a factitious disorder (a disorder in which the physical or psychological symptoms are under voluntary control), Munchausen's syndrome seems to be motivated by a need to assume the role of a patient. Unlike **malingering,** there does not seem to be any clear secondary gain (e.g., money) in Munchausen syndrome.

Individuals with Munchausen by proxy syndrome use their child (or another dependent person) to fulfill their need to step into the patient role. The disorder most commonly victimizes children from birth to 8 years old. Parents with MSBP may only exaggerate or fabricate their child's symptoms, or they may deliberately induce symptoms through various methods, including **poisoning,** suffocation, **starvation,** or infecting the child's bloodstream.

Causes & symptoms

The exact cause of Munchausen syndrome is unknown. It has been theorized that Munchausen patients are motivated by a desire to be cared for, a need for attention, dependency, an ambivalence toward doctors, or a need to suffer. Factors that may predispose an individual to Munchausen's include a serious illness in childhood or an existing personality disorder.

The Munchausen patient presents a wide array of physical or psychiatric symptoms, usually limited only by their medical knowledge. Many Munchausen patients are very familiar with medical terminology and symptoms. Some common complaints include **fevers, rashes, abscesses,** bleeding, and vomiting. Common Munchausen by proxy symptoms include apnea (cessation of breathing), fever, vomiting, and **diarrhea.** In both Munchausen and MSBP syndromes, the suspected illness

does not respond to a normal course of treatment. Patients or parents may push for invasive diagnostic procedures and display an extraordinary depth of knowledge of medical procedures.

Diagnosis

Because Munchausen sufferers often go from doctor to doctor, gaining admission into many hospitals along the way, diagnosis can be difficult. They are typically detected rather than diagnosed. During a course of treatment, they may be discovered by a hospital employee who encountered them during a previous hospitalization. Their caregivers may also notice that symptoms such as high fever occur only when the patient is left unattended. Occasionally, unprescribed medication used to induce symptoms is found with the patient's belongings. When the patient is confronted, they often react with outrage and check out of the hospital to seek treatment at another facility with a new caregiver.

Treatment

There is no clearly effective treatment for Munchausen syndrome. Extensive psychotherapy may be helpful with some Munchausen patients. If Munchausen syndrome co-exists with other mental disorders, such as a personality disorder, the underlying disorder is typically treated first.

Prognosis

The infections and injuries Munchausen patients self-inflict can cause serious illness. Patients often undergo countless unnecessary surgeries throughout their lifetimes. In addition, because of their frequent hospitalizations, they have difficulty holding down a job. Further, their chronic health complaints may damage interpersonal relationships with family and friends. Children victimized by sufferers of MSBP are at a real risk for serious injury and possible **death.** Those who survive physically unscathed may suffer developmental problems later in life.

Prevention

Because the cause of Munchausen syndrome is unknown, formulating a prevention strategy is difficult. Some medical facilities and healthcare practitioners have attempted to limit hospital admissions for Munchausen patients by sharing medical records. While these attempts may curb the number of hospital admissions, they do not treat the underlying disorder and may endanger Munchausen sufferers that have made themselves critically ill and require treatment. Children who are found to be victims of persons with Munchausen by proxy syndrome should be immediately removed from the care of the abusing parent or guardian.

Resources

BOOKS

American Psychiatric Association. *Diagnostic and Statistical Manual of Mental Disorders,* 4th ed. Washington, DC: American Psychiatric Press, Inc., 1994.

Feldman, Marc, and Charles Ford. *Patient or Pretender: Inside the Strange World of Factitious Disorders.* New York: John Wiley and Sons, 1994.

Goodman, Berney. *When the Body Speaks Its Mind: A Psychiatrist Probes the Mysteries of Hypochondria and Munchausen's Syndrome.* New York: Putnam, 1994.

PERIODICALS

Murray, John B. "Munchausen Syndrome/Munchausen Syndrome by Proxy." *The Journal of Psychology* 131, no. 3 (May 1997): 343-52.

Rosenberg, Janice. "Patient by Proxy." *American Medical News* 39, no. 47 (Dec 1996): 18-23.

ORGANIZATIONS

American Psychiatric Association (APA). Office of Public Affairs. 1400 K Street NW, Washington, DC 20005. (202) 682 6119. http://www.psych.org/.

American Psychological Association (APA). Office of Public Affairs. 750 First St. NE, Washington, DC 20002-4242. (202) 336-5700. http://www.apa.org/.

National Alliance for the Mentally Ill (NAMI). 200 North Glebe Road, Suite 1015, Arlington, VA 22203-3754. (800) 950-6264. http://www.nami.org.

National Institute of Mental Health (NIMH). 5600 Fishers Lane, Rm. 7C-02, Bethesda, MD 20857. (301) 443-4513. http://www.nimh.nih.gov/.

Paula Anne Ford-Martin

Mupirocin *see* **Antibiotics, topical**

Murine (endemic) typhus *see* **Typhus**

Muscle cramps *see* **Muscle spasms and cramps**

Muscle relaxants

Definition

Muscle relaxants are drugs that relax certain muscles in the body.

Purpose

Strains, sprains, and other muscle injuries can result in **pain,** stiffness, and muscle spasms. Muscle relaxants do not heal the injuries, but they do help ease the discomfort and stop muscle spasms. The muscle relaxant cyclobenzaprine (Flexeril) is also sometimes used to treat **fibromyalgia,** a condition that involves aches, stiffness, and fatigue.

Description

Muscle relaxants work by acting on the central nervous system. In the United States, they are available only with a physician's prescription. Some muscle relaxants are available in Canada without a prescription. Most come only in tablet form. However, methocarbamol (Robaxin) is available in both tablet and injectable forms. Examples of muscle relaxants are carisoprodol (Soma), chlorzoxazone (Parafon Forte DSC), cyclobenzaprine (Flexeril), and methocarbamol (Robaxin).

Recommended dosage

Recommended dosage depends on the patient and the type of drug. Check with the physician who prescribed the drug or the pharmacist who filled the prescription for the correct dosage. Always take muscle relaxants exactly as directed by your physician. Never take larger or more frequent doses, and do not take the drug for longer than directed.

Precautions

Muscle relaxants are usually prescribed along with rest, **exercise,** physical therapy, or other treatments. Although the drugs may provide relief, they should never be considered a substitute for these other forms of treatment. The drugs may make the injury feel so much better that one is tempted to go back to normal activity, but doing too much too soon can actually make the injury worse.

These drugs work quite well for relieving muscle pain due to injuries, but are not effective for other types of pain. They should not be used for any other purpose other than for what they were prescribed.

Some people feel drowsy, dizzy, confused, lightheaded, or less alert when using these drugs. The drugs may also cause blurred vision, clumsiness, or unsteadiness. For these reasons, anyone who takes these drugs should not drive, operate machinery, or do anything else that might be dangerous until they have found out how the drugs affect them.

Because muscle relaxants work on the central nervous system, they may add to the effects of alcohol and other drugs that slow down the central nervous system, such as **antihistamines,** cold medicine, allergy medicine, sleep aids, medicine for seizures, tranquilizers, some pain relievers, and other muscle relaxants. They may also add to the effects of anesthetics, including those used for dental procedures. Anyone taking muscle relaxants should check with his or her physician before taking any of the above.

Persons with diabetes should be aware that the metaxalone (Skelaxin) may cause false test results on one type of test for sugar in the urine.

Special conditions

People with certain medical conditions or who are taking certain other medicines can have problems if they take muscle relaxants. Before taking these drugs, be sure to let the physician know about any of these conditions:

ALLERGIES

Anyone who has had unusual reactions to muscle relaxants in the past should let his or her physician know before taking the drugs again. The physician should also be told about any **allergies** to foods, dyes, preservatives, or other substances.

BREASTFEEDING

One muscle relaxant, carisoprodol (Soma), passes into breast milk and may make nursing babies drowsy or upset their stomachs. Whether other muscle relaxants pass into breast milk is unknown, but no evidence exists

that they cause problems in nursing babies whose mothers take them. However, the physician should know whether any woman is pregnant or planning to get pregnant before she receives a prescription for this class of drugs.

OTHER MEDICAL CONDITIONS

Before using muscle relaxants, people with any of these medical problems should make sure their physicians are aware of their conditions:

* Kidney disease
* Heart or blood vessel disease or recent **heart attack**
* Irregular heartbeat
* Overactive thyroid gland
* Hepatitis or other liver disease
* Current or past alcohol or drug abuse
* Current or past blood disease caused by an allergy or a reaction to another drug
* **Glaucoma**
* Problems with urination.

In addition, people with epilepsy should be aware that taking the muscle relaxant methocarbamol may increase the likelihood of seizures.

USE OF CERTAIN MEDICINES

Taking muscle relaxants with certain other drugs may affect the way the drugs work or may increase the chance of side effects.

Side effects

The most common side effects are vision changes, such as double vision or blurred vision; **dizziness;** lightheadedness; drowsiness; and **dry mouth.** These problems usually go away as the body adjusts to the drug and do not require medical treatment. If dry mouth is bothersome, suck on sugarless hard candy or ice chips, chew sugarless gum, or use saliva substitutes, which come in liquid and tablet forms. Less common side effects, such as stomach cramps or pain, **nausea and vomiting, constipation, diarrhea, hiccups,** clumsiness or unsteadiness, confusion, nervousness, restlessness, irritability, flushed or red face, **headache, heartburn,** weakness, trembling, and sleep problems, also may occur and do not need medical attention unless they do not go away or they interfere with normal activities.

Methocarbamol and chlorzoxazone may cause harmless color changes in urine —orange or reddish-purple with chlorzoxazone and purple, brown, or green with methocarbamol. The urine will return to its normal color when the patient stops taking the medicine.

More serious side effects are not common, but may occur. If any of the following side effects occur, check with the physician who prescribed the medicine as soon as possible:

- Breathing problems
- Swelling of the face
- **Fainting**
- Unusually fast or unusually slow heartbeat
- **Fever**
- Tightness in the chest
- Rash, **itching, hives,** or redness
- Burning, stinging, red, or bloodshot eyes
- Stuffy nose
- Unusual thoughts or dreams.

The muscle relaxant chlorzoxazone (Parafon Forte DSC) has caused serious, life-threatening liver problems in some people. The reaction is rare, but anyone taking the drug should stop taking it and notify his or her physician immediately if any of these symptoms occur:

- Fever
- Rash
- Loss of appetite
- Nausea
- Vomiting
- Fatigue
- Pain in the upper right part of the abdomen
- Dark urine
- Yellow skin or eyes.

Additional, rare side effects may occur with any muscle relaxants. Anyone who has unusual symptoms after taking these drugs should get in touch with his or her physician.

Interactions

Muscle relaxants may interact with some other medicines. When this happens, the effects of one or both of the drugs may change or the risk of side effects may be greater. Anyone who plans to take muscle relaxants should let the physician know all other medicines he or she is taking. Among the drugs that may interact with muscle relaxants are:

- Central nervous system (CNS) depressants, such as antihistamines, tranquilizers, sedatives, sleep aids, some pain relievers, cold medicines, allergy medicines, and medicines for seizures.
- **Tricyclic antidepressants,** such as amitriptyline (Elavil), imipramine (Tofranil), and desipramine (Norpramin).

- **Monoamine oxidase inhibitors** (MAO), such as phenelzine (Nardil) or tranylcypromine (Parnate). Serious, life-threatening reactions are possible in patients who take the muscle relaxant cyclobenzaprine (Flexeril) within two weeks of taking MAO inhibitors.
- **Antispasmodic drugs,** such as belladonna alkaloids and phenobarbital (Donnatal) or dicyclomine (Bentyl)
- **Barbiturates,** such as phenobarbital
- High blood pressure drugs, that contain guanethidine such as Esimil or Ismelin.

Nancy Ross-Flanigan

Muscle spasms and cramps

Definition

Muscle spasms and cramps are spontaneous, often painful muscle contractions.

Description

Most people are familiar with the sudden pain of a muscle cramp. The rapid, uncontrolled contraction, or spasm, happens unexpectedly, with either no stimulation or some trivially small one. The muscle contraction and pain last for several minutes, and then slowly ease. Cramps may affect any muscle, but are most common in the calves, feet, and hands. While painful, they are harmless, and in most cases, not related to any underlying disorder. Nonetheless, cramps and spasms can be manifestations of many neurological or muscular diseases.

The terms cramp and spasm can be somewhat vague, and they are sometimes used to include types of abnormal muscle activity other than sudden painful contraction. These include stiffness at rest, slow muscle relaxation, and spontaneous contractions of a muscle at rest (fasciculation). Fasciculation is a type of painless muscle spasm, marked by rapid, uncoordinated contraction of many small muscle fibers. A critical part of diagnosis is to distinguish these different meanings and to allow the patient to describe the problem as precisely as possible.

Causes & symptoms

Causes

Normal voluntary muscle contraction begins when electrical signals are sent from the brain through the spinal cord along nerve cells called motor neurons. These include both the upper motor neurons within the brain and the lower motor neurons within the spinal cord and leading out to the muscle. At the muscle, chemicals released by the motor neuron stimulate the internal release of calcium ions from stores within the muscle cell. These calcium ions then interact with muscle proteins within the cell, causing the proteins (actin and myosin) to slide past one another. This motion pulls their fixed ends closer, thereby shortening the cell and, ultimately, the muscle itself. Recapture of calcium and unlinking of actin and myosin allows the muscle fiber to relax.

Abnormal contraction may be caused by abnormal activity at any stage in this process. Certain mechanisms within the brain and the rest of the central nervous system help regulate contraction. Interruption of these mechanisms can cause spasm. Motor neurons that are overly sensitive may fire below their normal thresholds. The muscle membrane itself may be over sensitive, causing contraction without stimulation. Calcium ions may not be recaptured quickly enough, causing prolonged contraction.

Interuption of brain mechanisms and overly sensitive motor neurons may result from damage to the nerve pathways. Possible causes include **stroke, multiple sclerosis, cerebral palsy,** neurodegenerative diseases, trauma, **spinal cord injury,** and nervous system poisons such as strychnine, **tetanus,** and certain insecticides. Nerve damage may lead to a prolonged or permanent muscle shortening called contracture.

Changes in muscle responsiveness may be due to or associated with:

• Prolonged **exercise.** Curiously, relaxation of a muscle actually requires energy to be expended. The energy is used to recapture calcium and to unlink actin and myosin. Normally, sensations of pain and fatigue signal that it is time to rest. Ignoring or overriding those warning signals can lead to such severe energy depletion that the muscle cannot be relaxed, causing a cramp. The familiar advice about not swimming after a heavy meal, when blood flow is directed away from the muscles, is intended to avoid this type of cramp. Rigor mortis, the stiffness of a corpse within the first 24 hours after **death,** is also due to this phenomenon.

• **Dehydration** and salt depletion. This may be brought on by protracted vomiting or **diarrhea,** or by copious sweating during prolonged exercise, especially in high temperatures. Loss of fluids and salts—especially so-dium, potassium, magnesium, and calcium—can disrupt ion balances in both muscle and nerves. This can prevent them from responding and recovering normally, and can lead to cramp.

• Metabolic disorders that affect the energy supply in muscle. These are inherited diseases in which particular muscle enzymes are deficient. They include deficiencies of myophosphorylase (McArdle's disease), phosphorylase b kinase, phosphofructokinase, phosphoglycerate kinase, and lactate dehydrogenase.

• Myotonia. This causes stiffness due to delayed relaxation of the muscle, but does not cause the spontaneous contraction usually associated with cramps. However, many patients with myotonia do experience cramping from exercise. Symptoms of myotonia are often worse in the cold. Myotonias include **myotonic dystrophy,** myotonia congenita, paramyotonia congenita, and neuromyotonia.

Fasciculations may be due to fatigue, cold, medications, metabolic disorders, nerve damage, or neurodegenerative disease, including **amyotrophic lateral sclerosis.** Most people experience brief, mild fasciculations from time to time, usually in the calves.

Symptoms

The pain of a muscle cramp is intense, localized, and often debilitating Coming on quickly, it may last for minutes and fade gradually. **Contractures** develop more slowly, over days or weeks, and may be permanent if untreated. Fasciculations may occur at rest or after muscle contraction, and may last several minutes.

Diagnosis

Abnormal contractions are diagnosed through a careful medical history, physical and neurological examination, and **electromyography** of the affected muscles. Electromyography records electrical activity in the muscle during rest and movement.

Treatment

Most cases of simple cramps require no treatment other than patience and stretching. Gently and gradually stretching and massaging the affected muscle may ease the pain and hasten recovery.

More prolonged or regular cramps may be treated with drugs such as carbamazepine, phenytoin, or quinine. Fluid and salt replacement, either orally or intravenously, is used to treat dehydration. Treatment of underlying metabolic or neurologic disease, where possible, may help relieve symptoms.

Alternative treatment

Cramps may be treated or prevented with Gingko (*Ginkgo biloba*) or Japanese quince (*Chaenomeles speciosa*). Supplements of vitamin E, niacin, calcium, and magnesium may also help. Taken at bedtime, they may help to reduce the likelihood of night cramps.

Prognosis

Occasional cramps are common, and have no special medical significance.

Prevention

The likelihood of developing cramps may be reduced by eating a healthy diet with appropriate levels of **minerals,** and getting regular exercise to build up energy reserves in muscle. Avoiding exercising in extreme heat helps prevent heat cramps. Heat cramps can also be avoided by taking salt tablets and water before prolonged exercise in extreme heat. Taking a warm bath before bedtime may increase circulation to the legs and reduce the incidence of nighttime leg cramps.

Resources

BOOKS

Bradley, Walter G., et al. *Neurology in Clinical Practice.* 2nd ed. Woburn, MA: Butterworth-Heinemann, 1995.

Muscular dystrophy

Definition

Muscular dystrophy is the name for a group of inherited disorders in which strength and muscle bulk gradually decline. Nine types of muscular dystrophies are generally recognized.

Description

The muscular dystrophies include:

- Duchenne muscular dystrophy (DMD): DMD affects young boys, causing progressive muscle weakness, usually beginning in the legs. It is the most severe form of muscular dystrophy. DMD occurs in about 1 in 3,500 male births, and affects approximately 8,000 boys and young men in the United States. A milder form occurs in very few female carriers.

KEY TERMS

Autosomal dominant—Diseases that occur when a person inherits only one flawed copy of the gene.

Autosomal recessive—Diseases that occur when a person inherits two flawed copies of a gene—one from each parent.

Becker muscular dystrophy (BMD)—A type of muscular dystrophy that affects older boys and men, and usually follows a milder course than DMD.

Contractures—A permanent shortening (as of muscle, tendon, or scar tissue) producing deformity or distortion.

Distal muscular dystrophy (DD)—A form of muscular dystrophy that usually begins in middle age or later, causing weakness in the muscles of the feet and hands.

Duchenne muscular dystrophy (DMD)—The most severe form of muscular dystrophy, DMD usually affects young boys and causes progressive muscle weakness, usually beginning in the legs.

Dystrophin—A protein that helps muscle tissue repair itself. Both DMD and BMD are caused by flaws in the gene that instructs the body how to make this protein.

Facioscapulohumeral muscular dystrophy (FSH)—This form of muscular dystrophy, also known as Landouzy-Dejerine disease, begins in late childhood to early adulthood and affects both men and women, causing weakness in the muscles of the face, shoulders, and upper arms.

Limb-girdle muscular dystrophy (LGMD)—This form of muscular dystrophy begins in late childhood to early adulthood and affects both men and women, causing weakness in the muscles around the hips and shoulders.

Myotonic dystrophy—This type of muscular dystrophy, also known as Steinert's disease, affects both men and women, causing generalized weakness first seen in the face, feet, and hands. It is accompanied by the inability to relax the affected muscles (myotonia).

Oculopharyngeal muscular dystrophy (OPMD)—This type of muscular dystrophy affects adults of both sexes, causing weakness in the eye muscles and throat.

- Becker muscular dystrophy (BMD): BMD affects older boys and young men, following a milder course than DMD. BMD occurs in about 1 in 30,000 male births.

- Emery-Dreifuss muscular dystrophy (EDMD): EDMD affects young boys, causing **contractures** and weakness in the calves, weakness in the shoulders and upper arms, and problems in the way electrical impulses travel through the heart to make it beat (heart conduction defects). Fewer than 300 cases of EDMD have been identified.

- Limb-girdle muscular dystrophy (LGMD): LGMD begins in late childhood to early adulthood and affects both men and women, causing weakness in the muscles around the hips and shoulders. It is the most variable of the muscular dystrophies, and there are several different forms of the disease now recognized. Many people with suspected LGMD have probably been misdiagnosed in the past, and therefore the prevalence of the disease is difficult to estimate. The number of people affected in the United States may be in the low thousands.

- Facioscapulohumeral muscular dystrophy (FSH): FSH, also known as Landouzy-Dejerine disease, begins in late childhood to early adulthood and affects both men and women, causing weakness in the muscles of the face, shoulders, and upper arms. The hips and legs may also be affected. FSH occurs in about 1 out of every 20,000 people, and affects approximately 13,000 people in the United States.

- Myotonic dystrophy: also known as Steinert's disease, affects both men and women, causing generalized weakness first seen in the face, feet, and hands. It is accompanied by the inability to relax the affected muscles (myotonia). Symptoms may begin from birth through adulthood. It is the most common form of muscular dystrophy, affecting more than 30,000 people in the United States.

- Oculopharyngeal muscular dystrophy (OPMD): OPMD affects adults of both sexes, causing weakness in the eye muscles and throat. It is most common among French Canadian families in Quebec, and in Spanish-American families in the southwestern United States.

- Distal muscular dystrophy (DD): DD begins in middle age or later, causing weakness in the muscles of the feet and hands. It is most common in Sweden, and rare in other parts of the world.

- Congenital muscular dystrophy (CMD): CMD is present from birth, results in generalized weakness, and usually progresses slowly. A subtype, called Fukuyama CMD, also involves **mental retardation.** Both are rare; Fukuyama CMD is more common in Japan.

Causes & symptoms

Causes

Several of the muscular dystrophies, including DMD, BMD, CMD, and most forms of LGMD, are due to defects in the genes for a complex of muscle proteins. This complex spans the muscle cell membrane to unite a fibrous network on the interior of the cell with a fibrous network on the outside. Current theory holds that by linking these two networks, the complex acts as a "shock absorber," redistributing and evening out the forces generated by contraction of the muscle, thereby preventing rupture of the muscle membrane. Defects in the proteins of the complex lead to deterioration of the muscle. Symptoms of these diseases set in as the muscle gradually exhausts its ability to repair itself. Both DMD and BMD are caused by flaws in the gene for the protein called dystrophin. The flaw leading to DMD prevents the formation of any dystrophin, while that of BMD allows some protein to be made, accounting for the differences in severity and onset between the two diseases. Differences among the other diseases in the muscles involved and the ages of onset are less easily explained.

The causes of the other muscular dystrophies are not as well understood:

- One form of LGMD is caused by defects in the gene for a muscle enzyme, calpain. The relationship between this defect and the symptoms of the disease is unclear.

- EDMD is due to a defect in the gene for a protein called emerin, which is found in the membrane of a cell's nucleus, but whose exact function is unknown.

- Myotonic dystrophy is linked to gene defects for a protein that may control the flow of charged particles within muscle cells. This gene defect is called a triple repeat, meaning it contains extra triplets of DNA code. It is possible that this mutation affects nearby genes as well, and that the widespread symptoms of myotonic dystrophy are due to a range of genetic disruptions.

- The gene for OPMD appears to also be mutated with a triple repeat. The function of the affected protein may involve translation of genetic messages in a cell's nucleus.

- The cause of FSH is unknown. Although the genetic region responsible for it has been localized on its chromosome, the identity and function of the gene or genes involved had not been determined as of 1997.

- The gene responsible for DD has not yet been found.

Genetics and patterns of inheritance

The muscular dystrophies are genetic diseases, meaning they are caused by defects in genes. Genes, which are linked together on chromosomes, have two functions: They code for the production of proteins, and they are the material of inheritance. Parents pass along genes to their children, providing them with a complete set of instructions for making their own proteins.

Because both parents contribute genetic material to their offspring, each child carries two copies of almost every gene, one from each parent. For some diseases to occur, both copies must be flawed. Such diseases are called autosomal recessive diseases. Some forms of LGMD and DD exhibit this pattern of inheritance, as does CMD. A person with only one flawed copy, called a carrier, will not have the disease, but may pass the flawed gene on to his children. When two carriers have children, the chances of having a child with the disease is one in four for each **pregnancy.**

Other diseases occur when only one flawed gene copy is present. Such diseases are called autosomal dominant diseases. Other forms of LGMD exhibit this pattern of inheritance, as do DM, FSH, OPMD, and some forms of DD. When a person affected by the disease has a child with someone not affected, the chances of having an affected child is one in two.

Because of chromosomal differences between the sexes, some genes are not present in two copies. The chromosomes that determine whether a person is male or female are called the X and Y chromosomes. A person with two X chromosomes is female, while a person with one X and one Y is male. While the X chromosome carries many genes, the Y chromosome carries almost none. Therefore, a male has only one copy of each gene on the X chromosome, and if it is flawed, he will have the disease that defect causes. Such diseases are said to be X-linked. X-linked diseases include DMD, BMD, and EDMD. Women aren't usually affected by X-linked diseases, since they will likely have one unaffected copy between the two chromosomes. Some female carriers of DMD suffer a mild form of the disease, probably because their one unaffected gene copy is shut down in some of their cells.

Women carriers of X-linked diseases have a one in two chance of passing the flawed gene on to each child born. Daughters who inherit the disease gene will be carriers. A son born without the disease gene will be free of the disease and cannot pass it on to his children. A son born with the defect will have the disease. He will pass the flawed gene on to each of his daughters, who will then be carriers, but to none of his sons (because they inherit his Y chromosome).

Not all genetic flaws are inherited. As many as one third of the cases of DMD are due to new mutations that arise during egg formation in the mother. New mutations are less common in other forms of muscular dystrophy.

Symptoms

All of the muscular dystrophies are marked by muscle weakness as the major symptom. The distribution of symptoms, age of onset, and progression differ significantly. **Pain** is sometimes a symptom of each, usually due to the effects of weakness on joint position.

DMD

A boy with Duchenne muscular dystrophy usually begins to show symptoms as a pre-schooler. The legs are affected first, making walking difficult and causing balance problems. Most patients walk three to six months later than expected and have difficulty running. Later on, the boy with DMD will push his hands against his knees to rise to a standing position, to compensate for leg weakness. About the same time, his calves will begin to swell, though with fibrous tissue rather than with muscle, and feel firm and rubbery; this condition gives DMD one of its alternate names, pseudohypertrophic muscular dystrophy. He will widen his stance to maintain balance, and walk with a waddling gait to advance his weakened legs. Contractures (permanent muscle tightening) usually begin by age five or six, most severely in the calf muscles. This pulls the foot down and back, forcing the boy to walk on tip-toes, called equinus, and further decreases balance. Frequent falls and broken bones are common beginning at this age. Climbing stairs and rising unaided may become impossible by age nine or ten, and most boys use a wheelchair for mobility by the age of 12. Weakening of the trunk muscles around this age often leads to **scoliosis** (a side-to-side spine curvature) and **kyphosis** (a front-to-back curvature).

The most serious weakness of DMD is weakness of the diaphragm, the sheet of muscles at the top of the abdomen that perform the main work of breathing and coughing. Diaphragm weakness leads to reduced energy and stamina, and increased lung infection because of the inability to cough effectively. Young men with DMD often live into their twenties and beyond, provided they have mechanical ventilation assistance and good respiratory hygiene.

About one third of boys with DMD experience specific learning disabilities, including trouble learning by ear rather than by sight and trouble paying attention to long lists of instructions. Individualized educational programs usually compensate well for these disabilities.

BMD

The symptoms of BMD usually appear in late childhood to early adulthood. Though the progression of symptoms may parallel that of DMD, the symptoms are usually milder and the course more variable. The same pattern of leg weakness, unsteadiness, and contractures occur later for the young man with BMD, often allowing independent walking into the twenties or early thirties.

Scoliosis may occur, but is usually milder and progresses more slowly. Heart muscle disease (cardiomyopathy), occurs more commonly in BMD. Problems may include irregular heartbeats (**arrhythmias**) and congestive **heart failure.** Symptoms may include fatigue, **shortness of breath,** chest pain, and **dizziness.** Respiratory weakness also occurs, and may lead to the need for mechanical ventilation.

EDMD

This type of muscular dystrophy usually begins in early childhood, often with contractures preceding muscle weakness. Weakness affects the shoulder and upper arm originally, along with the calf muscles, leading to foot-drop. Most men with EDMD survive into middle age, although a defect in the heart's rhythm (**heart block**) may be fatal if not treated with a pacemaker.

LGMD

While there are at least a half-dozen genes that cause the various types of LGMD, two major clinical forms of LGMD are usually recognized. A severe childhood form is similar in appearance to DMD, but is inherited as an autosomal recessive trait. Symptoms of adult-onset LGMD usually appear in a person's teens or twenties, and are marked by progressive weakness and wasting of the muscles closest to the trunk. Contractures may occur, and the ability to walk is usually lost about 20 years after onset. Some people with LGMD develop respiratory weakness that requires use of a ventilator. Lifespan may be somewhat shortened. (Autosomal dominant forms usually occur later in life and progress relatively slowly.)

FSH

FSH varies in its severity and age of onset, even among members of the same family. Symptoms most commonly begin in the teens or early twenties, though infant or childhood onset is possible. Symptoms tend to be more severe in those with earlier onset. The disease is named for the regions of the body most severely affected by the disease: muscles of the face (facio-), shoulders (scapulo-), and upper arms (humeral). Hips and legs may be affected as well. Children with FSH often develop partial or complete deafness.

The first symptom noticed is often difficulty lifting objects above the shoulders. The weakness may be greater on one side than the other. Shoulder weakness also causes the shoulder blades to jut backward, called scapular winging. Muscles in the upper arm often lose bulk sooner than those of the forearm, giving a "Popeye" appearance to the arms. Facial weakness may lead to loss of facial expression, difficulty closing the eyes completely, and inability to drink through a straw, blow up a balloon, or whistle. A person with FSH may not develop strong facial wrinkles. Contracture of the calf muscles may cause foot-drop, leading to frequent tripping over curbs or rough spots. People with earlier onset often require a wheelchair for mobility, while those with later onset rarely do.

MYOTONIC DYSTROPHY

Symptoms of Myotonic dystrophy include facial weakness and a slack jaw, drooping eyelids (**ptosis**), and muscle wasting in the forearms and calves. A person with this dystrophy has difficulty relaxing his grasp, especially if the object is cold. Myotonic dystrophy affects heart muscle, causing arrhythmias and heart block, and the muscles of the digestive system, leading to motility disorders and **constipation.** Other body systems are affected as well: Myotonic dystrophy may cause **cataracts,** retinal degeneration, low IQ, frontal balding, skin disorders, testicular atrophy, **sleep apnea,** and insulin resistance. An increased need or desire for sleep is common, as is diminished motivation. Severe disability affects most people with this type of dystrophy within 20 years of onset, although most do not require a wheelchair even late in life.

OPMD

OPMD usually begins in a person's thirties or forties, with weakness in the muscles controlling the eyes and throat. Symptoms include drooping eyelids, difficulty swallowing (dysphagia), and weakness progresses to other muscles of the face, neck, and occasionally the upper limbs. Swallowing difficulty may cause aspiration, or the introduction of food or saliva into the airways. **Pneumonia** may follow.

DD

DD usually begins in the twenties or thirties, with weakness in the hands, forearms, and lower legs. Difficulty with fine movements such as typing or fastening buttons may be the first symptoms. Symptoms progress slowly, and the disease usually does not affect life span.

CMD

CMD is marked by severe muscle weakness from birth, with infants displaying "floppiness" and very little voluntary movement. Nonetheless, a child with CMD may learn to walk, either with or without some assistive device, and live into young adulthood or beyond. In contrast, children with Fukuyama CMD are rarely able to walk, and have severe mental retardation. Most children with this type of CMD die in childhood.

Diagnosis

Diagnosis of muscular dystrophy involves a careful medical history and a thorough physical exam to determine the distribution of symptoms and to rule out other causes. Family history may give important clues, since all the muscular dystrophies are genetic conditions (though no family history will be evident in the event of new mutations).

Lab tests may include:

- Blood level of the muscle enzyme creatine kinase (CK). CK levels rise in the blood due to muscle damage, and may be seen in some conditions even before symptoms appear.

- Muscle biopsy, in which a small piece of muscle tissue is removed for microscopic examination. Changes in the structure of muscle cells and presence of fibrous tissue or other aberrant structures are characteristic of different forms of muscular dystrophy. The muscle tissue can also be stained to detect the presence or absence of particular proteins, including dystrophin.

- Electromyogram (EMG). This electrical test is used to examine the response of the muscles to stimulation. Decreased response is seen in muscular dystrophy. Other characteristic changes are seen in DM.

- Genetic tests. Several of the muscular dystrophies can be positively identified by testing for the presence of the mutated gene involved. Accurate genetic tests are available for DMD, BMD, DM, several forms of LGMD, and EDMD.

- Other specific tests as necessary. For EDMD and BMD, for example, an electrocardiogram may be needed to test heart function, and hearing tests are performed for children with FSH.

For most forms of muscular dystrophy, accurate diagnosis is not difficult when done by someone familiar with the range of diseases. There are exceptions, however. Even with a muscle biopsy, it may be difficult to distinguish between FSH and another muscle disease, **polymyositis.** Childhood-onset LGMD is often mistaken for the much more common DMD, especially when it occurs in boys. BMD with an early onset appears very similar to DMD, and a genetic test may be needed to accurately distinguish them. The muscular dystrophies may be confused with diseases involving the motor neurons, such as spinal muscular atrophy; diseases of the neuromuscular junction, such as **myasthenia gravis;** and other muscle diseases, as all involve generalized weakening of varying distribution.

Treatment

Drugs

There are no cures for any of the muscular dystrophies. Prednisone, a corticosteroid, has been shown to delay the progression of DMD somewhat, for reasons that are still unclear. Prednisone is also prescribed for BMD, though no controlled studies have tested its benefit. A related drug, deflazacort, appears to have similar benefits

with fewer side effects. It is available and is prescribed in Canada and Mexico, but is unavailable in the United States. Albuterol, an adrenergic agonist, has shown some promise for FSH in small trials; larger trials are scheduled for 1998. No other drugs are currently known to have an effect on the course of any other muscular dystrophy.

Treatment of muscular dystrophy is mainly directed at preventing the complications of weakness, including decreased mobility and dexterity, contractures, scoliosis, heart defects, and respiratory insufficiency.

Physical therapy

Physical therapy, in particular regular stretching, is used to maintain the range of motion of affected muscles and to prevent or delay contractures. Braces are used as well, especially on the ankles and feet to prevent equinus. Full-leg braces may be used in DMD to prolong the period of independent walking. Strengthening other muscle groups to compensate for weakness may be possible if the affected muscles are few and isolated, as in the earlier stages of the milder muscular dystrophies. Regular, nonstrenuous **exercise** helps maintain general good health. Strenuous exercise is usually not recommended, since it may damage muscles further.

Surgery

When contractures become more pronounced, tenotomy surgery may be performed. In this operation, the tendon of the contractured muscle is cut, and the limb is braced in its normal resting position while the tendon regrows. In FSH, surgical fixation of the scapula can help compensate for shoulder weakness. For a person with OPMD, surgical lifting of the eyelids may help compensate for weakened muscular control. For a person with DM, sleep apnea may be treated surgically to maintain an open airway. Scoliosis surgery is often needed in DMD, but much less often in other muscular dystrophies. Surgery is recommended at a much lower degree of curvature for DMD than for scoliosis due to other conditions, since the decline in respiratory function in DMD makes surgery at a later time dangerous. In this surgery, the vertebrae are fused together to maintain the spine in the upright position. Steel rods are inserted at the time of operation to keep the spine rigid while the bones grow together.

When any type of surgery is performed in patients with muscular dystrophy, anesthesia must be carefully selected. People with MD are susceptible to a severe reaction, known as malignant hyperthermia, when given halothane anesthetic.

Occupational therapy

The occupational therapist suggests techniques and tools to compensate for the loss of strength and dexterity.

Strategies may include modifications in the home, adaptive utensils and dressing aids, compensatory movements and positioning, wheelchair accessories, or communication aids.

Nutrition

Good nutrition helps to promote general health in all the muscular dystrophies. No special diet or supplement has been shown to be of use in any of the conditions. The weakness in the throat muscles seen especially in OPMD and later DMD may necessitate the use of a **gastrostomy** tube, inserted in the stomach to provide nutrition directly.

Cardiac care

The arrhythmias of EDMD and BMD may be treatable with antiarrhythmia drugs such as mexiletine or nifedipine. A pacemaker may be implanted if these do not provide adequate control. Heart transplants are increasingly common for men with BMD.

Respiratory care

People who develop weakness of the diaphragm or other ventilatory muscles may require a mechanical ventilator to continue breathing deeply enough. Air may be administered through a nasal mask or mouthpiece, or through a tracheostomy tube, which is inserted through a surgical incision through the neck and into the windpipe. Most people with muscular dystrophy do not need a tracheostomy, although some may prefer it to continual use of a mask or mouthpiece. Supplemental oxygen is not needed. Good hygiene of the lungs is critical for health and longterm survival of a person with weakened ventilatory muscles. Assisted cough techniques provide the strength needed to clear the airways of secretions; an assisted cough machine is also available and provides excellent results.

Experimental treatments

Two experimental procedures aiming to cure DMD have attracted a great deal of attention in the past decade. In myoblast transfer, millions of immature muscle cells are injected into an affected muscle. The goal of the treatment is to promote the growth of the injected cells, replacing the defective host cells with healthy new ones. Despite continued claims to the contrary by a very few researchers, this procedure is widely judged a failure. Modifications in the technique may change that in the future.

Gene therapy introduces good copies of the dystrophin gene into muscle cells. The goal is to allow the existing muscle cells to use the new gene to produce the dystrophin it cannot make with its flawed gene. Problems have included immune rejection of the virus used to introduce the gene, loss of gene function after several weeks, and an inability to get the gene to enough cells to make a functional difference in the affected muscle. Nonetheless, after a number of years of refining the techniques in mice, researchers are beginning human trials in 1998.

Prognosis

The expected lifespan for a male with DMD has increased significantly in the past two decades. Most young men will live into their early or mid-twenties. Respiratory infections become an increasing problem as their breathing becomes weaker, and these infections are usually the cause of **death.**

The course of the other muscular dystrophies is more variable; expected life spans and degrees of disability are hard to predict, but may be related to age of onset and initial symptoms. Prediction is made more difficult because, as new genes are discovered, it is becoming clear that several of the dystrophies are not uniform disorders, but rather symptom groups caused by different genes.

People with dystrophies with significant heart involvement (BMD, EDMD, Myotonic dystrophy) may nonetheless have almost normal life spans, provided that cardiac complications are monitored and treated aggressively. The respiratory involvement of BMD and LGMD similarly require careful and prompt treatment.

Prevention

There is no way to prevent any of the muscular dystrophies in a person who has the genes responsible for these disorders. Accurate genetic tests, including prenatal tests, are available for some of the muscular dystrophies. Results of these tests may be useful for purposes of family planning.

Resources

BOOKS

Brooke, Michael H. A Clinician's View of Neuromuscular Diseases, 2nd ed. Williams & Wilkins, 1986.

Emery, Alan. Muscular Dystrophy: The Facts. Oxford Medical Publications, 1994.

Swash, Michael, and Martin Schwartz. Neuromuscular Diseases: A Practical Approach to Diagnosis and Management, 3rd edition. Springer, 1997.

ORGANIZATIONS

Muscular Dystrophy Association. 3300 East Sunrise Drive, Tucson, AZ 85718. (520) 529-2000 or (800) 572-1717. http://www.mdausa.org.

Mushroom poisoning

Definition

Mushroom poisoning refers to the severe and often deadly effects of various toxins that are found in certain types of mushrooms. One type known as *Amanita phalloides*, appropriately called "death cap," accounts for the majority of cases. The toxins initially cause severe abdominal cramping, vomiting, and watery **diarrhea,** and then lead to liver and kidney failure.

Description

The highest reported incidences of mushroom poisoning occur in western Europe, where a popular pastime is amateur mushroom hunting. Since the 1970s, the United States has seen a marked increase in mushroom poisoning due to an increase in the popularity of "natural" foods, the use of mushrooms as recreational hallucinogens, and the gourmet qualities of wild mushrooms. About 90% of the deaths due to mushroom poisoning in the United States and western Europe result from eating *Amanita phalloides*. This mushroom is recognized by its metallic green cap (the color may vary from light yellow to greenish brown), white gills (located under the cap), white stem, and bulb-shaped structure at the base of the stem. A pure white variety of this species also occurs. **Poisoning** results from ingestion of as few as one to three mushrooms. Higher death (mortality) rates of more than 50% occur in children less than 10 years of age.

Causes & symptoms

Poisonous mushrooms contain at least two different types of toxins, each of which can cause death if taken in large enough quantities. Some of the toxins found in poisonous mushrooms are among the most potent ever discovered. One group of poisons, known as amatoxins, blocks the production of DNA, the basis of cell reproduction. This leads to the death of many cells, especially those that reproduce frequently such as in the liver, intestines, and kidney. Other mushroom poisons affect the proteins needed for muscle contraction, and therefore reduce the ability of certain muscle groups to perform.

Symptoms of *Amanita* poisoning occur in different stages or phases. These include:

- First phase. Abdominal cramping, nausea, vomiting, and severe watery diarrhea occur anywhere from 6-24 hours after eating the mushroom and last for about 24 hours. These intestinal symptoms can lead to **dehydration** and low blood pressure (**hypotension**).

- Second phase. A period of remission of symptoms that lasts 1-2 days. During this time, the patient feels better, but blood tests begin to show evidence of liver and kidney damage.

- Third phase. Liver and kidney failure develop at this point and either lead to death within about a week or recovery within 2-3 weeks.

Other symptoms are due to either a decrease in blood clotting factors that leads to internal bleeding or reduced muscle function, with the development of weakness and **paralysis.**

Diagnosis

In most cases, the fact that the patient has recently eaten wild mushrooms is the clue to the cause of symptoms. Moreover, the identification of any remaining mushrooms by a qualified mushroom specialist (mycologist) can be a key to diagnosis. When in doubt, the toxin known as alpha-amantin can be found in the blood, urine, or stomach contents of an individual who has ingested poisonous *Amanita* mushrooms.

Treatment

It is important to remember that there is no specific antidote for mushroom poisoning. However, several advances in therapy have decreased the death rate over the last several years. Early replacement of lost body fluids has been a major factor in improving survival rates.

Therapy is aimed at decreasing the amount of toxin in the body. Initially, attempts are made to remove toxins from the upper gastrointestinal tract by inducing vomiting or by gastric lavage (stomach pumping). After that continuous aspiration of the upper portion of the small intestine through a nasogastric tube is done and oral charcoal (every four hours for 48 hours) is given to prevent absorption of toxin. These measures work best if started within six hours of ingestion.

In the United States, early removal of mushroom poison by way of an artificial kidney machine (dialysis) has become part of the treatment program. This is combined with the correction of any imbalances of salts (electrolytes) dissolved in the blood, such as sodium or potassium. An enzyme called thioctic acid and **corticosteroids** also appear to be beneficial, as well as high doses of penicillin. In Europe, a chemical taken from the milk thistle plant, *Silybum marianum* , is also part of treatment. When liver failure develops, liver transplantation may be the only treatment option.

Prognosis

The mortality rate has decreased with improved and rapid treatment. However, according to some medical reports death still occurs in 20-30% of cases, with a higher mortality rate of 50% in children less than 10 years old.

Prevention

The most important factor in preventing mushroom poisoning is to avoid eating wild or noncultivated mushrooms. For anyone not expert in mushroom identification, there are generally no easily recognizable differences between nonpoisonous and poisonous mushrooms. It is also important to remember that most mushroom poisons are not destroyed or deactivated by cooking, canning, freezing, drying, or other means of food preparation.

Resources

BOOKS

Gitlin, Norman. "Clinical Aspects of Liver Disease Caused by Industrial and Environmental Toxins." In *Hepatology A Textbook of Liver Disease,* edited by David Zakim, et al. Philadelphia: W.B. Saunders, 1996, 1998.

PERIODICALS

"*Amanita phalloides* Mushroom Poisoning—Northern California, January 1997." *MMWR* 46(June 6, 1997): 489-492

O'Brien, Barbara L. and Linh Khuu. "A Fatal Sunday Brunch: Amanita Mushroom Poisoning in a Gulf Coast Family." *American Journal of Gastroenterology* 91(1996): 581-583.

OTHER

Alerts from the CDC. http://www.medsitenavigator.com/alerts/6_12_97.html.

Cyclopeptide-Containing Mushroom Toxicity. http://toxikon.er.uic.edu/mushroo.htm.

Mushroom Poisoning in Children from the AAFP. http://www.aafp.org/patientinfo/mushroom.html.

Mushroom Toxins from the FDA. http://vm.cfsan.fda.gov/~mow/chap40.html.

David S Kaminstein

Music therapy

Definition

Music therapy is the controlled use of music under the guidance of trained music therapists to help people overcome problematic conditions or behaviors and to achieve therapeutic ends.

Purpose

Music therapy is administered by a music therapist to individuals of all ages who require special services because of behavioral, social, learning, or physical disabilities. Music therapy can be found in hospitals, clinics, day care facilities, schools, community mental health centers, substance abuse facilities, nursing homes, hospices, **rehabilitation** centers, correctional facilities, and private practices.

Description

Music therapy is a treatment in which music is used within a therapeutic relationship to address cognitive, physical, psychological, and social needs in individuals. A qualified music therapist first assesses the strengths and needs of each client and then provides the appropriate treatment, including creating, singing, moving to, and/or listening to music. A client's abilities are strengthened and then transferred to other areas of their lives through their musical involvement in a therapeutic context. Research supports the effectiveness of music therapy in improving communication, facilitating movement and overall physical rehabilitation, providing emotional support for clients and their families, motivating people to cope with treatment, and providing an outlet for the expression of feelings. Clients can develop their auditory, visual, motor, communication, social, academic (cognitive), and self-help skills through many different types of music activities.

Music therapy sessions can be conducted in a group setting or in an individual one-on-one setting. The length of the sessions can vary, but are on average 30-60 minutes.

Preparation

A music therapist must prepare and carefully plan in order for music therapy treatment programs and intervention strategies to be effective for clients. The four basic steps for a music therapist to prepare for a new client are: (1) define the client's problem or area of need (assessment); (2) set a therapeutic goal for the client; (3) devise music activities that are related to the goal and appropriate to the client's level of functioning and capacity to respond; and (4) implement the procedure and evaluate the client's responses.

Assessment is the process of determining the client's individual strengths and weaknesses, including any particular problems or areas of need. This information can be obtained by observing the client in music activities that show the client's level of developmental, social, motor, auditory, and communication skills. Following assessment, the music therapist must create therapeutic goals and objectives that state what the client is to accomplish, and what changes in behavior the client will show if the therapy is successful. The final step in preparation for beginning therapy is deciding what types of music activities will be most beneficial in helping the client reach their goals and/or objectives.

Normal results

The client accomplishes the goals and/or objectives outlined by the music therapist.

Additionally, music therapy often elicits changes in non-target behaviors that may be just as significant as those initially sought. In the music therapy literature, positive "side effects" are almost always reported, as a result of the many influences of music. Frequently observed increases which often accompany musical experiences are: motivation to try new things, pride in self, and enhanced fine motor coordination.

Abnormal results

The client's maladaptive conditions and/or behavior patterns do not improve.

Resources

BOOKS

Hanser, S.B. *Music Therapist's Handbook.* St. Louis, Missouri: Warren H. Green, Inc., 1987, pp. 143-145.

Peters, J.S. *Music Therapy: An Introduction.* Springfield: Charles C. Thomas, 1987, pp. 52-57.

ORGANIZATIONS

American Music Therapy Association. 8455 Colesville Road, Suite 100, Silver Spring, MD 20910. (301)-589-3300. Http://www.amta.com/amta/

OTHER

NAMT Member Sourcebook. National Association for Music Therapy, 1996.

Kristy J. Layman

Mutism

Definition

Mutism is a rare childhood condition characterized by a consistent failure to speak in situations where talking is expected. The child has the ability to converse normally, and does so, for example, in the home, but consistently fails to speak in specific situations such as at school or with strangers. It is estimated that one in every 1,000 school-age children are affected.

Description

Experts believe that this problem is associated with **anxiety** and fear in social situations such as in school or in the company of adults. It is therefore often considered a type of social phobia. This is not a communication disorder because the affected children can converse normally in some situations. It is not a developmental disorder because their ability to talk, when they choose to do so, is appropriate for their age level. This problem has been linked to anxiety, and one of the major ways in which both children and adults attempt to cope with anxiety is by avoiding whatever provokes the anxiety.

Affected children are typically shy, and are especially so in the presence of strangers and unfamiliar surroundings or situations. However, the behaviors of children with this condition go beyond shyness.

Causes & symptoms

Mutism is believed to arise from anxiety experienced in social situations where the child may be called upon to speak. Refusing to speak, or speaking in a whisper, spares the child from the possible humiliation or embarrassment of "saying the wrong thing." When asked a direct question by teachers, for example, the affected child may act as if they are unable to answer. Some children may communicate via gestures, nodding, or very brief utterances. Additional features may include excessive shyness, oppositional behavior, and impaired learning at school.

Diagnosis

The diagnosis of mutism is fairly easy to make because the signs amd symptoms are clear-cut and easily observable. However, other social disorders effecting social speech, such as **autism** or **schizophrenia,** must be considered in the diagnosis.

Treatment

There are two recommended treatments for mutism: behavior modification therapy and antidepressant medication. Treatment is most effective when individualized to each patient. It has been suggested that speech pathologists may also be able to help these children.

Prognosis

The prognosis for mutism is good. Sometimes it disappears suddenly on its own. The negative impact on learning and school activities may, however, persist into adult life.

KEY TERMS

Behavior modification—A form of therapy that uses rewards to reinforce desired behavior. An example would be to give a child a piece of chocolate for grooming themselves appropriately.

Prevention

Mutism cannot be prevented because the cause is not known. However, family conflict or problems at school contribute to the seriousness of the symptoms.

Resources

BOOKS

Diagnostic and Statistical Manual of Mental Disorders, 4th ed. Washington, DC: American Psychiatric Association, 1994.

Donald Gardner Barstow

MVP *see* **Mitral valve prolapse**

Myalgic encephalomyelitis *see* **Chronic fatigue syndrome**

Myasthenia gravis

Definition

Myasthenia gravis is an autoimmune disease that causes muscle weakness.

Description

Myasthenia gravis (MG) affects the neuromuscular junction, interrupting the communication between nerve and muscle, and thereby causing weakness. A person with MG may have difficulty moving their eyes, walking, speaking clearly, swallowing, and even breathing, depending on the severity and distribution of weakness. Increased weakness with exertion, and improvement with rest, is a characteristic feature of MG.

About 30,000 people in the United States are affected by MG. It can occur at any age, but is most common in women who are in their late teens and early twenties, and in men in their sixties and seventies.

Causes & symptoms

Myasthenia gravis is an autoimmune disease, meaning it is caused by the body's own immune system. In MG, the immune system attacks a receptor on the surface of muscle cells. This prevents the muscle from receiving the nerve impulses that normally make it respond. MG affects "voluntary" muscles, which are those muscles under conscious control responsible for movement. It does not affect heart muscle or the "smooth" muscle found in the digestive system and other internal organs.

KEY TERMS

Antibody—An immune protein normally used by the body for combating infection and which is made by B cells.

Autoantibody—An antibody that reacts against part of the self.

Autoimmune disease—A disease caused by a reaction of the body's immune system.

Bulbar muscles—Muscles that control chewing, swallowing, and speaking.

Neuromuscular junction—The site at which nerve impulses are transmitted to muscles.

Pyridostigmine bromide (Mestinon)—An anticholinesterase drug used in treating myasthenia gravis.

Tensilon test—A test for diagnosing myasthenia gravis. Tensilon is injected into a vein and, if the person has MG, their muscle strength will improve for about five minutes.

Thymus gland—A small gland located just above the heart, involved in immune system development.

A muscle is stimulated to contract when the nerve cell controlling it releases acetylcholine molecules onto its surface. The acetylcholine lands on a muscle protein called the acetylcholine receptor. This leads to rapid chemical changes in the muscle which cause it to contract. Acetylcholine is then broken down by acetylcholinesterase enzyme, to prevent further stimulation.

In MG, immune cells create antibodies against the acetylcholine receptor. Antibodies are proteins normally involved in fighting infection. When these antibodies attach to the receptor, they prevent it from receiving acetylcholine, decreasing the ability of the muscle to respond to stimulation.

Why the immune system creates these self-reactive "autoantibodies" is unknown, although there are several hypotheses:

• During fetal development, the immune system generates many B cells that can make autoantibodies, but B cells that could harm the body's own tissues are screened out and destroyed before birth. It is possible that the stage is set for MG when some of these cells escape detection.

• Genes controlling other parts of the immune system, called MHC genes, appear to influence how susceptible a person is to developing autoimmune disease.

- Infection may trigger some cases of MG. When activated, the immune system may mistake portions of the acetylcholine receptor for portions of an invading virus, though no candidate virus has yet been identified conclusively.

- About 10% of those with MG also have **thymomas,** or benign tumors of the thymus gland. The thymus is a principal organ of the immune system, and researchers speculate that thymic irregularities are involved in the progression of MG.

Some or all of these factors (developmental, genetic, infectious, and thymic) may interact to create the autoimmune reaction.

The earliest symptoms of MG often result from weakness of the extraocular muscles, which control eye movements. Symptoms involving the eye (ocular symptoms) include double vision (diplopia), especially when not gazing straight ahead, and difficulty raising the eyelids **(ptosis).** A person with ptosis may need to tilt their head back to see. Eye-related symptoms remain the only symptoms for about 15% of MG patients. Another common early symptom is difficulty chewing and swallowing, due to weakness in the bulbar muscles, which are in the mouth and throat. **Choking** becomes more likely, especially with food that requires extensive chewing.

Weakness usually becomes more widespread within several months of the first symptoms, reaching their maximum within a year in two-thirds of patients. Weakness may involve muscles of the arms, legs, neck, trunk, and face, and affect the ability to lift objects, walk, hold the head up, and speak.

Symptoms of MG become worse upon exertion, and better with rest. Heat, including heat from the sun, hot showers, and hot drinks, may increase weakness. Infection and **stress** may worsen symptoms. Symptoms may vary from day to day and month to month, with intervals of no weakness interspersed with a progressive decline in strength.

''Myasthenic crisis'' may occur, in which the breathing muscles become too weak to provide adequate respiration. Symptoms include weak and shallow breathing, **shortness of breath,** pale or bluish skin color, and a racing heart. Myasthenic crisis is an emergency condition requiring immediate treatment. In patients treated with anticholinesterase agents, myasthenic crisis must be differentiated from cholinergic crisis related to overmedication.

Pregnancy worsens MG in about one third of women, has no effect in one third, and improves symptoms in another third. About 12% of infants born to women with MG have ''neonatal myasthenia,'' a temporary but potentially life-threatening condition. It is caused by the transfer of maternal antibodies into the fetal circulation just before birth. Symptoms include weakness, floppiness, feeble cry, and difficulty feeding. The infant may have difficulty breathing, requiring the use of a ventilator. Neonatal myasthenia usually clears up within a month.

Diagnosis

Myasthenia gravis is often diagnosed accurately by a careful medical history and a neuromuscular exam, but several tests are used to confirm the diagnosis. Other conditions causing worsening of bulbar and skeletal muscles must be considered, including drug-induced myasthenia, thyroid disease, Lambert-Eaton myasthenic syndrome, **botulism,** and inherited muscular dystrophies.

Edrophonium (Tensilon) blocks the action of acetylcholinesterase, prolonging the effect of acetylcholine and increasing strength. An injection of edrophonium rapidly leads to a marked improvement in most people with MG. An alternate drug, neostigmine, may also be used.

MG causes characteristic changes in the electrical responses of muscles that may be observed with an electromyogram, which measures muscular response to electrical stimulation. Repetitive nerve stimulation leads to reduction in the height of the measured muscle response, reflecting the muscle's tendency to become fatigued.

Blood tests may confirm the presence of the antibody to the acetylcholine receptor, though up to a quarter of MG patients will not have detectable levels. A **chest x ray** or chest **computed tomography scan** (CT scan) may be performed to look for thymoma.

Treatment

While there is no cure for myasthenia gravis, there are a number of treatments that effectively control symptoms in most people.

Pyridostigmine (Mestinon) is usually the first drug tried. Like edrophonium, pyridostigmine blocks acetylcholinesterase. It is longer-acting, taken by mouth, and well-tolerated. Loss of responsiveness and disease progression combine to eventually make pyridostigmine ineffective in tolerable doses in many patients.

Thymectomy, or removal of the thymus gland, has increasingly become standard treatment for MG. Up to 85% of people with MG improve after thymectomy, with complete remission eventually seen in about 30%. The improvement may take months or even several years to fully develop. Thymectomy is not usually recommended for children with MG, since the thymus continues to play an important immune role throughout childhood.

Immune-suppressing drugs are used to treat MG if response to pyridostigmine and thymectomy are not adequate. Drugs include **corticosteroids** such as prednisone, and the non-steroids azathioprine (Imuran) and cyclosporine (Sandimmune).

Plasma exchange may be performed to treat myasthenic crisis or to improve very weak patients before thymectomy. In this procedure, blood plasma is removed and replaced with purified plasma free of autoantibodies. It can produce a temporary improvement in symptoms, but is too expensive for long-term treatment. Another blood treatment, intravenous immunoglobulin therapy, is also used for myasthenic crisis. In this procedure, large quantities of purified immune proteins (immunoglobulins) are injected. For unknown reasons, this leads to symptomatic improvement in up to 85% of patients. It is also too expensive for long-term treatment.

People with weakness of the bulbar muscles may need to eat softer foods that are easier to chew and swallow. In more severe cases, it may be necessary to obtain nutrition through a feeding tube placed into the stomach (**gastrostomy** tube).

Prognosis

Most people with MG can be treated successfully enough to prevent their condition from becoming debilitating. In some cases, however, symptoms may worsen even with vigorous treatment, leading to generalized weakness and disability. MG rarely causes early **death** except from myasthenic crisis.

Prevention

There is no known way to prevent myasthenia gravis. Thymectomy improves symptoms significantly in many patients, and relieves them entirely in some. Avoiding heat can help minimize symptoms.

Some drugs should be avoided by people with MG because they interfere with normal neuromuscular function.

Drugs to be avoided or used with caution include:

- Many types of **antibiotics,** including erythromycin, streptomycin, and ampicillin

- Some cardiovascular drugs, including Verapamil, betaxolol, and propranolol

- Some drugs used in psychiatric conditions, including chlorpromazine, clozapine, and lithium.

Many other drugs may worsen symptoms as well, so patients should check with the doctor who treats their MG before taking any new drugs.

A Medic-Alert card or bracelet provides an important source of information to emergency providers about the special situation of a person with MG. They are available from health care providers.

Resources

BOOKS

Swash, Michael and Martin Schwarz. *Neuromuscular Diseases: A Practical Approach to Diagnosis and Management.* Springer, 1997.

PERIODICALS

Drachman, D.B. ''Myasthenia Gravis.'' *New England Journal of Medicine,* 330 (1994): 1797-1810.

Robinson, Richard. ''The Body At War with Itself.'' *Quest,* 4 (3)(1997): 20-24.

ORGANIZATIONS

Muscular Dystrophy Association. 3300 East Sunrise Drive, Tucson, AZ 85718. (520) 529-2000 or (800) 572-1717. www.mdausa.org.

Myasthenia Gravis Foundation of America. 222 S. Riverside Plaza, Suite 1540, Chicago, IL 60606. (800) 541-5454. www.med.unc.edu/mfga/.

Richard Robinson

Mycetoma

Definition

Mycetoma, or maduromycosis, is a slow-growing bacterial or fungal infection focused in one area of the body, usually the foot. For this reason—and because the first medical reports were from doctors in Madura, India—an alternate name for the disease is Madura foot. The infection is characterized by an abnormal tissue mass beneath the skin, formation of cavities within the mass, and a fluid discharge. As the infection progresses, it affects the muscles and bones; at this advanced stage, disability may result.

Description

Although the bacteria and fungi that cause mycetoma are found in soil worldwide, the disease occurs mainly in tropical areas in India, Africa, South America, Central America, and southeast Asia. Mycetoma is an uncommon disease, affecting an unknown number of people annually.

There are more than 30 species of bacteria and fungi that can cause mycetoma. Bacteria or fungi can be introduced into the body through a relatively minor skin wound. The disease advances slowly over months or years, typically with minimal **pain.** When pain is experienced, it is usually due to secondary infections or bone involvement. Although it is rarely fatal, mycetoma causes deformities and potential disability at its advanced stage.

KEY TERMS

Biopsy—A medical procedure in which a small piece of tissue is surgically removed for microscopic examination.

Grains—Flecks of hardened material such as bacteria or fungi spores.

Nodule—A hardened area or knot sometimes associated with infection.

Secondary infection—Illness caused by new bacteria, viruses, or fungi becoming established in the wake of an initial infection.

Sinuses—Cavities or hollow areas.

Tumor—A mass or clump of abnormal tissue, not necessarily caused by a cancer.

Causes & symptoms

Owing to a wound, bacteria or fungi gain entry into the skin. Approximately one month or more after the injury, a nodule forms under the skin surface. The nodule is painless, even as it increases in size over the following months. Eventually, the nodule forms a tumor, or mass of abnormal tissue. The tumor contains cavities—called sinuses—that discharge blood- or pus-tainted fluid. The fluid also contains tiny grains, less than two thousandths of an inch in size. The color of these grains depends on the type of bacteria or fungi causing the infection.

As the infection continues, surrounding tissue becomes involved, with an accumulation of scarring and loss of function. The infection can extend to the bone, causing inflammation, pain, and severe damage. Mycetoma may be complicated by secondary infections, in which new bacteria become established in the area and cause an additional set of problems.

Diagnosis

The primary symptoms of a tumor, sinuses, and grain-flecked discharge often provide enough information to diagnose mycetoma. In the early stages, prior to sinus formation, diagnosis may be more difficult and a biopsy, or microscopic examination of the tissue, may be necessary. If bone involvement is suspected, the area is x-rayed to determine the extent of the damage. The species of bacteria or fungi at the root of the infection is identified by staining the discharge grains and inspecting them with a microscope.

Treatment

Combating mycetoma requires both surgery and drug therapy. Surgery usually consists of removing the tumor and a portion of the surrounding tissue. If the infection is extensive, **amputation** is sometimes necessary. Drug therapy is recommended in conjunction with surgery. The specific prescription depends on the type of bacteria or fungi causing the disease. Common medicines include antifungal drugs, such as ketoconazole and **antibiotics** (streptomycin sulfate, amikacin, sulfamethoxazole, penicillin, and rifampin).

Prognosis

Recovery from mycetoma may take months or years, and the infection recurs after surgery in at least 20% of cases. Drug therapy can reduce the chances of a re-established infection. The extent of deformity or disability depends on the severity of infection; the more deeply entrenched the infection, the greater the damage. By itself, mycetoma is rarely fatal, but secondary infections can be fatal.

Prevention

Mycetoma is a rare condition that is not contagious.

Resources

PERIODICALS

Fahal, A.H., and M.A. Hassan. "Mycetoma." *British Journal of Surgery* 79(November 1992): 1138.

McGinnis, Michael R. "Mycetoma." *Dermatologic Clinics* 14(1)(January 1996): 97.

Welsh, Oliverio. "Mycetoma." *Seminars in Dermatology* 12(4)(December 1993): 290.

Julia Barrett

Mycobacterial infections, atypical

Definition

Atypical mycobacterial infections are infections caused by several types of mycobacteria similar to the germ that causes **tuberculosis.** These atypical mycobacterial infections are a frequent complication in patients with human **immunodeficiency** virus (HIV) infection or **AIDS.**

Description

Mycobacteria are a group of rod-shaped bacteria that cause several diseases, among them **leprosy** and tuberculosis. For some time, scientists have known of bacteria that are similar to *Mycobacterium tuberculosis,* the cause of tuberculosis, but that grow and act differently. When tuberculosis was a much more widespread problem and microbiology was much less able to tell the difference between similar microbes, these atypical mycobacteria were ignored. Today, they have been classified more precisely as members of the same species and called atypical (or nontuberculosis) mycobacteria.

Although the medical profession has known about these atypical infections for a long time, they were not considered a serious problem until the early 1980s. It was then that many of these atypical infections were noticed among homosexuals and intravenous drug users in New York City. These bacteria rarely cause infection in humans other than those with HIV or AIDS.

Causes & symptoms

Although there are more than a dozen species of atypical mycobacteria, the two most common are *Mycobacterium kansasii* and *M. avium-intracellulare.* These microbes are found in many places in the environment: tap water, fresh and ocean water, milk, bird droppings, soil, and house dust. The manner in which these bacteria are transmitted is not completely understood. There is no evidence that they are transmitted from person to person.

M. avium-intracellulare (MAC or MAI) is a rare cause of lung disease in otherwise healthy humans but a frequent cause of infection among those whose resistance has been lowered by another disorder (opportunistic infection). According to some experts, MAC infection is an almost inevitable complication of HIV. The infection is caused by one of two similar organisms, *M. avium* and *M. intracellulare.*

AIDS patients are almost always attacked by these mycobacteria. Once inside the body, the atypical myco-

bacterial organisms colonize and grow in the lungs like tuberculosis. Because AIDS patients have a poorly functioning immune system, the microbes multiply because they aren't stopped by the body's normal response to infection. Once they have colonized the lungs, the organisms enter the bloodstream and spread throughout the body, affecting almost every organ. These devastating infections can invade the lymph nodes, liver, spleen, bone marrow, gastrointestinal tract, skin, and brain.

Symptoms include **shortness of breath, fever,** night sweats, weight loss, appetite loss, fatigue, and progressively severe **diarrhea,** stomach **pain, nausea and vomiting.** If the infection spreads to the brain, the patient may experience weakness, **headaches,** vision problems, and loss of balance.

MAC and *M. kansasii* sometimes cause lung infections in middle-aged and elderly people with chronic lung conditions. MAC, *M. kansasii,* and *M. scrofulaceum* may cause inflammation of the lymph nodes in otherwise healthy young children. *M. fortuitum* and *M. chelonae* cause skin and wound infections and **abscesses** after trauma or surgical procedures. *M. marinum* causes a nodular inflammation, usually on the arms and legs. This infection is called "swimming pool granuloma" because it is associated with swimming pools, fish tanks, and other bodies of water. *M. ulcerans* infection causes chronic skin ulcerations, usually on an arm or leg. Atypical mycobacteria infections can also occur without causing any symptoms. In such cases, a **tuberculin skin test** may be positive.

Diagnosis

The diagnosis is made from the patient's symptoms and organisms grown in culture from the site of infection. In cases of lung infection, a diagnostic workup will include a **chest x ray** and tests on discharges from the respiratory passages (sputum).

Treatment

These nontypical mycobacteria are not easy to treat in any patient and the problem is complicated when the person has AIDS. **Antibiotics** aren't particularly effective, although rifabutin (a cousin of the anti-tuberculosis drug rifampin) and clofazimine (an anti-leprosy drug) have helped some patients. It is also possible to contain the infection to some degree by combining different drugs, including ethionamide, cycloserine, ethambutol, and streptomycin.

Prognosis

Because drug therapy is not easily effective, the overwhelming infections caused by these mycobacteria in AIDS patients can be fatal.

Prevention

People with HIV infection can prevent or delay the onset of MAC by taking disease-preventing drugs such as rifabutin.

AIDS patients and persons with tissue damage, such as skin **wounds** or pulmonary disease, can make a number of lifestyle changes to help prevent MAC infection. Since these mycobacteria are found in most city water systems, in hospital water supplies, and in bottled water, at-risk persons should boil drinking water. Persons at risk should also avoid raw foods, especially salads, root vegetables, and unpasteurized milk or cheese. Fruits and vegetables should be peeled and rinsed thoroughly. Conventional cooking (baking, boiling or steaming) destroys mycobacteria, which are killed at 176°F (80°C).

Finally, at-risk patients should avoid contact with animals, especially birds and bird droppings. Pigeons in particular can transmit MAC.

Resources

BOOKS

Gong, Victor and Norman Rudnick, eds. *AIDS: Facts and Issues.* New Brunswick: Rutgers University Press, 1996.

PERIODICALS

Rochell, Anne. "Hope and a Reality Check: Although a Cure Is Still a Distant Dream, New AIDS Treatments Invite Optimism." *Atlanta Journal and Constitution* 6 (July 1996): D1.

Wilson, Billie Ann. "Understanding Strategies for Treating HIV." *Medical Surgical Nursing* 6 (April 1, 1997): 109-111.

ORGANIZATIONS

National AIDS Treatment Advocacy Project. 580 Broadway, Rm. 403, New York NY 10012. (212) 219-0106 or (888) 26-NATAP. http://www.natap.org.

Carol A. Turkington

Mycobacterium avium complex (MAC) infection *see* **Mycobacterial infections, atypical**

Mycobacterium leprae infection *see* **Leprosy**

Mycobacterium tuberculosis infection *see* **Tuberculosis**

Mycoplasma infections

Definition

Mycoplasma are the smallest of the free-living organisms. (Unlike viruses, mycoplasma can reproduce outside of living cells.) Many species within the genus *Mycoplasma* thrive as parasites in human, bird, and animal hosts. Some species can cause disease in humans.

Description

Mycoplasma are found most often on the surfaces of mucous membranes. They can cause chronic inflammatory diseases of the respiratory system, urogenital tract, and joints. The most common human illnesses caused by mycoplasma are due to infection with *M. pneumoniae,* which is responsible for 10-20% of all **pneumonias.** This type of pneumonia is also called atypical pneumonia, walking pneumonia, or community-acquired pneumonia. Infection moves easily among people in close contact because it is spread primarily when infected droplets circulate in the air (that is, become aerosolized), usually due to coughing, spitting, or sneezing.

Causes & symptoms

Atypical pneumonias can affect otherwise healthy people who have close contact with one another. Pneumonia caused by *M. pneumoniae* may start out with symptoms of an upper respiratory infection, probably a **sore throat** progressing to a dry cough within a few days. Gradually, **fever,** fatigue, muscle aches, and a cough that produces thin sputum (spit or phlegm) will emerge. Nonrespiratory symptoms may occur too: abdominal **pain, headache,** and **diarrhea;** about 20% of patients may have ear pain.

Another mycoplasma species, *M. hominis,* is common in the mucous membranes of the genital area (including the cervix), and can cause infection in both males and females. Its presence doesn't always result in symptoms.

Diagnosis

Usually, mycoplasma pneumonia will be identified after other common diagnoses are set aside. For example,

KEY TERMS

Community-acquired—Refers to an infectious disease that is passed among individuals who have close contact with one another.

a type of antibiotic known as a beta-lactam might be prescribed for a respiratory infection producing fever and cough. If symptoms do not improve in 3-5 days, the organism causing the disease is not a typical one and not susceptible to these **antibiotics.** If a Gram's stain (a common test done on sputum) does not indicate a gram-positive pathogen, the doctor will suspect a gram-negative organism, such as mycoplasma. The actual underlying organism may not be identified (it isn't in almost 50% of cases of atypical pneumonia). Although it is rare, a rash may appear along with pneumonia symptoms. This should trigger suspicion of mycoplasma pneumonia, even if laboratory tests are inconclusive.

Standard x rays may reveal a patchy material that has entered the tissue; this can be evident for months. Laboratory tests include cold agglutinins, complement fixation, culture, and enzyme immunoassay. The presence of infection with *M. pneumoniae* would be indicated by a fourfold rise in *M. pneumoniae*-specific antibody in serum, during the illness or convalescence. Highly sophisticated and specific polymerase chain reaction methods (PCR) have been developed for many respiratory pathogens, including *M. pneumoniae*. They are not readily available and are very expensive.

Treatment

A 2-3 week course of certain antibiotics (erythromycin, azithromycin, clarithromycin, dirithromycin, or doxycycline) is generally prescribed for atypical pneumonia. This disease is infectious for weeks, even after the patient starts antibiotics. A persistent cough may linger for 6 weeks.

Prognosis

Mycoplasma pneumonia may be involved in the onset of **asthma** in adults; other rare complications include meningoencephalitis, **Guillain-Barré syndrome,** mononeuritis multiplex, **myocarditis,** or **pericarditis.** This may increase the risk of acute **arrhythmias** leading to **sudden cardiac death.** However, with proper treatment and rest, recovery should be complete.

Prevention

At this time, there are no vaccines for mycoplasma infection. It is difficult to control its spread, especially in a group setting. The best measures are still the simplest ones. Avoid exposure to people with respiratory infections whenever possible. A person who has a respiratory infection should cover the face while coughing or sneezing.

Resources

BOOKS

Cassell, Gail H., Gregory G. Gray, and K. B. Waites. "*Mycoplasma* Infections." In *Harrison's Principles of Internal Medicine,* edited by Anthony S. Fauci, et al. New York: McGraw-Hill, 1998.

"*Mycoplasma* Pneumonia." In *The Merck Manual,* 16th ed., edited by Robert Berkow. Rahyway, NJ: Merck Research Laboratories, Merck & Co., Inc., 1992.

Jill S. Lasker

Mycoplasmal pneumonia *see* **Mycoplasma infections**

Myelocytic leukemia, acute *see* **Leukemias, acute**

Myelocytic leukemia, chronic *see* **Leukemias, chronic**

. . . .

Myelodysplastic syndrome

Definition

Myelodysplastic syndrome (MDS) is a disease that affects the production of all three major types of human blood cells. Patients with MDS have a lack of red blood cells, white blood cells, and platelets. The disorder occurs because the blood cells do not develop into mature cells, but rather stay in an immature stage within the bone marrow.

Description

Overview

To understand MDS, a basic knowledge of blood cells is needed. Blood cells are used by the body for many important functions. For this reason, the spongy tissue inside large bones (the bone marrow) stores a supply of blood cells in case the body needs them. Specialized cells known as stem cells are stored here. Stem cells have the ability to develop into immature blast cells and eventually become different types of mature blood cells. The three main types of blood cells produced in the bone marrow are: red blood cells (to carry oxygen); white blood cells (to prevent and fight infection); and platelets (needed for blood clotting). When the body needs a specific type of blood cell, the bone marrow uses its stockpile of stem cells to produce the appropriate mature cell. Although several changes and stages are required

KEY TERMS

Acute myelogenous leukemia—A cancerous disease that involves high numbers (above 30%) of white cell blasts in the bone marrow. When MDS cases transform into acute leukemia, they usually belong to this type.

Anemia—A lack of red blood cells in the body that causes tiredness, shortness of breath, and weakness.

Blasts—Immature blood cells.

Bone marrow transplant—A form of therapy whereby patients are exposed to high doses of chemotherapy and/or radiation therapy to destroy all of their bone marrow. The destroyed marrow is then replaced with healthy bone marrow from another person.

Chemotherapy—The use of cell-killing drugs to destroy cancerous or rapidly dividing cells.

Chromosomes—The strands of DNA within a cell's nucleus that encode genetic information. Certain chromosomal abnormalities within bone marrow and blood cells are a sign of MDS.

Cytogenetics—An analysis of chromosomes that is used to diagnose specific types of MDS.

Growth factors—Natural protein substances made by the body that stimulate cell growth.

Leukemia—A cancerous disease that occurs when too many blood cells are produced and cannot function properly.

Monocyte—A white blood cell that works to fight infections.

Platelets—Small disk-shaped blood cells produced in the bone marrow. Platelets help to seal off cuts by forming clots that stop bleeding.

Red blood cells (RBCs)—Cells produced in the bone marrow that carry oxygen to all parts of the body in the blood circulation.

Stem cells—Cells that are able to develop into any type of mature blood cell.

White blood cells (WBCs)—Cells of the immune system that fight off invading germs and disease agents. WBCs are made in the bone marrow and lymph nodes.

during blood cell development, the process is carefully controlled and occurs rapidly to meet the body's demands.

In patients with MDS, blood cells fail to mature. They remain in various immature blast cell stages. Because the cells do not mature, they also do not leave the bone marrow. Eventually, the marrow becomes filled with blasts until there is no room for normal cells to develop. In addition, many of the cells that do mature cannot function correctly. MDS therefore causes a shortage of functional blood cells of all types.

Subtypes of MDS

There are five different subtypes of MDS that are classified according to the number and appearance of the blast cells in the bone marrow. It is important for doctors to know which type of MDS a patient has, because each subtype affects patients differently and requires specific treatment. The five subtypes of MDS are:

- Refractory anemia (RA). Less than 5% blasts. RA is characterized by an abnormal appearance of red cell blasts.

- Refractory anemia with ring sideroblasts (RAS). Less than 15% blasts. RAS is similar to RA but has additional abnormalities in the red cells.

- Refractory anemia with excess blasts (RAEB). 5-20% blasts. RAEB is characterized by abnormal white and platelet blast cells. This form of MDS may transform into acute myelogenous leukemia.

- Refractory anemia with excess blasts in transformation (RAEB-t). 21-30% blasts. RAEB is characterized by a bone marrow appearance similar to that seen in acute myelogenous leukemia, except that RAEB-t has slightly fewer blast cells. This form of MDS is most likely to become leukemic.

- Chronic myelomonocytic leukemia (CMML). 5-20% blasts. This form of leukemia is characterized by too many mature white cells (monocytes) in the blood. CMML is also considered a type of MDS because the bone marrow contains excess white cell blasts together with abnormal forms of red cell and platelet blasts.

Progression

MDS used to be called preleukemia because the blast cells can resemble certain leukemic cells or eventually become leukemic. Only about one-third of myelodysplastic cases, however, actually lead to leukemia. For this reason, most doctors today seldom use preleukemia as a name for the condition. The types of MDS most likely to turn into leukemia are RAEB and RAEB-t.

Incidence

Approximately 5,000 new cases of MDS are diagnosed each year in the United States. Most of these belong to the RA or RAS subtypes. Most MDS cases occur in the elderly; it is quite rare to have MDS before age 50. An estimated 0.1% of persons 65 years old have MDS; the median age for people with this disease is 70. In older patients, MDS is more common in males than in females.

Causes & symptoms

Causes of MDS

There is no clear cause for the majority of MDS cases, which are called primary myelodysplastic syndromes. In some cases, however, MDS results from earlier **cancer** treatments, such as radiation and/or **chemotherapy.** This type of MDS is called secondary or treatment-related myelodysplastic syndrome. It is often seen in patients under the age of 30. The time span between cancer therapy and the development of MDS is usually three to six years, with a range of 1.5 to 13 years.

Other possible causative agents for MDS include exposure to radiation, cigarette smoke, and such toxic chemicals as benzene. Children with preexisting chromosomal abnormalities such as those found in **Down syndrome** may also have a higher risk of developing MDS. MDS does not appear to run in families, nor can it be spread to other individuals.

Symptoms of MDS

MDS symptoms are related to the type of blood cells that the body is lacking. The earliest symptoms are usually due to anemia, which results from a shortage of mature red blood cells. Anemia causes patients to feel tired, weak, and out of breath, because there is a lack of cells transporting oxygen throughout the body. MDS may also lead to a shortage of white blood cells and cause immune system problems. These patients are more likely to get infections. Another symptom of MDS is abnormal bruising and bleeding (e.g., heavy periods, blood in the stool, bleeding gums, and nosebleeds). Excessive bleeding results from a low level of platelets. These symptoms can occur in any combination, depending on a given patient's specific subtype of MDS. For example, an enlargement of the spleen or lymph nodes is a characteristic symptom of CMML.

Diagnosis

Blood tests

The diagnosis of MDS requires a complete analysis of the patient's blood and bone marrow. This analysis is done by a doctor that specializes in blood diseases (a hematologist). But because the early symptoms of MDS are usually fatigue and difficulty breathing, patients with MDS often go first to their general practitioner. To test for anemia, the doctor takes a blood sample and sends it to a laboratory for analysis. A complete **blood count** (CBC) must be done first to determine the number of each blood cell type within the sample. Low numbers of red blood cells, white blood cells, or platelets are signs that the patient has MDS. In these cases, the hematologist also studies the blood cells under the microscope to find out if any of the cells are abnormal. This analysis is called a blood film report, and will usually show abnormal red blood cells in MDS patients.

Bone marrow biopsy

A bone marrow biopsy is required to confirm the diagnosis of MDS and determine the correct MDS subtype. This procedure involves using a needle to take a sample of marrow from inside the bone. The area on the skin where the needle is inserted is numbed or anesthetized, and sometimes the patient is also sedated. Patients may experience some discomfort, but the procedure is over fairly quickly. Marrow samples are usually taken from the back of the hip bone (the iliac crest) or from the breast bone (the sternum). A sample of the marrow, known as an aspirate, and a small piece of bone are both removed with the needle.

A hematologist or a specialist in diseases (a pathologist) will carefully examine the bone marrow samples through a microscope. Microscope examination allows the doctor to determine the number and type of blasts within the marrow in order to identify the MDS subtype. Cells from the bone marrow biopsy may also be used for cytogenetic testing, which analyzes the cells' chromosomes. Certain chromosomal abnormalities in bone marrow cells are common in MDS. In fact, 40-70% of MDS patients have changes within their bone marrow chromosomes as a result of the disease. The pattern of these changes can be used to predict how a patient will respond to treatment. Thus, the full set of information provided by a bone marrow biopsy ultimately allows the doctor to design the most effective treatment plan.

Treatment

Supportive care

Treatment for MDS is tailored to the patient's age, general health, and specific MDS subtype. Although treatment tends to vary for each patient, most treatment strategies are designed to control the symptoms of MDS. This approach is called supportive care; it aims to improve the patient's quality of life. Supportive care for MDS patients commonly includes red blood cell **transfusions** to relieve anemia symptoms. **Vitamins** may also be prescribed to increase red blood cell production. Platelet transfusions can also provide a way to control excessive bleeding. In patients with low white cell counts, **antibiotics** can be prescribed to combat infections.

Corrective treatment

BONE MARROW TRANSPLANTATION (BMT)

A variety of therapies are directed at providing MDS patients with a cure, although many of these approaches are still considered experimental. These strategies often require the patients to be in fairly good health and are therefore more likely to be used for younger patients. For example, **bone marrow transplantation** (BMT) has been found to be a successful treatment for MDS patients under the age of 50 (and some over 50 in good health). Following BMT, many patients are able to achieve long-term, disease-free survival. Unfortunately, most MDS patients cannot receive a bone marrow transplant because of their age, or because they do not have a suitable donor.

CHEMOTHERAPY

Chemotherapy has also been used to treat some MDS patients; however, the disease often recurs after a period of time. This type of therapy uses cell-killing (cytotoxic) drugs that are either taken orally or injected into the body. These drugs are standard chemotherapy agents, including cytarabine (ARA-C), idarubicin, daunorubicin (Cerubidine), 6-thioguanine (Lanvis), and mitoxantrone. The drugs primarily kill rapidly growing cells in the bone marrow and blood, but may also destroy healthy cells that are growing. For this reason, chemotherapy is generally not used until the MDS becomes aggressive. Chemotherapy is most successful in patients with the RAEB, RAEB-t and CMML subtypes of MDS.

Biological therapy agents are also being developed to treat MDS. One group of these agents, called growth factors, are natural protein substances that the body normally uses to control blood cell production. Growth factors have also been made in the laboratory and can be given to MDS patients. These substances stimulate the patient's bone marrow to produce healthy blood cells and platelets. Growth factors that stimulate white cell production are G-CSF (granulocyte colony stimulating factor, sold under the trade name Neupogen) and GM-CSF (granulocyte-macrophage colony stimulating factor, sold under the trade names Leukine or Prokine). In order to increase red blood cell production another growth factor, erythropoietin (EPO, Epogen), is used.

Alternative treatment

There are no alternative therapies that successfully treat MDS, as medical attention is required for this disease. A well-balanced diet and adequate rest, however, are helpful in managing the symptoms of anemia.

Prognosis

The prognosis for MDS patients depends on the subtype of their disease. Patients with the more common, lower-risk RA and RAS rarely develop leukemia and may live with the disease for some years, depending on when it is detected. The higher-risk subtypes—RAEB, RAEB-t, and CMML—progress more rapidly, and require intensive therapy to control the disease.

Managing MDS requires frequent doctor appointments to monitor disease progression and evaluate the patient's response to treatment. Fortunately for many patients, recent advances in therapy have significantly enhanced their ability to cope with MDS. Experimental drugs and a better understanding of the disease are likely to improve the quality of life for MDS patients.

Prevention

MDS is usually impossible to prevent, although avoiding exposure to radiation and benzene may decrease the risk of developing the disorder. Secondary complications of MDS such as bruising and bleeding may be prevented by being careful about daily activities and avoiding the use of aspirin-like products that thin the blood. Infections can also be prevented by practicing good hygiene and avoiding crowds or people with virus infections. A well-balanced diet is needed for the body to make red blood cells and avoid anemia.

Resources

BOOKS

Castro-Malaspina, Hugo, and Richard J. O'Reilly. "Aplastic Anemia and Myelodysplastic Syndromes." In *Harrison's Principles of Internal Medicine,* 14th ed., edited by Anthony S. Fauci, et al. New York: McGraw-Hill, 1998.

Nomura, Takeo, and Yataro Yoshida. *Myelodysplastic Syndromes: Advances in Research and Treatment.* Amsterdam: Elsevier Science, 1995.

ORGANIZATIONS

Aplastic Anemia Foundation of America. P.O. Box 613, Annapolis, MD 21404. (800)747-2820. http://www.aplastic.org.

Leukemia Society of America. 600 Third Avenue, New York, NY 10016. (800)955-4LSA. http://www.leukemia.org.

Myelodysplastic Syndromes Foundation. 464 Main Street, P.O. Box 477, Crosswicks, NJ 08515. (800)MDS-0839. http://www.mds-foundation.org.

Julie A. Gelderloos

Myelofibrosis

Definition

Myelofibrosis is a rare blood disorder of people over the age of 50.

Description

Myelofibrosis behaves like a leukemia and sometimes turns into one. However, instead of being a disease of white blood cells, it affects a more primordial cell type. Called progenitor cells, these cells retain their ability to become many different types of mature cells and tissues. In myelofibrosis, a progenitor cell begins to produce both immature blood cells and excess scar tissue. The scar tissue is mostly in the bone marrow, which hinders the production of normal blood cells. Extra blood cell production occurs all over the body, but it is most obvious in the spleen. As a consequence, the spleen can grow to an enormous size.

Causes & symptoms

The cause of myelofibrosis is unknown. Most patients are over 50 years old, but it can strike at any age. Symptoms may not appear for a year or more. A enlarged spleen discovered at an annual medical examination may be the first clue. Eventually, symptoms become prevalent.

- Anemia causes fatigue.

- An enlarged spleen can compromise digestion and lead to serious weight loss.

- Exuberant disease activity can hinder lung, bowel, kidney, heart, brain, and spinal cord function.

- General symptoms like **fever** and sweating are present.

Diagnosis

Since symptoms are similar to other diseases (mostly leukemias), myelofibrosis is not easy to diagnose. Correct diagnosis is imperative because the treatment of each type of disease is quite different. Blood tests and bone marrow biopsies are necessary, but more extensive testing may be required.

Treatment

There is no specific treatment for this disease, but there are many supportive measures that can be taken.

- Anemia is common and can be treated with androgens (male hormones, anabolic steroids). Hematinics may help briefly, but **transfusions** are required throughout the course of the disease.

- **Bone marrow transplantation** is also used to treat the anemia.

- **Cancer chemotherapy** and interferon-alpha have been used.

- Infections in the lung and other organs require **antibiotics.**

- Radiation or removal of an enlarged spleen is often helpful. A big spleen not only impairs digestion, parts of it can die (infarct) and hurt. It also destroys too many blood cells and causes anemia.

- Radiation may also help localized bone **pain,** tumors in certain places such as next to the spinal cord, and weeping fluid inside the abdomen.

Prognosis

Similar to many leukemias, this disease progresses rapidly, and requires intensive therapy to control the disease.

Resources

BOOKS

Bennett, J. Claude and Fred Plum, ed. *Cecil Textbook of Medicine.* Philadelphia: W. B. Saunders, 1996.

Lichtman, Marshall A. "Idiopathic Myelofibrosis." In *Williams Hematology,* edited by Ernest Beutler, et al. New York: McGraw-Hill, Inc., 1995, pp. 331-340.

Linker, Charles A. "Blood." In *Current Medical Diagnosis and Treatment,* edited by Lawrence M. Tierney Jr., et al. Stamford, CT: Appleton & Lange, 1996, pp. 502-503.

Spivak, Jerry L. "Polycythemia Vera and Other Myeloproliferative Disorders." In *Harrison's Principles of Internal Medicine,* edited by Kurt Isselbacher, et al. New York: McGraw-Hill, 1998, pp. 681-682.

J. Ricker Polsdorfer

Myelogram *see* **Myelography**

Myelography

Definition

Myelography is an x-ray examination of the spinal canal. A contrast agent is injected through a needle into the space around the spinal cord to display the spinal cord, spinal canal, and nerve roots on an x ray.

Purpose

The purpose of a myelogram is to evaluate the spinal cord and/or nerve roots for suspected compression. Pressure on these delicate structures causes **pain** or other symptoms. A myelogram is performed when precise detail about the spinal cord is needed to make a definitive diagnosis. In most cases, myelography is used after other studies, such as **magnetic resonance imaging** (MRI) or a **computed tomography scan** (CT scan), have not yielded enough information to be sure of the disease process. Sometimes myelography followed by CT scan is an alternative for patients who cannot have an MRI scan, because they have a pacemaker or other implanted metallic device.

A herniated or ruptured intervertebral disc, popularly known as a slipped disc, is one of the most common causes for pressure on the spinal cord or nerve roots. Discs are pads of fiber and cartilage that contain rubbery tissue. They lie between the vertebrae, or individual bones, which make up the spine. Discs act as cushions, accommodating strains, shocks, and position changes. A disc may rupture suddenly, due to injury, or a sudden straining with the spine in an unnatural position. In other cases, the problem may come on gradually as a result of progressive deterioration of the discs with aging. The lower back is the most common area for this problem, but it sometimes occurs in the neck, and rarely in the upper back. A myelogram can help accurately locate the disc or discs involved.

Myelography may be used when a tumor is suspected. Tumors can originate in the spinal cord, or in tissues surrounding the cord. **Cancers** that have started in other parts of the body may spread or metastasize in the spine. It is important to precisely locate the mass causing pressure, so effective treatment can be undertaken. Patients with known cancer who develop back pain may require a myelogram for evaluation.

Other conditions that may be diagnosed using myelography include arthritic bony growths, known as spurs, narrowing of the spinal canal, called **spinal stenosis,** or malformations of the spine.

Precautions

Patients who are unable to lie still or cooperate with positioning should not have this examination. Severe congenital spinal abnormalities may make the examination technically difficult to carry out. Patients with a history of severe allergic reaction to contrast material (x-ray dye) should report this to their physician. Pretreatment with medications to minimize the risk of severe reaction may be recommended.

Description

Myelograms can be performed in a hospital x-ray department or in an outpatient radiology facility. The patient lies on the x-ray table on his or her stomach. The radiologist first looks at the spine under fluoroscopy, where the images appear on a monitor screen. This is done to find the best location to position the needle. The skin is cleaned, then numbed with local anesthetic. The needle is inserted. Occasionally, a small amount of cerebrospinal fluid, the clear fluid which surrounds the spinal cord and brain, may be withdrawn through the needle and sent for laboratory studies. Then contrast material is injected. The contrast material (dye) is a liquid that shows up on x rays.

The x-ray table is tilted slowly. This allows the contrast material to reach different levels in the spinal canal. The flow is observed under fluoroscopy, then x rays are taken with the table tilted at various angles. A footrest and shoulder straps or supports will keep the patient from sliding.

In many instances, a CT scan of the spine will be performed immediately after a myelogram, while the contrast material is still in the spinal canal. This helps outline internal structures most clearly.

A myelogram takes approximately 30-60 minutes. A CT scan adds about another hour to the examination. If the procedure is done as an outpatient exam, some facilities prefer the patient to stay in a recovery area for up to four hours.

Preparation

Patients should be well hydrated at the time of a myelogram. Increasing fluids the day before the study is usually recommended. All food and fluid intake should be stopped approximately four hours before the myelogram.

Certain medications may need to be stopped for one to two days before myelography is performed. These include some antipsychotics, antidepressants, blood thinners, and diabetic medications. Patients should consult with their physician and/or the facility where the study is to be done.

Patients who smoke may be asked to stop the day before the test. This helps decrease the chance of nausea or **headaches** after the myelogram. Immediately before the examination, patients should empty their bowels and bladder.

Aftercare

After the examination is completed, the patient usually rests for several hours, with the head elevated. Extra fluids are encouraged, to help eliminate the contrast material and prevent headaches. A regular diet and routine medications may be resumed. Strenuous physical activity, especially any which involve bending over, may be discouraged for one or two days. The doctor should be notified if a **fever,** excessive **nausea and vomiting,** severe headache, or stiff neck develops.

Risks

Headache is a common complication of myelography. It may begin several hours to several days after the examination. The cause is thought to be changes in cerebrospinal fluid pressure, not a reaction to the dye. The headache may be mild and easily alleviated with rest and increased fluids. Sometimes, nonprescription medicine are recommended. In some instances, the headache may be more severe and require stronger medication or other measures for relief. Many factors influence whether the patient develops this problem. These include the type of needle used and the age and sex of the patient. Patients with a history of chronic or recurrent headache are more likely to develop a headache after a myelogram.

The chance of reaction to the contrast material is a very small, but potentially significant risk with myelography. It is estimated that only 5-10% of patients experience any effect from contrast exposure. The vast majority of reactions are mild, such as sneezing, nausea, or **anxiety.** These usually resolve by themselves. A moderate reaction, like **wheezing** or **hives,** may be treated with medication, but is not considered life threatening. Severe reactions, such as heart or **respiratory failure,** happen very infrequently. These require emergency medical treatment.

Rare complications of myelography include injury to the nerve roots from the needle, or from bleeding into the spaces around the roots. Inflammation of the delicate covering of the spinal cord, called arachnoiditis, or infections, can also occur. Seizures are another very uncommon complication reported after myelography.

Normal results

A normal myelogram would show a spinal canal of normal width, with no areas of constriction or obstruction.

Abnormal results

A myelogram may reveal a **herniated disk,** tumor, bone spurs, or narrowing of the spinal canal (spinal stenosis).

Resources

BOOKS

Daffner, Richard. *Clinical Radiology, The Essentials.* Baltimore: Williams and Wilkins, 1993.

Pagana, Kathleen and Timothy Pagana. *Mosby's Diagnostic and Laboratory Test Reference.* St. Louis: Mosby-Year Book, 1997.

Torres, Lillian. *Basic Medical Techniques and Patient Care in Imaging Technology.* Philadelphia: Lippincott, 1997.

ORGANIZATIONS

The Spine Center. 1911 Arch St., Philadelphia, PA 19103. (215) 665-8300. http://thespinecenter.org.

Ellen S. Weber

Myelomatosis *see* **Multiple myeloma**

. . . .

Myocardial biopsy

Definition

Myocardial biopsy is a procedure wherein a small portion of tissue is removed from the heart muscle for testing. This test is also known as endomyocardial biopsy.

Purpose

The main reason for a biopsy is to secure tissue samples that will be useful in the diagnosis, treatment,

KEY TERMS

Anticoagulant—Medication that thins the blood and slows clot formation.

Aplastic anemia—A greatly decreased production of all of the formed elements of the blood caused by a failure of the cell-generating capacity of the bone marrow.

Electrocardiography—A test that uses electrodes attached to the chest with an adhesive gel to transmit the electrical impulses of the heart muscle to a recording device.

Leukemia—A disease characterized by an increasing number of abnormal cells in the blood.

and care of heart muscle disorders. The test is also used to detect rejection after a **heart transplantation** procedure.

Precautions

This procedure is not used when the patient is taking blood-thinning medication (anticoagulant therapy). It should not be done when the patient has leukemia and **aplastic anemia** or if there is a blood clot on the interior wall of the heart.

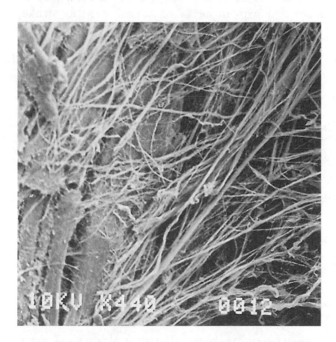

Once the catheter is threaded up into the heart, the surgeon will take several small samples of muscle for laboratory analysis. *(Custom Medical Stock Photo. Reproduced by permission.)*

Description

A long, flexible tube, called a catheter, is inserted into a vein and threaded up into the heart. The doctor can guide the catheter by watching its movement on a TV monitor showing an x-ray image of the area. The tip of the catheter is fitted with tiny jaws that the doctor can open and close. Once the catheter is in place, the doctor will take several small snips of muscle for microscopic examination.

Preparation

Preparation for myocardial biopsy is quite extensive. The patient will be asked not to eat for several hours before the procedure. A technician will shave the hair from the area of the incision and will also insert an intravenous line in the arm. The patient will be given a sedative to relax but will not be fully anesthetized. The patient will be connected to an electrocardiograph (ECG) to monitor the heart, and a blood-pressure cuff will be placed. Finally, the patient will be covered with sterile drapes, so that the area of the biopsy is kept free of germs. The cardiologist will numb the area where the catheter will be inserted.

Aftercare

At the end of the biopsy, the catheter will be removed and pressure will be applied at the site where it entered the blood vessel in order to encourage healing. The patient will then be taken to the recovery room. It is advisable to remain flat and not to move about for 6-8 hours. After that time, most people begin walking around. Swelling and bruising at the puncture site are common and usually go away without need for further attention.

Risks

The risks involved with myocardial biopsy are small because the patient is monitored closely and attended by well-trained staff. Racing of the heart (**palpitations**) and quivering of the heart muscles (atrial fibrillation) are both possible during the procedure.

Resources

BOOKS

McGoon, Michael D., ed. *Mayo Clinic Heart Book: The Ultimate Guide to Heart Health.* New York: William Morrow and Company, Inc., 1993

ORGANIZATIONS

American Heart Association. 7320 Greenville Avenue, Dallas, TX 75231. 1-800-889-7943. http://www.amhrt.org.

Dorothy Elinor Stonely

Myocardial infarction *see* **Heart attack**

Myocardial perfusion scan *see* **Thallium heart scan**

Myocardial resection

Definition

Myocardial resection is a surgical procedure in which a portion of the heart muscle is removed.

Purpose

Myocardial resection is done to improve the stability of the heart function or rhythm. Also known as endocardial resection, this open-heart surgery is done to destroy or remove damaged areas of the heart that cause life-threatening heart rhythms. This procedure is often performed in people who have had a **heart attack,** in order to prevent future rapid heart rates. It is also used in people who have **Wolff-Parkinson-White syndrome** (a condition resulting in abnormal heart rhythm).

Precautions

This is major surgery and should be the treatment of choice only after medications have failed and the use of an **implantable cardioverter-defibrillator** (a device that delivers electrical shock to control heart rhythm) has been ruled out.

Description

After receiving a general anesthetic, an incision will be made in the chest to expose the heart. When the exact source of the abnormal rhythm is identified, it is removed. If there are areas around the source that may contribute to the problem, they can be frozen with a special probe to further insure against dangerous heart rates. The amount of tissue removed is so small, usually only 2 or 3 millimeters, that there is no damage to the structure of the heart. On some occasions, aneurysms of the heart wall are removed as well.

Preparation

Prior to surgery, the physician will explain the procedure, routine blood tests will be completed, and consent forms will be signed.

KEY TERMS

. . . .

Implantable cardioverter-defibrillator—A device placed in the body to deliver an electrical shock to the heart in response to a serious abnormal rhythm.

Wolff-Parkinson-White syndrome—An abnormal, rapid heart rhythm, due to an extra pathway for the electrical impulses to travel from the atria to the ventricles.

Aftercare

Immediately after surgery, the patient will be moved to a recovery room until the affects of anesthesia have worn off. The patient will then be transferred to the intensive care unit for further recovery. In the intensive care unit, the heart will be monitored for any disturbances in rhythm and the patient will be watched for any signs of post-operative problems.

Risks

The risks of myocardial resection are based in large part on the person's underlying heart condition and, therefore, vary greatly. The procedure involves opening the heart, so the person is at risk for the complications associated with major heart surgery such as **stroke,** shock, infection, and hemorrhage.

Normal results

Anywhere from 5-25% of post-heart attack patients do not survive open-heart surgery. The survivors have a 90% arrhythmia-free one-year survival rate, (arrthymia is an irregular heart beat).

Resources

BOOKS

McGoon, Michael D., ed. *Mayo Clinic Heart Book: The Ultimate Guide to Heart Health.* New York: William Morrow and Company, Inc., 1993.

ORGANIZATIONS

American Heart Association. 7320 Greenville Avenue, Dallas, TX 75231. (800) 889-7943.

Dorothy Elinor Stonely

Myocarditis

Definition

Myocarditis is an inflammatory disease of the heart muscle (myocardium) that can result from a variety of causes. While most cases are produced by a viral infection, an inflammation of the heart muscle may also be instigated by toxins, drugs, and hypersensitive immune reactions. Myocarditis is a rare but serious condition that affects both males and females of any age.

Description

Most cases of myocarditis in the United States originate from a virus, and the disease may remain undiagnosed by doctors due to its general lack of initial symptoms. The disease may also present itself as an acute, catastrophic illness that requires immediate treatment. Although the inflammation or degeneration of the heart muscle that myocarditis causes may be fatal, this disease often goes undetected. It may also disguise itself as ischemic, valvular, or hypertensive heart disease.

An inflammation of the heart muscle may occur as an isolated disorder or be the dominating feature of a systemic disease (one that affects the whole body, like **systemic lupus erythematosus**).

Causes & symptoms

While there are several contributing factors that may lead to myocarditis, the primary cause is viral. Myocarditis usually results from the Coxsackie B virus, and may also result from **measles, influenza,** chicken pox, hepatitis virus, or the adenovirus in children. If an acute onset of severe myocarditis occurs, a patient may display the following symptoms:

- Rhythm disturbances of the heart

- Rapid heartbeat (**Ventricular tachycardia**)

- Left or right ventricular enlargement

- **Shortness of breath** (Dyspnea)

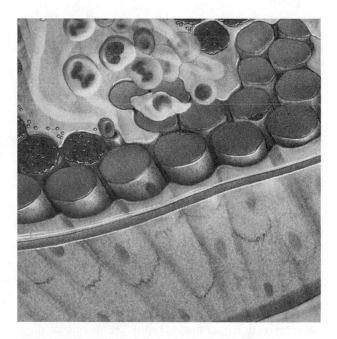

This illustration depicts the inflammation of the myocarditis, the middle muscular layer of the heart wall. *(Custom Medical Stock Photo. Reproduced by permission.)*

- **Pulmonary edema** (the accumulation of fluid in the lungs due to left-sided **heart failure**)

- Swollen legs.

Additional causes of myocarditis include:

- Bacterial infections, such as **tetanus, gonorrhea,** or **tuberculosis**

- Parasite infections, such as **Chagas' disease** (which is caused by an insect-borne protozoan most commonly seen in Central and South America)

- **Rheumatic fever**

- Surgery on the heart

- **Radiation therapy** for **cancer** that is localized in the chest, such as breast or **lung cancer**

- Certain medications.

As of 1996, research has shown that illegal drugs and toxic substances may also produce acute or chronic injury to the myocardium. These studies also indicate an increase in the incidence of toxic results from the use of cocaine. This illegal drug causes coronary artery spasm, myocardial infarction (**heart attack**), and **arrhythmias,** as well as myocarditis.

Further studies conducted in 1996 indicate that **malnutrition** encourages the Coxsackie B virus to flourish, leading to the potential development of myocarditis. Human **immunodeficiency** virus (HIV) is also now recognized as a cause of myocarditis, though its prevalence is not known.

Symptoms of myocarditis may start as fatigue, **shortness of breath, fever** and aching of the joints, all characteristic of a flu-like illness. In contrast to this type of mild appearance, myocarditis may also appear suddenly in the form of heart failure, or **sudden cardiac death** without any prior symptoms. If an inflammation of the heart muscle leads to congestive heart failure, symptoms such as swollen feet and ankles, distended neck veins, a rapid heartbeat, and difficulty breathing while reclining may all appear.

Diagnosis

The best way to diagnose myocarditis may be through a person's observation of his or her own symptoms, followed by a thorough medical history and physical exam conducted by a doctor. Further tests usually include laboratory blood studies and **echocardiography.** An electrocardiogram (ECG) is also routinely used due to its ability to detect a mild case of the disease. **Cardiac catheterization** and **angiography** are additional diagnostic tests used to determine the presence of myocarditis, or to rule out other possible heart diseases that may lead to heart failure.

Another measure used to diagnosis myocarditis is the endomyocardial biopsy procedure. This invasive catheterization procedure examines a biopsied, or "snipped," piece of the endocardium (the lining membrane of the inner surface of the heart). The tissue sample is examined to verify the presence of the disease, as well as to try to determine the infective cause. An approach used only with a patient's consent, this procedure may also confirm acute myocarditis, allowing close monitoring of potential congestive heart failure.

Treatment

While myocarditis is a serious condition, there is no medical treatment necessary if it results from a general viral infection. The only steps to recovery include rest and avoidance of physical exertion. Adequate rest becomes more important to recovery if the case is severe myocarditis with signs of dilated cardiomyopathy (disease of the heart muscles). In this case, medical treatment for congestive heart failure may include the following medications: angiotensin converting enzyme (ACE) inhibitors, **diuretics** to reduce fluid retention, digitalis to stimulate a stronger heartbeat, and low-dose beta-blockers.

If myocarditis is caused by a bacterial infection, the disease is treated with **antibiotics** to fight the infection. If severe rhythm disturbances are involved, cardiac assist devices, an "artificial heart," or **heart transplantation** may be the only option for complete recovery.

Prognosis

The outlook for a diagnosed case of myocarditis caused by a viral infection is excellent, with many cases healing themselves spontaneously. Severe or acute myocarditis may be controlled with medication to prevent heart failure. Because this disease may be mild or may be extreme and cause serious arrhythmias, the prognosis varies. Cases of myocarditis may vary from complete healing (with or without significant scarring), to severe congestive heart failure leading to death or requiring a heart transplant.

Inflammation of the myocardium may also cause acute **pericarditis** (inflammation of the outer lining of the heart). Due to the potential effects of the disease, including sudden death, it is imperative that proper medical attention is obtained.

Prevention

Although myocarditis is an unpredictable disease, the following measures may help prevent its onset. Individuals should:

- Take extra measures to avoid infections, and obtain appropriate treatment for infections.

- Limit alcohol consumption to no more than one or two drinks a day, if any.

- Maintain current immunizations against **diphtheria**, tetanus, measles, **rubella,** and **polio.**

- Avoid anything that may cause the abnormal heart to work too hard, including salt and vigorous **exercise.**

Resources

BOOKS

The Editors of Time-Life Books. ''Heart Disease.'' In *The Medical Advisor: The Complete Guide to Alternative & Conventional Treatments.* Richmond, VA: Time-Life Inc., 1996, p. 460.

Griffith, H. Winter. ''Myocarditis.'' In *Complete Guide To Symptoms, Illness & Surgery.* New York: The Putnam Berkley Group, Inc., 1995, p. 438.

''Myocarditis & The Cardiomyopathies.'' In *Currrent Medical Diagnosis & Treatment,* 35th ed., edited by Lawrence M. Tierney Jr., Stephen J. McPhee and Maxine A. Papdakis. Stamford, CT: Appleton & Lange, 1996, pp. 369-371.

PERIODICALS

''Viral Myocarditis.'' *Physician and Sportsmedicine* 23(July 1995): 63-66, 68.

Zeppilli, Paolo, et al. ''Role of Myocarditis in Athletes with Minor Arrhythmias and/or Echocardiographic Abnormalities.'' *Chest* 106(August 1994): 373.

ORGANIZATIONS

American Heart Association. 7272 Greenville Ave., Dallas, TX 75231-4596. (800) AHA-USA1. http://www.amhrt.org.

National Heart, Lung, and Blood Institute Information Center. PO Box 30105, Bethesda, MD 20824-0105. (800) 575-WELL.

Beth A. Kapes

Myoclonus *see* **Movement disorders**

Myoglobin test

Definition

Myoglobin is a protein found in muscle. Myoglobin tests are done to evaluate a person who has symptoms of a **heart attack** (myocardial infarction) or other muscle damage.

Purpose

Myoglobin holds oxygen inside heart and skeletal muscle (muscles that attach to and move bones). It is

---

KEY TERMS

Cardiac marker—A substance in the blood that rises following a heart attack.

Diagnostic window—A cardiac marker's timeline for rising, peaking, and returning to normal after a heart attack.

Myoglobin—A protein that holds oxygen in heart and skeletal muscle. It rises after damage to either of these muscle types.

---

continually released into the blood in small amounts due to normal turnover of muscle cells. Kidneys discard the myoglobin into urine.

When muscle is damaged, as in a heart attack, larger amounts of myoglobin are released and blood levels rise rapidly. Myoglobin is one of the first tests done to determine if a person with chest **pain** is having a heart attack, as it may be one of the first blood tests to become abnormal.

Damage or injury to skeletal muscle also causes myoglobin to be released into the blood.

Description

Heart attack must be diagnosed quickly. Medications to prevent heart damage are effective only within a limited number of hours. Yet, because of their risk for excessive bleeding, these medications are given only after a diagnosis of heart attack is made.

Myoglobin is one of several cardiac markers used to make the diagnosis. Cardiac markers are substances in blood whose levels rise in the hours following a heart attack. Increased levels help diagnose a heart attack; persistent normal levels rule it out.

Each cardiac marker rises, peaks, and returns to a normal level according to its own timeline, or diagnostic window. Myoglobin is useful because it has the earliest diagnostic window. It is the first marker to rise after chest pain begins. Myoglobin levels rise within two to three hours, and sometimes as early as 30 minutes. They peak after six to nine hours. The levels return to normal within 24-36 hours.

Although a rise in myoglobin supports a diagnosis of heart attack, it is not conclusive. Simultaneous skeletal muscle damage could also cause the increase. Myoglobin rules out, rather than proves, a diagnosis in the following way. If myoglobin levels have not risen after more than five hours, a heart attack in unlikely. Normal levels in the first two to three hours do not rule out an infarction.

The myoglobin test is sometimes repeated every one to two hours to watch for the rise and peak. Results are available within 30 minutes.

Myoglobin in large amounts is toxic to the kidney. When a person has high amounts of myoglobin in the blood, kidney function must be monitored.

Preparation

This test requires 5 ml of blood. Collection of the sample takes only a few minutes. A urine myoglobin test requires 1 ml of urine collected into a urine collection cup.

Aftercare

Discomfort or bruising may occur at the puncture site or the person may feel dizzy or faint. Pressure to the puncture site until the bleeding stops reduces bruising. Warm packs to the puncture site relieve discomfort.

Normal results

Normal results vary based on the laboratory and method used.

Abnormal results

Myoglobin levels and levels of other cardiac markers are usually considered before finally confirming a diagnosis of heart attack. A level that has doubled after one to two hours, even if the level is still in the normal range, indicates a significant rise that may be due to heart attack.

Increased levels are also found with skeletal muscle damage or disease, such as an injury, **muscular dystrophy,** or **polymyositis.** Myoglobin levels also rise during renal failure because kidneys lose their ability to clear myoglobin from blood.

Resources

BOOKS

Wu, Alan, ed. *Cardiac Markers.* Washington, DC: American Association of Clinical Chemistry (AACC) Press, 1998.

PERIODICALS

Chesebro, Marcia J. "Using Serum Markers in the Early Diagnosis of Myocardial Infarction." *American Family Physician,* (June 1997): 2667-2674.

Keffer, Joseph. "Myocardial Markers of Injury. Evolution and Insights." *American Journal of Clinical Pathology,* (March 1996): 305-320.

Mercer, Donald W. "Role of Cardiac Markers in Evaluation of Suspected Heart attack. Selecting the Most Clinically Useful Indicators." *Postgraduate Medicine* (November 1997): 113-117, 121-122.

Nancy J. Nordenson

Myomas *see* **Uterine fibroids**

Myomectomy

Definition

Myomectomy is the removal of fibroids (noncancerous tumors) from the wall of the uterus. Myomectomy is the preferred treatment for symptomatic fibroids in women who want to keep their uterus. Larger fibroids must be removed with an abdominal incision, but small fibroids can be taken out using **laparoscopy** or **hysteroscopy.**

Purpose

A myomectomy can remove **uterine fibroids** that are causing symptoms. It is an alternative to surgical removal of the whole uterus (**hysterectomy**). The procedure can relieve fibroid-induced menstrual symptoms that have not responded to medication. Myomectomy also may be an effective treatment for **infertility** caused by the presence of fibroids.

Precautions

There is a risk that removal of the fibroids may lead to such severe bleeding that the uterus itself will have to be removed. Because of the risk of blood loss during a myomectomy, patients may want to consider banking their own blood before surgery.

Description

Usually, fibroids are buried in the outer wall of the uterus and abdominal surgery is required. If they are on the inner wall of the uterus, uterine fibroids can be removed using hysteroscopy. If they are on a stalk (pedunculated) on the outer surface of the uterus, laparoscopy can be performed.

Removing fibroids through abdominal surgery is a more difficult and slightly more risky operation than a hysterectomy. This is because the uterus bleeds from the sites where the fibroids were, and it may be difficult or impossible to stop the bleeding. This surgery is usually performed under general anesthesia, although some patients may be given a spinal or epidural anesthesia.

The incision may be horizontal (the "bikini" incision) or a vertical incision from the navel downward. After separating the muscle layers underneath the skin, the surgeon makes an opening in the abdominal wall. Next, the surgeon makes an incision over each fibroid, grasping and pulling out each growth.

Every opening in the uterine wall is then stitched with sutures. The uterus must be meticulously repaired in order to eliminate potential sites of bleeding or infection. Then, the surgeon sutures the abdominal wall and muscle layers above it with absorbable stitches, and closes the skin with clips or nonabsorbable stitches.

When appropriate, a laparoscopic myomectomy may be performed. In this procedure, the surgeon removes fibroids with the help of a viewing tube (laparoscope) inserted into the pelvic cavity through an incision in the navel. The fibroids are removed through a tiny incision under the navel that is much smaller than the 4 or 5 inch opening required for a standard myomectomy.

If the fibroids are small and located on the inner surface of the uterus, they can be removed with a thin telescope-like device called a hysteroscope. The hysteroscope is inserted into the vagina through the cervix and into the uterus. This procedure does not require any abdominal incision, so hospitalization is shorter.

Preparation

Surgeons often recommend hormone treatment with a drug called leuprolide (Lupron) two to six months before surgery in order to shrink the fibroids. This makes the fibroids easier to remove. In addition, Lupron stops menstruation, so women who are anemic have an opportunity to build up their **blood count.** While the drug treatment may reduce the risk of excess blood loss during surgery, there is a small risk that temporarily-smaller fibroids might be missed during myomectomy, only to enlarge later after the surgery is completed.

Aftercare

Patients may need four to six weeks of recovery following a standard myomectomy before they can return to normal activities. Women who have had laparoscopic or hysteroscopic myomectomies, however, can leave the hospital the day after surgery and usually recovery completely within two to three days to one to three weeks.

Risks

The risks of a myomectomy performed by a skilled surgeon are about the same as hysterectomy (one of the most common and safest surgeries). Removing multiple fibroids is more difficult and slightly more risky.

Possible complications include:

• Infection.

• Blood loss.

• The wall of the uterus may be weakened if the removal of a large fibroid leaves a wound that extends the complete thickness of the wall. Special precautions may be needed in future pregnancies. For example, the delivery may need to be performed surgically (Caesarean section).

• Adverse reactions to anesthesia.

• Internal scarring (and possible infertility).

Since fibroids tend to appear and grow as a woman ages (until **menopause**), it is possible that new fibroids will appear after myomectomy.

Resources

BOOKS

Carlson, Karen J., Stephanie A. Eisenstat, and Terra Ziporyn. *The Harvard Guide to Women's Health* Cambridge, MA: Harvard University Press, 1996.

Youngson, Robert M. *The Surgery Book* New York: St. Martin's Press, 1993.

OTHER

Toaff, Michael E., M.D. *Alternatives to Hysterectomy: Myomectomy* http://www.netreach.net/~hysterectomyedu/myomecto.htm.

Carol A. Turkington

Myopathies

Definition

Myopathies are diseases of skeletal muscle which are not caused by nerve disorders. These diseases cause the skeletal or voluntary muscles to become weak or wasted.

Description

There are many different types of myopathies, some of which are inherited, some inflammatory, and some caused by endocrine problems. Myopathies are rare and not usually fatal. Typically, effects are mild, largely causing muscle weakness and movement problems, and many are transitory. Only rarely will patients become dependent on a wheelchair. However, **muscular dystrophy** (which is technically a form of myopathy) is far more severe. Some types of this disease are fatal in early adulthood.

KEY TERMS

Electromyogram (EMG)—A diagnostic test that records the electrical activity of muscles. In the test, small electrodes are placed on or in the skin; the patterns of electrical activity are projected on a screen or over a loudspeaker. This procedure is used to test for muscle disorders, including muscular dystrophy.

Inflammation—A protective response of injured tissues characterized by redness, increased heat, swelling, and/or pain in the affected area.

Voluntary muscles—Muscles producing voluntary movement.

Causes & symptoms

Myopathies are usually degenerative, but they are sometimes caused by drug side effects, chemical **poisoning,** or a chronic disorder of the immune system.

Genetic myopathies

Among their many functions, genes are responsible for overseeing the production of proteins important in maintaining healthy cells. Muscle cells produce thousands of proteins. With each of the inherited myopathies, a genetic defect is linked to a lack of, or problem with, one of the proteins needed for normal muscle cell function.

There are several different kinds of myopathy caused by defective genes:

• Central core disease

• Centronuclear (myotubular) myopathy

• Myotonia congenita

• Nemaline myopathy

• Paramyotonia congenita

• **Periodic paralysis** (hypokalemic and hyperkalemic forms)

• Mitochondrial myopathies.

Most of these genetic myopathies are dominant, which means that a child needs to inherit only one copy of the defective gene from one parent in order to have the disease. The parent with the defective gene also has the disorder, and each of this parent's children has a 50% chance of also inheriting the disease. Male and female children are equally at risk.

However, one form of myotonia congenita and some forms of nemaline myopathy must be inherited from both

parents, each of whom carry a recessive defective gene but who don't have symptoms of the disease. Each child of such parents has a 25% chance of inheriting both genes and showing signs of the disease, and a 50% chance of inheriting one defective gene from only one parent. If the child inherited just one defective gene, he or she would be a carrier but would not show signs of the disease.

A few forms of centronuclear myopathy develop primarily in males. Females who inherit the defective gene are usually carriers without symptoms, like their mothers, but they can pass on the disease to their sons. Mitochondrial myopathies are inherited through the mother, since sperm don't contain mitochondria. (Mitochondria play a key role in energy production in the body's cells.)

The major symptoms associated with the genetic myopathies include:

• Central core disease: mild weakness of voluntary muscles, especially in the hips and legs; hip displacement; delays in reaching developmental motor milestones; problems with running, jumping, and climbing stairs develop in childhood

• Centronuclear myopathy: weakness of voluntary muscles including those on the face, arms, legs, and trunk; drooping upper eyelids; facial weakness; foot drop; affected muscles almost always lack reflexes

• Myotonia congenita: voluntary muscles of the arms, legs, and face are stiff or slow to relax after contracting (myotonia); stiffness triggered by fatigue, **stress,** cold, or long rest periods, such as a night's sleep; stiffness can be relieved by repeated movement of the affected muscles

• Nemaline myopathy: moderate weakness of voluntary muscles in the arms, legs, and trunk; mild weakness of facial muscles; delays in reaching developmental motor milestones; decreased or absent reflexes in affected muscles; long, narrow face; high-arched palate; jaw projects beyond upper part of the face

• Paramyotonia congenita: stiffness (myotonia) of voluntary muscles in the face, hands, and forearms; attacks spontaneous or triggered by cold temperatures; stiffness made worse by repeated movement; episodes of stiffness last longer than those seen in myotonia congenita

• Periodic paralysis: attacks of temporary muscle weakness (muscles work normally between attacks); in the hypokalemic (low calcium) form, attacks triggered by vigorous **exercise,** heavy meals (high in carbohydrates), insulin, stress, alcohol, infection, **pregnancy;** in the hyperkalemic (normal/high calcium) form, attacks triggered by vigorous exercise, stress, pregnancy, missing a meal, steroid drugs, high potassium intake

- Mitochondrial myopathies: symptoms vary quite widely with the form of the disease and may include progressive weakness of the eye muscles (ocular myopathy), weakness of the arms and legs, or multisystem problems primarily involving the brain and muscles.

Endocrine-related myopathies

In some cases, myopathies can be caused by a malfunctioning gland (or glands), which produces either too much or too little of the chemical messengers called hormones. Hormones are carried by the blood and one of their many functions is to regulate muscle activity. Problems in producing hormones can lead to muscle weakness.

Hyperthyroid myopathy and hypothyroid myopathy affect different muscles in different ways. Hyperthyroid myopathy occurs when the thyroid gland produces too much thyroxine, leading to muscle weakness, some muscle wasting in hips and shoulders, and, sometimes, problems with eye muscles. The hypothyroid type occurs when too little hormone is produced, leading to stiffness, cramps, and weakness of arm and leg muscles.

Inflammatory myopathies

Some myopathies are inflammatory, leading to inflamed, weakened muscles. Inflammation is a protective response of injured tissues characterized by redness, increased heat, swelling, and/or **pain** in the affected area. Examples of this type include **polymyositis**, dermatomyositis, and myositis ossificans.

Dermatomyositis is a disease of the connective tissue that also involves weak, tender, inflamed muscles. In fact, muscle tissue loss may be so severe that the person may be unable to walk. Skin inflammation is also present. The cause is unknown, but viral infection and **antibiotics** are associated with the condition. In some cases, dermatomyositis is associated with rheumatologic disease or **cancer.** Polymyositis involves inflammation of many muscles usually accompanied by deformity, swelling, sleeplessness, pain, sweating, and tension. It, too, may be associated with cancer. Myositis ossificans is a rare inherited disease in which muscle tissue is replaced by bone, beginning in childhood.

Muscular dystrophy

While considered to be a separate group of diseases, the muscular dystrophies also technically involve muscle wasting and can be described as myopathies. These relatively rare diseases appear during childhood and adolescence, and are caused by muscle destruction or degeneration. They are a group of genetic disorders caused by problems in the production of key proteins.

The forms of muscular dystrophy (MD) differ according to the way they are inherited, the age of onset, the muscles they affect, and how fast they progress. The most common type is Duchenne MD, affecting one or two in every 10,000 boys. Other types of MD include Becker's, **myotonic dystrophy,** limb-girdle MD, and facioscapulohumeral MD.

Diagnosis

Early diagnosis of myopathy is important so that the best possible care can be provided as soon as possible. An experienced physician can diagnose a myopathy by evaluating a person's medical history and by performing a thorough physical exam. Diagnostic tests can help differentiate between the different types of myopathy, as well as between myopathy and other neuromuscular disorders. If the doctor suspects a genetic myopathy, a thorough family history will also be taken.

Diagnostic tests the doctor may order include:

- Measurements of potassium in the blood
- Muscle biopsy
- Electromyogram (EMG).

Treatment

Treatment depends on the specific type of myopathy the person has:

- Periodic paralysis: medication and dietary changes
- Hyperthyroid or hypothyroid myopathy: treatment of the underlying thyroid abnormality
- Myositis ossificans: medication may prevent abnormal bone formation, but there is no cure following onset
- Central core disease: no treatment
- Nemaline myopathy: no treatment
- Centronuclear (myotubular) myopathy: no treatment
- Paramyotonia congenita: treatment often unnecessary
- Myotonia congenita: drug treatment (if necessary), but drugs don't affect the underlying disease, and attacks may still occur.

Prognosis

The prognosis for patients with myopathy depends on the type and severity of the individual disease. In most cases, the myopathy can be successfully treated and the patient returned to normal life.

Muscular dystrophy, however, is generally a much more serious condition. Duchenne's MD is usually fatal by the late teens; Becker's MD is less serious and may not be fatal until the 50s.

Resources

BOOKS

Knowles, Anne. *Under the Shadow.* New York: Harper & Row, 1983.

ORGANIZATIONS

Muscular Dystrophy Association. 3300 East Sunrise Dr., Tucson, AZ 85718. (520) 529-2000.

National Arthritis and Musculoskeletal and Skin Diseases Information Clearinghouse. PO Box AMS, 9000 Rockville Pike, Bethesda, MD 20892. (301) 495-4484.

OTHER

Facts About Myopathies. Tucson, AZ: Muscular Dystrophy Association, 1993.

Carol A. Turkington

Myopia

Definition

Myopia is the medical term for nearsightedness. People with myopia see objects more clearly when they are close to the eye, while distant objects appear blurred or fuzzy. Reading and close-up work may be clear, but distance vision is blurry.

Description

Myopia affects about 30% of the population in the United States. To understand myopia it is necessary to have a basic knowledge of the main components involved in the eye's focusing system: the cornea, lens, and retina. The cornea is a tough, transparent, dome-shaped tissue that covers the front of the eye (not to be confused with the white, opaque sclera). The cornea lies in front of the iris (the colored part of the eye). The lens is a transparent, double-convex structure located behind the iris. The retina is a thin membrane that lines the rear of the eyeball. Light-sensitive retinal cells convert incoming light rays into electrical signals that are sent along the optic nerve to the brain, which then interprets the images. In people with normal vision, parallel light rays enter the eye and are bent by the cornea and lens (a process called refraction) to focus precisely on the retina, providing a crisp, clear image. In the myopic eye, the focusing power of the cornea (the major refracting structure of the eye) and the lens is too great with respect to the length of the eyeball. Light rays are bent too much, and they converge in front of the retina. This results in what is called a refractive error. In other words, an overly focused, fuzzy image is sent to the brain.

There are many types of myopia. Some common types include:

- Physiologic
- Pathologic
- Acquired.

By far the most common, physiologic myopia develops sometime between the ages of 5-10 years and gradually progresses until the eye is fully grown. This may include refractive myopia (cornea and lens-bending properties are too strong) and axial myopia (the eyeball is too long). Pathologic myopia is a far less common abnormality. This condition begins as physiologic myopia, but rather than stabilizing, the eye continues to enlarge at an abnormal rate (progressive myopia). This more advanced type of myopia may lead to degenerative changes in the eye (degenerative myopia). Acquired myopia occurs after infancy. This condition may be seen in association with uncontrolled diabetes and certain types of **cataracts. Antihypertensive drugs** and other medications can also affect the refractive power of the lens.

Causes & symptoms

Myopia is said to be caused by an elongation of the eyeball. This means that the oblong (as opposed to normal spherical) shape of the myopic eye causes the cornea and lens to focus at a point in front of the retina. A more precise explanation is that there is an inadequate correlation between the focusing power of the cornea and lens and the length of the eye.

Myopia is considered to be primarily a hereditary disorder, meaning that it runs in families. People are generally born with a small amount of **hyperopia** (farsightedness), but as the eye grows this decreases and myopia does not become evident until later. Because of this, it is sometimes argued that myopia is not inherited, but acquired. Some eyecare professionals believe that a tendency toward myopia may be inherited, but the actual disorder results from a combination of environmental and genetic factors. Environmental factors include close work, **stress,** and eye strain.

The symptoms of myopia are blurred distance vision, eye discomfort, squinting, and eye strain.

Diagnosis

The diagnosis of myopia is typically made during the first several years of elementary school when a teacher notices a child having difficulty seeing the chalkboard, reading, or concentrating. The teacher or school nurse often recommends an eye exam by an ophthalmologist or optometrist. An ophthalmologist—M.D. or D.O. (Doctor of Osteopathy)—is a medical doctor trained in the diagnosis and treatment of eye problems. Ophthalmologists

KEY TERMS

Accommodation—The ability of the lens to change its focus from distant to near objects. It is achieved through the action of the ciliary muscles which change the shape of the lens.

Cornea—The outer, transparent tissue that covers the front of the eye. The cornea is part of the eye's focusing system.

Diopter (D)—A unit of measure for describing refractive power.

Laser-assisted in-situ keratomileusis (LASIK)—A procedure that uses a cutting tool and a laser to modify the cornea and correct moderate to high levels of myopia. As of early 1998, the eximer laser is not approved by the FDA for this use.

Lens—The transparent, elastic, curved structure behind the iris (colored part of the eye) that helps focus light on the retina.

Ophthalmologist—A medical doctor (M.D or D.O.) who specializes in the diagnosis and medical and surgical treatment of eye diseases and disorders.

Optic nerve—A bundle of nerve fibers that carries visual messages in the form of electrical signals to the brain.

Optometrist—A doctor of optometry (O.D.) is trained and licensed to examine and test the eyes for disease and to treat visual disorders by prescribing corrective lenses and/or vision therapy. In many states, they are licensed to use diagnostic and therapeutic drugs, and if so, they can treat certain ocular diseases.

Orthokeratology—A method of reshaping the cornea using a contact lenses. Not considered a permanent method to reduce myopia.

Peripheral vision—The ability to see objects and movement to the side, outside of the direct line of vision.

Photorefractive keratectomy (PRK)—A procedure that uses a laser to make modifications to the cornea and permanently correct myopia. As of early 1998, only two lasers have been approved by the FDA for this purpose.

Radial keratotomy (RK)—A surgical procedure involving the use of a diamond-tipped blade to make several spoke-like slits in the peripheral (non-viewing) portion of the cornea to improve the focus of the eye and correct myopia by flattening the cornea.

Refraction—The bending of light rays as they pass from one medium through another. Used to describe the action of the cornea and lens on light rays as they enter they eye. Also used to describe the determination and measurement of the eye's focusing system by an optometrist or ophthalmologist.

Refractive eye surgery—A general term for surgical procedures that can improve or correct refractive errors by permanently changing the shape of the cornea.

Retina—The light-sensitive membrane that lines the back of the eye. The retinal cells process and send visual signals to the brain through the optic nerve.

Visual acuity—The ability to distinguish details and shapes of objects.

also perform eye surgery. An optometrist (O.D.) diagnoses and manages and/or treats eye and visual disorders. In many states, optometrists are licensed to use diagnostic and therapeutic drugs.

A patient's distance vision is tested by reading letters or numbers on a chart posted a set distance away (usually 20 ft). The doctor has the patient view images through a variety of lenses to obtain the best correction. The doctor also examines the inside of the eye and the retina. An instrument called a slit lamp is used to examine the cornea and lens. The eyeglass prescription is written in terms of diopters (D), which measure the degree of refractive error. Mild to moderate myopia usually falls between -1.00D and -6.00D. Normal vision is commonly referred to as 20/20 to describe the eye's focusing ability 20 ft away from an object. For example, 20/50 means that a myopic person must be 20 ft away from an eye chart to see what a normal person can see at 50 ft. The larger the bottom number, the greater the myopia.

Treatment

People with myopia have three main options for treatment: eyeglasses, contact lenses, and for those who meet certain criteria, refractive eye surgery.

Eyeglasses

Eyeglasses are the most common method used to correct myopia. Concave glass or plastic lenses are placed in frames in front of the eyes. The lenses are ground to the thickness and curvature specified in the eyeglass prescription. The lenses diverge the light rays so they focus further back, directly upon the retina, producing clear distance vision.

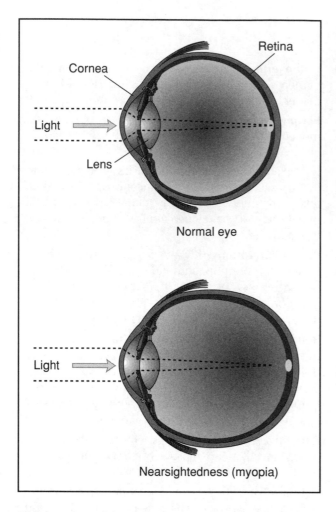

Cornea
Retina
Light
Lens

Normal eye

Light

Nearsightedness (myopia)

Myopia, or nearsightedness, is a condition of the eye in which objects are seen more clearly when close to the eye while distant objects appear blurred or fuzzy. *(Illustration by Electronic Illustrators Group.)*

Contact lenses

Contact lenses are a second option for treatment. Contact lenses are extremely thin round discs of plastic that are worn on the eye in front of the cornea. Although there may be some initial discomfort, most people quickly grow accustomed to contact lenses. Hard contact lenses, made from a material called PMMA, are virtually obsolete. Rigid gas permeable lenses (RGP) are made of plastic that holds its shape but allows the passage of some oxygen into the eye. Some believe that RGP lenses may halt or slow the progression of myopia because they maintain a constant, gentle pressure that flattens the cornea. A procedure called orthokeratology acts on this principle of "corneal molding"; however, when contact lenses are discontinued for a period of time, the cornea will generally go back to its original shape. Rigid gas permeable lenses offer crisp, clear, sight. Soft contact

lenses are made of flexible plastic and can be up to 80% water. Soft lenses offer increased comfort and the advantage of extended wear; some can be worn continuously for up to one week. While oxygen passes freely through soft lenses, bacterial contamination and other problems can occur, requiring replacement of lenses on a regular basis. It is very important to follow the cleaning and disinfecting regimens prescribed because protein and lipid buildup can occur on the lenses, causing discomfort or risking infection. Contact lenses offer several benefits over glasses, including: better vision, less distortion, clear peripheral vision, and cosmetic appeal. In addition, contacts don't steam up from changes in temperature or perspiration.

Refractive eye surgery

For people who find glasses and contact lenses inconvenient or uncomfortable, and who meet selection criteria regarding age, degree of myopia, general health, etc., refractive eye surgery is a third treatment alternative. Developed during the last two decades, there are three types of corrective surgeries available as of 1998: 1) **radial keratotomy,** 2) photorefractive keratectomy, and 3) laser-assisted in-situ keratomileusis, which is still under clinical evaluation by the Food and Drug Administration (FDA). Refractive eye surgery improves myopic vision by permanently changing the shape of the cornea so light rays focus properly on the retina. These procedures are performed on an out-patient basis and generally take 10-30 minutes.

RADIAL KERATOTOMY

Radial keratotomy (RK), the first of these procedures made available, is considered the riskiest. The surgeon uses a delicate diamond-tipped blade, a microscope, and microscopic instruments to make several spoke-like, "radial" incisions in the non-viewing (peripheral) portion of the cornea. The slits surgically alter the curve of the cornea, making it flatter, which may improve the focus of images onto the retina.

PHOTOREFRACTIVE KERATECTOMY

Photorefractive keratectomy (PRK) involves the use of a computer to measure the shape of the cornea. Using these measurements, the surgeon applies a computer-controlled laser to make modifications to the cornea. The PRK procedure flattens the cornea by vaporizing small amounts of tissue from the cornea's surface. As of early 1998, only two eximer lasers are approved by the FDA for PRK, although other lasers have been used. It is important to make sure the laser being used is FDA approved. Photorefractive keratectomy can be used to treat mild to moderate forms of myopia. The cost is approximately $2,000 per eye.

LASER-ASSISTED IN-SITU KERATOMILEUSIS

Laser-assisted in-situ keratomileusis (LASIK) is the newest of these procedures and, as of early 1998, is still under clinical investigation. It is recommended for moderate to severe cases of myopia. A variation on the PRK method, LASIK uses lasers and a cutting tool called a microkeratome to form a circular flap on the cornea. The flap is flipped back to expose the inner layers of the cornea. The cornea is treated with a laser to change the shape and focusing properties, then the flap is replaced.

All of these surgical procedures carry risks, the most serious being corneal scarring, corneal rupture, infection, cataracts, and loss of vision. Since refractive eye surgery doesn't guarantee 20/20 vision, it is important to have realistic expectations before choosing this treatment. In a 10-year study conducted by the National Eye Institute, over 50% of people with radial keratotomy gained 20/20 vision, and 85% passed a driving test (requiring 20/40 vision), after surgery, without glasses or contact lenses. Even if you gain near-perfect vision, however, there are potentially irritating side effects, such as postoperative **pain,** poor night vision, variation in visual acuity, light sensitivity and glare, and optical distortion. Refractive eye surgeries are considered elective procedures and are rarely covered by insurance plans.

Myopia treatments under research include corneal implants and permanent, surgically placed contact lenses.

Alternative treatment

Some eye care professionals recommend treatments to help improve circulation, reduce eye strain, and relax the eye muscles. It is possible that by combining **exercises** with changes in behavior, the progression of myopia may be slowed or prevented. Alternative treatments include: visual therapy (also referred to as **vision training** or eye exercises); discontinuing close work; reducing eye strain (taking a rest break during periods of prolonged near vision tasks); and wearing bifocals to decrease the need to accommodate when doing close-up work.

Prognosis

Glasses and contact lenses can (but not always) bring vision to 20/20. Refractive surgery can make permanent improvements for the right myopic candidate.

Prevention

Myopia is generally considered a hereditary condition, which means that it runs in families. From this perspective there is nothing that can be done to prevent this disorder. However, because the percentage of people with myopia in the United States has steadily increased over the last 50 years, some believe that the condition results from a combination of genetic and environmental factors. If this is true, then it may be possible to prevent or control myopia by: reducing close work; reading and working in good light; maintaining good nutrition; and practicing visual therapy (when recommended).

Try to prevent eye strain by using sufficient light for reading and close work, and by wearing corrective lenses as prescribed. Everyone should have regular eye exams to see if the prescription has changed or if any other problems have developed. This is particularly important for people with high (degenerative) myopia who may be at a greater risk of developing **retinal detachments** or other problems.

Resources

BOOKS

Birnbaum, Martin H. *Optometric Management of Nearpoint Vision Disorders.* Boston: Butterworth-Heinemann, 1993.

Curtin, Brian J. *The Myopias: Basic Science and Clinical Management.* Philadelphia: Harper & Row, 1985.

Rosanes-Berrett, Marilyn B. *Do You Really Need Eyeglasses?* Barrytown, NY: Station Hill Press, 1990.

Zinn, Walter J., and Herbert Solomon. *Complete Guide to Eyecare, Eyeglasses, and Contact Lenses.* Hollywood, FL: Lifetime Books, 1996.

PERIODICALS

Carey, Benedict. "Goodbye Glasses: New Surgery Can Deliver Sharp Vision to the Nearsighted—Without a Single Cut of the Scalpel (Photorefractive Keratotomy)." *Health* 10(September 1996): 46.

"Catching Your Eye (Photorefractive Keratotomy Evaluation." *People's Medical Society Newsletter* 15(August 1996): 6.

"Insight on Eyesight: Seven Vision Myths: Blind Spots About Vision Can Cause Needless Worry, Wasted Effort, and Unnecessary Treatment." *Consumer Reports on Health* 9(April 1997): 42.

"9 Ways to Look Better: If You Want to Improve Your Vision—Or Just Protect What You Have—Try These Eye Opening Moves." *Men's Health* 13(Jan.-Feb. 1998): 50.

Schwartz, Leslie. "Visionquest (Use of Lasers in Treatment of Nearsightedness or Myopia)." *Shape* 16(March 1997): 28.

ORGANIZATIONS

American Academy of Ophthalmology. P.O. Box 7424, San Francisco, CA 94120-7424. (415) 561-8500. http://www.eyenet.org.

American Optometric Association. 243 N. Lindbergh Blvd., St. Louis, MO 63141. (314) 991-4100. http://www.aoanet.org.

International Myopia Prevention Association. RD No. 5, Box 171, Ligonier, PA 15658. (412) 238-2101.

Myopia International Research Foundation. 1265 Broadway, Room 608, New York, NY 10001. (212) 684-2777.

National Eye Institute. NIH Bldg. 31, 9000 Rockville Pike, Bethesda, MD 20892. (301) 496-5248. http://www.nei.nih.gov/

Risa Palley Flynn

Myositis *see* **Myopathies**

Myotonia atrophica *see* **Myotonic dystrophy**

Myotonic dystrophy

Definition

Myotonic dystrophy is a progressive disease that keeps affected muscles from relaxing once they have been contracted or tightened.

Description

Myotonic dystrophy (DM), also called dystrophia myotonica, myotonia atrophica, or Steinert's disease, is a common form of **muscular dystrophy.** It affects more than 30,000 people in the United States. DM is an inherited disease, affecting men and women approximately equally. Symptoms may appear at any time from childhood to adulthood. DM causes general weakness, usually beginning in the muscles of the hands, feet, neck, or face. It slowly progresses to involve other muscle groups, including the heart. DM affects a wide variety of other organ systems as well.

A rare form of DM, congenital myotonic dystrophy, may appear in newborns of mothers who have DM. Congenital myotonic dystrophy is marked by severe weakness, poor sucking and swallowing responses, respiratory difficulty, delayed motor development, and **mental retardation.**

Causes & symptoms

Causes

Myotonic dystrophy is caused by an inherited gene defect, called a "triple repeat," on chromosome 19. The defective gene has not been positively identified as of early 1998. The triple repeat probably affects neighboring genes as well. Involvement of more than one gene would explain the multisystem effects of DM. The gene is inherited in an autosomal dominant pattern. In this pattern, one copy of the gene inherited from an affected parent is enough to cause the disease in the offspring. The chance of inheriting the DM gene from an affected parent

is 50% for each child. This percentage is not changed by results of other pregnancies.

The relation between the affected gene and the resulting myotonia, or inability to relax muscles, is not yet understood. The disease somehow blocks the flow of electrical impulses across the muscle membrane. Without proper flow of charged particles, the muscle cannot return to its relaxed state after it has contracted.

Symptoms

Myotonic dystrophy causes weakness and delayed muscle relaxation (myotonia). Symptoms of DM include facial weakness and a slack jaw, drooping eyelids (**ptosis**), and muscle wasting in the forearms and calves. A person with DM has difficulty relaxing his or her grasp, especially in the cold. DM affects heart muscle, causing irregularities in the heartbeat. It also affects the muscles of the digestive system, causing **constipation** and other digestive problems. DM may cause **cataracts,** retinal degeneration, low IQ, frontal balding, skin disorders, atrophy of the testicles, and insulin resistance. It can also cause **sleep apnea**—a condition in which normal breathing is interrupted during sleep. DM increases the need for sleep and decreases motivation. Severe disabilities do not set in until about 20 years after symptoms begin. Most people with myotonic dystrophy do not require a wheelchair, even late in life.

Diagnosis

Diagnosis of DM is not difficult, once the disease is considered. However, the true problem may be masked because symptoms can begin at any age, can be mild or severe, and can occur with a wide variety of associated complaints. Diagnosis of DM begins with a careful medical history and a thorough physical exam to determine the distribution of symptoms and to rule out other causes. A family history of DM or unexplained weakness helps to establish the diagnosis.

Lab tests may include:

• An electromyogram (EMG). This electrical test is used to examine the response of the muscles to stimulation. Characteristic changes are seen in DM that help distinguish it from other muscle diseases.

• A muscle biopsy. In this test, a small piece of muscle tissue is removed for microscopic examination. DM is marked by characteristic changes in the structure of muscle cells.

• DNA analysis. Examination of the DNA (genetic material) from blood or muscle cells conclusively demonstrates the presence of the disease. Prenatal **genetic testing** is also possible.

• An electrocardiogram. This electrical test may be used to detect characteristic abnormalities in heart rhythm associated with DM. These symptoms appear later in the course of the disease, however.

Treatment

Myotonic dystrophy cannot be cured, and no treatment can delay its progression. However, many of the symptoms it causes can be treated.

Physical therapy can help preserve or increase strength and flexibility in muscles. Ankle and wrist braces can be used to support weakened limbs. Occupational therapy is used to develop tools and techniques to compensate for loss of strength and dexterity. A speech-language pathologist can provide retraining for weakness in the muscles controlling speech and swallowing.

Irregularities in the heartbeat may be treated with medication or a pacemaker. A yearly electrocardiogram is usually recommended to monitor the heartbeat. **Diabetes mellitus** in DM is treated in the same way that it is in the general population. A high-fiber diet can help prevent constipation. Sleep apnea may be treated with surgical procedures to open the airways or with nighttime ventilation. Treatment of sleep apnea may reduce drowsiness. Lens replacement surgery is available for cataracts. Labor and delivery can be complicated by muscle weakness and require an obstetrician who knows about the particular problems of DM.

Wearing a medical bracelet is advisable. Some emergency medications may have dangerous effects on the heart rhythm in a person with DM. Adverse reactions to **general anesthesia** may also occur.

Prognosis

The course of myotonic dystrophy varies. When symptoms appear earlier in life, disability tends to become more severe. Some people with DM may require a wheelchair later in life. Children with congenital DM usually require special educational programs and physical and occupational therapy. For both types of DM, respiratory infections pose a danger when weakness becomes severe.

Prevention

Myotonic dystrophy cannot be prevented, because it is inherited. An accurate genetic test, including a prenatal test, is available. Results of these tests may be useful for purposes of family planning.

Resources

BOOKS

Brooke, Michael H. *A Clinician's View of Neuromuscular Diseases,* 2nd ed. Baltimore: Williams & Wilkins, 1986.

Swash, Michael and Martin Schwartz. *Neuromuscular Diseases: A Practical Approach to Diagnosis and Management,* 3rd ed. Springer, 1997.

ORGANIZATIONS

Muscular Dystrophy Association. 3300 East Sunrise Drive, Tucson, AZ 85718. (520) 529-2000. (800) 572-1717. http://www.mdausa.org.

Myringotomy and ear tubes

Definition

Myringotomy is a surgical procedure in which a small incision is made in the eardrum (the tympanic membrane), usually in both ears. The word comes from *myringa*, modern Latin for drum membrane, and *tomē*, Greek for cutting. It is also called myringocentesis, tympanotomy, tympanostomy, or **paracentesis** of the tympanic membrane. Fluid in the middle ear can be sucked out through the incision.

Ear tubes, or tympanostomy tubes, are small tubes, open at both ends, that are inserted into the incisions in the eardrums during myringotomy. They come in various shapes and sizes and are made of plastic, metal, or both. They are left in place until they fall out by themselves or until they are removed by a doctor.

Purpose

Myringotomy with the insertion of ear tubes is an optional treatment for inflammation of the middle ear with fluid collection (effusion), also called glue ear, that lasts more than three months (chronic **otitis media** with effusion) and does not respond to drug treatment. It is the recommended treatment if the condition lasts four to six months. Effusion is the collection of fluid that escapes from blood vessels or the lymphatic system. In this case, the fluid collects in the middle ear.

Initially, acute inflammation of the middle ear with effusion is treated with one or two courses of **antibiotics. Antihistamines** and **decongestants** have been used, but they have not been proven effective unless there is also hay fever or some other allergic inflammation that contributes to the problem. Myringotomy with or without the insertion of ear tubes is NOT recommended for initial treatment of otherwise healthy children with middle ear inflammation with effusion.

In about 10% of children, the effusion lasts for three months or longer, when the disease is considered chronic. In children with chronic disease, systemic steroids may help, but the evidence is not clear, and there are risks.

When medical treatment doesn't stop the effusion after three months in a child who is one to three years old, is otherwise healthy, and has **hearing loss** in both ears, myringotomy with insertion of ear tubes becomes an option. If the effusion lasts for four to six months, myringotomy with insertion of ear tubes is recommended.

The purpose of myringotomy is to relieve symptoms, to restore hearing, to take a sample of the fluid to examine in the laboratory in order to identify any microorganisms present, or to insert ear tubes.

KEY TERMS

Acute otitis media—Inflammation of the middle ear with signs of infection lasting less than three months.

Chronic otitis media—Inflammation of the middle ear with signs of infection lasting three months or longer.

Effusion—The escape of fluid from blood vessels or the lymphatic system and its collection in a cavity, in this case, the middle ear.

Middle ear—The cavity or space between the eardrum and the inner ear. It includes the eardrum, the three little bones (hammer, anvil, and stirrup) that transmit sound to the inner ear, and the eustachian tube, which connects the inner ear to the nasopharynx (the back of the nose).

Tympanic membrane—The eardrum. A thin disc of tissue that separates the outer ear from the middle ear.

Tympanostomy tube—Ear tube. A small tube made of metal or plastic that is inserted during myringotomy to ventilate the middle ear.

Ear tubes can be inserted into the incision during myringotomy and left there. The eardrum heals around them, securing them in place. They usually fall out on their own in 6-12 months or are removed by a doctor.

While they are in place, they keep the incision from closing, keeping a channel open between the middle ear and the outer ear. This allows fresh air to reach the middle ear, allowing fluid to drain out, and preventing pressure from building up in the middle ear. The patient's hearing returns to normal immediately and the risk of recurrence diminishes.

Parents often report that children talk better, hear better, are less irritable, sleep better, and behave better after myringotomy with the insertion of ear tubes.

Description

The procedure is usually done in an ambulatory surgical unit under general anesthesia, although some physicians do it in the office with sedation and local anesthesia, especially in older children. The ear is washed, a small incision made in the eardrum, the fluid sucked out, a tube inserted, and the ear packed with cotton to control bleeding.

There has been an effort to design ear tubes that are easier to insert or to remove, and to design tubes that stay in place longer. Therefore, ear tubes come in various shapes and sizes.

Preparation

The child may not have food or water for four to six hours before anesthesia. Antibiotics are usually not needed.

Aftercare

Use of antimicrobial drops is controversial. Water should be kept out of the ear canal until the eardrum is intact. A doctor should be notified if the tubes fall out.

Risks

The risks include:

• Cutting the outer ear

• Formation at the myringotomy site of granular nodes due to inflammation

• Formation of a mass of skin cells and cholesterol in the middle ear that can grow and damage surrounding bone (cholesteatoma)

• Permanent perforation of the eardrum.

The risk of persistent discharge from the ear (otorrhea) is 13%.

If the procedure is repeated, structural changes in the eardrum can occur, such as loss of tone (flaccidity), shrinkage or retraction, or hardening of a spot on the eardrum (typmanosclerosis). The risk of hardening is 51%; its effects on hearing aren't known, but they are probably insignificant.

It is possible that the incision won't heal properly, leaving a permanent hole in the eardrum, which can cause some hearing loss and increases the risk of infection.

It is also possible that the ear tube will move inward and get trapped in the middle ear, rather than move out into the external ear, where it either falls out on its own or can be retrieved by a doctor. The exact incidence of tubes moving inward is not known, but it could increase the risk of further episodes of middle-ear inflammation, inflammation of the eardrum or the part of the skull directly behind the ear, formation of a mass in the middle ear, or infection due to the presence of a foreign body.

The surgery may not be a permanent cure. As many as 30% of children undergoing myringotomy with insertion of ear tubes need to undergo another procedure within five years.

The other risks include those associated with sedatives or general anesthesia.

An additional element of post-operative care is the recommendation by many doctors that the child use ear plugs to keep water out of the ear during bathing or swimming, to reduce the risk of infection and discharge.

Resources

BOOKS

Lim, David J., et al., eds. *Recent Advances in Otitis Media: Proceedings of the Sixth International Symposium, June 4-8, 1995, Marriott Harbot Beach, Ft. Lauderdale, Florida.* Hamilton, Ontario: B. C. Decker Inc., 1996.

Middle Ear Fluid in Young Children. Consumer Version, Clinical Practice Guideline, Number 12. AHCPR Publication No. 94-0624. Rockville, MD: Agency for Health Care Policy and Research, Public Health Service, U.S. Department of Health and Human Services, July 1994. Available from AHCPR Publications Clearinghouse at (800) 358-9295, or POB 8547, Silver Spring, MD 20907.

Stool, Sylvan E., et al. *Managing Otitis Media with Effusion in Young Children. Quick Reference Guide for Clinicians, Number 12.* AHCPR Publication No. 94-0623. Rockville, MD: Agency for Health Care Policy and Research, Public Health Service, U.S. Department of Health and Human Services, July 1994. Available from AHCPR Publications Clearinghouse at (800) 358-9295, or POB 8547, Silver Spring, MD 20907.

Stool, Sylvan E., et al. *Otitis Media with Effusion in Young Children. Clinical Practice Guideline, Number 12.* AHCPR Publication No. 94-0622. Rockville, MD: Agency for Health Care Policy and Research, Public Health Service, U.S. Department of Health and Human Services, July 1994. Available from AHCPR Publications Clearinghouse at (800) 358- 9295, or POB 8547, Silver Spring, MD 20907.

Wiet, Richard J., Steven A. Harvey, and George P. Bauer. "Management of Complications of Chronic Otitis Media." In *Otologic Surgery,* edited by Derald E. Brackmann, Clough Shelton, and Moises A. Arriaga. Philadelphia: W. B. Saunders Company, 1994, 257-276.

PERIODICALS

Terris, Mark H., Anthony E. Magit, and Terence M. Davidson. "Otitis media with effusion in infants and children: Primary care concerns addressed from an otolaryngologist's perspective." *Postgraduate Medicine,* 97 (1) (January 1995): 137-151.

Mary Zoll

Myxedema *see* **Hypothyroidism**

Myxoma

Definition

A myxoma is a rare, usually noncancerous, primary tumor (a new growth of tissue) of the heart. It is the most common of all benign heart tumors.

Description

Myxoma is an intracardiac tumor; it is found inside the heart. Seventy five percent of all myxomas are found in the left atrium, and almost all other myxomas are found in the right atrium. It is very rare for a myxoma to be found in either of the ventricles. The tumor takes one of two general shapes: a round, firm mass, or an irregular shaped, soft, gelatinous mass. They are attached to the endocardium, the inside lining of the heart. The cells that make up the tumor are spindle-shaped cells and are embedded in a matrix rich in mucopolysaccharides (a group of carbohydrates). Myxomas may contain calcium, which shows up on x rays. The tumor gets its blood supply from capillaries that bring blood from the heart to the tumor. Thrombi (blood clots) may be attached to the outside of the myxoma.

There are three major syndromes linked to myxomas: embolic events, obstruction of blood flow, and constitutional syndromes. Embolic events happen when fragments of the tumor, or the thrombi attached to the outside of the tumor, are released and enter the blood stream. Gelatinous myxomas are more likely to embolize than the more firm form of this tumor.

Myxomas may also obstruct blood flow in the heart, usually at a heart valve. The mitral valve is the heart valve most commonly affected. Blood flow restrictions can lead to pulmonary congestion and heart valve disease. Embolization can lead to severe consequences. In cases of left atrial myxoma, 40-50% of patients experience embolization. Emboli usually end up in the brain, kidneys, and extremities.

The third syndrome linked to myxomas are called constitutional syndromes, nonspecific symptoms caused by the myxoma.

Causes & symptoms

There is no known causative agent for myxoma. The main symptoms, if any, produced by myxoma are generic and not specific. These include **fever,** weight loss, **anemia,** elevated white blood cell (WBC) count, decreased **platelet** count and Raynaud's phenomenon. Most patients with myxoma are between 30-60 years of age.

Diagnosis

Diagnosis is made following a suspicion that a myxoma might be present, and can usually be confirmed by echocardiogram

Treatment

Surgery is used to remove the tumor. Myxomas can regrow if they are not completely removed. The survival rate for this operation is excellent.

Prognosis

Successful removal of the tumor rids the patient of this disease. Emboli from a myxoma may survive in other areas of the body. However, there is no evidence that myxoma is truly metastatic (able to transfer disease from one area to another), causing tumors in other areas of the body.

Resources

BOOKS

Alexander, R.W., R. C. Schlant, and V. Fuster, eds. *The Heart,* 9th ed. New York, McGraw-Hill, 1998.

Berkow, Robert, ed. *Merck Manual of Medical Information.* Whitehouse Station, NJ: Merck Research Laboratories, 1997.

OTHER

''Myxoma, Intracardiac.'' http://www3.ncbi.nlm.nih.gov.

John T. Lohr